MW00851822

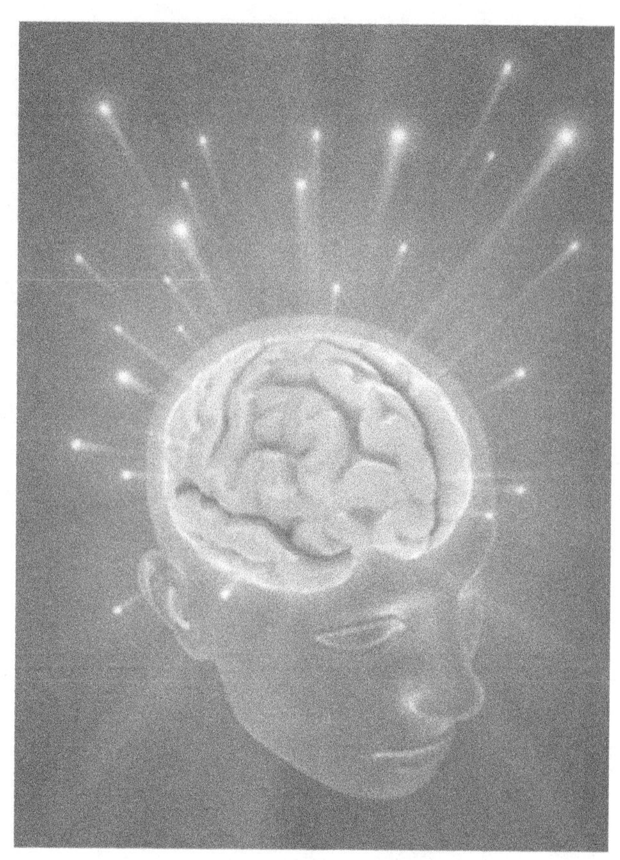

Psychiatric Advanced Practice Nursing

A Biopsychosocial Foundation for Practice

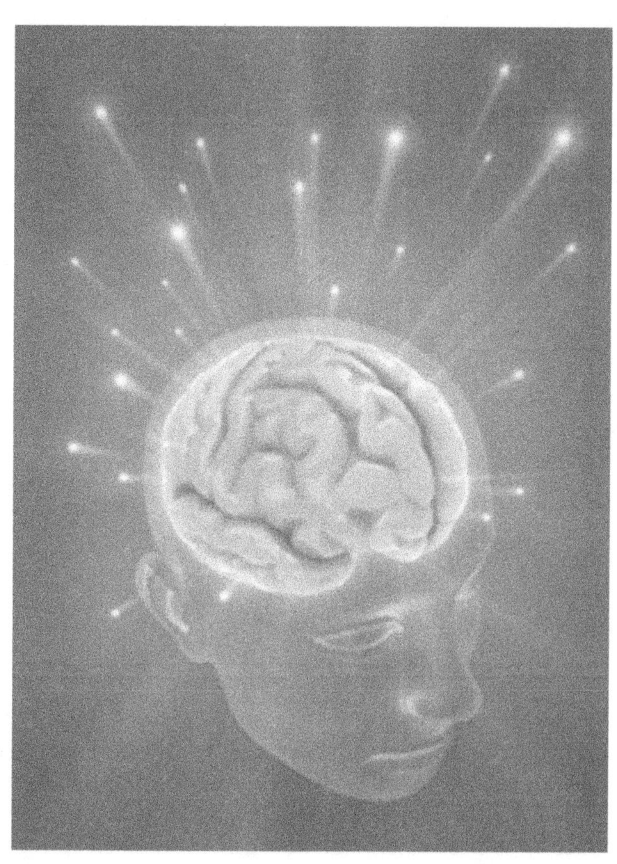

Psychiatric Advanced Practice Nursing

A Biopsychosocial Foundation for Practice

Eris Field Perese, APRN-PMH

F.A. Davis Company • Philadelphia

F. A. Davis Company
1915 Arch Street
Philadelphia, PA 19103
www.fadavis.com

Printed in the United States of America

Last digit indicates print number: 10 9 8 7 6 5 4

Publisher: Joanne P. DaCunha
Director of Content Development: Darlene D. Pedersen
Project Editor: Jamie M. Elfrank
Electronic Project Editor: Tyler Baber
Design & Illustration Coordinator: Carolyn O'Brien

Library of Congress Cataloging-in-Publication Data

Perese, Eris F.
Psychiatric advanced practice nursing : a biopsychosocial foundation for practice / Eris Field Perese. — 1st ed.
p. ; cm.
Includes bibliographical references and index.
ISBN 13: 978-0-8036-2247-0
ISBN 10: 0-8036-2247-3
I. Title.
[DNLM: 1. Mental Disorders—nursing. 2. Advanced Practice Nursing—methods. 3. Evidence-Based Nursing. 4. Psychiatric Nursing. WY 160]
616.89'0231--dc23 2011044445

To the memory of my mother, Emily Annis Wheeler, who was a psychiatric nurse at Vermont's Waterbury State Hospital, to my children—Dogan, Kerime Louise, Deniz, Eris Munevver, and San Emily—who provided the assistance, encouragement, and love that supported me during the many hours devoted to this project, and to my grandchildren who are the dividends of life.

EPIGRAPH

Once a disorder exists, and the brain has changed, the changes have to be dealt with in some way in order for a patient to recover. Drugs can induce adaptive changes in neural circuits, or put neural circuits in a state where adaptation and learning are promoted. But there's no guarantee that, left to its own devices, the brain will learn the right things. Patients, in other words, are likely to benefit most from drug therapy when the drug-induced adaptivity of their brains is directed in a meaningful way. This is probably best achieved by traveling down the pharmacological road to recovery with someone who understands not just the drug or the person, but the drug, the person and the life situation the person is experiencing (LeDoux, 2002, pp. 300-301).

PREFACE

One of the goals for improving the health of Americans is to ensure access to mental health care. Currently, less than half of the 26.2% of Americans with a psychiatric disorder receive care, and it is anticipated that with increased life expectancy and number of older Americans with psychiatric disorders, the gap between need for care and accessibility of care will widen dramatically. Achieving the nation's goal of greater accessibility of mental health services requires an increase in the nation's mental health workforce and a reduction of the incidence of psychiatric disorders.

Within the mental health work force, psychiatric advanced practice nurses have emerged as a vital and valued presence. *Psychiatric Advanced Practice Nursing* encompasses two groups of master's prepared psychiatric nurses—clinical specialists in psychiatric nursing and psychiatric nurse practitioners—who have added the knowledge, competencies, and expertise of these specialties to their baccalaureate nursing preparation. The roles of the two groups are similar and in some states are identical. Psychiatric advanced practice nurses are uniquely prepared through their educational programs and clinical experiences to provide care that is evidence-based and meets the needs of patients, families, care providing agencies, and society. One factor that limits the growth of this important segment of the mental health care workforce is the nationwide shortage of psychiatric nursing faculty. Another factor is the shortage of clinical teaching sites. A collateral but less studied problem is the limited number of textbooks that are available to meet the needs of faculty and students in psychiatric advanced practice nursing programs.

This textbook evolved in response to the lack of textbooks for psychiatric advanced practice nursing. It is designed to provide the information that will enable psychiatric advanced practice nursing students to build a biopsychosocial foundation for understanding the development of psychiatric disorders, for providing care for patients with psychiatric disorders, and for preventing the development of psychiatric disorders.

The textbook consists of nine units. The first unit presents an overview of the evolution of beliefs of causation of mental illnesses, practice of psychiatry, and psychiatric nursing activities. It describes traditional theories such as temperament, attachment, psychosocial development, needs, interpersonal relationships, and adaptation that are foundational to psychiatric advanced practice nursing. It also describes more recent theories of neural plasticity, resilience, and recovery that are part of current practice.

The second unit focuses on brain functioning, brain development and markers or indicators of abnormalities of brain development. The effects of compromised brain development and functioning are often manifested as symptoms of psychiatric disorders; e.g., deviations of cognition, inability to regulate mood, abnormal response to stressors, and maladaptive behaviors. This unit lays the foundation for understanding the development of psychiatric disorders. First, it provides information about normal brain development and functioning. Then it provides information about prenatal factors such as exposure to toxins or infections; perinatal factors such as adverse circumstances of birth; and postnatal factors or experienced factors such as childhood maltreatment that have the potential to disrupt normal brain development and thus contribute to the development of psychiatric disorders. The information in this unit provides the basis for the preventive, supportive, compensatory, remediative, restorative and recovery/resilience-building interventions that are used by psychiatric advanced practice nurses.

The third unit presents the Levers of Change—1) communication and assessment, 2) case formulation, diagnosis, and treatment planning, 3) psychotherapy, 4) pharmacotherapy, and 5) psychosocial interventions—that psychiatric advanced practice nurses use to help patients with psychiatric disorders move toward recovery.

Units four through eight focus on specific psychiatric disorders: the epidemiology including risk factors and protective factors, etiology including genetic influence, biological basis (abnormalities of structure, function and neurochemistry), clinical presentation of adults, older adults, and children, co-morbidities, differential diagnosis, treatment such as psychotherapy, pharmacotherapy, and psychosocial interventions, and course. The fourth unit is devoted to anxiety disorders, the fifth to mood disorders, the sixth to thought disorders (schizophrenia, dementia, and delirium), the seventh to dual diagnosis, and the eighth to personality disorders.

The ninth unit focuses on prevention of psychiatric disorders. Researchers have estimated that the incidence of psychiatric disorders, the number of new cases, could be reduced by at least 25% through the use of preventive interventions (Beekman, Cuijpers, Van Marwijk, et al., 2006). In Chapter 19, prevention is presented from the period of preconception to older adulthood. During the preconceptual period, the focus is on promoting the health of the mother and father before conception and on planning for their child. Preventive interventions that focus on the prenatal period of life are directed toward reducing risk factors, such as poor prenatal nutrition and the exposure of the fetus to maternally experienced toxins, infections, and illnesses including depression. During the postnatal period, the focus of prevention is on fostering protective factors, such as emotional self-regulation and secure attachment, and on preventing exposure to neglect and abuse. During childhood and adolescence, prevention is directed toward reducing specific childhood emotional and behavioral problems and psychiatric disorders that have their onset in childhood and adolescence and that have a high risk of persisting into adulthood, e.g., conduct disorder, oppositional defiant disorder, depression, anxiety disorders, and substance-related disorders (Andrews & Wilkinson, 2002). Among adults and older adults, the focus is on the prevention of anxiety disorders, depression, schizophrenia, personality disorders, substance-related disorders, and suicide. (Prevention of dementia is discussed in the chapter on dementia and delirium in Unit six.) Although prevention is addressed across the life span, the emphasis of this unit is on the urgent need to stop turning our nation's children from gold to lead through neglect and maltreatment (Felitti, 2002).

Although this textbook was developed to meet the needs of psychiatric advanced practice nurses whose focus is primarily on providing care for patients with psychiatric disorders, it is also appropriate for advanced practice nurses who manage the care of patients with medical problems and co-existing psychiatric disorders and for mental health care providers in other disciplines. This textbook takes the reader on a journey from the beginning of the development of the brain, within days of conception, to the factors that have the potential to disrupt brain development and impair brain functioning, to the psychiatric disorders that are the manifestations of impaired brain functioning and their treatment, and finally, to the prevention of psychiatric disorders starting in the preconception period. I hope that the readers will gain an appreciation of the complexity of the development of psychiatric disorders and the challenges of treatment and that they will find the textbook useful in building their foundation for practice.

Andrews, G. & Wilkinson, D. D. (2002). The prevention of mental disorders in young people. *Medical Journal of Australia, 177*, S97-S100.

Beekman, A. T., Cuijpers, P., van Marwijk, H. W., et al. (2006). The prevention of psychiatric disorders. *Nederlands Tijdschrift voor Geneeskunde, 150(8)*, 419-423.

Felitti, V. J. (2002). The relation between adverse childhood experiences and adult health: Turning gold into lead. *The Permantente Journal, Winter, 5*(1), 44-47.

ABOUT THE AUTHOR

Eris F. Perese has taught psychiatric nursing for twenty years. She was active in developing the psychiatric nurse practitioner program at the University at Buffalo School of Nursing and served as its first director. In addition to her interest in psychiatric nursing education, Eris has focused on the unmet needs of individuals with severe mental illness and on stigma and victimization. Her research includes the study of Assertive Community Treatment for voluntary and involuntary patients and the use of support groups by psychosocial club members. She has published and presented internationally on these topics, as well as on psychiatric nursing education. Prior to her career in psychiatric nursing, Eris served as a research assistant in neurosurgery where she developed an abiding interest in the brain and its functioning. Recently she was an advisor for the NOVA documentary, *Depression, Out of the Shadows,* that won the Peabody Award. She is Professor Emeritus at the University at Buffalo and a consultant for EPS Global Medical Development, Inc.

ACKNOWLEDGMENTS

I am deeply appreciative of the assistance and encouragement of both my developmental editor, Kim Mackey, and the staff of F.A. Davis, Joanne DaCunha, Publisher, Jamie Elfrank, Project Editor, Shirley Kuhn, Special Projects Manager, and others. This textbook would not have been possible without their help. They were the wind under my wings. I wish to express my gratitude to the contributors who gave so generously of their time to write chapters in their area of expertise and to my colleagues who contributed case studies.

And I am very thankful for the help of Sharon Murphy and other medical librarians, for the willingness to listen to Cathleen Getty and other colleagues, for the feedback of former students, and for the lessons that patients and families of the National Alliance on Mental Illness have taught me.

CONTRIBUTORS

Lora Humphrey Beebe, PhD, PMHNP-BC
Associate Professor and Coordinator, Psychiatric Mental Health Graduate Program
College of Nursing
University of Tennessee
Knoxville, Tennessee

Dessye Dee Clark, PhD, APRN, PMHCNS-BC
Psychiatric Clinical Nurse Specialist, Advanced Registered Nurse Practitioner
President & CEO, Sound View Counseling & Assoc. PS Inc.

Adjunct Assistant Professor
College of Nursing
Montana State University
Bozeman, Montana

Joan S. Grant, DSN, RN, CS
Professor
School of Nursing
University of Alabama at Birmingham
Birmingham, Alabama

Sharon R. Katz, PMH-APRN, BC
Executive Director
Collaborative Care of Abington
Abington, Pennsylvania

Norman L. Keltner, EdD, CRNP
Professor
School of Nursing
University of Alabama at Birmingham
Birmingham, Alabama

Ellen R. Portnoy, DNP, RN, PMHNP-BC
Administrative Director, Patient Services/Psychiatry
Detroit Medical Center Sinai-Grace Hospital
Detroit, Michigan

Kathleen A. H. Vertino, MSN, RN, PMHNP-BC, CARN-AP
VA Western New York Healthcare System at Buffalo
Behavioral Health Careline
Team Leader, Partial Hospital Program
Buffalo, New York

Adjunct Clinical Instructor
School of Nursing
University at Buffalo
Buffalo, New York

Diane M. Wieland, PhD, MSN, RN, PMHCNS-BC
Associate Professor
La Salle University
Philadelphia, Pennsylvania

Nurse Psychotherapist
Private Practice
Lansdale, Pennsylvania

CASE STUDY CONTRIBUTORS

Stefania Fynn-Aikins, MSN, RN, PMHNP-BC
Lake Shore Behavioral Health
Buffalo, New York

Sophie Knab, MS, RN
Professor
Niagara County Community College
Sanborn, New York

Lorraine A. Lopez, PMHNP-BC
Psychiatric Mental Health Nurse Practitioner
Private Practice
Amherst, New York

Nurse Practitioner and Consultant
Niagara Frontier Psychiatric Associates Pllc
Lockport, New York

Kerry Perese, MSN, RN
Adjunct Faculty
University at Buffalo
Buffalo, New York

Nurse Practitioner Women's Health
Planned Parenthood
Buffalo, New York

Cynthia Stuhlmiller, MS, RN, DNS
Professor of Rural Nursing
School of Health
University of New England
Armidale, New South Wales, Australia

Barry Tolchard, PhD, MSc, RNLD, RNM
Senior Lecturer
University of New England
Armidale, New South Wales, Australia

Ann Venuto, MSN, RN, PMHNP-BC
Clinical Instructor
School of Nursing
University at Buffalo
Buffalo, New York

REVIEWERS

Laurel Ash, DNP, CNP, RN
College of St. Scholastica
Duluth, Minnesota

Jennifer M. Boggs, MSN, PMHNP-BC
Frontier Health
Greeneville, Tennessee

Barbara Cornett, PhD, RN
Otterbein University
Westerville, Ohio

Diane Crayton, MSN, RNC, FNP
California State University Stanislaus
Turlock, California

M. Susan Dawson, EdD, PMHCNS/NP-BC
Allen College
Waterloo, Iowa

Maureen B. Doyle, PhD, PMHCNS-BC, CARN, NPP, APN-C, CNE, C
Fairleigh Dickinson University
Teaneck, New Jersey

Leslie A. Folds, EdD, PMHCNS-BC, CNE
Belmont University
Nashville, Tennessee

Melissa Garno, EdD, RN
Georgia Southern University
Statesboro, Georgia

Vaness Genung, PhD, RN, PMH-NP, LCSW-ACP, LMFT, LCDC
Midwestern State University
Wichita Falls, Texas

Masoud Ghaffari, PhD, MSN/RN, MEd (CHE), MT (ASCP), CMA
East Tennessee State University
Johnson City, Tennessee

Sheila Grossman, PhD, APRN-BC
Fairfield University
Fairfield, Connecticut

Glennena Haynes-Smith, DNP, APN-BC
Fairleigh Dickinson University
Teaneck, New Jersey

Patricia Hentz, EdD, PMHCNS-BC, CRNP
University of Pennsylvania
Philadelphia, Pennsylvania

Linda E. Jensen, PhD, RN, MN
Clarkson College
Omaha, Nebraska

Laura Kelly, PhD, APN
Monmouth University
West Long Branch, New Jersey

Jean M. Klein, PhD, PMHCNS-BC
Immaculata University
Immaculata, Pennsylvania

Laura G. Leahy, MSN, APN, PMH-CNS/FNP, BC
University of Pennsylvania
Philadelphia, Pennsylvania

Janet Merritt, PhD, RN, APRN-BC
The Catholic University of America
Washington, DC

Dale Muelle, EdD, MSN, MS, NEA-BC
California State University Dominguez Hills
Carson, California

Karen K. Paraska, PhD, CRNP, FNP-BC
Duquesne University
Pittsburgh, Pennsylvania

Geraldine S. Pearson, PhD, PMH-CNS, APRN, FAAN
University of Connecticut
Farmington, Connecticut

Paula Marie Pillone, MS, NP-P
Columbia University
New York, New York

Mechelle J. Plasse, MS, RN CS, NP, APRN
University of Massachusetts
Elmwood, Massachusetts

Carla E. Randall, PhD, RN
University of Southern Maine
Lewiston, Maine

Luann Richardson, PhD, CRNP
Duquesne University
Pittsburgh, Pennsylvania

Marcia Ellen Ring, PhD, APRN
George Washington University
Ashburn, Virginia

Nancy Scanlan, APRN, BC
Plattsburgh State University
Plattsburgh, New York

Renee Shell, EdD, MSN, ARNP-BC
Remington College
Lake Mary, Florida

Janet A. Sobczak, PhD, RN, NPP, PMHCNS-BC
Upstate Medical University
Syracuse, New York

TABLE OF CONTENTS

UNIT I

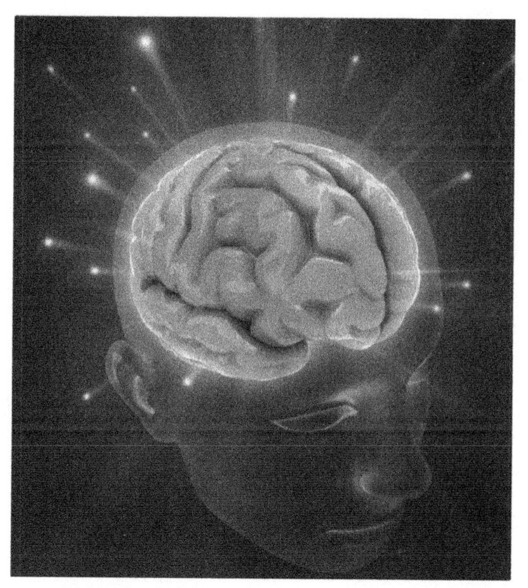

Foundational Theories That Support Advanced Practice Psychiatric Nurses' Practice

CHAPTER 1

Framework for Practice of Psychiatric Advanced Practice Nurses

Eris F. Perese, APRN-PMH

Psychiatric advanced practice nurses—both clinical specialists in psychiatric nursing and psychiatric nurse practitioners—fill the need in the nation's mental health care system for a biopsychosocial approach to managing the care of individuals diagnosed with psychiatric disorders. They also provide mental health teaching for patients and their families, promote self-care as a strategy for maximizing recovery and quality of life, and address mental health promotion and risk reduction of psychiatric disorders. The practice of psychiatric advanced practice nurses is founded on

- Information from neuroscience, such as research-derived information about normal brain development and functioning (Chapter 2), neurotransmitters and receptors (Chapter 2), and neuroplasticity (Chapter 1).
- Clinical knowledge of the epidemiology, risk and protective factors, etiology, biological basis, and clinical presentation of psychiatric disorders (Chapters 9 through 18).
- Clinical competencies to assess patients (Chapter 4), develop case formulation and generate diagnoses (Chapter 5), implement, monitor, and evaluate evidence-based treatment interventions such as psychopharmacotherapy (Chapter 6), psychotherapy (Chapter 7), and psychosocial interventions across the life span (Chapter 8).

Today's psychiatric advanced practice nurses use past and present research-generated information to build the knowledge base, skills, and competencies needed to meet the biopsychosocial health-care needs of their patients. They acquire skills in developing therapeutic relationships with patients and proficiency in communicating effectively with patients, their families, and care providers from other disciplines. They build assessment skills to use in obtaining a database for making a diagnosis, in formulating the case, and in generating treatment plans. In addition to their competencies in psychotherapy, pharmacotherapy, and psychosocial interventions, they have expertise in providing educational, supportive, remeditative, and compensatory nursing interventions such as anticipatory guidance and case management.

Evolution of Psychiatric Advanced Practice Nursing

The first psychiatric advanced practice nurses were clinical specialists in psychiatric nursing, and the first program to prepare clinical specialists in psychiatric nursing was developed in 1952 by Hildegarde Peplau, who is the founder of psychiatric nursing. At that time, most patients with psychiatric disorders received care in large, overcrowded, and inadequately staffed state hospitals (Smoyak & Skiba-King, 1998), where nursing care was at the custodial level (Shea,1999). Peplau's program was designed to prepare clinical specialists in psychiatric nursing who could provide care at more than the custodial level. Students were prepared to function in the role of psychotherapists (Shea). Peplau viewed the patient as a biopsychosocial being whose illness was based on disruptions of interpersonal relationships (Wheeler, 2008). Peplau believed that psychiatric nurses should be guided by patients' reactions to their problems and that changes in patients were brought about by the interaction between nurse and patient.

From 1953, when Hildegard Peplau developed the first master's program for psychiatric nursing, until the 1970s, all master's programs for clinical specialists in psychiatric nursing were based on the teachings of Peplau. Preparation of clinical specialists in psychiatric nursing focused on theories about human behavior and the role of the nurse as a psychotherapist. Early on, clinical specialists in psychiatric nursing functioned as psychotherapists, educators, consultants, researchers, and providers of treatment for patients with acute and chronic psychiatric disorders.

By the 1970s, while continuing to adhere to the theoretical framework of Peplau, programs for clinical specialists in psychiatric nursing began to change to incorporate newly generated neurobiological information. Courses in health assessment, pharmacology, pathophysiology, and neurophysiology were added (Delaney, Chisholm, Clement, et al., 1999; Naegle & Krainovich-Miller, 2001). Clinical specialists in psychiatric nursing began to change their view of their role. They saw the ability to prescribe medications and to discuss chronic medical issues as an expansion of the interpersonal relationship that clinical specialists in psychiatric nursing have with their patients. There was also a shift from their earlier psychodynamic model of orientation that was based on Freudian theory to greater acceptance of the biopsychosocial model (Engel, 1977, 1978, 1980).

With the 1990s came an astonishing growth of psychiatric mental health nurse practitioner (PMHNP) programs (Wheeler & Haber, 2004). For example, in 1992 there were 12 PMHNP programs in the United States (Nursing Data Review, 1992), and just 12 years later there were 36 PMHNP programs (National League for Nursing, 2004). Forces behind the development of PMHNP programs came both from within the profession and from without.

Forces within the Profession Promoting Psychiatric Nurse Practitioners

Within the profession, psychiatric nurses recognized the need to expand their role to meet the needs of the nation's mentally ill, who are among the most underserved citizens in terms of mental health care and basic health promotion (Bjorklund, 2003). Psychiatric nurses became advocates for more accessible care for underserved patients, especially for those with severe mental illness. They identified patients' unmet needs for mental health care and also their unmet personal needs. Aiken (1987) described unmet needs for care of individuals with chronic mental illness who were homeless, in shelters, in jails, and living on the streets, and she challenged nurses to meet those needs. Perese (1997) measured needs among individuals with chronic mental illness and found that the most frequently occurring unmet needs were the needs for a friend, for a role in life, for belonging to a group that accepted and claimed them, and for a sense of self-identity. Inability to meet their need for personal safety was reported by 30% of the study participants. Psychiatric nursing leaders urged members to prepare themselves to meet the challenges of integrating neuroscience into nursing practice (McBride & Austin, 1996).

Forces Outside the Profession Promoting Psychiatric Nurse Practitioners

Three outside influences promoted the psychiatric nurse practitioner profession:

1. Changes in delivery and reimbursement of mental health care
2. Changes in mental health care sites
3. The availability of information generated in the neurosciences during the Decade of the Brain (Sullivan, 1992)

With the movement toward managed care, state offices of mental health no longer provided direct patient care. Instead, they contracted with managed care organizations or managed behavioral health organizations to provide services for patients with psychiatric disorders and substance abuse disorders (Shea, 1999). With these changes in service provisions, the role of the psychiatric clinical nurse specialist was seen as not contributing directly to cost-effectiveness of care, and thus the demand shifted to psychiatric nurse practitioners, who were viewed as being able to provide cost-effective care within managed care organizations (Smoyak & Skiba-King, 1998).

Another factor that shaped the workforce was the shift of the primary site of treatment for individuals with psychiatric disorders from inpatient hospital units to community-based care. This shift required clinicians who could provide community-based care for patients with symptoms more severe than those of mental illnesses previously treated in community settings such as anxiety or depression. There was a need for clinicians who could provide care for patients with severe mental illnesses, functional disabilities, comorbid physical illnesses, and co-occurring substance related disorders, and for patients who had had very short hospitalizations and were discharged before being stabilized (Hanrahan, Stuart, Brown, et al., 2003). Four models of advanced practice psychiatric mental health nursing programs emerged:

1. The clinical specialists in psychiatric nursing model
2. The blended model, in which graduates had both clinical specialist competencies and nurse practitioner competencies
3. The additive model, in which nurse practitioner (NP) content was added after completion of a clinical specialist program
4. The primary care model, in which family nurse practitioners graduated with additional skills for the psychiatric population ("double NP" [Wheeler & Haber, 2004, p. 130])

Several leaders in psychiatric nursing supported the concept of the blended model because it kept the psychosocial traditions while incorporating the neuroscience perspectives and practitioner competencies (Bjorklund, 2003; Moller & Haber, 1996; Scharer, Boyd, Williams, et al., 2003). In the creation of curricula for blended PMHNP programs, selected competencies of the psychiatric mental health clinical specialist and nurse practitioner were combined (Wheeler & Haber, 2004). The trend was to develop programs that followed the American Nurses Association's (2000) *Scope and Standards of Psychiatric-Mental Health Nursing Practice,* which supports the blended role (Delaney, 2005), and *Psychiatric-Mental Health Nurse Practitioner Competencies* (National Panel for Psychiatric-Mental Health NP Competencies, 2003). which also serves as a guide for blended programs (Delaney).

Blended programs prepare psychiatric advanced practice nurses to practice in a variety of roles in the health-care system, in diverse settings, and in collaboration with members of other disciplines and with consumer groups; blended programs also prepare nurses to work with underserved populations—such as those with severe mental illness, the homeless, and those with comorbid health problems—and with those who are incarcerated (Williams, Pesut, Boyd, et al., 1998; Delaney, 2005). The preparation of psychiatric advanced practice nurses makes them a valued addition to the mental health care workforce (Naegle & Krainovich-Miller, 2001; Stark, 2006).

Other strong influences on psychiatric nursing were the advances in information and technology associated with the Decade of the Brain. A joint resolution of the United States Congress designated the decade beginning January 1, 1990, as the "Decade of the Brain" and called upon the citizens of the United States to work to generate knowledge of the disorders and disabilities that affect the brain in order to develop preventive and therapeutic interventions for brain disorders (Sullivan, 1992; Tandon, 2000). Knowledge generated during the Decade of the Brain provided a basis for integrating information about neurobiological processes and structural abnormalities with the manifested impairments of thinking, compromised modulation of emotions, and maladaptive behaviors that constitute the symptoms of psychiatric disorders (Hartman, 1993). The Decade of the Brain also produced conceptual advances, such as that of neuroplasticity (Laws, 2000), which is a conceptual framework that enables psychiatric advanced practice nurses to understand how the interventions that they provide—pharmacotherapy, psychotherapy, psychosocial interventions, and nursing interventions—bring about changes in their patients' perceptions, thinking, emotions, and behaviors (Kandel, 1998).

Information generated during the Decade of the Brain prompted families of those with mental illnesses to campaign for support of the view that psychiatric disorders are brain disorders. They advocated for care that was individualized, readily accessible, and evidence based. Information generated during the Decade of the Brain also stimulated new interest in psychiatric nursing (Shea, 1999), and programs for psychiatric advanced practice nurses began to integrate into their curricula new information from the neurosciences and new information about evidence-based care.

As a result of these changes, today the preparation and practice of the two types of psychiatric advanced practice nurses—clinical specialists in psychiatric nursing and psychiatric nurse practitioners—have a great deal in common. For example, in studying the tasks that were essential for clinical specialists in psychiatric nursing and the tasks that were essential for psychiatric nurse practitioners, Rice, Moller, DePascale, et al. (2007) found that 99% of the tasks were essential to both of their practices. The responsibilities of clinical specialists in psychiatric nursing and the responsibilities of psychiatric nurse practitioners are also similar, and in many states their practice is similar. In fact, 30 states and the District of Columbia recognize psychiatric clinical specialists and psychiatric nurse practitioners under the same title (Staten, Hamera, Hanrahan, et al., 2006).

Foundation of Practice of Psychiatric Advanced Practice Nurses

The practice of psychiatric advanced practice nurses is based on knowledge, skills, and competencies. Nursing values drive nursing practice, and evidence-based theory guides nurses in their treatment of patients.

Values Held by Psychiatric Advanced Practice Nurses

Nursing values are the force behind nursing practice. They are based on the beliefs that underlie the decisions that nurses make in the first days of their professional education and throughout their clinical experiences (Moore & Visovsky, 2000). The following nursing values have been identified by Liegeois (2001) as underlying mental health care:

- Individualizing care, e.g., addressing the unique needs, coping abilities, and resources of patients and families
- Fostering self-care, e.g., promoting and teaching self-care and healthy lifestyle practices
- Being vigilant, e.g., observing, assessing, and monitoring patients' health status and response to therapeutic interventions
- Maintaining caring interpersonal relationships, e.g., building trust that facilitates working together to promote biopsychosocial health
- Supporting patients' autonomy
- Treating each patient with respect
- Safeguarding patients' safety, dignity, and confidentiality
- Providing collaborative care
- Believing that nursing practice activities are based on the best available evidence (Cody, 2006; Mitchell & Bournes, 2006; Moore & Visovsky, 2000)

All of these values emphasize building a trusting relationship, respecting patients as individuals, providing for patient safety, and promoting patients' biopsychosocial health and patient self-care.

Theories Foundational to the Practice of Psychiatric Advanced Practice Nurses

Although information generated in the neurosciences and provided by new technology plays an important role in creating the knowledge base of psychiatric advanced practice nurses, the work of earlier researchers, psychiatrists, and psychiatric nurses continues to contribute to the foundation of their knowledge base and to support practice (Table 1-1).

TABLE 1-1 MENTAL ILLNESS ACROSS THE YEARS: THEORIES OF CAUSATION, RESEARCH/EVENTS, TREATMENT GOALS, TREATMENT, AND NURSING PRACTICE

Time	Theories of Causation	Research	Treatment Goals	Treatment	Nursing Practice
Early 1700s	Sin (people were punished for their sins). People were possessed by the devil.	Beginning interest in the relationship between case presentation and brain pathology on postmortem examination (Alexander & Selesnick, 1966).	Patients were viewed as unsafe to be in the community (Torrey & Miller, 2001).	Secluded at home. In 1727, the first workhouse was built for people whose families could not care for them.	
Mid 1700s	Mental illness was thought to be due to four humors, with melancholy being due to black humor (Alexander & Selesnick, 1966).	Specific brain regions were involved in motor functioning, e.g., paralysis following stroke or hemorrhage (Alexander & Selesnick, 1966). Nerve cells produced electricity, and electrical activity of one neuron affects the activity of other neurons (Kandel, Schwartz, & Jessell, 1995).	Restore balance of humors using bloodletting and purgatives (Alexander & Selesnick, 1966).	In 1748, the first hospital for the insane was built (Torrey & Miller, 2001).	
Late 1700s	Mental illness was thought to be caused by heredity and adverse life experiences (Alexander & Selesnick, 1966).	Mental illness could be localized to specific areas of the brain (Alexander & Selesnick, 1966).	In 1793, Pinel instituted moral treatment. Tuke built a therapeutic asylum based on the theory of moral treatment (Alexander & Selesnick, 1966). Moral treatment was instituted in Spain by the Moors, who in 1409 built hospitals for the mentally ill and in 1545, built a hospital with a unit for children (Alexander & Selesnick, 1966).	Moral treatment—kindness, respect, structured daily activities—could cure people.	
Early 1800s	It was thought that insanity was caused by factors in the environment and social stressors, e.g., reading agitating news (Torrey & Miller, 2001).	Golgi identified the cell body, axon, and dendrites of the neuron (Kandel et al., 1995). Cobb demonstrated that increased brain function is associated with increased blood flow to the brain. Cobb proposed that the mind was the output of brain activity (Bentinck-Smith & Stouffer, 1993).	Move patients from stressful environments to isolated asylums where patients could recover and return to society. Cure rate was 17%, with another 12% showing improvement (Torrey & Miller, 2001).	Custodial care in large state asylums that were run by superintendents. They quickly became overcrowded.	

Mid 1800s	There was a beginning belief of biological basis of mental illness.	American psychiatrist Benjamin Rush taught that mental illness was caused by somatic conditions. There was a trend to explain mental illness in terms of disruption of nervous system structures and functioning (Alexander & Selesnick, 1966).	The 1840s and 1850s were periods of construction of large state hospitals. New York's Pilgrim State Hospital had 14,000 patients (Torrey & Miller, 2001).	Custodial care	In 1843, a nurse, Dorothea Dix, addressed state legislators and advocated for better treatment for the insane. She described insane asylums as overcrowded, dirty, and lacking in light and air and reported that patients were kept in cages and beaten (Torrey & Miller, 2001). Psychiatric nursing in the 1860s was similar to that of other nursing with an emphasis on clean wards, patient hygiene, food, sleep, fresh air, exercise, and kindness (Boyd, 2005).
Late 1800s	Heredity was believed to be a cause of mental illness.	Mental illness was thought to be due to brain pathology and alterations of brain chemistry (Alexander & Selesnick, 1966).	Treatment goal was to prevent mental illness by restricting marriage and by sterilization of patients with mental illness (Clarke, 1912; Faulke, 1911; Reilly, 1987).	To gain support to build more asylums, superintendents reported cure rates of 90%. In 1876, Pliny Earle published a paper saying that the cure rate was a myth. This exposé resulted in the end of building of large institutions. In 1876, chloral hydrate was synthesized and used for sedation of agitated patients (Alexander & Selesnick, 1966).	In 1882, the first program for psychiatric nurses was on initiated at McLean Hospital. Emphasis was on hygiene, nutrition, and ward activities. In 1885, Buffalo State Hospital became the first state hospital to offer instruction for nurses (Buckley, 1938).
Early 1900s	Psychoanalytical theory: psychopathology is due to disturbed development caused by childhood experiences and faulty parenting.	1930s research began to focus on heredity. Congenital features (deafness and blindness) were believed to be due to genetics; congenital was equated with hereditary (Webster, 1998). National League of Nurses recommended inclusion of psychiatric nursing content in curricula (Kneisl & Wilson, 2004).	Goals of treatment in the 1930s were to restore functioning through the use of somatic treatments (Alexander & Selesnick, 1966).	Psychoanalysis Nonspecific medications and somatic treatments: e.g., electroconvulsive therapy, insulin shock therapy, cold baths, wet sheet wraps. Surgical treatment with lobotomies.	Role of the nurse was to be subservient to physicians. Nursing interventions included prolonged baths, wet packs, tube feedings, suicide precautions, socialization, leisure activities, and sleep promotion (Poston, 1928).

Continued

TABLE 1-1 MENTAL ILLNESS ACROSS THE YEARS: THEORIES OF CAUSATION, RESEARCH/EVENTS, TREATMENT GOALS, TREATMENT, AND NURSING PRACTICE—continued

Time	Theories of Causation	Research	Treatment Goals	Treatment	Nursing Practice
Mid 1900s	Psychoanalytical theory. Prevalence of mental illness among soldiers raised awareness of the extent of mental illness. Sullivan (1953) viewed psychopathology as a lack of awareness of interpersonal relationships; anxiety resulted from social insecurity. Erikson (1950) believed that individuals built strengths and coping attributes by successfully resolving life's developmental tasks. Insecure attachment early in life influences later development of psychopathology.	Medications such as chlorpromazine (Thorazine), a first-generation antipsychotic, became available to reduce agitation and psychotic symptoms. Psychiatry began to move toward biological psychiatry (Martin, 2002). Peplau's (1952) nursing theory, the Interpersonal Model. Maslow's (1970) hierarchy of needs theory, which stated that people are motivated by unmet needs. Attachment theory developed by Bowlby (1969, 1973). 1960's Community Mental Health Act.	Control of symptoms. 1940s: Insulin shock and electroconvulsive therapy. Discharge of patients from institutions to community.	Antipsychotic medications controlled symptoms and made release from hospital possible. Community-based care was insufficient and inadequate. Lack of community resources. Emergence of patient self-help organizations; e.g., Fountain House. Focus was on symptom control; prevention of hospitalization; compliance with medications to prevent relapse; adaptation to limitations of illness and disabilities (Drake, Green, Mueser, et al., 2003).	Nurses assisted with electroconvulsive therapy and insulin shock therapy, supervised patients' hygiene and smoking breaks, monitored arts and crafts, and administered medications such as paraldehyde (McCrone, 1996). Psychiatric nursing included using interpersonal psychotherapy.
Late 1990s	Adaptation theories; maladaptation to adversities or life influence development of psychopathology.	Hansell (1976a) theory: adaptation achieved through essential attachments to the environment (basic needs). Newer, second-generation antipsychotics with fewer side effects. Roger's (1970) nursing theory: unitary human beings (patient as a whole interacting with environment to achieve change). Roy (1976) developed nursing theory: the Adaptation Model. Erickson, Tomlin, and Swain (1983) developed nursing theory of biopsychosocial adaptation—Modeling and Role-modeling.	Community mental health centers required to provide 11 essential services/supports. Treatment goal was to help people function in adult societal roles (Drake et al., 2003).	Medications and psychiatric rehabilitation. Skills training to improve functioning.	Medication management; social skills implementation; groups for social skills acquisition.
2000	Biopsychosocial model: Impairments of patients' physical, psychological, and social functioning cause psychopathology.	Plasticity of the brain (Kandel, 1998). Development of psychotropic medications with targeted actions and fewer side effects than the older medications but with other side effects.	Treatment goal is recovery and development of resilience (Drake et al., 2003).	Psychopharmacotherapy, psychotherapy, and psychosocial interventions; e.g., patient and family education, appropriate housing, supported work, social skills training, case management, peer support. Repeat transcranial magnetic stimulation. Vagal nerve stimulation, alternative interventions.	Managing medical and mental health care; implementing evidence-based practices and preventive interventions, e.g., weight control, prevention of diabetes, and fostering resilience. Prescribing and monitoring medications by psychiatric mental health nurse practitioners.

Some of the theories that have contributed to the knowledge base of psychiatric nursing and continue to do so are as follows: moral treatment, temperament theory, attachment theory, psychosocial developmental theory, needs theory, Freud's drive theory, interpersonal relations theory, adaptation theory, and biopsychosocial theory. More recently, psychiatric advanced practice nurses have been influenced by the theories of neuroplasticity and resilience and the theory of recovery, and they are incorporating these theories into their knowledge base and practice. The theories of neuroplasticity, resilience, and recovery are discussed later in the chapter.

Moral Treatment

The origin of moral treatment dates back to 1793 and is attributed to the French psychiatrist Philippe Pinel and to an English nonpsychiatrist Quaker, William Tuke. Moral treatment was based on the principles of kindness, respect for the patient, and providing a refuge and controlled environment that would guide the patient toward habits and values that conform to those of the outside world (Edginton, 1997). Daily structured routines and activities such as exercise, playing games, animal care, gardening, sports, field trips to places of interest, art, and music were used to distract patients from the symptoms of their illness and to refocus them on the environment that was designed to move them toward mainstream life and toward recovery (Edginton). The principles and some of the strategies of moral treatment underlie many of the psychosocial interventions, nursing interventions, and promotion of recovery that psychiatric advanced practice nurses use in their practice today.

Temperament Theory

Temperament is a concept that helps us to understand personality and psychopathology. Childhood temperament traits are viewed as an early form of personality (Caspi, Roberts, & Shiner, 2005; Whittle, Allen, Lubman, et al., 2006) and as possible predictors of later development of psychopathology; so, for example, childhood temperament traits have been used to predict attention deficit-hyperactivity disorder and pediatric bipolar disorder (West, Schenkel, & Pavuluri, 2008). Temperament is considered to be a combination of genetically influenced responses to external stimuli, such as new experiences, and the behaviors that reflect those biological responses, such as avoidance behaviors or approach behaviors (West et al.). Some of the first researchers of temperament, Thomas, Chess, and Birch (1963), identified early-appearing temperament qualities including activity, rhythmicity, adaptability, intensity, responsiveness, positive and negative mood, distractibility, and persistence. They hypothesized that these qualities interacted with environmental influences—such as caring and nurturing—to form individuals' patterns of adapting to stimuli and eventually to form personality characteristics. Based on their study of traits of temperament, Chess and Thomas (1987) developed three categories to describe infants' temperaments: easy, slow-to-warm-up, and difficult. Chess and Thomas (p. 280) said that difficult babies account for 10% of the population, that slow-to-warm-up babies account for 15% of the population, and that easy babies account for 40% of the population. Mixed-temperament babies account for 35% of the population (Karen, 1994; Thomas, Chess, & Birch, 1970).

Easy Babies

Easy babies respond positively to new things, tend to have regular sleep and eating patterns, and smile easily. Later, they make easy adjustments to going to school, to being left with babysitters, and to a new home. Because of their easy adjustments to new situations, people tend to respond positively to them and also to their parents (Chess & Thomas, 1986). As children, they are capable of self-control. They are self-confident and do not become upset when meeting new people or encountering new situations (Caspi, Moffitt, Newman, et al., 1996).

Slow-To-Warm-Up Babies

Kagan (1978, 1990) studied slow-to-warm-up children and found that, as babies, they tended toward fretfulness, anxiety, and inhibition and were difficult to soothe. In childhood, they were reluctant to interact with others, shy, timid, and fearful. They were afraid to speak in class, to attend summer camp, to be alone at home, and to go to their bedrooms alone at night. When new or unfamiliar events occurred, they were anxious and clung to their mothers. At age 7, 75% of slow-to-warm-up babies retained the same pattern, e.g., they were afraid to go to camp, to watch violent television shows, and to sleep over at a friend's house. At age 10, they still preferred to play alone rather than in a group. At age 13, the anxious profile remained. As adults, they tended to select secure jobs in which they could work alone, to show few spontaneous smiles, and to express few positive feelings.

Difficult Babies

Difficult temperament appears to be due to underlying biological abnormalities. Characteristics of a difficult temperament include high levels of activity, distractibility, and intensity; poor adaptability (difficulty accepting change); and crankiness or irritability. Behaviors include withdrawal from new or unfamiliar situations or persons; overreactivity to noises, lights, and hunger; restlessness; irregular eating and sleeping habits; and difficulties in settling down (West et al., 2008). In infancy, difficult temperament is seen as hyperactivity; in childhood, it is seen as aggressive conduct. The symptoms of aggressiveness, hyperactivity, and impulsivity suggest disruption of executive functioning of the frontal lobe. Parents may lose faith in their parenting skills and may decrease their involvement with the child. This decrease in involvement may lead to failure of the child to learn rules and to internalize standards that inhibit antisocial behavior.

Mixed-Temperament Babies

Mixed-temperament babies have characteristics of more than one of the above categories or have characteristics from all three categories. They may appear moody, and their response to a new situation is unpredictable. In some situations their response is similar to that of the easy baby, and in other situations it is similar to that of a difficult baby. Parents must read their babies' cues, such as facial expression and level of activity, and be flexible in their responses.

Social and Cultural Influences on Temperament

Both genes and culture are passed from parents to children. It has been found that children with difficult temperaments often have parents with similar temperaments who use inconsistent methods of discipline; likewise, children with easy temperaments tend to have warm, confident parents (Caspi, 2000). Thus, parents may reinforce temperament traits. Furthermore, throughout life, people tend to choose partners and situations that reinforce their earlier determined interactional styles; as Caspi wrote, "The child thus becomes the father of the man" (p. 170).

Gemelli (2008) pointed out that the infant's characteristics of temperament develop in the context of the socializing environment that the parents provide and that environment is shaped by the parents' culture. Culture defines health and illness, delineates acceptable from nonacceptable behavior, influences living situations, and provides support. The two main categories of culture—individualism/independence and collectivism/interdependence—have different expectations for family life, parenting, and children's behaviors. Each culture has a set of beliefs, attitudes, practices, and behaviors related to childrearing, family roles and activities, and interpersonal relationships that shape individuals' adaptation to the challenges and stressors of life (Feldman & Masalha, 2007).

In cultures that stress individualism, parenting goals are to foster autonomy and self-competence. Children often live in a nuclear family where the mother provides most of their care. Time is often set aside for face-to-face interactions with the child to build vocalization skills and play skills.

In contrast, in collectivistic cultures, parenting goals are to teach deference to authority and that the goals of the family take precedence over the goals of the individual. There is an emphasis on compliance, reduction of aggression, and politeness. Interactions with the child take place within the work activities of the family, and early on, there is nearly constant physical contact between the child and parents and with members of the extended family, who provide care and social support and who take an active part in modulating problematic behaviors.

By age 18 months, infants develop an awareness of their own characteristics of temperament and of their parents' support for certain characteristics and nonsupport for others. Infants are innately motivated to seek repetition of pleasurable experiences, such as parents' approval, and to avoid unpleasant experiences. Through this process, the interactions between the child and parents and members of the extended family modify and reinforce characteristics of temperament.

Temperament Over Time

Types of temperament identified in early childhood provide some clues to behavioral problems in childhood, emotions and behavior in early adulthood, and later development of psychopathology (Caspi, 2000). Children who have been identified as having been difficult infants have more externalizing problems such as fighting, bullying, lying, and disobeying; others described them as unreliable and untrustworthy. At age 18, children who had been identified as difficult babies describe themselves as danger-seeking, impulsive, aggressive, and having adversarial relationships. They also describe feeling mistreated, deceived, and betrayed by others (Caspi). At age 18, the inhibited (slow-to-warm-up) children were found to lack friends and interests, to be cautious and nonassertive, and to tend to avoid harm. They were submissive and lacking in leadership skills. Easy children at 18 years of age were confident, self-controlled, and well adjusted. They tended to use active coping skills.

At age 21 years, inhibited children were likely to have smaller social networks; to have lower levels of social support, guidance, or mentoring; and to be more likely to meet the criteria for depression. At age 21 years, difficult children were more likely to be unemployed, to meet criteria for antisocial personality disorder, to have alcohol dependence, and to be involved in criminal activities. Adults who had been difficult children or inhibited children were more likely than easy children to have psychiatric disorders. Those who had been inhibited children were more likely to have depression, and those who had been difficult children were more likely to have developed antisocial personality disorder. Adults who had been inhibited or difficult children were more likely to commit suicide than those who had been easy children (Caspi, 2000; Caspi et al., 1996).

Attachment Theory

Attachment is an emotional bond to an individual who is special and whose place cannot be filled by another individual (Karen, 1994). Attachment is characterized by the need to stay close to that one special individual. Individuals experience distress when separated from that individual, joy when reunited, and grief at the loss of the individual. In infancy, attachment figures are usually parents. Later, attachment figures tend to be close friends, peers, and romantic partners. Among older adults, attachment figures may be their own children (Ainsworth, 1989), or their attachment may be to pets, values, or causes.

Development of Attachment Theory

Attachment is hard-wired in humans: it is an innate biological drive that fosters closeness to the caregiver (Daniel, 2006). It provides young children with protection from danger and a sense of comfort and security (Wilson, 2009). Attachment enables defenseless infants and children to survive and thrive. Attachment theory developed from early studies of children who had experienced lack of attachment through neglect and maternal deprivation.

Maternal Deprivation

In the early 1900s, there were reports of extremely high mortality rates among maternally deprived children in children's wards, such as in the asylums of Bellevue, where the death rate was 32% to 75% by the end of the child's second year in the asylum. Children in Bellevue's asylums were listless and unhappy; failed to gain weight; slept less than babies cared for at home; and had infections that lasted for months rather than improving in a few days despite rigid aseptic care (Bakwin, 1942). In an effort to improve outcomes, the signs that reminded staff to wash their hands before entering the children's ward were replaced with signs that read, "Do not enter this ward without picking up a baby" (Bakwin, p. 31). As the nurses began to hold and cuddle the babies, the infection rates went down.

In addition to affecting a child's physical health, maternal deprivation has a negative effect on intelligence, language development, and ability to form relationships. As early as 1937, Levy described children who lacked maternal care in their early life as follows:

- Unable to bond with their adoptive parents
- Unresponsive to affection; rejecting fondling
- Unmanageable
- Pleasant on the surface but indifferent underneath
- Having frequent behavior problems, such as stealing and temper tantrums
- Failing to make meaningful relationships

In search of ways to remedy these deficits, child psychiatrist Harold Skeels placed 13 maternally deprived institutionalized 2-year-old toddlers in the care of teenage girls who were in a residential setting for feeble-minded girls; each toddler was assigned to an older girl, who provided mothering for the child. Over a period of 1 to 5 years, when compared with 13 toddlers who received standard care in the orphanage (limited adult contact and opportunities for play), the toddlers placed with the teenage girls improved overall and their intelligence scores rose while the intelligence scores of the other toddlers declined (Skeels & Dye, 1939).

The effects of maternal deprivation were also evidenced by children in England who had been removed from their parents to protect them from the bombings of London during the Second World War. Despite warnings by Bowlby and other child psychiatrists of the danger of separating children from their mothers, children were sent to families in Canada and Ireland. Children who remained with their parents, even though they were exposed to nightly air raids and had to seek safety with their families in shelters, did better than those removed from their families (Freud & Burlingham, 1943).

Bowlby's Theory of Attachment

Based on evidence of the detrimental effect of maternal deprivation, Bowlby (1973) concluded that attachment—which he defined as a warm, continuous interaction between the mother or a permanent mother substitute and the infant—provides a sense of security, comfort, calmness, and peace that is essential for long-term mental health (Bowlby, 1988b). Bowlby (1973) believed that early childhood interactions with a primary caregiver form patterns of attachment: if the primary caregiver provided supportive, comforting care, then secure patterns formed; if the caregiver was unpredictable, nonresponsive, harsh, or abusive, then insecure patterns—avoidant, inhibited, or disorganized—formed (Bowlby, 1973; Main & Solomon, 1986).

Although Bowlby (1973) described attachment as taking place between the infant and one individual, which is known as the *dyadic* model of attachment, later researchers (Herzog, 1982; Lamb, 1981) described attachment as taking place between mother, father, and infant, the *triadic* model. It is now accepted that fathers can fulfill the attachment role that was once thought to be a mother's-only role and that infants can form multiple attachments (Sadock & Sadock, 2007).

Attachment accrues from the quality and quantity of interactions with both parents. Attachment provides a "secure base" from which children and adolescents can explore, learn new things, and gain mastery over their environment (Bowlby, 1988b, p. 11).

Bowlby (1973, 1988a) believed that early childhood attachment experiences become transformed during the end of the first year of life into inner working models of self and mother. By the end of the fifth year of life, the child uses a complex model of self and mother that includes the mother's interests, moods, and intentions. The inner working models are made up of the child's view of himself/herself as part of the relationship with the attachment figure; the child's view of the adult in the attachment/caregiver relationship; and the behaviors used by the child to keep the caregiver in the attachment relationship. These models are used constantly and influence the child's feelings, thoughts, and behaviors. These working models of the world influence other attachment relationships all through life, e.g., they serve as a template for other relationships (Bowlby, 1973, 1988a).

The specific behaviors that are designed to promote survival are called attachment behaviors. In infants and children, attachment behaviors include crying, calling, clinging, strong protesting if left alone, and temper tantrums. These childhood attachment behaviors may be seen in adults when they are distressed, afraid, or ill. Later, attachment behaviors become organized into patterns of behavior that are designed to keep the caregiver available to provide comfort, security, and protection. Patterns of attachment behaviors develop in response to the type of attachment—secure or insecure—that the child has with the attachment figures in his or her life, and they are thought to persist into adulthood.

Attachment Patterns

Based on Ainsworth's research with children in strange situations, which were test situations in which the child's responses were observed when the mother left for a short time and then returned (Ainsworth, Bell, & Stayton, 1971), Bowlby (1988b) identified a secure attachment pattern and two patterns of insecure attachment: ambivalent and avoidant. Main and Solomon (1986) observed that children who had been maltreated did not fit the insecure categories of ambivalent or avoidant, and they developed another category of insecure attachment: the disorganized pattern. For more information on these attachment patterns, see Table 1-2.

Implications for Psychiatric Advanced Practice Nurses

In summary, children with secure attachment patterns know that their caregiver will keep them safe. Children with insecure attachment patterns are not certain that their caregiver will keep them safe, and they do not derive soothing comfort from their caregiver.

Bowlby (1988a) said that a child's pattern of attachment determines whether the child will have resiliency or vulnerability to stressful events later in life. However, before the age of 3, the child's pattern of attachment can be changed if the parents treat the child differently (Bowlby). For example, among children with disorganized pattern of attachment, parents or caregivers have been found to have unresolved losses or to have experienced trauma. They have inappropriate expectations of their child's abilities and high expressed emotions, often shouting intense, angry words at the child. If there is no change in how the parents treat the child, then the child's pattern of attachment becomes more difficult to change with time, and the child imposes it on new relationships.

Psychiatric advanced practice nurses can promote the development of more secure attachment patterns by helping parents or caregivers learn about infants' and children's developmental needs, learn how the parents or caregivers can meet those needs, and learn what are realistic expectations for the child. The goal is to increase caregivers' caring, empathetic responses that modulate children's emotional distress so that the children develop the ability to modulate their own emotional responses. Early researchers believed that attachment patterns determined the development of later social relationships, but more recent researchers point out that attachment is only one of many influences that determine social interactions and relationships (Rutter, Kreppner, & Sonuga-Barke, 2009). However, Bowlby's theory of attachment is still a core topic in nursing curricula and still guides mental health care of children, hospital policies about parents' staying with their children, and world opinion about how children should be treated (MacDonald, 2001). Bowlby's theory of attachment contributes to the foundation underlying prevention of psychiatric disorders (Bowlby, 1988a; Green, Stanley, & Peters, 2007; Wilson, 2009). More information on the prevention of psychiatric disorders can be found in Chapter 19.

Psychosocial Developmental Theory

Eight Ages of Man

Erikson (1950) believed that individuals develop within a social setting of family and cultural heritage, and he described this process of development as the "Eight Ages of Man" (pp. 248-250) (Table 1-3). Erikson believed that the cycle of life contains certain stages that have specific tasks that individuals must master in order to build moral virtues or internal resources that they use to adapt to the challenges of life. It is not the life cycle that shapes individuals' virtues; rather, it is the interaction of individuals' biology, culture, demographics, history, social structure, and patterns of family life as they meet the challenges or tasks of each stage in the life cycle.

Individuals' personalities continue to develop across the life span as a result of their responses to challenges. How successfully the challenges of one stage are met influences success or failure in the next stage. Failure is reflected in compromised physical, cognitive, social, and emotional functioning, and success in the accruement of internal strengths or virtues, adaptive coping resources, and well-being.

Proposed Ninth Age of Man: Beyond the Life Cycle

It has been proposed that there should be a ninth age of man: the age beyond the life cycle. Cole (2004) wrote, "For the first time in modern history, mass longevity became the norm in developed countries" (p. 3). Earlier, Erikson (1950) had foreseen future problems with identity as a result of our Western civilization's view of life as a straight line from one success or achievement to another and then an abrupt end—alive but with no further identified tasks or accomplishments. Although there is little written about the tasks that older adults face in the time beyond the eighth stage, it is generally known that they must overcome the challenges of life transitions, e.g., loss of loved ones, retirement, limitation of activities, poorer health, relocation, and financial hardships. They must face the fact that their identity has changed, accept their obligations and place in the cycle of generations, and find a meaning or purpose to life.

In the past, society's expectations for the life cycle were schooling for the young, jobs for middle-aged adults, and retirement or patienthood for the aged. More recently, the health-care industry has responded to the growing number of older adults with an emphasis on maintaining middle-age functioning and the unrealistic promotion of aging as an option or a treatable, preventable condition. The leisure-time industry has responded with programs and products to help older adults satisfy their desire to travel and participate in games and sports. Society has not identified roles for older adults beyond the roles of retirees, patients, and consumers.

TABLE 1-2 TYPES OF ATTACHMENT, CHARACTERISTICS OF MOTHER/CHILD INTERACTION, AND CHARACTERISTICS OF MOTHER, CHILD, AND ADULTS

Types of Attachment		Characteristics of Mother/ Child Interaction	Characteristics of Mother	Characteristics of Child	Characteristics of Adults
TYPE	OCCURRENCE				
Secure pattern of attachment	Present in 59% of U,S, population (Mickelson, Kessler, & Shaver, 1997).	Under stress, child may stop exploring, seek proximity to the primary caregiver, and appear confident of the attachment figure's accessibility and responsiveness (Carlson, Jacobvitz, & Sroufe, 1995; Parkes, Stevenson-Hinde, & Morris, 1991).	Sensitive, lovingly responsive, accessible, and cooperative as the child tries new experiences.	Secure, self-reliant, trusting, cooperative, and helpful toward others.	Able to cope with stress; take risks; face challenges Open to new things Able to play, work, and seek help (Parkes, Stevenson-Hinde, & Morris, et al., 1991). Has happy love relationships, trusted friends, fewer divorces, and more stable employment (Hazan & Shaver, 1987).
Insecure attachment: Ambivalent or inhibited, anxious pattern	Present in 11% of U.S. population (Mickelson, Kessler, & Shaver, 1997)	In both safe and stressful situations, the child is uncertain of the caregiver's response. Child focuses on the caregiver and uses attachment-seeking behaviors to keep the caregiver close and attentive (Parkes et al., 1991).	Unpredictable and uses threats of abandonment as means of control. Rebuffs the child (Bowlby, 1988a, 1988b).	As an infant, is fretful, anxious, clinging. As a toddler, does not feel secure enough to explore or try new things (Galderisi & Mucci, 2000). As a child, may be clinging, anxious, and overly dependent on teachers. He/she tends to have separation anxiety. He/she is often bullied by other children.	Tends to: • Struggle with loneliness, have intense rollercoaster romances; fall in love easily • Be hypervigilant about separations • Becomes anxious, clinging; feels impotent rage • Feel that his/her attachment needs will never be met • Use guilt and blame to hold attachment figures • Have work problems such as procrastination, difficulty concentrating; easily distracted by interpersonal concerns • Have care-soliciting behaviors, e.g., histories of suicide attempts, anorexia (Sroufe, Carlson, Levy, et al., 1999). • His/her children tend to have ambivalent/anxious attachment patterns (Hazan & Shaver, 1987; Sroufe et al., 1999).

Continued

TABLE 1-2 TYPES OF ATTACHMENT, CHARACTERISTICS OF MOTHER/CHILD INTERACTION, AND CHARACTERISTICS OF MOTHER, CHILD, AND ADULTS—continued

Types of Attachment		Characteristics of Mother/ Child Interaction	Characteristics of Mother	Characteristics of Child	Characteristics of Adults
TYPE	OCCURRENCE				
Insecure attachment: Avoidant	Present in 25% of U.S. population (Mickelson, Kessler, & Shaver, 1997)	Under stress, the child may expect the caregiver to reject him/her and may reduce his/her reaction to the caregiver and direct his/her attention toward objects (Parkes et al., 1991). Early experiences have taught the child that he/she is unworthy of care (Sroufe et al., 1999).	Angry, rejecting, rigid, hostile. Averse to physical contact with the child. Behavior is threatening (mocking the infant, speaking sarcastically to the infant; staring the infant down; and handling the infant roughly).	Child avoids the mother on reunion after separation. If picked up, the child indicates a desire to be put down, e.g., may point to a toy. The child shows no distress, anger, or fear. Child does not seek love and care from others and may have odd behaviors—hand flapping, fears, and attachment to objects.	May have difficulties in social situations and avoid adults who are trying to make friends (Main & Weston, 1982). Tries to live without love and support from others and frequently complains of depression and somatic symptoms. Tends to be dismissive, hostile, distant, condescending, dissociated from loneliness. May be addicted to work, power, acquisitions, and achievements; have obsessive rituals; feel too ashamed to approach anyone for love; believes that he/she will be rejected. High rates of divorce and promiscuity and, under stress, may develop depression and psychosomatic symptoms (Hazan & Shaver, 1985; Sroufe et al., 1999).
Insecure attachment: Disorganized	Present among maltreated children (Bakermans-Kranenburg, van Ijzendoorn & Juffer, 2005). No rates of occurrence available.	Child is apprehensive of caregiver (Wilson, 2009). In response to stressful situations, child does not use attachment-seeking behaviors because the protector is also the source of fear. "Fright without solution" (Hesse & Main, 2000, p. 310).	Caregiver has frightening manner toward the infant, such as abusing the infant physically or sexually. Or, the mother may be frightened, not secure. The mother may be suffering physical, sexual, or verbal abuse and is viewed by the child as unable to provide protection.	Absence of an organized strategy for managing the stress of separation or a strange situation. Fearful of the caregiver. Child freezes and is disoriented with a desire to seek proximity but also to avoid it (Parkes et al., 1991).	Shows unresolved mourning. Child has a high rate of social and cognitive difficulties and psychopathology during childhood and adolescence, e.g., conduct disorder and oppositional defiant disorder (Green & Goldwyn, 2002). Among those who later experience trauma, the risk for dissociation in early adulthood is high (Sroufe et al., 1999).

TABLE 1-3 ERIKSON'S STAGES OF PSYCHOSOCIAL DEVELOPMENT, WITH TASKS, OUTCOMES, AND ACCRUED ATTRIBUTES

Life Stages	Task	Successful Outcome	Unsuccessful Outcome	Attributes Accrued With Successful Task Completion
Trust vs. mistrust (0–18 months)	To accept comforting and need satisfaction from mother (caregiver); to develop ability to internalize image of mother, e.g., let her out of sight.	Self-confidence; optimism; a faith that needs will be met; hope for the future. As an adult, is optimistic, confident, self-reliant.	Suspiciousness; difficulty with relationships. Never satisfied emotionally. Bitterness toward others.	**Drive and hope.*** Ability to trust self and others; feeling of worthiness; foundation of acceptance of religion.
Autonomy vs. shame and doubt (18 months–3 years)	To achieve balance between love and hate, cooperation and willfulness, freedom of self-expression and suppression.	Sense of self-control; ability to delay gratification; self-confidence in one's ability to perform. As an adult, is self-directed, persistent, able to control own life.	Lack of self-confidence; shame and doubt; lack of pride in the ability to perform; sense of being controlled by others; anger against self.	**Self-control and willpower.** Self-confidence; sense of justice.
Initiative vs. guilt (3–5 years)	To use energy to learn roles, functioning, and beginning skills to perform work.	Ability to exercise restraint and self-control of behavior; assertiveness and dependability; enjoyment of learning; development of a sense of conscience. As an adult, can delay gratification, solve problems.	Feelings of inadequacy; sense of defeat, guilt, rage.	**Direction and purpose.** Self-modulation; ability to work toward goals. Sense of self-responsibility and purpose.
Industry vs. inferiority (5–13 years)	To prepare for adult life; e.g. to work, parent, and provide. To work with others.	Sense of satisfaction and pleasure in interactions with others; reliable work habits; attitudes of trustworthiness; conscientiousness; pride in achievement and ability to enjoy play. As an adult, able to set goals, use problem-solving.	Feelings of inadequacy; unable to cooperate and compromise with others in group activities; unable to problem-solve or complete tasks successfully; may become passive and meek; or may become overly aggressive to cover up feelings of inadequacy. May develop unrealistic expectations for personal achievement.	**Method and competence.** Diligence and perseverance. A sense of competence.
Identity vs. role-diffusion (13–21 years)	To integrate emotions, preparedness for adulthood, expectations of others, and opportunities of diverse roles, e.g., to form a solid sense of self-identity and a life plan such as a career plan.	Secure sense of confidence; emotional stability; view of self as a unique individual; commitment to values, a career, and relationships.	Self-doubt and confusion about role in life; lack of personal values or goals; superficial and brief relationships; delinquent and rebellious behavior; fear of adult responsibilities.	**Devotion and fidelity.** Stable sense of self-identity. Commitment to values and ideals.

Continued

TABLE 1-3 ERIKSON'S STAGES OF PSYCHOSOCIAL DEVELOPMENT, WITH TASKS, OUTCOMES, AND ACCRUED ATTRIBUTES—continued

Life Stages	Task	Successful Outcome	Unsuccessful Outcome	Attributes Accrued With Successful Task Completion
Intimacy vs. isolation (21–40 years)	To commit to affiliations and partnerships. Has warm, sharing relationships with adults; able to commit to others.	Early years: capacity for mutual love and respect between two people; ability to make total commitment to another individual. Later years: having one partner and creating a family; establishing a career; accepting aging process.	Social isolation; aloneness; inability to form lasting relationships; frequent, superficial sexual contacts; frequent occupational changes; lack of a career.	**Affiliation and love.** Ability to love and work, to commit to others. Development of an ethical sense.
Generative lifestyle vs. stagnation or self-absorption (40–60 years)	To establish and guide the next generation. Accepts self in totality.	Sense of gratification from personal and professional achievements; able to provide caring and pass on knowledge and skills. Is satisfied with this stage of life.	Preoccupation with self; lack of concern for welfare of others; withdrawn, isolated, and self-indulgent.	**Production and caring.** Empathy; ability to experience gratification from a task completed.
Integrity vs. despair (60 years–death) Erikson (1964, 1968)	To defend the dignity of his/her own life despite physical and financial threats; to establish order and meaning to life; to establish world order and spirituality.	Sense of self-worth and self-acceptance; sense of dignity; does not fear death.	Sense of self-contempt and disgust with how life has progressed; feels worthless and helpless to change; anger, depression, and loneliness; death is feared or denied; may have ideas of suicide. There may be a sense that time has run out, no more time to get things done that should have been done.	**Renunciation and wisdom.** Ability to accept self; leadership.

*Attributes in **bold** are Erikson's and are defined as "basic virtues" (Erikson, 1963, p. 274).

Adapted from Erikson, E. E. (1963). Eight ages of man. In **Childhood and society** *(pp. 247-274). New York: W. W. Norton & Company; & Erickson, H. (2006).* **Modeling and role-modeling: A view from the client's world.** *Cedar Park, TX: Unicorns Unlimited.*

With long life spans as the norm, individuals need to learn how to be aged. Although the course has not been charted for them, many older adults continue to follow the course that they have followed all their lives, seeking to be all that they can be. They use the supporting structure, norms, and standards of conduct of their family, their religion, and their community. They create a new identity by making sense of the life they have lived through the use of life-review, reminiscence, storytelling, writing, or working to help their families and others. They secure their identities through interactions with others and through their commitment to meeting the needs of others and to supporting their communities. One view of the contribution of older adults to society is called the "grandmother hypothesis" that proposes that older women who maintain cognitive functioning such as communication and memory create intergenerational social support networks that contribute to the survival and success of their grandchildren (Allen, Bruss, & Damasio, 2006; Fox, Sear, Beise, et al., 2010, p. 567). Cole (2004) said that the most valuable contribution of older adults is modeling the last stage of life—the stage after the life cycle—for younger people.

Through their accomplishments, older adults achieve virtues beyond wisdom, which is the virtue of Erikson' eighth age of man. They acquire the virtue of courage to adapt to continuing losses and the certainty of death. They develop public virtue: the pursuit of the common good rather than self-interest. They acquire patience and humility, the capacity to forgive, let go, and adjust. And they achieve a state of wise independence, or the ability to plan and control one's life as well as possible and to accept help when necessary in ways that are gratifying to the giver (Ruddick, 2000).

Needs Theory

According to Maslow (1943), human needs motivate behavior and they are arranged in order of powerfulness of need, with each need resting on prior satisfaction of a more urgent or powerful need. However, Maslow added that "no need or drive can be treated as though isolate or discrete; every drive is related to the state of satisfaction or dissatisfaction of other drives" (Maslow, p. 370). Boyd (2005, p. 79) presented Maslow's hierarchy of needs as follows:

- Physiological needs: air, water, food, shelter, sleep, exercise, elimination, sexual expression, health care
- Safety and security needs: shelter from harm, predictable social and physical environment
- Love and belonging needs: affection and acceptance from family and friends, enduring intimacy
- Esteem needs: self-worth, positive self-image, sense of competence
- Self-actualization needs: development of full personal potential

Maslow believed that the first four needs, survival needs, had to be met before self-actualization could be met. Maslow described people who were self-actualizers as being reality- and problem-centered and viewing their life journey as being as important as the destination (Boeree, 2006). However, Boeree provided examples of artists, authors, handicapped individuals, and prisoners of war who could be thought of as meeting self-actualization who had not met the basic survival needs of food, housing, and safety (Boeree).

Freud's Psychoanalytical Theory: Drive Theory

The early psychiatrist Sigmund Freud believed that humans have two main drives: to survive, obtaining supplies often by using aggression, and to reproduce, which is a sexual drive (Dilts, 2001). According to Freud, the id is unconscious and is the seat of drives, wishes, desires, and fantasies. The ego is half conscious and half unconscious and is involved in awareness of consequences of actions, judgment, reality testing, impulse control, and formation of relationships (Sadock & Sadock, 2007). The ego is also involved in conflict-free activities—thinking, learning, perception, motor control, and language (Gabbard, 2005). The superego, also half conscious and half unconscious, is the individual's moral conscience that develops through the internalization of the values of parents and society, a process that takes place at 5 to 6 years of age.

According to Gabbard (2005), "The superego, the ego and the id battle among themselves as sexuality and aggression strive for expression and discharge" (p. 33). The battle causes anxiety, and the ego develops defense mechanisms to reduce the anxiety. Examples of early or immature primitive defense mechanisms are denial, blocking, splitting, or acting out. Less primitive defense mechanisms include repression, suppression, and rationalization. Mature defense mechanisms include altruism, anticipation, and sublimation.

Freud believed (1) that the mostly unconscious aggressive and sexual drives influence every organ of the body and (2) that humans regulate aggressive and sexual drives in order to achieve greater pleasure and to avoid danger. Freud also believed that thoughts, feelings, behaviors, and symptoms were all outcomes of unconscious mental activities (Sadock & Sadock, 2007). Based on the knowledge that the ego's defense mechanisms regulate anxiety, psychiatric advanced practice nurses encourage patients to use mature anxiety-defense mechanisms such as humor, sublimation, and altruism because mature defense mechanisms are more likely to help patients on their road to recovery than immature defense mechanisms such as acting out, splitting, and passive-aggression. (For descriptions of specific defense mechanisms, see Gabbard, 2005.)

Interpersonal Relations Theory

Sullivan (1953) believed that individuals were motivated by (1) the pursuit of satisfying biological needs such as food, sleep, sex, rest, and physical closeness to other humans and (2) the pursuit of security, which is a state of well-being, of belonging, and of being accepted. Psychopathology was viewed as the result of problems with interpersonal relationships in which anxiety results when an individual experiences barriers to the satisfaction of his or her needs or to social insecurity. Sullivan believed that individuals adapted their behavior to reduce anxiety in order to obtain satisfaction and security.

Psychiatric nursing was strongly influenced by Sullivan's Interpersonal Relations Theory (Sullivan, 1953). In the 1950s, Hildegarde Peplau developed a model for psychiatric nursing that was based on the Interpersonal Relations Theory of Sullivan, and that model guided psychiatric nursing for 20 years. Peplau believed that change was brought about by the interaction of the nurse and the patient (Scharer et al., 2003). She viewed the role of nursing as helping patients to reduce their anxiety by improving their functioning (Peplau, 1952). She believed that through their interpersonal relationship, the patient and the nurse became collaborators in problem-solving and that the process would promote reduction of the patient's anxiety (Keltner, Schwecke, & Bostrom, 2003). Peplau also believed that nurses should help patients to gain competencies beyond those that they had before they became ill (Gastmans, 1998). In that regard, Peplau was an early advocate for the promotion of resilience that would enable patients not only to overcome their present problems but also to use their newly acquired skills to adapt more successfully to future challenges and stressors.

Adaptation Theory

Adaptation refers to the ability of an individual to cope with new or changed situations.

Hansell's Theory of Adaptation

Psychiatrist Norris Hansell's Theory of Adaptation provides an approach for understanding the dynamics of adaptation and the characteristics of individuals who are in distress. It also provides strategies that facilitate distressed individuals' connection or reconnection with resources that will help them in adaptation. In his theory of adaptation, Hansell said that everyone faces "life's flow of adaptive challenges" (1976a, p. 13). He believed that as individuals meet their basic needs, they are able to make adaptations to changing circumstances that enable them to survive. Hansell (1976b) defined basic human needs as an individual's life-supporting transactions with the environment. Hansell's basic human needs can be conceptualized as follows:

1. Food and other essentials for survival, including information and safety
2. A clear concept of self-identify
3. One individual in persisting interdependent contact
4. A group to belong to that claims the individual as a member
5. A role in life
6. Money or purchasing power
7. A sense of meaning to life (Perese, 1997)

In contrast to Maslow, who is known for his belief that an individual's needs are hierarchical, Hansell (1976b) believed that an individual's essential transactions with the environment are cantilevered. The effect of one uncompleted transaction or unmet need affects all needs and thus the well-being of the individual.

Nursing Theories of Adaptation

Roy's Adaptation Model and Erickson, Tomlin, and Swain's Modeling and Role-Modeling (M & RM) Theory of Adaptation focus on the role of nursing as key in helping patients to improve their potential for adaptation.

Roy's Adaptation Model

In Roy's (1976) Adaptation Model, the main feature is the response of an individual's adaptive system to a constantly changing environment. The role of the nurse is to use scientific knowledge to help patients adapt to challenging life problems while promoting positive health and lifestyle practices (Patton, 2004). Adaptation takes place by way of two coping mechanisms: the short-loop, in which stimuli from the environment and internal stimuli are processed through neural-chemical-endocrine channels and produce immediate responses, and the long-loop, in which external and internal stimuli are processed through cognitive/emotional pathways that are involved with learning, emotions, and judgment and produce more delayed responses. Nursing practice focuses on promoting adaptation in four domains: physiological (basic needs), self-concept (image of physical, psychological, and spiritual self), role functioning, and interdependence (love, respect, and valuing of others).

Modeling and Role-Modeling (M & RM) Theory of Adaptation

Nursing theorists Erickson, Tomlin, and Swain (1983) developed a nursing theory of adaptation called Modeling and Role-Modeling (M & RM) that integrates needs theory, attachment theory, and psychosocial developmental theory. When needs are met through attachment, individuals are better able to accomplish the developmental tasks of life; by accomplishing these tasks, they acquire internal strengths that can be used in coping with the challenges and stressors of life (Bray, 2005).

M & RM theory (Case Study 1-1) assumes the wholeness of the individual, and it proposes that individuals' potential for adapting to changes or stressors, such as illness, is determined by their ability to mobilize internal and external resources. Internal resources include both the patient's unique innate attributes, such as genetically influenced temperament, and acquired strengths or virtues, such as self-efficacy (Erickson et al., 1983). External resources include social networks, social support, health care, information, finances, and other services and supplies (Erickson et al.). Capacity for mobilizing external resources is influenced by patients' store of internal resources and the degree to which their basic needs are met through attachments with others (Erickson et al.; Leidy, Ozbolt, & Swain, 1990). The focus of nursing is on building and restoring resources and helping patients to cope with stressors, resolve losses, choose healthy lifestyles, and find meaning in their lives. More information on the whole individual's attachment sources, basic needs, internal and external resources, and potential biopsychosocial outcomes can be found in Table 1-4.

Biopsychosocial Theory

Traditionally, there have been three models of mental illness—the biological, the psychological, and the social. The *biological* model of mental illness proposes that mental illnesses are caused by abnormalities of brain structures, functioning, and neurochemistry. The *psychological* model proposes that mental illnesses are the result of previous conflicts, e.g., earlier patterns of perceiving, thinking, feeling, and behaving. The *social* model proposes that mental illnesses are caused by dysfunctional interpersonal interactions (Dilts, 2001). The *biopsychosocial* model proposes that impairments of physical, psychological, and social functioning cause mental illness.

Before the 1970s, physicians focused on the diseases for which patients sought treatment. There was little emphasis on the human side of illness or the psychosocial dimension of health care: how one feels about the illness, how one carries out family and work roles, how the illness affects patient and family finances, and how one makes choices related to the future (Engel, 1978). Based on his observation that the end product—heart disease—was due to the effects of cultural, social, spiritual, and psychological influences on the cardiovascular system, Engel (1977, 1978) developed the biopsychosocial model in which health, disease, and disability are conceptualized in terms of the relative intactness and functioning of each component system on each hierarchical level—cells, tissues, organs, organ systems, the individual, the family, the community, and society. The model is based on the belief that the interaction of biological factors, psychological factors, and social and cultural factors underlies both health and disease (Gilbert, 2002; Green & Shellenberger, 1991). Biological factors include genetics; abnormalities of brain development related to prenatal exposure to nutritional deficits, infections, traumas, and toxins; adverse circumstances of birth such as extreme prematurity; temperament; lifestyle practices such as smoking, substance use, and lack of exercise; and physical illnesses and disabilities (Engel, 1980; MacDonald & Mikes-Liu, 2009). Psychological factors include an individual's personality, his or her ability to modulate emotional responses and responses to new experiences or stress, and resilience. Social and cultural factors include positive factors such as family support, social

CASE STUDY 1-1

Application of M & RM Theory: Young Adult Male With Schizophrenia

Demir is a 20-year-old first-year college student from Turkey. He is the first member of his family to attend college and has taken out student loans to make it possible. Police brought Demir to the psychiatric emergency room of a general hospital after he smashed the TV in his parent's home. Two days prior to this incident, his roommate, Jonathan, had driven him home, an 8-hour trip. Jonathan said that he was very worried about Demir because he had been skipping all of his classes except philosophy. It had been Demir's custom to pray five times a day, but on that day and evening he had paced the floor instead. For the past several weeks, he would eat only food in sealed containers that he had bought. During the drive home, Demir had talked in a stream of jumbled words, but some were clear: "They are coming after me. They will kill me."

Demir's parents were astonished by the changes in their son in the 2 months since they had last seen him. He had lost weight, was disheveled, and was shivering in the thin shirt he was wearing. His father had taken charge of the situation saying, "There's nothing wrong with him that a good night's sleep won't fix." His mother wrung her hands and cried, "They aren't feeding him right at that place!"

Using M & RM theory, the psychiatric advanced practice nurse determines that the following needs are unmet:

- Safety for self and others
- Health care for medical problems and psychiatric disorder
- Food, warm clothing, and sleep
- Information about his illness and treatment options
- Connectedness to friends, social support networks, religious groups, and academic counselors

The internal resources that Demir has to use in adaptation include

- Intelligence, as indicated by academic achievement and ability to speak three languages (Turkish, English, and French)
- Ability to form a friendship
- Sense of self-identity
- Perseverance in accomplishing tasks
- Resourcefulness, as seen in obtaining financial assistance
- Love for family
- A sense of purpose in life
- Religious faith

The external resources that he has to use in adaptation include

- Financial resources
- Housing (college and parents' home)
- Transportation (parents and friend)
- Support from his family and his roommate
- Student health insurance
- Academic counseling from college

Demir's adaptation is dependent on meeting his needs through the use of internal and external resources. Nurses facilitate the patient's use of available resources and the development and acquisition of additional needed resources.

TABLE 1-4 NURSING THEORY OF ADAPTATION: MODELING AND ROLE-MODELING

Attachment sources	Basic Needs	Patient's Internal Resources	External Resources	Promotion of Biopsychosocial Health: Outcomes
1. Close family (parents, spouse, partner, siblings) 2. Extended family 3. Neighbors 4. Coworkers 5. Community, e.g., clergy, health-care providers 6. Service providers; e.g., meals-on-wheels, traveling libraries, home care 7. Pets 8. Valued causes; e.g., political, environmental, global	1. Food, water, clothing, safe housing and other essentials for survival including information 2. Money or purchasing power 3. A clear concept of self-identity 4. One individual in a persisting interdependent contact 5. A group to belong to that claims the individual as a member 6. A role in life 7. A sense of meaning to life	1. Trust 2. Hope 3. Love 4. Fidelity 5. Ability to care for others 6. Self-identity 7. Self-competence 8. Willpower 9. Wisdom (Walsh, VandenBosch, & Boehm, 1989)	1. Information 2. Social support 3. Health care 4. Transportation 5. Financial assistance 6. Case management 7. Rehabilitation services 8. Spiritual support 9. Legal aid 10. Advocacy	1. Reduction of distressful symptoms 2. Improvement of functioning 3. Prevention of disabilities 4. Development of resilience 5. Attainment of optimal level of recovery 6. Enhancement of quality of life

Adapted from Erickson, H., Tomlin, E., & Swain, M. (1983). **Modeling and role-modeling: A theory and paradigm for nursing**. *Englewood Cliffs, NJ: Prentice-Hall, Inc.*

networks, community resources, culture, and religion and negative factors such as poverty, stigma, victimization, bullying, poor schools, and undesirable living situations (Green & Shellenberger; Perese, 2007).

Over time, the biopsychosocial model has evolved to the concept of domains of functioning: biological, psychological or intrapsychic, and sociocultural functioning (MacDonald & Mikes-Liu, 2009). A disruption of functioning can occur at any level of any system and may result in a cascade of disruptions involving many systems. For example, a disruption of functioning of the individual's social network may impact several physiological systems such as cardiovascular, immune, and hormonal (Gilbert, 2002). If the disruption is contained at the level involved, then adaptation takes place and the disruption may not involve other systems. All living creatures adapt and change in order to survive, and every disruption and adaptation becomes part of the history of each system. In the biopsychosocial model, there is no return to the health status prior to an illness. Health restored represents a different harmony between the systems that incorporates all the changes in all the systems during the illness. The individual is changed and so are family, friends, coworkers, and others. Even society may be changed by the illness, disease, traumatic event, or disability.

The biopsychosocial model provides a framework for understanding the development of health problems, for formulating a case, for selecting interventions that promote recovery, and for guiding research (Cummings & Cassie, 2008). The biopsychosocial model also provides a framework for prevention of psychiatric disorders.

Diagnosing and Case Formulation

In the medical approach, there is emphasis on differential diagnoses and systematic consideration of different possible causes of the patient's problem. In the biopsychosocial approach, data obtained during the comprehensive psychiatric interview, laboratory data, history of medical disorders and treatment, presence of current stressors, and current and remote functioning are used in generating a biopsychosocial case formulation. Specific biological, psychological, and social contributions can be found in Box 1-1.

Treatment

In the biopsychosocial model, psychiatric advanced practice nurses think in terms of patients experiencing both symptoms of distress and impairment of functioning, and they accept that psychotherapeutic principles should be followed in every interaction with patients, including 15-minute medication management sessions (Gabbard, 2007; Gabbard & Kay, 2001). Although pharmacotherapy often provides rapid relief of symptoms of distress, psychotherapy brings about changes that encompass broader areas than the symptoms of distress (Gabbard & Kay). Psychotherapy is a form

BOX 1-1 Information Gathered in a Biopsychosocial Patient History

Biological Contributions
- Genetic influences
- Prenatal and postnatal influences
- Adverse obstetrical circumstances
- Medical conditions
- Substance use

Psychological Contributions
- History of neglect
- Abandonment or abuse
- Cognitive deficits
- Problems with regulation of emotions
- Dysfunctional behaviors

Social Contributions
- Deficits of social support
- Lack of social, cultural/religious, spiritual networks
- Unemployment
- Undesirable living situations
- Bullying, discrimination, and poverty

of learning that produces changes in thinking, perceptions, emotions, and behavior through changes in neural connectivity in response to changes in gene expression (Kandel, 1998, 1999). Combined treatment—psychotherapy, pharmacotherapy, and psychosocial interventions—has been found to be more effective than any one alone for some patients, e.g., for those with schizophrenia (Hogarty, Anderson, Reiss, et al., 1991) and for those with depression, panic disorder, and social phobia (Keller, McCullough, Klein, et al., 2000). However, only 55% of patients treated by psychiatrists receive combined treatment (Pincus, Zarin, Tanielian, et al., 1999).

Research

The biopsychosocial model has been used to measure the perception of met and unmet needs among older adults with severe mental illness (Cummings & Cassie, 2008). Patients identified biological needs as the need for help with their physical illnesses, medications, mobility, and hearing and vision problems; their psychological needs as the need for help with symptoms of distress, memory, hallucinations, and delusions; and their social needs as the need for help with social relationships, money management, benefits, and housing. The most frequently unmet needs occurred across the three domains: physical illness, symptoms of distress, and social contact.

In summary, patients with psychiatric disorders often experience distressful symptoms, have impairment of functioning in several domains, and are socially embedded in a "sea of interactions and values" (Gilbert, 2002, p. 13). The biopsychosocial model is well suited as a guide for psychiatric advanced practice nurses in assessing patients, developing case formulations, and generating plans of appropriate treatment interventions (Green & Shellenberger, 1991; MacDonald & Mikes-Liu, 2009).

Box 1-2 illustrates how the biopsychosocial model may be adapted to clinical practice.

BOX 1-2 Adapting the Biopsychosocial Model to Practice

Assessment of Risk Factors

- Biological: genetic vulnerability, abnormalities of brain functioning, temperament, medical illnesses and their treatment, physical disabilities, exposure to toxins, use of alcohol and other drugs
- Psychological: cognitive distortions, maladaptive coping styles, stressors, depressive and anxious symptoms, danger to self or others, violent relationships, suicide ideation
- Social: poverty; unsafe or undesirable housing situation; disruptions of family structure such as divorce, military deployment, or death; loss of social support networks; relocation of housing, schools, or work; disconnection with religious institutions

Assessment of Protective Factors

- Biological: good health, regular physical activity, adequate sleep, healthy diet, low or moderate use of alcohol, abstinence from smoking and drugs
- Psychological: low levels of stress, good intimate relationships, good problem-solving skills, resilience
- Social: adequate financial resources and housing, supportive social network, belonging and participating in social groups, connection to religion or religious institutions

Treatment

The treatment approach is based on the principle that biopsychosocial systems, including systems at the level of genes, are flexible. Therapeutic interventions and social interactions have the capacity to bring about structural and physiological changes in the brain that may be evidenced in changes in functioning.

BOX 1-3 Decade of the Brain Findings

Mental disorders/ psychiatric disorders are brain disorders.
Over half of human genome is composed of brain-related cells.
Stem cells can grow into neurons.
Brains can create new brain cells.
Genetic vulnerability was identified for some psychiatric disorders.
Learning/experience modifies brain function by altering synaptic strength through the regulation of gene expression (Kandel, 2001).
Advances in brain imaging provided information about the links between structural and functional changes in the brain and psychiatric symptoms, neurotransmitters, and neuronal receptors.

Neuroscience's Influence on Psychiatric Advanced Practice Nursing

The 1980s and 1990s brought fulfillment of early psychiatrists' hopes that advances in neuroscience would provide a foundation for understanding the connection between the brain and psychiatric disorders. During the 1990s (the Decade of the Brain), the Genome Project that began to map human genes provided support for previous observations and studies that suggested that there were family patterns for psychiatric disorders: a genetic loading or vulnerability (Begley, Katz, & Drew, 1987). Other findings that emerged from the Decade of the Brain are presented in Box 1-3.

During the decade that followed the Decade of the Brain, described as the "Decade of Discovery" (Insel, 2006, p. 4), data obtained through advances in the neurosciences and accompanying advances in technology indicated that psychiatric disorders are brain disorders characterized by genetic vulnerability and abnormalities of brain development and neural circuitry. (Neural developmental abnormalities are discussed in Chapter 2.) Examples of advances in neuroscience are present in Box 1-4.

BOX 1-4 Decade of Discovery Findings

- Mental illnesses/psychiatric disorders are disorders of the development of brain circuitry and synaptic connections and functioning.
- Epigenetics: the study of changes in gene activity that do not involve alterations of the genetic code.
- External stimuli such as early life stressors can modify the expression of genes.
- Mirror neurons are associated with mimicry and empathy.
- Deep brain stimulation was found to be effective treatment for severe depression and obsessive-compulsive disorder.
- Human brain is plastic and highly responsive to environmental stimuli across the life span.
- Connections between neurons can change within minutes of stimulation.
- Neurogenesis (birth of new neurons) takes place in certain brain regions such as the hippocampus throughout life.
- Cognitive activation is associated with neuroplasticity, i.e., cognitive activation alters brain structures.
- Acquiring a second language even late in life increases the size of brain area associated with language.
- Cognitive exertion slows cognitive decline.

The advances generated during the Decade of the Brain and the Decade of Discovery support the emerging theories of neuroplasticity/brain plasticity, resilience, and recovery.

Theory of Neuroplasticity/Brain Plasticity

The brain is plastic, which means that it is able to change constantly as it accomplishes its activities, e.g., thinking, planning, learning, remembering, emotional responses, motor and behavioral responses, and other activities that ensure survival. May, Hajak, Ganssbauer, et al. (2007) wrote, "Brain plasticity refers to the brain's ability to undergo functional and structural alterations in response to internal and external environmental changes" (p. 205). Whenever an individual is learning a new skill, practicing to perfect previously acquired skills, or participating in a therapeutic intervention, physical changes take place in the brain's structure and functioning (Kujala & Naatanen, 2010). The brain has a lifelong capacity for physical changes, e.g., changes of brain structures and their functioning, changes in the rate of birth or death of neurons, changes in the dendrites of neurons, changes in density and functioning of neuron receptors, and changes of neuronal circuits (Jancke, 2009; Mahncke, Bronstone, & Merzenich, 2006).

The concept of neuroplasticity had been proposed as early as 1884 by Cajal, who believed that through an individual's mental activity, nerve connections within the brain could be expanded and strengthened (Albright, Jessell, Kandel, et al., 2000). In 1948, the Polish neuroscientist Jerzy Konorski introduced the term "neuroplasticity" to explain the reorganization of the brain as a result of experience. At about the same time, the Canadian neuropsychologist Donald C. Hebb (1949) proposed that synapses were strengthened with use. Much later, Kandel's research with the Aplysia snail demonstrated that memory is stored as changes in the strength of synaptic connections. This finding, for which Kandel won a Nobel Prize, provides support for Cajal's early hypothesis and an explanation for the biological changes that take place in the brain when an individual is exposed to new experiences such as learning, musical and sports training, or psychotherapy (Kandel & Spencer, 1968; Schlaug, 2001). It is believed that the dendrites, the branches of neurons, are covered with a membrane that contains an enzyme called calpain. When an electrical stimulus that is generated by new information travels through the neuron, the calpain weakens an area of the membrane and allows a new spur of the dendrite to form, thus creating new synapses or strengthening existing synaptic connections ("Memory," 1986) (Fig. 1-1).

Brain plasticity is an innately determined characteristic. That is, although plasticity is present in all individuals, there are varying levels of plasticity among individuals (LeDoux, 2002). Thus, each individual's brain has its own capacity and limit for learning and adapting to new experiences. It has recently been found that shared genes influence brain plasticity and intellectual ability. The brain's cognitive functioning ability—such as learning and memory—depends on brain plasticity that is controlled in part by genetic influences (Brans, Kahn, Schnack, et al., 2010).

While genetics has a strong influence on brain development (see Chapter 2), interactions of individuals with

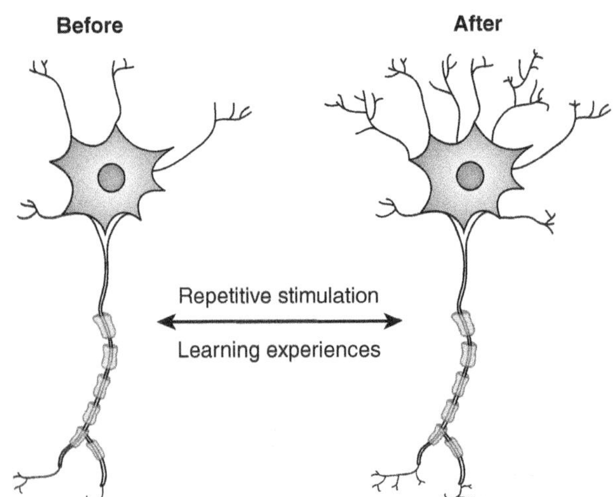

FIGURE 1-1: Brain Plasticity. The brain is plastic across the life span. In response to stimuli (learning, experiences, interactions, and changes in interpretation of past experiences), the brain remodels itself by reorganizing existing neuronal circuits, by generating new neuronal circuits, and by dendritic growth. This figure shows that, in response to learning, there was new growth of dendrites on neurons. New dendrites make new connections with other neurons, which increases the brain's capacity for processing information.

others and with the environment also influence brain development (Black, Jones, Nelson, et al., 1998); that is, experiences shape the brain. Experiences are conveyed to the brain by sensory processes and result in physical changes in the brain structures and functioning (Huttenlocher, 2002). The process of brain plasticity is continuous across the life span, with the brain responding to experiences with changes in the underlying neural substrate, which consists of neurons and neuronal connections (Cicchetti, 2002; Curtis & Cicchetti, 2003; Jancke, 2009; Kujala & Naatanen, 2010). Experiences that shape the brain can be internal—through aging, hormones, and psychopathological processes such as stress or depression—or external—through learning, playing, maltreatment, and psychotherapy. Both positive external experiences such as loving and nurturing and negative external experiences such as abuse and traumatic events shape the brain. The therapeutic interventions that psychiatric advanced practice nurses use—psychotherapy, pharmacotherapy, milieu therapy, psychosocial interventions, and nursing interventions—also shape the brain (Bavelier & Neville, 2002; Cicchetti, 2003).

In discussing brain plasticity, Andreasen (2001) said that the brain remodels itself by changing the connections between the cells. The brain can also change by reorganizing neuronal circuits, by generating new neuronal circuits, by growth or death of dendrites, and by formation or elimination of synapses (Kolb & Gibb, 2001). Kandel (1998) proposed that although genes are important determinants of the pattern of interconnections between neurons in the brain, it is behaviors and social factors that modify the expression of genes and thus the function of nerve cells; that is, alterations in gene expression induced by learning and experiences can cause changes in patterns of neuronal and synaptic connections and changes in functioning and behavior. Therefore, nurture (parenting, caring, and teaching) is ultimately expressed as a biological process that shapes the brain. Similarly, psychotherapy or counseling brings about long-term changes in behavior by producing changes in gene expression that alter synaptic connections and produce structural changes in the interconnections between nerve cells of the brain (Nasrallah, 2006). In brief, when a patient learns a new skill or takes an active part in an intervention, plastic changes take place in the brain (Kujala & Naatanen, 2010).

Evidence Supporting Neuroplasticity

Evidence supporting neuroplasticity comes out of both the Decade of the Brain (the 1990s) and the Decade of Discovery (the 2000s). Cochlear implants have illustrated brain plasticity, as have studies of institutionalized Romanian children without caregivers and studies of taxi drivers who had to learn their routes. Musical training and meditation also reveal the brain's neuroplasticity, and early interventions for children with autism have shown that the brain can develop and improve in function with extensive therapy.

Cochlear Implants

One example that supports the theory of neuroplasticity is the change that occurs following a cochlear implant. After cochlear implantation, the wiring of the brain changes to accommodate for the sounds (electrical impulses) that travel through the auditory nervous system, and the individual's ability to understand sounds develops as speech develops. Neuronal circuits form in response to repeated patterns of sound that are presented to the cortex of the brain (White, Ochs, Merzenich, et al., 1990).

Institutionalized Romanian Children

Another example that proves brain plasticity is the United Kingdom's study on the health of Romanian children who had suffered severe deprivation in institutions. The study observed the children both before and after they were adopted into functional families. The effect of caring parenting on severely neglected children resulted in improvement of both physical health and cognitive functioning.

Before adoption, the Romanian children had been confined to cots, they had few playthings, and their caregivers had not talked to them or given them individual attention. They were in poor physical condition, were malnourished, and had chronic infections. They were developmentally impaired on physical measures (51% were below the third percentile at adoption), and cognitive measures also showed impairment. Among those adopted before 6 months of age, there was a dramatic "catch-up" of cognitive functioning by age 4. The adopted children's cognitive functioning was normal, although physical growth caught up to about 90% of normal. Cognitive and physical "catch-up" was less for those children who were adopted after 6 months (Rutter & The English and Romanian Adoptees [ERA] study team, 1998).

Musical Training

Research has shown that the acquisition of musical expertise has an effect on the anatomy and functioning of the brain (Gaab, Gaser, & Schlaug, 2006; Munte, Altenmuller, & Jancke, 2002; Schlaug, 2001). Neuroimaging studies of adult musicians have shown that anatomical changes of the brain include enlargement of the anterior half of the corpus callosum, which integrates information from the right hemisphere of the brain with that of the left hemisphere; enlargement of motor areas; and increased volume of the cerebellum, which is involved in movement coordination and sequencing (Gaser & Schlaug, 2003; Schlaug, 2001). It is thought that these structural changes are due to brain growth in response to repeated use (Gaser & Schlaug). The areas of increased brain volume are parts of networks that are involved in acquiring the skills needed by performing musicians. Musicians use the right hemisphere and the left hemisphere of the brain simultaneously to process and play music (Schlaug, Forgeard, Zhu, et al., 2009, p. 205).

The increased size of the corpus callosum is more marked among musicians who started their musical training early in life and is linked to intensity of practicing (Schlaug et al., 2009). For example, in a study of children who had had 4 years of musical training, it was found that there was increased gray matter volume in several brain areas (Schlaug, Norton, Overy, et al., 2005) and that increased gray matter volume was positively associated with amount of musical practice (Gaser & Schlaug, 2003). In another study of children 7 years old or younger who had 15 months of musical training, it was found that structural changes in the brain occurred in motor and auditory areas and that there were functional changes in music-related motor and auditory behaviors (Hyde, Lerch, Norton, et al., 2009). The researchers concluded that training produces structural changes in young brains. This finding supports the use of long-term interventions based on the theory of neuroplasticity to help children with developmental disorders.

Recently, in a study to examine transfer effects between music and language, it was found that children who have as little as 6 months of musical training have improved ability to process pitch in music and better pitch discrimination in speech. They also had improved reading skills (Moreno, Marques, Santos, et al., 2009). Among children with dyslexia who have impaired pitch discrimination, it has been found that (1) visual-auditory multimedia training using reading and (2) writing training with pitch and tone training resulted in improved writing performance (Kast, Meyer, Vogeli, et al., 2007). Musical training also has positive effects on understanding and learning foreign languages (Marques, Moreno, Castro, et al., 2007).

Meditation

Meditation as an intervention to alter higher cognitive functioning through its effect on neuroplasticity is receiving growing attention. Meditation has the benefits of being self-administered and having no reported adverse side effects (Green & Turner, 2010). Research supports the beneficial effects of meditation in improving psychological and physiological well-being (Luders, Toga, Lepore, et al., 2009). More specifically, active meditation and mindfulness practice has been found to beneficially affect autonomic nervous system activity (Green & Turner) and to foster emotional self-regulation and greater flexibility of behavioral responses (Wenk-Sormaz, 2005). The changes in brain structures associated with mindfulness and meditation include more gray matter volume (more neurons) in brain areas that are associated with meditation. For example, in a study comparing individuals who had meditated 2 hours a day for about 8 years with individuals who had never meditated, brain imaging showed that the brain structures involved in meditation—the right anterior insula (an area of the brain involved in mindfulness and empathy) and the right hippocampus (a brain structure involved in learning, memory, and modifying arousal)—were larger in those who meditated than in nonmeditators (Holzel, Ott, Gard, et al., 2008; Lazar, Kerr, Wasserman, et al., 2005). Green and Turner suggest that meditation brings about changes in brain structures and functioning that result in stress reduction and increased sense of well-being.

Taxi Drivers

Taxi drivers in London who train for about 2 years to acquire extensive knowledge of the streets of London before they are able to obtain a license show a change in the hippocampus compared to a control group (males of the same age who did not drive taxis). Whereas the overall volume of the hippocampus was the same for both taxi drivers and controls, the trained drivers had increased volume of the posterior part of the hippocampus, which is an area of the brain that stores spatial representation of the environment and learned information about the environmental space and a decreased volume of the anterior part of the hippocampus (Maguire, Gadian, Johnsrude, et al., 2000). The researchers suggest that in response to the need to store more spatial representations of the environment, the brain reorganized the circuitry of the hippocampus; that is, learning to meet the challenge of their job caused plastic reorganization of the brain.

Autism: Early Interventions

Autism is a neurodevelopmental disorder that has a strong genetic component (Dawson, 2008). It is characterized by impairments in social and communication behaviors and limited interests and interactions with others. Some researchers believe that autism is a disorder of plasticity of synapses where information is passed from one neuron to another. It is thought that genetic influences cause postnatal disruption of synaptic ability to process experiences, such as parents' social interactions with their infant (Garber, 2007; Zoghbi, 2003). Early intensive interventions that start as soon as possible—preferably by 12 months, or at least before age 4 years—are used to remediate synaptic plasticity, i.e., to correct faulty wiring (Altemeier & Altemeier, 2009). Interventions focus on imitation, language, playing with toys, social interaction, and motor and adaptive behavior. Interventions are provided 25 hours a week or more for at least 2 years (Dawson, p. 790). Studies of early intervention treatment have shown that a substantial number of children with autism have gains in IQ, language, and educational placement (less time in special education classes) (Cohen, Amerine-Dickens, & Smith, 2006). Children with milder forms of autism have a better response to early interventions than children with more severe forms of autism (Smith, Mirenda, & Zaidman-Zait, 2007).

To summarize, the term "brain plasticity" refers to the ability of learning and experience to remodel the brain at the level of cells and circuits of cells, thus changing their structure and functioning (Carter, 2009). Carter wrote, "Brain tissue can be 'strengthened' and built up like a muscle according to how much it is exercised" (p. 38).

Theory of Resilience

Resilience is the capacity to deal with, overcome, learn from, or even gain from adversities of life (Grotberg, 2003; Wagnild & Collins, 2009). It comprises inner strength, acquired competencies, a sense of optimism and hope, flexibility, the ability to cope with adversity, and forgiveness (Wagnild & Collins). Resilience is also considered to be a dynamic process, a process by which individuals bounce back from adversity (Luthar, Cicchetti, & Becker, 2000). The consequence or byproduct of resilience is a sense of mastery over one adversity that can be transferred to other situations.

Resilience differs from adapting to a situation. *Adapting* is accepting something you cannot change, whereas *resilience* implies something good emerging from adversity. The core elements of resilience are

- Competencies in thinking, communication, problem-solving, and coping
- Attitudes such as optimism, hope, faith, and positive self-concept
- Behaviors such as planning, using foresight, helping others, and participating in religious activities (Werner, 2006)

Resilience connotes hope and involves the use of personal strengths and skills (Dyer & McGuinness, 1996; Wright & Masten, 2006). Resilience is a protective factor that reduces an individual's vulnerability to adverse events. It is associated with the ability to function well in many roles, with a positive self-concept, and with good mental health (Goldstein & Brooks, 2006).

Resilience in Childhood

Cicchetti (2004) said that resilience represents the child's capacity either to adapt successfully despite experiencing multiple adversities such as poverty and maltreatment, or to adapt successfully to a chronic illness or severe trauma. Resilience arises from the child's systems of adaptive processes that are made up of the child's unique attributes, such as genetic vulnerabilities and temperament, brain functioning, relationships with parents, capacity to regulate emotions and behaviors, and readiness to interact with the environment. However, the child's adaptive processes are embedded in systems of interactions—family, school, neighborhood, and culturally sanctioned rituals, beliefs, and supports (Werner, 2006). Thus, failure to develop resilience may be caused by influences, forces, or events that injure or do not protect the systems that carry out adaptive processes.

Attributes of Resilient Children

Children with resilience tend to have been easy babies (cuddly, slept well, ate well, and were even-tempered) and to elicit positive responses from adults. Their attributes include

- Having a high activity level and sociability level and a low level of excitability and distress
- Good school performance
- Good communication skills, reading skills, and problem-solving skills
- Ability to self-regulate their emotions and behaviors
- Possession of a special hobby that they can share with a friend

Resilient children tend to come from families with four or fewer children and from families in which there is space of 2 or more years between the children. In spite of poverty, family discord, and parental mental illness, resilient children are able to establish a close bond with at least one caretaker from whom they received positive attention during the first years of life. The nurturing individual might be from within the family (grandparent, older sibling, aunt, or uncle) or outside of the family (a favorite teacher, church group leader, YMCA counselor, neighbor, or babysitter). Structured activities, routines, and assigned chores have been found to be part of resilient children's lives (Masten, 2001; Werner & Smith, 1992).

Resilience Among Children in Severe Adverse Situations

In Apfel and Simon's (1996) book *Minefields in Their Hearts,* which describes the experiences of children exposed to war, persecution, and violence, the authors identified characteristics or attributes of children who were resilient. These children were able to hold on to good, sustaining memories and use them. They were resourceful and had the ability to marshal resources for survival. These children were able to get some support and kindness out of someone even in the worse circumstances. They were able to turn to adults for support and help if their parents were unable to provide it, and they knew how to reciprocate and thus maintain the supportive relationship. They tended to learn as much as they could about the circumstances in which they found themselves and to use that information to get help. They had the ability to see the adverse experience as something that happens to others also, not just to them. They strongly believed that they had the right to survive and could help others to survive.

Promoting Resilience

At one time it was thought that resilience was inborn (Shenfeld, 2007); now it is accepted that resilience is not static. Resilience can be changed by new experiences and by creating new meaning to prior adverse experiences (Curtis & Chicchetti, 2003). Kandel (1998) found that learning new information and being exposed to different experiences produce alterations in gene expression that promote changes in neuronal and synaptic connections. Thus, social and psychological experiences, including therapeutic interventions, can alter gene expression, brain structures, and brain functioning; they can build resilience (Kandel; Kolb & Whishaw, 1998). Promoting the development of resilience includes reducing risks to the development of resilience, mobilizing protective factors, and increasing external resources that foster the development of resilience.

Risk Factors Associated With Failure to Develop Resilience

Risk factors for failure to develop resilience to stressors include

- Family poverty or lack of income
- Parental psychopathology, such as depression or substance-related disorders
- Parental criminality
- Family conflict, discord, or violence
- Family disruptions (abandonment; separations, divorce, foster care)
- Large family size, more than four children
- Living in high-crime neighborhoods (Werner & Smith, 1992)

Protective Processes and Factors That Promote Resilience

There are protective processes that promote resilience. Rutter (1987) wrote, "It is protective to have a well established feeling of one's own worth as a person together with a confidence and conviction that one can cope successfully with life's challenges" (p. 327). He added, "Two types of experiences are most influential: secure and harmonious love relationships and successful accomplishment of tasks important to the individuals" (p. 327). He continued, "It appears that good intimate relationships, even in adult life, can do much to bolster individuals' positive concepts about themselves and their worth in other individuals' eyes" (p. 328).

The protective processes of resilience are strongly influenced by the presence of specific protective factors, e.g., an individual's attributes and competencies (Dyer & McGuiness, 1996). These attributes and competencies include

- Easy temperament
- Secure attachment patterns
- High intelligence
- Academic achievement
- Ability to self-regulate thinking, emotions, and behavior
- Hope, faith, and optimism
- Health-promoting skills, such as effective communication skills and problem-solving skills
- Ability to rebound
- Strong sense of self-efficacy
- Determination to overcome obstacles (Dyer & McGuiness, 1996; Fraley, Fazzari, Bonanno, et al., 2006; Wright & Masten, 2006)

These protective factors are often associated with the development of secondary protective factors. For example, individuals who are optimistic are able to generate more social support and tend to use a greater number of positive adaptive coping strategies in adapting to stressful situations (Brissette, Scheler, & Carver, 2002). Protective factors can also be external resources, with social support being one of the most effective protective factors against stressor-generated anxiety (Muller & Lemieux, 2000). Other external protective resources include good relationships with extended family and neighbors, participation in cultural and spiritual traditions and social network activities, and availability of community services.

Resilience Can Be Built

The brain's attribute of lifelong plasticity enables an individual's interactions with the environment to alter the brain's development and functioning and thus produce resilient or less resilient outcomes (Curtis & Cicchetti, 2003). Therefore, because resilience is modifiable, it can be promoted as a buffer to stressful events; psychiatric advanced practice nurses can teach families how to nurture resilience in their children and in the family. Shenfeld (2007) suggested the following strategies to build resilience:

- Teaching the family to use effective communication
- Helping families to develop and use problem-solving skills
- Advocating for the use of an authoritative parenting style (warm, nurturing; firm rules; appropriate expectations for children's age; praise for efforts and accomplishments)
- Showing families how to spend time together in pleasurable activities
- Supporting involvement with extended family and neighbors
- Helping the family to strengthen a sense of belonging and security through the regular routines and participation in celebrations and rituals
- Encouraging the family to share their faith, beliefs, and spiritual connections

In summary, resilience is a protective factor against stressors. It comprises innate attributes and learned attitudes, skills, and behaviors. Because of brain plasticity, it is possible to promote resilience in individuals and families.

Recovery

Significance and Requirements of Recovery

For a long time, patients with psychiatric disorders and their families were led to believe that their future was bleak: a lifelong sentence to a chronic illness (Spaniel, Gagne, & Koehler, 2003). They were expected to adjust to the illness and give up hope of being able to be a productive member of society. Treatment goals included compliance with medications, reduction of hospital admissions, and adaptation to a chronic illness (Marder & Rehm, 2005). Individuals with psychiatric disorders have repudiated those treatment goals (Deegan, 1996). Now, they are advocating for the same treatment goal as individuals with medical illnesses—recovery (Ahern & Fisher, 2001). Within the model of recovery, the objectives are that the individual will

- Acquire or return to a meaningful social role
- Develop relationships
- Reclaim a sense of self-identity
- Become a member of the community (Ahern & Fisher, 2001)

Recent studies from Japan, Germany, Switzerland, and the United States have shown that over time, one-half to two-thirds of people with severe mental illness achieve significant recovery, which provides support for patients' insistence upon recovery as their goal (Harding, 1989; Harding & Keller, 1998; Harding & Zahniser, 1994; Harding, Zubin, & Strauss, 1992).

Recovery is viewed as a process, a way of life, and an outcome (Egeland, Carlson, & Stroufe, 1993). For patients, recovery means being responsible for their lives; it means accepting what they cannot do or be, discovering what they can do and be, and accepting responsibility for pursuing all that they can be (Deegan, 1996). A national research project on recovery states that recovery is the product of the interaction between individuals' unique attributes—self-esteem, self-care, self-determination, independence, personal resourcefulness, sense of hope, a purpose in life, and meaning to life—and the environment, which includes health care; resources for meeting basic needs and living and work situations; and being accepted in the community (National Research Project on Recovery, 2003).

Mental illnesses, especially severe mental illnesses such as schizophrenia, bipolar disorder, depression, substance-related disorders, and some anxiety disorders and personality disorders, affect all aspects of individuals' lives—physical and emotional well-being, social relations, work, sense of self, and core identity (Roe, 2005). Individuals with mental illnesses must recover from the multiple traumas associated with having a psychiatric disorder: the effects of psychotropic medications, negative professional attitudes, devaluating mental health programs, stigma, societal discrimination, and victimization (Perese, 2007).

Individuals with psychiatric disorders also experience multiple losses—loss of roles such as partner, parent, and coworker; loss of hope; loss of a sense of purpose in life; loss of a sense of self; and loss of connectedness with others (Davidson, Stayner, & Haglund, 1998). Roe (2005) found that loss of a basic sense of self-identity caused a diminished sense of self. Sense of self includes a sense of self-esteem, self-efficacy, and a sense of being worthy of love and support (Muller & Lemieux, 2000). A diminished sense of self was associated with feeling discouraged and pessimistic about the future, with being afraid of failure and rejection, with giving up, and with protecting oneself from failure and rejections by withdrawing and not being involved in anything. Roe concluded that the course of severe mental illness is influenced not only by characteristics of the psychiatric disorder and response to treatment, but also by the patient's sense of self.

A sense of self-identity is tied to the social position or the social roles that individuals fulfill. Social roles are sets of behavioral expectations that provide a sense of predictability to life. Social roles provide information about how individuals are supposed to behave; when individuals meet these role expectations, they experience an increase in their self-esteem. Social roles provide a purpose to life and provide other people with information about who they are (Thoits, 1983). The more roles that an individual is able to fulfill successfully, the more accumulated role identities they have, which in turn is associated with increased self-esteem, greater personal control, and healthier lifestyle practices (Cohen, Doyle, Skoner, et al., 1997).

One agent in recovery for patients with psychiatric disorders may be the rediscovery and reconstruction of a sense of self. The reconstruction of self requires that patients take an active and collaborative part in the process of recovery (Davidson & Strauss, 1992). The process may take place in treatment centers, but more often it takes place in community settings that do not provide mental health care. These community settings are called "arenas of recovery" by Sells, Borg, Marin, et al. (2006, p. 3). For example, patients have described feeling known, understood, accepted, and cared for in psychosocial clubs. Others have described community places such as bowling alleys where they could be with people, watch what was going on, bowl on a team, and be accepted as a bowler and not a patient. Some patients believed that fellowship found in community activities—such as visiting museums, shopping, going for coffee—was helpful. Some patients thought that meaningful routines, employment, and spirituality had helped them in their recovery process. Many patients said that their perception of their roles had shifted as they became engaged in community activities. Sells et al. (2006) studied the events that patients believed had helped them on the road to recovery and found a common theme of community arenas helping patients in "developing alternative understandings of the self" (p. 14).

Recovery can be viewed as a process and an outcome (Spaniel, Gagne, & Koehler, 2003). Spaniel et al. described the process of recovery as moving toward self-discovery, self-renewal, transformation, and healing physically and emotionally, i.e., "of adjusting one's attitudes and feelings, perceptions, beliefs, roles and goals in life" (p. 38). They described the desired outcomes of recovery as working, living independently, having meaningful relationships, and contributing to the community.

Individuals with psychiatric disorders have identified what they need to move toward recovery. The first step is meeting their basic needs—health care, housing, finances adequate for living, transportation, means of communication (telephone), personal safety from abuse and victimization, social connectedness, a job, a sense of self-identity, and a purpose in life. These needs are frequently unmet among individuals with psychiatric disorders who are living in the community (Aiken, 1987; Perese, 1997; Perese & Wu, 2010). The second step toward recovery is hope: a hope that is shared by the ill individual, his or her family, care providers, and the community. Third, individuals with psychiatric disorders ask for a holistic approach to promoting total health while allowing for their independence and participation in the planning process for care that will enable them to move toward recovery. They specifically ask that "best practice" program elements such as psychosocial interventions, health care, supported work, and self-help resources be available for them (National Research Project on Recovery, 2003). Although it is known that psychosocial interventions are effective in facilitating recovery, very few patients—as few as 10%—receive the psychosocial interventions that would help them (Torrey, Drake, Dixon, et al., 2001).

Programs that have adopted the philosophy of recovery understand the need to keep the values of recovery foremost while using evidence-based practices that may have traditional outcomes such as community tenure, employment, decreased hospital admissions, and decreased use of mental health services. Programs that value the concept of recovery for patients with mental illness have four key features: "person orientation, person involvement, self determination/choice, and growth potential" (Farkas, Gagne, Anthony, et al., 2005, p. 146).

The Psychiatric Advanced Practice Nurse's Role in Recovery

How can psychiatric advanced practice nurses help patients achieve the goal of recovery? Individuals with psychiatric disorders need to rebuild their personal, social, environmental, and spiritual connections; to reclaim a sense of self, i.e., self-efficacy, self-esteem, and self-control; and to actively take care of themselves by doing things that make their life work better, such as getting up on time, keeping appointments, preparing healthy meals for themselves, and planning activities. Patients with severe mental illness who are in the process of recovery suggest that care providers do the following:

- Focus on how the individual feels, what the individual is experiencing, and what the individual wants, rather than on symptoms and diagnoses
- Share information about self-help skills and strategies
- Break tasks down into the smallest steps
- Recognize even the smallest indications of progress
- Listen to the individual in the process of recovery
- Encourage connections with peer or self-help groups (Mead & Copeland, 2000)

The role of psychiatric advanced practice nurses in the process of recovery includes working with patients to develop a plan of care that will facilitate movement toward recovery; prescribing and monitoring medications and managing their side effects; providing psychotherapy; providing or referring the individual for psychosocial interventions such as case management and supported work; using nursing interventions such as anticipatory guidance and coping enhancement; and identifying community resources. They can also encourage the use of the strategies that Mead and Copeland (2000) have identified as helpful for individuals in recovery:

- Stress reduction and relaxation techniques
- Exercise: walking, climbing stairs, running, biking, swimming
- Creative and fun activities: crafts, listening to music, gardening, and woodworking
- Writing in a journal
- Reducing coffee intake
- Getting outdoors for at least 30 minutes a day
- Self-help, mutual-help, and peer support groups; psychosocial clubs
- Having a generic daily plan of activities to use when it is hard to make decisions
- Developing a plan of symptoms identification and response: a list of what has to be done each day to maintain wellness; triggers that may increase symptoms and how to prevent that response; early signs of an increase of symptoms and how to prevent further increase; crisis planning for possibility of loss of control

Recovery is the personal goal of most patients with psychiatric disorders, and it is the treatment goal that psychiatric advanced practice nurses have for their patients.

Practice of Psychiatric Advanced Practice Nurses

The practice of psychiatric advanced practice nurses consists of specific activities that are intended to benefit individuals, groups, or society. Practice activities are chosen from a variety of options with the choice predicated upon the nursing value of providing the best care available for each individual patient. Provision of such care is structured by evidence.

Evidence-Based Care

Evidence-based interventions are characterized by research that demonstrates effectiveness in assisting patients to achieve outcomes (Mueser, Torrey, Lynde, et al., 2003); uses an experimental design; obtains similar research findings by different researchers; and achieves widely accepted outcomes such as decrease of symptoms and increase of social and vocational functioning (Mueser, Corrigan, Hilton, et al., 2002). However, sometimes studies of comparison groups that have not been randomized may be the best available research evidence: a quasi-experimental design.

There is a wide array of evidence-based pharmacological interventions that are detailed in textbooks of psychopharmacology and that are included in guidelines for treatment; additionally, there are many documented evidence-based psychotherapeutic interventions (Nathan & Gorman, 1998). However, there is less information available about evidence-based psychosocial interventions. Mueser et al. (2002) summarized the evidence supporting the use of six psychosocial interventions as follows:

1. Psychoeducation programs: Result in increased knowledge of mental illness but no improvement in other outcomes measured. Psychoeducation may serve as the foundation for other interventions and may increase patients' ability to make informed decisions about treatment.
2. Behavioral tailoring: Incorporates taking medications into patients' daily life; e.g., provides cues for taking medications. Results in improvement in taking their medications.
3. Relapse prevention: Teaches patients and families to recognize environmental triggers of relapse and early warning signs or symptoms and how to take steps to prevent exacerbation of symptoms. Relapse prevention programs result in a decrease of relapses and rehospitalizations.
4. Coping skills training: The goal is to increase patients' ability to deal with symptoms, stress, and persistent symptoms. Results show effectiveness in reducing symptom severity.
5. Comprehensive programs: Programs include different components such as psychoeducation, relapse prevention, goal setting, stress management, coping strategies, and problem-solving. Results vary from program to program, but the results suggest fewer relapses, better social adjustment, and improved quality of life.
6. Cognitive behavioral treatment for psychosis: Teaches coping skills such as distraction to reduce focusing on symptoms and to modify dysfunctional beliefs about mental illness, themselves, and the environment. Results show cognitive behavioral treatment is more effective than supportive counseling or standard care in reducing psychotic symptoms. There are also beneficial effects on social withdrawal and lack of pleasure in activities.

Among the subgroups of patients for whom psychiatric advanced practice nurses will provide care are those with severe mental illness such as schizophrenia, schizoaffective disorder, bipolar disorder, and major depression. Mueser et al. (2003) described the evidence that supports the use of six interventions for this population:

- Pharmacological interventions (see Chapter 6 for information about psychopharmacotherapy and neurotransmission; see Chapters 9 through 18 for disorder-specific psychopharmacotherapy interventions): They reduce symptoms and prevent relapses.
- Assertive Community Treatment (ACT) (see Chapter 8): ACT provides treatment for patients in their own living situation rather than in a clinic. ACT supplies direct services rather than having multiple service providers; offers 24-hour coverage; uses a team approach; and ensures that case managers have small caseloads so that they can provide individualized, immediate service. Research-derived evidence shows reduced hospitalizations, stable housing in the community, reduced severity of symptoms, lower treatment costs, and improved quality of life.
- Family psychoeducation (see Chapter 8): There are different models of family psychoeducation. Effective programs last at least 6 months and provide information about the psychiatric illness and its management; reduce tension and stress in the family; give social support and empathy to the family; focus on hope for the future; and aim to improve functioning of all family members. With short-term family psychoeducation programs (6 months or less), there is improvement in family knowledge and family sense of burden of care but limited effect on severity or course of the illness. In some studies, longer programs are associated with reduced rates of relapse and rehospitalization and improved family relationships.
- Supported employment (see Chapter 8): In supported employment, the patient is assisted with a rapid job search and placement. Vocational training and clinical services are integrated, and jobs are matched to patients' preferences. Research-generated evidence shows improved rates of competitive employment.
- Illness self-management (Mueser et al., 2002): Patients are encouraged to be active in managing their symptoms, getting their basic needs met, and defining their desired outcomes. Strategies used include psychoeducation about psychiatric disorders and treatment; promotion of effective use of medications; and teaching relapse-prevention skills and how to cope with symptoms.
- Integrated dual-disorders treatment (treatment provided simultaneously for psychiatric disorder and substance abuse): Comprehensive integrated treatment programs are effective in reducing substance abuse. Reduced substance use correlates with improved functioning and stability of housing.

Knowing the effectiveness of interventions to bring about desired outcomes is important for both patients and clinicians. For example, when surveyed, patients with severe mental illness asked that "best practice" program elements be available for them (Recovery, 2003, p. 9). Psychiatric advanced practice nurses use knowledge about evidence-based interventions to select ones that target their patients' treatment needs.

Summary

Psychiatric advanced practice nurses have emerged as a valued presence in the mental health care workforce. They have a knowledge base that encompasses the restoration and maintenance of physical and mental health and the clinical expertise to provide comprehensive, cost-effective, ongoing quality mental health care for culturally diverse persons with psychiatric disorders across the life span (Merwin & Fox, 1999). They also are able to integrate time-honored theories of attachment, psychosocial development, need satisfaction, and adaptation with the newer theories of neuroplasticity and resilience to guide care for individuals with psychiatric disorders that will facilitate recovery (Ryff & Singer, 2000).

Key Points

- Temperament is a genetically influenced early form of personality.
- Temperament in babies is categorized as easy, slow-to-warm up, difficult, and mixed.
- Risk for psychopathology is greater among individuals who had a difficult temperament as a child.
- Attachment is an innate biological drive that fosters closeness to a caregiver and promotes a sense of security.
- Warm nurturing parenting produces secure patterns of attachment that are associated with healthy outcomes.
- Neglectful or abusive parenting produces insecure attachment patterns that are associated with higher rates of psychopathology.
- Through attachment, individuals meet their needs and are able to successfully accomplish age-related tasks that build inner virtues or strengths.
- Brain plasticity refers to the ability of learning and experience to remodel the brain.
- Brain plasticity takes place at the level of gene expression, neurons, synapses, brain structures, and brain functioning.
- Brain plasticity outcomes are changes in perception, thinking, emotions, and behavior.
- Resilience is the capacity to deal with, overcome, learn from, or even gain from adversities of life.
- Resilience can be built.
- Recovery is the goal of patients with psychiatric disorders, their families, and care providers.
- Recovery goals include having a meaningful social role, relationships, a sense of self-identity, and respected membership in the community.
- Because of brain plasticity, the levers of change that psychiatric advanced practice nurses use—psychotherapy, pharmacotherapy, milieu therapy, psychosocial interventions, and nursing interventions—can change the brain.

References

Ahern, L., & Fisher, D. (2001). Recovery at your own pace (Personal assistance in community existence). *Journal of Psychosocial Nursing and Mental Health Services, 39*(4), 22-32.

Aiken, L. (1987). Unmet needs of the chronically mentally ill: Will nursing respond. *Image, 19*(3), 121-125.

Ainsworth, M. D. (1989). Attachments beyond infancy. *American Psychologist, 44*(4), 709-716.

Ainsworth, M. D., Bell, S. M., & Stayton, D. J. (1971). Individual differences in strange-situation behaviour of one-year olds. In H. R. Schaffer (Ed.), *The origins of human social relations* (pp. 17-32). New York: Academic Press.

Albright, T. D., Jessell, T. M., Kandel, E. R., et al. (2000). Neural science: A century of progress and the mysteries that remain. *Cell, 100, 25*, S1-S55.

Alexander, F. G., & Selesnick, S. T. (1966). The history of psychiatry: An evaluation of psychiatric thought and practice from prehistoric times to the present. New York: Harper and Row Publishers.

Allen, J. S., Bruss, J., & Damasio, H. (2005). The aging brain: The cognitive reserve hypothesis and hominid evolution. *American Journal of Human Biology, 17*(6), 673-689.

Altemeier, W. A., & Altemeier, L. E. (2009). How can early, intensive training help a genetic disorder? *Pediatric Annals, 38*(3), 167-172.

American Nurses Association (2000). *Scope and standards of psychiatric-mental health nursing practice.* Washington, DC: American Nurses Association.

Andreasen, N. (2001). *Brave new brain: Conquering mental illness in the era of the genome.* Oxford, UK: Oxford University Press.

Apfel, R. J., & Simon, B. (Eds.). (1996). *Minefields in their hearts: The mental health of children in war and communal violence.* New Haven: Yale University Press.

Bakermans-Kranenburg, M. J., van Ijzendoorn, M. H., & Juffer, F. (2005). Disorganized infant attachment and preventive interventions: A review and meta-analysis. *Infant Mental Health Journal, 26*(3), 191-216.

Bakwin, H. (1942). Loneliness in infants. *American Journal of Diseases of Children, 63*, 30-40.

Bavelier, D., & Neville, H. J. (2002). Cross-modal plasticity: Where and how? *Nature Reviews. Neuroscience, 3*(6), 443-452.

Begley, S. Katz, S. E., & Drew, L. (1987, August 31). The genome initiative. *Newsweek*, 58-60.

Bentinck-Smith, W., & Stouffer, E. (1993). *Harvard University history of named chairs: Sketches of donors and donations: Professorships of the Faculties of Medicine and Public Health.* Cambridge, MA: Harvard University Press.

Bjorklund, P. (2003). The certified psychiatric nurse practitioner: Advanced practice psychiatric nursing reclaimed. *Archives of Psychiatric Nursing, 17*(2), 77-87.

Black, J., Jones, T. A., Nelson, C. A., et al. (1998). Neuronal plasticity and the developing brain. In N. E. Alessi, J. T. Coyle, S. I. Harrison, & S. Eth (Eds.), *Handbook of child and adolescent psychiatry* (pp. 31-53). New York: John Wiley & Sons.

Boeree, G. C. (2006). Personality theories: Abraham Maslow. Retrieved from http://www.ship.edu/~cgboeree/maslow.html

Bowlby, J. (1969). Attachment and loss (Vol. I. *Attachment.*) London: Hogarth Press.

Bowlby, J. (1973). Attachment and loss (Vol. II. *Separation anxiety and anger.*) London: Hogarth Press.

Bowlby, J. (1988a). Developmental psychiatry comes of age. *The American Journal of Psychiatry, 145*(1), 1-10.

Bowlby, J. (1988b). The role of attachment in personality development. In J. Bowlby (Ed.), *A secure base: Clinical implications of attachment theory.* London: Routledge.

Boyd, M. A. (2005). *Psychiatric nursing: Contemporary practice.* Philadelphia: Lippincott Williams & Wilkins.

Brans, R. G. H., Kahn, R. S., Schnack, H. G., et al. (2010). Brain plasticity and intellectual ability are influenced by shared genes. *The Journal of Neuroscience, 10*(16), 5519-5524.

Bray, C. O. (2005). *The relationship between psychosocial attributes, self-care resources, basic need satisfaction and measures of cognitive and theory* (Doctoral dissertation). The University of Texas Graduate School of Biomedical Sciences. Galveston, TX.

Brissette, J., Scheler, M. F., & Carver, C. S. (2002). The role of optimism in social network development, coping and psychological adjustment during a life transition. *Journal of Personality and Social Psychology, 82*(1), 102-111.

Buckley, A. (1938). *Nursing mental and nervous diseases.* Philadelphia: J. B. Lippincott Company.

Carlson, E., Jacobvitz, D., & Sroufe, L. A. (1995). A developmental investigation of inattentiveness and hyperactivity. *Child Development, 66*(1), 37-54.

Carter, R. (2009). *The human brain book: An illustrated guide to its structure, function, and disorders.* London: Dorling Kindersley Limited (DK).

Caspi, A. (2000). The child is father of the man: Personality continuities from childhood to adulthood. *Journal of Personality and Social Psychology, 78*(1), 158-172.

Caspi, A., Moffitt, T., Newman, D., et al. (1996). Behavioral observations at age 3 years predict adult psychiatric disorders. *Archives of General Psychiatry, 53,* 1033-1039.

Caspi, A., Roberts, B. W., & Shiner R. L. (2005). Personality development: Stability and change. *Annual Review of Psychology, 56,* 453-484.

Chess, S., & Thomas, A. (1986). *Temperament in clinical practice.* New York: Guilford Press.

Chess, S., & Thomas, A. (1987). *Origins and evolution of behavior disorders.* Cambridge, MA: Harvard University Press.

Cicchetti, D. (2002). How a child builds a brain: Insights from normality and psychopathology. In W. Hartup & R. Weinberg (Eds.), *Minnesota symposia on child psychology. Vol. 32: Child psychology in retrospect and prospect* (pp. 23-71). Mahwah, NY: Erlbaum.

Cicchetti, D. (2003). Neuroendocrine functioning in maltreated children. In D. Cicchetti & E. Walker (Eds.), *Neurodevelopmental mechanisms in psychopathology* (pp. 345-365). Cambridge, UK: Cambridge University Press.

Cicchetti, D. (2004). An odyssey of discovery: Lessons learned through three decades of research on child maltreatment. *American Psychologist, 59*(8), 731-741.

Clarke, G. (1912). Sterilization from the eugenic standpoint. *Journal of Mental Science, 58,* 48-49.

Cody, W. K. (2006). *Philosophical and theoretical perspectives for advanced nursing practice.* Boston: Jones and Bartlett Publishers.

Cohen, H., Amerine-Dickens, M., & Smith, T. (2006). Early intensive behavioral treatment: Replication of the UCLA model in a community setting. *Journal of Development and Behavioral Pediatrics, 27,* S145-S155.

Cohen, S., Doyle, W. J., Skoner, D. P., et al. (1997). Social ties and susceptibility to the common cold. *Journal of American Medical Association, 277,* 1940-1944.

Cole, T. (2004, June). *After the life cycle: The moral challenges of later life.* Paper presented at the June 2004 meeting of The President's Council on Bioethics, Washington, DC.

Cummings, S. M., & Cassie, K. M. (2008). Perceptions of biopsychosocial services needs among older adults with severe mental illness: met and unmet needs. *Health & Social Work, 33*(2), 133-143.

Curtis, W. J., & Cicchetti, D. (2003). Moving research on resilience into the 21st century: Theoretical and methodological considerations in examining the biological contributors to resilience. *Development and Psychopathology, 15,* 773-810.

Daniel, S. J. F. (2006). Adult attachment patterns and individual psychotherapy: A review. *Clinical Psychology Review, 26,* 968-984.

Davidson, L., Stayner, D. A., & Haglund, K. E. (1998). Phenomenological perspectives on the social functioning of people with schizophrenia. In K. T. Mueser & N. Tarrier (Eds.), *Handbook of social functioning in schizophrenia* (pp. 97-120). Needham Heights, MA: Allyn & Bacon Publishers.

Davidson, L., & Strauss, J. S. (1992). Sense of self in recovery from severe mental illness. *British Journal of Medical Psychology, 65,* 131-145.

Dawson, G. (2008). Early behavioral intervention, brain plasticity, and the prevention of autism spectrum disorder. *Development and Psychopathology, 20,* 775-803.

Deegan, P. E. (1996). *Recovery and the conspiracy of hope.* Presented at the Sixth Annual Mental Health Services Conference of Australia and New Zealand, Brisbane, Australia.

Delaney, K. R. (2005). The psychiatric nurse practitioner 1993-2003: A decade that unsettled a specialty. *Archives of Psychiatric Nursing, 19*(3), 107-115.

Delaney, K. R., Chisholm, M., Clement, J., et al. (1999). Trends in psychiatric mental health nursing education. *Archives of Psychiatric Nursing, 13*(2), 67-73.

Dilts, S. L. (2001). *Models of the mind: A framework for biopsychosocial psychiatry.* York, PA: Wellspan Health System.

Drake, R. E., Green, A. I., Mueser, K. T., et al. (2003). The history of community mental health treatment and rehabilitation for persons with severe mental illness. *Community Mental Health Journal, 39*(5), 427-440.

Dyer, J. G., & McGuinness, T. M. (1996). Resilience: Analysis of the concept. *Archives of Psychiatric Nursing, 10*(5), 276-282.

Edginton, B. (1997). Moral architecture: The influence of the York Retreat on asylum design. *Health & Place, 3*(2), 91-99.

Egeland, B., Carlson, E., & Stroufe, L. A. (1993). Resilience as process. *Development and Psychopathology, 5,* 517-528.

Engel, G. L. (1977). The need for a new medical model: A challenge for biomedicine. *Science, 196,* 129-136.

Engel, G. L. (1978). The biopsychosocial model and the education of health professionals. *Annals of the New York Academy of Sciences, 310*(1), 169-187.

Engel, G. L. (1980). The clinical application of the biopsychosocial model. *The American Journal of Psychiatry, 137*(5), 535-544.

Erickson, H. (2006). *Modeling and Role-modeling: A view from the client's world.* Cedar Park, TX: Unicorns Unlimited.

Erickson, H., Tomlin, E., & Swain, M. (1983). *Modeling and role-modeling: A theory and paradigm for nursing.* Englewood Cliffs, NJ: Prentice-Hall, Inc.

Erikson, E. (1950). *Childhood and society* (35th ed.). New York: W. W. Norton & Company.

Farkas, M., Gagne, C., Anthony, W., et al. (2006). Implementing recovery oriented evidence based programs: Identifying the critical dimensions. *Community Mental Health Journal, 41*(2), 141-158.

Faulks, E. (1911). The sterilisation of the insane. *Journal of Mental Science, 57,* 36-74.

Feldman, R., & Masalha, S. (2007). The role of culture in moderating the links between early ecological risk and young children's adaptation. *Development and Psychopathology, 19,* 1-21.

Fox, M., Sear, R., Beise, J., et al. (2010). Grandma plays favourites: X-chromosome relatedness and sex-specific childhood mortality. *Proceedings of the Royal Society, 277,* 567-573.

Fraley, C., Fazzari, D. A., Bonanno, G. A., et al. (2006). Attachment and psychological adaptation in high exposure survivors of the September 11th attack on the World Trade Center. *Personality and Social Psychology Bulletin, 32*(4), 538-551.

Freud, A., & Burlingham, D. (1943). *Infants without families.* London: G. Allen and Unwin.

Gaab, N., Gaser, C., & Schlaug, G. (2006). Improvement-related functional plasticity following pitch memory training. *NeuroImage, 31*(3), 255-263.

Gabbard, G. O. (2005). *Psychodynamic psychiatry in clinical practice* (4th ed.). Washington, DC: American Psychiatric Publishing, Inc.

Gabbard, G. O. (2007). Psychotherapy in psychiatry. *International Review of Psychiatry, 19*(1), 5-12.

Gabbard, G. O., & Kay, J. (2001). The fate of integrated treatment: Whatever happened at the biopsychosocial psychiatrist? *American Journal of Psychiatry, 158,* 1956-1963.

Galderisi, S., & Mucci, A. (2000). Emotions, brain development, and psychopathologic vulnerability. *CNS Spectrums, 5*(8), 44-48.

Garber, K. (2007). Autisms' cause may reside in abnormalities at the synapse. *Science, 317,* 190-191.

Gaser, C., & Schlaug, G. (2003). Gray matter differences between musicians and non-musicians. *Annals of the New York Academy of Sciences, 999,* 514-517.

Gastmans, C. (1998). Interpersonal relations in nursing: A philosophical-ethical analysis of the work of Hildegard E. Peplau. *Journal of Advanced Nursing, 28*(6), 1312-1319.

Gemelli, R. J. (2008). Normal child and adolescent development, In R. E. Hales, S. C. Yudofsky, & G. O. Gabbard (Eds.), *The American psychiatric publishing textbook of psychiatry* (5th ed.) (pp. 245-300). Washington, DC: American Psychiatric Publishing, Inc.

Gilbert, P. (2002). Understanding the biopsychosocial approach: Conceptualization. *Clinical Psychology, 14*, 13-17.

Goldstein, S., & Brooks, R. B. (2006). Why study resilience? In S. Goldstein & R. B. Brooks (Eds.), *Handbook of resilience in children* (pp. 3-15). New York: Springer Science & Business Media, Inc.

Green, J., & Goldwyn, R. (2002). Annotation: Attachment disorganization and psychopathology: New findings in attachment research and their potential implications for developmental psychopathology in childhood. *Journal of Child Psychology and Psychiatry, 43*(7), 835-846.

Green, J., & Shellenberger, R. (1991). *The dynamics of health & wellness: A biopsychosocial approach.* Fort Worth, TX: Holt, Rinehart and Winston, Inc.

Green, J., Stanley, C., & Peters, S. (2007). Disorganized attachment representation and atypical parenting in young school age children with externalizing disorder. *Attachment & Human Development, 9*(3), 207-222.

Green, R., & Turner, G. (2010). Growing evidence for the influence of meditation on brain and behaviour. *Neuropsychological Rehabilitation, 20*(2), 306-311.

Grotberg, E. H. (2003). Promoting resilience. *New York State Office of Mental Health Quarterly, 8*(4), 6-7.

Hanrahan, N., Stuart, G. W., Brown, P., et al. (2003). The psychiatric-mental health nursing workforce: Large numbers, little data. *Journal of the American Psychiatric Nurses Association, 9*, 111-114.

Hansell, N. (1976a). Enhancing adaptational work during service. In R. G. Hirschowitz & B. Levy (Eds.), *The changing mental health scene* (pp. 94-114). New York: Spectrum.

Hansell, N. (1976b). *The person-in-distress.* New York: Human Sciences Press.

Harding, C. M. (1989). Long-term follow-up studies of schizophrenia: Recent findings and surprising implications. *Yale Psychiatric Quarterly, 11*(3), 3-5.

Harding, C. M., & Keller, A. B. (1998). Long-term outcome of social functioning. In K. T. Mueser & N. Tarrier (Eds.), *Handbook of social functioning in schizophrenia.* Boston: Allyn & Bacon.

Harding, C. M., & Zahniser, J. H. (1994). Empirical correction of seven myths about schizophrenia with implications for treatment. *Acta Psychiatrica Scandinavica, 90*(Suppl 384), 140-146.

Harding, C. M., Zubin, J., & Strauss, J. S. (1992). Chronicity in schizophrenia revisited. *British Journal of Psychiatry*, 161, 27-37.

Hartman, D. (1993). Critical thinking in psychiatric nursing in the decade of the brain. *Holistic Nurse Practitioner, 7*(3), 55-63.

Hazan, C., & Shaver, P. (1987). Romantic love conceptualized as an attachment process. *Journal of Personality and Social Psychology, 52*, 511-524.

Hebb, D. C. (1949). *The organization of behavior: A neuropsychological theory.* New York: John Wiley & Sons.

Herzog, J. M. (1982). On father hunger: The father's role in the modulation of aggressive drive and fantasy. In S. W. Cath, A. R. Gurwitt, & J. M. Ross (Eds.), *Father and child* (pp. 163-174). Boston: Little Brown.

Hesse, E., & Main, M. (2000). Disorganized infant, child and adult attachment: Collapse in behavioral and attentional strategies. *Journal of the American Psychoanalytic Association, 48*, 1097-1127.

Hogarty, G. E., Anderson, C. M., Reiss, D. J., et al. (1991). Family psychoeducation, social skills training, and maintenance chemotherapy in the aftercare treatment of schizophrenia. II. Two-year effects of a controlled study on relapse and adjustment. Environmental-Personal Indicators in the Course of Schizophrenia (EPICS) Research Group. *Archives of General Psychiatry, 48*(4), 340-347.

Holzel, B. K., Ott, U., Gard, T., et al. (2008). Investigation of mindfulness meditation practitioners with voxel-based morphometry. *SCAN, 3*, 55-61.

Huttenlocher, P. R. (2002). *Neural plasticity: The effects of experience on the development of the cerebral cortex.* Cambridge, MA: Harvard University Press.

Hyde, K. I., Lerch, J., Norton, A., et al. (2009). Musical training shapes structural brain development. *The Journal of Neuroscience, 29*(10), 3019-3025.

Insel, T. R. (2006). Introduction. In *The 2006 progress report on brain research* (pp. 1-4). New York: The Dana Alliance for Brain Initiatives.

Jancke, L. (2009). The plastic human brain. *Restorative Neurology & Neuroscience, 27*(5), 521.

Kagan, J. (1978). *The growth of the child: Reflections on human development.* New York: W. W. Norton & Company.

Kagan, J. (1990). Temperament and social behavior. *The Harvard Mental Health Letter, 6*(10), 4-5.

Kandel, E. (1998). A new intellectual framework for psychiatry. *American Journal of Psychiatry, 155*, 469-475.

Kandel, E. (1999). Biology and the future of psychoanalysis: A new intellectual framework for psychiatry revisited. *American Journal of Psychiatry, 156*, 505-524.

Kandel, E. (2001). The molecular biology of memory storage: A dialogue between genes and synapses. *Science, 294*(5544), 1030-1038.

Kandel, E. R., Schwartz, J. H., & Jessell, T. M. (1995). *Essentials of neural science and behavior.* Norwalk, CT: Appleton & Lange.

Kandel, E. R., & Spencer, W. A. (1968). Cellular neurophysiology approaches in the study of learning. *Physiologic Review, 48, 65-134.*

Karen, R. (1994). *Becoming attached.* New York: Warner Books, Inc.

Kast, M., Meyer, M., Vogeli, C., et al. (2007). Computer-based multisensory learning in children with developmental dyslexia. *Restorative Neurology and Neuroscience, 25*, 355-369.

Keller, M. B., McCullough, J. P., Klein, D. N., et al. (2000). A comparison of nefazodone, the cognitive behavioral-analysis system of psychotherapy, and their combination for the treatment of chronic depression. *The New England Journal of Medicine, 342*, 1462-1470.

Keltner, N., Schwecke, L., & Bostrom, C. (2003). *Psychiatric nursing* (4th ed.). St. Louis: Mosby.

Kneisl, C. R., & Wilson, H. S. (2004). The psychiatric-mental health nurse's personal integration and professional role. In C. R. Kneisl, H. S. Wilson, & E. Trigoboff (Eds.), *Contemporary psychiatric-mental health nursing.* Upper Saddle River, NJ: Pearson Prentice Hall.

Kolb, B., & Gibb, R. (2001). Early brain injury, plasticity and behavior. In C. A. Nelson & M. Luciana (Eds.), *Handbook of developmental cognitive neuroscience* (pp. 175-190). Cambridge, MA: MIT Press.

Kolb, B., & Whishaw, I. Q. (1998). Brain plasticity and behavior. *Annual Review of Psychology,* 49, 43-64.

Konorski, J. (1948). *Conditioned reflexes and neuron organization.* Cambridge, UK: Cambridge University Press.

Kujala, T., & Naatanen, R. (2010). The adaptive brain: A neurophysiological perspective. *Progress in Neurobiology, 91*(1), 55-67.

Lamb, M. E. (Ed.). (1981). *The role of the father in child development* (2nd ed.). New York: John Wiley.

Laws, E. R. Jr. (2000). The decade of the brain: 1990 to 2000. *Neurosurgery, 47*(6), 1257-1260.

Lazar, S., Kerry, C. E., Wasserman, R. H., et al. (2005). Meditation experience is associated with increased cortical thickness. *Neuroreport, 16*(17), 1893-1897.

LeDoux, J. (2002). *Synaptic self: How our brains become who we are.* New York: Viking Press.

Leidy, N., Ozbolt, J., & Swain, M. (1990). Psychophysiological processes of stress in chronic physical illness: A theoretical perspective. *Journal of Advanced Nursing, 15*, 478-480.

Levy, D. (1937). Primary affect hunger. *American Journal of Psychiatry, 94*, 643-652.

Liegeois, A. (2001). Ethical aspects of deinstitutionalization in mental healthcare. Lecture presented at the European Conference on Mental Health, Rotterdam, Netherlands.

Luders, E., Toga, A. W., Lepore, N., et al. (2009). The underlying anatomical correlates of long-term meditation: Larger hippocampal and frontal volumes of gray matter. *NeuroImage, 45*(3), 672-678.

Luthar, S. S., Cicchetti, D., & Becker, B. (2000). The construct of resilience: A critical evaluation and guidelines for future work. *Child Development, 71*(3), 543-562.

MacDonald, C., & Mikes-Liu, K. (2009). Is there a place for biopsychosocial formulation in a systemic practice? *The Australian and New Zealand Journal of Family Therapy, 39*(4), 269-283.

MacDonald, S. (2001). The real and the researchable: A brief review of the contribution of John Bowlby (1907-1990). *Perspectives in Psychiatric Care, 37*(2), 60-64.

Maguire, E. A., Gadian, D. G., Johnsrude, I. S., et al. (2000). Navigation-related structural change in the hippocampi of taxidrivers. *Proceedings of the National Academy of Science, USA*, 97(8), 4398-4403.

Mahncke, H. W., Bronstone, A., & Merzenich, M. M. (2006). Brain plasticity and functional losses in the aged: Scientific basis for a novel intervention. *Progress in Brain Research, 157,* 81-109.

Main, M., & Solomon, J. (1986). Discovery of an insecure disorganized/disoriented attachment pattern. In T. B. Brazelton & M. W. Yogman (Eds.), *Affective development in infancy* (pp. 95-124). Norwood, NJ: Ablex.

Main, M., & Weston, D. (1982). Avoidance of the attachment table in infancy: Disruptions and interpretations. In Parkes, C, M., & Stevenson-Hinde, J. (Eds.), *The place of attachment in human behavior* (pp. 31-59). London: Tavistock.

Marder, E., & Rehm, K. J. (2005). Development of central pattern generating circuits. *Current Opinion in Neurobiology, 15*(1), 86-93.

Marques, C., Moreno, S., Castro, S., et al. (2007). Musicians detect pitch violation in a foreign language better than non-musicians: Behavioural and electrophysiological evidence. *Journal of Cognitive Neuroscience, 19,* 1453-1463.

Martin, J. (2002). The integration of neurology, psychiatry and neuroscience in the 21st century. *The American Journal of Psychiatry, 159*(5), 695-704.

Maslow, A. H. (1943). A theory of human motivation. *Psychological Review, 50*(4), 370-396.

Maslow, A. (1970). *Motivation and personality* (revised ed.). New York: Harper & Brothers.

Masten, A. S. (2001). Ordinary magic: Resilience processes and development. *American Psychologist, 56,* 227-238.

May, A., Hajak, G., Ganssbauer, S., et al. (2007). Structural brain alterations following 5 days of intervention: Dynamic aspects of neuroplasticity. *Cerebral Cortex, 17,* 205-210.

McBride, A., & Austin J. (1996). Integrating the behavioral and biological sciences: Implications for practice, education and research. In A. B McBride & J. K. Austin (Eds.), *Psychiatric-mental health nursing: Integrating the behavioral and biological sciences* (pp. 425-434). Philadelphia: W. B. Saunders Company.

McCrone, S. H. (1996). The impact of the evolution of biological psychiatry on psychiatric nursing. *Journal of Psychosocial Nursing, 34*(1), 38-46.

Mead, S., & Copeland, M. E. (2000). What recovery means to us. NY: Plenum Publishers. Retrieved from http://www.mentalhealthpeer.com/pdfs/Whatrecoverymeanstous.pdf

Memory (1986, September 29). *Newsweek,* 48-52.

Merwin, E. I., & Fox, J. C. (1999). Trends in psychiatric nursing graduate education. *Psychiatric Services, 50*(7), 905.

Mickelson, K. D., Kessler, R. C., & Shaver, P. R. (1997). Adult attachment in a nationally representative sample. *Journal of Personality and Social Psychology, 73*(5), 1092-1106.

Mitchell, G. J., & Bournes, D. A. (2006). Challenging the theoretical production of nursing knowledge; a response to Reed and Rolfe's column. *Nursing Science Quarterly, 19*(2), 116-119.

Moller, M. D., & Haber J. (1996, August 1). Advanced practice psychiatric nursing. *On-line Journal of Issues in Nursing,* 1-9. Retrieved from www.nursingworld.org/OJIN

Moore, S. M., & Visovsky, C. (2000). Nursing in the new millennium: Touching patients' lives through computers. *Proceedings of the IEA 2000/HFES 2000 Congress.*

Moreno, S., Marques, C., Santos, A., et al. (2009). Musical training influences linguistic abilities in 8-year-old children: More evidence for brain plasticity. *Cerebral Cortex, 19,* 712-723.

Mueser, K. T., Corrigan, P. W., Hilton, D., et al. (2002). Illness management and recovery for severe mental illness: A review of the research. *Psychiatric Services, 53,* 1272-1284.

Mueser, K. T., Torrey, W. C., Lynde, D., et al. (2003). Implementing evidence-based practices for people with severe mental illness. *Behavior Modification, 27*(3), 387-411.

Muller, R. T., & Lemieux, K. E. (2000). Social support, attachment and psychopathology in high risk formerly maltreated adults. *Child Abuse and Neglect, 24*(7), 883-900.

Munte, T. F., Altenmuller, E., & Jancke, L. (2002). The musician's brain as a model of neuroplasticity. *Nature Reviews Neuroscience, 3*(6), 473-478.

Naegle, M. A., & Krainovich-Miller, B. (2001). Shaping the advanced practice psychiatric-mental health nursing role: A futuristic model. *Issues in Mental Health Nursing, 22,* 461-482.

Nasrallah, H. A. (2006). Medications with psychotherapy: A synergy to heal the brain. *Current Psychiatry, 5*(10), 11-12.

Nathan, P. E., & Gorman, J. M. (Eds.). (1998). *A guide to treatments that work.* New York: Oxford Press.

National League for Nursing. (2004). *Official guide to undergraduate and graduate nursing programs* (2nd ed.). Boston: Jones and Bartlett Publishers.

National Panel for Psychiatric-Mental Health NP Competencies. (2003). *Psychiatric-mental health nurse practitioner competencies.* Washington, DC: National Organization of Nurse Practitioner Faculties.

National Research Project on Recovery. (2003). *OMH Quarterly, 8*(4), 8, 9, 15.

Nursing Data Source, 1992: Volume III: Leaders in the Making: Graduate Education in *Nursing* (1992). Division of Research, Pub. No. 19-2482, i-vi, 1-45. New York: National League for Nursing Press.

Parkes, C. M., Stevenson-Hinde, J., & Morris, P. (1991). *Attachment across the life cycle.* London: Tavistock/Routledge.

Patton, D. (2004). An analysis of Roy's Adaptation Model of Nursing as used within acute psychiatric nursing. *Journal of Psychiatric and Mental Health Nursing, 11,* 221-228.

Peplau, H. (1952). *Interpersonal relations in nursing.* New York: G. P. Putnam.

Perese, E. (1997). Unmet needs of persons with chronic mental illnesses: Relationship to their adaptation to community living. *Issues in Mental Health Nursing, 18*(1), 18-34.

Perese, E. (2007). Stigma, poverty and victimization: Roadblocks to recovery for individuals with severe mental illness. *Journal of the American Psychiatric Nurses Association, 13*(5), 285-295.

Perese, E., & Wu, B. (2010). Shortfalls of treatment of patients with schizophrenia: Unmet needs, obstacles to recovery. *International Journal of Psychosocial Rehabilitation, 14*(2), 43-56.

Pincus, H. A., Zarin, D. A., Tanielian, T. L., et al. (1999). Psychiatric patients and treatments in 1997: Findings from the American Psychiatric Practice Research Network. *Archives of General Psychiatry, 56*(5), 441-449.

Poston, A. (1928). Psychiatric nursing. In G. W. Henry (Ed.), *Essentials of psychiatry.* Baltimore: Williams & Wilkins Company.

Recovery (2003). New York State Office of Mental Health News Letter (p. 9.)

Reilly, P. R. (1987). Involuntary sterilization in the United States: A surgical solution. *Quarterly Review of Biology, 62*(2), 153-170.

Rice, M. J., Moller, M. D., DePascale, C., et al. (2007). APNA and ANCC collaboration: Achieving consensus on future credentialing for advanced practice psychiatric and mental health nursing. *Journal of American Psychiatric Nurses Association, 13*(3), 153-159.

Roe, D. (2005). Recovering from severe mental illness: Mutual influences of self & illness. *Journal of Psychosocial Nursing and Mental Health Services, 43*(2), 34-40.

Roger, M. (1970). *The theoretical basis in nursing.* Philadelphia: F. A. Davis.

Roy, C. (1976). *Introduction to nursing: An adaptation model.* New York: Prentice Hall.

Ruddick, S. (2000). Virtues and age. In M. U. Walter (Ed.), *Mother time.* New York: Rowman & Littlefield.

Rutter, M. (1987). Psychosocial resilience and protective mechanisms. *American Journal of Orthopsychiatry, 57,* 316-331.

Rutter, M., & The English and Romanian Adoptees (ERA) Study Team (1998). Developmental catch-up, and deficit, following adoption after severe global early privation. *Journal of Child Psychiatry, 39*(4), 465-476.

Rutter, M., Kreppner, J., & Sonuga-Barke, E. (2009). Emanuel Miller Lecture: Attachment insecurity, disinhibited attachment, and attachment disorders: Where do research findings leave the concepts? *The Journal of Child Psychology and Psychiatry, 50*(5), 529-543.

Ryff, C. D., & Singer, B. H. (2000). Biopsychosocial challenges of the new millennium. *Psychotherapy and Psychosomatics, 69,* 170-177.

Sadock, B. J., & Sadock, V. A. (2007). *Kaplan & Sadock's synopsis of psychiatry: Behavioral sciences/clinical psychiatry* (10th ed.). Philadelphia: Wolters Kluwer.

Scharer, K., Boyd, M., Williams, C., et al. (2003). Blending specialist and practitioner roles in psychiatric nursing: Experiences of graduates. *Journal of the American Psychiatric Nurses Association, 9*(4), 136-144.

Schlaug, G. (2001). The brain of musicians: A model for functional and structural adaptation. *Annals of the New York Academy of Sciences, 930,* 281-299.

Schlaug, G., Forgeard, M., Zhu, L., et al. (2009). Training-induced neuroplasticity in young children. *Annals of the New York Academy of Sciences, 1169*, 205-208.

Schlaug, G., Norton, A., Overy, K., et al. (2005). Effects of music training on brain and cognitive development. *Annals of the New York Academy of Sciences, 1060*, 219-230.

Sells, D., Borg, M., Marin, I., et al. (2006). Arenas of recovery for persons with severe mental illness. *American Journal of Psychiatric Rehabilitation, 9*, 3-16.

Shea, C. (1999). Graduate nursing education for advanced practice. In C. Shea, L. Pelletier, E. Poster, et al. (Eds.), *Advanced practice nursing in psychiatric and mental health care* (pp. 437-465). St. Louis: Mosby.

Shenfeld, K. (2007). CrossCurrents: From deficits to strengths: How to help families nurture resilient children. Centre for Addiction and Mental Health. Retrieved from http://www.camh.net/Publications/Cross_Currents/Summer_%202007/deficitsstrengths_crcusummer07.htm. Retrieved 3/14/2009

Skeels, H. M., & Dye, H. B. (1939). A study of the effects of differential stimulation on mentally retarded children. *Proceedings and Addresses of the American Association on Mental Deficiency, 44*(1), 114-136.

Smith, V., Mirenda, P., Zaidman-Zait, A. (2007). Predictors of expressive vocabulary growth in children with autism. *Journal of Speech, Language and Hearing Research. 50*(1), 149-161.

Smoyak, S. A., & Skiba-King, E. W. (1998). Historical influences on today's education and practice. In A. W. Burgess (Ed.), *Advanced practice psychiatric nursing* (pp. 15-26). Stanford, CT: Appleton & Lange.

Spaniel, L., Gagne, C. Koehler, M. (2003). The recovery framework in rehabilitation: Concepts and practices from the field of serious mental illness. In. J. J. R. Finch & D. Moxley (Eds.), *Source book of rehabilitation and mental health services* (pp. 37-50). New York: Plenum Press.

Sroufe, L. A., Carlson, E. A., Levy, A. K., et al. (1999). Implications of attachment theory for developmental psychopathology. *Development and Psychopathology, 11*, 1-13.

Stark, S. W. (2006). The effects of master's degree education on the role choices, role flexibility, and practice settings of clinical nurse specialists and nurse practitioners. *Journal of Nursing Education, 45*(1), 7-15.

Staten, R. R., Hamera, E., Hanrahan, N. P., et al. (2006). Advanced practice psychiatric nurses: 2005 Legislative update. *Journal of the American Psychiatric Nurses Association, 11*(6), 371-380.

Sullivan, H. S. (1953). *Interpersonal theory of psychiatry.* New York: W. W. Norton & Company.

Sullivan, L. (1992). The decade of the brain. *The National Alliance for the Mentally Ill, 3*(3), 1-2.

Tandon, P. N. (2000). The decade of the brain: A brief review. *Neurology India, 48*(3), 199-207.

Thoits, P. A. (1983). Multiple identities and psychological well-being: A reformulation of the social isolations hypothesis. *American Sociological Review, 48*(2), 174-187.

Thomas, A., Chess, S., Birch, H. G., et al. (1963). *Behavioral individuality in early childhood.* New York: New York University Press.

Thomas, A., Chess, S., & Birch, H. G. (1970). The origin of personality. *Scientific American, 223*(2), 102-109.

Torrey, E. F., & Miller, J. (2001). *The invisible plague: The rise of mental illness from 1750 to the present.* New Brunswick, NJ: Rutgers University Press.

Torrey, W. C., Drake, R. E., Dixon, L., et al. (2001). Implementing evidence-based practices for persons with severe mental illnesses. *Psychiatric Services, 52*(1), 45-50.

Wagnild, G. M., & Collins, J. A. (2009). Assessing resilience. *Journal of Psychosocial Nursing, 47*(12), 28-33.

Walsh, K., VandenBosch, T., & Boehm, S. (1989). Modeling and role-modeling: Integrating nursing theory into practice. *Journal of Advanced Nursing, 14*, 755-761.

Webster, W. S. (1998). Teratogen update: Congenital rubella. *Teratology, 58*, 13-23.

Wenk-Sormaz, H. (2005). Meditation can reduce habitual responding. *Alternative Therapies in Health and Medicine, 11*(2), 32-58.

Werner, E. E. (2006). What can we learn about resilience from large-scale longitudinal studies? *Handbook of resilience in children* (pp. 91-105). New York: Springer Science & Business Media, Inc.

Werner, E. E., & Smith, R. S. (1982). *Vulnerable but invincible.* New York: McGraw-Hill.

Werner, E. E., & Smith, R. S. (1992). *Overcoming the odds: High risk children from birth to adulthood.* Ithaca, NY: Cornell University Press.

West, A. E., Schenkel, L. S., & Pavuluri, M. N. (2008). Early childhood temperament in pediatric bipolar disorder and attention deficit hyperactivity disorder. *Journal of Clinical Psychology, 64*(4), 402-421.

Wheeler, K. (2008). *Psychotherapy for the advanced practice psychiatric nurse.* St. Louis: Mosby/Elsevier.

Wheeler, K., & Haber, J. (2004). Development of psychiatric-mental health nurse practitioner competencies: Opportunities for the 21st century. *Journal of the American Psychiatric Nurses Association, 10*(3), 129-138.

White, M. W., Ochs, M. T., Merzenich, M. M., et al. (1990). Speech recognition in analog multichannel cochlear prosthesis: Initial experiments in controlling classifications. IEEE. *Transactions on Biomedical Engineering, 37*, 1002-1010.

Whittle, S., Allen, N. B., Lubman, D. I., et al. (2006). The neurobiological basis of temperament: Towards a better understanding of psychopathology. *Neuroscience and Biobehavioral Reviews, 30*, 511-525.

Williams, C. A., Pesut, D. J., Boyd, M., et al. (1998). Toward an integration of competencies for advanced practice mental health nursing. *Journal of the American Nurses Association, 4*, 48-56.

Wilson, S. L. (2009). Understanding and promoting attachment. *Journal of Psychosocial Nursing, 47*(8), 23-27.

Wright, M. O., & Masten, A. S. (2006). Resilience processes in development. In *Handbook of resilience in children* (pp. 17-47). New York: Springer Science & Business Media, Inc.

Zoghbi, H. Y. (2003). Postnatal neurodevelopmental disorders: Meeting at the synapse? *Science, 302*, 826-830.

UNIT II

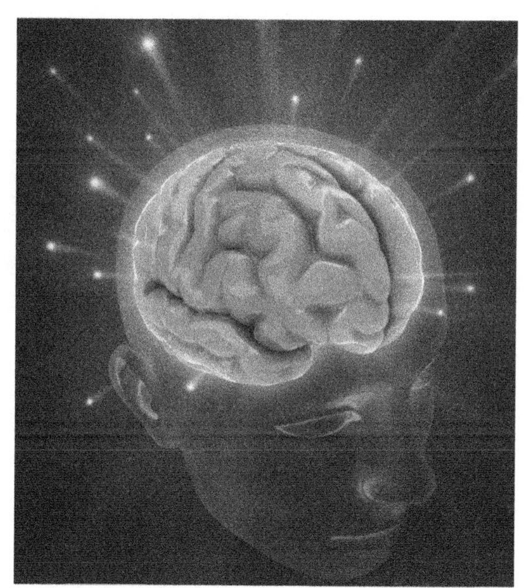

Understanding the Development of Psychiatric Disorders: The Why of Clinical Presentation and Response to Treatment

CHAPTER 2

Brain Functioning and Brain Development

Eris F. Perese, APRN-PMH

PART ONE: Brain Functioning

While the human brain has been shaped by evolution (Gaze, 1989), each individual's brain is shaped by genetic influences, prenatal factors, and postnatal experiences and interactions with the environment (Bartley, Jones, & Weinberger, 1997; Toga & Thompson, 2005). Each uniquely molded brain produces the individual's behaviors—motor activities, thinking, speaking, planning, creating, and loving—with different regions of the brain having different functions (Andreasen & Black, 2006; Bear, Connors, & Paradiso, 2007). The brain gathers information about the individual's internal and external worlds, analyzes the information, and responds with the best adaptation, whether it is to an opportunity, a challenge, or a stressor (Higgins & George, 2007; McEwen, 2009). Compromised brain functioning is manifested in symptoms or in clusters of symptoms that form the basis for the diagnosis of psychiatric disorders (Hedaya, 1996; Kandel, Schwartz, & Jessell, 2000). As LeDoux (2002) said, "The essence of who we are is encoded in our brains and brain changes account for the alterations of thought, mood, and behavior that occur in mental illness" (p. 260).

Psychiatric advanced practice nurses study the brain and its functioning in order to understand how the brain regulates emotions, thoughts, and behaviors. With this information, psychiatric advanced practice nurses are able to recognize impairments of patients' functioning; they are also able to plan interventions that promote restoration of optimal functioning and compensate for compromised functioning. In studying the brain, psychiatric advanced practice nurses build a foundation for understanding the brain's plasticity and the brain's ability to change throughout the lifetime in response to learning and experiences (Kandel, 1998; Kujala & Naatanen, 2010). They create a framework for understanding the biopsychosocial treatment interventions of psychotherapies, psychopharmacotherapy, and psychosocial interventions, all of which bring about change at the biological level by altering synaptic connections and gene expression; these alterations lead to new patterns of behavior (Kandel, 2005; McEwen, 2009).

To understand the brain and how it functions, psychiatric advanced practice nurses must look at both the nervous system and neurotransmission.

Nervous System

"The nervous system is the body's major communication and control network" (Carter, Aldridge, Page, et al., 2009, p. 40). It is a complex system of structures, circuits, and cells that regulates an individual's responses to internal and external stimuli. The human nervous system has two parts: the peripheral nervous system (PNS), which consists of ganglia and peripheral nerves, and the central nervous system (CNS), which consists of the brain and spinal cord (Nolte, 2010).

Peripheral Nervous System

The brain (Fig. 2-1) processes a stream of information about the environment, both the external environment of the world and the internal environment of the body. This information is supplied to the brain by the PNS, which is functionally intertwined with the CNS. The PNS lies outside the brain and spinal cord and is composed of 12 pairs of cranial nerves and 31 pairs of spinal nerves. The primary neurotransmitter of the PNS is acetylcholine. The PNS has both somatic and autonomic divisions (Bear et al., 2007; Nolte, 2010).

Somatic Division of the Peripheral Nervous System

The somatic division of the PNS includes neurons that send stimuli to the skin, muscles, and joints. Neuron receptors in this division provide information to the CNS about muscle and limb position, touch, and pressure and about the environment outside the body (Higgins & George, 2007).

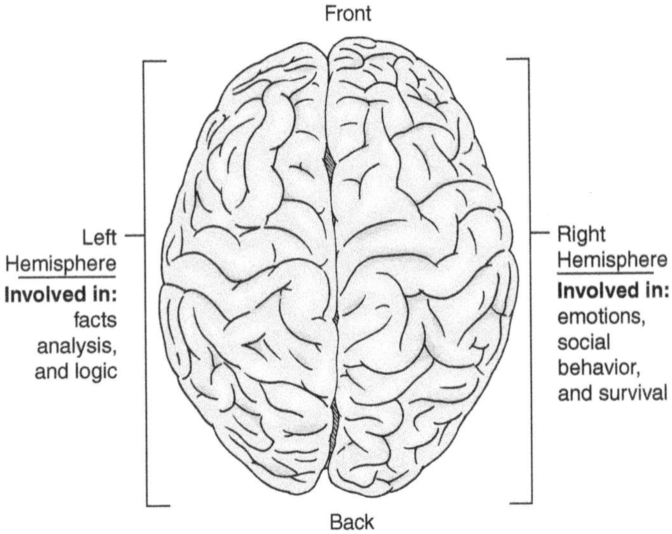

Front

Left Hemisphere
Involved in:
facts
analysis,
and logic

Right Hemisphere
Involved in:
emotions,
social
behavior,
and survival

Back

FIGURE 2-1: **Human Brain.** The human brain is a pinkish gray organ that weights approximately 3 lb and has the consistency of tofu. The surface of the brain is convoluted with sulci (grooves) and gyri (ridges). The brain is divided into two hemispheres that have different functions. The left hemisphere is for factual, analytical, and logical tasks. The right hemisphere is for emotional, social, and survival tasks (Carter et al., 2009; Joseph, 2000; Pincus & Tucker, 2002).

Autonomic Division of the Peripheral Nervous System

The autonomic division of the PNS consists of neurons that send stimuli to the internal organs, blood vessels, and glands. The autonomic division is influenced by the cerebral cortex, amygdala, reticular activating system, and most strongly by the hypothalamus (Higgins & George, 2007; Kandel, Schwartz, & Jessell, 1995; Nolte, 2010); these brain structures will be discussed later in the chapter. The autonomic division of the PNS regulates temperature, pulse, blood pressure, and water and food intake (Kandel et al.; Nolte). The functions of the autonomic nervous system are usually carried out without conscious thought; for example, blushing is an involuntary autonomic system activity. The autonomic division includes the sympathetic nervous system, the parasympathetic nervous system, and the enteric nervous system. The sympathetic and parasympathetic systems function in a parallel manner but with opposite effects.

Sympathetic System

The sympathetic system is involved with the response of the body to emergencies, e.g., the responses of excitement, apprehension, fear, rage, and panic. Activation of the sympathetic nervous system stimulates the neurotransmitters norepinephrine and epinephrine, which are involved in the fight-or-flight response. The sympathetic system responds to emergencies by increasing the heart rate; redistributing the blood supply to the brain, heart, and skeletal muscles; and restricting the blood supply to the skin and intestines (England & Wakely, 2006). The sympathetic system also controls other physical responses, including dilation of the pupils, salivation, and breathing (Higgins & George, 2007).

Parasympathetic System

The parasympathetic system is involved with conserving the body's resources and restoring homeostasis, which is a steady state of the internal environment of the body. The parasympathetic system is involved with rest and digestion (Kandel et al., 2000; England & Wakely, 2006). It constricts pupils, stimulates salivation, constricts the airway, slows the heartbeat, stimulates digestion, and causes the bladder to contract (Higgins & George, 2007).

Enteric System

The enteric system is a neural system that is located in the lining of the esophagus, stomach, intestines, pancreas, and gallbladder. It controls the transportation and digestion of food (Bear et al., 2007).

Central Nervous System

The CNS consists of the parts of the nervous system that are encased in bone, which are the cerebrum, cerebellum, brainstem, and spinal cord (Higgins & George, 2007; Nolte, 2010) (Fig. 2-2).

Cells of the Central Nervous System

There are two main types of cells in the CNS: neurons and glial cells (Kandel et al., 2000; McAllister, Usrey, Noctor, et al., 2008). Neurons convey and receive messages. Glial cells protect the neurons, bring nourishment to the neurons, remove debris, and support the neurons (Nolte, 2010; Snyder & Ferris, 2000).

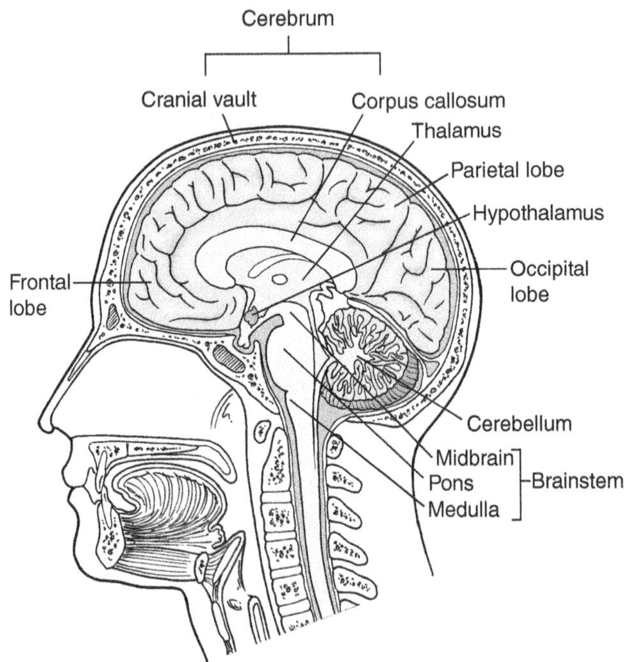

FIGURE 2-2: **Central Nervous System.** The CNS consists of the parts of the nervous system that are encased in bone: cerebrum, cerebellum, brainstem, and spinal cord (Higgins & George, 2007; Nolte, 2010). The CNS is the controller of the body.

Neurons

The function of the neuron is to receive, process, and transmit information to other neurons, to muscles, and to secretory cells (McAllister et al., 2008; Yu & Rasenick, 2009). The human brain contains more than 23 billion neurons (Howard, 2006). Brains of males have 2 billion more neurons than brains of females, and brains of females have more neuropil, which is the substance that makes up dendrites, axons, and synapses, which facilitate interneuron communications (Howard, p. 50). Each neuron maintains about 1,000 connections—or synapses—with other neurons, though some neurons have 200,000 synapses. Knowledge of the structure and function of the neuron (Fig. 2-3) is essential for psychiatric advanced practice nurses' understanding of the action of psychotropic medications.

The cell membrane of the neuron contains receptors, ion channels, and reuptake pumps. The cell body of the neuron contains the nucleus, which contains the DNA; the DNA is the double helix that transmits information from generation to generation and codes for gene expression (Yu & Rasenick, 2009). Extensions from the cell body include axons, axon terminals, and dendrites. The axon is a thin tube-like extension from the cell body that carries information to other neurons. The end of the axon, the presynaptic ending, contains synaptic vesicles that are filled with neurotransmitters. The terminal end of the axon, the axon terminal, forms the synapse with the dendrites of another neuron (Bear et al., 2007). Dendrites are parts of a neuron that sprout off; they are similar to branches of a tree. There are spines along the dendrites that are postsynaptic receptors for incoming signals. They pick up information from other neurons and relay it to the cell body of their neuron (Higgins & George, 2007). Dendritic abnormalities are often found in individuals with schizophrenia and mental retardation, in whom the neurons have less dendritic branching and the dendrites have fewer spines (Higgins & George). The synapse is the communication site where one neuron passes information to another neuron (Daube & Stead, 2009) (Fig. 2-4). Neurons do not touch: they are separated by a very thin space called the synaptic cleft (Carter et al., 2009). Neurons play a very specific role in brain communication, which will be discussed later in this chapter.

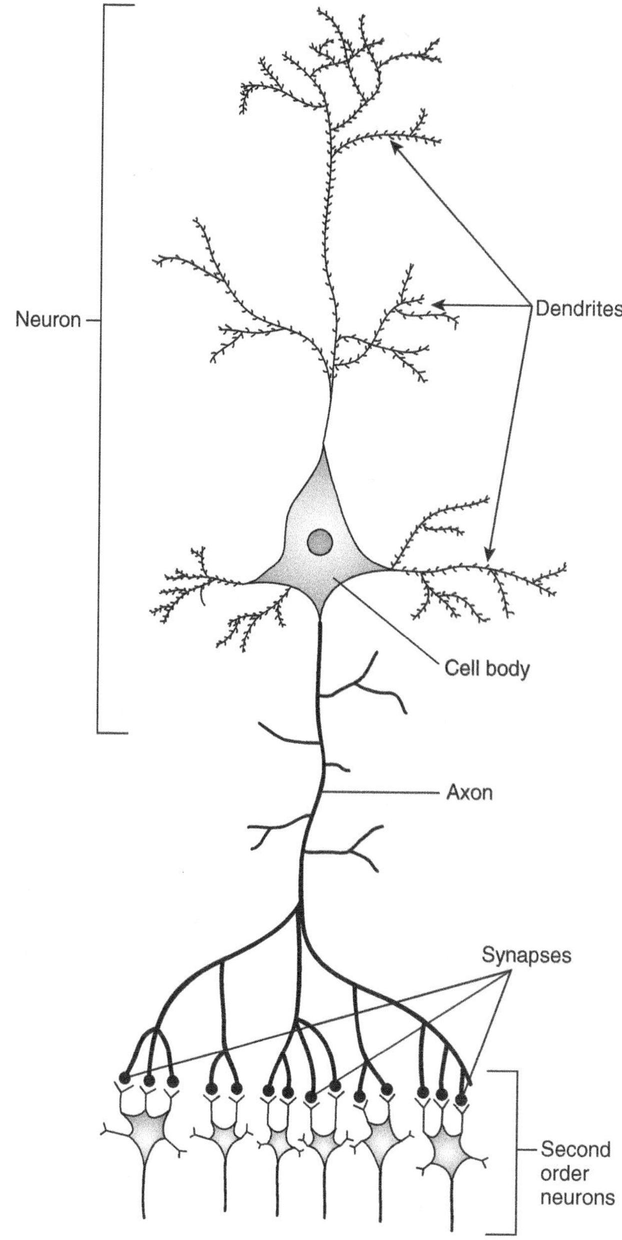

FIGURE 2-3: Neuron. The neuron is a brain cell that transmits information to other cells. The nucleus of the neuron contains the DNA that provides instructions for functioning of the cell and codes for gene expression (Yu & Rasenick, 2009). Extensions from the cell body include axons, axon terminals, and dendrites. The axon is a thin, tube-like extension that carries information to other neurons. The end of the axon, the presynaptic ending, contains synaptic vesicles that are filled with neurotransmitters. The cell membrane of the neuron contains receptors, ion channels, and reuptake pumps.

Glial Cells

There are four main types of glial cells—oligodendrocytes, Schwann cells, astrocytes, and microglia. Oligodendrocytes produce myelin to insulate the neurons in the brain. Myelinization is the spiral wrapping of myelin around the neuron's axon, and it speeds the conduction of the action potential along the axon (Carter et al., 2009). The process of myelinization starts prenatally, but myelinization of the neurons in the neocortex is not completed until the second decade of life (Morrell & Quarles, 1999). Myelinization of corticolimbic areas that are involved in emotional intensity and sociability—the hippocampus, parahippocampal structures, and cingulum—continues into the sixth decade of life (Benes, Turtle, Khan, et al., 1994). Thus, older adults may feel things more intensely although they may appear to be less emotional (Hotz, 2002).

Schwann cells produce myelin to insulate the neurons in the PNS. Astrocytes have three functions: they provide the scaffolding over which the neurons migrate during early development of the brain, they nourish neurons, and they form the blood-brain barrier that prevents toxic substances in the blood from entering the brain. Microglia cells remove

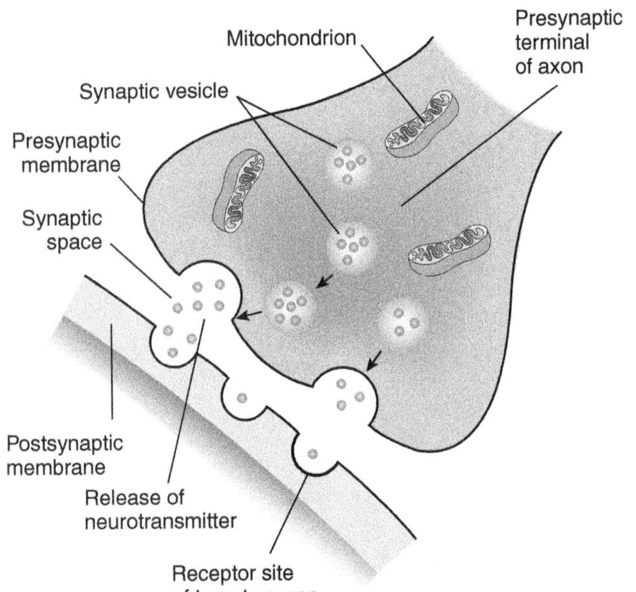

FIGURE 2-4: **Synapses.** Synapses are spaces between two neurons where information is transmitted. The synaptic cleft has a width of 20 billionths of a meter. Neurons sending information release into synapses neurotransmitters that are received by neurons on the other side of the space, completing the transmission of information.

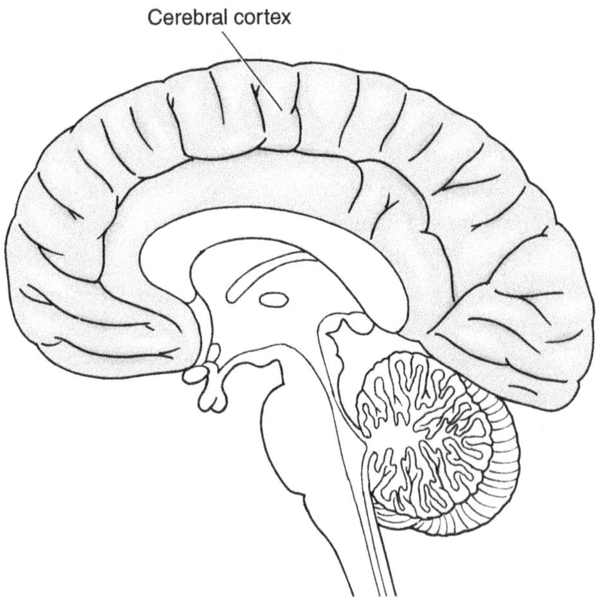

FIGURE 2-5: **Cerebral Cortex.** The cerebral cortex, also called the neocortex, is the outer wrinkled area that covers the hemispheres of the brain. It receives information from sensory systems, processes the information, analyses it, compares it with previously stored information, and determines the response. The cerebral cortex is the part of the brain involved in higher mental functioning.

debris following injury to the brain (Higgins & George, 2007; Kandel et al., 2000; McAllister et al., 2008; Nolte, 2010).

In clinical practice, abnormalities of glial cell functioning are seen when glial cells are destroyed, such as during the destruction of oligodendrocytes in the demyelinating disease of multiple sclerosis, or when glial cells grow out of control and form brain tumors that are called gliomas. The most common of the gliomas arise from astrocytes. Recent studies suggest that astrocytes may be involved in neuronal cell death through their control of the synthesis, reuptake, and disposal of the excitatory neurotransmitter glutamate (Hertz & Zielke, 2004; Snyder & Ferris, 2000).

Brain Structures and Their Functioning

The brain lies protected within the bony cranial cavity that is formed by the frontal, occipital, parietal, temporal, sphenoid (located at base of the skull) and ethmoid (located between the nasal cavity and the brain cavity) bones (Carter et al., 2009; Sugarman, 2002). Within that cavity, the brain is suspended in cerebrospinal fluid (Carter et al.; England & Wakely, 2006).

The largest part of the brain is the cerebrum, which consists of the cerebral cortex and basal ganglia. The cerebral cortex is a thick layer that covers the two hemispheres of the brain (Fig. 2-5), and it is composed of gray matter (neurons) and white matter (glial cells) (Higgins & George, 2007; Nolte, 2010). The neurons in the cerebral cortex number in the billions, and the glial cells in the trillions (Taber & Hurley, 2008). The cerebral cortex is where information is processed and interpreted; where plans are made, evaluated, and kept or discarded; and where responses that control movement and behaviors are selected (Bear et al., 2007; Nolte). The basal ganglia (Fig. 2-6) are located below the cortex and are involved in movement and motor control. The structures in the basal ganglia are the caudate nucleus, the putamen, and the globus pallidus. They are interconnected nuclei, which means that they are clusters of neurons that work together to perform specialized functions (Higgins & George; Nolte).

Laterality of the Brain

The brain is divided into a right hemisphere and a left hemisphere. The two hemispheres are connected by the corpus callosum, which enables communication between the two hemispheres, and by the anterior commissure, which is

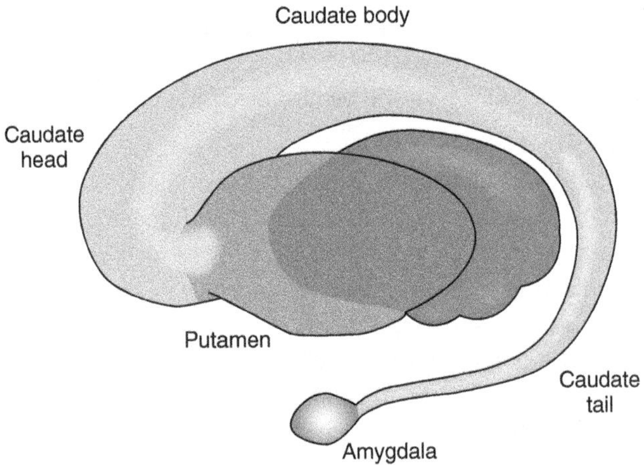

FIGURE 2-6: **Basal Ganglia.** The basal ganglia are composed of clusters of nerve cells (interconnected nuclei) that work together to perform specialized functions such as movement and coordination (Higgins & George, 2007; Nolte, 2010).

a band of fibers that connects the basal areas of the hemispheres (Campbell, 2005; Todd, Swarzenski, Rossi, et al., 1995). The corpus callosum can be seen in Figure 2-7.

Although both hemispheres are involved in perceptual, cognitive, emotional, memory, and motor functions (Kandel et al., 2000), they have specialized functions. The left hemisphere encodes and recalls verbal memories and positive memories (Carter et al., 2009). It is involved in cheerfulness and approach behaviors, such as a willingness to try new things (Howard, 2006). The right hemisphere encodes and recalls nonverbal memories and negative memories (Carter et al; Joseph, 2000; Pincus & Tucker, 2002). It is involved in avoidance behaviors such as avoiding new situations that might cause discomfort, anxiety, fear, or rejection (Howard).

Right Hemisphere

The right hemisphere develops first and is involved with functioning that ensures survival (Chiron, Jambaque, Nabbout, et al., 1997). It is involved with emotions, recognition of facial expressions, body image, music, visual imagery, REM sleep, daydreams, and perception of nonverbal sounds (Carter et al., 2009; Joseph, 1990). Damage to the right hemisphere that may be related to deficits in development, lesions, tumors, or injury results in compromised functioning that may be manifested as

- Problems with interpretation of speech, such as how something is said or what the speaker feels (anger, happiness, sadness, sarcasm, or empathy)
- A flat, monotone speech

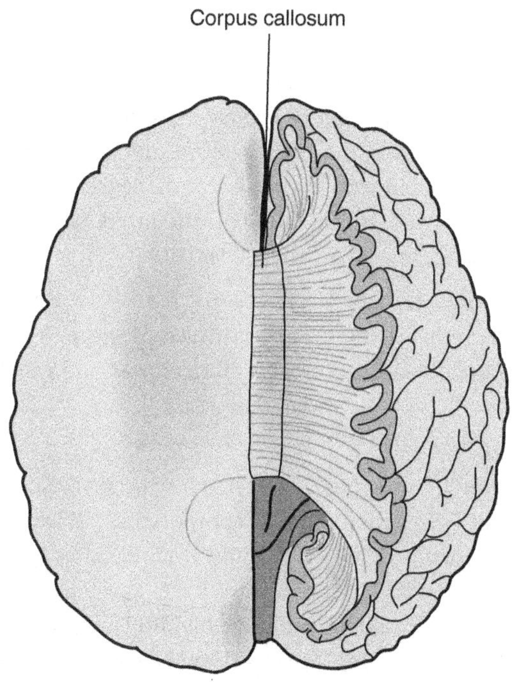

FIGURE 2-7: Corpus Callosum. The corpus callosum is made up of millions of axons crossing between the two hemispheres. The corpus callosum connects broad regions of the cortex in all the lobes of the two hemispheres.

- Impaired ability to recognize nonverbal cues, such as missing the point, or very concrete interpretations of what was said
- Lack of ability to sing or recognize music or to take pleasure in music
- Visuospatial and perceptual function disturbances such as deficits in judgments that involve visual relationships; misplacing things; difficulty in balance, such as walking into things; and becoming lost, confused, or disoriented
- Disturbances in drawing, such as drawing the face of a clock
- Problems with reading and mathematics
- Memory deficits
- Disturbance of body image
- Deficits in pain perception or distortions concerning sensation in various parts of the body
- Problems with recognizing faces of friends or even one's own face
- Mania or lability of moods, pressured speech, ideas of reference, irritability, euphoria, impulsivity, or promiscuity

If there is damage to the right hemisphere in the temporal parietal area, there may be impairment of ability to comprehend or produce appropriate emotional speech as well as impaired ability to distinguish between different emotional qualities of speech. If there is damage to the right frontal area, there may be confabulation (making up experiences to fill in memory gaps), excessive speech, and tangentiality (not getting to the point) (Joseph, 1990).

Left Hemisphere

The left hemisphere of the brain is involved with speech, knowledge of language, and thinking as it is involved in communication, mathematics, and reasoning (Dimberg & Petterson, 2000; Joseph, 1990). In contrast to right hemisphere speech, which is social, melodic, and emotional, the left hemisphere speech is factual. It describes and explains things by placing them in time and sequence (Carter et al., 2009; Joseph).

In the left frontal hemisphere, an area called *Broca's area* is involved in production of speech (Andreasen & Black, 2006) (Fig. 2-8). Damage to Broca's area results in disorders of language that are characterized by expressive aphasia, which is the limited ability to speak (Black & Andreasen, 2011). Damage to Broca's area may also affect the individual's ability to write, and patients may have difficulty performing three-step commands such as hitting the table with the palm of the hand, then the edge of the hand, then a fist. Patients with Broca's aphasia may become depressed, irritated, frustrated, sad, and tearful.

Patients with left frontal and medial damage that spares Broca's area may appear apathetic, hypoactive, and poorly motivated. They may experience anomia, which is a word-finding difficulty; e.g., anomia patients may have problems

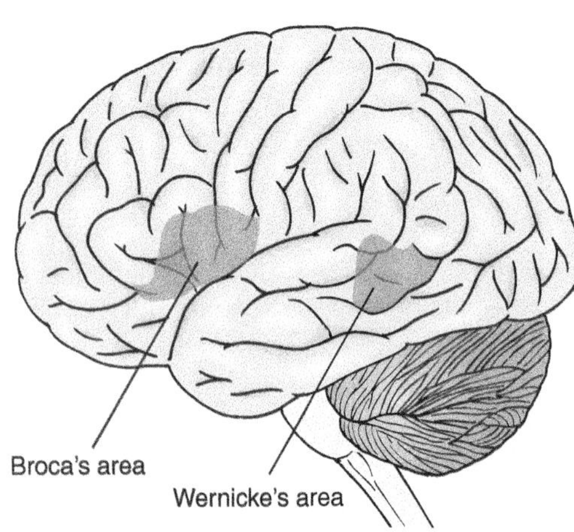

FIGURE 2-8: **Broca's Area and Wernicke's Area.** Language areas of the brain include Broca's area, which is involved in speaking, and Wernicke's area, which is involved in understanding language.

naming objects or describing pictures and are unable to do so even with hints. These patients may also substitute another word for a word that they cannot remember, e.g., using the word "cutter" for "scissors." They often are unable to repeat the phrase, "no ifs, ands, or buts" (Joseph, 1990).

Wernicke's area, an area in the left hemisphere in the posterior part of the temporal lobe near the inferior parietal area, is involved with comprehension of language (Black & Andreasen, 2011) (*see* Fig. 2-8). Damage to Wernicke's area may result in difficulty comprehending spoken or written language so that naming, reading, writing, and ability to repeat are impaired. Patients with damage to Wernicke's area may be able to talk, but their speech is usually abnormal, lacking content (Carter et al., 2009).

Corpus Callosum

As the cerebral cortex develops, bundles of fibers called commissures connect the corresponding areas of the two hemispheres. The largest of the cerebral commissural systems is the corpus callosum (see Fig. 2-7). The corpus callosum contains 200 million nerve fibers, which are the axons of neurons; it connects the neocortical areas of the two hemispheres (Campbell, 2005; Moore & Persaud, 1993; Nolte, 2010). The back part of the corpus callosum, the splenium, is larger in females and allows for greater communication between the two hemispheres (Blank, 1999). A much smaller commissure, the anterior commissure, connects parts of the temporal lobes and parts of the olfactory system (Nolte, 2010).

Before the age of 3 years, there is no ability to recall memories or events because the hippocampus has not matured sufficiently to retain memories (Carter et al., 2009) and the linkage between the two hemispheres by the corpus callosum is not complete ("Memory," 1986). Communication between the right and left hemispheres is present by age 5 years and continues to develop as the corpus callosum develops. Interestingly, researcher Joy Hirsch found that when children learn to speak more than one language during early childhood, the same part of the brain is used for all languages ("Memory"); however, when children or adults learn languages later on, after age 7 or 8 years, then additional, separate areas of the brain within Broca's area are established for each language learned ("Memory"). Individuals who learn to speak two languages as children speak both languages as their native tongue (Winslow, 1997).

The corpus callosum continues to develop and mature until the early twenties (Joseph, 2000; Park, 2004). It is interesting that although a driver's license may be obtained by teenagers, car rental agencies require that a renter be 25 or 26 years of age, an age at which the corpus callosum's linkage of the emotional right hemisphere and the thinking left hemisphere is more developed.

Increases in corpus callosum size are believed to be reflective of increased ability for more abstract thinking (Giedd, 1999). Similarly, damage to the corpus callosum or failure of the corpus callosum to develop is manifested by impaired ability to transfer information—such as emotional, tactile, cognitive, or visual information—from one hemisphere to the other. Agenesis, or lack of development, during the prenatal stage of the corpus callosum is associated with childhood developmental delays, intellectual disabilities, and neurological deficits (Campbell, 2005; Sztriha, 2005). In adulthood, individuals with agenesis of the corpus callosum may perform normally on a standardized intelligence test but may show deficits in social functioning; that is, they may not be aware of subtle social interactions and may not understand humor, jokes, stories, or nonliteral language (Brown, Paul, Symington, et al., 2005). For example, individuals with schizophrenia who often display concrete thinking or literal interpretation of questions have been found to have several brain abnormalities, including agenesis of the corpus callosum that results in a smaller corpus callosum (Gur & Arnold, 2004). Additionally, the corpus callosum has been found to be smaller in men who as boys had experienced neglect and in women who as girls had experienced sexual abuse (Teicher, Dumont, Ito, et al., 2004).

Major Brain Structures

The structures of the brain that have prominent roles in psychiatric disorders are the cerebral cortex and the limbic system.

Cerebral Cortex

The cerebral cortex (see Fig. 2-5) covers the surface of the two brain hemispheres and is composed of a layer of gray matter that is made up of neurons. It participates in various functions, including memory storage and recall; music; mathematics; speaking and understanding language; paying attention; interpreting sensory input; recognizing people, places, and emotional expressions; and planning goal-directed behaviors (Nolte, 2010). About one-third of the cortex is on the surface of the brain, and the remainder of the cortex is buried in the sulci and fissures of the brain, which are the valleys of the brain. An island of cerebral cortex, the insula, is buried underneath the lateral sulcus, which is a deep groove or fissure between the frontal and temporal lobes. The insula is involved in autonomic functions and also in emotional responses (England & Wakely, 2006). The cerebral cortex develops in layers:

- The neocortex, which is the latest part of the brain to evolve, has six layers (Fig. 2-9).
- The allocortex, also known as the limbic cortex, has three layers.
- The mesocortex, which is the area between the neocortex and allocortex, varies from three to six layers.

The six-layered neocortex provides an efficient way for organizing input and output of cortical neurons by allowing for feedback of information to different structures during the processing and integrating of the information (Campbell, 2005; Kandel et al., 2000; Nolte, 2010). Fibers from the six layers form connections *between* the hemispheres through the corpus callosum and connections *within* the hemispheres through association areas, which are groupings of neurons that are involved in the same function, e.g., in vision (Box 2-1).

The cerebral cortex is organized so that each hemisphere controls the sensory and motor processes of the opposite side. For example, information or stimuli that enter the spinal cord from the left side of the body cross over to the right side of the CNS before they are carried to the cerebral cortex. It is the same for motor functioning: the left side of the cerebral cortex controls the motor functioning on the right side of the body (Kandel et al., 2000).

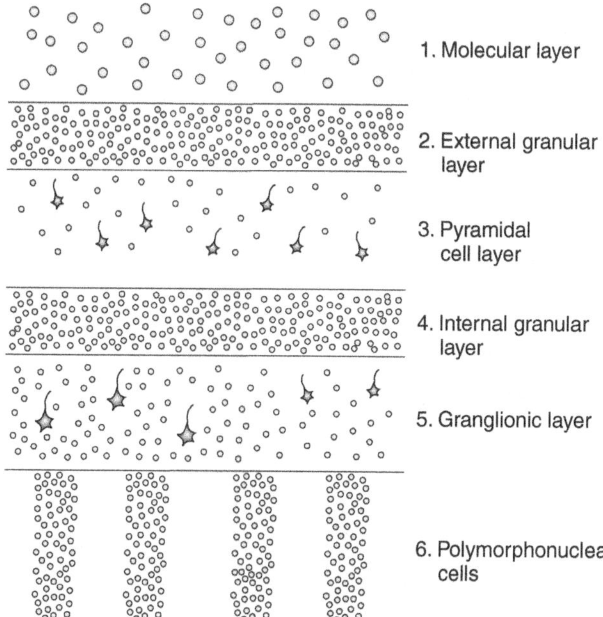

FIGURE 2-9: Layers of the Neocortex. The neocortex of the brain is composed of six layers. Fibers from the six layers form connections *between* the hemispheres through the corpus callosum and connections *within* the hemispheres through association areas, which are groupings of neurons that are involved in the same function. The six-layered neocortex provides efficient processing of information by different brain structures (Campbell, 2005; Kandel et al., 2000; Nolte, 2010).

BOX 2-1 Association Areas of the Cerebral Cortex

The association areas of the cerebral cortex have integrative functioning. They interpret sensory information, link perceptions with previous experience, focus attention, and integrate information about the environment (Kandel et al., 2000). There are two types of association areas: the unimodal, and the heteromodal or multimodal. Unimodal association areas process only one sensory modality, e.g., the visual, auditory, or somatosensory association area. Multimodal association areas receive input from many unimodal association areas. There are three multimodal association areas:

1. The posterior association area, which is located at the edge of the parietal, temporal, and occipital lobes. It links information related to perception and language.
2. The limbic association area, which is located in the limbic area. It is involved with emotional and memory storage.
3. The anterior association area, which is located in the prefrontal cortex. It is involved in planning movements (Kandel et al., 2000; Nolte, 2010).

Damage to unimodal association areas is associated with impairment of sensory perception in a specific area and loss of function such as loss of the ability to recognize faces (Nolte, 2010). Damage to the multimodal areas is associated with more complex impairment of cognitive and emotional functioning (Gilman & Newman, 2003; Nolte, 2010).

The cerebral cortex of each hemisphere is divided into four lobes (Fig. 2-10) named after the frontal, parietal, temporal, and occipital bones that cover them. Each lobe of the brain has foldings or elevations; the crests of these foldings are called gyri, the grooves between the foldings are called sulci, and deeper grooves are called fissures (Nolte, 2010). Kandel et al. (2000) noted that sulci are "a favored evolutionary strategy for packing in more cells in a limited space" (p. 9). The four lobes and other structures of the cerebral cortex—including the cingulate cortex and the insular cortex, and the limbic system—have specialized functions (Kandel et al.; Tamminga, 2004).

The cingulate cortex and the insular cortex are involved in responding to pain; i.e., both cortexes integrate sensory, emotional, and cognitive components of pain. In addition, the insular cortex is involved in processing information related to tactile memory, called stereognosis (Kandel et al., 2000), and is involved in processing information relating to heat, cold, hunger, thirst, disgust for repulsive objects, and cravings such as for cigarettes or drugs (Blakeslee, 2007).

Limbic System

Andreasen (2001) said that "While the frontal system is the phylogenetically newest cortical region, the limbic system is the oldest and most primitive" (p. 70). The limbic system is involved in learning, memory, emotions, aggression,

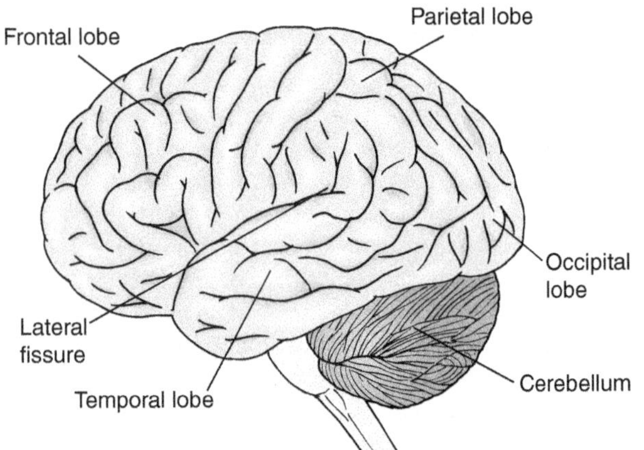

FIGURE 2-10: Lobes of the Brain. Each hemisphere of the brain contains a frontal lobe, parietal lobe, occipital lobe, and temporal lobe. The frontal lobe is involved in thinking, judging, making plans, and weighing consequences; the parietal lobe is involved in spatial and body orientation and attention; the occipital lobe is involved in visual processing; and the temporal lobe is involved in hearing, language, and memory.

submissive behavior, and generating emotional response to external stimuli (England & Wakely, 2006). The limbic system is made up of the medial portions of the frontal, parietal, and temporal lobes, which are the innermost parts of the brain, located closest to the ventricles. Although there is no consensus on which structures are part of the limbic system, it is generally accepted that the limbic system consists of five parts (Fig. 2-11): the hypothalamus, which receives stimuli from the brainstem and spinal cord, controls the autonomic nervous system, and is involved in drive-related behaviors; the thalamus, which gaits information and relays it to different brain structures such as the cerebral cortex; the hippocampus, which is involved in learning and autobiographical memory; the amygdala, which is involved in fear and anger; and the septal nuclei, which are involved in attachment and reward (Nolte, 2010).

Although brain structures are usually described as having different functions, many functions are performed by several structures (Carter et al., 2009; Sugarman, 2002). Table 2-1 presents the function of specific brain structures, the effects if damaged, and the association with psychopathology.

Coverings of the Brain: Meninges

The meninges are protective coverings of the brain and the spinal cord (Fig. 2-12). They enclose the CNS and prevent it from being injured by sudden movements (England & Wakely, 2006). Discussion of meninges will be limited to the brain and will not include the spinal cord.

There are three separate layers to the meninges: dura mater, arachnoid, and pia mater (Carter et al., 2009). The *dura mater* is a thick, tough layer that is also the periosteum (a vascular membrane covering the bones) of the inside of the skull bones. Trauma to the head may result in bleeding below the dura, known as a subdural hematoma, or in bleeding between the dura and the skull bone, known as an extradural hematoma or epidural hematoma. The *arachnoid* and *pia mater* are thinner, collagenous membranes. The arachnoid is attached to the inside of the dura with no space between them. It is attached to the pia mater by strands of arachnoid tissue forming a suspension cradle for the brain; cerebrospinal fluid fills the space between the arachnoid and the pia mater. The arachnoid also functions as a barrier by preventing diffusion of extracellular substances from the dura into the cerebrospinal fluid.

The pia mater is attached to the surface of the brain and follows the brain into the folds and deep fissures. The top surface of the pia is connected to the arachnoid by strands of arachnoid tissue, and the bottom surface of the pia is attached to ". . . astrocyte end feet that carpet the surface of the CNS" (Nolte, 2010, p. 27). The pia mater is involved in maintaining the blood supply to the brain (England & Wakely, 2006).

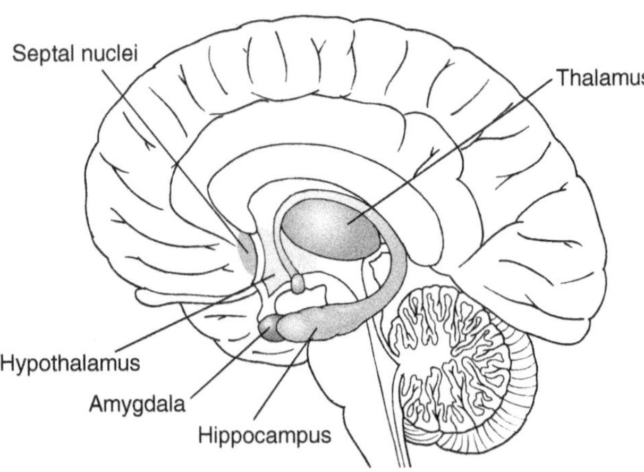

FIGURE 2-11: Limbic System. The limbic system is made up of the medial areas of the frontal, parietal, and temporal lobes. Structures within the limbic system include the hypothalamus, thalamus, hippocampus, amygdala, and septal nuclei (Nolte, 2010). The limbic system is involved in instinctive survival behaviors; basic impulses such as sex, anger, and pleasure; attachment; processing information; memory; emotions; and reward.

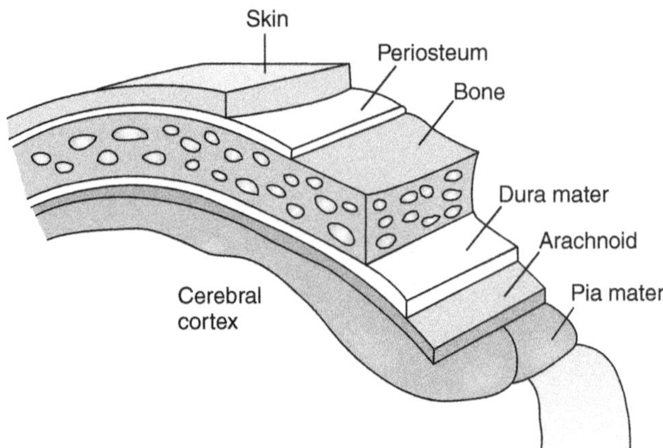

FIGURE 2-12: Meningeal Layers. The brain is protected by three meningeal layers: the dura mater, the arachnoid, and the pia mater. The tough dura mater protects the brain. The arachnoid supports the brain in cerebrospinal fluid. The pia mater is involved in maintaining the blood supply to the brain.

TABLE 2-1 BRAIN STRUCTURES AND THEIR FUNCTIONS, DAMAGE EFFECTS, AND PSYCHOPATHOLOGIES

Brain Structure	Function	Damage Effect	Psychopathology
Frontal lobe	**Executive functioning and personality** Maintain and focus attention. Organize thinking, planning, speech, and motor activities. Weigh consequences. Set goals. Modulate emotions. Integrate ideas, emotions, and perceptions. Shape personality (Joseph, 1990; Taber & Hurley, 2008).	Left side: depression, reduced speech, apathy. Right side: impulsivity, confabulation, verbosity, grandiosity, and mania (Hedaya, 1996). Medial area: difficulty speaking, motor abnormalities, agraphia, and catatonia. Damage to Broca's area results in aphasia (Taber & Hurley, 2008). Orbital frontal area: emotional unresponsiveness and lack of inhibition (Campbell, 2005); euphoric, overtalkative, irresponsible, tactless, grandiose, promiscuous (Joseph, 1990); and disruptions of social conduct, deficits in planning, judgment, and decision making (Taber & Hurley).	Frontal lobe syndrome (Luria, 1969; Sadock & Sadock, 2007). "Executive dysfunction syndrome" (Lyketsos, Rosenblatt, & Rabins, 2004, p. 252). Schizophrenia (Belger & Dichter, 2006). Depression (Mayberg, 2006). Anxiety (Mayberg).
Parietal lobe	**Body sensations** Motor activities; attention and perception of spatial relations (Joseph, 1990; Taber & Hurley, 2008). Processes sensory impulses from the thalamus (Campbell, 2005). Maintains focused attention. Registers acts of aggression (Joseph, 2000). Left temporoparietal junction contains Wernicke's area, which is involved in comprehension of speech (Taber & Hurley).	Impairment of attention, concentration, language, grammar, ability to do numerical calculations, visual-spatial relations, body image, motor activity, recognition of people and objects, and ability to learn from past experiences. Misjudgment of speed of objects, distance or position of body (Carter et al., 2009).	Aphasia, agnosia, and apraxia (Campbell, 2005). Out-of-body experiences such as looking down at one's self (Carter et al., 2009).
Temporal lobe	**Emotion and memory circuits** Hearing, learning, memory circuits, emotions, sexual identity, and processing of auditory stimuli (Taber & Hurley, 2008). Gives emotional tone to memories. Is involved in making moral judgments (Carter et al., 2009).	Fear, anxiety, anger and paranoia. Hyper-religiosity (Rubia-Vila, 2001). Temporal lobe seizures are associated with depersonalization (Campbell, 2005). Prosopagnosia (disturbed ability to recognize faces).	Auditory hallucinations and delusions that are associated with depression, mania, and schizophrenia (First & Tasman, 2004; Post, 2000). Involved in experiencing intense fear, feelings of ecstasy, and perceiving ghosts (Carter et al., 2009).
Occipital lobe	**Vision** Vision and visual memory (Campbell, 2005); reading; language formation; and reception of vestibular, acoustic, and tactile stimuli.	Visual loss; visual hallucinations, such as sparks, tongues of flames, and flashes of lights. Difficulty understanding the meaning of the written word (Joseph, 1990).	Blindness, color blindness, impaired visual orientation, impaired depth perception (Taber & Hurley, 2008).
Cerebellum (sits on top of the brainstem)	**Functions as an auxiliary structure for the entire cerebral cortex (Taber & Hurley, 2008).** Posture and balance in walking. Sequential movements required in eating and writing. Controls speed and acceleration of movement. Involved in smooth eye movement (Nolte, 2010). Cognition and language (Gilman & Newman, 2003). Memory and impulse control (Taber & Hurley).	Impairment of balance, standing, and walking. Ataxia, tremors, and nystagmus. Abnormalities of executive functioning. Emotional blunting. Depression. Lack of inhibition and inappropriate behaviors. Impaired ability to multitask. Psychotic symptoms.	Thought to be involved in autism (Munson, Dawson, Abbott, et al., 2006; Sokol & Edwards-Brown, 2004) and attention deficit-hyperactivity disorder (Taber & Hurley, 2008). Abnormalities found in some patients with schizophrenia (Belger & Dichter, 2006). Tremors, impaired fine timing of movements (Carter et al., 2009). In children: clumsiness; delayed milestones. Language problems, inability to read social cues, and tactile defensiveness (Schmahmann, 2004).

Continued

TABLE 2-1 BRAIN STRUCTURES AND THEIR FUNCTIONS, DAMAGE EFFECTS, AND PSYCHOPATHOLOGIES—continued

Brain Structure	Function	Damage Effect	Psychopathology
Brainstem (medulla oblongata, pons, and midbrain) (Gilman & Newman, 2003)	Medulla oblongata: regulating blood pressure, respiration, and digestion. Reflex center for vomiting, coughing, sneezing, swallowing, and hiccupping (Gilman & Newman, 2003). Pons: relays information from the cerebral hemispheres to the cerebellum. Midbrain: controls many sensory and motor functions including eye movements (Kandel et al., 2000).	Pons damage is associated with disinhibition, anxiety, depression, and personality changes (Taber & Hurley, 2008). Midbrain damage may cause tics or block voluntary movement (Carter et al., 2009).	Post-traumatic stress disorder (Post, 2000). Although not a psychiatric disorder, "locked-in syndrome" does involve the CNS nerves (Gilman & Newman, 2003, p. 118). Bilateral lesions of ventral pons can interrupt corticobulbar and corticospinal tracts. Patient is aware of his/her surroundings and able to see and hear but cannot activate any voluntary muscles. Becomes totally paralyzed, unable to speak but with some eye movement. Psychosis, coma, and death (Taber & Hurley, 2008).
Locus ceruleus (a brainstem nucleus located within the reticular activating system) (Howard, 2006; Joseph, 2000)	Produces norepinephrine. Activity maintains arousal and inactivity allows for sleep (Hedaya, 1996).	Arousal and impairment of memory.	Panic disorder; anxiety and post-traumatic stress disorder.
Dorsal raphe (nuclei on top of brainstem)	Produces serotonin. Controls sleep/wake cycles.	Alteration of gene expression of serotonin (Goswami et al., 2010)	Depression and mood disorders.
Reticular activating system (RAS) (begins in the upper brainstem and continues into the lower part of the cerebral cortex)	**Involved in arousal and sleep; e.g., the "toggle switch" (Howard, 2006, p. 47).** Integrates responses of the central nervous system. Switches cerebral cortex on when individual is relaxed. Switches limbic system on when there is a threat (Howard). Regulates thalamus and cortex activities that are involved in emotions. Involved in arousal, attention, intention, and emotion (Kandel et al., 2000). Involved in processing pain and in regulation of heartbeat and breathing, perspiration, swallowing, coughing, salivation, urination, and sexual arousal (Carter et al., 2009; Gilman & Newman, 2003).	Sedation, state of unresponsiveness. Anesthesia acts on neurons in RAS, suppressing alertness and awareness (Carter et al., 2009).	Tumors may prevent switching from limbic system functioning to cortical functioning, with resulting persistence of rage behaviors (Howard, 2006). Attention deficit-hyperactivity disorder and anxiety disorders (Hedaya, 1996).
Olfactory bulb	Sense of smell; crucial for survival. Involved in fight-or-flight response and sexuality (survival of species); triggers past memories.	Loss of a sense of smell (anosmia) and increased olfactory sensitivity (hyperosmia).	Hyperosmia may occur in some psychoses (Gilman & Newman, 2003).
Hypothalamus (most primitive part of limbic system; the location of Freud's Id) (Joseph, 2000)	**Bridges internal homeostasis and outside environment.** **Newborn infants function at the level of the hypothalamus until other brain structures develop (Joseph, 2000).** Involved with raw emotions of pleasure, reward, aversion, and rage. Regulates the autonomic nervous system and secretion of hormones by pituitary. Involved in hunger, thirst, water balance, regulation of temperature, circadian rhythms, and stress response (Joseph, 1990; Joseph, 2000; Taber & Hurley, 2008).	Results in increased eating, emotional instability with episodes of rage, changes in body temperature, disturbed sleep and sexual functioning, uncontrollable laughter and crying (Joseph, 1990). Inflammation, tumors, and compression of hypothalamus may result in hypothalamic rage (growling, baring teeth, biting, and attacking moving objects) (Joseph, 2000).	Aggression Violence Anorexia Depression Altered sleep-wake cycles Gelastic seizures (laughing) (Taber & Hurley, 2008).

TABLE 2-1 BRAIN STRUCTURES AND THEIR FUNCTIONS, DAMAGE EFFECTS, AND PSYCHOPATHOLOGIES—continued

Brain Structure	Function	Damage Effect	Psychopathology
Thalamus (key relay station that is buried in the temporal lobe)	Gaits information to the neocortex (Andreasen, 2001; Nolte, 2010). Processes information coming from the five senses and information coming from the amygdala and cerebellum before it goes to the neocortex. Involved in wakefulness, sleep, and pain perception.	Impairment of ability to gait information; e.g., individuals are flooded with information. Apathy, drowsiness, and disturbed perception.	Negative symptoms of schizophrenia (Bogerts, 1993). Decreased volume in schizophrenia (Andreasen, 1997).
Amygdala Connected to hypothalamus and controls impulses of hypothalamus. Connected to hippocampus and controls memory functioning (Joseph, 2000)	**Anxiety and anger** Generates rudimentary emotions—fear, rage, religious ecstasy, sexual desire (Joseph, 2000). Surveys the environment. Regulates fear and response to stress (Gilman & Newman, 2003). Evaluates expressions of friendliness, fear, love, affection, distrust, and anger (Joseph, 1990; LeDoux, 2007). Contributes to establishing emotional memories, especially fear related (Shirtcliff et al., 2009). Seeks attachments indiscriminately.	Tumors or injury are associated with irritability, anger, rage, and aggression. There may be hyper-religiosity and sexual preoccupation. Bilateral damage: docility, inability to recognize anyone, putting things in the mouth to identify them, and insatiable appetite.	Involved in: Post-traumatic stress disorder, phobias, panic disorder, depression, schizophrenia, and autism (LeDoux, 2007). Kluver-Bucy syndrome (Hedaya, 1996).
Insula (cerebral cortex buried underneath the frontal, parietal, and temporal lobes) Considered by some to be part of limbic system (Saze, Hirao, Namiki, et al., 2007)	Involved in negative emotions: disgust, pain, hunger, empathy, and callousness (Shirtcliff et al., 2009).	Neuroplasticity of insula is involved in meditation. Thicker cortical volume of insula has been found in individuals who have meditated for many years (Lazar, Kerr, Wasserman, et al., 2005).	Abnormalities of insula are thought to be linked with lack of insight and misinterpretation of sensory inputs that are found in patients with schizophrenia (Saze, Kazuyuki, Namiki, et al., 2007). Reduced volume of insula found in children with conduct disorder (Sterzer, Stadler, Poustka, et al., 2007).
Cingulate cortex (ACC) (the part of the cortex closest to the limbic system) (Carter et al., 2009)	**Links emotions to actions and predicts the consequences of actions.** Involved in experiencing intense love, anger, or lust. Activated when mother hears her infant cry. Involved in detecting how others feel and reacting to others' emotions. Registers social rejection. Adjusts behavior to social context (Carter et al., 2009).	Reduced cingulated activity may contribute to akinetic mutism (individual does not move or speak), diminished self-awareness, neglect, reduced response to pain, and inappropriate social behaviors (Devinsky, 1994).	Obsessive-compulsive disorder. Addictions. Tics (Black & Andreasen, 2011; Devinsky, 1994). Depression (Pizzagalli, Oakes, Fox, et al., 2004).
Hippocampus and parahippocampal gyrus	**"Memory Structures" (Taber & Hurley, 2008, p. 177).** Regulates information coming to the neocortex. Involved in memory, learning, long-term memories, and retrieval of information (Joseph, 2000). Builds "cognitive maps" of individual in relation to time, place, and past and present experiences (Gilman & Newman, 2003). Assigns the time and place to an event (Van der Kolk, 1996).	Impaired ability to pay attention, learn new things, and remember or alter pre-existing learning memory deficits (Taber & Hurley, 2008).	Post-traumatic stress disorder (decreased hippocampal volume) (Post, 2000). Reduced volume in depression that may be reversible (Campbell, Marriott, Nahmias, et al., 2004; Mayberg, 2006). Reduced volume in individuals with low self-esteem (Pruessner, Baldwin, Dedovic, et al., 2005).
Septal nuclei (Attachment matures at 7 months of age.) (Joseph, 1990)	Quiets and dampens down responses of rage. Involved in socialization and development of enduring emotional attachments. Regulates hippocampal memory-related activity (Joseph, 2000). Involved in pleasure and reward; sexual pleasure.	Impairment may be due to lack of nurturing of primary caretaker during the time the septal area is building attachment connections.	Hypersexuality (Gorman & Cummings, 1992). Social stickiness (intrusive, repeated, inappropriate contact with anyone nearby) (Joseph, 1990).

Continued

TABLE 2-1 BRAIN STRUCTURES AND THEIR FUNCTIONS, DAMAGE EFFECTS, AND PSYCHOPATHOLOGIES—continued

Brain Structure	Function	Damage Effect	Psychopathology
Nucleus accumbens (part of the basal ganglia)	Modulates the limbic system. Involved in reward and pleasure circuit (LeDoux, 2002).	Impaired functioning following repeated methamphetamine use (Jefferson, 2005). Flat affect, social isolation, and loss of interest in activities.	Substance abuse/addictions.
Cingulate gyrus (part of the cerebral cortex located in the paralimbic area; surrounds the surface of the corpus callosum) (Kandel et al., 2000)	Integrates emotional information and cognition before conveying that information to the hypothalamus and neocortex (Benes, 1995). Assigns emotional value to stimuli. Involved in mother-child interactions, long-term attachments. Regulates autonomic, endocrine functioning and motor functions. Involved in retrieval of short-term memories (Devinsky, Morrell, & Vogt, 1995).	Impairment of ability to read facial expressions/cues and to express emotions. Apathy, flat affect, indifference. Obsessive-compulsive symptoms. Deviant social behavior. Stuttering related to reduced blood flow in the area (Joseph, 1990).	Increased cingulate activity: tics, obsessive-compulsive behaviors, and deviant social behaviors. Decreased cingulate activity: depression, reduced response to pain (Devinsky et al., 1995; Post, 2000). Symptoms similar to those of schizophrenia (Mayberg, 2006).
Basal ganglia Four ganglia: 1. Striatum (caudate nucleus, putamen) 2. Pallidum 3. Substantia nigra 4. Subthalamic nucleus) (Hedaya, 1996; Taber & Hurley, 2008)	Brings together: emotion, executive function, motivation, and motor activity (Taber & Hurley, 2008). Involved in posture, walking and eye movements. Moderates motor expression of emotional states (hitting, biting, licking). Also involved in memory, cognition, and emotion (Andreasen, 2001). Controls extrapyramidal motor tract.	Impairments of basal ganglia overall: slowness of movement, rigidity, cogwheel rigidity, and dystonias. Impairment of specific ganglia: 1. Striatum: obsessive-compulsive behaviors, tics, and symptoms of Tourette's syndrome (Hedaya, 1996; Sadock & Sadock, 2007). 2. Pallidum: flapping movement of arms and legs. 3. Substantia nigra: impairment of production of dopamine; e.g., rigidity. 4. Subthalamic nucleus: jerky movements.	Obsessive-compulsive disorder (Post, 2000). (Also neurological disorders: Parkinson's disease and Huntington's disease) (Andreasen, 2001). Cognitive and emotional dysfunction (Taber & Hurley, 2008). Extrapyramidal tract symptoms.

Ventricular System of the Brain

The ventricles are four cavities inside the cerebral hemispheres: two lateral ventricles are inside the cerebral hemispheres, the third ventricle lies within the diencephalon (thalamus and hypothalamus), and the fourth ventricle is in the caudal part of the brainstem in the pons and medulla oblongata. Inside each ventricle is a choroid plexus that produces the cerebrospinal fluid that fills the ventricles (England & Wakely, 2006). Cerebrospinal fluid regulates the neurochemical environment of the brain and provides protection for the brain from impact against the bones of the skull. The cerebrospinal fluid flows from the ventricles into the subarachnoid space, where it covers the surface of the brain and spinal cord. It passes through arachnoid villi, which are small projections of the arachnoid covering of the brain that protrude through the dura, and into the venous bloodstream (Gilman & Newman, 2003; Nolte, 2010). Obstruction of the normal passage of cerebrospinal fluid causes cerebrospinal fluid to accumulate in the ventricles, which is what occurs in hydrocephalus. Increased pressure from the accumulated fluid causes swelling of the optic nerve or papilledema. The most common cause of obstruction of the flow of cerebrospinal fluid is a brain tumor. Other causes are infections, drug intoxication, and trauma (England & Wakely; Gilman & Newman).

Vascular System of the Brain

Blood flows through the brain via two interconnected systems—the internal carotid system and the vertebral-basilar system. The internal carotid arteries supply blood to most of the cerebral hemispheres with the exception of the medial surface of the occipital lobe and the inferior surface of the temporal lobe, which are supplied with blood by the vertebral-basilar system. There are two branches of internal carotid arteries: the anterior cerebral arteries and the middle cerebral arteries. Both the anterior and middle arteries supply the cortex and also the hypothalamus, basal ganglia, and internal capsule with blood. The vertebral-basilar system supplies the midbrain, brainstem, and cerebellum with blood. The total amount of blood to the brain stays constant, but more blood goes to areas of the brain that are engaged in greater activity (Nolte, 2010).

Neurotransmission

The brain communicates using neurotransmission, which is the process of transferring information from one neuron to another neuron. Recall the neuron anatomy discussed earlier in this chapter. Neurotransmission involves (1) electrical impulses or action potentials to move the message down the axon, (2) the release of neurochemicals (neurotransmitters) into the synapse to relay the message, (3) receptors to receive the message, and (4) termination of neurotransmitter exertion by transport of excess neurotransmitter back into the presynaptic neuron or by metabolism of the neurotransmitter in the synaptic cleft (Carter et al., 2009). Thus, the process of neurotransmission can be thought of as four S's:

- Spark (electrical action potential)
- Spray (release of neurotransmitter into the synaptic cleft)
- Slide (into the receptors),
- Scoop-up (transport of unused neurotransmitter from the synaptic cleft back into the presynaptic neuron for reuse)

Figure 2-13 illustrates neurotransmission.

Synapses are the sites where information is transmitted (Daube & Stead, 2009). Optimal functioning of synapses is maintained by the neurotransmitter calpain, which is derived from calcium found in dairy products and green leafy vegetables. Calpain facilitates functioning of the synapses by removing protein debris from the synaptic cleft. Optimal functioning of the synapses is also maintained by lifestyle practices: interacting with an enriched environment of art, music, crafts, and games; exercising; eating a healthy diet that includes fats; and making new learning a part of daily activities (Howard, 2006). Synapses are the most important part of neurotransmission; synapses are where the brain does its work (LeDoux, 2002). Decker and Butcher (1992, p. 12) state in their ode to neurotransmission,

We may live without conscience, we may live without heart.
We may live without poetry, music and art.
We may live without politics or nuclear fission.
But no one can live without neurotransmission.

Likewise, LeDoux (2002) believed that ". . . self, the essence of who you are, reflects patterns of interconnectivity between neurons in your brain" (p. 2). We are the sum of information that has been encoded by transmission across synapses.

Transmitting Information

Processes of Transmission

Electrical and chemical processes carry out CNS communication (Daube & Stead, 2009). Electrical signals, called action potentials, are usually charged sodium, potassium, or chloride ions; the signals start where the axon emerges from the cell body, and the signal travels down the length of the axon (Bear et al., 2007). An action potential is like a rolling wave down the axon toward the terminal (Daube & Stead). LeDoux (2002) described the process as a "neurodomino effect" (p. 44).

The axon is wrapped in myelin, which is an electrical insulator that increases the efficiency and speed of the electrical conduction of information (Nolte, 2010). Small spaces of the axon are not covered with myelin. These spaces are called the *nodes of Ranvier*, and electrical impulses are able to jump from node to node of myelinated neurons (Fig. 2-14). In unmyelinated neurons, electrical impulses are carried by circuits of ion currents that flow into the membrane of the axon, through the axon, and out through other sections of the membrane. Morrell and Quarles (1999, p. 70) said that if nerves were not myelinated, the human spinal cord would have to be the size of a large tree trunk.

Near the end of the axon, the axon divides and forms fine branches that form synapses with the dendrites at the end of other neurons. Recall that synapses are the spaces between neurons in which one neuron transmits information to another neuron.

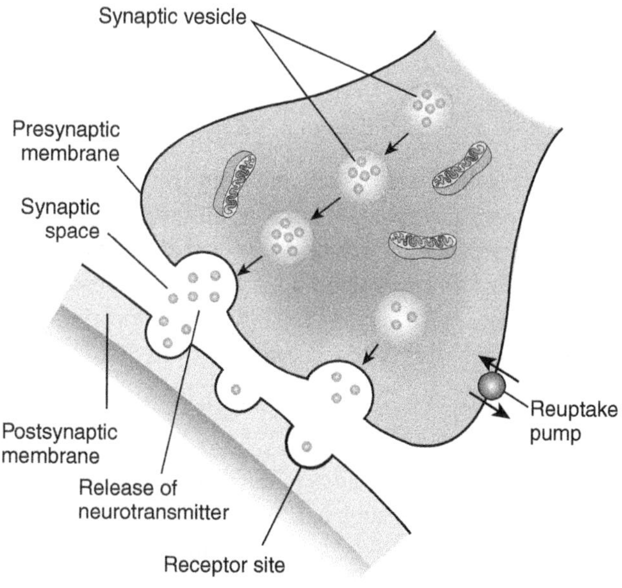

FIGURE 2-13: Neurotransmission. Information is transmitted by electrical impulses and neurochemicals, called neurotransmitters. Electrical impulses force neurotransmitters that are stored in neurons to be released into the synaptic cleft. The neurotransmitters fit into the receptors on a postsynaptic neuron and thus carry information from one neuron to another.

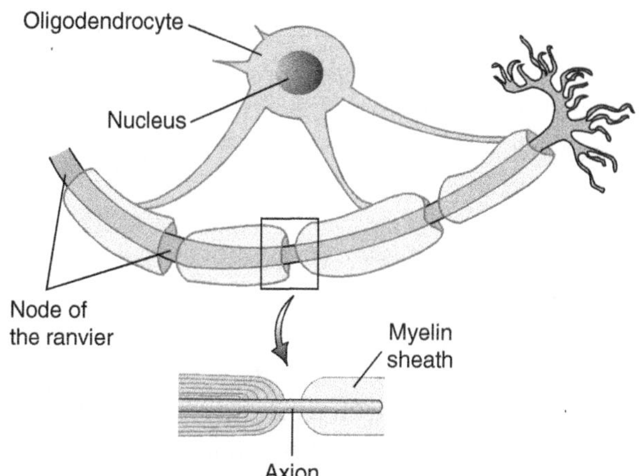

FIGURE 2-14: Myelinated Neuron. Myelination is the spiral wrapping of a myelin sheath produced by glial cells around the neuron's axon to insulate it and speed the flow of information along the axon. The nodes of Ranvier are breaks in the myelin sheath that allow impulses to skip from node to node, speeding impulses along the axon (Carter et al., 2009).

Synapses

Synaptic transmission involves the release of informational substances, which are chemicals such as neurotransmitters, from vesicles, which are storage sites in the presynaptic axon terminal. When the action potential reaches the terminal, it causes the vesicles to fuse with the presynaptic membrane of the neuron in a process called exocytosis (Daube & Stead, 2009, p. 90). Neurotransmitters that were stored in the vesicles are then sprayed into the synaptic cleft (Daube & Stead), thereby transmitting information to be picked up by receptors on another neuron.

Receiving Information

If the information from one neuron travels through the synapatic cleft and is picked up by the receptors of the next neuron, then the goal of producing an electrical response in the postsynaptic receivers of another neuron is achieved (Higgins & George, 2007; LeDoux, 2002) and the message is received. The receptors of neurons are thus key to receiving information that is transmitted across the synapses.

Receptors

Receptors are protein molecules located on the dendrites of neurons that recognize and respond to specific neurotransmitters or drug molecules (Andreasen, 2001). They are microscopic, folded protein structures that are transmembranal, which means that they extend across the cell membrane from the outside to the inside of the cell (Fig. 2-15). There are four major groups of receptors:

- The *ion-gated receptors,* also called ionotropic receptors, which are activated by smaller, faster neurotransmitters such as glutamate and gamma-aminobutyric acid (GABA).
- The *G protein receptors,* which constitute 80% of all receptors in the body, regulate cellular activity by generating "second messengers" (Szabo, Gould, & Manji, 2009, p. 5). They are the receptors for neurotransmitters such as dopamine, norepinephrine (NE), serotonin, cannabinoids, and enkephalins (Kandel et al., 2000; Sadock & Sadock, 2007; Szabo et al.) and for acetylcholine, neuropeptides, and sensory signals such as light and odors (Szabo et al.).
- *Tyrosine kinases and phosphatase receptors,* which contain enzyme activity and are used by growth factors (such as neurotropic factors) and by cytokines (such as interleukins and lymphokines) that are involved in the generation of an immune response.
- *Nuclear receptors,* which regulate gene expression. They are transcription factors that activate genes and regulate gene expression in response to steroid hormones and other chemicals.

There are also autoreceptors and heteroreceptors. *Autoreceptors* are receptors located on neurons that produce the ligand (binding chemical compound) for that neuron, e.g., a serotonin receptor on a serotonin-producing neuron. *Heteroreceptors* are receptors on neurons that do not produce the ligand for that receptor, e.g., a serotonin receptor on a dopamine neuron (Szabo et al., 2009). The functioning of receptors in pharmacotherapy can be seen in Box 2-2.

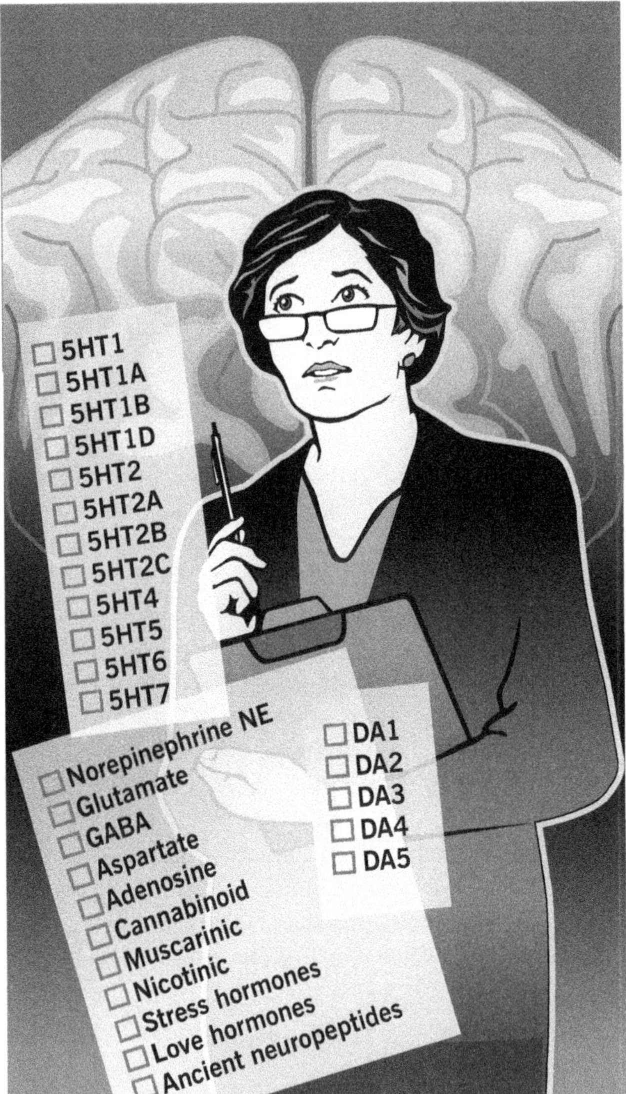

FIGURE 2-15: Receptors. Receptors are the targets of neurotransmitters that have been released into the synaptic cleft.

Processes of Reception: Synaptic Neurotransmission

Synaptic neurotransmission takes place through both a rapid, direct process and a longer process that involves modulatory changes in the actual structure and functioning of the neuron.

Neurotransmission that is rapid involves brief changes in activation or inhibition of the neuron by way of binding of the neurotransmitter with ion-gated (ionophore) receptors. When a neurotransmitter's receptor is ion gated, the process is as follows: (1) the receptor is activated; (2) gates

BOX 2-2 Functioning of Receptors in Pharmacotherapy

The activities of receptors in response to the administration of psychotropic medication include

1. *Receptor agonists:* The medication fits the receptor the same as the naturally occurring neurotransmitter and thus activates the receptor in the same way as the neurotransmitter.
2. *Receptor antagonists:* The medication blocks the receptor function so that a neurotransmitter cannot bind with the receptor.
3. *Autoreceptors:* Autoreceptors are receptors located on neurons that produce the neurotransmitter for that neuron. They serve as a feedback mechanism to stimulate or inhibit the release of a neurotransmitter into the synaptic cleft and are usually found on the presynaptic neuron. Medications can enhance or suppress action of autoreceptors.
4. *Inhibition of enzymes:* The medication binds to the enzyme and thus prevents the enzyme from binding to the neurotransmitter and metabolizing it thereby keeping more of the neurotransmitter available.
5. Receptor *downregulation:* The medication acts to decrease the rate of neurotransmitter receptor synthesis (takes days to weeks).
6. Receptor *upregulation:* The medication acts to increase receptor synthesis.

Bear et al., 2007; Stahl, 2000; Szabo et al., 2009.

of ion channels are either opened or closed to the flow of potassium, chloride, sodium, or calcium ions; and (3) the result of the ion flow determines whether the neuron is activated to fire (pass a signal to the next neuron) or inhibited (dormant) (Bear et al., 2007; Daube & Stead, 2009). Examples of neurotransmission that involves ionophore receptors is the action of the neurotransmitters glutamate and GABA.

In contrast to the rapid process of neurotransmission that takes place in ion-gated receptors, the longer process of neurotransmission occurs in G protein–coupled receptors and involves modulatory changes in the actual structure and functioning of the neuron. According to Andreasen (2001), "G-protein receptors wind in and out across the fatty sandwich of the neuronal membrane seven times" (p. 78). When a neurotransmitter, the first messenger, occupies a G protein receptor, the G protein receptor changes its shape. This process leads to the release of a "second messenger" in the neuron (Andreasen, p. 79). According to Andreasen, "the second messengers help create the proteins that regulate the expression of genes, the structural components of the cell, and the enzymes that aid in the synthesis of neurotransmitters" (p. 79). Third-messenger molecules—proto-oncogenes, such as *c-fos* genes—code for proteins that regulate gene expression. When neurotransmitters (first messengers) communicate with other neurons, a cascade of events via the second and third messengers inside the cell occurs to convey information from the outside environment to the cell. This process is slow, and the effects last a long time (Daube & Stead, 2009; Kandel et al., 2000).

Informational Substances

Informational substances are neurochemicals that carry the message from one neuron to another (McGeehan, http://www.greenteacher.com/articles/McGeehan.pdf). Knowledge of informational substances and the properties and functioning of their receptors in the CNS enables psychiatric advanced practice nurses to understand the role that receptors have in psychiatric symptoms, the action of newer psychotropic medications that affect multiple receptor types, and the side effects associated with the action of medications at different receptor sites. Information about receptors is increasing rapidly, and at the same time, research findings are suggesting that some psychiatric disorders (for instance, schizophrenia), pervasive developmental disorders (for instance, autism), and the learning disorders (for instance, dyslexia) may result from impaired functioning of the synapses, primarily impaired functioning of receptors. The main informational substances are neurotransmitters, neurotropins, neurohormones, neuropeptides, and protein ligands (ligands are chemical compounds that bind to a specific site on a receptor).

Neurotransmitters

In the past, there was a trend to view psychiatric disorders as being neurotransmitter based; that is, psychiatric disorders were caused by a chemical imbalance. This early view was accepted eagerly by families of the mentally ill because it was a movement away from blaming them for causing the illness and it created hope that finding the right balance of neurotransmitters would cure their family member. However, it has since been determined that neurotransmitters have defined actions at specific receptors and that emotions, cognition, and behaviors are the result of the integrated activities of large circuits of neurons, *not* the result of the activity of one or more chemicals (Melchitzky & Lewis, 2009).

Traditionally, neurotransmitters have been thought to share the following characteristics:

1. Neurotransmitters are manufactured by a cell.
2. Neurotransmitters are stored in presynaptic terminals.
3. Neurotransmitters are released into the synaptic cleft in response to stimulation, where they create an action in the postsynaptic receptor.
4. Neurotransmitters have a specific mechanism for termination of action (Kandel et al., 2000, p. 281).

About 50 substances present in the brain appear to be neurotransmitters (Szabo et al., 2009). However, because more molecules such as neuropeptides and more gases such as nitric oxide and carbon monoxide are being identified as neurotransmitters, Snyder and Ferris (2000) suggested that the definition of a neurotransmitter be broadened thus: "A transmitter is a molecule, released by neurons or glia, that physiologically influences the electrochemical state of adjacent cells" (p. 1748).

Neurotransmitters include classic neurotransmitters, amino acid neurotransmitters, cholinergic neurotransmitters, neuropeptides, and neurohormones (Szabo et al., 2009). In addition, molecules that have an effect on nerve cells—such as nitric oxide gas, carbon monoxide gas, and prostaglandins (metabolites of arachidonic acid, a component of fatty acids)—have recently been identified as neurotransmitters. These molecules are not stored in vesicles and released like the other neurotransmitters; rather, they cross cell membranes by diffusion and act as second messengers at G protein–coupled receptors (Kandel et al., 2000; McAllister et al., 2008). Nitric oxide and carbon monoxide are thought to be involved in neuronal activity related to learning and memory (Szabo et al.).

Categories of agents that act as neurotransmitters include

1. Classic neurotransmitters, which are monoamines. Monoamines are also called the biogenic amines, and they include the catecholamines (dopamine, NE, and epinephrine), the indoleamines (serotonin and melatonin), and histamine.
2. Amino acids, such as glutamate, aspartate, GABA, glycine, and adenosine.
3. Cholinergic neurotransmitters, or acetylcholine (which is sometimes included with the monoamines).
4. Neuropeptides, which are short chains of amino acids (Hedaya, 1996).
5. Neurohormones, such as cortisol.

Although the neurotransmitters are discussed in this chapter as separate neurochemicals with separate actions and pathways, it is now accepted that most neurons contain a monoamine neurotransmitter, at least one amino acid neurotransmitter, and more than one neuropeptide (Daube & Stead, 2009; Snyder & Ferris, 2000). For example, serotonin and the neuropeptide substance P coexist in the dorsal raphe neurons of the brain (Sergeyev, Hokfelt, & Hurd, 1999).

Classic Neurotransmitters: Monoamines

There are two classes of monoamines: catecholamines (dopamine, NE, and epinephrine) and indoleamines (serotonin and melatonin) (Higgins & George, 2007). These neurotransmitters are implicated in disorders such as mania, depression, schizophrenia, Parkinson's disease, attention deficit-hyperactivity disorder, and tics. The monoamines are influenced by antidepressant medications such as selective serotonin reuptake inhibitors (SSRIs) and tricyclic antidepressants, by antipsychotics, and by cocaine, amphetamines, and other drugs. For example, lysergic acid diethylamide (LSD) acts on serotonin receptors (LeDoux, 2002). The monoamine neurotransmitters are found primarily in the frontal lobes and limbic system and are involved in higher brain functions. The monoamines are taken back into the neuron through the action of a transporter such as an NE transporter, a serotonin transporter, or a dopamine transporter. (The relationship of neurotransmitters with psychotropic medications and psychiatric disorders is discussed in Chapter 6.)

Dopamine

Dopamine is an inhibitory neurotransmitter that is synthesized in the substantia nigra in the brainstem from the amino acid tyrosine. It is first converted to L-dopa and then transformed to dopamine by the enzyme L-aromatic amino acid decarboxylase (Melchitzky & Lewis, 2009). Dopaminergic neurons appear after the NE and serotonin neurons. They are not as widespread as NE or serotonin neurons and are found in discrete circuits. The dopamine neurotransmitter system is illustrated in Figure 2-16.

Dopamine is involved in thinking, decision making, ability to respond with reward-seeking behaviors, integration of thoughts and emotions, emotional responses, and fine muscle movements. Dopamine plays a role in stimulating the hypothalamus to release sex hormones and hormones affecting thyroid and adrenal glands. Dopamine is found in neural pathways from the frontal lobe to the spinal cord (Bear et al., 2007).

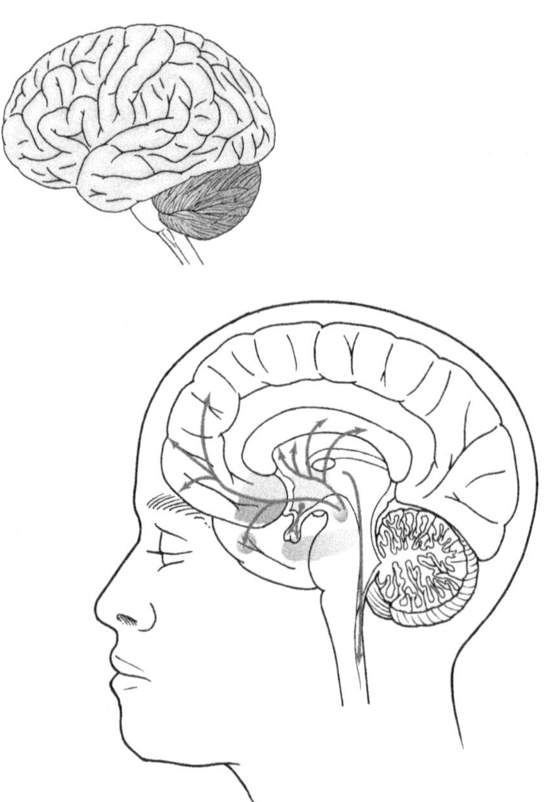

FIGURE 2-16: Dopamine Neurotransmitter System. Dopamine is involved in thinking, decision making, ability to respond with reward-seeking behaviors, integration of thoughts and emotions, emotional responses, muscle movements, and endocrine functioning. There are four main dopamine pathways—mesolimbic, nigrostriatal, mesocortical, and tuberoinfundibular (Szabo et al., 2009).

Dopamine Pathways

There are four main dopamine pathways—mesolimbic, nigrostriatal, mesocortical, and tuberoinfundibular (Szabo et al., 2009).

1. *Mesolimbic dopamine pathway.* The mesolimbic pathway is involved in feelings of reward. It consists of dopamine neurons in the ventral tegmental area that go to the hypothalamus, nucleus accumbens, olfactory bulb, septum, thalamus, amygdala, hippocampus, and frontal and cingulate regions of the cerebral cortex. The mesolimbic pathway is implicated in mood disorders, psychoses, and drug abuse (Cooper, Bloom, & Roth, 2001); in the positive symptoms (hallucinations and delusions) of schizophrenia (Higgins & George, 2007); and in motor and reward pathways (Szabo et al., 2009).
2. *Nigrostriatal dopamine pathway.* The nigrostriatal pathway is the largest of the dopaminergic pathways and is involved in voluntary movement and involuntary movement such as in motor tics and movement disorders. It is also involved in making decisions about actions that will bring rewards and in goal-directed activities that are often excessive in patients with bipolar disorder (Szabo et al., 2009).
3. *Mesocortical dopamine pathway.* The mesocortical dopaminergic pathway projects to the cerebral cortex, cingulate cortex, and entorhinal cortex. These areas are sensitive to stress and are involved in functions such as cognition, planning, and modulating behavior. Some researchers believe that abnormalities of the mesocortical dopamine pathway underlie the negative symptoms of schizophrenia, which are apathy, anhedonia, and lack of motivation (Higgins & George, 2007; Melchitzky & Lewis, 2009).
4. *Tuberoinfundibular dopamine pathway.* The tuberoinfundibular pathway sends projections to the hypothalamus and pituitary, where it regulates the secretions of hormones such as prolactin. Use of drugs that interrupt the action of dopamine in this tract may be associated with hyperprolactinemia, which is an increase of prolactin that may result in amenorrhea, galactorrhea, and gynecomastia.

Dopamine Receptors

There are five types of dopamine receptors, and all belong to the G protein–coupled receptor family. The receptors can be grouped into two main classes: D1 and D2. D1 class includes D1 and D5 receptors. D1 receptors are present in the frontal cortex and in the extrapyramidal system; they are thought to be involved in higher cognitive functioning and in the antipsychotic effects of medications. D5 receptors are located in the prefrontal region of the brain, the premotor region, the hippocampus, the limbic system, and the nucleus accumbens. The D5 receptor has a ten times greater affinity for dopamine than the D1 receptor, but the D1 receptor is more prevalent (Melchitzky & Lewis, 2009).

D2 class includes D2, D3, and D4 receptors (Cooper et al., 2001; Szabo et al., 2009). The highest levels of D2 receptors are found in the caudate nucleus, putamen, nucleus accumbens, ventral tegmetal area, and substantia nigra. Lower levels of D2 receptors are found in the septal region, amygdala, hippocampus, thalamus, cerebellum, and cerebral cortex (Melchitzky & Lewis, 2009). D2 receptors, which are the targets of many antipsychotic medications, are thought to be involved with the positive symptoms of schizophrenia (hallucinations and delusions), with extrapyramidal symptoms, and with increased levels of prolactin (Szabo et al.). Dopamine receptor D3 is located in the limbic region of the brain, particularly in the nucleus accumbens. Overstimulation of D3 receptors may result in negative symptoms of schizophrenia. Dopamine receptor D4 is located on cortical neurons that influence thought processes. Clozapine has a stronger affinity for D4 receptors than for D2 receptors, and this may account for improvement of both positive and negative symptoms of schizophrenia.

The dopamine transporters act as pumps to clear dopamine from the synaptic cleft. Drugs of abuse may alter the action of the dopamine transporters. For example, amphetamine may act on the dopamine transporters so that they release dopamine instead of carrying it back to the vesicles for storage, resulting in high levels of available dopamine with increases in alertness, irritability, paranoia, and violence (Szabo, Gould, & Manji, 2004).

Alterations in the dopamine system are believed to be associated with schizophrenia, with other psychiatric disorders, with neurological disorders such as Parkinson's disease, and with movement disorders (Bear et al., 2007; Sadock & Sadock, 2007).

Epinephrine and Norepinephrine (NE)

Both epinephrine and NE are part of the noradrenergic neurotransmitter system, Epinephrine is a monoamine neurotransmitter that is not prevalent in the brain but is prevalent in the PNS. NE, which is prevalent in the brain, is involved in alertness, arousal, learning, the formation of memories, the ability to focus attention, the ability to be oriented, and the storage and retrieval of traumatic memories (Charney, Grillon, & Bremmer, 1998). NE receptors are involved in the fight-or-flight response.

Noradrenergic Neurotransmitter System

The noradrenergic system (NE and epinephrine) is the first of the neurotransmitter systems to develop in the embryo. In the locus ceruleus of the brainstem, the precursor tyrosine synthesizes NE into L-dihydroxyphenylalanine (L-dopa), which is transformed into dopamine and then into NE by the enzyme dopamine beta-hydoxylase (Kandel et al., 2000; Melchitzky & Lewis, 2009) (Fig. 2-17). The action of NE is terminated by either (1) reuptake by the NE transporter, a

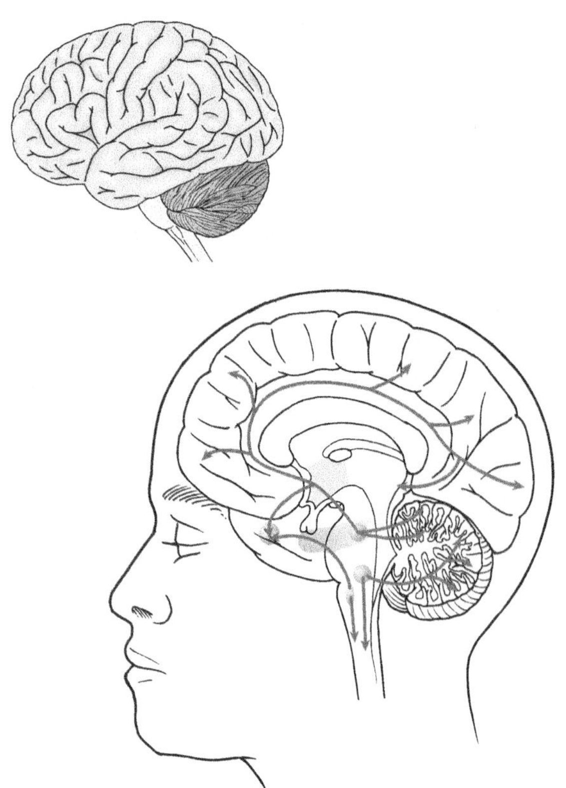

FIGURE 2-17: **Norepinephrine System.** NE is an excitatory neurotransmitter that is involved in alertness, arousal, learning, the storage and retrieval of traumatic memories, and the fight-or-flight response (Charney, Grillon, & Bremmer, 1998).

structure in the nerve cell membrane that scoops up NE from the synaptic cleft and returns it to the vesicles in the neuron where it is stored for future use, or (2) degradation of NE by two enzymes in the synaptic cleft—monoamine oxidase (MAO) and catechol-O-methyltransferase (COMT) (Higgins & George, 2007). The NE transporter also takes up dopamine. Thus, use of medications that act as NE reuptake inhibitors may increase availability of dopamine as well as NE in the prefrontal cortex (Higgins & George).

Melchitzky, Austin, & Lewis (2004) described two NE systems. One is in the locus ceruleus, which connects to the hippocampus and cortex and is involved in learning, memory, and attention. The other is in the brainstem, in the medulla oblongata. From the medulla oblongata, NE fibers go to the spinal cord, cerebellum, limbic system, and cortex. Thus, NE activates the sympathetic nervous system (Kandel et al., 2000), priming it for fight or flight.

Norepinephrine Receptors

The receptors for NE are G protein–mediated second-messenger systems. NE α_1 and NE β_1 receptors are located throughout the cerebrum and in the thalamus and hypothalamus. Decreased availability of NE results in an increase of α_1 and β_1 receptor sites. Long-term use of antidepressants results in downregulation of α_1 and β_1 receptor sites; it is also associated with a decrease in both the number and the sensitivity of the NE α_2 receptors located in the cortex, limbic system, and locus ceruleus that serve as autoreceptors. Stimulation of the NE α_2 receptors causes a decrease in the release of NE. Medications that serve as antagonists at α_2 receptors block the receptors, thus increasing the availability of NE (Melchitzky & Lewis, 2009).

Based on animal studies, it is thought that environmental influences, such as maltreatment or emotionally stressful experiences in early childhood, may adversely affect the noradrenergic system and that deviations of the noradrenergic system may alter synaptic plasticity of the cortex and the development of other neurotransmitter systems (McEwen, 1998; Sood & Koziol, 1994). Thus, alterations of development of the NE neurotransmitter system may be manifested in the compromised functioning associated with certain psychiatric disorders such as mood disorders, generalized anxiety disorder, panic disorder, posttraumatic stress disorder, and depression (Higgins & George, 2007; Stahl, 2000) and in attention deficit-hyperactivity disorder (Anderson, 1998). The level of NE in the locus ceruleus drops between the ages of 40 and 60 years, and that decrease may account for the mellowing often described in people in this age group.

Serotonin

Serotonergic System

Serotonin (5-hydroxytryptamine, 5-HT) is the second neurotransmitter system to appear in the fetus. The serotonin neurotransmitter system can be seen in Figure 2-18. Serotonin is synthesized in the raphe nucleus of the brainstem. The precursor for serotonin is the amino acid tryptophan, which is found in dairy products, poultry, barley, brown rice, soybeans, and peanuts. Tryptophan is hydroxylated by the enzyme tryptophan hydroxylase to form serotonin. Serotonin fibers project to the cortex (especially the frontal and prefrontal cortex), limbic system, thalamus, and hypothalamus. Serotonin has a role in inhibiting activity and behavior. It tends to increase sleep time and to reduce aggression and sexual activity. It mediates eating, mood, and pain perception and is involved in neuroendocrine function and release of prolactin and adrenocorticotropic hormone (ACTH). Alterations in the serotonin system that result in deficits of serotonin are associated with irritability, hostility, sleep dysregulation, loss of appetite, loss of sexual interest, and anxiety disorders including obsessive-compulsive disorder, depression, and suicidality (Sadock & Sadock, 2007). Serotonin is a precursor of melatonin, which plays a role in maintaining circadian rhythms and in depression, sleep disruptions, and jet lag (Melchitzky et al., 2004).

Serotonin Receptors

There are seven subfamilies of serotonin receptors—5HT1, 5HT2, 5HT3, 5HT4, 5HT5, 5HT6, and 5HT7—with distinctive features and responses to medications. The subfamilies

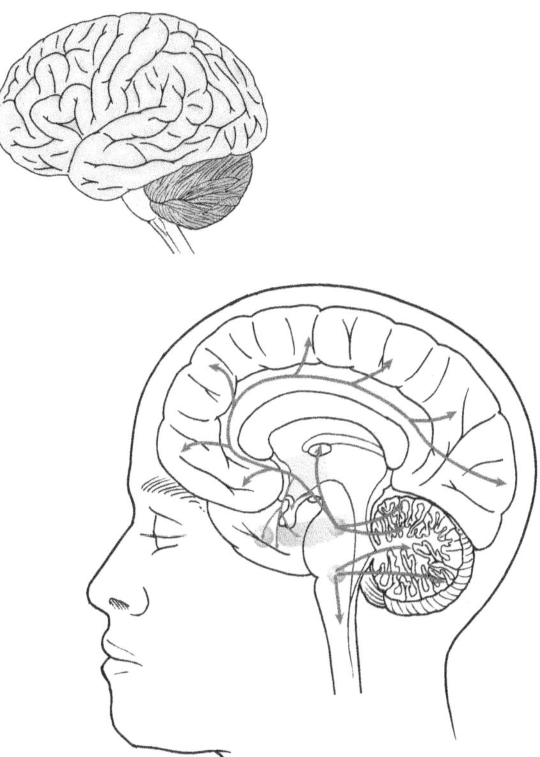

FIGURE 2-18: Serotonin Neurotransmitter System. Serotonin fibers project to the cortex (especially the frontal and prefrontal cortexes), limbic system, thalamus, and hypothalamus. Serotonin has an inhibiting action and tends to increase sleep time and to reduce aggression, sexual activity, and eating. It mediates depression and pain perception and is involved in neuroendocrine functioning.

have subtypes of serotonin receptors (Szabo et al., 2009). All serotonin receptors are G protein–coupled receptors, with the exception of the 5HT3 receptor, which is an ionotropic receptor.

1. *Subfamily 5HT1 receptors.* The 5HT1 receptors are found in high concentrations in the limbic area. They are also located on serotonergic neuron cell bodies, where they serve as autoreceptors that regulate the activity of the serotonin neuron, and they are located at postsynaptic receptors on astrocytes and other glial cells (Szabo et al., 2009). Reduced 5HT1 functioning, possibly in response to stress, may be associated with depression. Subtypes of the 5HT1 receptor include (Melchitzky & Lewis, 2009)
   a. Subtype 5HT1A: These receptors are involved in regulation of body temperature, eating, and sexual behavior and are implicated in depression and anxiety. Blockage of subtype 5HT1A receptors is associated with an antidepressant, anxiolytic, and antiaggressive action. Blockage of 5HT1A receptors that function as autoreceptors postsynaptically cuts the feedback that shuts off serotonin. Thus, using a medication that blocks the 5HT1A receptors will prevent the feedback that shuts off serotonin, making more serotonin available.
   b. Subtype 5HT1B: These receptors are involved in anxiety, movement disorders, food intake, sexual activity, and aggressive behavior.
   c. Subtype 5HT1C: The 5HT1C classification is no longer used because it is similar in structure and function to the 5HT2 receptor class (Szabo et al., 2009).
   d. Subtype 5HT1D: These receptors are involved in motor action, vasoconstriction, migraine headaches, and appetite. These receptors are located in the cortex, caudate nucleus, limbic system, hypothalamus, basal ganglia, and spinal cord.
2. *Subfamily 5HT2 receptors.* The 5HT2 receptors are located in the cortex, striatum, nucleus accumbens, olfactory bulb and hippocampus. They are involved in affect (emotion), cognition, movement, reward, memory, and reactions to smell. There are three subtypes of 5HT2 receptors:
   a. Subtype 5HT2A: This is often referred to as "the 5HT2 receptor" and is involved in smooth muscle contraction, control of release of hormones and neurotransmitters, sexual activity, regulation of sleep, and motor behaviors. It is implicated in epilepsy, migraine headaches, anxiety, depression, schizophrenia, and hallucinations.
   b. Subtype 5HT2B: This subtype is involved in smooth muscle contraction and cognition.
   c. Subtype 5HT2C: This subtype is involved with the choroid plexus, which produces cerebrospinal fluid. It is also involved in motor behavior and appetite. It may be involved in weight gain associated with psychotropic medications (Szabo et al., 2009).

   Clozapine, one of the atypical antipsychotic medications, binds to 5HT2 receptors. Medications such as mirtazapine (Remeron) that block this serotonin receptor may also balance the dopamine antagonism effect on the striatum, thus producing fewer extrapyramidal side effects and less sexual dysfunction. Some of the atypical antipsychotics block both dopamine 2 receptors and 5HT2 receptors, and this balancing action may be what gives them their special properties (Szabo et al., 2009).
3. *Subfamily 5HT3 receptors.* The 5HT3 serotonin receptors are located in the intestines and are implicated in gastrointestinal distress. Medications that are 5HT3 receptor antagonists such as mirtazapine are used to treat irritable bowel syndrome. The 5HT3 receptors that are located in the brainstem are associated with vomiting. Medications such as ondansetron (Zofran ODT) that are antagonists for 5HT3 receptors are being used to control vomiting in patients with cancer who are receiving chemotherapy (Szabo et al., 2009).

4. *Subfamily 5HT4 receptors.* The 5HT4 receptors are located in basal ganglia, hippocampus, and neocortex. 5HT4 receptors are involved in cardiac, adrenal, bladder, and gastrointestinal tract activity. They modulate release of GABA and are believed to be involved in cognition.
5. *Subfamily 5HT5 receptors.* The 5HT5 receptors are located in the hypothalamus, hippocampus, corpus callosum, ventricles and glial cells. They have a high affinity for LSD. They are also believed to be involved in brain development.
6. *Subfamily 5HT6 receptors.* The 5HT6 receptors are located in the cerebral cortex and in the limbic system. They have a high affinity for tricyclic antidepressant medications and for some antipsychotics.
7. *Subfamily 5HT7 receptors.* The 5HT7 receptors are located in the cerebral cortex, hippocampus, thalamus, and caudate nucleus. They are involved in smooth muscle relaxation and play a role in sensory processes, circadian rhythms, and behaviors related to mood (Gerhardt & van Heerikhuizen, 1997; Melchitzky & Lewis, 2009; Szabo et al., 2009).

The effect of serotonin is terminated in the synaptic cleft by serotonin's metabolism by enzymes in the synaptic cleft or by a reuptake process that is carried out by the serotonin transporter. The serotonin transporter scoops up serotonin from the synaptic cleft and transports it back to the presynaptic neuron, where it is stored for reuse. One class of antidepressants, the MAO inhibitors, blocks the metabolism of serotonin in the synaptic cleft, and other antidepressant medications block the reuptake of serotonin, thus keeping more serotonin available in the synaptic cleft (Szabo et al., 2009).

Histamine

Histamine is involved in regulating brain function, stimulating gastric secretions, and regulating biorhythms, neuroendocrine functioning, and immune and inflammatory responses. It influences arousal, attention, food and water intake, sleep-wake cycles, response to pain, and the release of oxytocin, prolactin, and ACTH (Higgins & George, 2007). Neurons that release histamine are located in the hypothalamus and project to the cerebral cortex, limbic system, and thalamus.

Amino Acid Neurotransmitters

The amino acid neurotransmitters are the most widely used neurotransmitters in the brain (Szabo et al., 2009). The major *excitatory* amino acid neurotransmitters are glutamate and aspartate. The major *inhibitory* amino acid neurotransmitters are GABA and glycine. Amino acids are made from the foods that we eat. Thus, patients with depression, severe psychosis, and anorexia, whose diets are often insufficient, lack the essential amino acids needed to produce neurotransmitters, and that deficiency may affect the patients' response to medications such as antidepressants (Hedaya, 1996).

Glutamate

Glutamate Pathways

Glutamate is an excitatory neurotransmitter that exerts stimulating effects on neural activity by affecting almost all neurons. It is "the major work horse of the brain. It gets the brain started" (Higgins & George, 2007, p. 38). Found in the cortex, hippocampus, thalamus, striatum, cerebellum, and spinal cord, it is a calcium channel regulator and is thought to play a role in neural plasticity, learning, and memory (Szabo et al., 2009). The glutamate system is believed to be involved in epilepsy and schizophrenia (Coyle, Tsai, & Goff, 2002; Keltner, Hogan, & Knight, et al., 2001). Trauma, ischemia, and severe stress increase levels of glutamate in the hippocampus (Szabo et al.). Clinical data suggest that, in excess, glutamate can function as an excitotoxin, causing neuronal cell death. For example, "reduced reuptake by a glial glutamate transporter appears to be an important mechanism underlying excitotoxicity in amyotrophic lateral sclerosis (also known as Lou Gehrig's disease)" (Gilman & Newman, 2003, p. 219; Knott & Bossy-Wetzel, 2007).

Glutamate Receptors

Glutamate receptors include AMPA (α-amino-3-hydroxy-5-methyl-4-isoxazolepropionic acid) receptors, NMDA (*N*-Methyl-D-aspartic acid) receptors, and kainite receptors (Szabo et al., 2009). Glutamate and glycine act together to open NMDA receptors that are involved in memory storage (Szabo et al.). NMDA receptors are found in the cortex, hippocampus, cerebellum, and spinal cord. Excessive NMDA receptor activity may lead to excess calcium influx and may result in neuronal death.

AMPA receptors are stimulated by glutamate and produce a fast excitatory synaptic signal. It is thought that drugs of abuse alter AMPA receptors in the ventral tegmental area (the reward center of the brain), producing permanent changes in the response of the brain to drugs of abuse (Szabo et al., 2009). Kainite receptors are involved with synaptic plasticity and with regulation of mood, risk-taking behaviors, and behaviors associated with mania (Szabo et al.). It is thought that a hypoglutamate state may be present in individuals with schizophrenia (Gao, Sakai, Roberts, et al., 2000) and that increased levels may be associated with the nerve cell death of amyotrophic lateral sclerosis (Kwak & Kawahara, 2005).

Aspartate

Aspartate is an excitatory neurotransmitter very similar to glutamate. It is found primarily in the spinal cord (Snyder & Ferris, 2000).

Gamma-Aminobutyric Acid (GABA)

GABA is the major inhibitory neurotransmitter in the CNS, and it is located in every area of the brain (Szabo et al., 2009). The precursor for GABA is glutamate. GABA is synthesized through the enzyme glutamate decarboxylase and requires vitamin B6 for its synthesis. GABA is involved in the reduction of aggression and anxiety, and in working memory, sleep, and muscle relaxation. Figure 2-19 provides an illustration of GABA pathways.

GABA inhibits neuronal activity by inhibiting action potentials (LeDoux, 2002; Melchitzky & Lewis, 2009). It causes an influx of chloride into the cell, resulting in a hyperpolarization or inhibition. It also acts as a guard to prevent glutamate from excessive stimulation of neurons, preventing the constant firing that could result in death of the neuron. GABA agonists—such as benzodiazepines—that have anxiolytic, muscle relaxant, anticonvulsant, and sedative properties also induce the inflow of chloride. Without inhibition, neurons become excitable and can produce rapid thoughts, excessive anxiety, and even seizure activity.

GABA transmission in the prefrontal cortex is increased by serotonin. This action partly explains the effectiveness of selective serotonin reuptake inhibitors (SSRIs) in anxiety disorders (Keltner et al., 2001). GABA neurons are vulnerable to stress-related elevated levels of cortisol and to excitotoxicity associated with glutamate (First & Tasman, 2004). Psychiatric disorders associated with GABA include the anxiety disorders and possibly schizophrenia (Melchitzky & Lewis, 2009).

Glycine

Glycine is an inhibitory transmitter. It acts primarily in the brainstem and spinal cord (Szabo et al., 2009) and inhibits neuronal firing by gating chloride channels. It is believed that glycine has the ability to change NMDA functioning. The NMDA agonists, glycine-D-serine and D-cycloserine, have been found to improve cognition and to decrease negative symptoms of patients with schizophrenia who are receiving antipsychotic medications (Coyle, Tsai, & Goff, 2002).

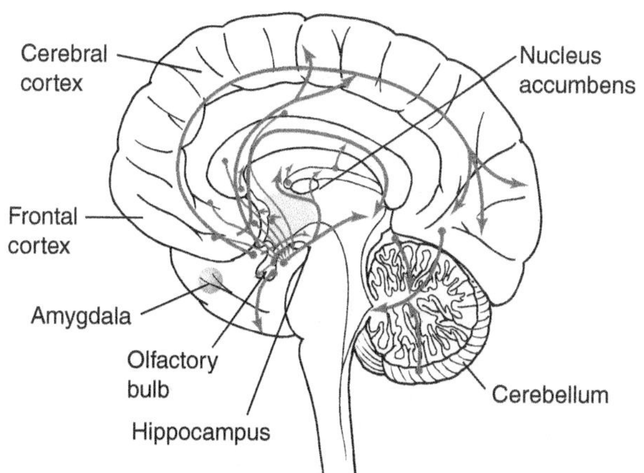

FIGURE 2-19: GABA Pathways. The GABA neurotransmitter is the major inhibitory neurotransmitter in the CNS and is located in every area of the brain (Szabo et al., 2009). GABA is involved in the reduction of aggression and anxiety and also in working memory, sleep, and muscle relaxation.

Adenosine Triphosphate (ATP)

Adenosine is a inhibitory neurotransmitter (Olsen & Delorey, 1999). It is involved in neuromodulation through its activity in regulating sodium/potassium ion channels. It is also involved in the reuptake of neurotransmitters such as glutamate. When the adenosine system does not work effectively, glutamate may accumulate, causing damage to neurons (Daube & Stead, 2009). The action of adenosine is blocked by caffeine.

Cholinergic Neurotransmitters: Acetylcholine

Cholinergic neurons are the last of the neurotransmitters to appear during gestation. Acetylcholine is synthesized from choline—which is a component of lecithin, which is found in egg yolks, liver, and soybeans—and from acetyl coenzyme A (Wurtman, 1982). Acetylcholine is the primary neurotransmitter of motor neurons of the PNS (Higgins & George, 2007). It is involved in preparation for action and for defensive or aggressive behaviors; it is also involved in attention, learning, and memory. Acetylcholine controls salvation, gastrointestinal motility, pupil size, shape of the lens of the eye, and mucus secretion. It is found in the caudate nucleus, hippocampus, thalamus, striatum, cerebellum, limbic system, and cerebral cortex (Higgins & George, 2007). The thalamus and hippocampus—which are the brain structures involved in filtering information, learning, and memory—are densely innervated by cholinergic neurons (Kandel et al., 2000). Acetylcholine pathways can be found in Figure 2-20.

Acetylcholine neurons balance the dopamine input in the striatum, thus coordinating extrapyramidal motor control. When dopamine-blocking medications result in extrapyramidal side effects (motor side effects), anticholinergic medications are used to restore the balance of acetylcholine and dopamine and thus restore normal movements (Higgins & George, 2007). The action of acetylcholine is terminated by metabolism by the enzyme acetylcholinesterase. Impairment of the acetylcholine system is associated with Alzheimer's disease and other dementias (Davis, Lah, & Levey, 2009). Medications for Alzheimer's disease have focused on inhibiting the action of the cholinesterases in order to keep more acetylcholine available (Melchitzky & Lewis, 2009).

Acetylcholine receptors are divided into two main types: muscarinic and nicotinic. Muscarinic receptors are G protein–coupled, and they act by regulating ion channels, particularly potassium or calcium ion channels, or by being linked to second-messenger systems (Melchitzky & Lewis, 2009; Szabo et al., 2004). Muscarinic receptors are associated with attention, learning, and memory, and also with cardiac, gastrointestinal, and salivary gland functioning (Keltner et al., 2001). Medications that block muscarinic receptors—such as atropine—cause memory

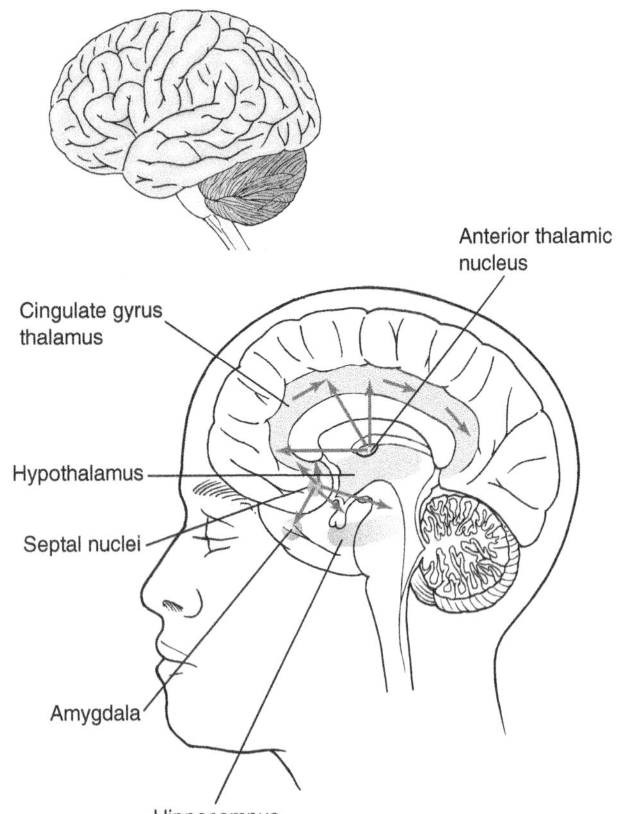

FIGURE 2-20: Acetylcholine Pathways. Acetylcholine is the primary neurotransmitter of motor neurons of the PNS (Higgins & George, 2007). It is also involved in attention, learning, and memory.

problems and confusion and also dry mouth, constipation, and blurred vision, which are known as anticholingeric side effects. Nicotinic receptors are ionotropic receptors and are thought to be involved in epilepsy, Alzheimer's disease, Parkinson's disease, and schizophrenia (Melchitzky & Lewis; Stahl, 2000). There are two types of nicotinic receptors: nicotinic N at ganglion synapses, and nicotinic M at neuromuscular synapses. There are many subtypes of receptors within these two types. The nicotinic receptors at the neuromuscular synapses are blocked irreversibly by snake alpha toxins, which is the venom from certain poisonous snakes (Siegel, Agranoff, Albers, et al., 1999).

LeDoux (2002) described the action of a chemical agent used in World War I on acetylcholine receptors: "Nerve gas works by disrupting acetylcholine transmission at muscles, especially muscles required for normal breathing. Many insecticides have similar effects in bugs" (p. 59). Drugs are also used therapeutically to block the action of acetylcholine. For example, the muscle relaxant succinylcholine (Anectine) is used for reduction of muscle contractions during electroconvulsive therapy, and the neuromuscular blocker pancuronium (Pavulon) is used with patients receiving mechanical ventilation (Keltner et al., 2001, p. 142).

Neuropeptides

Neuropeptides are phylogenetically ancient biochemical messengers, having existed for longer than 2 billion years (Hokfelt, Xu, Broberger, et al., 2000; Nemeroff, 1988). They are so old that neuropeptides such as insulin, somatostatin, ACTH, and neurostatin have been found in single-cell organisms such as bacteria. They were first identified in the intestine and much later in the CNS.

Neuropeptides are short chains of amino acids that fulfill the functions of neurotransmission (Higgins & George, 2007); that is, they inhibit or excite neurotransmitters and receptors. They regulate body homeostatic behaviors such as food and water consumption, sexual behavior, sleep, and body temperature (Panksepp & Harro, 2004). They are produced in a restricted number of neurons and endocrine cells and are not subject to reuptake mechanisms. Neuropeptides that are thought to be involved in psychiatric disorders such as depression, dementia, and schizophrenia include but are not limited to vasopressin, cholecystokinin (CCK), corticotropin-releasing factor (CRF), neurotensin, galanin, somatostatin (SRIF), substance P, bombesin (BOM), calcitonin (CT), neuropeptide Y, and the opioids enkephalins, endorphins, and dynorphins (Szabo et al., 2009). Neuropeptide Y has high concentrations in the limbic area. It plays a role in neuroendocrine regulation and circadian rhythms. It is implicated in Huntington's disease, Alzheimer's disease, Parkinson's dementia, and major depression. The location of various neuropeptides, their actions, and their implications for psychiatric disorders can be found in Table 2-2.

Neurohormones

Neurohormones have an *organizational effect* on the developing prenatal brain and an *activational effect* on postnatal brain functioning. Neurohormones act as modulators. Higgins and George (2007) said that "Hormones change the function of the target cell by stimulating changes in gene expression" (p. 631). They also act directly on other neurotransmitters. They alter the effectiveness of glutamate or GABA transmission by binding to specific receptors. For example, cortisol, a steroid hormone released from the pituitary during stress, alters information processing in the circuits involved with memory and learning by altering the ability of GABA to inhibit glutamate (LeDoux, 2002).

Cortisol

Cortisol is called the stress hormone. In response to stress, cortisol elevates blood glucose, suppresses inflammatory response, increases gastric secretions, and has a catabolic effect, breaking down muscle, lymphoid tissue, adipose tissue, skin, and bones into their components in order to produce energy (Shelby & McCance, 2002). Cortisol stimulates the urge to ingest "comfort" foods (high in calories, fat, and sugar); these energy sources may then be stored as abdominal

TABLE 2-2 NEUROPEPTIDES: LOCATION, ACTION, AND IMPLICATIONS FOR PSYCHIATRIC DISORDERS

Neuropeptide	Location	Action	Implications for Psychiatric Disorders
Vasopressin (known as antidiuretic hormone) (Panksepp & Harro, 2004)	Multiple systems of the brain.	Regulates anterior pituitary gland. Potentates release of ACTH. Involved in memory, biological rhythms, reward, tolerance, adaptation, and aggression (Ferris, 2005).	Decreased in depression and increased in mania.
Cholecystokinin (CCK)	Throughout CNS including spinal cord, limbic system, hippocampus, and prefrontal cortex.	Regulates emotional systems. Modulates feeding (satiety), sex, and pain. Involved in learning associated with adverse events.	Anxiety disorders, panic attacks, and depression (Hebb, Poulin, Roach, et al., 2005).
Corticotropin-releasing factor (CRF)	Hypothalamus.	Stimulates ACTH release from the pituitary; e.g., increases production of cortisol. Is involved in cognition, adaptation to stress, mood, and memory (Aborelius, Owens, Plotsky, et al., 1999; DeSouza & Grigoriadis, 2002).	Increased CRF is linked with depression. Reduced CRF is linked with mania. It may be involved with Alzheimer's disease (Nemeroff, 1988).
Neurotensin (endogenous neuroleptic) (Sharma, Janicak, Bissette, et al., 1997, p. 294)	Amygdala, hypothalamus, and basal ganglia.	Acts as antagonist at dopamine receptors.	Low levels of neurotensin among nonmedicated individuals with schizophrenia. Increased levels in neurotensin following treatment with antipsychotic medications (Sharma et al., 1997).
Galanin	Locus ceruleus, prefrontal cortex, and limbic system.	Involved in learning, memory, pain control, food intake, reward, neuroendocrine control, cardiovascular regulation, and modulation of anxiety (Brewer, Echevarria, Langel, et al., 2005).	Deficits of galanin are associated with increase of anxiety-like behaviors (Bonne, Drevets, Neurmeister, et al., 2004). There is an increase of galanin over the course of Alzheimer's disease (Counts, Perez, Kahli, et al., 2001).
Somatostatin (SRIF) (known as growth hormone release inhibiting hormone)	Limbic system, hypothalamus.	Regulated by acetylcholine, norepinephrine, dopamine, and serotonin; linked with GABA.	Reduced SRIF in patients with depression, acute multiple sclerosis, Parkinson's disease, and Alzheimer's disease and in maternally deprived children (Kellaway & Noebels, 1989). Increased SRIF in patients with mania, depression, schizophrenia, and schizoaffective disorder. Highest in patients with mania (Sharma, Bissette, Janicak, et al., 1995).
Substance P	Throughout the CNS; co-localized with serotonin (Sergeyev et al., 1999).	Pain perception, anxiety, memory, neurochemical response to stress.	Increased in patients with schizophrenia and depression (Rimon, LeGreves, Nybert, et al., 2002).
Bombesin (BOM)	Hypothalamus, periaqueductal gray matter (gray matter surrounding cerebral aqueduct), cingulate gyrus, and hippocampus (Olry & Haines, 2003).	Increases gastric acid secretion. Involved in satiety and pain.	Decreased in patients with schizophrenia.
Calcitonin (CT)	Secreted by C-cells in thyroid.	Controls serum and calcium levels.	Increased calcium levels are associated with lethargy, severe depression. Decreased calcium levels are associated with hyperactivity, excitability, instability.

Continued

TABLE 2-2 NEUROPEPTIDES: LOCATION, ACTION, AND IMPLICATIONS FOR PSYCHIATRIC DISORDERS—continued

Neuropeptide	Location	Action	Implications for Psychiatric Disorders
Opioid: Endorphins	Limbic system and hypothalamus. Released in response to pain, exercise, and hot chili peppers (Howard, 2006).	Regulate the hypothalamus-pituitary-adrenal axis.	Epilepsy, Parkinson's disease, addiction, and anorexia.
Opioid: Enkephalins	Released from adrenal medulla. Found in limbic system, hippocampus, thalamus, and amygdala.	Inhibit transmission of pain impulses in the spinal cord and brain.	Low levels of enkephalins have been found to be associated with anxiety and post-traumatic stress disorder.

fat (Esch & Stefano, 2010). In response to stress, cortisol may alter perceptual and emotional functioning as well as decrease the recall of short-term memories, and its effect on the brain may last for hours or even days (Shirtcliff, Vitacco, Graf, et al., 2009). Cortisol can directly change gene expression and increase programmed neuronal cell death.

Thyrotropin-Releasing Hormone (TRH)

The thyrotropin-releasing hormone (TRH) releases thyroid-stimulating hormone (TSH), which stimulates the release of thyroid T4 and T3. TRH is regulated, in part, by conventional neurotransmitters—acetylcholine, NE, dopamine, and serotonin (Nemeroff, 1988). TSH blunting occurs in 26% of persons with depression, in about 35% of people with alcohol abuse, and in 47% of persons with borderline personality disorder. Hypothyroidism is associated with reduced brain activity, depressed mood, psychomotor retardation, poor memory, and, in severe forms, with hallucinations and delusions; hyperthyroidism is associated with anxiety, irritability, emotional instability, and psychomotor agitation (Higgins & George, 2007).

Growth Hormone

Growth hormone is produced in the anterior pituitary gland. It controls height and weight gain. Physical and psychological stressors influence growth hormone. It has been found to be depressed in maternally deprived children and deficient in some patients with major depressive disorder and with dysthymia (Sadock & Sadock, 2007).

Prolactin

Prolactin is secreted from the anterior pituitary gland. The hypothalamus controls prolactin secretion, whereas GABA and opioids control prolactin regulation. Hyperprolactinemia is associated with anxiety, irritability, depression, decreased libido, and difficulty tolerating stress (Sadock & Sadock, 2007).

Oxytocin

Oxytocin is called the love hormone. Synthesized in the hypothalamus, it regulates fluid balance, carbohydrate metabolism, food intake, temperature, immunity, and reproduction. It is involved in learning and memory and promotes social bonding and attachment (Ferris, 2005; Szabo et al., 2009). It can facilitate the intensity of reward from natural occurring social interactions and can relieve the distress of the loss of loved ones (Panksepp, 2003). Higher levels of oxytocin have been found to be associated with trust and trustworthiness in humans (Zak, Kurzban, & Matzner, 2005).

Unconventional Neurotransmitters

Two types of unconventional neurotransmitters are gases and endocannabinoids.

One gas, nitric oxide, signals other cells to increase activity. It is formed in glutamate neurons when arginine is converted to citrulline and nitric oxide. Another gas, carbon monoxide, is involved in long-term alterations of the neurons that are involved in learning and memory (Szabo et al., 2009).

Endocannabinoids are endogenous cannabinoids. Cannabinoid receptors, which are the receptors to which marijuana binds, are widespread in the brain. Activation of cannabinoid receptors results in inhibition of neurons, resulting in a sense of euphoria or calmness, distorted thoughts, and the desire to eat, known as the "munchies" (Higgins & George, 2007, p. 47); conversely, blocking cannabinoid receptors has been found to help with losing weight (Higgins & George).

Neurotropins

Neurotropins are regulatory factors that are involved in the survival of neurons, in synaptic plasticity, and in modulating synaptic transmission (Szabo et al., 2009). They include nerve growth factor (NGF), brain-derived neurotropic factor (BDNF), neurotropin-3 (NT3), and neurotropin-6 (NT6). BDNF is believed to be involved in mood disorders, Parkinson's disease, and Alzheimer's disease. The neurotropins are released in response to activity of the neuron. Neurons that are active call for and receive more neurotropins that nourish and protect them.

Part One: Summary

The brain carries out a vast array of functions, from ensuring survival to enabling individuals to love, to learn, to move, and to create. Specific components of brain functioning are carried out by two very different hemispheres, by complex brain structures and primitive brain structures, and by electricity and neurochemicals working together. Understanding the functioning of the brain is the cornerstone of the knowledge base of psychiatric advanced practice nurses.

Part One: Key Points

- The nervous system has two parts: the peripheral nervous system and the central nervous system (brain and spinal cord).
- Brain functioning includes thinking, planning, evaluating, learning, emotional responses, motor functioning, and behavioral responses.
- The brain is divided into right and left hemispheres that have specialized functions.
- Brain hemispheres are connected by the corpus callosum.
- The cerebral cortex covers the hemispheres and is made up of neurons that convey information and glial cells that support the neurons.
- The cerebral cortex is divided into four lobes—frontal, temporal, parietal, and occipital—that have specialized functions.
- The limbic system is a more primitive part of the brain that is involved with emotions of fear, rage, love, and reward.
- Meninges are three layers of coverings that protect the brain.
- Ventricles are cavities inside the cerebral hemispheres that are filled with cerebrospinal fluid.
- Brain communication is carried out by neurons using electrical impulses and neurotransmitters.
- Neurotransmitters include classic neurotransmitters, amino acids, cholinergic neurotransmitters (acetylcholine), neuropeptides, and neurohormones.
- Neurons are insulated with glial-produced myelin that improves transmission of information.
- Receptors receive information sent by neurons.
- Ion channel receptors have a direct action and are fast; G protein receptors are slower and change their structure to process the information.
- Knowledge of brain functioning and brain structures provides the basis for understanding the symptoms and treatment of psychiatric disorders.
- Psychiatric advanced practice nurses use psychotherapy, psychotropic medications, and psychosocial interventions to promote new neuronal connections.
- Treatment can change gene expression that can result in changes in behavior; conversely, changes in behavior can result in changes in gene expression.
- New information, learning, psychotherapy, pharmacotherapy, different experiences, and changes in patients' life situations can change gene expression and change the course of psychiatric disorders.

PART TWO: Brain Development

The symptoms of psychiatric disorders are manifestations of impaired brain functioning that may be due to compromised brain development (Bear et al., 2007; Post, 2000). Common symptoms associated with psychiatric disorders include impairments or deviations in perceptions, thoughts, feelings, emotions, and behaviors.

Early psychiatrists, well aware of the link between the brain and psychiatric disorders, hoped that the time would come when technology would be available to study the relationship of brain development, brain functioning, and psychiatric disorders. The 1990s, known as the Decade of the Brain, fulfilled the early psychiatrists' hopes: advances in the neurosciences laid the foundation for understanding the connection between the brain and psychiatric disorders. For example, the Genome Project began to map human genes, and its findings supported both previous observations and family studies that showed a family pattern for many of the psychiatric disorders, known as a genetic loading or vulnerability; however, the Genome Project also revealed that gene expression may have more influence on individual differences in development than genetic variations (Kramer, 2005). (Gene expression will be discussed later in this chapter.) In addition, computed tomography (CT scans) and magnetic resonance imaging (MRIs) provided information about the structures and developmental abnormalities of the brain. Data obtained through these advances in the neurosciences and through technology indicate that genetic influences and abnormalities of brain development are involved in the development of psychiatric disorders.

Factors in Normal Brain Development

The human brain develops in a complex sequence of processes, guided by genetic influences, which are internal neurodevelopmental factors that are unique to each individual, and influenced by external experiences. Gottesman and Hanson (2005) called brain development a "dance among partners of neuron, glia, vascular supply, and experience" (p. 273). The success of each step of development rests on the successful achievement of the previous step (Kennedy, 2006). Therefore, abnormalities of early brain development influence later maturation of the brain and brain functioning throughout the life span (Kandel et al., 2000; Kennedy; Waddington, 1993). Abnormalities of early development may manifest as cognitive impairment, impaired modulation of emotional arousal, problems with impulsivity, and motor deficits that adversely affect functioning and ability to adapt to the challenges of life (Rees & Inder, 2005).

Genetic Influence on Brain Development

Genes influence development of the brain because they provide the memory of humankind; i.e., they provide a genetic blueprint for human brain development that unfolds as soon as the egg is fertilized (LeDoux, 2002). Although the basic systems are the same for all humans, genes also give each brain its unique qualities (LeDoux) and strongly influence brain size (Bartley et al., 1997; Pennington, Filipick, Lefly, et al., 2001).

Genes shape the brain by several mechanisms. Very early on, genes guide the development of the brain by creating a map in the ventricular zone, which is the area within the neural tube where all cells are generated. Glial cells follow that map as they build the scaffolding along which neurons migrate to form the layers of the brain (Bear et al., 2007; Hu, 2006; Jones & Murray, 1991). Genes control which ectodermal cells will become neuroblasts (embryonic nerve cells) and which will not. Genes influence the production of proteins and enzymes that trigger chemical reactions in the brain, which in turn controls certain genes that induce other genes to make additional proteins. They regulate brain development through their effect on proliferation of cells, on molecules that guide migration such as the cell adhesive molecule, and on molecules that determine programmed cell death. Genes also influence the connectivity of neurons, a crucial part of brain development, by making proteins that shape how neurons get wired together (Bear et al.; LeDoux, 2000).

Epigenesis

Genetic influence on brain development is subject to a mechanism that produces changes in genetic expression, a process called epigenesis. As quoted by Kuehn (2008), Jirtle said, "Epigenetic changes may be thought of as chemical switches that can turn on and off the expression of genes in response to environmental factors" (p. 1249), and Gottesman and Hanson (2005) said that epigenesis refers to "the mechanisms by which cells change form or function and then transmit that form or function to future cells in that cell line" (p. 267). Genes are turned off or on by cellular material, called the epigenome, which sits on top of the gene. Researcher Randy Jirtle described the difference between the gene and the epigenome as the difference between the hardware and software of a computer: the gene, like hardware, determines the basic properties of the cell/computer; the epigenome, like software, largely determines how the cell's/computer's capabilities are used, e.g., which features you activate and which you do not (Dolinoy, Weidman, & Jirtle, 2007).

The epigenome is dysregulated by environmental factors such as poor prenatal nutrition and viral infections, poor diet, stress, damaging developmental processes, inadequate parenting, and maltreatment (Gottesman & Hanson, 2005; Kramer, 2005). The epigenome is most susceptible to dysregulation during gestation, neonatal development, puberty, and old age (Dolinoy et al., 2007). However, gene expression operates continuously throughout life (Kramer). The altered epigenome makes a mark or imprint on the gene, and that mark is passed on from one generation to the next. There is evidence that epigenetics is associated with cancer (Das, Hampton, & Jirtle, 2009). Evidence suggests that epigenetic dysregulation may be involved in susceptibility to certain disorders, including adult disorders such as Alzheimer's disease and schizophrenia; childhood disorders such as autism (Dolinoy et al., 2007); and imprinting disorders such as Beckwith-Wiedemann syndrome, transient neonatal diabetes, Angelman's syndrome, and Prader-Willi syndrome (European Society for Human Reproduction and Embryology, 2005).

The study of epigenetics has shown that changes in gene activity and changes in how genes are expressed do not involve changes in the genetic code (the DNA); nevertheless, the genetic changes are passed down to following generations. Cloud (2010) wrote, "Epigenetic changes represent a biological response to an environmental stressor" (p. 51). An example of the relationship between alterations of gene expression and psychiatric disorders is provided by the study of Mayfield, Lewohl, Dodd, et al. (2002) of a group of individuals with chronic alcoholism. The researchers found that 191 genes in the frontal and motor areas of the brain were altered in comparison to those of a control group. The altered genes were involved in activities such as myelin production, neurotransmission, neuroprotection, and neurodegeneration. The researchers suggest that the alterations of gene expression were associated with the symptoms and behavioral changes seen in chronic alcoholism.

According to Cloud (2010), "[A biological] response can be inherited through many generations via epigenetic marks, but if you remove the environmental pressure, then the epigenetic marks will eventually fade and the DNA code will—over time—begin to revert to its original programming" (p. 51). Epigenetic changes also occur as part of the aging process. Molecules that have silenced genes earlier in life tend to melt away, allowing previously unexpressed genes to be expressed (Begley, 2004).

Nongenetic Factors' Influence on Brain Development

Gottesman and Hanson (2005) stated that "Everything that is genetic is biological, but not all things biological are genetic" (p. 265). The developing embryo is linked to the outside world through what the mother eats, drinks, breathes, and experiences. The embryo also is in contact with maternal viral infections and is exposed to maternally experienced toxins such as alcohol, drugs, lead, mercury, and ionizing radiation (Jones & Murray, 1991). Even the stressors that the mother experiences affect the stress hormone levels of the embryo. Note that all of these factors are biological, but not genetic.

Prenatal factors that have an adverse effect on the developing brain include maternal deficiencies in nutrition, maternal infections, and maternal exposure to toxins, radiation, and stress. Prenatal factors will be discussed in the first section of Chapter 3. Postnatal factors, which are experienced factors (also called environmental factors), such as poor nutrition, exposure to toxins, lack of sensory stimuli, inadequate parenting, poverty, conflicted family situations, stress, neglect, and abuse, exert an adverse effect on continuing brain development by influencing the activity of nerve cells and the development of connections between neurons. Postnatal factors will be discussed in the second section of Chapter 3.

Process of Brain Development

The development of the human brain retraces the process of evolution. According to the study of phylogeny (the history, origin, and evolution of a species), the first brains were those of lizards and reptiles, and their functioning was limited to maintenance of survival through respiration, digestion, circulation, and reproduction, all of which are brainstem functions in humans (Bear et al., 2007). Vaillant (2008) described the functioning of the lizard brain as focusing on ". . . the four F's: fight, fright, feeding, and fornication" (p. 28). The second stage of brain to develop from the lizard brainstem was the leopard brain or limbic system, which added the function of experiencing emotion and coordinating it with movement, e.g., the fight-or-flight response. The third phase of brain development was the learning brain, which added the ability to learn, develop memory, use language, solve problems, and be creative (Howard, 2006, p. 46).

The processes of prenatal development of the brain include neural induction, neurulation, cell proliferation, differentiation of neurons, production of neural crest cells, and migration of neurons to form the structures of the brain.

Neural Induction: Formation of the Neural Plate

Every cell in the nervous system has a history that can be traced back through successive cell divisions from the fertilized egg (Kandel et al., 1995, p. 91). The first step in development after conception is the formation of the zygote. The zygote divides to form cells through a process called cleavage. In humans, about 14 days after conception, chemical signals cause ectodermal cells to divide and form a sheet, the neural plate. This process is called neural induction (LeDoux, 2002) (Fig. 2-21).

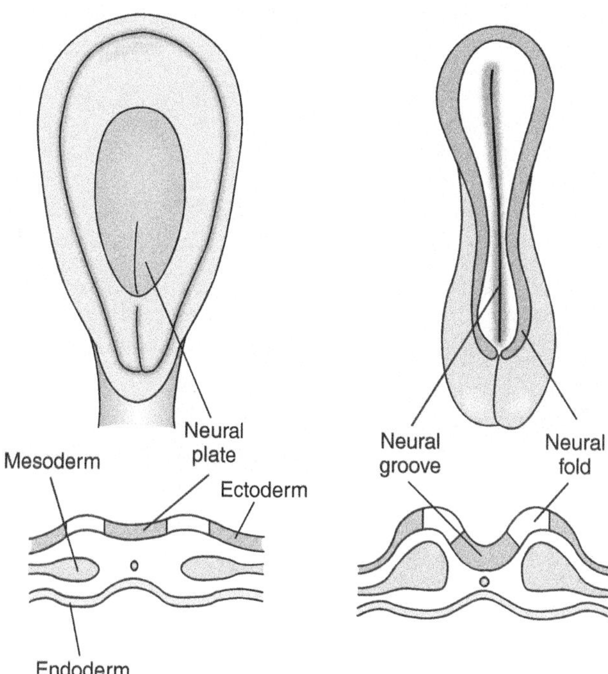

FIGURE 2-21: Neural Induction: Formation of the Neural Plate. In humans, about 14 days after conception, chemical signals cause ectodermal cells to divide and form a sheet, the neural plate. The neural plate develops distinct areas designated to become the structures of the brain, and the cells of the neural plate begin to develop into glial cells and neuronal cells. The entire nervous system comes from the ectodermal layer of the neural plate (Kandel et al., 2000).

At 17 days after conception, the brain is still a flat sheet of cells (Bear et al., 2007); however, between 18 and 24 days after conception, the cells multiply, divide, and form three layers—the ectoderm, mesoderm, and endoderm (Carter et al., 2009). The ectoderm, the outermost layer, is the source of the entire nervous system; the PNS develops from the ectodermal layer of the neural crest, which is the edges of the neural plate (Kandel et al., 2000). Ectodermal cells that do not differentiate as neurons or glial cells become the epidermis of the skin (Kandel et al.). The mesoderm, which is the middle layer of the developing embryo, forms bone, connective tissue, muscle, blood, vascular and lymphatic tissue, and pleura and peritoneum. The endoderm, the innermost layer of the developing embryo, forms the epithelium of the trachea, bronchi, lungs, gastrointestinal tract, liver, pancreas, bladder, and thyroid gland (Bear et al.; Moore & Persaud, 1993; Nelson, 2004). During this time, the neural plate becomes regionally patterned; that is, distinct areas are designated to become structures and specific areas of functioning (Copp, 1997), and the cells of the neural plate begin to develop different properties, creating both glial and neuronal cells (Kandel et al.).

Defects of Neural Induction

Global defects of neural induction are not usually seen in humans because they are often associated with early pregnancy loss, such as first trimester abortion. One defect of neural induction that may be seen is malformation caused by a local deficit of forebrain induction, known as holoprosencephaly. A mild form of holoprosencephaly is fetal alcohol syndrome; more severe forms of holoprosencephalies include cyclopia and arrhinencephaly, the latter of which is a lack of the olfactory bulb (Thorogood, 1997). Defects of induction are also associated with agenesis (lack of development) of the corpus callosum.

Defects in nervous system patterning or in the specification of regional identity to craniocaudal, dorsoventral, and mediolateral axes may result in cerebellar agenesis, which is the lack of part or all of the cerebellum, and Dandy-Walker syndrome, which is the cystic malformation of the fourth ventricle (Copp, 1997).

Neurulation: Formation of the Neural Tube

Neurulation refers to the process of the formation of the neural plate, the development of the neural folds, and the closure of the neural folds to form the neural tube (Kandel et al., 1995). Formation of the neural plate is illustrated in Figure 2-21. The process of neurulation does not occur all at once (Copp, 1997). By the 18th day of gestation, the neural plate has formed the neural groove with neural folds on each side; these folds will close to form the neural tube. The formation of the neural tube (Fig. 2-22) begins at the end of the third week of gestation and is completed by the end of the fourth week (Carter et al., 2009; Copp; Moore & Persaud, 1993). Thus, the formation of the neural tube begins even before a woman knows that she is pregnant (Bear et al., 2007).

One end of the neural tube will become the brain and the other end will become the spinal cord (Carter et al., 2009; Moore & Persaud, 1993). Development of the brain precedes that of the spinal cord (Copp, 1997; Gottesman & Hanson, 2005; Kandel et al., 1995; LeDoux, 2002). The end of the neural tube that will become the brain forms three bulges: forebrain, midbrain, and hindbrain. The forebrain divides into two parts by the 36th day—the telencephalon and the diencephalon. The telencephalon will form the two cerebral hemispheres, the cerebral cortex, the basal ganglia, the hippocampal formation, the amygdala, and the olfactory bulb. The diencephalon will become the thalamus and hypothalamus. The midbrain includes the optic and auditory areas and the cerebral aqueduct. The hindbrain includes the pons, medulla, and cerebellum. During the fifth week of gestation, the hindbrain partly divides into the metencephalon and the myelencephalon. The metencephalon becomes the pons and cerebellum, and the myelencephalon becomes the medulla oblongata (Bear et al., 2007; Moore & Persaud, 1993).

Defects of Neural Tube Formation

Defects of neural tube formation during the third and fourth weeks of gestation may result in structural abnormalities, such as anencephaly (the congenital absence of major portions of the brain), spina bifida (the incomplete closure of the vertebral column), or myelomeningocele (protrusion of a portion of spinal cord through a defect in vertebral column) (Copp, 1997). Disruptions of neural tube formation may result in disturbed functioning such as epilepsy, mental retardation, and behavioral disturbances (Thorogood, 1997, p. 133).

Cell Proliferation

After closure of the neural tube, cells proliferate (reproduce) very rapidly within the tube. Glial cells develop from the earliest cells in the wall of the neural tube. Starting around the fifth week of gestation and continuing until the 18th week, precursor cells divide and give rise to neurons that will build the cerebral cortex of the brain and other brain structures (Bear et al., 2007; Todd et al., 1995). The birth of neurons is the foundation of brain development. LeDoux (2002) wrote, ". . . at the peak production point, about 250,000 neurons are generated per minute" (p. 67).

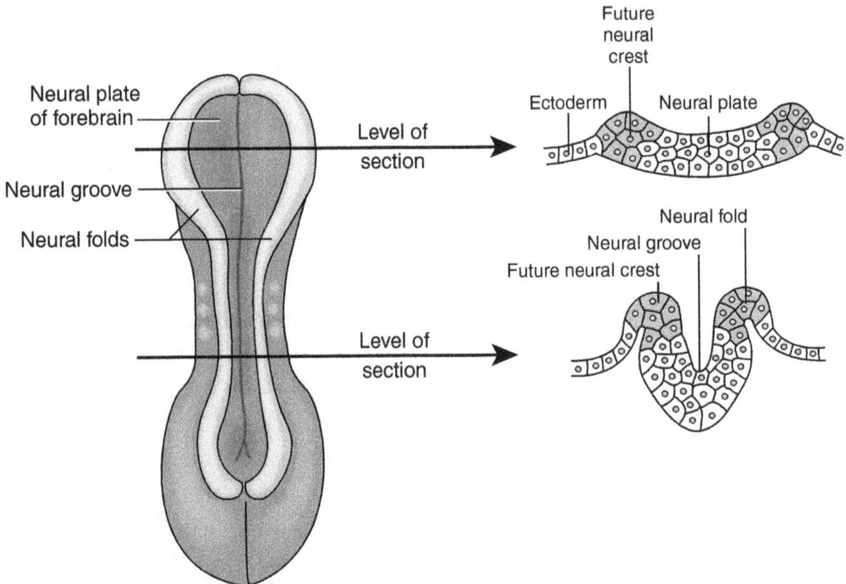

FIGURE 2-22: Formation of the Neural Tube. By the 18th day of gestation, the neural plate forms the neural groove with neural folds on each side; these folds will close to form the neural tube. One end of the neural tube will become the brain and the other end will become the spinal cord.

Cell proliferation is regulated by genetic influences and other factors such as growth factors, hormones, and neurotransmitters. These factors increase or decrease the generation of neurons (Suter & Bhide, 2006). Soon after the neurons are formed, they take up separate places in the neural tube, where neurons destined to be part of the hindbrain, midbrain, or forebrain cluster together (LeDoux). This segregation is under the control of special genes, called homeotic genes, that make proteins that provide boundaries for the neurons, guide their movement, and create the adhesive surfaces that allow cells to stay together (Bear et al.; Rodier, 2000).

Defects in Neuronal Proliferation

Defects in neuronal proliferation reduce the number of neurons produced and hence overall head size and brain volume. The result is microencephaly, which is associated with mental retardation and epilepsy (Copp, 1997; Francis, Meyer, Fallet-Bianco, et al., 2006). Too few neurons to build the cortex of the brain may also be due to an increase in programmed cell death, which is the planned pruning of cells (Rakic, 2005). The resulting conditions are microlissencephaly (small brain with smooth surface), agyria (smooth brain surface with no gyri or folds), and hypoplasia (arrested growth) of the cerebellum, brainstem, and spinal cord (Francis et al., 2006; Hong, Shugart, Huang, et al., 2000).

Neuronal Differentiation

Neurons that come from inside the neural tube are differentiated before they leave the ventricular zone, which is the inner layer of vesicles within the neural tube that will later become the ventricles of the brain (Bear et al., 2007). Cell differentiation is the result of the expression of specific genes in a cell. Inducing factors are the molecules provided by other cells that provide signals; these inducing factors influence gene expression. Thus, a cell's fate is determined by signals from the area where the cell is located in the embryo and by the cell's ability to respond to the signals.

Neural Crest Cell Proliferation and Migration

Neural crest cells are derived from the ectoderm and form from the cells of the folded edges of the neural tube, which is also known as the neural crest. Neural crest cells are undifferentiated at first; however, as they migrate out of the neural tube, they receive signals from the cells in the environment through which they migrate that determine what type of neuron they will become (Moore & Persaud, 1993). Neural crest cells are involved in the development of the PNS, craniofacial skeleton, thalamus, thyroid, parathyroid, cardiac structures, pigment cells in the skin, meningeal coverings of the brain, glial cells, and neurons (Copp, 1997; Hu, 2006).

Defects in Neural Crest Cell Proliferation

Defects in neural crest cell development, differentiation, and migration are believed to be involved in the development of craniofacial defects such as clefts of the lip or palate; skin hypopigmentation such as lack of skin color; hearing loss; aplasia (absence of tissue) of the thymus, thyroid, and parathyroid; heart defects; and Hirschsprung's disease, which is the absence of autonomic ganglia in the smooth muscle wall of the colon (Copp, 1997; Moore & Persaud, 1993).

Neuronal Migration

Cells that will form the brain are already destined in the neural tube to form specific brain structures, and they will migrate from the neural tube to form those structures.

Tangential and Radial Neuronal Migration

There are two methods of migration: tangential and radial. In tangential migration, the neurons travel parallel to the surface of the developing brain by adhering to the surface of the axons of other neurons (Gottesman & Hanson, 2005; Rakic, 1990). Tangential migration is involved in the development of the more primitive parts of the brain, e.g., the pons and the medulla oblongata.

The hypothesis of radial migration is based on the understanding "that the ventricular zone contains a protomap of the prospective cytoarchitechtonic areas and that glial grids serve to assure reproduction of this map onto the expanding and curving cortical mantle" (Rakic, 1988a, p. 25). In radial migration, the first wave of migrating cells from the neural tube consists of glial cells that are guided by local genetically determined chemical cues. The glial cells move out between the fifth and seventh weeks of gestation (England & Wakely, 2006) and build a scaffolding of radial fibers; this scaffolding creates a perpendicular bridge from the ventricular area to the pia mater (Howard, Zhicheng, Filipovic, et al., 2008). Later, waves of migrating neurons climb along the glial radial fibers to form the structures of the brain, the connections between the structures, and the cortex of the brain where higher thought processes occur. Neurons are programmed to glide along the glial radial fibers, to stop at their targeted destination, to drop off the glial radial fiber at their targeted area, and then to form precise columnar arrangements and layers that eventually become the structures of the brain. Radial migration is primarily involved in the development of the neocortex and the hippocampus, but it is also involved in the development of some parts of the limbic system. Figure 2-23 illustrates radial neuronal migration.

All brain functioning—cognitive, emotional, motor, and behavioral—depends on interconnections between neurons (LeDoux, 2002). Formation and nurturing of these

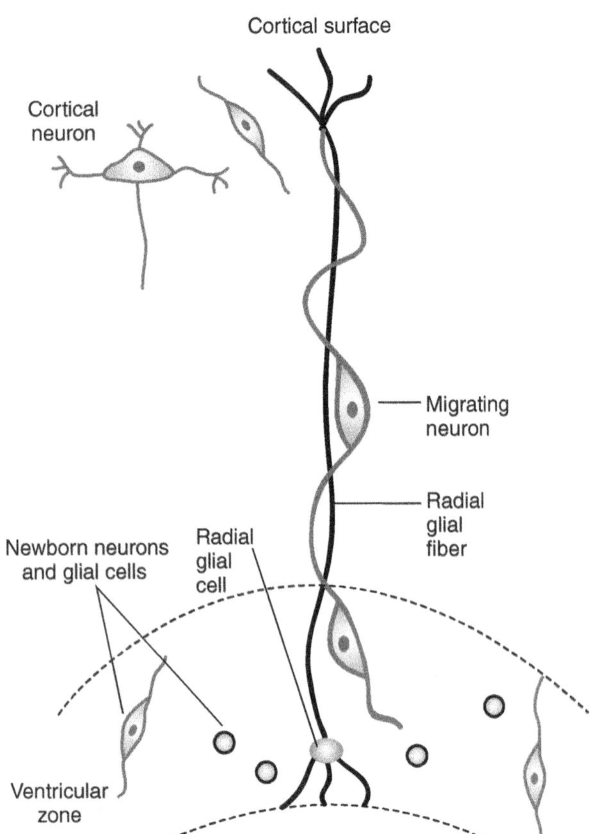

FIGURE 2-23: Radial Neural Migration. In radial neural migration, glial cells build a scaffolding of radial fibers, which neurons climb to build the structure of the brain.

Development of Cortical Structures

Waves of migrating neurons are involved in the development of cortical structures. The first wave of neuronal migration to the developing cortex begins between the 13th and 15th weeks of gestation. The neurons move out of the area near the ventricles and climb the glial scaffold to build the cortex of the brain. During the process of migration (Fig. 2-24), the neuron adds new membrane to the leading process of the neuron that is advancing along the glial guide wires; then, the rest of the neuron flows into the leading process, dragging the axon behind. These trailing axons will eventually form all cortical and subcortical connections, including the corpus callosum (Bear et al., 2007). The process is similar to a hand-over-hand rope climb during which the climber wraps around the rope, pulls up, lets go, moves higher, and pulls up again.

At the leading tip of the neuron is the growth cone, a "highly specialized and versatile navigational machine" (Hynes & Lander, 1992, p. 312). The growth cone moves toward its target destination dragging the extending axon behind it. Growth cones have specific chemical affinities and must find a target area with similar chemical affinities (Bear et al., 2007; Kandel et al., 2000). Tessier-Lavigne and

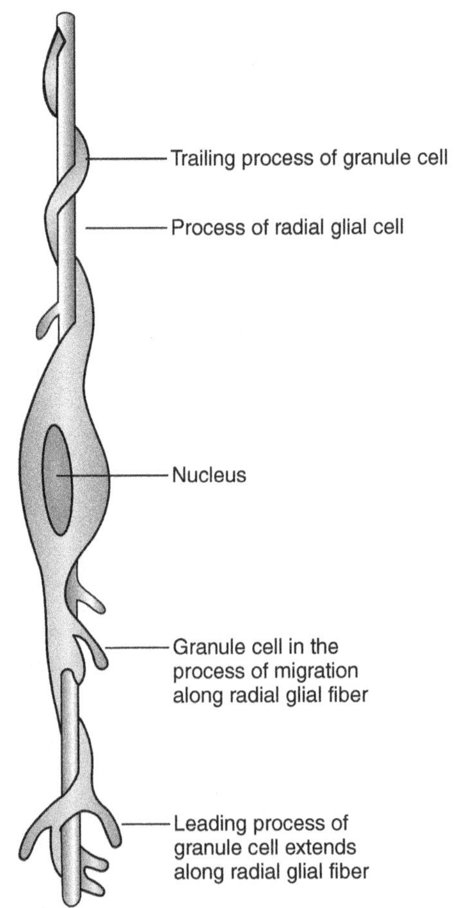

FIGURE 2-24: Neuronal Migration Along Glial Scaffolding. Migrating neurons crawl along the glial radial fibers, stop at their targeted destination, drop off the glial radial fiber, and form precise columnar arrangements and layers that eventually become the structures of the brain.

connections starts during embryonic development of the brain and continues throughout life.

Development of Subcortical Structures

As early as 4 weeks after conception, neurons begin to migrate to form the cerebellum (Rakic, 1988b, p. 631). From the fourth through the seventh weeks, neurons are generated and migrate to form the amygdala and hypothalamus. From the fifth through the seventh weeks, neurons migrate to form the brainstem and the midbrain, including the area that will produce dopamine (substantia nigra) and serotonin (raphe nuclei). From the fifth through the ninth weeks, neurons are generated and migrate to form the septal nuclei. In the seventh week and up to the 18th week, neurons that will form the caudate nucleus and putamen of the basal ganglia are generated. The corpus callosum begins to develop in the 10th to 11th weeks. The hippocampus—which is the primary structure involved in learning and memory—develops based on the migration of neurons during the second trimester. The hippocampus continues to develop up to the 16th week. The developing hippocampus is extremely sensitive to lack of oxygen and infections (Thorogood, 1997). The development of brain gyri, which is under both genetic and nongenetic influences (Biondi, Nogueira, Dormont, et al., 1998), starts at 26 weeks of gestation (England & Wakely, 2006).

Goodman (1996) described the process as "push, pull and hem" (p. 1124). The traveling neuron is pushed from behind by chemical repellants, pulled toward its destination by chemoattractants, and kept within boundaries or hemmed in by attractive and repulsive chemical cues such as netrins, semaphorin 3As, slits, and ephrins (Bear et al.).

Specific molecules guide axons toward their target through a mechanism of cueing, which is a chemical matching of axon and target. The survival of migrating neurons is regulated by signals from the neuronal target. Target cells secrete neurotropic factors such as nerve growth factor and brain-derived neurotropic factor that promote the survival of the neurons (Rehen & Chun, 2006). Once neurons have migrated to their correct location, they send out axons and dendrites to form more connections (Bear et al., 2007; Webb, Monk, & Nelson, 2001) (Fig. 2-25).

Neuronal cells migrate in a series of waves, and the cortical plate expands as each wave arrives to form the six layers of the cerebral cortex (Howard et al., 2008). Each wave of neurons must push its way through layers formed by earlier arriving neurons (Kandel et al., 2000). Thus, neurons born earliest end up in the deepest layers of the brain, nearest to the ventricles, and neurons born later end up in the more superficial layers of the brain, closest to the meninges. Nash (1997) quoted Rakic's description of the process: "It's as if the entire population of the East Coast decided to move en masses to the West Coast [...] and marched through Cleveland, Chicago and Denver to get there" (p. 53). The six-layered cortex of the brain (see Fig. 2-5) is therefore the product of waves of neuronal migration, and the position of the neurons in each layer is determined before they migrate.

Each cortical layer has specific types of neurons and different neurochemistry (Bear et al., 2007; Nelson, 2004). The types of neurons that make up the six layers are the pyramidal cells, stellate cells, and fusiform cells. The pyramidal cells are shaped like pyramids: they have long axons that leave the cortex to reach other cortical areas or subcortical areas. They are the main output neurons. Stellate cells are small, have short axons, and do not leave the cortex. Fusiform cells are found in the deepest cortical layer. They are spindle shaped with a tuft of dendrites at each end, and they have an axon that leaves the cortex.

The layers of the cortex are listed in Box 2-3. The six layers of the cortex subserve the brain's inputs, local circuits, and outputs (Tamminga, 2001). To summarize, layers two and four are receiving layers: they receive information from

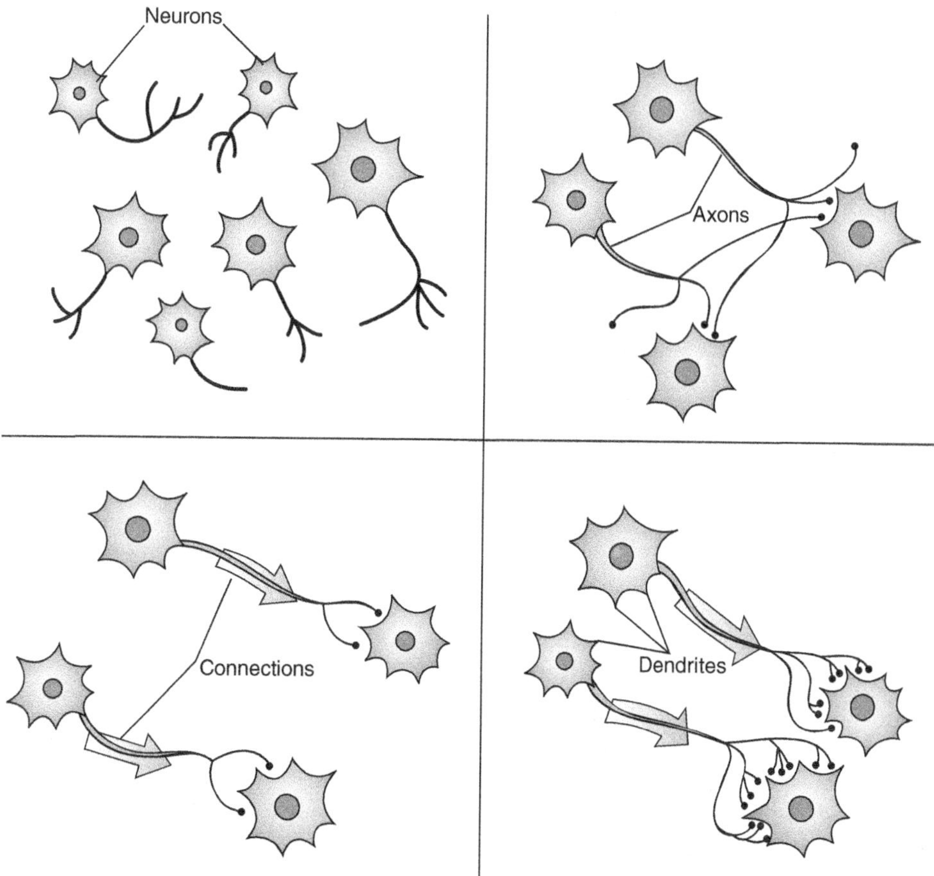

FIGURE 2-25: Formation of Neuronal Connections: Synaptogenesis. Each neuron makes connections with over a thousand target cells to form the circuits that are necessary for functioning of the brain and nervous system (Tessier-Lavigne & Goodman, 1996). Synaptic connections are shaped and reshaped constantly across the life span (Gottesman & Hanson, 2005). What individuals think, value, understand, interpret, and learn and how they behave are the products of patterns of interconnections between nerve cells in the brain (Kandel et al., 2000).

BOX 2-3 The Six Layers of the Cortex

1. The *molecular layer* is the uppermost layer, closest to the meningeal layers and the bones of the skull. It contains few neurons.
2. The *external granular layer* contains pyramidal cells. The neurons in this layer receive stimuli or information from sensory and association areas.
3. The *external pyramidal layer* contains pyramidal cells that send fibers to association areas of the cerebral cortex and to commissures that connect brain structures such as the corpus callosum.
4. The *internal granular layer* receives input from the thalamus. It contains stellate cells that are the interneurons of the cerebral cortex.
5. The *internal pyramidal layer* contains pyramidal cells that project to subcortical structures and send fibers to the brainstem and spinal cord.
6. The *multiform layer* contains fusiform cells that project primarily to the thalamus.

the sensory and association areas and have the highest density of synaptic connections (Huttenlocher & Dabholkar, 1997). Layers three, five, and six send fibers to the rest of the cortex: layer three sends fibers to the association areas and to the corpus callosum, layer five sends fibers to the spinal cord and brainstem, and layer six sends fibers to the thalamus (Kandel et al., 2000). Layer one does not have cell bodies. It consists of the dendrites and axons from lower layers.

Disruptions of Migration

Because the brain forms according to a prototype that is stored in the ventricles, bleeding into the ventricles during gestation may distort the prototype and compromise normal brain development. For example, in a follow-up study of children who had experienced prenatal intraventricular hemorrhage, 22.4% had cerebral palsy, 10.2% had mental retardation, and 11.3% had borderline intelligence. The higher rates of adverse effects were among those with a higher grade of intraventricular bleeding (Futagi, Toribe, Ogawa, et al., 2006).

Deviations of Migration

Deviations in migration include failure of the neurons to migrate, possibly due to absence of a signal to migrate; neurons left along the pathway, possibly due to failure of mechanisms that propel the neuron to the next position; and malplacement of the neurons within their targeted structure, possibly due to neurons' not recognizing the target or the target's not recognizing the neurons (Rakic, 1988a). Rakic (1988a) believes that defects of migration are due to environmental factors and that, during migration, the neurons are especially vulnerable to exposure to factors such as heat (maternal fever), ionizing radiation, various drugs, alcohol, and viruses.

Failure to Migrate

Failure to migrate can result in fewer neurons in the targeted area or in ectopic neurons, which are neurons located outside of the targeted place that make connections and survive. Abnormalities due to too few neurons or ectopic neurons may result from fetal exposure to agents such as ionizing irradiation. For example, among individuals who were exposed in utero to the irradiation following the atomic bombing of Hiroshima and Nagasaki in 1945, many were born with smaller heads. Evaluation of this population showed neurological and psychiatric disorders and higher rates of mental retardation among those irradiated between 8 and 15 weeks of gestation (Otake & Schull, 1984), which is the time period of the second migration of neurons that supplies neurons to the superficial layers of the cerebral cortex. Postmortem examination showed that the neurons did not migrate; rather, they stayed as a band of ectopic neurons near the lateral ventricle. Because the neurons did not move out to form their targeted structures, a decreased number of cells in some structures and a reduced size of some structures were evident.

Abnormalities of the cerebral cortex that may be due to defective proliferation or to failure to migrate at 12 to 13 weeks of gestation include lissencephaly (smooth cerebral surface and smaller area); pachygyria (a broadening and flattening of the gyri of the brain); polymicrogyria (thinner cortex and a highly convoluted cerebrum); and Zellweger syndrome, marked by failure of the brain to develop, craniofacial abnormalities, and liver and kidney defects (Francis et al., 2006). Abnormalities of migration may be responsible for severe mental retardation, epilepsy, and learning disabilities (Burgaya, Garcia-Frigola, Andres, et al., 2006). For example, abnormalities of migration and formation of neuronal connections are thought to be associated with dyslexia (Gleeson, 2006). Other abnormalities of migration include periventricular heterotopia—in which neurons are in abnormal positions near the ventricles (Francis et al.)—and heterotopic neurons that have been found in layer three instead of their targeted layer two. Heterotopic neurons have been found on postmortem examination of the brains of individuals with schizophrenia, individuals with bipolar disorder (Beckmann & Jakob, 1991), and individuals with dyslexia (LoTurco, Wang, & Paramasivam, 2006).

Cell Adhesive Molecules

Neurons are able to cling to the glial scaffolding because of cell adhesive molecules. Cell adhesive molecules determine how the neurons move, where they will stop, and if they will align properly (Hynes & Lander, 1992; Mintz, Bekirov, Anderson, et al., 2006). There are many different types of cell adhesive molecules that assist in the process of neuronal migration, and all contain sialic acid (which contains sugar) (Kandel et al., 2000). Early-stage cell adhesive molecules have more stickiness than adult adhesive molecules.

Lack of or alteration of the cell adhesive molecules may cause migratory defects; for example, neurons may drop off too soon.

Cell Adhesive Molecules and Migration Disruption

Animal studies exploring the role of cell adhesive molecules and migration disruption have shown abnormal development of neuronal wiring when the change from embryonic sialic acid to adult sialic acid does not take place. Because neuronal alignment must occur within a window of time, if the sialic acid is affected by viruses and the adhesive quality is weakened, as happens in the presence of influenza virus (Conrad & Scheibel, 1987), then the neurons may not arrive at their destined area or may not align correctly when they do arrive (Fig. 2-26).

Cell adhesive molecules are also affected by alcohol (Miller & Luo, 2002). Prenatal exposure to alcohol is associated with an increased stickiness of the cell adhesive molecules. The neurons are stranded, unable to complete migration (Siegenthaler & Miller, 2006).

Neurotransmitter Systems Development

Neurotransmitter systems develop from the first trimester onward, with the circuits of the same neurotransmitter developing at different rates in different structures of the brain (Levitt, 2003). The process of neurotransmitter development continues after birth, with different neurotransmitters reaching maturity at different postnatal ages through puberty. Thus, injuries or exposure to adverse factors at different times of brain development will affect developing neurotransmitter systems differently in different areas of the brain (Levitt).

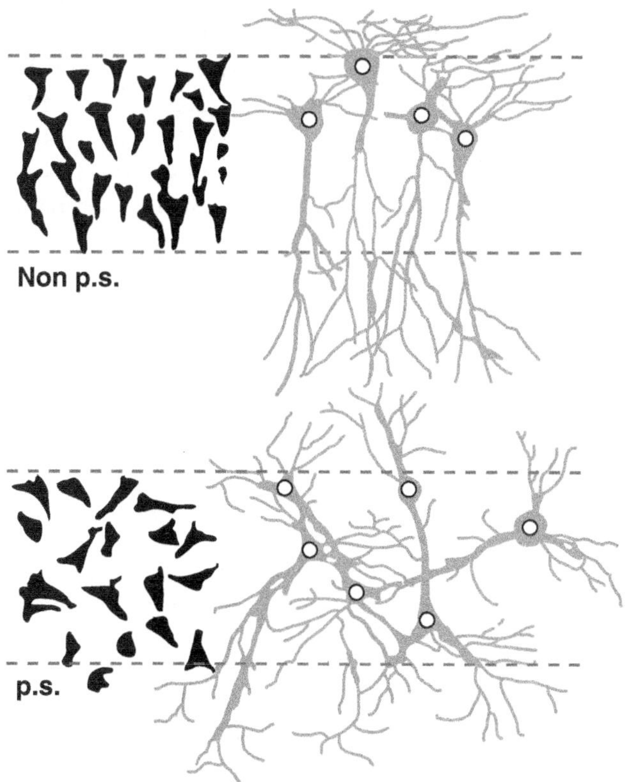

FIGURE 2-26: Deviation in Migration. Neurons are programmed to form precise columnar arrangements that facilitate transmission of information. In individuals without psychotic disorders (NPS), the neurons are aligned normally in columns; in individuals with psychosis (PS), the neurons are malpositioned.

Formation of Connections: Synaptogenesis

Brain functioning—processing information, modulating emotions, learning and memory, planning and evaluating, motor activity, and behaviors—depends on the connections or synapses between different types of neurons. The ability of the brain to process information depends on the formation of a network of connections between neurons.

Synaptogenesis is the creation of new synapses: the formation of a new neurotransmitter release site in the presynapatic neuron and a new neurotransmitter receptive site in the postsynaptic neuron. Each neuron among the trillion neurons in human adults makes connections with over a thousand target cells to form the circuits that are necessary for functioning of the brain and nervous system (Tessier-Lavigne & Goodman, 1996). Synaptic connections that are not integrated into a neuronal circuit are gradually eliminated (Bear et al., 2007; Huttenlocher & Dabholkar, 1997). Early synaptogenesis is controlled by internal factors such as genetic influence, whereas later synaptogenesis is responsive to experiences and environmental factors; later on, use will determine which synaptic connections survive. Synaptic connections are shaped and reshaped constantly as they function to enable individuals to adapt to challenges across their life spans (Gottesman & Hanson, 2005). What we think, value, understand, interpret, and learn and how we behave are the products of patterns of interconnections between nerve cells in the brain (Kandel et al., 2000). LeDoux (2002) put it succinctly: "you are your synapses" (p. IX).

Connectivity Disorders

Abnormalities of cortical networks may be thought of as "miswiring" or connectivity disorders (Francis et al., 2006, p. 878). Connectivity disorders are thought to be involved in cognitive impairment, autism, schizophrenia, language disorders such as dyslexia, attention deficit-hyperactivity disorder, obsessive-compulsive disorder, and certain forms of epilepsy (Francis et al., 2006). For example, in autism, it is thought that areas of the brain that integrate information may not be connected with areas that receive incoming information (Belmonte, Allen, Beckel-Mitchener, et al., 2004).

Plasticity

Synaptic connections can change and areas of the brain that represent the increased synaptic connections can expand because of the brain's plasticity, its "capacity for being formed or molded" (Higgins & George, 2007, p. 83). (Brain plasticity is discussed in Chapter 1.) Whereas previously it was believed that the brain was "hard-wired" early in life (Woodruff-Pak, 1993), now it is believed that the brain has a life-long capacity for physical and functional change (Mahncke, Bronstone, & Merzenich, 2006). Brain plasticity is foundational for learning, memory, skill acquisition, and recovery from trauma and addiction (Gottesman & Hanson, 2005).

Both negative factors and therapeutic interventions influence plasticity. Negative factors include prenatal events, genetic influences, insufficient diet, disease, stress, drugs, and aging (Kolb, Gibb, & Robinson, 2003). For example, research has shown that chronic stress is associated with a reduction in plasticity of frontal cortical activity (Kuipers, Trentani, Den Boer, et al., 2003) and, according to Gottesman and Hanson (2005), "Repeated exposure to amphetamines and cocaine alters the cytoarchitecture of the nucleus accumbens and frontal cortex..." (p. 273). Therapeutic factors include pleasurable cognitive, emotional, physical, or interpersonal experiences; exercise (Fabel & Kempermann, 2008); psychotherapy; psychopharmacotherapy (Nasrallah, 2006); and meditation (Vaillant, 2008).

Cell Death

Survival of developing neurons depends on essential protective substances that are supplied by cells near the developing neuron. These protective substances are called neurotropic substances or, to quote Howard (2006), "fertilizers for nerve cells" (p. 122). Target cells secrete a limited amount of neurotropic substances, and neurons compete for the neurotropic substances (Pettmann & Henderson, 1998). There are more neurons seeking to make a connection with a target cell than there are target cells. Neurons that fail to make connections die; in fact, approximately one-third of all neurons die due to lack of access to these neurotropic factors (Rehen & Chun, 2006). Neurotropic factors that are able to promote survival of neurons include the neuropeptide nerve growth factor that is specific for peripheral nerves; interleukin C–related cytokines, which are involved in immune responses; fibroblast growth factor, which is involved in homeostasis and wound healing; sonic hedgehog, which is involved in motor neurons of the spinal cord (Reichardt & Farinas, 1997); and brain-derived neurotropic factor (Rehen & Chun), which is implicated in neurodegenerative disorders such as Huntington's, Parkinson's, and Alzheimer's diseases (Higgings & George, 2007). Neurotropic factors modulate neurotransmission and synaptic plasticity. They also suppress cell suicide, as cells without neurotropic factors will shrink and disintegrate. However, cell death may also be due to other causes such as increased levels of the stress hormone cortisol, which increases the amount of calcium flowing into a cell, thus causing cell death (Bear et al., 2007; Margolis, Chuang, & Post, 1994; McEwen, 2002; Sapolski, 1994). Interestingly, animal studies suggest that physical exercise increases the production of neurotropic factors (Neeper, Gómez-Pinilla, Choi, et al., 1996).

Programmed Cell Death

Neuronal death is a normal part of the development of the nervous system (Bear et al., 2007; Margolis et al., 1994; Oppenheim, 1991; Rakic, 2005). In contrast to necrosis, which is cell death in response to a toxin, programmed cell death refers to a genetically controlled process of pruning cells and synaptic connections (Bear et al.; Kandel et al., 1995). Programmed cell death is the mechanism that determines the size and shape of the CNS (Kuan, Roth, Flavell, et al., 2000; Rakic).

Programmed cell death is not the result of external cues; rather, it results from internal cues or stimuli (Pettmann & Henderson, 1998). Errors in the stimuli that control programmed cell death may result in an abnormal amount of pruning of neurons or inappropriate pruning with regard to time and place; these errors may result in compromised brain development and functioning (Margolis et al., 1994). Too much pruning is thought to have occurred in persons with schizophrenia, who have a reduction of neurons in the cerebral cortex, hippocampus, thalamus, and amygdala. It is also thought that too much pruning may have occurred in the cerebellum of persons with autism and in the entorhinal area linked to the hippocampus in persons with bipolar disorder (Kandel et al., 2000).

Cerebral Dysgenesis

Cerebral dysgenesis is the disruption of the process of brain development. Causes may include genetic influences or factors such as maternal use of alcohol; maternal infections like rubella; maternal diabetes; or maternal folic acid deficiency (Schaefer, Sheth, & Bodensteiner, 1994). One marker of cerebral dysgenesis is hypoplasia of the corpus callosum, which is thought to be the result of disturbances of neuronal migration. Severe forms of cerebral dysgenesis include microencephaly, lissencephaly (smooth brain), pachygyria (four-layer instead of six-layer formation of the cortex), thickened gyri, and ectopic neurons (displaced neurons found in the subcortical white matter). The more immature the brain is at the time of injury, the more widespread and serious will be the consequences.

Indicators of Compromised Brain Development

Observable physical markers and markers that are evident during a neurological assessment indicate compromised brain development. These markers include neurointegrative defects, minor physical anomalies (MPAs), hand and fingerprint abnormalities, impairment of smooth pursuit eye movements, and soft neurological signs.

Neurointegrative Defects

Fish (1992) believed that some infants at high risk for developing schizophrenia had identifiable neurological deviations that indicated impairment of brain development that were evident from the first day of life. She believed that what was inherited was a "subtle neuro-integrative defect" (Fish, 1977, p. 1306). The features of the neurointegrative defect seen in infancy (birth to 4 weeks) that Fish (1977) identified include

- Continuous visual alertness for 15 to 80 minutes, versus the normal 2 to 5 minutes
- Marked decrease in spontaneous crying.
- No crying with postural manipulation of the body or extremities
- Normal or increased responses to visual, auditory, and tactile stimuli
- Muscles "doughy" to palpation (as in Down's syndrome)
- Flaccid overextension at the joints

She described impairments of functioning seen later in childhood as decreased hand-to-hand skills, delayed developmental milestones (walking, sitting, and standing), posture abnormalities, speech irregularities, sensitivity to stimuli, and problems getting along with peers.

Minor Physical Anomalies (MPA)

MPAs are mild defects of morphogenesis, which is the process of structure development. MPAs are found in many areas of the body—head and face, eyes, ears, mouth, hands, feet, and torso (Compton & Walker, 2009). MPAs have been described as

- Hair whorls and fine hair that will not comb down
- Widened nose base
- Wide-spaced eyes and eyes with mongoloid slant or inner epicanthic folds
- Fused eyebrows and abnormalities of eyebrows
- Bossing of the forehead
- Asymmetrical or low-seated ears or earlobe adherence
- Narrow or steepled palate
- Little finger curvature
- Single transverse palm crease
- Partial syndactyly of the feet, large gap between the first and second toes, and third toes longer than second toes
- Café-au-lait spots (Compton & Walker; Gourion, Goldberger, Bourdel, et al., 2003).

MPAs are quite common and usually cause no problems in functioning; for example, one to four MPAs occur among individuals in the general population. Higher rates of MPAs are associated with prenatal alcohol and drug exposure, low birth weight, and obstetrical complications. MPAs are thought to originate from inherited genetic influences, from noninherited genetic influences resulting from epigenetic activity that alters gene expression, and from influences arising from the uterine environment such as exposure to toxins like alcohol or drugs (Compton & Walker, 2009).

MPAs are indicators of ectodermal abnormalities, and because the CNS is also derived from ectodermal tissue, it is thought that the development of MPAs may be associated with impaired brain development during the first trimester of pregnancy and during the early part of the second trimester of pregnancy (Compton & Walker, 2009; Gourion et al., 2003). For example, the palate, which is often abnormal in patients with schizophrenia and in children with autism, develops during the 9th to 15th weeks of gestation. Researchers, reasoning that a large number of MPAs might indicate a parallel maldevelopment of the brain, have studied MPAs among persons with psychiatric disorders and have found increased numbers of MPAs among individuals with schizophrenia (Lohr & Flynn, 1993; O'Callaghan, Buckley, Madigan, et al., 1995), and among individuals with attention deficit-hyperactivity disorder, cerebral palsy, epilepsy, fetal alcohol syndrome, mental retardation, hyperactivity, and autism (Compton & Walker; Human Brain Informatics, 2005; Tripi, Roux, Canziani, et al., 2008). Among children with autism spectrum disorders, MPAs most commonly occur in the head, ears, mouth (abnormal palate), and hands (Tripi et al.). Among patients with schizophrenia and schizophrenia spectrum disorders, the most common MPAs are craniofacial anomalies, high steepled palate, fine electric hair, large gap between the first and second toes, epicanthus, tongue with rough and smooth spots, and third toe equal in length or longer than second toe (Akabaliev, Sivkov, & Baltadjiev, 2001).

Hand and Fingerprint Abnormalities

Hand Abnormalities

Hands are formed from ectodermal cells during the second trimester at the same time that neurons are migrating to form the brain. Dermal cell migration is sensitive to ischemic events (insufficient blood supply to an organ) and to exposure to infections such as rubella and cytomegalovirus. It is thought that an event such as an infection or exposure to a toxin that disrupts migration of cells to form the hand may disrupt migration of cells destined to form the layers of the brain. Thus, abnormalities of hand development may be an observable indication of abnormalities of brain development (Bracha, Torrey, Gottesman, et al., 1992). Following that line of reasoning, Bracha et al. studied hand abnormalities among identical twins, one having schizophrenia and the other not, and found that maldevelopment of the hand occurred more frequently in the twin who had developed schizophrenia and that there was a more frequent occurrence of abnormalities on the right hand, implicating left brain damage. They reported the presence of the following hand abnormalities among patients with schizophrenia: smaller thumbs, broken proximal palmar lines, smaller little fingers (also seen in Down's syndrome), single palmar crease, and curving of the little fingers.

Fingerprint Abnormalities

In the second trimester, at the same time that neuronal cells migrate to the cortex, fingertip dermal cells also migrate to form the ridges that make up fingerprints

(Bracha et al., 1992). Abnormalities of fingertip ridge count have been found in individuals with developmental reading disorder and fetal alcohol syndrome and in those exposed in utero to viral infections such as rubella and cytomegalovirus.

Dermatoglyphic Asymmetries

Dermatoglyphic asymmetries are differences in right- and left-hand finger ridge counts. Researchers (Weinstein, Diforio, Schiffman, et al., 1999) have described dermatoglyphic asymmetries in individuals with schizotypal personality disorder and other personality disorders. Because the development of finger ridges and palm creases begins during the second month of gestation and continues through the fourth month, researchers suggest that abnormalities in the ridges may be evidence of disruptions of brain development (Bracha et al., 1992; Gutierrez, Guerra, Arias, et al., 2001). Abnormalities of finger ridges and palm creases have been associated with maternal exposure to infections, alcohol, and stress, and with later intellectual disabilities in the child (Gutierrez et al.).

Impairment of Smooth Pursuit Eye Movements

Another form of MPA is impaired smooth pursuit eye movement, a condition that often is impaired in persons with schizophrenia and in their relatives who do not have schizophrenia, indicating a genetic influence. The development of smooth eye tracking parallels the development of neurointegrative development, especially in the frontal lobe (Kandel et al., 2000).

Soft Neurological Signs

The term "soft neurological sign" refers to nondiagnostic abnormalities in sensory and motor performance that are found on a neurological examination (Dazzan & Murray, 2002). Unlike hard neurological signs, which are localized to the corticospinal, extrapyramidal, and cerebellar components of the motor system, soft neurological signs do not indicate a focal neurological disorder or evidence of trauma to specific nerves or nerve tracts (Rossi, De Cataldo, Di Michele, et al., 1990; Woods, Kinney, & Yurgelun-Todd, 1991). Instead, they indicate diffuse or nonlocalized abnormalities and are concentrated in the functional areas of sensory integration, coordination, and sequential motor acts. Soft neurological signs have been found to be associated with decreased volume of subcortical structures—putamen, globus pallidus, and thalamus—and decreased volume of the cerebral cortex (Dazzan, Morgan, Orr, et al., 2004).

In his classic work on neurological soft signs, Quitkin believed that they were due to intrauterine injury or anoxia (Quitkin, Rifkin, Kane, et al., 1976). He described positive neurological signs as difficulties with mirror movements, speech (tested using tongue twisters), finger-to-thumb opposition, and fist–edge of hand–palm tasks. Other researchers have expanded on Quitkin et al.'s identification of soft neurological signs. Additional signs include

- Slow, clumsy alternating movements
- Balance abnormality: sense of imbalance without vertigo, stumbling, or falling
- Asymmetrical reflex hyperactivity
- Babinski's sign, indicating upper pyramidal tract injury or upper motor neuron damage
- Whole-body clumsiness
- Asymmetrical facial weakness: motor weakness on one side of the face, e.g., Bell's palsy
- Unilateral motor weakness
- Gait ataxia: lack of coordination, staggering gait or broad-based gait, difficulty making turns (indicative of cerebellum damage)
- Unilateral sensory loss: loss of sensation on one side such as loss of pain or temperature sensation
- Unilateral cogwheel rigidity: muscle cannot be relaxed smoothly, relaxation occurs in steps
- Unilateral agraphesthesia: inability to feel or identify writing on the skin
- Resting tremor: an involuntary tremor that occurs when the patient is at rest; seen in patients with Parkinson's disease
- Intention tremor: tremor during movement when the patient tries to stop the movement, which may indicate cerebellar damage
- Grasp reflex: a pathologic reflex in which fingers flex when the palm of the hand is stroked (Donaghy, 2005; Duus, 1998; Gourion et al., 2003).

Soft neurological signs are concentrated in the functional areas of sensory integration, coordination, and sequential motor acts, possibly indicating impairment in the subcortical areas of the brain (Gourion et al., 2003). Soft neurological signs have been found in patients with schizophrenia (Flashman, Flaum, Gupta, et al., 1996; Minzenberg, Yoon, & Carter, 2008; Venkatasubramanian, Jayakumar, Gangadhar, et al., 2008), among adults with bipolar disorder (Goswami, Sharma, Kastigir, et al., 2006), and in children with tic disorders, attention deficit-hyperactivity disorder, learning disorders, and autism (Ursano, Kartheiser, & Barnhill, 2008). In the past, the value of soft neurological signs was thought to be limited to their indication of diffuse brain involvement; now, evidence suggests that soft neurological signs are a manifestation of connectivity impairment of the frontal and subcortical circuits, both of which are involved in motor speed and in coordinating and sequencing actions (Dazzan et al., 2004; Hollander, Schiffman, Cohen, et al., 1990).

Structural Abnormalities of the Brain: Manifestations of Abnormal Brain Development

Structural abnormalities of the brain have been most frequently studied in patients with schizophrenia. The following abnormalities have been found on postmortem examination of brains of individuals with schizophrenia in comparison to those of individuals without a psychiatric disorder:

- Brains weighed 6% to 8% less.
- Brains had reduced temporal lobe matter (18% to 21% less) on the left, particularly at the level of the amygdala and the anterior hippocampus.
- Cells in the hippocampus showed structural disarray.
- There were fewer neural cells (less cell density), especially on the left side.
- Brain length was reduced (4% less).
- Cerebral volume was reduced (8% less).
- Gray matter was decreased (6% less).
- Ventricles were enlarged, especially the third ventricle (Roberts, 1991).

Previous to 1992, the enlarged ventricles found in some patients with schizophrenia and in some patients with other psychiatric disorders were thought to occur after the onset of the illness. It was assumed that the illness caused atrophy of the brain with resulting enlargement of the ventricles. Now it is known that abnormalities in brain development result in smaller brain structures that fail to compress the ventricles to normal size (Gaser, Nenadic, Buchsbaum, et al., 2004; Roberts).

Part Two: Summary

Abnormalities of early brain development affect the development of brain structures, circuitry, and neurochemistry and thus affect brain functioning across the life-span (Kandel et al., 1995). Because the structures of the brain develop at different times, the time at which the damage occurs determines the area of the brain that is affected and the sequential compromised functioning. The effects of damage may not be evident until the CNS matures or until the individual must meet more complex challenges in adolescence or early adulthood, at which time impairment of brain functioning may be manifested as symptoms of psychiatric disorders. Evidenced-based knowledge of normal brain development and of the consequences of disrupted brain development is crucial for psychiatric advanced practice nurses.

Part Two: Key Points

- Symptoms of psychiatric disorders reflect impaired brain functioning that often reflects compromised brain development.
- Early brain development is influenced by genetic, epigenetic, and nongenetic factors.
- Brain development after birth is shaped by the interaction of the brain and experienced and environmental factors.
- Brain development starts with the formation of the neural plate and then of the neural tube.
- Defects of neural tube formation are seen in anencephaly, spina bifida, mental retardation, epilepsy, and behavioral disturbances.
- Neurons and glial cells are produced and proliferate in the neural tube.
- Disruptions of proliferation may result in a smaller brain or abnormal development of the brain.
- Neurons and glial cells migrate from the neural tube by tangential migration or radial migration.
- Glial cells migrate out of the neural tube first to form the scaffolding for the neurons to use in building the brain.
- Neurons migrate to form six layers of the cerebral cortex and other brain structures.
- Disruptions of migration may result in smaller brains, severe mental retardation, epilepsy, and learning disabilities.
- Neurotransmitter systems (the neurochemical systems of the brain) develop at different times.
- After migration, neurons form synapses (connections with other neurons) to survive.
- Synapses form circuits, connections for communication.
- Disruptions of synapses' circuits may result in schizophrenia, autism, language difficulties, obsessive-compulsive disorder, and epilepsy.
- Evidence of compromised brain development is suggested by minor physical anomalies that are more common in individuals with schizophrenia, autism, mental retardation, and fetal alcohol syndrome.
- Soft neurological signs indicate abnormal functioning in subcortical areas—limbic system and basal ganglia.
- The brain is plastic. It has life-long ability to make new connections.
- Adverse events, such as trauma, and positive events, such as attachment, affect brain plasticity.

Resources

DVD

Joseph, R. (Director). (2009). *Brain Lectures: Brain, Mind, Emotion, Memory, Language, Consciousness, Insanity, Frontal Lobes, Limbic System* [DVD]. United States: UniversityPress.info, BrainMind.com.

References

Aborelius, L., Owens, M. S., Plotsky, P. M., et al. (1999). The role of corticotrophin-releasing factor in depression and anxiety disorders. *Endocrinology, 160*, 1-12.

Akabaliev, V. H., Sivkov, S. T., Baltadjiev, G. A., et al. (2001). Discriminant analysis of minor physical anomalies as dysontogenetic markers of schizophrenia. *Folia Medica (Plovdiv), 43*(3), 21-26.

Anderson, S. (1998). The biological basis of mental illness. In C. Glod (Ed.), *Contemporary psychiatric-mental health nursing: The brain-behavior connection* (pp. 73-90). Philadelphia: F. A. Davis Company.

Andreasen, N. (1997). The role of the thalamus in schizophrenia. *Canadian Journal of Psychiatry, 42*, 27-33.

Andreasen, N. (2001). *Brave new brain: Conquering mental illness in the era of the genome.* Oxford: Oxford University Press.

Andreasen, N. C., & Black, D. W. (2006). *Introductory textbook of psychiatry* (4th ed.). Washington, DC: American Psychiatric Publishing, Inc.

Bartley, A. J., Jones, D. W., & Weinberger, D. R. (1997). Genetic variability of human brain size and cortical gyral patterns. *Brain, 120*(Pt. 2), 257-269.

Bear, M. F., Connors, B. W., & Paradiso, M. A. (Eds.). (2007). *Neuroscience: Exploring the brain.* Baltimore: Lippincott, Williams & Wilkins.

Beckmann, H., & Jakob, H. (1991). Prenatal disturbances of nerve cell migration in the entorhinal region: A common vulnerability factor in functional psychosis? *Journal of Neural Transmission, 84*, 155-164.

Begley, S. (2004, July 23). How a second, secret genetic code turns genes on and off. *The Wall Street Journal*, p. A9.

Belger, A., & Dichter, G. (2006). Structural and functional neuroanatomy. In J. Lieberman, T. S. Stroup, & D. O. Pickens (Eds.), *The American psychiatric publishing textbook of schizophrenia* (pp. 167-185). Washington, DC: American Psychiatry Publishing, Inc.

Belmonte, M. K., Allen, G., Beckel-Mitchener, A., et al. (2004). Autism and abnormal development of brain connectivity. *The Journal of Neuroscience, 24*(42), 9229-9231.

Benes, F. M. (1995). A neurodevelopmental approach to the understanding of schizophrenia and other mental disorders. In D. Cicchetti & D. Cohen (Eds.), *Developmental psychopathology: Theory & methods* (pp. 227-253). New York: John Wiley & Sons, Inc.

Benes, F. M., Turtle, M., Khan, Y., et al. (1994). Myelination of a key relay zone in the hippocampal formation occurs in the human brain during childhood, adolescence and adulthood. *Archives of General Psychiatry, 51*, 477-484.

Biondi A., Nogueira H., Dormont D., et al. (1998). Are the brains of monozygotic twins similar? A three-dimensional MR study. *American Journal of Neuroradiology, 19*, 1361-1367.

Black, D. W., & Andreasen, N. C. (2011). *Introductory textbook of psychiatry* (5th ed.). Washington, DC: American Psychiatric Publishing, Inc.

Blakeslee, S. (2007, February 6). A small part of the brain, and its profound effects. *The New York Times.* Retrieved from http://www.nytimes.com/2007/02/06/health/psychology/06/brain.html?)r=1

Blank, R. (1999). *Brain policy: How the new neurosciences will change your lives and your politics.* Washington, DC: Georgetown University Press.

Bogerts, B. (1993). Recent advances in the neuropathology of schizophrenia. *Schizophrenia Bulletin, 19*(2), 431-445.

Bonne, O., Drevets, W. C., Neurmeister, A., et al. (2004). Neurobiology of anxiety disorders. In A. F. Schatzberg & C. B. Nereroff (Eds.), *The American psychiatric publishing textbook of psychopharmacology* (3rd ed.) (pp. 775-792). Washington, DC: American Psychiatric Publishing, Inc.

Bracha, H. S., Torrey, E. F., Gottesman, I. I., et al. (1992). Second-trimester markers of fetal size in schizophrenia: A study of monozygotic twins. *American Journal of Psychiatry, 149*(10), 1355-1361.

Brewer, A., Echevarria, D. J., Langel, U., et al. (2005). Assessment of new functional roles for galanin in the CNS. *Neuropeptides, 39*(3), 323-326.

Brown, W. S., Paul, L. K., Symington, M., et al. (2005). Comprehension of humor in primary agenesis of the corpus callosum. *Neuropsychologia, 43*(6), 906-916.

Burgaya, F., Garcia-Frigola, C., Andres, R., et al. (2006). New genes involved in cortical development. In G. D. Rosen (Ed.), *The dyslexic brain* (pp. 143-165). Mahwah, NJ: Lawrence Erlbaum Associates Publishers.

Campbell, S., Marriott, M., Nahmias, C., et al. (2004). Lower hippocampal volume in patients suffering from depression: A meta-analysis. *American Journal of Psychiatry, 161*, 598-607.

Campbell, W. W. (2005). *The neurologic examination.* Philadelphia: Lippincott Williams & Wilkins.

Carter, R., Aldridge, S., Page, M., et al. (2009). *The human brain book: An illustrated guide to its structure, function, and disorders.* London: DK Books.

Charney, D., Grillon, C., & Bremmer, D. (1998). The neurobiological basis of anxiety and fear: Circuits, mechanisms and neurochemical interactions (part II). *The Neuroscientist, 4*(2), 122-132.

Chiron, C., Jambaque, I., Nabbout, R., et al. (1997). The right brain hemisphere is dominant in human infants. *Brain, 120*, 1057-1065.

Cloud, J. (2010, January 18). Why genes aren't destiny. *Time*, pp. 49-53.

Compton, M. T., & Walker, E. F. (2009). Physical manifestations of neurodevelopmental disruption: Are minor physical anomalies part of the syndrome of schizophrenia? *Schizophrenia Bulletin, 35*(2), 425-436.

Conrad, A., & Scheibel, A. (1987). Schizophrenia and the hippocampus: The embryological hypothesis extended. *Schizophrenia Bulletin, 13*(4), 577-587.

Cooper, J. R., Bloom, F. E., & Roth, R. H. (2001). *The biochemical basis of neuropharmacology.* New York: Oxford University Press.

Copp, A. J. (1997). The neural tube. In P. Thorogood (Ed.), *Embryos, genes and birth defects* (pp. 133-152). New York: John Wiley & Sons, Inc.

Counts, S. E., Perez, S. E., & Kahli, U., et al. (2001). Galantin: Neurobiologic mechanisms and therapeutic potential for Alzheimer's disease. *CNS Drug Review, 7*, 445-470.

Coyle, J. T., Tsai, G., & Goff, D. C. (2002). Ionotropic glutamate receptors as therapeutic targets in schizophrenia. *Current Drug Targets CNS Neurological Disorders, 1*(2), 183-189.

Cramer, D. A. (2005). Commentary: Gene-environment interplay in the context of genetics, epigenetics, and gene expression. *Journal of American Academy of Child and Adolescent Psychiatry, 44*(1), 19-27.

Das, R., Hampton, D. D., & Jirtle, R. L. (2009). Imprinting evolution and human health. *Mammalian Genome, 29*, 563-572.

Daube, J. R., & Stead, S. M. (2009). Basics of neurophysiology. In J. R. Daube & D. I. Rubin (Eds.), *Clinical neurophysiology* (3rd ed.) (pp. 69-96). Oxford: Oxford University Press.

Davis, A. A., Lah, J. J., & Levey, A. I. (2009). Neurobiology of Alzheimer's disease. In A. F. Schatzberg & C. B. Nemeroff (Eds.), *The American psychiatric publishing textbook of psychopharmacology* (4th ed.) (pp. 987-1005). Washington, DC: American Psychiatric Publishing, Inc.

Dazzan, P., Morgan, K. D., Orr, K. G., et al. (2004). The structural brain correlates of neurological soft signs in AESOP first-episode psychoses study. *Brain, 127*(Pt 1), 143-153.

Dazzan, P. A., & Murray, R. M. (2002). Neurological soft signs in first-episode psychosis: A systematic review. *British Journal of Psychiatry, 18*(Suppl 43), s50-s57.

Decker, M., & Butcher, L. (1992). *Neurotransmitter interactions and cognitive function.* Boston: Birkhauser.

DeSouza, S., & Grigoriadis, E. B. (2002). Corticotropin-releasing factor: Physiology, pharmacology and role in central nervous system disorders. In K. L. Davis, D. Charney, J. T. Coyle, & C. Nemeroff (Eds.), *Neuropsychopharmacology: The fifth generation of progress* (pp. 91-107). Philadelphia; Lippincott, Williams & Wilkins.

Devinsky, O. (1994). Contributions of anterior cingulated cortex to behaviour. *Human Molecular Genetics, 18*(1), 279-306.

Devinsky, O., Morrell, M., & Vogt, B. A. (1995). Contributions of anterior cingulated cortex to behaviour. *Brain, 118*, 279-306.

Dimberg, U., & Petterson, M. (2000). Facial reactions to happy and angry facial expressions: Evidence for right hemisphere dominance. *Psychophysiology, 37*(5), 693-696.

Dolinoy, D. C., Weidman, J. R., & Jirtle, R. L. (2007). Epigenetic gene regulation: Linking early developmental environment to adult disease. *Reproductive Toxicology, 23*(3), 297-307.

Donaghy, M. (2005). *Neurology* (2nd ed.). Oxford: Oxford University Press.

Duus, P. (1998). *Topical diagnosis in neurology.* Stuttgart: Thieme.

England, M. A., & Wakely, J. (2006). *Color atlas of the brain and spinal cord* (2nd ed.). Philadelphia: Mosby Elsevier, Ltd.

Esch, T., & Stefano, G. B. (2010). The neurobiology of stress management. *Neuroendocrinology Letters, 31*(1), 19-39.

European Society for Human Reproduction and Embryology (2005, June 22). Imprinting disorders and assisted reproduction.

Fabel, K., & Kempermann, G. (2008). Physical activity and the regulation of neurogenesis in the adult and aging brain. *Neuromolecular Medicine, 10*(2), 59-66.

Fabel, K. & Kempermann, G. (2008). Physical activity and the regulation of neurogenesis in the adult and aging brain. *Neuromolelcular Medicine, 10*(2), 59-66.

Ferris, C. F. (2005). Vasopressin/oxytocin and aggression. *Novartis Foundation Symposium, 268*, 190-198.

First, M. B., & Tasman, A. (2004). *DSM-IV-TR mental disorders: Diagnosis, etiology, and treatment.* West Sussex, England: John Wiley & Sons, Ltd.

Fish, B. (1977). Neurobiologic antecedents of schizophrenia in children: Evidence for an inherited congenital neurointegrative defect. *Archives of General Psychiatry, 34*, 1297-1313.

Flashman, L. A., Flaum, M., Gupta, S., et al. (1996). Soft signs and neuropsychological performance in schizophrenia. *American Journal of Psychiatry, 153*(4), 527-532.

Francis, F., Meyer, G., Fallet-Bianco, C., et al. (2006). Human disorders of cortical development: From past to present. *European Journal of Neuroscience, 23*, 877-893.

Futagi, Y., Toribe, Y., Ogawa, K., et al. (2006). Neurodevelopmental outcome in children with intraventricular bleeding. *Pediatric Neurology, 34*(3), 219-224.

Gao, X. M., Sakai, K., Roberts, R. C., et al. (2000). Ionotropic glutamate receptors and expression of N-methyl-D-aspartate receptor subunits in subregions of human hippocampus: Effects of schizophrenia. *American Journal of Psychiatry, 157*, 1141-1149.

Gaser, C., Nenadic, I., Buchsbaum, B. R., et al. (2004). Ventricular enlargement in schizophrenia related to volume reduction of the thalamus, striatum and superior temporal cortex. *American Journal of Psychiatry, 161*, 154-156.

Gaze, S. B. (1989). Biological psychiatry: Is there any other kind? *Psychological Medicine, 19*, 315-323.

Gerhardt, C. C., & van Heerikhuizen, H. (1997). Functional characteristics of heterologously expressed 5-HT receptors. *European Journal of Pharmacology, 334*, 1-23.

Giedd, J. (1999). Human brain growth. *American Journal of Psychiatry, 156*(1), 4.

Gilman, S., & Newman, S. W. (2003). *Manter and Gatz' essential of clinical neuroanatomy and neurophysiology* (10th ed.). Philadelphia: F. A. Davis Company.

Gleeson, J. (2006). Genetic disorders of neuronal migration and brain wiring. In G. D. Rosen (Ed.), *The dyslexic brain* (pp. 129-142). Mahwah, NJ: Lawrence Erlbaum Associates Publishers.

Gorman, D. G., & Cummings, J. L. (1992). Hypersexuality following septal injury. *Archives of Neurology, 49*, 308-310.

Goswami, D. B., May, W. L., Stockmeier, C. A., et al. (2010). Transcriptional expression of serotonergic regulators in laser-captured microdissected dorsal raphe neurons of subjects with major depressive disorder: sex specific differences. *Journal of Neurochemistry, 112*, 397-409.

Goswami, U., Sharma, A., Kastigir, U., et al. (2006). Neuropsychological dysfunction, soft neurological signs, and social disability in euthymic patients with bipolar disorder. *British Journal of Psychiatry, 188*, 366-373.

Gottesman, I. I., & Hanson, D. R. (2005). Human development: Biological and genetic processes. *Annual Review of Psychology, 56*, 263-286.

Gourion, D., Goldberger, C., Bourdel, M., et al. (2003). Neurological soft-signs and minor physical anomalies in schizophrenia: Differential transmission within families. *Schizophrenia Research, 63*(1-2), 181-187.

Gur, R. E., & Arnold, S. E. (2004). Neurobiology of schizophrenia. In A. F. Schatzberg & C. B. Nemeroff (Eds.), *The American psychiatric publishing textbook of psychopharmacology* (3rd ed.) (pp. 765-774). Washington, DC: American Psychiatric Publishing, Inc.

Gutierrez, A. R., Guerra, A., Arias B., et al. (2001). Dermatoglyphics and abnormal palmar flexion creases as markers of early prenatal stress in children with idiopathic intellectual disability. *Journal of Intellectual Disability Research, 45*(5), 416-423.

Hebb, A. L., Poulin, J. F., Roach, S. P., et al. (2005). Cholecystokinin and endogenous opioid peptides: Interactive influence on pain, cognition and emotion. *Progress in Neuro-Psychopharmacology & Biological Psychiatry, 29*, 1225-1238.

Hedaya, R. J. (1996). *Understanding biological psychiatry.* New York: W. W. Norton & Company , Inc.

Hertz, L., & Zielke, H. R. (2004). Astrocytic control of glutamatergic activity: Astrocytes as stars of the show. *Trends in Neuroscience, 27*(12), 735-743.

Higgins, E. S., & George, M. S. (2007). *The neuroscience of clinical psychiatry: The pathophysiology of behavior and mental illness.* Philadelphia: Wolters Kluwer-Lippincott Williams & Wilkins.

Hokfelt, T., Xu, A., Broberger, C., et al. (2000). Neuropeptides—an overview. *Neuropharmacology, 39*(8), 1337-1356.

Hollander, E., Schiffman, E., Cohen, B., et al. (1990). Signs of central nervous system dysfunction in obsessive-compulsive disorder. *Archives of General Psychiatry, 47*, 27-32.

Hong, S. E., Shugart, Y. Y., Huang, D. T., et al. (2000). Autosomal recessive lissencephaly with cerebellar hypoplasia is associated with human RELN mutations. *National Genetics, 26*, 93-96.

Hotz, R. L. (2002, November 17). A scientific exploration of emotion. *Los Angeles Times.*

Howard, B. M., Zhicheng, M., Filipovic, F., et al. (2008). Radial glia cells in the developing human brain. *The Neuroscientist, 14*, 459-473.

Howard, P. J. (2006). *The owner's manual for the brain* (3rd ed.). Austin, TX: Bard Press.

Hu, H. (2006). Neuronal migration. In M. W. Miller (Ed.), *Brain development: Normal process and the effects of alcohol and nicotine* (pp. 27-44). New York: Oxford University Press.

Human Brain Informatics (2005). Retrieved from http://www.hubin.org/about/projects/min_phys)anomalies)en.html

Huttenlocher, P. R., & Dabholkar, A. S. (1997). Regional differences in synaptogenesis in human cerebral cortex. *The Journal of Comparative Neurology, 387*, 167-178.

Hynes, R., & Lander, A. (1992). Contact and adhesive specificities in the associations, migrations, and targeting of cells and axons. *Cell, 68*, 308-322.

Jefferson, D. J. (2005, September 9). America's most dangerous drug. *Newsweek*, pp. 41-48.

Jones, P., & Murray, R. M. (1991). The genetics of schizophrenia is the genetics of neurodevelopment. *British Journal of Psychiatry, 158*, 615-623.

Joseph, R. (1990). *Neuropsychology, neuropsychiatry and behavioral neurology.* New York: Plenum Press.

Joseph, R. (1999). Frontal lobe psychopathology: Mania, depression, confabulation, catatonia, perseveration, obsessive compulsions and schizophrenia. *Psychiatry, 62*(2), 138-172.

Joseph, R. (2000). The limbic system, hypothalamus, septal nuclei, amygdala and hippocampus. In R. Joseph (Ed.), *Neuropsychiatry, neuropsychology, clinical neuroscience.* New York: Academic Press.

Kandel, E. R. (1998). A new intellectual framework for psychiatry. *American Journal of Psychiatry, 155*, 457-469.

Kandel, E. R. (2005). *Psychiatry, psychoanalysis, and the new biology of mind.* Washington, DC: American Psychiatric Publishing, Inc.

Kandel, E. R. , Schwartz, J. H., & Jessell, T. M. (1995). *Essentials of neural science and behavior.* Norwalk, CT: Appleton & Lange.

Kandel, E. R., Schwartz, J. H., & Jessell, T. M. (2000). *Principles of neural science* (4th ed.). New York: McGraw-Hill.

Kellaway, P., & Noebels, J. (Eds.). (1989). Maternally deprived children and somatostatin. In *Problems and concepts in developmental neurophysiology.* Baltimore: The Johns Hopkins University Press.

Keltner, N., Hogan, B., Knight, T., et al. (2001). Adrenergic, cholinergic, GABAergic and glutaminergic receptor function in the CNS. *Perspectives in Psychiatric Care, 37*(4), 140-145.

Kennedy, D. N. (2006). MRI-based morphometry in human developmental disorders: Looking back in time. In G. D. Rosen (Ed.), *The dyslexic brain: New pathways in neuroscience discovery* (pp. 291-305). Mahwah, NJ: Lawrence Erlbaum Associates Publishers.

Knott, A. B., & Bossy-Wetzel, E. (2007). ALS: Astrocytes take center stage, but must they share the spotlight? *Cell Death and Differentiation, 14*, 1985-1988.

Kolb, B., Gibb, R., & Robinson, T. (2003). Brain plasticity and behavior. *Current Direction of Psychological Science, 12*, 1-5.

Kramer, D. A. (2005). Commentary: Gene-environment interplay in the context of genetics, epigenetics, and gene expression. *Journal of American Academy of Child and Adolescent Psychiatry, 44*(1), 19-27.

Kuan, C. Y., Roth, K. A., Flavell, R. A., et al. (2000). Mechanisms of programmed cell death in the developing brain. *Trends in Neurosciences, 23*(7), 291-297.

Kuehn, B. M. (2008) [interview]. Randy L. Jirtle, PhD: epigenetics a window on gene dysregulation, disease. *Journal of the American Medical Association, 299*(11), 1249-1250.

Kuipers, S. D., Trentani, A., Den Boer, J. A., et al. (2003). Molecular correlates of impaired prefrontal plasticity in response to chronic stress. *Journal of Neurochemistry, 85,* 1312-1323.

Kujala, T., & Naatanen, R. (2010). The adaptive brain: A neurophysiological perspective. *Progress in Neurobiology, 91,* 55-67.

Kwak, S., & Kawahara, Y. (2005). Deficient RNA editing of GluR2 and neuronal death in amyotrophic lateral sclerosis. *Journal of Molecular Medicine, 83*(2), 110-120.

Lazar, C. E., Kerr, R. H., Wasserman, J. R., et al. (2005). Meditation experience is associated with increased cortical thickness. *Neuroreport, 16,* 1893-1897.

LeDoux, J. (2000). Emotion circuits in the brain. *American Review of Neuroscience, 23,* 155-184.

LeDoux, J. (2002). *Synaptic self: How our brains become who we are.* New York: Viking Press.

LeDoux, J. (2007). The amygdala [Review]. *Current Biology, 17*(20), R868-R874.

Levitt, P. (2003). Structural and functional maturation of the developing primate brain. *The Journal of Pediatrics, 143*(4) (Suppl, October 2003), S35-S45.

Lohr, J., & Flynn, K. (1993). Minor physical anomalies, schizophrenia and mood disorders. *Schizophrenia Bulletin, 19*(3), 551-556.

LoTurco, J. J., Wang, Y, & Paramasivam, M. (2006). Neuronal migration and dyslexia susceptibility. In G. D. Rosen (Ed.), *The dyslexic brain* (pp. 107-127). Mahwah, NJ: Lawrence Erlbaum Associates Publishers.

Luria, A. R. (1969). Frontal lobe syndrome. In P. J. Vinken & G. W. Bruun (Eds.), *Handbook of Clinical Neurology* (Vol. 2). Philadelphia: Elsevier.

Lyketsos, C. G., Rosenblatt, A., & Rabins, P. (2004). Forgotten frontal lobe syndrome or "Executive Dysfunction Syndrome." *Psychosomatics, 45*(3), 247-255.

Mahncke, H. W., Bronstone, A., & Merzenich, M. M. (2006). Brain plasticity and functional losses in the aged: Scientific bases for a novel intervention. *Progress in Brain Research, 157,* 81-109.

Margolis, R., Chuang, D., & Post, R. (1994). Programmed cell death: Implications for neuropsychiatric disorders. *Biological Psychiatry, 35,* 946-956.

Mayberg, H. S. (2006). Brain imaging. In D. J. Stein, D. J. Kupfer, & A. F. Schatzberg (Eds.), *The American psychiatric publishing textbook of mood disorders* (pp. 219-234). Washington, DC: American Psychiatric Publishing, Inc.

Mayfield, R. D., Lewohl, J. M., Dodd, P. R., et al. (2002). Patterns of gene expression are altered in the frontal and motor cortices of human alcoholics. *Journal of Neurochemistry, 81,* 802-813.

McAllister, A. K., Usrey, W. M., Noctor, S. C., et al. (2008). Cellular and molecular biology of the neuron. In R. E. Hales, S. C. Yudofsky, & G. O. Gabbard (Eds.), *The American psychiatric publishing textbook of psychiatry* (5th ed.) (pp. 113-155). Washington, DC: American Psychiatric Publishing, Inc.

McEwen, B. S. (1998). Protective and damaging effects of stress mediators. *The New England Journal of Medicine, 338,* 171-179.

McEwen, B. S. (2002). Sex, stress and the hippocampus: Allostasis, allostatic load and the aging process. *Neurobiological Aging, 23*(5), 921-939.

McEwen, B. S. (2009). The brain is the central organ of stress and adaptation. *NeuroImage, 47*(3), 911-913.

McGeehan, J. (n.d.). Brain-compatible learning. Retrieved from http://www.greenteacher.com/articles/McGeehan.pdf

Melchitzky, D. S., Austin, M. C., & Lewis, D. (2004). Chemical neuroanatomy of the primate brain. In A. F. Schatzberg & C. B. Nemeroff (Eds.), *The American psychiatric publishing textbook of psychopharmacology* (3rd ed.) (pp. 69-87). Washington, DC: American Psychiatric Publishing, Inc.

Melchitzky, D. S., & Lewis, D. A. (2009). Chemical neuroanatomy of the primate brain. In A. F. Schatzberg & C. B. Nemeroff (Eds.), *The American psychiatric publishing textbook of psychopharmacology* (4th ed.) (pp. 105-134). Washington, DC: American Psychiatric Publishing, Inc.

Memory (1986, October 29). *Newsweek,* pp. 48-54.

Miller, M. W., & Luo, J. (2002). Effects of ethanol and transforming growth factor (TGFB) on neuronal proliferation and NCAM expression. *Alcohol Clinical Experience and Research, 26,* 1281-1285.

Mintz, C. D., Bekirov, I. H., Anderson, T. R., et al. (2006). Neuronal differentiation: From axons to synapses. In M. W. Miller (Ed.), *Brain development: Normal processes and the effects of alcohol and nicotine* (pp. 45-72). Oxford: Oxford University Press.

Minzenberg, M. J., Yoon, J. H., & Carter, C. S. (2008). Schizophrenia. In R. E. Hales, S. C. Yudofsky, & G. O. Gabbard (Eds.), *The American psychiatric publishing textbook of psychiatry* (5th ed.) (pp. 407-456). Washington, DC: American Psychiatric Publishing, Inc.

Moore, K., & Persaud, T. (1993). The nervous system. In K. L. Moore & T. V. N. Persaud (Eds.), *The developing human: Clinically oriented embryology* (pp. 385-422). Philadelphia: W. B. Saunders Company.

Morrell, P., & Quarles, R. H. (1999). Myelin formation, structure and biochemistry. In G. J. Siegel, B. W. Agranoff, R. W. Albers, et al. (Eds.), *Basic neurochemistry: Molecular, cellular, and medical aspects* (6th ed.) (pp. 69-93). Philadelphia: Lippincott, Williams & Wilkins.

Munson, J., Dawson, G., Abbott, R., et al. (2006). Amygdalar volume and behavioral development in autism. *Archives of General Psychiatry, 63*(6), 686-693.

Nash, M. J. (1997, February 3). Fertile minds. *Time,* pp. 49-62.

Nasrallah, H. A. (2006). Medication with psychotherapy: Asynergy to heal the brain. *Current Psychiatry, 5*(10), 11-12.

Neeper, S. A., Gómez-Pinilla, F., Choi, J., et al. (1996). Physical exercise increases mRNA for brain-derived neurotropic factor and nerve growth factor in rat brain. *Brain Research, 726,* 49-56.

Nelson, C. A. (2004). Brain development during puberty and adolescence: Comments on Part II. *Annals of the New York Academy of Science, 1021,* 105-109.

Nemeroff, C. (1988). *Neuropeptides in psychiatric and neurological disorders.* Baltimore: The John Hopkins University Press.

Nolte, J. (2010). *Essential of the human brain.* Philadelphia: Mosby Elsevier.

O'Callaghan, E., Buckley, P., Madigan, C., et al. (1995). The relationship of minor physical anomalies and other putative indices of developmental disturbance in schizophrenia to abnormalities of cerebral structure on magnetic resonance imaging. *Schizophrenia Bulletin, 38,* 516-524.

Olry, R., & Haines, D. E. (2003). Give a kiss to a frog and it will turn into. . . A neuropepetide: The genealogy of the bombesin-like family. *Journal of the History of the Neurosciences, 12*(4), 411-412.

Olsen, R. W., & Delorey, T. M. (1999). GABA and glycine. In G. J. Siegel, B. W. Agranoff, R. W. Albers, et al. (Eds.), *Basic neurochemistry: Molecular, cellular, and medical aspects* (6th ed.) (pp. 336-346). Philadelphia: Lippincott, Williams & Wilkins.

Oppenheim, R. W. (1991). Cell death during development of the nervous system. *Annual Review of Neuroscience, 14,* 453-501.

Organization of the cerebral cortex. Retrieved from http://psychmemlab2.lakeheadu.ca/Psy5111/Cortical%20layers.html

Otake, M., & Schull, W. J. (1984). In utero exposure to A-bomb radiation and mental retardation: A reassessment. *British Journal of Radiology, 57,* 409-414.

Panksepp, J. (2003). Can anthromorphic analysis of "separation cries" in other animals inform us about the nature of social loss in humans. *Psychology Review, 110,* 376-388.

Panksepp, J., & Harro, J. (2004). Future of neuropeptides in biological psychiatry and emotional psychopharmacology goals and strategies. In J. Panksepp (Ed.), *Textbook of biological psychiatry* (pp. 627-659). Hoboken, NJ: John Wiley-Liss Inc.

Park, A. (2004, May 10). What makes teens tick. *Time,* pp. 56-65.

Pennington, B. F., Filipick, P. A., Lefly, D., et al. (2001). A twin MRI study of size variations in human brain. *Journal of Cognitive Neuroscience, 12,* 223-232.

Pettmann, B., & Henderson, C. E. (1998). Neuronal cell death. *Neuron, 20,* 633-647.

Pincus, J. H., & Tucker, G. J. (2002). *Behavioral neurology.* New York: Oxford University Press.

Pizzagalli, D. A., Oakes, T. R., Fox, A. S., et al. (2004). Functional but not structural subgenual prefrontal cortex abnormalities in melancholia. *Molecular Psychiatry, 9,* 392-405.

Post, R. (2000). Neural substrates of psychiatric syndromes. In M. M. Mesulam (Ed.), *Principles of behavioral and cognitive neurology* (2nd ed.) (pp. 406-438). Oxford: Oxford University Press.

Pruessner, M. W., Baldwin, K., Dedovic, R. M. N. K., et al. (2005). Self-esteem, locus of control, hippocampal volume, and cortisol regulation in young and old adulthood. *NeuroImage, 28,* 815-826.

Quitkin, F. N., Rifkin, A., Klein D. F., et al. (1976). Neurological soft signs in schizophrenia and character disorders. *Archives of General Psychiatry, 33,* 845-853.

Rakic, P. (1988a). Defects of neuronal migration and the pathogenesis of cortical malformations. In G. J. Boer, M. G. P. Feenstra, M. Mirmiran, et al. (Eds.), *Progress in brain research* (Vol. 73) (pp. 15-37). Philadelphia: Elsevier Science Publishers.

Rakic, P. (1988b). Specification of cerebral cortex areas. *Science, 241,* 170-176.

Rakic, P. (1990). Principles of neural cell migration. *Experientia, 46,* 882-891.

Rakic, P. (2005). Less is more: progenitor death and cortical size. *Nature Neuroscience, 8*(8), 981-982.

Rees, S., & Inder, T. (2005). The making of the nervous system and neonatal origins of altered brain development. *Early Human Development, 81*(9), 753-761.

Rehen, S. K., & Chun, J. J. M. (2006). Cell death. In M. W. Miller (Ed.), *Brain development: Normal processes and the effects of alcohol and nicotine* (pp. 73-90). Oxford: Oxford University Press.

Reichardt, L. F., & Farinas, L. (1997). Neurotropic factors and their receptors. In W. M. Gowan, T. M. Jessell, & S. L. Zipurskky (Eds.), *Molecular and cellular approaches into neural developmental* (pp. 220-263). New York: Oxford University Press.

Rimon, R., LeGreves, P., Nyberg, F., et al. (2002). Elevation of substance-P like peptides in the CSF of psychiatric patients. *Biological Psychiatry, 19,* 509-516.

Roberts, G. W. (1991). Schizophrenia: A neuropathological perspective. *British Journal of Psychiatry, 158,* 8-17.

Rodier, P. M. (2000, February). The early origins of autism. *Scientific American, 282*(2), 56-63.

Rossi, A., De Cataldo, S., Di Michele, V., et al. (1990). Neurological soft signs in schizophrenia. *British Journal of Psychiatry, 157,* 735-739.

Rubia-Vila, F. J. (2001). The remarkable symptoms of the temporal lobe dysfunction (Spanish). *Anoles de la Real Academia Nacional de Medicina, 118*(3), 583-590.

Sadock, B., & Sadock, V. (2007). *Kaplan and Sadock's synopsis of psychiatry* (10th ed.). New York: Lippincott Williams & Wilkins.

Sapolski, R. M. (1994). *Why zebras don't get ulcers: A guide to stress, stress-related diseases and coping.* New York: W.H. Freeman.

Saze, T., Hirao, K., Namiki, C., et al. (2007). Insular volume reduction in schizophrenia. *European Archives of Psychiatry and Clinical Neuroscience, 257*(8), 473-479.

Schaefer, G. B., Sheth, R. D., & Bodensteiner, J. B. (1994). Cerebral dysgenesis. An overview. *Neurologic Clinics, 12*(4), 773-788.

Schmahmann, J. D. (2004). Disorders of the cerebellum: Ataxia, dysmetria of thought, and the cerebellar cognitive affective syndrome. *Journal of Neuropsychiatry & Clinical Neurosciences, 16*(3), 367-378.

Sergeyev, V., Hokfelt, T., & Hurd, Y. (1999). Serotonin and substance P co-exist in dorsal raphe neurons of the human brain. *Neuroreport, 10*(18), 3967-3970.

Sharma, R. P.¡ Bissette, G., Janicak, P. G., et al. (1995). Elevation of CSF somatostatin concentrations in mania. *American Journal of Psychiatry, 152*(12), 1807-1809.

Sharma, R. P., Janicak, P. G., Bissette, G., et al. (1997). CSF neurotensin concentrations and antipsychotic treatment in schizophrenia and schizoaffective disorder. *American Journal of Psychiatry, 154,* 1019-1021.

Shelby, J., & McCance, K. L. (2002). Stress and disease. In K. L. McCance & S. E. Huether (Eds.), *Pathophysiology: the biologic basis for disease in adults and children* (4th ed.) (pp. 272-289). St. Louis,: Mosby.

Shirtcliff, E. A., Vitacco, M. J., Graf, A. R., et al. (2009). Neurobiology of empathy and callousness: Implications for the development of antisocial behavior. *Behavioral Sciences and the Law, 27,* 137-171.

Siegel, G. J., Agranoff, B. W., Albers, R. W., et al. (1999). *Basic neurochemistry: Molecular, cellular and medical aspects* (6th ed.). Philadelphia: Lippincott Williams & Wilkins.

Siegenthaler, J. A., & Miller, M. W. (2006). Mechanisms of ethanol-induced alterations in neuronal migration. In M. W. Miller (Ed.), *Brain development: Normal process and the effects of alcohol and nicotine* (pp. 216-229). Oxford, UK: Oxford University Press.

Snyder, S., & Ferris C. (2000). Novel neurotransmitters and their neuropsychiatric relevance. *The American Journal of Psychiatry, 157*(11), 1738-1751.

Sokol, D. K., & Edwards-Brown, M. (2004). Neuroimaging in autistic spectrum disorder. *Journal of Neuroimaging, 14*(1), 8-15.

Sood, A., & Koziol, L. (1994). The integration of psychopharmacological treatment with psychotherapy. In L. F. Kosiol & C. E. Stout (Eds.), *The neuropsychology of mental disorders: A practical guide* (pp. 220-241). Springfield, Il: Charles C Thomas.

Stahl, S. (2000). *Essential psychopharmacology* (2nd ed.) (pp. 1-133). Cambridge, UK: Cambridge University Press.

Sterzer, P., Stadler, C., Poustka, F., et al. (2007). A structural neural deficit in adolescents with conduct disorder and its association with lack of empathy. *NeuroImage, 37*(1), 335-342.

Sugarman, R. S. (2002). Structure and function of the neurologic system. In K. L. McCance & S. E. Huether (Eds.), *Pathophysiology: The biologic basis for disease in adults and children* (pp. 363-400). St. Louis: Mosby.

Suter, B., & Bhide, P. G. (2006). Cell proliferation. In M. W. Miller (Ed.), *Brain development: Normal processes and the effects of alcohol and nicotine* (pp. 9-26). Oxford: Oxford University Press.

Szabo, G., Gould, T. D., & Manji, H. (2004). Neurotransmitters, receptors, signal transduction and second messengers in psychiatric disorders. In A. F. Schatzberg & C. B. Nemeroff (Eds.), *The American psychiatric publishing textbook of psychopharmacology* (3rd ed.) (pp. 3-52). Washington, DC: American Psychiatric Publishing, Inc.

Szabo, G., Gould, T. D., & Manji, H. (2009). Neurotransmitters, receptors, signal transduction, and second messengers in psychiatric disorders. In A. F. Schatzberg & C. B. Nemeroff (Eds.), *The American psychiatric publishing textbook of psychopharmacology* (4th ed.) (pp. 3-58). Washington, DC: American Psychiatric Publishing, Inc.

Sztriha, L. (2005). Spectrum of corpus callosum agenesis. *Pediatric Neurology, 32*(2), 94-101.

Taber, K. H., & Hurley, R. A. (2008). Neuroanatomy for the psychiatrists. In R. E. Hales, S. C. Yudofsky, & G. O. Gabbard (Eds.), *The American psychiatric publishing textbook of psychiatry* (5th ed.) (pp. 157-189). Washington, DC: American Psychiatric Publishing, Inc.

Tamminga, C. A. (2001). The human brain. In D. Purves, G. J. Augustine, D. Fitzpatrick, et al. (Eds.), *Neuroscience.* Sunderland, MA: Sinauer Associates.

Tamminga, C. A. (2004). Frontal cortex function. *The American Journal of Psychiatry, 161*(12), 2178.

Teicher, M. H., Dumont, N. L., Ito, Y., et al. (2004). Childhood neglect is associated with reduced corpus callosum area. *Biological Psychiatry, 56,* 80-85.

Tessier-Lavigne, M., & Goodman, C. (1996). The molecular biology of axon guidance. *Science, 274,* 1123-1133.

Thorogood, P. (1997). *Embryos, genes and birth defects.* New York: John Wiley & Sons, Inc.

Todd, R., Swarzenski, B., Rossi, R., et al. (1995). Structural and functional development of the human brain. In D. Cicchetti & D. Cohen (Eds.), *Developmental psychopathology* (Vol. I: Theory & methods). New York: John Wiley & Sons, Inc.

Toga, A. W., & Thompson, P. M. (2005). Genetics of brain structure and intelligence. *Annual Review of Neuroscience, 28,* 1-28.

Tripi, G., Roux, S., Canziani, T., et al. (2008). Minor physical anomalies in children with autism spectrum disorder. *Early Human Development, 84*(4), 217-223.

Ursano, A. M., Kartheiser, P. H., & Barnhill, L. J. (2008). Disorders usually first diagnosed in infancy, childhood or adolescence. In R. E. Hales, S. C. Yudofsky, & G. O. Gabbard (Eds.), *The American psychiatric publishing textbook of psychiatry* (5th ed.) (pp. 861-920). Washington, DC: American Psychiatric Publishing, Inc.

Vaillant, G. E. (2008). *Spiritual evolution: A scientific defense of faith.* New York: Broadway Books.

Van der Kolk, B. A. (1996). The body keeps the score: Approaches to the psychobiology of posttraumatic stress disorder. In F. A. van der Kolk, A.

C. McFarlane, & W. Lars (Eds.), *Traumatic stress: The effects of overwhelming experience on mind, body and society* (pp. 214-241). New York: Guilford Press.

Venkatasubramanian, G., Jayakumar, P., Gangadhar, B. N., et al. (2008). Neuroanatomical correlates of neurological soft signs in antipsychotic-naïve schizophrenia. *Psychiatry Research, 164*(3), 215-222.

Waddington, J. L. (1993). Neurodynamics of abnormalities in cerebral metabolism and structure in schizophrenia. *Schizophrenia Bulletin, 19*(1), 55-68.

Webb, S. J., Monk, C. S., & Nelson, C. A. (2001). Mechanisms of postnatal neurobiological development: Implications for human development. *Developmental Neuropsychology, 19*(2), 147-171.

Weinstein, D. D., Diforio, D., Schiffman, J., et al. (1999). Minor physical anomalies, dermatoglyphic asymmetries, and cortisol levels in adolescents with schizotypal personality disorder. *American Journal of Psychiatry, 156*(4), 617-623.

Winslow, R. (1997, July 10). How language is stored in brain depends on age. *Wall Street Journal*, p. B1.

Woodruff-Pak, D. S. (1993). Neural plasticity as a substrate for cognitive adaptation in adulthood and aging. In J. Cerella, J. Rybash, W. Hover, et al. (Eds.), *Adult information processing: Limits on loss.* San Diego, CA: Academic Press.

Woods, B., Kinney, D., & Yurgelun-Todd, D. (1991). Neurological "Hard" signs and family history of psychosis in schizophrenia. *Biological Psychiatry, 30*(8), 806-816.

Wurtman, R. S. (1982). Nutrients that modify brain function. *Scientific America, 246*, 42-51.

Young, S. N., & Ghadirian, A. M. (1989). Folic acid and psychopathology. *Neuropsychopharmacology & Biological Psychiatry, 13*, 841-863.

Yu, J-Z, & Rasenick, M. M. (2009). Basic principles of molecular biology and genomics. In A. F. Schatzberg & C. B. Nemeroff (Eds.), *The American psychiatric publishing textbook of psychopharmacology* (4th ed.) (pp. 59-80). Washington, DC: American Psychiatric Publishing, Inc.

Zak, P. J., Kurzban, R., & Matzner, W. T. (2005). Oxytocin is associated with human trustworthiness. *Hormones & Behavior, 48*(5), 522-527.

CHAPTER 3

Prenatal, Perinatal, and Postnatal Influences on Brain Development and Functioning

Eris F. Perese, APRN-PMH

This chapter focuses on prenatal, perinatal, and postnatal factors that are risks for less than optimal brain development. Chapters 9 through 18 identify many of these factors as risk factors for the development of specific psychiatric disorders. Chapter 19 is devoted to preventive interventions across the life span—from preconception to older adulthood—and it presents interventions that both reduce the risk factors for impaired brain development and increase protective factors that promote optimal brain development.

As discussed in Chapter 2, different parts of the brain develop at different times, with each developing brain structure dependent on the processes of cell proliferation, cell differentiation, neuronal migration, and synaptogenesis (Costa, Aschner, Vitalone, et al., 2004). Prenatal exposure to hypoxia, malnutrition, infections, toxins, and stress interferes with these processes and may compromise the development of brain structures, alter brain neurochemistry, and impair brain functioning. Disturbances of early brain development are now thought to be one of the etiological factors associated with the development of psychiatric disorders throughout the life span (Grossman, Churchill, McKinney, et al., 2003; Rees & Inder, 2005).

Early researchers used the term "minimal brain dysfunction" to describe organic damage to brain development. They thought that minimal brain dysfunction was caused by prenatal, perinatal, or immediate postnatal hypoxia and that hypoxia was the cause of later development of psychiatric disorders (Handford, 1975; Hortocollis, 1978). Today's researchers believe that the development of psychiatric disorders is related to the interaction of multiple factors over time. Factors currently under investigation include genetic vulnerability, compromised neurodevelopment of the brain, adverse circumstances of birth, the compatibility of the infant's temperament and the caregiver's temperament, and experienced factors like neglect and abuse.

Genetic Influence on Brain Development

Genes influence how the brain develops during the early prenatal stage; however, the strength of genetic influence on development varies among different areas of the brain (Thompson, Levitt, & Stanwood, 2009). There is a *strong* genetic influence on the development of the frontal areas of the brain, which are the areas involved in cognition, intelligence (IQ), verbal and spatial abilities, perceptual speed, and emotional reaction to stress (Eley & Plomin, 1997). There is a *moderate* genetic influence on language-related areas of the cerebral cortex (Broca's and Wernicke's language areas) and on the sensorimotor regions. There is *some* genetic influence on the size of the brain (Tramo, Loftus, Stukel, et al., 1998), the corpus callosum, and the ventricles (Biondi, Nogueira, Dormont, et al., 1998; Oppenheim, Skerry, Tramo, et al., 1989). The strong genetic influence on the frontal brain region may be the basis of individual differences in cognition. Genetic influence on the development of the frontal area of the brain, and thus its functioning, may be the basis of the known genetic vulnerability to some psychiatric disorders, such as schizophrenia, which is manifested in deficits of frontal brain functioning, cognitive deficits, and deficits of information processing (Thompson et al., 2009). The genetic influence associated with each psychiatric disorder and with each of the ten personality disorders is discussed in Chapters 9 through 18, which focus on specific psychiatric disorders.

Studies of identical twins are often used to sort out genetic influences from nongenetic influences on the development of a disorder (Plomin, 1990). For example, the monozygotic (identical) Genain quadruplets—four girls known by the names of Nora, Iris, Myra, and Hester (the initials of the National Institute of Mental Health)—were born in 1930 in the United States. According to Mirsky & Quinn (1988) the word "Genain" was selected by Rosenthal (1963) and means "dreadful gene" (p. 595). Although their father had no specific psychiatric diagnosis, he was described as suspicious, domineering, destructive, and abusive; he was also said to abuse alcohol. The mother was described as viewing the girls as an extension of herself rather than as individuals. There was a history of psychiatric disorders among several members of the father's family. The quadruplets were delivered by internal podalic version (shifting of the fetus so that the feet present during delivery) (Nora's birth weight was 2041 g; Myra, 1928 g; Iris, 1503 g; and Hester, 1361 g). Later, in a 1981 follow-up evaluation using newly developed neurological testing procedures, all four of the quadruplets showed soft neurological signs indicating diffuse abnormalities of brain development (Mirsky & Quinn) (see Chapter 2). The parents prevented the girls from having any socializing experiences during their infancy and preschool years and used harsh methods of discipline. All four girls developed schizophrenia, but the illness differed in severity, time of onset, symptoms, and course. Nora was the last to become ill and did the best in school. Myra's disease was under control. Iris' illness was more severe than that of the others. Hester, who was the smallest, did not walk until age 20 months, showed strange behaviors as a preschool child, was the first to develop schizophrenia, and had the poorest clinical course (Mirsky & Quinn; Rosenthal). It appears that the interaction of the Genain quadruplets' shared genetic factors and their individual obstetrical complications, low birth weights, and experienced factors resulted in the unique characteristics and course of schizophrenia that each developed.

Although genes provide the template of each individual's neural circuitry and capacity for plasticity and functioning, this template is molded by the individual's prenatal and postnatal experiences, which in turn influence how genes will be expressed (Blank, 1999). In brief, genes contain information to make proteins such as receptors, ion channels, neuropeptides, enzymes, and neurotropic factors (which are essential for neuronal survival). Experience modulates proteins that control gene expression. Gene expression regulates the functioning of individual cells, circuits of cells, structures, and systems, which is essentially the functional capacity of the entire organism (Blank). Thus, it is the interaction of genetically influenced brain development and functioning, genetically influenced temperament (early personality traits), and—some researchers say—genetically influenced life experiences that underlie an individual's thinking, emotions, responses, and behaviors that determine health or psychopathology. Tamminga (1999) summarized: "Ultimately, the mechanisms of all human diseases must be understood in terms of changes in gene expression within pertinent cell groups of the body" (p. XIII).

Prenatal Factors Influencing Brain Development and Functioning

For the developing fetal brain to reach its potential, there must be an optimal intrauterine environment (Rees & Harding, 2004). Unfortunately, there are many factors and mechanisms that may adversely influence the environment that the fetus experiences. These adverse factors, known as neurotoxic factors, are chemical, biological, or physical agents that cause structural changes or functional alterations to the developing brain (Rees & Inder, 2005).

Neurobehavioral Teratology

Neurobehavioral teratology is the study of the developmental impact of exposure to exogenous agents or events during the development of the brain. *Teratogens* are substances, agents, or processes that interfere with normal prenatal development, causing one or more developmental abnormalities (Pollard, 2007). Exposure to teratogens may result in death, physical malformation, growth abnormalities, and disruption of developing organs and systems including the central nervous system (Fawcett & Brent, 2006; Mayes & Ward, 2003).

Teratogens that appear to affect the central nervous system—and particularly prenatal brain development—include exposure through the mother's exposure to or use of

- Prescription and nonprescription drugs: benzodiazepines, carbamazepine, valproic acid, phenobarbital, phenytoin, retinoids, and cocaine
- Alcohol
- Nicotine
- Marijuana
- Industrial chemicals, e.g., methylmercury
- Environmental pollutants, e.g., polychlorobiphenyls, lead
- Irradiation, e.g., ionizing radiation
- Viral infections
- Nutritional deprivations
- Hyperthermia
- Stress (Mayes & Ward, 2003; Peters & Schaefer, 2001; Pollard, 2007)

Cell Processes and Teratogens

Damage to the developing brain may occur during the division, differentiation, proliferation, or migration of cells; during synaptogenesis (the formation of neuronal connections); or during periods of programmed cell death (Arndt, Stodgell, & Rodier (2005). These processes occur at different times, with cell proliferation occurring 2 to 4 months after conception; migration 3 to 5 months after conception; and brain organization, connection building, and programmed cell death occurring from 6 months after conception through several postnatal years. Thus, there are "windows of vulnerability" (Mayes & Ward, 2003, p. 11) during which time exposure to teratogens has different effects on the developing brain. The researched effects of teratogens on specific cell processes are listed below:

- *Cell division.* An example of an agent with antimitotic properties (inhibition of cell division) is methylmercury (Costa et al., 2004); animal studies have shown that exposure to methylmercury interferes with cell division (Li, Dong, Proschel, et al., 2007). Other agents that affect cell division are lead, arsenic, ethanol, and herbicides such as paraquat (Li et al.).
- *Cell differentiation.* Agents such as retinoic acid and the antiseizure medication valproic acid have been found to disrupt differentiation of cells into neurons and glial cells, and exposure to lead induces premature differentiation of cells (Crumpton, Atkins, Zawia, et al., 2001).
- *Cell proliferation.* Agents that adversely affect proliferation include radiation (Schull & Otake, 1999), methylmercury (Mundy, Radio, & Freudenrich, 2010; Takizawa & Kitamura, 2001), and ethanol (Goodlett, Horn, & Zhou, 2005; Miller, 1993, 1996). The overall outcome of adverse effects on cell proliferation is a reduction in volume or size of the brain structures that the cells were destined to form. Diminished size of brain structures is reflected in a smaller than normal head size and impairment of functioning that is related to the involved structures, including impaired cognitive, affective, motor, and behavioral functioning.
- *Cell migration.* Prenatal exposure to teratogens may also lead to disruption of normal migration and result in ectopic neurons, which are neurons that are present in destinations other than the one where they would be expected to be (Arndt et al., 2005). Agents that adversely affect migration include radiation (Schull & Otake, 1999), methylmercury (Takizawa & Kitamura, 2001), and ethanol (Miller, 1993, 1996).
- *Cell synaptogenesis.* The processes that neurons use to establish connections are susceptible to many forms of damage. Animal studies have shown that the number of connections formed by neurons during development is affected by agents such as malnutrition (Bedi, Thomas, Davies, et al., 1980), hypoxia (Rees & Harding, 2004), and exposure to lead (Averill & Needleman, 1980; Winneke & Krämer, 1997).
- *Programmed cell death.* Genetically controlled cell death, which is called apoptosis, is a normal part of the development of the brain. Teratogens cause apoptosis in some cells and not others and at different windows of time during brain development. Teratogens associated with apoptosis that have been well studied include alcohol (Goodlett et al., 2005), lead and methylmercury (Oberto, Marks, Evans, et al., 1996), and hyperthermia (Edwards, Saunders, & Shiota, 2003). Maternal hyperthermia may be due to fever of 38.9°C (102.02°F) for 24 hours or longer (Chambers, Johnson, Dick, et al., 1998) or to exposure to hot tubs or saunas (Milunsky, Ulcickas, Rothman, et al., 1992).

The sequelae of adverse influences on the process of brain development are determined primarily by the stage of brain development when the adverse effect occurs. In humans, the second half of gestation is a time of rapid, continuous growth of the brain (Pollard, 2007). During this time, the developing cerebral hemispheres and cerebellum are especially vulnerable to teratogens.

The sequelae are evidenced in different ways throughout an individual's life (Ornoy, 2006). The effects may be evident at birth, or they may be "sleepers," showing little or no effect in childhood and becoming apparent only under the more challenging life situations of adolescence or early adulthood (Mayes & Ward, 2003; Pollard, 2007; Rees & Inder, 2005). These later effects have been called the "deferred legacy of developmental neurotoxicity" (Weiss, 1996, p. 327).

Specific Neurotoxic Factors

Specific neurotoxic factors that affect the fetus' developing brain include cerebral hypoxia; nutritional deficiencies; and maternal infections, hyperthermia, exposure to neurotoxic drugs and environmental neurotoxicants, and stress (Moretti, Bar-Oz, & Fried, 2005; Pollard, 2007).

Cerebral Hypoxia

Fetal response to hypoxia includes edema, rupture of blood vessels, hemorrhage, formation of blood-filled blisters, and necroses of affected tissues. These responses may result in loss or distortion of structures that are in the process of forming or that have already formed (Rees, Breen, Loeliger, et al., 1999). Cerebral hypoxia has been found to be associated with the presence of anomalies such as club feet, syndactyly, and anencephaly (Fawcett & Brent, 2006).

Lack of oxygen to the developing fetal brain leads to different injuries depending on the duration of hypoxia and the stage of gestation. Brief periods of fetal hypoxia may result in neuronal cell death in the cerebellum, hippocampus, and cerebral cortex. It may also result in damage to glial cells and glial processes and in reduced synaptic connectedness (Rees & Inder, 2005). Chronic mild placental insufficiency that causes reduced levels of oxygen and restriction of nutrients may result in fetal growth restriction, deficits in neuronal connectivity, and diminished myelinization (Rees & Harding, 2004). Under hypoxic conditions, reduced uptake of glutamate by glial cells leads to an excess of glutamate in the synaptic cleft. Excessive glutamate allows more calcium to enter the cells and may result in neuronal cell death or in damage to glial matter or to the axons of neurons (Rees & Harding, 2004). Increased cell death associated with hypoxemia may reduce the total number of neurons in the hippocampus, cerebellum, and cerebral cortex, with resulting impairments of neural connectivity and postnatal brain functioning (Rees & Harding, 2004).

Nutritional Deficiencies

Effect of Deficiencies on Neurological Development

Good fetal nutrition means that the fetus has a consistent supply of amino acids, glucose, trace elements, and vitamins (Morgane, Austin-LaFrance, Bronzino, et al., 1993). Maternal malnutrition before conception and during pregnancy has an adverse effect on fetal brain development and the development of neurotransmitter systems (Rao & Georgieff, 2003). In the developing brain, it is the neurotransmitters that regulate neurogenesis, neuronal migration, and synaptogenesis (Wainwright & Martin, 2005). Thus, the effect of malnutrition on the development of neurotransmitter systems is seen in abnormalities of brain development and diminished capacity of neurons to communicate.

The effects of prenatal nutritional deficiencies are seen as neurodevelopmental defects of the central nervous system, for example, spina bifida (a neural tube defect involving the spine), anencephaly (absence of part of the brain), and microencephaly (abnormally small head), and with increased rates of psychopathology. Nutritional defects have also been found to be associated with impaired verbal and spatial abilities and reduced IQ (Rao & Georgieff, 2003).

Famine suffered by civilian populations during World War II had devastating effects on fetal brain development. During the Dutch "Hunger Winter" of 1944-1945, the Nazi blockade resulted in severe famine in the western part of Holland. Babies conceived at the height of the famine had small heads, anencephaly, and neural tube defects. Later, among the adults who had been exposed to prenatal famine in early gestation, there was a twofold increase in the rate of schizophrenia and increased rates of schizoid and schizotypal personality disorders (Hoek, Susser, Buck, et al., 1996). There was also an increase in major depressive disorder in males (Brown, Susser, Lin, et al., 1995). Similarly, during the siege of Leningrad, which lasted from August 1941 to January 1943, including an extremely cold winter of 1942, the citizens suffered severe deprivation of food, heat, and medical care. Among the babies born during the siege, there was a very high rate of stillbirths (26%), premature births (30%), low birth weight babies (50%), and babies with many anomalies of the head (Antonov, 1947).

Famine is not the only cause of prenatal nutritional deficits. Brain development can be affected by either insufficient quantity or insufficient supply of specific nutrients such as essential fatty acids, folic acid, vitamins, and minerals (Greenblatt, Huffman, & Reiss, 1994; Saugstad, 2004; Scott, Weir, Molloy, et al., 1994; Wainwright, 2002). Nutritional deficiency can also be due to protein energy malnutrition, which may be related to starvation, as seen in developing countries, and which may be found in women with poor nutritional status, poor prenatal care, and poor socioeconomic status and among those who smoke (Rao & Georgieff, 2003). Protein energy malnutrition alters the processes of synaptogenesis and myelinization that are involved in communication and information processing.

Effect of Specific Nutritional Deficiencies

Polyunsaturated Fatty Acids

There is increasing evidence that polyunsaturated fatty acids play a role in brain development and functioning through their involvement in neuronal survival and plasticity. They give flexibility to neuronal cell membranes, thus allowing the membranes to quickly change and form new connections (Wainwright & Martin, 2005).

In addition, the brain is largely composed of long-chain polyunsaturated fatty acids, primarily docosahexaenoic acid (one of the omega-3 fatty acids) and arachidonic acid (a component of lecithin) (Saugstad, 2004). Saugstad added that "normal brain development before birth, in infancy, and later on, cannot be accomplished if the fatty acids are deficient during pregnancy and lactation" (p. 5). In support of her view, she pointed out that East African Digo infants, whose mothers have a diet rich in fatty acids during pregnancy, are 3 to 4 weeks ahead of European and American infants in sensorimotor measures at birth and during the first year of life.

Deficiency of alpha-linolenic acid, one of the omega-3 fatty acids, alters the course of brain development by disturbing the composition and chemical properties of brain cell membranes, neurons, and two of the classes of glial cells—the oligodendrocytes that form myelin, and the astrocytes that link the neuron with its blood supply (Bourre, 2004; Scott et al., 1994) (see Chapter 2). The disruption of brain cell membrane formation and functioning results in neurosensory and behavioral impairments.

Folic Acid

Folic acid is an essential vitamin for brain development. Folate deficiency is known to result in neural tube defects such as anencephaly, which is absence of the cranial vault, and spina bifida, which is a defect in closure of the bony encasement that encloses the spinal cord (Simpson, Bailey, Pietrzik, et al., 2010). Animal studies have shown that folic acid is involved in neurogenesis, cell growth, and myelinization (Scott et al., 1994).

Zinc

Zinc is a trace element that is involved in gene transcription, in the activity of other enzymes involved in cellular metabolism, and in the synthesis of serotonin and melatonin (Johnson, 2001). Zinc deficiencies that cause abnormal brain development by altering protein synthesis are thought to be associated with impairments of learning and altered attention (Rao & Georgieff, 2003).

Iron

Iron is essential for lipid metabolism in the developing brain. It is involved in the process of myelinization. Prenatal iron deficiency is associated with alterations of neuronal proliferation and is believed to be associated with impairment of learning and memory tasks and with reduced IQ (Rao & Georgieff, 2003).

Vitamins

Vitamins are essential co-factors in the synthesis of neurotransmitters. For example, ascorbic acid and vitamin B_{12} are required for the synthesis of dopamine, and thiamin, glucose, and choline are essential for the synthesis of acetylcholine. Vitamins are also essential for energy metabolism by the brain, for maintaining the brain's blood supply, for receptor binding of neurotransmitters, and for nerve conduction (Haller, 2005). Animal studies suggest that prenatal deprivation of vitamin D_3 causes impaired brain development owing to abnormalities of cell proliferation (McGrath, Feron, Burne, et al., 2004).

Maternal Infections

Prenatal exposure to maternal infections may damage the migrating neurons or cause cell death. It is believed that intrauterine infections cause fetal brain damage by producing proinflammatory cytokines in the fetal systemic circulation. The cytokines then pass through the blood-brain barrier into the fetal brain where they cause the death of glial cells—specifically astrocytes—and damage to the neural axons (Rees & Harding, 2004). During different windows of time, exposure to the same infections results in different forms of damage to the brain. For example, exposure to maternal rubella during the sixth week of gestation is associated with fetal cataracts; during the ninth week, with deafness; and during the fifth through tenth weeks, with cardiac defects and dental anomalies. Table 3-1 lists maternal infections and their effects on prenatal brain development and long-term sequelae.

Maternal Exposure to Neurotoxic Drugs

Adverse effects of prenatal exposure to certain drugs, prescribed and illegal, are presented in Table 3-2. However, maternal exposure to one neurotoxic drug is often concurrent with exposure to other neurotoxic drugs, infections, nutritional deficiencies, and stress. In addition, women who abuse drugs while pregnant tend to have poorer prenatal care, increased rates of sexually transmitted diseases, and more comorbid psychiatric disorders than those who do not abuse drugs (Bishai & Koren, 2001). Therefore, it is difficult to determine the effect of one neurotoxic drug on the developing embryonic/fetal brain (Kosofsky & Hyman, 2001).

Although the focus of this section of the chapter is the effect of agents on brain development, the presence of facial dysmorphic features is included in the table when it occurs. Ornoy (2006) said that most children who have been exposed to agents such as antiepileptic medications that cause intellectual or learning deficits also have facial dysmorphic features. He pointed out that the brain development is closely interrelated with the development of craniofacial structures and that disruption of development of craniofacial structures may be paralleled by disruptions of brain development.

TABLE 3-1 MATERNAL INFECTIONS: THEIR EFFECTS ON BRAIN DEVELOPMENT AND LONG-TERM SEQUELAE

Maternal Infections	Effect on Brain Development	Long-term Sequelae
Chlamydia trachomatis	Premature delivery; low birth weight (Geist & Koren, 2001)	Information not available
Cytomegalovirus (a member of the herpesvirus family) (1%–4% of pregnancies)	Microencephaly (Geist & Koren, 2001)	Mental retardation
Influenza	Neural tube defects, preterm delivery (possibly due to fetal exposure to the fever associated with the illness) (Rasmussen, Jamieson, & Bresee, 2008)	Increased risk for schizophrenia and major depressive disorder (Machon, Mednick, & Huttenen, 1997; Watson et al., 1999)
Malaria	Prematurity; low birth weight; growth retardation (Geist & Koren, 2001)	Information not available
Rubella (German measles)	Damage to developing brain occurs after rubella infection only in first 16 weeks of gestation Adverse effect on neuron proliferation Microencephaly (Webster, 1998)	Cerebral palsy; mental retardation; developmental deficits, e.g., intellectual, motor. and behavioral (Geist & Koren, 2001)
Syphilis	Multiple central nervous system problems; hydrocephalus (Geist & Koren, 2001)	Mental retardation
Toxoplasma gondii (parasite in feces of cats and undercooked or raw meat)	Hydrocephalus and microencephaly (Geist & Koren, 2001)	Learning disorders, movement problems, vision loss, and mental retardation (Geist & Koren, 2001) Increased risk for schizophrenia and schizophrenia spectrum disorders (Brown, Schaefer, Quesenberry, et al., 2005)
Varicella	Low birth weight, microencephaly, brain atrophy, growth retardation (Geist & Koren, 2001; Robert, Reuvers, & Schaefer, 2001)	Mental retardation

TABLE 3-2 NEUROTOXIC DRUGS: THEIR PUTATIVE MECHANISMS OF ACTION, EFFECTS ON FETAL BRAIN DEVELOPMENT, AND LONG-TERM SEQUELAE

Neurotoxic Drugs	Putative Mechanism of Action	Effect on Fetal Brain Development	Long-term Sequelae
Alcohol	Alterations in proliferation and migration of neurons (Miller, 1986; Miller & Potempa, 1990)	Microencephaly, brain malformations, mental retardation, and behavioral abnormalities (Costa et al., 2004; Moore & Persaud, 1993) Deficits of development of cerebellum, basal ganglia, caudate nucleus, brainstem, and corpus callosum (Costa et al., 2004; Fryer, McGee, Spandoni, et al., 2005) Abnormalities of hypothalamic-pituitary-adrenal axis with resulting elevated cortisol levels (Huizink et al., 2004)	Mental retardation; abnormal development of attention, memory, executive functioning, motor skills, learning, and judgment (Barr, Bookstein, O'Malley, et al., 2006; Costa et al., 2004) In adolescence, alcohol and drug use problems (Baer, Sampson, Barr, et al., 2003; Streissguth, Bookstein, Barr, et al., 2004) Antisocial behavior (Carmichael-Olson, Streissguth, Sampson, et al., 1997) Dysthymia, anxiety, and substance abuse (Mathew, Wilson, Blazer, et al., 1993)
Amphetamine	Causes vasoconstriction	Premature birth, growth retardation (Garbis & McElhatton, 2001) Brain abnormalities, microencephaly, neural tube defects (Nulman, Atanackovic, & Koren, 2001)	Hyperexcitability; impaired functioning in language, mathematics, and sports (Cernerud, Eriksson, Jonsson, et al., 1996)
Benzodiazepines (used by 2% of pregnant women) (Bergman, Wilholm, Rosa, et al., 1992)	Different benzodiazepines are associated with different risks of teratology (Iqbal, Sobhan, & Ryals, 2002); evidence is not conclusive but suggests that exposure during 2 weeks to 8 weeks of gestation should be avoided; benzodiazepines target the GABA system receptors, and GABA is associated with early migration of neurons to form the brain (Thompson et al., 2009)	Case reports of oral clefts, but research is inconclusive; reports of central nervous system defects Microencephaly (Garbis & McElhatton, 2001) Studies of abnormalities are not conclusive (Dolovich, Addis, & Vaillancourt, 2001)	Floppy infant syndrome (sedation, apnea, tremors, cyanosis) (Garbis & McElhatton, 2001)
Carbamazepine	Use during first trimester is associated with neural tube defects (Matalon, Schechtman, Goldzweig, et al., 2002; Stahl, 2005)	Low birth weight, craniosynostosis, cleft palate (Diav-Citrin, Shechtman, Arnon, et al., 2001) Microencephaly (Robert et al., 2001) Possible risks of neural tube defects (spina bifida) (Stahl, 2005; Ornoy, 2006)	Slight reduction of cognitive functioning in school-age children (Ornoy, 2006)
Cocaine	Impairment of cell differentiation and formation of the neural tube (Volpe, 1992) Disruption of neuronal migration (Kosofsky & Hyman, 2001) Impairs maternal reuptake of norepinephrine and epinephrine that is associated with vasoconstriction and uterine vasoconstriction and increases excitatory effect of dopamine	Microencephaly, agenesis of the corpus callosum, neuronal heterotopia, abnormal development of layers of cortex Premature birth, intrauterine growth retardation (Bishai & Koren, 2001)	Functional impairment: motor, emotional stability, attention, cognition language, and relationships (Lester, LaGasse, & Seifer, 1998; Thompson et al., 2009) Language delays (Nulman et al., 2001)
Heroin	Intrauterine growth restriction, e.g., smaller head circumference indicating smaller brain size (Bandstra, Morrow, Mansoor, et al., 2010)	Preterm delivery (Bishai & Koren, 2001) Low birth weight (Schneiderman, 2001) Smaller head (Persaud et al., 1990)	Increased risk for sudden infant death (Schaefer, 2001) Hyperactivity, brief attention span, temper outbursts (Persaud et al., 1990)
Lithium	Increased risk for birth defects (Stahl, 2005), but not all researchers agree	Reduced head size (Ornoy, 2006)	Floppy infant syndrome (sedation, apnea, tremors, cyanosis) (Garbis & McElhatton, 2001)

TABLE 3-2 NEUROTOXIC DRUGS: THEIR PUTATIVE MECHANISMS OF ACTION, EFFECTS ON FETAL BRAIN DEVELOPMENT, AND LONG-TERM SEQUELAE—continued

Neurotoxic Drugs	Putative Mechanism of Action	Effect on Fetal Brain Development	Long-term Sequelae
Marijuana (fat soluble; remains in bloodstream for 30 days)	Increased blood levels of carbon monoxide and decreased levels of oxygen Thought to affect neural adhesive molecules that are involved in cell proliferation, migration, and synaptogenesis (Gomez, Hernandez, Johansson, et al., 2003)	Affects developing amygdala and systems that regulate emotional behavior (Wang, Dow-Edwards, Anderson, et al., 2004)	In infants, tremors, sleep disturbances, and increased startle response (Huizink & Mulder, 2006) Increased hyperactivity, impulsivity, and inattention; increased externalizing problems (Goldschmidt, Day, & Richardson, 2000) Impaired executive functioning (planning, problem-solving, analyzing, and modification of behavior in response to feedback) (Fried, 2002)
Nicotine	Constriction of blood flow; reduced fetal uptake of serotonin; alterations of dopamine and norepinephrine systems; altered cholinergic brain cell growth (Marret, 2005; Wakschlag, Lahey, Loeber, et al., 1997) Disruption of cell differentiation; reduced dendritic branching	Premature birth, intrauterine growth retardation, low birth weight (Lindsay, Thomas, Catalano, et al., 1997)	Sudden infant death syndrome (Shah et al., 2006) Increased rates of hyperactivity, conduct disorder in boys (Ernst, Moolchan, & Robinson, 2001; Fergusson, Woodward, & Horwood, 1998; Wakschlag et al., 1997) Increased rates of substance abuse (Maughan, Taylor, Tallor, et al., 2001) Learning, language, reading problems (Fried, O'Connell, & Watkinson, 1992a; Fried, Watkinson, & Gray, 1992b) Attention deficit- hyperactivity disorder (Huizink & Mulder, 2006; Linnet, Dalsgaard, Obel, et al., 2003; Thaper, O'Donovan, & Owen, 2003) Lower IQ, poorer impulse control, impaired visual-perceptual performance in adolescents (Fried, 2002)
Phenobarbital	Abnormalities of ridge patterns of fingers indicating early damage to developing brain (Bokhari, Coull, & Holmes, 2002) (see Chapter 2 for discussion of abnormalities of finger ridges and brain development)	Facial anomalies, growth deficiencies (Costa et al., 2004) Low birth weight Small head circumference and decreased intellectual functioning (Ornoy, 2006)	Reduced head size (Ornoy, 2006) Developmental delays and impaired cognitive functioning (Costa et al., 2004)
Phenytoin	(Same as for Phenobarbital)	Prenatal growth retardation Microencephaly (Costa et al., 2004)	Learning disabilities and decreased IQ scores (Costa et al., 2004) Not conclusive (Ornoy, 2006)
Retinoids (Retin A)	(Same as above)	Increased abortion and stillbirths. CNS defects, microencephaly, absent cerebellar vermis, abnormalities of head and ears	Intelligence deficits (Peters & Schaefer, 2001)
Toluol; chlorinated hydrocarbons (sniffing substances; e.g., glues, paints, paint thinners)	Results suggest that exposure to PCBs and/or hexachlorobenzene at background levels may affect thyroid function during pregnancy; e.g., maternal thyroid hormones play an essential role in fetal neurodevelopment (Chevrier, Eskenazi, Holland, et al., 2008)	Symptoms similar to fetal alcohol syndrome Microencephaly (Schneiderman, 2001)	Attention deficits, central nervous system dysfunction (Schneiderman, 2001) Fetal solvent syndrome (Bentur & Koren, 2001, p. 533)
Valproic acid	Antagonist for folic acid receptors (blocks) and causes depletion of vitamin K (Ornoy, 2006)	Severe neural tube deficits such as spina bifida and microencephaly (Costa et al., 2004; Stahl, 2005)	Developmental delays, mental retardation, cognitive impairment, and behavioral deficits (Costa et al., 2004; Wyszynski, Nambisan, Surve, et al., 2005) Autism (Rodier, 2000) Hyperactivity (Moore, Turnpenny, Quinn, et al., 2000) Fetal anticonvulsant syndrome may be associated with brain dysfunction and autistic disorder (Ornoy, 2006; Rasalam, Hailey, Williams, et al., 2005; Thompson et al., 2009)

Continued

TABLE 3-2 NEUROTOXIC DRUGS: THEIR PUTATIVE MECHANISMS OF ACTION, EFFECTS ON FETAL BRAIN DEVELOPMENT, AND LONG-TERM SEQUELAE—continued

Neurotoxic Drugs	Putative Mechanism of Action	Effect on Fetal Brain Development	Long-term Sequelae
Vitamin A	In animal studies, doses of vitamin A resulted in abnormalities of migration of neural crest cells that form craniofacial structures (Mulder, Manley, Grant, et al., 2000)	Central nervous system malformations with maternal dosage in excess of 25,000 IU daily (Peters & Schaefer, 2001)	Mental retardation (Jain, 2011)

Maternal Health Conditions

Certain maternal health conditions—including diabetes, epilepsy, hypothyroidism, phenylketonuria, folic acid deficiency, and binge drinking—and their effects on fetal brain development and long-term sequelae are discussed in Table 3-3.

Maternal Exposure to Environmental Neurotoxicants

Maternal exposure to the environmental neurotoxicants methylmercury, lead, ionizing radiation, polychlorinated biphenyls (PCB), carbon monoxide, and hazardous waste landfill sites can affect embryonic/fetal development. More information on these effects can be found in Table 3-4.

Maternal Stress and Stressful Events

It is common folklore that maternal emotions and distressing experiences affect the developing fetus. Although those early views were later disavowed for lack of scientific evidence, it is now known that maternal stress has the potential to adversely affect brain development through its influence on the development of the fetal autonomic nervous system and central nervous system (McEwen, Gould, Sakai, 1992; Wadhwa, Dunkel-Schetter, Chicz-DeMet, et al., 1996). Prenatal exposure to maternal stress has also been found to be associated with a smaller head circumference (Lou, Hansen, Nordentoft, et al., 1994), suggesting compromised brain development and a smaller brain, which increase the risk of cognitive deficits and neuropsychiatric disorders in adulthood (Spauwen, Krabbendam, Lieb, et al., 2004; Weinstrock, 2001).

The effect of stress on the developing brain may be related to cortisol. Maternal stress is associated with elevated plasma levels of cortisol, and chronic stress appears to affect the fetus more than episodic stress (Huizink, Robles de Medina, Mulder, et al., 2002; van den Bergh, 1990). Exposure to maternal stress-induced elevated levels of cortisol may adversely affect later functioning of the child's hypothalamic-pituitary-adrenal (HPA) axis, behavior, cognition, and response to stressors (Welberg & Seckl, 2001).

In animal studies, early exposure to glucocorticoids—which are similar to cortisol—modified the development of neurotransmitter systems including the norepinephrine, serotonin, dopamine, and gamma-aminobutyric acid (GABA) systems (Diaz, Fuxe, & Ogren, 1997; Lewis, 2000); in addition, prenatal exposure to elevated levels of glucocorticoids resulted in hippocampal damage (Uno, Lohmiller, Thierme, et al., 1990) and alteration of dendrites in the hippocampus (Lawrence & Sapolsky, 1994; Wooley, Gould, &

TABLE 3-3 MATERNAL HEALTH CONDITIONS: THEIR EFFECTS ON FETAL BRAIN DEVELOPMENT AND LONG-TERM SEQUELAE

Maternal Health Conditions	Effect on Fetal Brain Development	Long-term Sequelae
Binge drinking (5 or more drinks on one occasion) (Barr, Bookstein, O'Malley, et al., 2006)	Inhibition of central nervous system development (Schaefer, 2001)	In preschool children, distractibility (Schaefer, 2001) Increased substance abuse, dependence, passive-aggressive disorder, and antisocial disorders and traits (Barr, Bookstein, O'Malley, et al., 2006)
Diabetes (1% of pregnancies) (Geist & Koren, 2001)	Neural tube defects, anencephaly, spina bifida, microencephaly (Geist & Koren, 2001)	No information available
Epilepsy (0.3%–0.5% of pregnancies)	Neural tube defects (Geist & Koren, 2001)	Mental disorders, mild developmental deficits and lower IQ scores among adult males (Ehrenstein, Sorensen, & Pedersen, 2011)
Folic acid deficiency (1 in 3 women worldwide) (Geist & Koren, 2001)	Neural tube defects (Schaefer & Peters, 2001)	No information available
		Cerebral palsy and mental retardation
Hypothyroidism	Low birth weight (Geist & Koren, 2001)	Learning difficulties (Morreale de Escobar, Obregón, & Escobar del Rey, 2000)
Phenylketonuria	Microencephaly	Mental retardation

TABLE 3-4 MATERNAL EXPOSURE TO ENVIRONMENTAL NEUROTOXICANTS: PUTATIVE MECHANISMS OF ACTION, EFFECTS ON FETAL BRAIN DEVELOPMENT, AND LONG-TERM SEQUELAE

Environmental Neurotoxicants	Putative Mechanism of Action	Effect on Fetal Brain Development	Long-term Sequelae
Carbon monoxide	Hypoxic ischemic injuries	Central nervous system abnormalities, encephalopathy (Bailey, 2001)	Mental and motor impairments, seizures, involuntary movements (Bailey, 2001)
Hazardous waste landfill sites (living within 3 km of site)	Information not available	Neural tube defects Growth retardation (McElhatton, Garbis, & Schaeuer, 2001)	Information not available
Ionizing radiation (exposure to atomic bomb)	Disruption of neuronal proliferation and migration; ectopic neurons (Mole, 1982)	Microencephaly, thinning of the thalamus and cerebral cortex (Peters & Schaefer, 2001)	Mental retardation and 20% increase in psychotic disorders (Mole, 1982; Miller, 1956; Otake & Schull, 1984)
Ionizing radiation (exposure to Chernobyl nuclear reactor accident) (Chernobyl, 2003)	Information not available	Low birth weight babies, increased rate of babies born with Down's syndrome and neural tube defects (Harjulehto, Aro, Rita, et al., 1989; Little, 1993; McElhatton, Garbis, Schaefer, et al., 2001b)	Motor learning deficits (Ericson & Källén, 1994) Impairment of cognitive functioning (Gamache, Levinson, Reeves, et al., 2005)
Methylmercury (70% of mercury in environment comes from man-made sources, e.g., coal-fired electric power generators, waste dumps; exposure is primarily through seafood contaminated by mercury but also airborne vapors)	Disrupts cell proliferation and migration by affecting cell adhesive molecules (Lewandowski, Ponce, Charleston, et al., 2003; Takizawa & Kitamura, 2001)	Microencephaly, spina bifida (Davidson, Myers, & Weiss, 2004; Feldstein & Singer, 1997)	Minamata disease—increased rates of cerebral palsy, seizures, and mental retardation (Harada, 1995) Sensory and motor disturbances, cerebral palsy, seizures, blindness, deafness, impaired language and cognition, and mental retardation (Bakir, Rustam, Tikriti, et al., 1980; Burbacher, Rodier, & Weiss, 1990; Debes, Budtz-Jorgensen, Weihe, et al., 2006; Oken, Wright, Kleinman, et al., 2005)
Polychlorinated biphenyls (PCB)	PCBs can disrupt dopamine levels and dopaminergic functioning in the brain (dopamine regulates dendritic growth) and can reduce circulating levels of thyroid hormones that are important for brain development (Sagiv, Thurston, Bellinger, et al., 2010)	Smaller heads (thought to reflect a smaller brain); low birth weight (Bentur, Zalzatien, & Koren, 2001)	Increased impulsivity, impaired memory (Jacobson & Jacobson, 2003) Mental retardation (Peters & Schaefer, 2001) Increased risk of attention deficit-hyperactivity disorder (Sagiv et al., 2010)

McEwen, 1990). These findings have implications for the common practice of administering synthetic corticosteroids such as betamethasone to women at risk for premature delivery (Ng, Wong, Lam, et al., 1999). Repeated antenatal courses of corticosteroids have been found to be associated with aggressive-destructive behaviors and greater distractibility and hyperactivity in children (French, Hagan, Evans, et al., 2004; Velisek, 2005). Other studies have shown that children who had been exposed to dexamethasone prematurely because of the mothers' risk of congenital adrenal hyperplasia had increased emotionality, unsociability, avoidance, and behavioral problems and reduced head circumference (Trautman, Meyer-Bahlburg, Postelnek, et al., 1995).

Maternal stress can be caused by everyday factors—such as financial problems, family conflict, caregiving burden, or social isolation (Kofman, 2002)—or by extreme political or natural events, such as wars, earthquakes, and snow and ice storms.

- *War.* In an early study, children of mothers whose husbands died during the pregnancy (mostly during World War II) had increased rates of schizophrenia and other psychiatric disorders (Huttenen & Niskanen, 1978). In another study, both male and female offspring of women who were in the first trimester of their pregnancy during the 5-day 1940 invasion of the Netherlands in World War II had increased rates of schizophrenia (van Os & Selten, 1998), but among mothers in their second trimester, only male offspring had increased rates of schizophrenia. Among children whose mothers were pregnant during the Arab-Israel War, there were increased rates of developmental delays and behavioral problems (Meijer, 1985).

- *Earthquake.* Exposure to earthquakes early in pregnancy has been found to be associated with a shorter gestational period (Glynn, Wadhwa, Dunkel-Schetter, et al., 2001). Among adults who were exposed prenatally to a severe earthquake in China, there was a significant increase in unipolar depression among males who had been exposed during the second trimester of pregnancy, but not among females (Watson, Mednick, Huttunen, et al., 1999).
- *Snow and ice.* Among 2-year-old children born to mothers who had been pregnant during the 1998 ice storm in Canada that affected 1.5 million people and lasted from hours to 5 weeks, there was impairment of language and general intelligence in comparison to those whose mothers had not experienced the ice storm. The more severe the mother's stress, the greater was the child's impairment. The damage was greatest for exposure to maternal stress during the first and second trimesters of pregnancy and least for exposure during the third trimester (Laplante, Barr, Brunet, et al., 2004).

New epidemiological and neurohormonal evidence suggests a relationship between a stressful intrauterine environment and preterm delivery (Pike, 2005). According to Pike (2005), maternal cues are delivered to the fetus through glucocorticoids, which are stress hormones in the mother's blood. These cues signal to the developing fetus that the intrauterine environment is insufficient due to nutritional stress or maternal psychosocial stress. The fetus responds with accelerated organ maturation and hormonal changes that lead to an early expulsion from the stressful environment. In addition to premature birth, there is also evidence that prenatal stress may be associated with low birth weight and smaller head circumference (Copper, Goldenberg, Das, et al., 1996; Hedegaard, Hendriksen, Sabroe, et al., 1996). Exposure to chronic gestational stress can have long-term effects on neuronal development that may be associated with impaired adaptation to new experiences, altered attention and cognition, increased emotionality, and retarded motor development (Huizink, Mulder, & Buitelaar, 2004). The effect of prenatal exposure to maternal stress may also be revealed by different types of childhood behavioral disorders (Kofman, 2002; Weinstrock, 2001) and possibly by onset of psychopathology in later life (Austin, Leader, & Reilly, 2005; Koubovec, Geerts, Odendaal, et al., 2005).

Perinatal Factors Influencing Brain Development and Functioning

Perinatal factors that influence brain development and functioning include hypoxia, prematurity, and Rh incompatibility. Maternal psychiatric disorders also affect perinatal brain development and functioning, as does being born "unwanted" by the parents.

Hypoxia

Hypoxia depletes cell energy, which in turn activates neuroexcitatory processes that can lead to cell death (Rees & Inder, 2005; Reiss, Plomin, & Hetherington, 1991). In premature infants, cerebral white matter that is made up of glial cells is most likely to be injured following hypoxia. The resulting damage, called periventricular leukomalacia, includes cystic infarcts near the lateral ventricles and widespread gliosis, which is an indication of glial healing processes after central nervous system injury. It is thought that injury to neurons in the cerebral cortex, hippocampus, and cerebellum is secondary to injury of glial cells.

Prematurity

Premature birth disrupts pregnancy during the time when the brain is developing most rapidly (Marlow, 2004). Premature birth is associated with reductions in brain volume in specific regions: the sensorimotor cortex, cerebellum, basal ganglia, amygdala, hippocampus, and corpus callosum (Peterson, Vohr, Staib, et al., 2000). These abnormalities in development are associated with poorer cognitive functioning and lower levels of intelligence. Involvement of the motor area of the cortex, basal ganglia, and corpus callosum is thought to be associated with the high rates of cerebral palsy and motor disturbances seen in children who are born preterm. The sequelae of preterm birth are seen later in childhood as learning disabilities, deficits in executive function, language impairment, difficulties in visual-motor integration, motor coordination disorders, behavioral problems, attention deficit-hyperactivity disorder, and reduced educational achievement (Salt & Redshaw, 2006).

Low Birth Weight and Preterm Infants

Most studies of infants born before term use birth weight as the identifying factor, but others use gestational age as the identifying factor. Studies based on birth weight are not directly comparable to studies based on gestational age because they may include infants of older gestational age with restriction of intrauterine growth.

Low birth weight infants are considered to have a birth weight between 1501 g and 2500 g; *very low birth weight infants* are considered to have a birth weight between 1001 g and 1500 g; and *extremely low birth weight infants* weigh 1000 g or less (Marlow, 2004; Salt, D'Amore, Ahluwalia, et al., 2006). *Very preterm infants* are infants born at 30 weeks or less, whereas *extremely preterm infants* are infants born before 26 weeks of gestation (Marlow). Although the terms "extremely low birth weight" and "extremely preterm birth" are sometimes used interchangeably, they will be discussed separately because extremely preterm birth reflects the stage of development of the brain more accurately than does extremely low birth weight.

The developing fetal brain is most vulnerable in the late second and early third trimesters. Although the survival rate for very preterm infants is improving, the incidence of neurodevelopmental problems in very preterm infants and very low birth weight infants is still high (Ment, Vohr, Allan, et al., 1999). The most frequent abnormalities involve reduced brain volume (Nosarti, Al-Asady, Frangou, et al., 2002) and abnormalities of the ventricles, the corpus callosum, and the white matter of the brain (Nosarti, Rushe, Woodruff, et al., 2004). Infants born very prematurely have a high risk of intraventricular and periventricular hemorrhage and of hypoxic-ischemic damage. In response to metabolic and hemodynamic stress, the capillaries involved in the process of producing neurons and glial cells may bleed, sometimes into the adjacent ventricle. This response has been reported to occur in 40% of very low birth weight babies (Whitaker, Van Rossem, Feldman, et al., 1997, pp. 847-848).

The effects of abnormal brain development on very low birth weight children and very preterm children are manifested across the life span. Table 3-5 lists the early, childhood, adolescent, and early adulthood outcomes of very low birth weight and extremely low birth weight infants, and Table 3-6 lists the early and childhood outcomes of very preterm and extremely preterm infants and the adolescent outcomes of very preterm infants.

To summarize Tables 3-5 and 3-6, in comparing the outcomes of children born preterm to those born at full term, children born preterm have been found to have four to five times the rate of attention deficit-hyperactivity disorder. The number requiring special educational services was more than twice that of full-term infants (61% vs. 23%). In childhood, those born preterm have higher rates of

- Impaired cognitive functioning
- Academic problems
- Behavioral problems, such as hyperactivity
- Problems with social skills
- Attention problems
- Shyness and withdrawn behavior
- Asthma
- Visual and hearing impairments
- Cerebral palsy (Hack & Klein, 2006; Watts & Saigal, 2006)

As adults, they have lower IQs and lower levels of academic achievement. They are more likely to be employed in less skilled occupations, to have more health problems, and to have fewer risk-taking behaviors. Among men, there was increased risk of thought or attention problems; among women, there were more anxiety and depressive symptoms (Hack, Flannery, Schluchter, et al., 2002; Hack & Klein, 2006).

TABLE 3-5 OUTCOMES OF VERY LOW BIRTH WEIGHT AND EXTREMELY LOW BIRTH WEIGHT INFANTS

Birth Weight	Early Outcomes (to Age 2 Years)	Childhood Outcomes	Adolescent Outcomes	Early Adulthood Outcomes
Very low birth weight (less than 1500 g)	Cerebral palsy (6.2%); developmental delays (13.7%) (Salt & Redshaw, 2006) Smaller head (24% smaller circumference thought to reflect a smaller brain) (Peterson, Taylor, Minich, et al., 2006)	Special education (19%–22%); held back one year (22%–26%); received special help in regular class (11%–15%) (Hille, Den Ouden, & Bauer, 1994); Difficulties with social behaviors, cognition, and attention (Hille, Den Ouden, & Saigal, 2001) 28% of those between 750 g and 1499 g had IQ less than 85 (Hack, Taylor, Klein, et al., 1994)	Growth abnormalities (49%); mental or emotional problems (58%); limitation of physical activity (32%); visual impairment (31%) (Hack, Taylor, Klein, et al., 2000) Increased rates of psychiatric symptoms such as attention deficits, anxiety symptoms, and problems with relationships (Indredavik, Vik, Heyerdahl, et al., 2004) Attention deficit-hyperactivity disorder (28%) (Botting, Powls, Cooke, et al., 1997)	Less likely to have graduated from high school; lower mean IQ (87 vs. 92) Men: less likely to be enrolled in college; have less risk-taking behaviors, less use of alcohol and drugs, and less contact with police Women: fewer had ever had intercourse, been pregnant, or delivered a live baby (Hack et al., 2002) Less advanced educational achievement, poorer physical abilities, higher blood pressures, and poorer respiratory functioning (Hack, Flannery, & Schluchter, 2002) Age 20 years: Men: more thought problems (attention) Women: more anxiety and depressive symptoms (Hack, Youngstrom, Carter, et al., 2004)

Continued

TABLE 3-5 **OUTCOMES OF VERY LOW BIRTH WEIGHT AND EXTREMELY LOW BIRTH WEIGHT INFANTS—continued**

Birth Weight	Early Outcomes (to Age 2 Years)	Childhood Outcomes	Adolescent Outcomes	Early Adulthood Outcomes
Extremely low birth weight (less than 1000 g)	Cerebral palsy (10%–14%); developmental delays (21.5%) (Hack, Taylor, Drotar, et al., 2005; Marlow, 2004; Salt, D'Amore, Ahluwalia, et al., 2006)	Social, cognitive, and attention problems (Hille et al., 2001; Wolke, 1997) 50% of those born at less than 750 g had IQ less than 85 (Hack et al., 1994) More chronic conditions and functional limitations; poor motor skills and poor adaptive functioning (Hack et al., 2005) Learning problems (41%); impairment of visual short-term memory and fine and gross motor functioning; problems working independently; poor social skills and withdrawal from challenging tasks (Whitfield, Grunau, & Holsti, 1997) Impaired executive functioning (Salt & Redshaw, 2006)	Information not available	Self-reported: functional limitations of cognition, mobility, self-care; less likely to go to college or be employed (Saigal, Stoskopf, Pinelli, et al., 2006)

TABLE 3-6 **OUTCOMES OF VERY PRETERM AND EXTREMELY PRETERM INFANTS**

Gestational Age	Early Outcomes (to Age 2 Years)	Childhood Outcomes	Adolescent Outcomes
Very preterm (30 weeks or less gestational age)	Developmental or cognitive impairment; cerebral palsy (6.9%) (Salt & Redshaw, 2006) Blindness; deafness; transient dystonia; feeding difficulties; delayed language skills (Marlow, 2004) Cognitive handicaps (2%–5%) (McCarton, Brooks-Gunn, Wallace, et al., 1997; McCormick, Workman-Daniels, & Brooks-Gunn, 1996)	Cognitive impairment; motor impairment; visual-spatial-perceptual problems; attention deficit-hyperactivity disorder; psychiatric symptoms; ocular impairments; poor auditory discrimination; special education needs (Marlow, 2004) More than 50% require special assistance in school. with nearly 20% requiring special education classrooms and 16% repeating at least one grade (McCarton et al., 1997; McCormick et al., 1996) Impaired executive functioning (Salt & Redshaw, 2006) Risk for psychiatric disorders was 23%, nearly three times greater than for children of normal birth weight children; e.g., attention deficit-hyperactivity disorder (12%); emotional disorders (9%); and autism septum disorders (8%) (Johnson, Hollis, Kochhar, et al., 2010).	Reduced volume of cerebellum; cognitive deficits (Allin, Matsumoto, Santhouse, et al., 2001) Impairment of verbal fluency and intellectual functioning (Allin, Walshe, Fern, et al., 2008)
Extremely preterm (26 weeks or less gestational age)	Head size was smaller at 30 months (thought to reflect a smaller brain) (Wood, Marlow, Costeloe, et al., 2000) Cognitive impairment most common disability (Marlow, Wolke, Bracewell, et al., 2005) About half had disability (severe, 23%, and less severe, 26%) Impaired mental and psychomotor development, neuromotor function, or sensory (hearing and vision) and communication function (7% had no speech at 30 months) (Wood et al., 2000)	Cognitive impairment (41%); cerebral palsy (20%) (Barclay, 2005; Marlow et al., 2005) At age 8 years: Cognitive, educational, and behavioral impairments (Andersen, Nielsen, & Grandjean, 2003)	Information not available

Rh Incompatibility

Another perinatal factor that may influence brain development and functioning is Rh compatibility. The plus or minus following a blood type represents the presence or absence of the Rh factor, which is a protein found on the red blood cell's surface. Most individuals produce this protein and thus are Rh positive. However, about 15% of whites and 7% of blacks do not produce it and are Rh negative.

One example of when Rh status becomes important is when the mother is Rh negative and the father is Rh positive. If the baby inherits the father's Rh-positive blood, during pregnancy, red blood cells from the fetus may enter the mother's bloodstream. If the mother is Rh negative, her system cannot tolerate the Rh-positive red blood cells, and her immune system responds by making antibodies against the red blood cells of the fetus. In a first pregnancy, there is little risk of Rh-induced hemolytic disease because the baby is born before the mother's antibodies are produced and can harm the baby. In later pregnancies, however, the mother's antibodies can reach the fetus and destroy fetal red blood cells, causing the release of free hemoglobin into the fetus' circulation. Hemoglobin is converted into bilirubin that causes the infant to become jaundiced.

Hydrops fetalis is a severe form of Rh incompatibility. It is characterized by massive fetal red blood cell destruction, anemia, fetal heart failure, total body swelling, enlarged liver, respiratory distress, and circulatory collapse. Death can occur as early as 17 weeks of gestation and results in spontaneous abortion.

Because maternal antibodies remain in the infant's circulatory system, destruction of red blood cells can continue after birth, causing hyperbilirubinemia. Without a replacement transfusion, *kernicterus*—deposits of bilirubin in the brain—may occur. Kernicterus occurs several days after delivery and is characterized by a high-pitched cry, opisthotonos, bulging fontanel, and seizures. Among those who survive, there may be muscle rigidity, speech disorders, movement disorders, and mental retardation. Rh incompatibility has also been found to be associated with the development of schizophrenia in second-born male adults (Hollister, Laing, & Mednick, 1996).

Maternal Psychiatric Disorders

Prenatal maternal depression may slow fetal growth and increase risk for preterm delivery (Hoffman & Hatch, 2000). Maternal depression has been found to be associated with neurobiological alterations in children, such as elevated cortisol levels (Lundy, Jones, Field, et al., 1999). Infants born to mothers who experienced anxiety or depression during their pregnancy demonstrate excessive crying, fussiness, and irritability at birth (Austin et al., 2005). Later, the children show abnormal regulation of emotions, decreased motor development, and problems with social interactions, fear, and anxiety (Cohn & Campbell, 1992). Children of depressed mothers are at higher risk for emotional instability, depression, suicidal behaviors, and behavioral problems (van den Bergh & Marcoen, 2004), and they require more psychiatric treatment (Lyons-Ruth, Wolfe, & Lyubchik, 2000). There is less evidence of the effects of other maternal psychiatric disorders.

Born "Unwanted"

In a study of children born unwanted (defined as born to a mother who had twice been denied an abortion for the pregnancy), it was found that they were rated by teachers and mothers as having more negative qualities, lacking maturity, having problems in socializing, and being rejected by classmates in comparison to a control group of children of wanted pregnancies (David, 2006). As teenagers, the children did not achieve academically as well as the controls, and they dropped out of school more often (Myhrman, Olsen, Rantakallio, et al., 1995). In early adulthood (age 21 to 23 years), those born unwanted reported less job satisfaction, less satisfying social relationships, and more disappointments in love. They sought more psychiatric treatment than the controls, and twice as many had been incarcerated (David). Between ages 28 to 31 years, the differences between men born unwanted and the controls narrowed overall. However, within that age group, the differences for women who had been born unwanted increased. They were more likely to be unmarried or divorced, having problems with parenting, and unemployed. They tended to be depressed and to have received more psychiatric treatment than the controls. By age 35, 8.5% of those born unwanted had received inpatient psychiatric care in comparison to 1.2% of the controls. Anxiety and depression were the most common psychiatric disorders (David).

Other researchers reported that individuals born of unwanted pregnancies are at increased risk for developing schizophrenia (Myhrman, Rantakallio, Isohanni, et al., 1996) and, among women, for criminality (Kemppainen, Jokelainen, Isohanni, et al., 2002). In summary, there is evidence that the effects of being born unwanted continue through childhood and into adulthood and include impairment of cognitive, social, interpersonal, and academic/vocational functioning and increased rates of psychiatric disorders (David, 2006; David, Dytych, & Matejcek, 2003; Forssman & Thuwe, 1966; Kubicka, Roth, Dytrych, et al., 2002). Chapter 19 provides a discussion of interventions to prevent psychiatric disorders that can be implemented in the preconception period and prenatal period.

Postnatal Factors Influencing Brain Development and Functioning

The foundation of a child's physical and emotional health forms from the interaction of the prenatally developed brain and its neuronal circuits with postnatal experienced factors; in other words, the brain that has been shaped by genetic influences and prenatal factors continues to be molded by the child's interactions with the postnatal environment (Rutter & Silberg, 2002).

The child's first environment, or the context in which he or she experiences life, is primarily within the family. Health promoting families provide a safe environment, a sense of emotional security and belonging, and experiences that will help the child to acquire self-regulation and social competence. Conversely, families characterized by unsupportive, neglectful relationships, family conflict, violence, and abuse are considered to be "risky families" because they place their children at increased risk for mental and physical health problems (Repetti, Taylor, & Seeman, 2002, p. 330).

Recall Chapter 1's discussions of temperament, attachment, and psychosocial development. These attributes are unique to each child and play a vital role in postnatal brain development that continues through the second and third years (Pollard, 2007). The combined effect of genetically influenced temperament, secure or insecure attachments, internal strengths built through accomplishing psychosocial developmental tasks, social and cultural environment, and positive or negative experiences influences brain development, brain functioning, and brain plasticity after birth. Experienced factors and factors in the postnatal environment play a crucial role in determining the trajectory of a child's brain development, with some factors reinforcing normal development and some factors influencing deviations from normal development (Grossman et al., 2003).

Temperament

Temperament (see Chapter 1) is an early indicator of personality and personality traits such as inhibition, novelty seeking, and harm avoidance. Temperament is a unique individual attribute present at birth that interacts over time with experienced factors to either increase or decrease the risk of an individual's developing psychopathology (Rutter, 2002). Higher rates of depression have been found among adults who had been inhibited or slow-to-warm-up babies, and higher rates of antisocial personality disorder and criminal activities have been found among adults who had been difficult babies. As adults, those who had been difficult babies or inhibited babies had higher rates of suicide than adults who had been easy babies (Caspi, Moffit, Newman, et al., 1996).

Attachment

Attachment theory (see Chapter 1) offers an explanation of the way human infants make strong bonds to another person in order to survive (Bowlby, 1969, 1973, 1988; Sroufe, Carlson, Levy, et al., 1999). Attachment provides for the infant's survival by meeting the infant's needs, reducing distress, and regulating the infant's perceptual, sensory, cognitive, and emotional systems (Fries, Ziegler, Kurian, et al., 2005; Gunnar, Broderson, Nachmias, et al., 1996; Nachmias, Gunnar, Mangelsdorf, et al., 1996). Patterns of attachment influence the child's capacity for emotional modulation through their effect on the development of the limbic circuitry of the brain that is involved in emotional reactivity (Galderisi & Mucci, 2000; Gunnar, 1998). Prolonged and elevated levels of emotional distress in the infant may be linked with HPA axis activation and neurotransmitter alterations that appear to be detrimental to the maturation of these circuits. Without external modulation of emotional reactivity by the caregiver, the infant's brain does not learn to self-regulate (Fries et al., 2005; Glazer, 2000). Later in life, self-regulation of emotional reactivity is key to establishing social relationships, interacting with peers, enabling successful cognitive performance, pursuing long-term goals, and managing the stressful experiences of daily living (Fries et al; Galderisi & Mucci). Thus, intense and persistent psychosocial distress that is not modulated through attachment may produce permanent changes in the brain that may result in reduced adaptive regulation of the stress response in adult life. If the child does not develop a secure pattern of attachment with his or her caregiver early in life, he or she may have a reduced ability to adapt to stress in adulthood (Galderisi & Mucci).

Ability to Accomplish Psychosocial Development Tasks

Erikson's (1964, 1968) theory of psychosocial development (see Chapter 1) identifies tasks or challenges that people face across the life span in their adaptation to the expectations and requirements of society. Successful achievement of the tasks of each stage generates internal strengths or assets such as trust, hope, and work skills; failure is reflected in compromised physical, cognitive, social, and emotional functioning. Failure is also associated with increased risk for the development of psychopathology such as depression, schizoid personality disorder, substance-related disorders, and paranoid or delusional disorders (Sadock & Sadock, 2007).

Experience and Brain Plasticity

Following neuronal migration (see Chapter 2), the neurons begin to form the synapses and circuits that are common to the human species (Grossman et al., 2003). In this process, neurons generate an excess of synaptic connections. Experience strengthens the synaptic connections that are needed for survival, thus determining which synaptic connections survive and which do not. Nelson and Bosquet (2000) described this characteristic of brain plasticity as "the process whereby the structure of experience is incorporated into the structure of the brain" (p. 42). Whereas early prenatal brain development is primarily guided by genetic influences, postnatal brain development is shaped by the interactions of the brain with environmental factors and experiences (Rutter, 2002). There are windows of time when two different types of experience are needed for the brain to develop to its full capacity (Dawson, Ashman, & Carver, 2000). One is the early experience-expectant process, which has narrow windows of time, and the other is the experience-dependent process, which occurs later and has broader windows of time (Galderisi & Mucci, 2000; Greenough & Black, 1992; Greenough, Black, & Wallace, 1987).

Experience-Expectant Plasticity

Experience-expectant plasticity refers to the brain's readiness at specific windows of time to receive information from the environment (Curtis & Cicchetti, 2003; Greenough et al., 1987; Grossman et al., 2003). The process associated with experience-expectant information storage is thought to have evolved as a way for the human species to prepare for incorporating specific information that is essential for survival: for example, vision and language (Dawson et al., 2000; Eliassen, Souza, & Sanes, 2003).

The key feature of experience-expectant plasticity is that the synapses have formed but require exposure to experience at specific windows of time to survive (Nelson & Bosquet, 2000). Strengthening and survival of those synaptic connections will not happen unless an experience occurs within that window of time (Greenough & Black, 1992). For example, if an eye is deprived of visual stimuli, reduction in visual acuity may occur (Grossman et al., 2003). Thus, if connections are not strengthened by experience during these periods, the connections do not survive, and permanent deficits of functioning result (Nelson & Bosquet, 2000).

However, although lack of stimuli is associated with impaired development and functioning, there is no evidence that more stimuli "applying a full-court developmental press" is better (Bruer, 1999, p. 123). Bruer said, "the key is balance and overall timing of neural activity among competing axons and synapses" (p. 123). Experience-expectant plasticity can be thought of as the "hardwiring" of the brain, strengthening connections already in place that are common to humans.

Experience-Dependent Plasticity

In contrast, the connections among neurons that modulate thinking, learning, memory, emotions, social behaviors, and functioning are not hardwired. Rather, the formation of these connections depends on experience (Black, Jones, Nelson, et al., 1998; Curtis & Cicchetti, 2003). Experiences from the environment that are unique for each individual are involved in storing information that is specific for the individual, such as sources of food, safety, security, and comfort (Grubb & Thompson, 2004). The experiences can be health promoting, for example, what results from exposure to a nurturing, caring environment, or they can be health impairing, as with exposure to deprivation, neglect, and abuse.

Experience-dependent plasticity is associated with promoting the formation of new synapses, not just strengthening existing ones (Greenough et al., 1987). New synapses create pathways for attention, memory, modulation of emotions, language, and formation of affiliation. For example, it is thought that the experience of receiving maternal care may modify responses to stress by altering gene expression, thus altering the effects of a stressful event on the HPA system. In this way, effects of maternal caregiving become "biologically embedded" and are carried on into adulthood (Meaney & Szyf, 2005, p. 461).

Through the process of brain plasticity, experience also shapes the hemispheres of the brain, which develop at different rates and have different functions (Galderisi & Mucci, 2000). Whereas the functions of the left hemisphere are specialized for cognitive tasks requiring analytical sequential processing, the right hemisphere is highly involved in responding to novel stimuli or emotional experiences, with bonding and attachment, and with emotional reactivity (Henry, 1993) (see Chapter 2).

Emotional reactivity is involved in the regulation of behaviors such as individuals' social interactions and their ability to delay gratification, to inhibit behavior, to pursue long-term goals, and to cope with stressful situations (Galderisi & Mucci, 2000). Emotional reactivity is molded by the interaction between genetic influences and experienced factors such as parenting.

There has been a tendency in the media and among policy-makers to accept the unfounded premise that the first 3 years of life determine the child's long-term outcomes, a premise that Bruer (1999) called the "myth of the first three years" (p. 27). He said that the windows of time for experience-dependent plasticity are much wider than generally thought. The human brain continues to strengthen connections and to make new connections in response to experience throughout the life span.

Adverse Experiences

Early adverse experiences—poverty, prolonged separation from the primary caregiver, parental conflict, divorce, parental psychopathology, neglect or abuse, and violence—have a negative effect on the child's developing brain (Nemeroff, 2004) and thus on later functioning. All adverse experiences increase the child's exposure to stress, and it is the response to stress that is believed to affect brain development and functioning and the later development of psychopathology such as major depression, anxiety disorders, and other psychiatric disorders (Kaufman, Plotsky, Nemeroff, et al., 2000; Nemeroff).

Biological Effects of Adverse Experiences on the Brain

The effects of adverse experiences are global in that they alter brain structures, neurotransmitters, and stress circuits. Adverse experiences are associated with smaller brain volume and larger ventricles (DeBellis, 1998), atrophy of the hippocampus (Bremmer, Randall, Vermetten, et al., 1997; McNeil, Cantor-Graae, & Weinberger, 2000; Stein, Koverola, Hanna, et al., 1997), and a smaller corpus callosum (Teicher, Dumont, Ito, et al., 2004). Adverse experiences also affect the brain at the cellular level. Adverse experiences lead to neurobiological changes in the noradrenergic and serotonergic neurotransmitter systems, which are two neurotransmitter systems involved in anxiety and depression (Nemeroff, 2004). Experience-generated stress also affects the HPA axis, starting a cascade of events that leads to increased levels of the stress hormone cortisol (Gutman & Nemeroff, 2002; LeDoux, 2000), which inhibits the ability of the hippocampus to produce new neurons throughout adult life (Karten, Olariu, & Cameron, 2005).

Studies of severe childhood adversity have shown that early life stressful experiences such as maternal deprivation affect the development of neuroendocrine, cognitive, and behavioral systems by producing persistent changes in the neural circuits that coordinate autonomic, endocrine, immune, and behavioral responses to stress (Gutman & Nemeroff, 2002).

Adverse Experiences and Development of Psychopathology

The development of psychopathology appears to be related to disruptions of normal brain development that may be due to genetic influences, prenatal factors, postnatal experienced factors, or an interaction of these factors. For example, genetic influence is the primary cause of fragile X syndrome, and prenatal exposure to alcohol is the primary cause of fetal alcohol syndrome (Grossman et al., 2003). However, in contrast to having a single factor as cause, psychiatric disorders such as anxiety disorders, depression, schizophrenia, substance-related disorders, and personality disorders are associated with the interaction of genetic influences, prenatal factors, perinatal factors, and postnatal environmental and experienced factors (Buka, Goldstein, Seidman, et al., 1999; Grossman et al., 2003; Jones, Rantakallio, Hartikaienen, et al., 1998). Evidence suggests that individuals who are exposed to early-life adverse experiences are at increased risk for developing psychiatric disorders later in life (Debellis, Keshavan, Shifflett, et al., 2002; Heim & Nemeroff, 2001).

Specific Adverse Experiences

Poverty, prolonged separation from the primary caregiver, family conflict, divorce, parental psychopathology, violence, and childhood maltreatment are all adverse experiences that affect postnatal brain development and functioning.

Poverty

In the United States, children living in poverty are more than twice as likely as children living in middle-income families to be exposed to multiple family stressors; poverty has also been found to be associated with higher levels of cortisol, the stress hormone (Evans & English, 2002). Poverty affects the physical, emotional, and cognitive well-being of children and their academic functioning through the effects of

- Poor living conditions
- Greater family conflict and chaotic households
- Early and frequent separations from the family
- Increased risk for development of insecure attachment patterns
- Exposure to violence
- Harsh discipline
- Lack of predictability, structure, and stability in daily life
- Less social support
- Fewer stimulating resources or experiences that lead to greater school readiness
- Poorer schools and day-care facilities (Brooks-Gunn & Duncan, 1997; Dawson et al., 2000; Evans, 2004; McLeod & Shanahan, 1996; Schoon, Sacker, & Bartley, 2003)

The multiple demands required of a child to adapt to living in persistent poverty—defined as 4 consecutive years of poverty—foster the development of medical and mental illnesses. For example, children living in persistent poverty are twice as likely to have poor biopsychosocial health as children of middle-income families (Evans, 2004; Schoon et al., 2003). They have higher rates of asthma, upper respiratory infections, AIDS, and injuries (Aber, Jones, & Cohen, 2000). They are almost twice as likely to have had a low birth weight and four times as likely to experience lead poisoning with resulting stunted growth and impaired cognitive functioning. Children living in persistent poverty are also more likely to have experienced developmental delays and learning problems, and they are twice as likely to repeat a grade and are more than twice as likely to drop out of school (Brooks-Gunn & Duncan, 1997).

The longer a child lives in poverty, the greater the adverse effect on the child's mental health (Evans & English, 2002; McLeod & Shanahan, 1996), and persistent poverty has twice the effect as transient poverty (Duncan, Brooks-Gunn, & Klebanov, 1994). Among 4- to 8-year-old children, persistent poverty is associated with increased levels of *internalizing* symptoms such as dependency, anxiety, and unhappiness; in contrast, current poverty (poverty of 1 year) is associated with an increased level of *externalizing* symptoms such as hyperactivity, peer conflicts, and behavioral problems (Aber et al., 2000; Brooks-Gunn & Duncan, 1997; Costello, Compton, Keeler, et al., 2003; McLeod & Shanahan, 1996). Among older children, persistent poverty is associated with depression, increased antisocial behavior, substance abuse problems, poor academic achievement, and violent behavior (Fergus & Zimmerman, 2005; McLeod & Shanahan, 1996). Chapter 19 includes a discussion of poverty as a risk factor for psychopathology.

Prolonged Separation from the Primary Caregiver

Prolonged separation of a child from the primary caregiver can have numerous causes, such as the caregiver's need for treatment of physical or psychiatric disorders, the caregiver's leaving the family to migrate ahead of the family, the caregiver's leaving to serve in the military, or the removal of the child from the family because of unsafe conditions. Studies of adults who had been separated from their families as infants for an average of 7 months owing to tuberculosis in the family reveal that the rate of depression was higher for the separated subjects than for matched controls and that mortality rates were higher among the separated subjects, mainly due to suicides and accidents (Veijola, Maki, Joukamaa, et al., 2004). Children who experienced prolonged separation from their parents owing to migration have difficulties with school performance and have symptoms of psychological distress (Pottinger, 2005). Protective factors for these children include living in a supportive family and being able to talk about the migration. Removal from the family and placement in foster care before the age of 6 years is associated with feelings of hopelessness, negative expectation of relationships with others, and not seeking interpersonal connectedness (Hagino, 2002). Bowlby (1969) believed that any disruption of the attachment relationship of the child and primary caregiver would cause distress in the child, would be experienced as a threat to security and survival, and had the potential to adversely affect the psychosocial development of the child.

Family Conflict

Families in conflict are characterized by anger and aggression and often by neglect of the child's needs and welfare (Hanson, 1999). Families in conflict may not provide the environment in which the child can develop various skills, including self-regulatory competencies (e.g., regulation of emotional arousal); a repertoire of coping skills that might help them adapt to later stressors; and mastery of age-appropriate tasks (Essex, Klein, Cho, et al., 2003; Grych & Fincham, 1990).

Parental conflict appears to be associated with increased risk of insecure attachment in infants and toddlers (Essex et al., 2003). In children, exposure to marital conflict is associated with a higher risk for both physical health problems (Nicolotti, el-Sheikh, & Whitson, 2003) and psychological problems such as aggression, hostility, anxiety, depression, and suicide (Essex et al.; Grych & Fincham, 1990). It is the level of conflict to which children are exposed that is related to their development of problems (Hetherington, Cox, & Cox, 1985). Children who are exposed to unhappy, hostile, and tense marital situations have more adjustment and behavioral problems than children exposed to unhappy marriages in which the parents are apathetic or indifferent to each other (Hetherington, 2006). A child's high level of self-blame with regard to the parental conflict is associated with internalizing behaviors such as depression and anxiety; a child's high level of perceived threat to himself or herself is associated with externalizing behaviors such as aggression and behaviors associated with oppositional defiant disorder and conduct disorder (El-Sheikh, Harger, & Whitson, 2001; Essex et al.). Conflict that the children are unaware of (encapsulated conflict) is not associated with behavioral problems.

Divorce

In the early 1900s, 25% of the children in the United States experienced the death of a parent before they were 15 years old, but only 7% to 9% experienced divorce. Today, about 5% of children in the United States experience the death of a parent, and 40% experience divorce before the age of 16 years (Wallerstein & Blakeslee, 1989). Approximately 50% of all marriages in the United States end in divorce (Rodgers & Rose, 2002), and among divorced families with children, about half of the children are 6 years old or younger (Wallerstein & Lewis, 2004); among children ages 14 to 18 years, only 42% live in a first marriage, defined as an intact two-biological parent family (Fagan & Rector, 2000).

In times of crises—such as fires, floods, and war—parents save the children first; in divorce, the welfare of the children is often put on hold and parents may be less aware and less responsive to their children's needs. They may have a diminished capacity for parenting, that is, for providing consistent discipline, physical care, playtime, and emotional support. In other kinds of crises, such as with death, people offer help to the family: neighbors bring food and help out in other ways, clergy offer consolation, and the role of the grandparents is clear: they are there to help. After a divorce, there are no established norms for offering help. The family is often disorganized, and living situations, employment, and financial resources may change dramatically (Kaplan & Pruett, 2000). Each member of the family takes on a changed role and a changed identity (Wallerstein & Blakeslee, 1989).

The adverse effects of divorce, once thought to heal with time, are now believed to continue to influence the lives of children through the associated losses and changes that occur (Wallerstein & Blakeslee, 1989; Wallerstein & Lewis, 2004). Children of divorce suffer many losses. They lose the fundamental structure of the family that would have otherwise provided them with support and modeled adult ways of facing problems, reconciling differences, and managing relationships. After divorce, children must try to unify the structure of two families, two worlds. Children of divorce must adjust to changes in parenting, such as less support, fewer rules, harsher discipline, less supervision, and greater dependence on the child (Hetherington, 2006). They also must adjust to social changes, such as economic hardships (50% move into poverty), moving to a less desirable neighborhood, changing schools, and disruption of religious practices (Fagan & Rector, 2000).

Thus, children who experience divorce face multiple adversities. The greater the number of adversities experienced in childhood, the stronger the association with later development of depressive disorders, substance-use disorders, and suicidality (Afifi, Enns, Cox, et al., 2008). For adolescents, divorce is very frightening. They feel rejected and may see the divorce as a collapse of their whole world. They lose the family control that may have helped them to control their own sexual and aggressive impulses and often fear that they will repeat their parents' failures in relationships (Hetherington & Kelly, 2002; Wallerstein & Blakeslee, 1989; Wallerstein & Lewis, 2004). More effects of divorce on children, adolescents, young adults, and adults can be seen in Box 3-1.

In early research on the effect of divorce on children, divorce was thought of as a static event without a history of prior conflict, coexisting problems, and ongoing conflict after the divorce. More recent studies consider the effect of divorce in relation to the developmental stage of the child, the presence of mediating or protective factors (Amato, 2006), and the concurrence of other adversities (Afifi, Boman, Fleisher, et al., 2009). For example, when a child experiences abuse in addition to parental divorce, the rate of impairment of function and psychopathology is greater than the rate associated with divorce or abuse alone (Afifi et al.).

Certain factors modulate the effect of divorce on children, adolescents, and adults (Box 3-2). For example, one intervention that has recently been found to reduce mental health problems among adolescents of divorced parents is a manualized program that focuses on improving the mother's relationship with the child and her use of effective discipline, increasing the father's access to the child, and

BOX 3-1 Effects of Parents' Divorce in Children, Adolescents, Young Adults, and Adults

Effects of Parents' Divorce in Children

Infants

- Respond to parents' mood with loss of appetite, upset stomach, and spitting up

Preschoolers

- Fear being left alone; fear abandonment, fear being forgotten
- Cling and cry more often
- Seek familiar toys
- May be angry, uncooperative
- May be cranky and have periods of crying
- May regress to earlier behaviors

Early Childhood

- Feel loss, rejection, guilt, and conflict over loyalty
- May have nightmares
- May think that they should be punished
- May be accident prone

School-Age Children

- Experience grief, embarrassment, resentment, intense anger, and divided loyalty
- Blame themselves for the divorce
- Experience sadness and loss, loneliness, concern for the welfare of one or both parents
- Have feelings of rejection and fears for their future
- Feel less protected and less cared for
- Feel that they do not get the same support as children from intact families
- Have difficulty concentrating and have a decline in school performance (math, reading, and spelling)
- Repeat grades more often
- Complain of stomachaches or headaches
- Have more internalizing and externalizing psychiatric symptoms (Fagan & Rector, 2000; Kelly, 2000)
- Hope parents will get back together
- Worry about the future
- Have a lower standard of living
- Are at risk for delinquency
- Are at higher risk for abuse
- Among girls, risk for sexual abuse from stepfather or cohabitor is 6 times (Russell, 1984) to 40 times (Wilson & Daly, 1987) higher than in intact families (Fagan & Rector, 2000)

Additional sources: Fagan & Rector, 2000; Wallerstein & Lewis, 2004.

Effect of Parents' Divorce in Adolescents

- Feel anger, fear, grief, loneliness, powerlessness, guilt, anxiety, depression, and disillusionment
- Feel abandoned by the parent who left

BOX 3-1 Effects of Parents' Divorce in Children, Adolescents, Young Adults, and Adults—continued

- Exhibit disruptive and aggressive behaviors
- Have greater use of alcohol, cigarettes, and marijuana
- Have more teenage pregnancies
- Show slightly poorer academic achievement
- Have higher dropout rates (McLanahan & Sandefur, 1994)
- May feel that they have to take over control of the family, e.g., care for younger siblings
- Doubt their ability to get married and stay married
- Worry about family finances

Additional sources: Amato, 2000; Hetherington, 2006.

Effect of Parents' Divorce in Young Adults

- Have poor relationships with both parents
- Show more emotional distress
- Exhibit more behavioral problems
- Are more likely to have received psychological help
- Have lower rates of attending college
- Are less likely to have received financial aid to complete college
- Have higher rates of medical problems, illnesses, and physician visits than children from intact families as young adults (Zill, Morrison, & Coiro, 1993)
- Have lower earning capacity (Fagan & Rector, 2000)
- Have a high risk for suicide (Garnefski & Diekstra, 1997)
- Grieve for the loss of their family and question the value of family traditions (Temke & Douglas, 2006)

Effect of Parents' Divorce in Older Adults

- Exhibit greater social isolation
- Have poor subjective well-being
- Have a lower level of academic achievement (Amato, 2006)
- Exhibit more marital problems (Amato, 2006)
- Describe less satisfying sex lives and more negative life events (Amato, 2000, 2006)
- Have a lower standard of living
- Have less wealth and greater economic hardships (more so for women) (Amato, 2000)
- Have an increased likelihood of undergoing divorce (Amato, 2000, 2006; Tucker, Friedman, Schwartz, et al., 1997)
- Have a higher risk for premature mortality (Tucker et al., 1997)

BOX 3-2 Divorce-Related Protective Factors for Children, Adolescents, and Adults

Children

- Support from adults, family, and friends
- Therapeutic interventions, e.g., school-based programs
- Ability to use active coping skills
- Limited amount and intensity of conflict between parents
- Parental agreement on discipline and childrearing

Adolescents

- Support from parents, neighbors, and friends
- Close relationship with nonparental adult
- Positive school experience and school connectedness

Adults

- Higher levels of education
- Employment
- Support from a new partner, relatives, and friends
- Being the spouse who initiated the divorce
- Receiving material assistance reduced distress, but when given in conjunction with advice, it increased distress (Amato, 2000)

Sources: Amato, 2000, 2006; Rogers & Rose, 2002.

reducing parental conflict. The program reduced externalizing problems such as aggression; hostility; delinquency; mental symptoms; use of alcohol, marijuana, and other drugs; and high-risk sexual behaviors (Wolchik, Sandler, Millsap, et al., 2002).

Psychiatric advanced practice nurses should be aware that despite the reduction of the stigma of divorce and the increase of services such as therapeutic interventions for children and divorce mediation, children with divorced parents are at risk for lower levels of success at school, more behavioral and emotional problems, lower levels of self-esteem, and more difficulties with social relationships than children with nondivorced parents (Amato, 2003). Factors that may influence outcomes for children of divorced parents include level of conflict between parents, quality of parenting from both parents, changes in the child's standard of living, parental remarriage or presence of new cohabiting partners, and number of stressors such as changing schools or moving (Amato). Chapter 19 describes programs related to divorce that are designed for children and parents.

Parental Psychopathology

Parental mental health has an influence on a child's early brain activity, immediate behavior, and long-term behaviors (Dawson et al., 2000). Whereas parents' good mental health is a protective factor that reduces the risk of their children's developing problems with cognitive functioning, adaptation, and delinquency (Seifer & Dickstein, 2000), parental psychopathology increases the risk of their children's developing psychiatric disorders (Sameroff, 2006).

Parents with psychopathology tend to be more authoritarian and hostile and to have lower expectations for their children's achievements (Seifer & Dickstein, 2000). The effect of exposure to parental psychopathology is manifested differently at each stage of a child's development. For example, in infants, the effects are seen in insecure patterns of attachment, problems with language development and accomplishment of milestones, and lack of regulation of sleeping and eating. Seifer and Dickstein made the point that not all studies of maternal psychopathology have found differences in the infants and children when compared with infants and children of mothers without psychopathology. They also noted that maternal psychopathology often exists in a context of marital discord, low socioeconomic situations, and other stressors and that these factors may contribute to the child's development of psychopathology.

Common parental psychopathologies include maternal depression, maternal schizophrenia, and parental alcohol abuse and substance-related disorders. Parental psychopathology is associated with increased rates of mental illness in their children, indicating genetic influence (Kendler, Neale, Kessler, et al., 1992), and with the development of other problems—poor social adaptations, cognitive deficits, and delinquency (Shaw, Owens, Vondra, et al., 1996).

Maternal Depression

Mothers who are depressed are less responsive to their infants (Cohn & Campbell, 1992), are less likely to interact with their infants (Dawson et al., 2000), and display more negative emotions (Seifer & Dickstein, 2000). Because infancy may be the optimal window of time for development of regulation of emotion, the failure of a depressed mother to respond to her infant may increase the risk of the child's developing internalizing problems, such as anxiety and depression (Essex et al., 2003).

Infants of depressed mothers have been found to be less active, more withdrawn, and likely to show more negative emotions than infants of nondepressed mothers (Dawson et al., 2000). Young children whose mothers are depressed are more likely to have insecure patterns of attachment than those whose mothers are not depressed (Essex et al., 2003) and are more likely to have cognitive and language delays and higher levels of hostile and aggressive behaviors (Dawson et al.). Because depression often occurs in the presence of other adverse family circumstances—stressful life events, lack of social support, and family conflict—children of depressed mothers may be at increased risk of poor parenting from both caregivers (Cicchetti, Rogosch, & Toth, 1998). Older children of depressed mothers are more likely to have problems with mood and anxiety, poor self-esteem, and academic and conduct problems (Cicchetti & Rogosch, 1996; Essex et al.; Kim-Cohen, Moffitt, Taylor, et al., 2005). Chapter 19 includes a discussion of parental depression and increased risk of depression in children. Early preventive interventions, such as the treatment of maternal depression, have the potential to decrease the risk of children's developing anxiety and depressive disorders (Essex et al.).

Maternal Schizophrenia

According to Seeman (2004), approximately half of women with schizophrenia become mothers. The ability of a mother who has schizophrenia to parent may be affected by the difficulties she experiences in comforting others, the trouble she has determining what others need, and the symptoms of her own illness. About one-third of mothers with schizophrenia lose custody of their children. Tienari, Sorri, Lathi, et al. (2004) found that children of mothers with schizophrenia had more developmental and behavioral problems than children of healthy mothers and showed more psychopathology as adults. After reviewing studies of mothers with schizophrenia, Seifer and Dickstein (2000) found that the mothers tended to be less affectionate, to have greater anger and hostility, and to live in poor home environments. Their infants had problems with regulation of responses to social stimuli and distractibility and tended to have insecure attachment patterns (Seifer & Dickstein). However, not all studies reviewed by Seifer and Dickstein found that the infants differed from infants of mothers without schizophrenia.

Alcohol Abuse

Parents who are abusing alcohol may neglect their children by not providing the warm, supportive care that would enable them to develop secure attachments (Kelley, Cash, Grant, et al., 2004). Among children in families with alcohol abuse, younger children—ages 4 to 5 years—are aware of the problem and feel responsible for causing it. Older children feel rage, disillusionment, or resignation. They are afraid that their parents will die, that their parents do not love them, or that society will brand them because of their parent's alcoholism. They feel that they cannot talk to anyone about the problem. As adults, they are more apprehensive about adult relationships and have higher lifetime rates of dysthymia, generalized anxiety disorder, panic disorder, simple phobia, agoraphobia, and antisocial symptoms in comparison with adults who did not have alcoholic parents (Kelley et al.).

Substance-Related Disorders

Parents with substance-related disorders may not be able to provide a safe environment for their children, give nurturing care, set limits on the child's behavior, or help the child regulate eating, sleeping, and emotions. In addition, their lives may involve domestic violence and partner or family substance use to which the child is exposed (Lester, Boukydis, & Twomey, 2000). There is little information about the effect of substance use by the mother on child development. What information is available suggests that there may be adverse effects on intelligence (IQ), language development, and academic problems, but these effects may also reflect prenatal exposure and related brain damage (Lester et al.).

To summarize, children of parents with psychopathology are likely to

- Have increased rates of mental health problems
- Demonstrate more negative interactions
- Have insecure attachment patterns
- Have conflicted relationships with parents
- Be more impulsive
- Have difficult peer and social interactions (Seifer & Dickstein, 2000, pp. 156-157)

Violence

Family violence, exposure to war and terrorism, and viewing violence in the media all affect child development.

Family Violence

Factors associated with family violence include poverty, stressors, family disorganization, parental substance use, parental psychopathology, and neighborhood characteristics (e.g., high rates of juvenile delinquency, drug trafficking, and violent crime) (Cicchetti & Toth, 1995; Emery & Laumann-Billings, 1998).

Children who witness family violence experience symptoms similar to those of children who have been abused (Centerwell, 1992; Jaffe, Hurley, & Wolfe, 1990). Among children who witness abuse, 34% of the boys and 20% of the girls have been found to have a level of adjustment problems that reaches clinical significance. They are unable to calm themselves enough to do their work and may display both internal and external symptoms. Conflict and violence before divorce, and maternal battering are two forms of family violence that have an enduring adverse effect on children.

- *Conflict and violence before divorce.* In the time before divorce, children often witness conflict between their parents, and half of the children witness actual physical violence between their parents (Wallerstein & Blakeslee, 1989). Childhood exposure to parental conflict increases the child's risk for developing psychological problems, for having weak ties to the father, for perceiving a lack of social support, and for discord in their own marriages later on (Amato, 2006). In a study of family violence described in the book *Behind Closed Doors,* men who had observed family violence in childhood had a higher rate of wife beating than men who did not have such experiences (Straus, Gelles, Steinmetz, 1980).
- *Maternal battering.* Among women, wife battering accounts for more injuries than car accidents, muggings, and rapes by strangers. Many times the children are in the room where the violence takes place or in the next room. Children of battered women are at increased risk of being abused (Emery & Laumann-Billings, 1998); in fact, one study reveals that nearly half of the children of battered mothers are abused by their fathers (McCloskey, 2001). McCloskey suggested that the fathers may abuse the children in order to control or get back at their wives. Children who have been exposed to maternal battering appear to be sad, cautious, and unhappy and to have somatic complaints. Their reaction to other stressful situations is one of fear (Christensen, 1995).

Chronic exposure to family violence prevents the child from integrating sensory, emotional, and cognitive information into a positive inner model of how the world works. Children exposed to family violence have no organized way of responding to stressors in their lives and many lack the capacity for emotional self-regulation, resulting in poor sense of self, deficits of impulse control, aggressive behaviors, and lack of trust in what others will do (Streeck-Fischer & van der Kolk, 2000). After controlling for possible confounding factors such as child abuse and neglect, socioeconomic status, the child's cognitive ability, and life stressors, childhood exposure to family violence has been found to be related to externalizing problems among boys and internalizing problems among girls (Kashani, Daniel, Dandoy, et al., 1992; Yates, Egeland, & Sroufe, 2003). As adolescents, they are more likely to engage in drug abuse and aggressive behaviors than adolescents who have not been exposed to family violence (Fergusson & Horwood, 1998; Kendall-Tackett, Williams, & Finkelhor, 1993). As adults, they have increased rates of depression, anxiety, nicotine dependence, alcohol abuse, cannabis abuse, and criminal offenses (Emery & Laumann-Billings, 1998).

Exposure to War and Terrorism

The effect of exposure to war and terrorism on children is influenced by the severity of the trauma, the child's developmental stage, and the situation within the family and community (Williams, 2006). Severity of trauma ranges from experiencing shelling, being separated from parents, or losing parents to acts of violence, suffering torture, or being forced to witness death of parents. Protective circumstances for children include being with parents and families, having contact with peers, attending school and religious services, and maintaining daily routines (Macksoud, Aber, & Cohn, 1996). Negative outcomes of exposure to war and terrorism include anxiety, social withdrawal, aggression toward others, delinquency, depression, and post-traumatic stress disorder.

Having the attribute of resilience (see Chapter 1) appears to serve as a buffer (Masten & Schaffer, 2006). For example, children who had grown up in stable, problem-free families had more severe responses to exposure to violence than children growing up in families that had prior experience in responding to problems. That is, children of families that had not encountered and adapted successfully to problems were less able to confront the conflict and stress of war and terrorism (Macksoud et al., 1996). Psychiatric advanced practice nurses can help children who have been exposed to war and terrorism to rebuild their world by helping them to meet their basic needs for food, shelter, safety, and information and their developmental needs for routines, structure, friendship, and social support (Williams, 2006). (See Chapter 8 for a discussion of psychological first aid.)

Exposure to Media Violence

To put the impact of exposure to media violence in perspective, it is necessary to be aware of the vastness of the exposure. The average American child between the ages of 2 and 5 years spends about 32 hours a week using media (television, videos, movies, video games, recorded music, computer, and Internet), and children ages 6 to 11 years spend 28 hours a week watching television (McDonough, 2009). Excessive use of the media affects the physical, mental, and social health of children. Watching 2 hours of media a day has been found to be associated with being overweight in children ages 3 and 4 (Rich, Woods, Goodman, et al., 1998), and among adults age 26 years, being overweight was linked to having watched television for more than 2 hours a day in childhood and adolescence (Hancox, Milne, & Poulton, 2004).

Researchers have found that media violence causes intense fear in children that often lasts for weeks or months (Hoekstra, Harris, & Helmick, 1999; Zillmann & Weaver, 1999). Very young children who are between ages 2 and 6 years tend to be frightened by scary images of animals, natural disasters, and monsters; they tend to be calmed by nonverbal or physical strategies. Older children are more likely to be frightened by realistic threats to their personal well-being; they tend to be calmed by gaining information about why the event is not likely to happen to them and learning how they can prevent it (Canto, 1998, 2000). Television-watching reduces time available for other activities such as reading, sports, homework, socializing, and community projects. Excessive television-watching as a child has also been found to be associated with dropping out of school and poor academic achievement in young adults (van der Molen & Bushman, 2008), and it increases the child's exposure to observed violence (Bickham & Rich, 2006).

A large amount of media time includes exposure to acts of violence (Yokota & Thompson, 2000). American media tends to portray heroes using violence as a way to solve problems or conflicts and to triumph over others (Comstock & Strasburger, 1993). The average American child will witness 8,000 murders on TV before finishing elementary school and by age 18 will have seen 200,000 acts of violence, including 40,000 murders (Herr, 2007). The amount of time spent watching violent programs has been found to be associated with less time spent playing with friends (Bickham & Rich, 2006) and with inactivity and increased consumption of snack foods (Herr, 2007).

Among more than 3,500 research studies that examined the association between media violence and violent behavior, all but 18 have shown a positive relationship (Grossman & DeGaetano, 1999). Taken together, the evidence suggests that exposure to media violence promotes an increase of violent attitudes and aggressive and antisocial behaviors (Johnson, Cohen, Smailles, et al., 2002; Meyers, 2003; Paik & Comstock, 1994; Willis & Strasburger, 1998). Children tended to model their behavior after violent scenes in which they identified with the perpetrator of the violence, in which the perpetrator is rewarded for the violence, and in which the children consider the scene to be like real life.

The most compelling evidence of the antisocial effects of television comes from longitudinal studies (Browne & Hamilton-Giachritsis, 2005). In a 22-year longitudinal study of media violence viewing in childhood and adult behavior, habitual exposure of boys and girls between the ages of 6 and 9 years to violence in the media—after controlling for socioeconomic status, IQ, and various parenting factors—was associated with more aggressive and violent adult behaviors (Huesmann, Moise-Titus, Podolski, et al., 2003).

The American Academy of Pediatrics, American Academy of Child & Adolescent Psychiatry, American Psychological Association, American Medical Association, American Academy of Family Physicians, and American Psychiatric Association warn of potential adverse effects of exposure to media violence on children. These adverse effects are increased antisocial and aggressive behavior, less sensitivity to violence and those who suffer from violence, increased desire to see more violence in entertainment and real life, and viewing violence as an acceptable way to settle conflicts (American Academy of Pediatrics. Committee on Public Education, 2001; Congressional Public Health Summit, 2000).

Childhood Maltreatment

In the United States, 3.3 million cases of child abuse or neglect involving 6 million children were reported in 2006, and it is estimated that twice as many cases go unreported each year (U.S. Department of Health and Human Services Agency on Children, Youth and Families, 2008). According to the Center for Disease Control's research that was released in April 2008, an estimated 14% of U.S. children have experienced some form of child maltreatment such as neglect, physical abuse, and sexual abuse (Journalism Center on Children & Families, 2008), and approximately 33% of maltreated children experience a combination of neglect, physical abuse, emotional abuse, and sexual abuse (Edwards, Holden, Felitti, et al., 2003).

Children are more affected by maltreatment than by all serious illnesses combined (Theodore & Runyan, 1999).

Child maltreatment represents a failure of the child's environment—parents, family, community, and society—to provide for the child's normal development (Chicchetti, 2004). Failure of normal development in which a child masters the emotional, cognitive, social, and functional challenges of each age-specific phase of life increases the child's risk for later maladaptive behaviors, psychopathology, and substance abuse (Cicchetti). Felitti (2002) has asked how the nation can turn the gold of newborn children into the lead of biopsychosocial health–impaired adults.

The child's response to maltreatment is determined by his or her temperament, the severity and duration of the trauma, and the child's stage of development. Responses to maltreatment include the fight-or-flight response, accommodating or compliant behavior, frozen stillness, and dissociation (Streeck-Fischer & van der Kolk, 2000).

- The *fight-or-flight response* may include hyperarousal, fighting, and destructive behaviors. The child may experience feelings of rage, anger, or sadness and may have impaired ability to pay attention, learn, or control impulsive behaviors.
- In the *accommodating or compliant pattern of response*, the superficial compliant behavior allows the child to maintain some relationship with the caregiver. Later, the child may have problems with knowing his or her own feelings and with feeling empathy for others.
- In the *frozen stillness response*, the child may be disoriented and may react inappropriately or even show regressive behaviors. The child may have poor coordination, speak incoherently, and make facial grimaces.
- *Dissociation* describes a compartmentalization of experiences, a failure to integrate them. Some compartments of the self contain pain or fear associated with the maltreatment, and other compartments of the self continue to function in everyday activities, although the child may have learning difficulties and lack the ability to play. Maltreated children may use several mechanisms of dissociation such as daydreaming, avoidance, derealization, and depersonalization.

Maltreatment and the resulting adverse effects on the child's development depend on a balance between risk factors for maltreatment and factors that protect the developmental process (Chicchetti & Lynch, 1993). Compromised development may occur when the risk factors for maltreatment and the vulnerability of the child are greater than available protective factors (Bernat & Resnick, 2006).

- *Risk factors.* According to the report, *Risk and Protective Factors for Child Abuse and Neglect* (National Clearinghouse for Child Abuse and Neglect, 2004), factors that place children at risk for neglect and abuse can be divided into child-related factors, parental or family risk factors, and social risk factors. These factors are discussed in more detail in Box 3-3.

BOX 3-3 Child, Family, and Social Risk Factors for Childhood Maltreatment

Child Factors That Increase Risk of Childhood Maltreatment

- Premature birth
- Low birth weight
- Physical, cognitive, emotional disabilities
- Chronic illnesses or injuries
- Age
- Difficult temperament
- Behavior problems
- Being a stepchild
- Being an unwanted child

Family Factors That Increase Risk of Childhood Maltreatment

- Parental attributes: poor impulse control, depression, anxiety, lack of trust
- Childhood history of abuse
- Family conflict
- Violence
- Family structure: single parent and/or large family
- Lack of social support
- Substance abuse
- Separation or divorce
- Age
- Poor child-parent interactions
- Inaccurate knowledge of child development

Social Factors That Increase Risk of Childhood Maltreatment

- Low socioeconomic status; poverty
- Stressful life events
- Lack of resources, e.g., medical care, insurance, child care
- Unemployment
- Homelessness
- Social isolation
- Discrimination
- Poor schools
- Dangerous/violent neighborhoods

Sources: Brown, Cohen, Johnson, et al., 1998; National Clearinghouse on Child Abuse and Neglect, 2004.

- *Protective factors.* Factors that reduce the risk of developing psychiatric disorders following adversities have been defined as protective factors (Fraser, Richman, & Galinsky, 1999; Garmezy, 1974; Hetherington & Blechman, 1996; Rutter, 1979; Sameroff, 2006). Protective factors can be categorized at the level of the child, the level of the family, and the level of the community or society (Mash & Dozois, 1996). Box 3-4 describes these protective factors in more detail.

Specific Types of Childhood Maltreatment

Specific types of childhood maltreatment include neglect, abuse, and sexual abuse. Potential interventions for those who have experienced childhood maltreatment can be found at the end of this chapter and in Chapter 19.

BOX 3-4 Factors Protective Against Maltreatment at the Child, Family, and Community Levels

Protective Factors at the Child Level

- Easy temperament
- Ability to seek help
- Ability to work alone
- High intelligence
- Competence in school
- Good communication skills
- Good problem-solving skills
- Positive self-esteem
- High level of self-efficacy
- Good health
- Appealing to others, particularly adults
- A talent valued by others
- Sense of connectedness to family and school

Protective Factors at the Family Level

- A close relationship with at least one person in the family
- Positive, warm, effective parenting
- Parents with a high level of education
- Good child care
- Household structure with rules and supervision
- Parents have prosocial behavior expectations
- Spirituality or religion in the family (provides stability in times of hardship)

Protective Factors at the Community Level

- Good relationships between family and caring neighbors
- Presence of respected elders in the community who serve as role models
- Good schools
- Opportunities for adult education and community participation
- Supportive friends
- Connectedness with adults beyond family; e.g., neighbors, housekeepers, teachers, librarians

Sources: Bernat & Resnick, 2006; Mash & Dozois, 1996; Massie & Szajnberg, 2006; National Clearinghouse on Child Abuse and Neglect, 2004; Weiner & Smith, 1992; Werner, 1989.

Neglect

Childhood neglect is experienced by approximately 2.3 million American children each year, which is about 4% of the nation's children (Theodore & Runyan, 1999), and it is estimated to be three times more common than childhood abuse (Streeck-Fischer & van der Kolk, 2000). It is the form of maltreatment most strongly linked with poverty (Emery & Laumann-Billings, 1981). The home situation is often characterized by poor parenting skills, poverty, inadequate parental supervision, deliberate withholding of basic supplies that the child needs, parental substance abuse, and parental abandonment. Child neglect results from both acts of omission and acts of commission and includes active physical neglect, passive physical neglect, active emotional neglect, and passive emotional neglect (Berkowitz, 2001).

- *Active physical neglect* describes acts on the part of the parent that are not accidental and that cause the child to be harmed.
- *Passive physical neglect* describes parental failure to meet the child's physical needs and thus endangering of the child's health.
- *Active emotional neglect* describes acts of the parent that cause the child harm even though it is not physical.
- *Passive emotional neglect* describes the parent's inability or actions that lead to failure to provide security, care, and attention that would promote the child's development (Christensen, 1995).

Early child neglect is usually associated with the medical diagnosis of failure to thrive, which is characterized by an abnormal retardation of growth and development. The child's failure to thrive may be due to poor parenting skills, lack of resources, and other factors (Theodore & Runyan, 1999). Older children can also fail to thrive physically, academically, and socially. They may have behavioral problems, school failure, poor hygiene, and injuries. In follow-up studies of children who have experienced emotional neglect, the children are described as being socially withdrawn and experiencing academic problems (Erickson & Egeland, 1996).

Neglect is an extremely important factor in the health and well-being of children. It is involved in 30% to 40% of all child maltreatment deaths, which include deaths from lack of basic needs such as food and medical care, from withholding or refusing medical care, and from inadequate parental supervision that results in drowning, burns, or shootings (Berkowitz, 2001).

Abuse

Thirty percent of children seen for treatment in outpatient psychiatric settings have a history of childhood abuse, and 55% of children receiving inpatient psychiatric treatment have a history of childhood abuse. Emery and Laumann-Billings (1998) suggested that there has been an increase in child abuse. Although the number of cases involving moderate abuse—such as abuse that leaves an observable bruise, causes pain, or causes emotional distress for up to 48 hours—has remained stable, the number of cases with more severe abuse—abuse that causes long-term impairment of physical, mental, or emotional capacities such as loss of consciousness, broken bones, and serious burns—has increased (Emery & Laumann-Billings; Theodore & Runyan, 1999). The increase of serious abuse is believed to be linked to increased use of illegal drugs, greater poverty, and increased violence in the United States (Garbarino, 1995; Lung & Daro, 1996; Sedlak & Broadhurst, 1996). Confounding the problem of determining the prevalence of childhood abuse is the high rate of concurrence of different forms of abuse. For example, among children who are exposed to marital violence, 40% to 75% also experience physical abuse and are at high risk of being sexually abused (McCloskey, Figueredo, & Koss, 1995).

Sexual Abuse

The reported rate of childhood sexual abuse varies, with Molnar, Buka, and Kessler (2001) reporting a rate of 13.5% in women and 2.5% in men, and Frankelor (1994) and Dube, Felitti, Dong, et al. (2003b) estimating a much higher rate of 20% to 25% in women and 5% to 16% in men. There are more than 100,000 known cases of childhood sexual abuse each year in the United States, and the actual rate is believed to be much higher (Botash, 2000). Frankelor (1994) found that children who experienced inadequate or unavailable parenting, harsh punishment, and emotional deprivation were more likely to also have experienced sexual abuse; Frankelor also found that most sexual abuse is committed by someone known to the child 70% to 90% of the time. The years of greatest likelihood for sexual abuse are between the ages of 7 and 13 (Frankelor). In one European study of female children who had experienced sexual abuse, the perpetrator was from within the family in 52% of the cases (a father or stepfather in 40% of the instances). Occurrence is highest in summer, in the afternoon, and in the home (Csorba, Lampé, Borsos, et al., 2006). Risk factors for sexual abuse include

- Parent abused as a child
- Multiple caretakers for the child
- Caretaker or parent who has multiple sexual partners
- Drug and/or alcohol abuse
- Stress associated with poverty
- Social isolation and family secrecy
- Child with poor self-esteem or other vulnerable state
- Other family members abused
- Parent or caretaker having gang-member associations (American Psychological Association)

Effects of Maltreatment

Cicchetti (2004) has said that all forms of maltreatment create a risk that the child will not be able to move successfully through each stage of biological and psychosocial development. Failure to succeed in mastering developmental tasks places the child at increased risk of developing impairments of functioning and psychopathology. Isolated events of maltreatment are likely to cause conditioned behavioral and biological responses to reminders or triggers of the trauma. Chronic maltreatment has a broader impact on children's development: it affects their ability to integrate emotional, cognitive, and sensory information about the maltreatment; without integration of that information into their inner working models of themselves and their world, their ability to respond to other stressors or developmental challenges is compromised and likely to result in poor control of emotions, poor impulse control, and problems with socializing and with sense of self (Cicchetti, 2002; Putnam, 2003; Streeck-Fischer & van der Kolk, 2000).

The effect of maltreatment is cumulative. More abuse is associated with greater risk for physical illnesses, unhealthy lifestyle practices, and psychiatric disorders such as depression, alcoholism, and repeated suicide attempts (Box 3-5).

BOX 3-5 Effects of Childhood Maltreatment in Children, Adolescents, and Adults

Effects of Childhood Maltreatment in Children

- Malnutrition, bruises, burns, and fractures (Cicchetti, 2004)
- Impaired physiological and emotional regulation
- Failure to develop a secure attachment relationship with the primary caregiver (Massie & Szajnberg, 2006)
- Fears, anxiety, and sadness (Massie & Szajnberg, 2006)
- Anger (Massie & Szajnberg, 2006)
- Inability to develop a stable self-system of self-esteem and sense of self-efficacy
- Deficits in cognitive and language skills (Cicchetti, 2004)
- Failure to achieve Erikson's psychosocial tasks (Massie & Szajnberg, 2006)
- Poor impulse control; depression (Massie & Szajnberg, 2006)

Effects of Childhood Maltreatment in Adolescents

- Unplanned pregnancies (Dietz, Spitz, Anda, et al., 1999)
- Sexually transmitted diseases (Felitti, Anda, Nordenberg, et al., 1998; Hillis, Anda, Felitti, et al., 2000)
- Problems with peer relationships and school performance
- Behavioral problems
- Conduct disorder
- Suicide attempts (Ystgaard, Hestetun, Loeb, et al., 2004)
- Substance use
- Trouble with the police; e.g., running away from home, prostitution (Hettler & Greenes, 2003; Streeck-Fischer & van der Kolk, 2000)

Effects of Childhood Maltreatment in Adults

- Increased rates of health problems, cancer, chronic lung disease, skeletal fractures, and liver disease (Felitti et al., 1998; Felitti, 2002)
- Problems with intimate relationships
- Higher rates of disruptions of relationships; leaving or divorce
- Take longer to commit to intimate relationships if one is terminated (Colman & Widom, 2004)
- Psychiatric disorders: depression, anxiety disorders, personality disorders (Cicchetti & Manly, 2001)
- Alcohol abuse (Dube, Anda, Felitti, et al., 2002)
- Substance abuse (Dube, Felitti, Dong, et al., 2003a)
- Suicide attempts (Curtis, 2006; Dube, Anda, Felitti, et al., 2001)
- Abuse of the next generation (25% abuse their own children) (Streeck-Fischer & van der Kolk, 2000)

Maltreatment and Development of Psychopathology

Maltreated children who have experienced multiple traumas may develop anxiety disorders, such as overanxious disorder or separation anxiety, and other psychiatric disorders, such as attention deficit-hyperactivity disorder, oppositional defiant disorder, and conduct disorder. Among children who have been physically or sexually abused, one-fourth to one-half may experience post-traumatic stress disorder; this risk is higher for those children who experience more severe abuse (Famularo, Fenton, Kinscherff, et al., 1994).

In addition, adults who have a history of childhood abuse and neglect have higher rates of psychopathology (Dube et al., 2003b; Horwitz, Widom, McLaughlin, et al., 2001). For example, a childhood history of abuse has been found to be associated with depression and suicide attempts among young adults (Brown, Cohen, Johnson, et al., 1999). In fact, childhood abuse makes a young adult three to four times more likely to experience depression and to attempt suicide.

Childhood sexual abuse doubles the risk of an individual's later developing psychopathology. Childhood sexual abuse is associated with later development of:

- Conduct disorder (Fergusson, Horwood, & Lynskey, 1996)
- Depression (Fergusson et al., 1996; Nelson, Heath, Phil, et al., 2002)
- Panic disorder (Dumas, Katerndahl, & Burge, 1995)
- Substance abuse (Walker, Scott, & Koppersmith, 1998)
- Eating disorders (DeGroot, Kennedy, Rotin, et al., 1992; Vize & Cooper, 1995)
- Post-traumatic stress disorder (Rowan, Foy, Rodriguez, et al., 1994; Wolfe, Sas, & Wekerle, 1994)
- Borderline personality disorder (Guzder, Paris, Zelkowitz, et al., 1996)
- Suicide attempts (Nelson et al., 2002; Sfoggia, Pacheco, & Grassi-Oliveira, 2008)

Severity of psychopathology associated with sexual abuse correlates with the severity of the abuse. That is, as adults, those who experienced childhood sexual abuse without physical contact had higher rates of anxiety and depression than those with no childhood sexual abuse; however, they did not have higher rates of alcohol use, substance use, or suicide. Adults who had experienced childhood sexual abuse that involved contact but no attempted or completed intercourse had higher rates of anxiety, depression, alcohol use, substance use, and suicide attempts than those without any experienced childhood sexual abuse. Finally, adults who had experienced childhood sexual abuse with attempted or completed intercourse had the highest rates of anxiety, depression, alcohol use, substance use, and suicide attempts (Nelson et al., 2002). Buffering factors that reduce the likelihood that psychiatric disorders will develop among children who have experienced sexual abuse include positive school experiences, involvement in school sports, parental support, good relationship with the father, establishing stable relationships, and social support networks (Hetherington, 2006; Mullen & Fleming, 1998).

Retrospective studies imply a direct causal effect between childhood maltreatment and later development of psychiatric disorders; however, the effect of maltreatment is not direct. Childhood abuse often takes place in an environment with multiple stressors such as poverty and alcohol abuse that are known to be associated with increased risk for psychiatric disorders (Horwitz et al., 2001; Widom, 2000). Also, the effects of maltreatment vary from child to child and may be manifested differently over the life span (Cohen, Brown, & Smailes, 2001). For example, it has been found that among children who had been identified as being neglected or abused, rates of disruptive behaviors remain high across the life span. On the other hand, these children have very high rates of anxiety disorders in early adolescence that decline in late adolescence and decline even further in adulthood. Children who experienced physical abuse have high rates of disruptive disorders (attention deficit-hyperactivity disorder, oppositional defiant disorder, and conduct disorder), substance use, and major depressive disorder later on, and children who have experienced sexual abuse have an earlier incidence of substance abuse, mainly alcohol abuse. Thus, the effects of maltreatment differ over the life span and according to type of maltreatment.

In addition, other events that occur across the life span of those who have been maltreated as children influence the development of psychiatric disorders. For example, adults who have experienced childhood maltreatment have a greater number of lifetime stressors—for example, unemployment, being fired, birth of a child, death of a parent, divorce, poverty, homelessness, and arrests—than those who have not experienced childhood maltreatment. Horwitz et al. (2001) accurately summarized this finding when they wrote: "The long-term mental health impacts of childhood victimization unfold within the context of a lifetime of stressors" (p. 197).

Maltreatment and Resilience

Although there are strong correlations between childhood maltreatment and later development of psychiatric disorders, many individuals who experience childhood maltreatment do not develop psychopathology (Lynskey & Fergusson, 1997). Researchers have reported that at least 22% of children exposed to childhood maltreatment have few after-effects (Fergusson & Mullen, 2002; McGloin & Widom, 2001). Even among those who experience childhood sexual abuse, one of the most severe forms of maltreatment, about one-fourth do not develop psychiatric disorders. They appear to demonstrate *resilience* when facing the adversity of maltreatment.

In the classic longitudinal study of resilience in which all infants born on the island of Kauai were followed for 30 years, Werner (1989) identified high-risk children (i.e., the children at risk for developing psychopathology) as those who had experienced prenatal or perinatal stress such as birth complications and whose families were characterized by poverty, discord, alcohol, divorce, low education levels, and parental mental illness. Among the 129 high-risk children (defined as those with four risk factors before the age of 2), two-thirds had developed serious learning or behavioral problems by the age of 10 years or, as adolescents, had mental health problems, teenage pregnancies, or contact with the police. However, one-third of the high-risk children developed into well-functioning young adults. Werner described the difference between the resilient children who had not developed problems and those who had developed problems in terms of characteristics (Box 3-6).

Early researchers of resilience, Garmezy (1971) and Werner and Smith (1982), thought that learning what enabled exceptional children—or those who were viewed as invulnerable or resilient—to overcome the effects of adversity, develop normally, and avoid psychopathology would guide interventions to help other children to become resilient. Early researchers thought that resilience was rare. Now, resilience is viewed as a normative process involving the child's system of adaptation that brings about good outcomes in response to risks or actual adversities (Masten, 2001). In fact, Masten (p. 227) has referred to resilience as "ordinary magic" that arises from the child's adaptive processes. If the adaptation system is in good working order, the child's normal development will continue without being compromised, even in the face of adversities.

The systems that carry out adaptive processes are made up of the child's unique attributes, brain functioning, relationship with caregivers, capacity to regulate emotions and behaviors, and readiness to interact with the environment. Influences, forces, or events that damage or fail to protect the systems that carry out adaptive processes will endanger the child's development. A child's adaptive system may be adequate to interact with one adversity to produce resilience, but it may not be adequate to interact with a different adversity or with co-occurring adversities (Fraser et al., 1999).

BOX 3-6 Characteristics of Resilient Infants, Toddlers, School-Age Children, and Their Families

Infants
- Active
- Good-natured
- Easy to take care of
- Few sleeping and eating problems

Toddlers
- Active participants in interactions with adults
- Liked new experiences
- Good communication skills

School-Age Children
- Got along well with classmates
- Good reading skills and reasoning ability
- Had hobbies and outside activities
- Had social network of relatives, neighbors, church leaders, and teachers to whom they could turn to for help

Families
- Four or fewer children in the family
- Children were at least 2 years apart in age
- Children had close attachment with at least one adult caregiver
- No long separations during first year of life

Sources: Werner & Smith, 1992; Wright & Masten, 2006.

Resilience is rare among children who experience multiple adversities such as poverty, poor parental care, and neglect or abuse (Fraser et al.).

There are different predictors of resilience in maltreated children in comparison with nonmaltreated children (Cicchetti, 2004). Among maltreated children, positive self-esteem, self-efficacy, and an attitude of *interpersonal reserve* predict resilience, whereas in nonmaltreated children, *interpersonal relationships* are strong predictors. In general, promoting resilience includes reducing known risk factors, maximizing protective factors, and promoting competence and self-efficacy in children in order for their systems of adaptation to function in response to adversities (Masten, 2001). For maltreated children, promoting self-confidence, autonomy, mastery, and self-determination may be more effective than relationship building (Cicchetti). It should be noted that resilience for maltreated children may come at the price of a life of joylessness, unfulfilled dreams, and diminished self-confidence (Massie & Szajnberg, 2006).

Interventions for Those Exposed to Childhood Maltreatment

Interventions that psychiatric advanced practice nurses can use for children who have suffered from early maltreatment that may have caused structural and functional changes in the brain include fostering secure positive attachments, promoting positive coping, and providing psychotherapy and pharmacotherapy (Rick & Douglas, 2007).

According to Kaufman and Henrich (2000), positive attachment relationships can decrease the negative effects of childhood abuse. Kaufmann et al. (2000) believed that providing permanent and secure placements for maltreated children can optimize the likelihood of good long-term outcomes. Positive coping can be promoted through the use of interventions such as teaching impulse control, effective coping strategies, relaxation techniques, social skills, communication skills, and how to use diversional activities (Rick & Douglas, 2007, p. 52). Psychotherapy—cognitive behavioral therapy, cognitive restructuring, exposure therapy, play therapy, and combinations of therapy—has been found to be beneficial in reducing the effects of abuse (Campbell & Humphreys, 2003; Rasmussen & Charney, 2000). Pharmacotherapy has been found to be beneficial in treating anxiety disorders, such as post-traumatic stress disorder and depression, which are frequently associated with exposure to maltreatment (Teicher, Andersen, Polcari, et al., 2003). Chapter 19 describes programs that focus on preventing maltreatment of children.

There is also a need for interventions for adults who experienced childhood maltreatment. Recently, two nurse researchers reported on a study of women who considered themselves to be successful despite childhood maltreatment (Roman & Bolton, 2008). The women described the main after-effects of childhood maltreatment as depression, anxiety, problems with memory and sleep, flashbacks, mood swings, substance abuse, and suicidal episodes. These women also described people or events—sometimes the tiniest ray of hope—that helped them to see the possibilities of what they could become. It was people outside the immediate family—grandparents, aunts, siblings, teachers, husbands, partners, and neighbors—who offered a glimpse of a world of ordinary things that they had never experienced. These people showed the women that they were individuals with interests, talents, and worthiness. The main finding of the study was that the women underwent a process called "becoming resolute" (Roman & Bolton, p. 187), which is defined as "a transitional process demonstrating a steely will for de-centering abuse in one's life trajectory and achieving success in work and relationships" (Roman & Bolton, p. 187).

Summary

For psychiatric advanced practice nurses, knowledge of adverse influences on brain development provides a basis for understanding impaired brain functioning associated with certain psychiatric disorders. Knowledge of adverse influences on brain development also builds a foundation for promotion of mental health and prevention of psychiatric disorders, and it provides a basis for developing psychotherapy, psychopharmacology, psychosocial, and nursing interventions that will mitigate, remediate, and compensate for the sequelae of compromised brain development and will move patients with compromised brain development toward recovery.

Key Points

- Genes influence how the brain develops during the early prenatal stage.
- Prenatal exposure to hypoxia, malnutrition, infections, toxins, and stress may compromise brain development.
- Prenatal neurotoxic factors that affect the developing brain include cerebral hypoxia, nutritional deficiencies, and exposure through the mother's exposure to infections, neurotoxic drugs, health conditions, environmental neurotoxicants, and stress.
- Perinatal factors that influence brain development and functioning include hypoxia, prematurity, Rh incompatibility, maternal psychiatric disorders, and being born "unwanted."
- The brain is plastic; it is shaped by experiences across the life span.
- Postnatal factors that shape the brain include temperament, attachment, and achievement of psychosocial tasks and experienced factors.
- Early adverse experiences—poverty, prolonged separation from the primary caregiver, parental conflict, divorce, parental psychopathology, neglect/abuse, and violence—have a negative effect on the developing brain.
- Psychopathology appears to be related to disruptions of normal brain development that may be due to an interaction of genetic influences, prenatal factors, perinatal factors, and postnatal experienced factors.
- Factors that prevent the development of psychopathology are present at the level of the child, the family, and the community.
- Systems for adaptation develop from the child's unique characteristics, brain functioning, relationship with caregivers, ability to regulate emotions and behaviors, and readiness to interact with the environment.
- Optimally functioning systems of adaptation build resilience.

Resources

Organizations

European Network of Teratology Information Services (ENTIS)
http://www.entis.org
Organization of Teratology Information Services (OTIS)
http://www.otis.pregnancy.org
REPROTOX
http://www.reprotox.org
The Society for Neuroscience
http://www.sfn.org
The International Neurotoxicology Association
http://www.neurotoxicology.org
Teratology Society
http://www.teratology.org/

References

Aber, J. L., Jones, S., & Cohen, J. (2000). The impact of poverty on the mental health and development of very young children. In C. H. Zeanah, Jr. (Ed.), *Handbook of infant mental health* (2nd ed.) (pp. 113-128). New York: Guilford Press.

Afifi, T. O., Boman, J., Fleisher, W., et al. (2009). The relationship between child abuse, parental divorce, and life time mental disorders and suicidality in a nationally representative adult sample. *Child Abuse & Neglect, 33,* 139-147.

Afifi, T. O., Enns, M. W., Cox, B. J., et al. (2008). Population attributable fractions of psychiatric disorders and suicidal ideation and attempts associated with diverse childhood events in the general population. *American Journal of Public Health, 98,* 946-952.

Allin, M., Matsumoto, H., Santhouse, A. M., et al. (2001). Cognitive and motor function and the size of the cerebellum in adolescents born very pre-term. *Brain, 124*(Pt 1), 60-66.

Allin, M., Walshe, M., Fern, A., et al. (2008). Cognitive maturation in preterm and term born adolescents. *Journal of Neurology, Neurosurgery, and Psychology, 79*(4), 381-386.

Amato, P. R. (2000). The consequences of divorce for adults and children. *Journal of Marriage and the Family, 62,* 1269-1287.

Amato, P. R. (2003). Children of divorce in the 1990's: An update of the Amato and Keith (1991) meta-analysis. *Journal of Family Psychology, 15*(3), 355-370.

Amato, P. R. (2006). Marital discord, divorce and children's well-being: Results from a 20 year longitudinal study of two generations. In A. Clarke-Stewart & J. Dunn (Eds.), *Families count: Effects on child and adolescent development* (pp. 179-202). Cambridge, UK: Cambridge University Press.

American Academy of Pediatrics. Committee on Public Education. (2001). Media violence. *Pediatrics, 108*(5), 1222-1226.

American Psychological Association. Child sexual abuse: What parents should know. Retrieved from www.apa.org/pi/families/resources/child_sexual_abuse.aspx. Retrieved October 5, 2011.

Andersen, H. R., Nielsen, J. B., & Grandjean, P. H. (2003). Toxicologic evidence of developmental neurotoxicity of environmental chemicals. *Toxicology, 144*, 121-127.

Antonov, A. N. (1947). Children born during the siege of Leningrad in 1942. *The Journal of Pediatrics, 30*(3), 250-259.

Arndt, T. L., Stodgell, C. J., & Rodier, P. M. (2005). The teratology of autism. *International Journal of Developmental Neuroscience, 23*(2-3), 189-199.

Austin, M. P., Leader, L. R., & Reilly, N. (2005). Prenatal stress, the hypothalamic-pituitary-adrenal axis, and fetal and infant. *Early Human Development, 81*(11), 917-926.

Averill, D. R., & Needleman, H. L. (1980). Neuronal lead exposure retards cortical synaptogenesis in the rat. In H. L. Needleman (Ed.), *Low level lead exposure: The clinical implications of current research* (pp. 201-210). New York: Raven Press.

Baer, J. S., Sampson, H. M., Barr, P. D., et al. (2003). A 21-year longitudinal analysis of the effects of prenatal alcohol exposure on your adult drinking. *Archives of General Psychiatry, 60*, 377-385.

Bailey, B. (2001). Carbon monoxide poisoning during pregnancy. In G. Koren (Ed.), *Maternal-fetal toxicology* (3rd ed.) (pp. 257-268). New York: Marcel Dekker, Inc.

Bakir, F., Rustam, H., Tikriti, S., et al. (1980). Clinical and epidemiological aspects of methylmercury poisoning. *Postgraduate Medical Journal, 56*(651), 1-10.

Bandstra, E., Morrow, C. E., Mansoor, E., et al. (2010). Prenatal drug exposure: Infant and toddler outcomes. *Journal of Addictive Diseases, 29*(2), 245-258.

Barclay, L. (2005). Extreme prematurity linked to cognitive impairment at school age. *Medscape Medical News.* Retrieved from http://www.medscape.com/viewarticle/496847. Retrieved January 6, 2005.

Barr, H. M., Bookstein, F. L., O'Malley, K. D., et al. (2006). Binge drinking during pregnancy as a predictor of psychiatric disorders on the Structured Clinical Interview for DSM-IV in young adult offspring. *American Journal of Psychiatry, 163*(6), 1061-1065.

Bedi, K. S., Thomas, Y. M., Davies, C. A., et al. (1980). Synapse to neuron ratios of the frontal and cerebellar cortex of 30-day-old and adult rats undernourished during postnatal life. *Journal of Comparative Neurology, 193*, 49-56.

Bentur, Y., & Koren, G. (2001). The common occupational exposures encountered by pregnant women. In G. Koren (Ed.) *Maternal-fetal toxicology* (3rd ed.) (pp. 529-546). New York: Marcel Dekker, Inc.

Bentur, Y., Zalzatien, E., & Koren, G. (2001). Occupational exposures known to be human reproductive toxins. In G. Koren (Ed.), *Maternal-fetal toxicology* (3rd ed.) (pp. 529-546). New York: Marcel Dekker, Inc.

Bergman, U., Wilholm, B. E., Rosa, F., et al. (1992). Effects of exposure to benzodiazapines during fetal life. *Lancet, 346(*88210), 694-696.

Berkowitz, C. D. (2001). Fatal child neglect. *Advances in Pediatrics, 48*, 331-361.

Bernat, D. N., & Resnick, M. D. (2006). Health youth development: Science and strategies. *Journal of Public Health Management and Practice, 12*, S10-S16.

Bickham, D. S., & Rich, M. (2006). Is television viewing associated with social isolation? Roles of exposure time, viewing context and violent content. *Archives of Pediatrics & Adolescent Medicine, 160*(4), 387-392.

Biondi, A., Nogueira, H., Dormont, D., et al. (1998). Are the brains of monozygotic twins similar: A three-dimensional MR study. *American Journal of Neuroradiology, 19*, 1361-1367.

Bishai, R., & Koren, G. (2001). Maternal and obstetrical effects on prenatal drug exposure. In G. Koren (Ed.), *Maternal-fetal toxicology* (3rd ed.) (pp. 335-346). New York: Marcel Dekker, Inc.

Black, J., Jones, T. A., Nelson, C. A., & Greenough, W. T. (1998). Neuronal plasticity and the developing brain. In N. E. Alessi, J. T. Coyle, S. I. Harrison, & S. Eth (Eds.), *Handbook of child and adolescent psychiatry* (pp. 31-53). New York: John Wiley & Sons.

Blank, R. (1999). *Brain policy: How the new neurosciences will change our lives and our politics.* Washington, DC: Georgetown University Press.

Bokhari, A., Coull, B. A., & Holmes, L. B. (2002). Effect of prenatal exposure to anticonvulsant drugs on dermal ridge patterns of fingers. *Teratology, 66*, 19-23.

Botash, A. S. (2000). Pediatrics, child sexual abuse. *eMedicine.* Retrieved from http://www.emedicine.com/emerg/topoic369.htm. Retrieved November 23, 2006.

Botting, N., Powls, A., Cooke, R. W., et al. (1997). Attention deficit hyperactivity disorders and other psychiatric outcomes in very low birthweight children at 12 years. *Journal of Child Psychology and Psychiatry, 38*(8), 931-941.

Bourre, M. (2004). Roles of unsaturated fatty acids (especially omega 3 fatty acids) in the brain at various ages and during aging. *Journal of Nutrition, Health, and Aging, 8*(3), 163-174.

Bowlby, J. (1969). *Attachment and loss* (Vol. 1. Attachment). London: Hogarth.

Bowlby, J. (1973). *Attachment and loss* (Vol. II: Separation, anger and loss). New York: Basic Books Incorporated.

Bowlby, J. (1988). The role of attachment in personality development. In *A secure base: Clinical implications of attachment theory.* London: Routledge.

Bremmer, J. D., Randall, P., Vermetten, E., et al. (1997). Magnetic resonance imaging-based measurement of hippocampal volume in posttraumatic stress disorder related to childhood physical and sexual abuse: A preliminary report. *Biological Psychiatry, 41*, 23-32.

Brooks-Gunn, J., & Duncan, G. J. (1997). The effects of poverty on children. *The Future of Children: Children and Poverty, 7*(2), 55-71.

Brown, A. S., Schaefer, C. A., Quesenberry, C. P., Jr., et al. (2005). Maternal exposure to toxoplasmosis and risk of schizophrenia in adult offspring. *The American Journal of Psychiatry, 162*(4), 767-773.

Brown, A. S., Susser, E. S., Lin, S. P., et al. (1995). Increased risk of affective disorders in males after second trimester prenatal exposure to the Dutch Hunger Winter of 1944-1945. *British Journal of Psychiatry, 166*, 601-606.

Brown, J., Cohen, P., Johnson, J. G., et al. (1998). A longitudinal analysis of risk factors for child maltreatment findings from a seventeen-year prospective study of self-reported and officially recorded child abuse and neglect. *Child Abuse and Neglect, 22*, 1065-1078.

Brown, J., Cohen, P., Johnson, J. G., et al. (1999). Childhood abuse and neglect: Specificity of effects on adolescent and young adult depression and suicidality. *Journal of the American Academy of Child & Adolescent Psychiatry, 38*(2), 1490-1496.

Browne, K. D., & Hamilton-Giachritsis, C. (2005). The influence of violent media on children and adolescents: A public-health approach. *Lancet, 365*, 702-710.

Bruer, J. T. (1999). *The myth of the first three years: A new understanding of early brain development and lifelong learning.* New York: Free Press.

Buka, S. L., Goldstein, J. M., Seidman, L. J., et al. (1999). Prenatal complications, genetic vulnerability, and schizophrenia: The New England Longitudinal Studies of Schizophrenia. *Psychiatric Annals, 29*(3), 151-156.

Burbacher, T. M., Rodier, P. M., & Weiss, B. (1990). Methylmercury developmental neurotoxicity. A comparison of effects in humans and animals. *Neurotoxicity and Teratology, 12*, 191-202.

Campbell, J. C., & Humphreys, J. C. (2003). *Family violence and nursing practice.* Philadelphia: Lippincott Williams & Wilkins.

Canto, J. (1998). *Mommy, I'm scared: How TV and movies frighten children and what we can do to protect them.* San Diego, CA: Harcourt Brace.

Canto, J. (2000). Media violence. *Journal of Adolescent Health, 27*(2), 30-44.

Carmichael-Olson, A. P., Streissguth, P., Sampson, H. M., et al. (1997). Association of prenatal alcohol exposure with behavioral and learning problems in early adolescence. *Journal of the American Academy of Child and Adolescent Psychiatry, 36*, 1187-1194.

Caspi, A., Moffit, T., Newman, D., et al. (1996). Behavioral observations at age 3 years predict adult psychiatric disorders. *Archives of General Psychiatry, 53*, 1033-1039.

Centerwell, B. (1992). TV and violence. *Journal of the American Medical Association, 267*(2), 3059.

Cernerud, L., Eriksson, M., Jonsson, B., et al. (1996). Amphetamine addiction during pregnancy: 14-year follow-up of growth and school performance. *Acta Paediatrica, 85*(2), 204-208.

Chambers, C. D., Johnson, K. A., Dick, L. M., et al. (1998). Maternal fever and birth outcome: A prospective study. *Teratology, 58*(6), 251-257.

Chernobyl (2003). Nuclear Energy Agency. Retrieved from http://www.nea.fr/html/reports/2003/nea3508-Chernobyl.pdf. Retrieved January 18, 2005.

Chevrier, J., Eskenazi, B., Holland, N., et al. (2008). Effects of exposure to polychlorinated biphenyls and organochlorine pesticides on thyroid function during pregnancy. *American Journal of Epidemiology, 168*(3), 298-310.

Christensen, E. (1995). Families in distress, the development of children growing up with alcohol and violence. *Arctic Medical Research, 54*(Suppl 1), 53-59.

Cicchetti, D. (2002). The relationship of adverse childhood experiences to adult health: Turning gold into lead. English translation of Felitti, V. J. (2002). Belastungen in der Kindheit und Gesundheit im Erwachsenenalter: die Verwandlung von gold in Blei. *Z Psychosomatic Medicine Psychotherapy, 48*(4), 359-369.

Cicchetti, D. (2004). An odyssey of discovery: Lessons learned through three decades of research on child maltreatment. *American Psychologist, 59*(8), 731-741.

Cicchetti, D., & Lynch, M. (1993). Toward an ecological/transactional model of community violence and child maltreatment. *Psychiatry, 56,* 96-118.

Cicchetti, D., & Manly, J. T. (2001). Operationalizing child maltreatment: Developmental processes and outcomes. *Special Issue: Developmental and Psychopathology, 13*(4), 755-1048.

Cicchetti, D., & Rogosch, F. A. (1996). Eqifinality and multifinality in developmental psychopathology. *Development and Psychopathology, 8,* 597-600.

Cicchetti, D., Rogosch, F. A., & Toth, S. L. (1998). Maternal depressive disorder and contextual risk: Contributions to the development of attachment insecurity and behavior problems in toddlerhood. *Development and Psychopathology, 10,* 283-300.

Cicchetti, D., & Toth, S. L. (1995). A developmental psychopathology perspective on child abuse and neglect. *Journal of the American Academy of Child and Adolescent Psychiatry, 34,* 541-565.

Cohen, P., Brown, J., & Smailes, E. (2001). Child abuse and neglect and the development of mental disorders in the general population. *Development and Psychopathology, 13,* 981-999.

Cohn, J., & Campbell, S. (1992). Influence of maternal depression on infant affect regulation. In D. Cicchetti & S. Toth (Eds.), *Developmental perspectives on depression* (Vol. 4) (pp. 103-130). Rochester, NY: University of Rochester Press.

Colman, R. A., & Widom, C. S. (2004). Childhood abuse and neglect and adult intimate relationships: A prospective study. *Child Abuse & Neglect, 28,* 1133-1151.

Comstock, G., & Strasburger, V. C. (1993). Media violence: Q & A. *Adolescent Medicine, 4,* 495-510.

Congressional Public Health Summit (2000, July 26). Joint statement on the impact of entertainment violence on children. Retrieved from www.aap.org/advocacy/releases/jusmtevc.htm

Copper, R. L., Goldenberg, R. I., Das, A., et al. (1996). The preterm prediction study: Maternal stress is associated with spontaneous preterm birth at less than thirty-five weeks gestation. National Institute of Child Health and Human Development Maternal-Fetal Medicine Units Network. *American Journal of Obstetrics and Gynecology, 175,* 1286-1292.

Costa, L. G., Aschner, M., Vitalone, A., et al. (2004). Developmental neuropathology of environmental agents. *Annual Review of Pharmacology and Toxicology, 44,* 87-110.

Costello, E. J., Compton, S. N., Keeler, G., et al. (2003). Relationships between poverty and psychopathology: A natural experiment. *Journal of the American Medical Association, 290*(15), 2023-2029.

Crumpton, T., Atkins, D. S., Zawia, N. H., et al. (2001). Lead exposure in pheochromocytoma (PC12) cells alters neural differentiation and Sp1 DNA-binding. *Neurotoxicology, 22,* 49-62.

Csorba, R., Lampé, L., Borsos, A., et al. (2006). Female child sexual abuse within the family in a Hungarian county. *Gynecologic & Obstetric Investigation, 61*(4), 188-193.

Curtis, C. (2006). Sexual abuse and subsequent suicidal behavior. Exacerbating factors and implications for recovery. *Journal of Child Sexual Abuse, 15*(2), 1-21.

Curtis, W. J., & Cicchetti, D. (2003). Moving research on resilience into the 21st century: Theoretical and methodological considerations in examining the biological contributors to resilience. *Development and Psychopathology, 15,* 777-810.

David, H. P. (2006). Born unwanted: 35 years later: The Prague Study. *Reproductive Health Matters, 14*(27), 181-190.

David, H. P., Dytrych, Z., & Matejcek, Z. (2003). Born unwanted. Observations from the Prague Study. *The American Psychologist, 58*(3), 224-229.

Davidson, P., Myers, G., & Weiss, B. (2004). Mercury exposure and child development outcomes. *Pediatrics, 111*(4), 1023-1029.

Dawson, G., Ashman, S. B., & Carver, L. J. (2000). The role of early experience in shaping behavioral and brain development and its implications for social policy. *Development and Psychopathology, 12,* 695-712.

DeBellis, M. (1998). Brain development and stress. *NARSAD Research Newsletter, 10*(3), 12-21.

DeBellis, M. D., Keshavan, M. S., Shifflett, H., et al. (2002). Brain structures in pediatric maltreatment-related posttraumatic stress disorder: A sociodemographically matched study. *Biological Psychiatry, 52,* 1066-1078.

Debes, F., Budtz-Jorgensen, E., Weihe, P., et al. (2006). Impact of prenatal methylmercury exposure on neurobehavioral function at age 14 years. *Neurotoxicology & Teratology, 28*(3), 363-375.

DeGroot, J. M., Kennedy, S., Rotin, G., et al. (1992). Correlates of sexual abuse in women with anorexia nervosa and bulimia nervosa. *Canadian Journal of Psychiatry, 37,* 516-518.

Diav-Citrin, O., Shechtman, S., Arnon, J., et al. (2001). Is carbamazepine teratogenic? A prospective controlled study of 210 pregnancies. *Neurology, 57*(2), 321-324.

Diaz, R., Fuxe, K., & Ogren, S. O. (1997). Prenatal corticosterone treatment induces long-term changes in spontaneous and apomorphine-mediated motor activity in male and female rats. *Neuroscience, 81*(1), 129-140.

Dietz, P. M., Sptiz, A. M., Anda, V. J., et al. (1999). Unintended pregnancies among adult women exposed to abuse or household dysfunction during their childhood. *Journal of the American Medical Association, 282,* 1359-1364.

Dolovich, L. R., Addis, A., & Vaillancourt, J. M. (2001). Benzodiazepine use in pregnancy and major malformations or oral clefts: Meta analysis of cohort and case-control studies. In G. Koren (Ed.), *Maternal-fetal toxicology* (3rd ed.) (pp. 105-114). New York: Marcel Dekker, Inc.

Dube, S. R., Anda, R. F., Felitti, V. J., et al. (2001). Childhood abuse, household dysfunction and the risk of attempted suicide throughout the life span: Findings from Adverse Childhood Experiences Study. *Journal of American Medical Association, 286,* 3089-3096.

Dube, S. R., Anda, R. F., Felitti, V. J., et al. (2002). Adverse childhood experiences and personal alcohol abuse as an adult. *Addict Behavior, 7,* 713-725.

Dube, S. R., Felitti, V. J., Dong, M., et al. (2003a). Childhood abuse, neglect and household dysfunction and the risk of illicit drug use: The Adverse Childhood Experiences Study. *Pediatrics, 111*(31), 564-572.

Dube, S. R., Felitti, V. J., Dong, M., et al. (2003b). The impact of adverse childhood experiences on health problems: Evidence from four birth cohorts dating back to 1900. *Preventive Medicine, 37*(3), 268-277.

Dumas, C. A., Katerndahl, D. A., & Burge, S. K. (1995). Familial patterns in patients with infrequent panic attacks. *Archives of Family Medicine, 4,* 863-867.

Duncan, G., Brooks-Gunn, J., & Klebanov, P. (1994). Economic deprivation and early childhood development. *Child Development, 65,* 296-318.

Edwards, M. J., Saunders, R. D., & Shiota, K. (2003). Effects of heat on embryos and foetuses. *International Journal of Hyperthermia, 19*(3), 295-324.

Edwards, V. J., Holden, G. W., Felitti, V. J., et al. (2003). Relationship between multiple forms of childhood maltreatment and adult mental health in community respondents: Results from the adverse childhood experiences study. *The American Journal of Psychiatry, 160*(8), 1453-1460.

Ehrenstein, V., Sorensen, H.T., & Pedersen, L. (2011). Maternal epilepsy and cognitive/psychiatric status of sons. *Epidemiology, 22,* 280-282.

Eley, T. C., & Plomin, R. (1997). Genetic analyses of emotionality. *Current Opinion in Neurobiology, 7,* 279-284.

Eliassen, J. C., Souza, T., & Sanes, J. N. (2003). Experience-dependent activation patterns in human brain during visual-motor associative learning. *The Journal of Neuroscience, 23*(33), 10540-10547.

El-Sheikh, M., Harger, J., & Whitson, S. (2001). Exposure to parental conflict and children's adjustment and physical health: The moderating role of vagal tone. *Child Development, 72,* 1617-1636.

Emery, R. E., & Laumann-Billings, L. (1998). An overview of the nature, causes and consequences of abusive family relationships: Toward differentiating maltreatment and violence. *American Psychologist, 53*(2), 121-135.

Erickson, M. F., & Egeland, B. J. (1996). Child neglect. In J. Briere, L. Berliner, J. Bulkley, et al. (Eds.), *The APSAC handbook on child maltreatment* (pp. 4-20). Thousand Oaks, CA: Sage.

Ericson, A., & Källén, B. (1994). Pregnancy outcome in Sweden after the Chernobyl accident. *Environmental Research, 67*(2), 149-159.

Erikson, E. (1964). *Insight and responsibility.* New York: W. W. Norton & Company.

Erikson, E. (1968). *Identity: Youth and crisis.* New York: W. W. Norton & Company.

Ernst, M., Moolchan, E. T., & Robinson, M. L. (2001). Behavioral and neural consequences of prenatal exposure to nicotine. *Journal of the American Academy of Child and Adolescent Psychiatry, 6,* 630-641.

Essex, M. J., Klein, M. H., Cho, E., et al. (2003). Exposure to maternal depression and marital conflict: Gender differences in children's later mental health symptoms. *Journal of the American Academy of Child & Adolescent Psychiatry, 42*(6), 728-737.

Evans, G. W. (2004). The environment of childhood poverty. *American Psychologist, 59*(2), 77-92.

Evans, G. W., & English K. (2002). The environment of poverty: Multiple stressor exposure, psychophysiological stress, and socioemotional adjustment. *Child Development, 73*(4), 1238-1248.

Fagan, P. F., & Rector, R. (2000). The effects of divorce on America. *The Heritage Foundation Backgrounder: Executive Summary, 1373,* 1-23.

Famularo, R., Fenton, T., Kinscherff, R., et al. (1994). Maternal and child posttraumatic disorder in cases of child maltreatment. *Child Abuse & Neglect, 18,* 27-36.

Fawcett, L. B. Y., & Brent, R. L. (2006). Pathogenesis of abnormal development. In R. Hood (Ed.), *Developmental and reproductive toxicology: A practical approach* (2nd ed.) (pp. 61-92). Boca Raton, FL: Taylor & Francis.

Feldman, R. G., & White, R. F. (1992). Lead neurotoxicity and disorders of learning. *Journal of Child Neurology, 7,* 354-359.

Feldstein, M., & Singer, S. (1997, May 26). The border babies (pp. 72-74). *Time Magazine.*

Felitti, V. J. (2002). The relationship of adverse childhood experiences to adult health: Turning gold into lead. *Zeitschrift fur Psychosomatische Medizin und Psychotherapie, 48*(4), 359-369.

Felitti, V. J., Anda, R. F., Nordenberg, D., et al. (1998). Relationship of childhood abuse and household dysfunction to many of the leading causes of death in adults. *American Journal of Preventive Medicine, 14*(4), 245-258.

Fergus, S., & Zimmerman, M. A. (2005). Adolescent resilience: A framework for understanding healthy development in the face of risk. *Annual Review of Public Health, 26,* 399-419.

Fergusson, D. M., & Horwood, L. J. (1998). Exposure to interparental violence in childhood and psychosocial adjustment in young adulthood. *Child Abuse & Neglect, 22*(5), 339-357.

Fergusson, D. M., Horwood, J., & Lynskey, M. (1996). Childhood sexual abuse and psychiatric disorder in young adulthood, II: Psychiatric outcomes of childhood sexual abuse. *Journal of American Academy of Child & Adolescent Psychiatry, 35,* 1365-1374.

Fergusson, D. M., & Mullen, P. E. (2002). Review of childhood sexual abuse: An evidence-based perspective. *Child and Family Behavioral Therapy, 24*(3), 78-85.

Fergusson, D. M., Woodward, L. J., & Horwood, L. J. (1998). Maternal smoking during pregnancy and psychiatric adjustment in late adolescence. *Archives of General Psychiatry, 55*(88), 721-727.

Finkelstein, Y., Markowitz, M. E., & Rosen, J. F. (1998). Low-level lead-induced neurotoxicity in children: An update on central nervous system effects. *Brain Research. Brain Research Review, 27,* 168-176.

Forssman, H., & Thuwe, I. (1966). One hundred and twenty children born after application for therapeutic abortion refused. Their mental health, social adjustment and educational level up to the age of 21. *Acta Physiologica Scandinavica, 42*(1), 71-88.

Frankelor, D. (1994). Current information on the scope and nature of child sexual abuse. *Future of Children, 4*(2),31-53.

Fraser, M. W., Richman, J. M., & Galinsky, M. J. (1999). Risk, protection and resilience: Toward a conceptual framework for social work practice. *Social Work Research, 23*(3), 131-142.

French, N. P., Hagan, R., Evans, S. F., et al. (2004). Repeated antenatal corticosteroids: Effects on cerebral palsy and childhood behavior. *American Journal of Obstetrics and Gynecology, 190*(3), 588-595.

Fried, P. A. (2002). Conceptual issues in behavioral teratology and their application in determining long-term sequelae of prenatal marihuana exposure. *Journal of Child Psychology and Psychiatry, 43,* 81-102.

Fried, P. A., O'Connell, C. M., & Watkinson, B. (1992a). 60- and 72-month follow-up of children prenatally exposed to marijuana, cigarettes, and alcohol: Cognitive and language assessment. *Journal of Developmental and Behavioral Pediatrics, 13,* 383-391.

Fried, P. A., Watkinson, B., & Gray, R. (1992b). A follow-up study of attentional behavior in 6-year-old children exposed prenatally to marihuana, cigarettes, and alcohol. *Neurotoxicology and Teratology, 14,* 299-311.

Fries, A. B., Ziegler, T. E., Kurian, J. R., et al. (2005). Early experience in humans is associated with changes in neuropeptides critical for regulating social behavior. Retrieved from www.pnas.org/cgi/doi/10.1073/pnas.0504767102

Fryer, S. L., McGee, C. L., Spandoni, A. D., et al. (2005). Influence of alcohol on the structures of the developing brain. In M. M. Miller (Ed.), *Development of the mammalian central nervous system: Lessons learned from studies on alcohol and nicotine exposure.* Oxford, UK: Oxford University Press.

Galderisi, S., & Mucci, A. (2000). Emotions, brain development, and psychopathologic vulnerability. *CNS Spectrums, 5*(8), 44-48.

Gamache, G. L., Levinson, D. M., Reeves, D. L., et al. (2005). Longitudinal neurocognitive assessments of Ukrainians exposed to ionizing radiation after the Chernobyl nuclear accident. *Archives of Clinical Neuropsychology, 20*(1), 81-93.

Garbarino, J. (1995). Growing up in a socially toxic environment: Life for children and families in the 1990's. In B. Melton (Ed.), *Nebraska symposium on motivation. Vol. 42. The individual, the family and the social good: Personal fulfillment in times of change* (pp. 1-20). Lincoln, NE: University of Nebraska.

Garbis, H., & McElhatton, P. R. (2001). Psychotropic, sedative-hypnotic and Parkinson drugs. In C. Schaefer, P. Peters, & R. Miller (Eds.), *Drugs during pregnancy and lactation: Handbook of prescription drugs and comparative risk assessment with updated information on recreational drugs* (pp. 182-191). New York: Elsevier.

Garmezy, N. (1971). Vulnerability research and the issue of primary prevention. *American Journal of Orthopsychiatry, 41*(1), 101-116.

Garmezy, N. (1974). The study of competence in children at risk for severe psychopathology. In E. J. Anthony & C. Koupernik (Eds.), *The child in his family. Vol.3. Children at psychiatric risk* (pp. 77-97). New York: John Wiley & Sons.

Garnefski, N., & Diekstra, R. F. W. (1997). Adolescents from one parent, stepparent and intact families: Emotional problems and suicide attempts. *Journal of Adolescence, 20,* 201-208.

Geist, R., & Koren, G. (2001). Maternal disorders leading to increased reproductive risk. In G. Koren (Ed.), *Maternal-fetal toxicology* (3rd ed.) (pp. 697-732). New York: Marcel Dekker, Inc.

Glazer, D. (2000). Child abuse and neglect and the brain: A review. *Journal of Child Psychology and Psychiatry, 41*(1), 97-116.

Glynn, L. M., Wadhwa, P. D., Dunkel-Schetter, C., et al. (2001). When stress happens matters: Effects of earthquake timing on stress responsivity in pregnancy. *American Journal of Obstetrics and Gynecology, 184,* 637-642.

Goldschmidt, L., Day, N. L., & Richardson, G. A. (2000). Effects of prenatal marijuana exposure on child behavior problems at age 10. *Neurotoxicology and Teratology, 22*(3), 325-336.

Gomez, M., Hernandez, M., Johansson, B., et al. (2003). Prenatal cannabinoid and gene expression for neural adhesion molecule L1 in the fetal rat brain. *Brain Research Developmental Brain Research, 30*(147), 201-207.

Goodlett, C. R., Horn, K., & Zhou, F. C. (2005). Alcohol teratogenesis: Mechanisms of damage and strategies for intervention. *Experimental Biology and Medicine, 230,* 394-406.

Greenblatt, J. M., Huffman, L. C., & Reiss, A. L. (1994). Folic acid in neurodevelopment and child psychiatry. *Progress in Neuro-psychopharmacology & Biological Psychiatry, 18*(3), 647-659.

Greenough, W., & Black, J. (1992). Induction of brain structure by experience: Substrate for cognitive development. In M. R. Gunnar & C. A. Nelson (Eds.), *Minnesota symposia on child psychology 24: Developmental behavioral neuroscience* (pp. 155-200). Hillsdale, NJ: Lawrence Erlbaum.

Greenough, W., Black, J., & Wallace, C. S. (1987). Experience and brain development. *Child Development, 58,* 539-559.

Grossman, A. W., Churchill, J. D., McKinney, B. C., et al. (2003). Experience effects on brain development: Possible contributions to psychopathology. *Journal of Child Psychology and Psychiatry, 44*(1), 33-63.

Grossman, A. W., & DeGaetano G. (1999). *Stop teaching our children to kill: A call to action against TV, movie and video game violence.* New York: Random House, Inc.

Grubb, M. S., & Thompson, I. D. (2004). The influence of early experience on the development of sensory systems. *Current Opinion in Neurobiology, 14,* 503-512.

Grych, J. H., & Fincham, F. D. (1990). Marital conflict and children's adjustment: A cognitive-contextual framework. *Psychological Bulletin, 108,* 267-290.

Gunnar, M. (1998). Quality of early care and buffering of neuroendocrine stress reactions: Potential effects on the developing human brain. *Preventive Medicine, 27,* 208-211.

Gunnar, M. R., Broderson, L., Nachmias, M., et al. (1996). Stress reactivity and attachment security. *Developmental Psychobiology, 29,* 191-204.

Gutman, D. A., & Nemeroff, C. B. (2002). Neurobiology of early life stress: Rodent studies. *Seminars in Clinical Neuropsychiatry, 7,* 89-95.

Guzder, J., Paris, J., Zelkowitz, P., et al. (1996). Risk factors for borderline pathology in children. *Journal of American Academy of Child and Adolescent Psychiatry, 35,* 26-33.

Hack, M., Flannery, D. J., Schluchter, M., et al. (2002). Outcomes in young adulthood for very-low-birth-weight infants. *The New England Journal of Medicine, 346,* 149-157.

Hack, M., & Klein, N. (2006). Young adult attainments of preterm infants. *Journal of the American Medical Association, 295*(6), 695-696.

Hack, M., Taylor, H. G., Drotar, D., et al. (2005). Chronic conditions, functional limitations, and special health care needs of school-aged children born with extremely low birth weight in the 1990s. *Journal of the American Medical Association, 294,* 318-325.

Hack, M., Taylor, H. G., Klein, N., et al. (1994). School-age outcomes in children with birth weights under 750 g. *The New England Journal of Medicine, 331,* 753-759.

Hack, M., Taylor, H. G., Klein, N., et al. (2000). Functional limitations and special health care needs of 10 to 14 year old children weighing less than 750 grams at birth. *Pediatrics, 106,* 554-560.

Hack, M., Youngstrom, E., Cartar, L., et al. (2004). Behavioral outcomes and evidence of psychopathology among very low birth weight infants at age 20 years. *Pediatrics, 114*(4), 932-940.

Hagino, K. (2002). Early separation from primary caretakers: Effects of foster care on perceptions and expectations of interpersonal relationships. *Dissertation Abstracts International: Section B: The Sciences and Engineering, 63*(2-B), 1027.

Haller, J. (2005). Vitamins and brain function. In H. R. Lieberman, R. B. Kanarek, & C. Rasad (Eds.), *Nutritional neuroscience* (pp. 207-233). Boca Raton, FL: CRC Press.

Hancox, R. J., Milne, B. J., & Poulton, R. (2004). Association between child and adolescent television viewing and adult health: A longitudinal birth cohort study. *Lancet, 364,* 257-262.

Handford, H. A. (1975). Brain hypoxia, minimal brain dysfunction, and schizophrenia. *American Journal of Psychiatry, 132*(2), 192-194.

Hanson, T. L. (1999). Does parental conflict explain why divorce is negatively associated with child welfare? *Social Forces, 77,* 1283-1316.

Harada, M. (1995). Minamata disease—methylmercury poisoning in Japan caused by environmental pollution. *Critical Reviews in Toxicology, 25,* 1-24.

Harada, M., & Smith, A. (1975). Minamata disease: A medical report. In W. E Smith & A. M. Smith (Eds.), *Minamata* (pp. 180-192). New York: Holt, Rinehardt, & Winston.

Harjulehto, T., Aro, T., Rita, H., et al. (1989). The accident of Chernobyl and outcome of pregnancy in Finland. *British Medical Journal, 298,* 995.

Hedegaard, M., Henriksen, T. B., Sabroe, S., et al. (1996). The relationship between psychological distress during pregnancy and birth weight for gestational age. *Acta Obstetricia et Gynecologica Scandinavica, 75*(1), 32-39.

Heim, C., & Nemeroff, C. B. (2001). The role of childhood trauma in the neurobiology of mood and anxiety disorders: Preclinical and clinical studies. *Biological Psychiatry, 49,* 1023-1039.

Henry, J. P. (1993). Psychological and physiological responses to stress: The right hemisphere and the hypothalamic-pituitary-adrenal axis, an inquiry into problems of human bonding. *Integrated Physiological Behavioral Science, 28,* 369-387.

Herr, N. (2007). Television and health. The Source Book for Teaching Science. Retrieved from www.csun.edu/science/health/docs/tv+health.html

Hetherington, E. M. (2006). The influence of conflict, marital problem solving and parenting on children's adjustment in non-divorced, divorced and remarried families. In A. Clarke-Stewart & J. Dunn (Eds.), *Families count: Effects on children and adolescent development* (pp. 203-272). Cambridge, UK: Cambridge University Press.

Hetherington, E. M., & Blechman, E. A. (1996). *Stress, coping and resiliency in children and families.* New York: Cambridge University Press.

Hetherington, E. M., Cox, M., & Cox, R. (1985). Long-term effects of divorce and remarriage on the adjustment of children. *Journal of the American Academy of Child Psychiatry, 24,* 518-530.

Hetherington, E. M., & Kelly, J. (2002). *For better or for worse: Divorce reconsidered.* New York: W. W. Norton & Company.

Hettler, J., & Greenes, D. S. (2003). Can the initial history predict whether a child with a head injury has been abused? *Pediatrics, 111*(3), 602-607.

Hille, E., Den Ouden, A. L., & Bauer, L. (1994). School performance at nine years of age in very premature and very low birth weight infants: Perinatal risk factors and predictors at five years of age. *Journal of Pediatrics, 125,* 426-434.

Hille, E., Den Ouden, A. L., Saigal, S., et al. (2001). Behavioural problems in children who weight 1000 g or less at birth in four countries. *Lancet, 357,* 1641-1643.

Hillis, S. D., Anda, R. F., Felitti, V. J., et al. (2000). Adverse childhood experiences and sexually transmitted diseases in men and women: A retrospective study. *Pediatrics, 106*(1), E11.

Hoek, H. W., Susser, E., Buck, K. A., et al. (1996). Schizoid personality disorder after prenatal exposure to famine. *American Journal of Psychiatry, 153,* 1637-1639.

Hoekstra, S. J., Harris, R. J., & Helmick, A. L. (1999). Autobiographical memories about the experience of seeing frightening movies in childhood. *Media Psychology, 1,* 117-140.

Hoffman, S., & Hatch, M. C. (2000). Depressive symptomatology during pregnancy: Evidence for an association with decreased fetal growth in pregnancies of lower social class women. *Health Psychology, 19*(6), 535-543.

Hollister, J. M., Laing, P., & Mednick, S. A. (1996). Rhesus incompatibility as a risk factor for schizophrenia in male adults. *Archives of General Psychiatry, 53,* 19-24.

Hortocollis, P. (1978). Minimal brain dysfunction in young adults. In L. Bellak (Ed.), *Psychiatric aspects of minimal brain dysfunction in adults* (pp. 103-112). New York: Grune & Stratton.

Horwitz, A. V., Widom, C. S., McLaughlin, J., et al. (2001). The impact of childhood abuse and neglect on adult mental health: A prospective study. *Journal of Health & Social Behavior, 42*(2), 184-201.

Huesmann, L. R., Moisse-Titus, J., Podolski, C., et al. (2003). Longitudinal relations between children's exposure to TV violence and their aggressive and violent behavior in young adulthood: 1977-1992. *Developmental Psychology, 39*(2), 201-221.

Huizink, A. C., & Mulder, E. J. (2006). Maternal smoking, drinking or cannabis use during pregnancy and neurobehavioral and cognitive functioning in human offspring. *Neuroscience Behavioral Review, 30*(1), 24-41.

Huizink, A. C., Mulder, E. J., & Buitelaar, J. K. (2004). Prenatal stress and risk for psychopathology: Specific effects or induction of general susceptibility? *Psychology Bulletin, 130*(1), 115-142.

Huizink, A. C., Robles de Medina, P. G., Mulder, E. J. H., et al. (2002). Psychological measures of prenatal stress as predictors of infant temperament. *Child & Adolescent Psychiatry, 41*(9), 1078-1085.

Huttenen, M. O., & Niskanen, P. (1978). Prenatal loss of father and psychiatric disorders. *Archives of General Psychiatry, 35,* 429-431.

Indredavik, M. S., Vik, T., Heyerdahl, S., et al. (2004). Psychiatric symptoms and disorders in adolescents with low birth weight. *Archives of Disease in Childhood. Fetal and Neonatal Edition, 89*(5), F445-450.

Iqbal, M. M., Sobhan, T., & Ryals, T. (2002). Effects of commonly used benzodiazepines on the fetus, the neonate, and the nursing infant. *Psychiatric Services, 53*(1), 3-49.

Jacobson, J., & Jacobson, S. (2003). Prenatal exposure to polychlorinated biphenyls and attention at school age. *Journal of Pediatrics, 143*(6), 780-788.

Jaffe, P., Hurley, D., & Wolfe, D. (1990). Children's observations of violence: 1. Critical issues in child development and intervention planning. *Canadian Journal of Psychiatry, 35,* 466-470.

Jain, U. D. (2011). Psychosocial and environmental pregnancy risks. Medscape. Retrieved from emedicine.medscape.com/article/259346_overview#AW2AAbcb5. Retrieved November 15, 2011.

Johnson, J. G., Cohen, P., Smailes, E. M., et al. (2002). Television viewing and aggressive behavior during adolescence and adulthood. *Science, 295*(5564), 2468-2471.

Johnson, S. (2001). Micronutrient accumulation and depletion in schizophrenia, epilepsy, autism and Parkinson's disease? *Medical Hypotheses, 56*(5), 641-645.

Johnson, S., Hollis, C., Kochhar, P., et al. (2010). Psychiatric disorders in extremely preterm children: Longitudinal finding at age 11 years in the EPICure Study. *Journal of the American Academy of Child & Adolescent Psychiatry, 49*(50), 453-463.

Jones, P. B., Rantakallio, P., Hartikaienen, A., et al. (1998). Schizophrenia as a long-term outcome of pregnancy, delivery, and perinatal complications: A 28-year follow-up of the 1966 North Finland general population birth cohort. *American Journal of Psychiatry, 155*(3), 355-364.

Journalism Center on Children & Families. (2008). *Child welfare.* Retrieved from http://www.journalismcenter.org/resources/childneglect.cfm. Retrieved January 1, 2009

Kaplan, M. D., & Pruett, K. D. (2000). Divorce and custody: Developmental implications. In C. H. Zeanah, Jr. (Ed.), *Handbook of infant mental health* (2nd ed.) (pp. 533-547). New York: Guilford Press.

Karten, Y. J., Olariu, O., & Cameron, H. A. (2005). Stress in early life inhibits neurogenesis in adulthood. *Trends in Neurosciences, 28*(4), 171-172.

Kashani, J. H., Daniel, A. E., Dandoy, A. C., et al. (1992). Family violence: Impact on children. *American Academy of Child and Adolescent Psychiatry, 32*(2), 181-189.

Kaufman, J., & Henrich, C. (2000). Exposure to violence and early childhood trauma. In C. H. Zeanah, Jr. (Ed.), *Handbook of infant mental health* (pp. 195-207). New York: Guilford Press.

Kaufman, J., Plotsky, P. M., Nemeroff, C. B., et al. (2000). Effects of early adverse experiences on brain structures and function: Clinical implications. *Biological Psychiatry, 48,* 778-790.

Kelly, J. B. (2000). Children's adjustment in conflicted marriage and divorce: A decade review of research. *Journal of the American Academy of Child & Adolescent Psychiatry, 39*(8), 963-973.

Kelley, M. L., Cash, T. F., Grant, A. R., et al. (2004). Parental alcoholism: Relationships to adult attachment in college women and men. *Addictive Behaviors, 29*(8), 1633-1636.

Kemppainen, L., Jokelainen, J., Isohanni, M., et al. (2002). Predictors of female criminality: Findings from the Northern Finland 1966 birth cohort. *Journal of American Academy of Child and Adolescent Psychiatry, 41*(7), 854-859.

Kendall-Tackett, K. A., Williams, L. M., & Finkelhor, D. (1993). Impact of sexual abuse on children: A review and synthesis of recent empirical studies. *Psychology Bulletin, 113*(1), 164-180.

Kendler, K. S., Neale, M. C., & Kessler, R. C. (1992). Major depression and generalized anxiety disorder: Same genes, (partly) different environments? *Archives of General Psychiatry, 49*(9), 716-722.

Kim-Cohen, J., Moffitt, T., Taylor, A., et al. (2005). Maternal depression and children's antisocial behavior: Nature and nurture effects. *Archives of General Psychiatry, 6292,* 173-181.

Kofman, O. (2002). The role of prenatal stress in the etiology of developmental behavioural disorders. *Neuroscience and Biobehavioral Reviews, 26,* 457-470.

Kosofsky, B. E., & Hyman, S. E. (2001). No time for complacency: The fetal brain on drugs. *Journal of Comparative Neurology, 435,* 259-262.

Koubovec, D., Geerts, L., Odendaal, H., et al. (2005). Effects of psychological stress on fetal development and pregnancy outcome. *Current Psychiatry Reports, 7*(4), 274-280.

Kubicka, L., Roth, Z., Dytrych, Z., et al. (2002). The mental health of adults born of unwanted pregnancies, their siblings, and matched controls: A 35-year follow-up study from Prague, Czech Republic. *The Journal of Nervous and Mental Disease, 190*(10), 653-662.

Laplante, D., Barr, R., Brunet, A., et al. (2004). Stress during pregnancy affects general intellectual and language functioning in human toddlers. *Pediatric Research, 56*(3), 400-410.

Lawrence, M. S., & Sapolsky, R. M. (1994). Glucocorticoids accelerate ATP loss following metabolic insults in cultured hippocampal neurons. *Brain Research, 646,* 303-306.

LeDoux, J. E. (2000). Emotion circuits in the brain. *Annual Review of Neuroscience, 23,* 155-182.

Lester, B., Boukydis, C. F. Z., & Twomey, J. E. (2000). Maternal substance abuse and child outcome. In C. H. Zeanah, Jr. (Ed.), *Handbook of infant mental health* (2nd ed.) (pp. 161-175). New York: Guilford Press.

Lester, B. M., LaGasse, L. L., & Seifer, R. (1998). Cocaine exposure and children: The meaning of subtle effects. *Science, 282,* 633-634.

Lewandowski, T. A., Ponce, R. A., Charleston, J. S., et al. (2003). Effect of methylmercury on midbrain cell proliferation during organogenesis: Potential cross-species differences and implications for risk assessment. *Toxicological Sciences, 75,* 124-133.

Lewis, D. A. (2000). GABAergic local circuit neurons and prefrontal cortical dysfunction in schizophrenia. *Brain Research Brain Research Review, 31,* 270-276.

Li, Z., Dong, T., Proschel, C., et al. (2007). Chemically diverse toxicants converge on Fyn and c-Cbl to disrupt precursor cell function. *PLoS Biology, 5*(2), e35, 0212-0231.

Lindsay, C. A., Thomas, A. J., & Catalano, P. M. (1997). The effect of smoking tobacco on neonatal body composition. *American Journal of Obstetrics and Gynecology, 177*(5), 1124-1128.

Linnet, K. M., Dalsgaard, S., Obel, C., et al. (2003). Maternal life style factors in pregnancy risk of attention deficit hyperactivity disorder and associated behaviors: Review of the current evidence. *The American Journal of Psychiatry, 160,* 1028-1040.

Little, J. (1993). The Chernobyl accident, congenital anomalies and other reproductive outcomes. *Paediatric and Perinatal Epidemiology, 7*(2), 121-151.

Lou, H. C., Hansen, D., Nordentoft, M., et al. (1995). Prenatal stressors of human life affect fetal brain development. *Developmental Medicine & Child Neurology, 36*(9), 826-832.

Lundy, V. L., Jones, N. A., Field, T., et al. (1999). Prenatal depression effects on neonates. *Infant Behavior and Development, 22,* 119-129.

Lung, C. T., & Daro, D. (1996). *Current trends in child abuse reporting and fatalities: The results of the 1995 annual fifty state survey.* Chicago: National Committee to Prevent Child Abuse.

Lynskey, M. T., & Fergusson, D. M. (1997). Factors protecting against the development of adjustment difficulties in young adults exposed to childhood sexual abuse. *Child Abuse & Neglect, 21*(12), 1177-1190.

Lyons-Ruth, K., Wolfe, R., & Lyubchik, A. (2000). Depression and the parenting of young children: Making the case for early preventive mental health services. *Harvard Review of Psychiatry, 8,* 148-153.

Machon, R., Mednick, S., & Huttunen, M. (1997). Adult major affective disorder after prenatal exposure to an influenza epidemic. *Archives of General Psychiatry, 54,* 322-328.

Macksoud, M., Aber, L., & Cohn, I. (1996). Assessing the impact of war on children. In R. J. Apfel & B. Simon (Eds.), *Minefields in the heart* (pp. 218-231). New Haven, CT: Yale University Press.

Marlow, N. (2004). Neurocognitive outcome after very preterm birth. *Archives of Disease in Childhood. Fetal and Neonatal Edition, 89*(3), 224-228.

Marlow, N., Wolke, D., Bracewell, M. A., et al. (2005). Neurologic and developmental disability at six years of age after extremely preterm birth. *The New England Journal of Medicine, 352*(1), 9-19.

Marret, S. (2005). Effects of maternal smoking during pregnancy on fetal brain development. *Journal de Gynecologie, Obstetrique et Biologie de la Reproduction, 34,* Spec No. 1:3S230-233.

Mash, E., & Dozois, D. (1996). Child psychopathology: A development systems perspective. In E. Mash & R. Barkley (Eds.), *Child psychopathology* (pp. 3-60). New York: Guilford Press.

Massie, H., & Szajnberg, N. (2006). My life is a longing: Child abuse and its adult sequelae. *International Journal of Psychoanalysis, 87,* 471-496.

Masten, A. S. (2001). Ordinary magic: Resilience processes in development. *American Psychologist, 56*(3), 227-238.

Masten, A. S., & Shaffer, A. (2006). How families matter in child development: Reflections from research on risk and resilience. In A. Clarke-Stewart & J. Dunn (Eds.), *Families Count: Effects on child and adolescent development* (pp. 5-25). Cambridge, UK: Cambridge University Press.

Matalon, S., Schechtman, S., Goldzweig, G., et al. (2002). The teratogenic effect of carbamazepine: A meta-analysis of 1255 exposures. *Reproductive Toxicology, 16*(9), 9-17.

Mathew, R. J., Wilson, W. H., Blazer, D. G., et al. (1993). Psychiatric disorders in adult children of alcoholics: Data from the Epidemiologic Catchment Area Project. *American Journal of Psychiatry, 150*(5), 793-800.

Maughan, B., Taylor, C., Tallor, A., et al. (2001). Pregnancy smoking and childhood conduct problems: A causal association? *Journal of Child Psychology and Psychiatry and Allied Disciplines, 42,* 1021-1028.

Mayes, L. C., & Ward, A. (2003). Principles of neurobehavioral teratology. In D. Cicchetti & E. F. Walker (Eds.), *Neurodevelopmental mechanisms in psychopathology* (pp. 3-34). Cambridge, UK: Cambridge University Press.

McCarton, C., Brooks-Gunn, J., Wallace, I., et al. (1997). Results at age 8 years of early intervention for low-birth-weight premature infants. *Journal of the American Medical Association, 277,* 126-142.

McCloskey, L. A. (2001). The "Media complex" among men: The instrumental abuse of children to injure wives. *Violence and Victims, 16*(1), 19-37.

McCloskey, L. A., Figueredo, A. J., & Koss, M. P. (1995). The effects of systemic family violence on children's mental health. *Child Development, 66*(5), 1239-1261.

McCormick, M., Workman-Daniels, K., & Brooks-Gunn, J. (1996). The behavioral and emotional well-being of school-age children with different birth weights. *Pediatrics, 94,* 700-708.

McDonough, P. (2009). TV viewing among kids at an eight-year high. Nielseriwire (October 26, 2009). Retrieved from http://blog.nielsen.com/nielseriwire/media/entertainment/tv-viewing-among-kids-at-an-eight-yhear-high/

McElhatton, P., Garbis, H., & Schaefer, C. (2001). Industrial and environmental chemicals. In C. Schaefer (Ed.), *Drugs during pregnancy and lactation: Handbook of prescription drugs and comparative risk* (pp. 225-245). Amsterdam: Elsevier.

McEwen, B. S., Gould, E. A., & Sakai, R. R. (1992). The vulnerability of the hippocampus to protective and destructive effects of glucocorticoids in relation to stress. *British Journal of Psychiatry Suppl.,* Feb, 18-23.

McGloin, J. M., & Widom, C. S. (2001). Resilience among abused and neglected children grown up. *Developmental Psychopathology, 13*(4), 1021-1058.

McGrath, J. J., Feron, F. P., Burne, T. H. J., et al. (2004). Vitamin D3—implications for brain development. *The Journal of Steroid Biochemistry & Molecular Biology, 89-90,* 557-560.

McLanahan, S., & Sandefur, G. D. (1994). *Growing up with a single parent: What hurts, what helps* (p. 67). Cambridge, MA: Harvard University Press.

McLeod, J. D., & Shanahan, M. J. (1996). Trajectories of poverty and children's mental health. *Journal of Health and Social Behavior, 37*(3), 207-220.

McNeil, T. F., Cantor-Graae, E., & Weinberger, D. R. (2000). Relationship of obstetric complications and differences in size of brain structures in monozygotic twin pairs discordant for schizophrenia. *American Journal of Psychiatry, 157,* 203-212.

Meaney, M. J., & Szyf, M. (2005). Maternal care as a model for experience-dependent chromatin plasticity? *Trends in Neurosciences, 28*(9), 456-463.

Meijer, A. (1985). Child psychiatric sequelae of maternal war stress. *Acta Psychiatrica Scandinavia, 72,* 505-511.

Ment, L. R., Vohr, B., Allan, W., et al. (1999). The etiology and outcome of cerebral ventriculomegaly at term in very low birth weight preterm infants. *Pediatrics, 104*(2), Part 1 of 2, 243-248.

Meyers, K. S. (2003). Television and video game violence: Age differences and the combined effects of passive and interactive violent media. *The Sciences and Engineering, 63*(11-B), 5551.

Miller, M. W. (1986). Effects of alcohol on the generation and migration of cerebral cortical neurons. *Science, 233,* 1308-1311.

Miller, M. W. (1993). Migration of cortical neurons is altered by gestational exposure to ethanol. *Alcohol Clinical Experience Research, 17,* 304-314.

Miller, M. W. (1996). Limited ethanol exposure selectively alters the proliferation of precursor cells in the cerebral cortex. *Alcohol Clinical Experience Research, 20,* 139-143.

Miller, M. W., & Potempa, G. (1990). Number of neurons and glia in mature rat somatosensory cortex: Effects of prenatal exposure to ethanol. *Journal of Comparative Neurology, 293,* 92-102.

Miller, R. W. (1956). Delayed effects occurring within the first decade after exposure of young individuals to the Hiroshima atomic bomb. *Pediatrics, 18*(1), 1-18.

Milunsky, A., Ulcickas, M., Rothman, K. J., et al. (1992). Maternal heat exposure and neural tube defects. *Journal of the American Medical Association, 268,* 882-885.

Mirsky, A. F., & Quinn, O. W. (1988). The Genain quadruplets. *Schizophrenia Bulletin, 14*(4), 595-612.

Mole, R. H. (1982). Consequences of pre-natal radiation exposure for post-natal development: A review. *International Journal of Radiation Biology, 42*(1), 1-12.

Molnar, B. E., Buka, S. L., & Kessler, R. C. (2001). Child sexual abuse and subsequent psychopathology: Results from the National Comorbidity Survey. *American Journal of Public Health, 91*(5), 753-760.

Moore, K. L., & Persaud, T. V. N. (1993). *The developing human: Clinically oriented embryology.* Philadelphia: W. B. Saunders Company.

Moore, S. J., Turnpenny, P., Quinn, A., et al. (2000). A clinical study of 57 children with fetal anticonvulsant syndrome. *Journal of Medical Genetics, 37,* 489-497.

Moretti, M. E., Bar-Oz, B., Fried, S. (2005). Maternal hyperthermia and the risk for neural tube defects in offspring: systematic review and meta-analysis. *Epidemiology, 16*(2), 216-219.

Morgane, P. J., Austin-LaFrance, R., Bronzino, J., et al. (1993). Prenatal malnutrition and development of the brain. *Neuroscience and Biobehavioral Reviews, 17,* 91-128.

Morreale de Escobar, G., Obregón, M. J., & Escobar del Rey, F. (2000). Is neuropsychological development related to maternal hypothyroidism or to maternal hypothyroxinemia? *Journal of Clinical Endocrinology and Metabolism, 85*(11), 3975-3987.

Mulder, G. B., Manley, N., Grant, J., et al. (2000). Effects of excess vitamin A on development of cranial neural crest-derived structures: A neonatal and embryologic study. *Teratology, 62,* 214-226.

Mullen, P. E., & Fleming, J. (1998). Long-term effects of child sexual abuse. *Issues in Child Abuse Prevention, 9,* 1-19.

Mundy, W. R., Radio, N. M., & Freudenrich, T. M. (2010). Neuronal models for evaluation of proliferation in vitro using high content screening. *Toxicology, 270,* 121-130.

Myhrman, A., Olsen, P., Rantakallio, P., et al. (1995). Does the wantedness of a pregnancy predict a child's educational attainment? *Family Planning Perspectives, 27*(3), 116-119.

Myhrman, A., Rantakallio, P., Isohanni, M., et al. (1996). Unwantedness of a pregnancy and schizophrenia in the child. *The British Journal of Psychiatry, 169*(5), 637-640.

Nachmias, M., Gunnar, M. R., Mangelsdorf, S., et al. (1996). Behavioral inhibition and stress reactivity: Moderating role of attachment security. *Child Development, 67,* 508-522.

National Clearinghouse on Child Abuse and Neglect (2004). *2004 Child Abuse Prevention Community Resource Packet* (2nd ed.). Washington, DC: U.S. Department of Health and Human Services.

Nelson, E. C., & Bosquet, M. (2000). Neurobiology of fetal and infant development: Implications for infant mental health. In C. H. Zeanah, Jr. (Ed.), *Handbook of infant mental health* (2nd ed.) (pp. 37-59). New York: Guilford Press.

Nelson, E. C., Heath, A. C., Phil, D., et al. (2002). Association between self-reported childhood sexual abuse and adverse psychosocial outcomes. *Archives of General Psychiatry, 59,* 139-145.

Nemeroff, C. B. (2004). Neurobiological consequences of childhood trauma. *Journal of Clinical Psychiatry, 65*(Suppl 1), 18-28.

Nicolotti, L., el-Sheikh, M., Whitson, S. M. (2003). Children's coping with marital conflict and their adjustment and physical health: Vulnerability and protective functions. *Journal of Family Psychology, 17*(3), 315-326.

Ng, P. C., Wong, G. W., Lam, C. W., et al. (1999). Effect of multiple courses of antenatal corticosteroids on pituitary-adrenal function in preterm infants. *Archives of Disease in Childhood. Fetal & Neonatal Edition, 80*(3), F213-216.

Nosarti, C., Al-Asady, M. H., Frangou, S., et al. (2002). Adolescents who were born very preterm have decreased brain volumes. *Brain, 125*(Pt 7), 1616-1623.

Nosarti, C., Rushe, T. M., Woodruff, P. W., et al. (2004). Corpus callosum size and very preterm birth: Relationship to neuropsychological outcome. *Brain, 127*(Pt 9), 2080-2089.

Nulman, I., Atanackovic, G., & Koren, G. (2001). Teratogenic drugs and chemicals in humans. In G. Koren (Ed.), *Maternal-fetal toxicology: A clinician's guide* (3rd ed.) (pp. 57-71). New York: Marcel Dekker, Inc.

Oberto, A., Marks, N., Evans, H. L., et al. (1996). Lead (Pb + 2) promotes apoptosis in newborn rat cerebellar neurons: Pathological implications. *The Journal of Pharmacology and Experimental Therapeutics, 279*, 435-442.

Oken, E., Wright, R. O., Kleinman, K. P., et al. (2005). Maternal fish consumption, hair mercury and infant cognition. *Environmental Health Perspectives, 113*(10), 1376-1380.

Oppenheim, J. S., Skerry, J. E., Tramo, M. J., et al. (1989). Magnetic resonance imaging morphology of the corpus callosum in monozygotic twins. *Annals of Neurology, 26*, 100-104.

Ornoy, A. (2006). Neuroteratogens in man: An overview with special emphasis on the teratogenicity of antiepileptic drugs in pregnancy. *Reproductive Toxicology, 2292*, 214-226.

Otake, M., & Schull, J. W. (1984). In utero exposure to A-bomb radiation and mental retardation: A reassessment. *British Journal of Radiology, 57*, 409-414.

Paik, H., & Comstock, G. (1994). The effects of television violence on antisocial behavior: A meta-analysis. *Communication Research, 2*, 516-546.

Persaud, T. V. N., Path, F. R., & Path, P. F. (1990). *Environmental causes of human birth defects.* Springville, IL: Charles C. Thomas.

Peters, P., & Schaefer, C. H. (2001). General commentary to drug therapy and drug risks in pregnancy. In C. H. Schaefer (Ed.), *Drugs during pregnancy and lactation* (pp. 1-13). Amsterdam: Elsevier.

Peterson, B., Vohr, B., Staib, L. H., et al. (2000). Regional brain volume abnormalities and long-term cognitive outcome in preterm infants. *Journal of the American Medical Association, 284*(15), 1939-1947.

Peterson, J., Taylor, H. G., Minich, N., et al. (2006). Subnormal head circumference in very low birth weight children: Neonatal correlates and school-age consequences. *Early Human Development, 82*(5), 325-334.

Pike, I. L. (2005). Maternal stress and fetal responses: Evolutionary perspectives on preterm delivery. *American Journal of Human Biology, 17*(1), 5-21.

Plomin, R. (1990). The role of inheritance in behavior. *Science, 248*, 183-188.

Pollard, I. (2007). Neuropharmacology of drugs and alcohol in mother and fetus. *Seminars in Fetal & Neonatal Medicine, 12*, 106-113.

Pottinger, A. M. (2005). Children's experience of loss by parental migration in inner-city Jamaica. *American Journal of Orthopsychiatry, 75*(4), 485-496.

Putnam, F. W. (2003). Ten-year research update review: Child sexual abuse. *Journal of the American Academy of Child & Adolescent Psychiatry, 42*(3), 269-278.

Rao, R., & Georgieff, M. K. (2003). Early nutrition and brain development. In C. Nelson (Ed.), *The effects of early adversity on neurobehavioral development: The Minnesota Symposia on Child Psychology* (Vol. 3) (pp. 1-30). Mahwah, NJ: Lawrence Erlbaum Associates Publishers.

Rasalam, A. D., Hailey, H., Williams, J. H. G., et al. (2005). Characteristics of fetal anticonvulsant syndrome associated autistic disorder. *Developmental Medicine & Child Neurology, 47*(88), 551-555.

Rasmussen, S., & Charney, D. (2000). Posttraumatic therapy. In G. Fink (Ed.), *Encyclopedia of Distress* (Vol. 3) (pp. 192-200). San Diego, CA: Academic Press.

Rasmussen, S. A., Jamieson, D. J., & Bresee, J. S. (2008). *Pandemic influenza and pregnant women, Emerging Infectious Diseases* (serial on the internet) 14(1). Retrieved from http://www.cdc.gov/EID/content/14/1/95.htm

Rees, S., Breen, S., Loeliger, M., et al. (1999). Hypoxemia near mid-gestation and long term effects on fetal brain development. *Journal of Neuropathology & Experimental Neurology, 58*(9), 932-945.

Rees, S., & Harding, R. (2004). Brain development during fetal life: Influences of the intra-uterine environment. *Neuroscience Letters, 361*, 111-114.

Rees, S., & Inder, T. (2005). Fetal and neonatal origins of altered brain development. *Early Human Development, 81*, 753-761.

Reiss, D., Plomin, R., & Hetherington, E. M. (1991). Genetics and psychiatry: An unheralded window on the environment. *The American Journal of Psychiatry, 148*(3), 283-291.

Repetti, R. L., Taylor, S. E., & Seeman, T. E. (2002). Risky families: Family social environments and the mental and physical health of offspring. *Psychological Bulletin, 128*, 330-336.

Rich, M., Woods, E. R., Goodman, E., et al. (1998). Aggressors or victims: Gender and race in music video violence. *Pediatrics, 101*(4 Pt 1), 669-674.

Rick, S., & Douglas, D. H. (2007). Neurobiological effects of childhood abuse. *Journal of Psychosocial Nursing, 45*(4), 47-52.

Risk and Protective Factors for Child Abuse and Neglect. (2004). National Clearinghouse for Child Abuse and Neglect Information. Retrieved from http://nccanch.acf.hhs.gov/topics/prevention/emerging/report.pdf. Retrieved May 8, 2011.

Robert, E., Reuvers, M., & Schaefer, C. (2001). Antiepileptics. In C. Schaefer (Ed.), *Drugs during pregnancy and lactation: Handbook of prescription drugs and comparative risk* (pp. 46-57). Amsterdam: Elsevier.

Rodier, P. M. (2000). The early origins of autism. *Scientific American, 282*(2), 56-63.

Rodgers, K. B., & Rose, H. A. (2002). Risk and resiliency factors among adolescents who experience marital transitions. *Journal of Marriage and Family, 64*, 1024-1037.

Roman, M. W., & Bolton, K. S. (2008). Nurturing natural resources: The ecology of interpersonal relationships in women who have thrived despite childhood maltreatment. *Advances in Nursing Science, 31*(3), 184-197.

Rosenthal, D. (1963). *The Genain quadruplets: A study of heredity and environment in schizophrenia.* New York: Basic Books.

Rowan, A. B., Foy, D. W., Rodriguez, N., et al. (1994). Posttraumatic stress disorder in a clinical sample of adults sexually abused as children. *Child Abuse and Neglect, 18*, 51-61.

Russell, D. E. H. (1984). The prevalence and seriousness of incestuous abuse: Stepfathers vs. biological fathers. *Child Abuse and Neglect, 8*, 15-22.

Rutter, M. (1979). Separation experiences: A new look at an old topic. *Journal of Pediatrics, 95*, 147-154.

Rutter, M. (2002). The interplay of nature, nurture, and developmental influences: The challenge ahead for mental health. *Archives of General Psychiatry, 59*, 996-1000.

Rutter, M., & Silberg, J. (2002). Gene-environment interplay in relation to emotional and behavioral disturbance. *Annual Reviews of Psychology, 53*, 463-490.

Sadock, B. J., & Sadock, V. A. (2007). *Kaplan & Sadock's synopsis of psychiatry* (10th ed.). Philadelphia: Lippincott, Williams & Wilkins.

Sagiv, S. K., Thurston, S. W., Bellinger, D. C., et al. (2010). Prenatal organochlorine exposure and behaviors associated with attention deficit hyperactivity disorder in school-aged children. *American Journal of Epidemiology, 171*(5), 593-610.

Saigal, S., Stoskopf, B., Pinelli, J., et al. (2006). Self-perceived health-related quality of life of former extremely low birth weight infants at young adulthood. *Pediatrics, 118*(3), 1140-1148.

Salt, A., D'Amore, A., Ahluwalia, J., et al. (2006). Outcome at 2 years for very low birthweight infants in a geographical population: Risk factors, cost, and impact of congenital anomalies. *Early Human Development, 82*(2), 125-129.

Salt, A., & Redshaw, M. (2006). Neurodevelopmental follow-up after preterm birth: Follow up after two years. *Early Human Development, 82*(3), 185-197.

Sameroff, A. (2006). Identifying risk and protective factors for healthy child development. In A. Clarke-Stewart & J. Dunn (Eds.), *Families count: Effects on child and adolescent development* (pp. 53-76). Cambridge, UK: Cambridge University Press.

Saugstad, L. F. (2004). From superior adaptation and function to brain dysfunction: The neglect of epigenetic factors. *Nutrition and Health, 18*(1), 3-27.

Schaefer, C. (2001). Recreational drugs. In C. Schaever (Ed.), *Drugs during pregnancy and lactation: Handbook of prescription drugs and comparative risk* (pp. 214-224). Amsterdam: Elsevier.

Schneiderman, J. F. (2001). The approach to the mother on nonmedicinal and chemical use in pregnancy. In G. Koren (Ed.), *Maternal-fetal toxicology* (3rd ed.) (pp. 321-334). New York: Marcel Dekker, Inc.

Schoon, I., Sacker, A., & Bartley, M. (2003). Socio-economic adversity and psychosocial adjustment: A developmental-contextual perspective. *Social Science & Medicine, 57,* 1001-1015.

Schull, W. J., & Otake, M. (1999). Cognitive function and prenatal exposure to ionizing radiation. *Teratology, 59*(4), 222-226.

Scott, J. M., Weir, D. G., Molloy, A., et al. (1994). Folic acid metabolism and mechanisms of neural tube defects. *Ciba Foundation Symposium, 181,* 180-187.

Sedlak, A. J., & Broadhurst, D. D. (1996). *Third national incidence study on child abuse and neglect.* Washington, DC: U.S. Department of Health and Human Services.

Seeman, M. V. (2004). Schizophrenia and motherhood. In M. Gopfert, J. Webster, & M. V. Seeman (Eds.), *Parental psychiatric disorder* (2nd ed.). Cambridge, UK: Cambridge University Press.

Seifer, R., & Dickstein, S. (2000). Parental mental illness and infant development. In C. H. Zeanah, Jr. (Ed.), *Handbook of infant mental health* (2nd ed.). (pp. 176-194). New York: Guilford Press.

Sffogia, A., Pacheco, M. A., & Grassi-Oliveira, R. (2008). History of childhood abuse and neglect and suicidal behavior at hospital admission. *Journal of Crisis Intervention & Suicide, 29*(3), 154-158.

Shah, T., Sullivan, K., & Carter, J. (2006). Sudden infant death syndrome and reported maternal smoking during pregnancy. *American Journal of Public Health, 96*(10), 1757-1759.

Shaw, D. S., Owens, E., Vondra, K., et al. (1996). Early risk factors and pathways in the development of early disruptive behavioral problems. *Development and Psychopathology, 4,* 679-700.

Simpson, J. L., Bailey, L. B., Pietrzik, K., et al. (2010). Micronutrients and women of reproductive potential, required dietary intake and consequences of dietary deficiencies or excess: Part 1. Folate, Vitamin B12, Vitamin B6. *Journal of Maternal, Fetal & Neonatal Medicine, 23*(13), 1323-1343.

Spauwen, J., Krabbendam, L., Lieb, R., et al. (2004). Early maternal stress and health behaviours and offspring expression of psychosis in adolescence. *Acta Psychiatrica Scandinavica, 10*(5), 356-364.

Sroufe, L. A., Carlson, E. A., Levy, A. K., et al. (1999). Implications of attachment theory for developmental psychopathology. *Development and Psychopathology, 11,* 1-13.

Stahl, S. (2005). *Essential psychopharmacology: The prescriber's guide.* Cambridge, UK: Cambridge University Press.

Stein, M. B., Koverola, C., Hanna, C., et al. (1997). Hippocampal volume in women victimized by childhood sexual abuse. *Psychological Medicine, 27,* 951-959.

Straus, M. A., Gelles, R. J., & Steinmetz, S. K. (1980). *Behind closed doors: Violence in the American family.* Garden City, NY: Anchor.

Streeck-Fischer, A., & van der Kolk, B. A. (2000). Down will come baby, cradle and all: Diagnostic and therapeutic implications of chronic trauma on child development. *Australian and New Zealand Journal of Psychiatry, 34*(6), 903-918.

Streissguth, A. P., Bookstein, F. L., Barr, H. M., et al. (2004). Risk factors for adverse life outcomes in fetal alcohol syndrome and fetal alcohol effects. *Journal of Developmental and Behavioral Pediatrics, 25*(4), 228-238.

Takizawa, Y., & Kitamura, S. (2001). Estimation of the incidence of mercury exposure in the Minamata and Niigata areas using mathematical model from Iraqi poisoning. In Y. Takizawa & M. Osame (Eds.), *Understanding Minamata disease: Methylmercury poisoning in Minamata and Niigata, Japan* (pp. 27-32). Japan Public Health Association.

Tamminga, C. A. (1999). *Schizophrenia in a molecular age.* Washington, DC: American Psychiatric Publishing, Inc.

Teicher, M. H., Andersen, S. L., Polcari, A., et al. (2003). The neurobiological consequences of early stress and childhood maltreatment. *Neuroscience & Biobehavioral Reviews, 27,* 33-44.

Teicher, M. H., Dumont, N. L., Ito, Y., et al. (2004). Childhood neglect is associated with reduced corpus callosum area. *Biological Psychiatry, 56,* 80-85.

Temke, M., & Douglas, E. (2006). *The effects of divorce on children.* University of New Hampshire Cooperative Extension. Family & Consumer Resources. Retrieved from http://extension.unh.edu/family/documents/divorce.pdf

Thaper, A., O'Donovan, M., & Owen, M. J. (2005). The genetics of attention deficit hyperactivity disorder. *Human Molecular Genetics, 14,* R275-R282.

The Henry J. Kaiser Family Foundation (1999). *Kids and Media at the New Millennium: A Kaiser Family Foundation Report.* Merlo Park, CA: The Henry J. Kaiser Family Foundation.

Theodore, A. D., & Runyan, D. K. (1999). A medical research agenda for child maltreatment: Negotiating the next steps. *Pediatrics, 104* (1S-II) supplement, 168-177.

Thompson, B. L., Levitt, P., & Stanwood, G. D. (2009). Prenatal exposure to drugs: Effects on brain development and implications for policy and education. *Nature Reviews and Neuroscience, 10,* 303-312.

Tienari, P., Sorri, A., Lathi, I., et al. (2004). Genotype-environment interaction in schizophrenia-spectrum disorder: Long-term follow-up study of Finnish adoptees. *British Journal of Psychiatry, 184,* 216-222.

Tramo, M. J., Loftus, W. C., Stukel, T. A., et al. (1998). Brain size, head size, and intelligence quotient in monozygotic twins. *Neurology, 50*(5), 1246-1252.

Trautman, P. D., Meyer-Bahlburg, H. F., Postelnek, J., et al. (1995). Effects of early prenatal dexamethasone on the cognitive and behavioral development of young children: Results of a pilot study. *Psychoneuroendocrinology, 20*(4), 439-449.

Tucker, J. S., Friedman, H. S., Schwartz, J. E., et al. (1997). Parental divorce: Effects on individual behavior and longevity. *Journal of Personality and Social Psychology, 73*(2), 381-391.

Uno, H., Lohmiller, L., Thieme, C., et al. (1990). Brain damage induced by prenatal exposure to dexamethasone in fetal rhesus macaques 1. Hippocampus. *Brain Research Brain Developmental Research, 58*(2), 157-167.

U.S. Department of Health and Human Services Agency on Children, Youth and Families. (2008). *Child Maltreatment 2006.* Washington, DC: Government Printing Office.

van den Bergh, B. (1990). The influence of maternal emotion during pregnancy on fetal and neonatal behavior. *Pre and Peri-natal Psychology, 5*(2), 119-130.

van den Bergh, B. R., & Marcoen, A. (2004). High antenatal maternal anxiety is related to ADHD symptoms, externalizing problems, and anxiety in 8- and 9-year-olds. *Child Development, 75*(4), 1085-1097.

van der Molen, J. H., & Bushman, B. J. (2008). Children's direct fright and worry reactions to violence in fiction and news television programs. *Journal of Pediatrics, 153*(3), 420-424.

van Os, J., & Selten, J. P. (1998). Prenatal exposure to maternal stress and subsequent schizophrenia. The May 1940 invasion of The Netherlands. *British Journal of Psychiatry, 172,* 324-326.

Veijola, J., Maki, P., Joukamaa, M., et al. (2004). Parental separation at birth and depression in adulthood. A long-term follow-up of the Finnish Christmas Seal Home Children. *Psychological Medicine, 34*(2), 357-362.

Velisek, L. (2005). Prenatal corticosteroid impact on hippocampus: Implications for postnatal outcomes. *Epilepsy & Behavior, 7*(1), 57-67.

Vize, C. M., & Cooper, P. J. (1995). Sexual abuse in patients with eating disorders, patients with depression and normal controls. *British Journal of Psychiatry, 167,* 80-85.

Volpe, J. (1992). Effect of cocaine use in the fetus. *The New England Journal of Medicine, 327*(6), 399-407.

Wadhwa, P. D., Dunkel-Schetter, C., Chicz-DeMet, A., et al. (1996). Prenatal psychosocial factors and the neuroendocrine axis in human pregnancy. *Psychosomatic Medicine, 58*(5), 432-446.

Wainwright, P. E. (2002). Dietary essential fatty acids and brain function: A developmental perspective on mechanisms. *Proceedings of the Nutrition Society, 61,* 61-69.

Wainwright, P. E., & Martin, D. (2005). Role of dietary polyunsaturated fatty acids in brain and cognitive function: Perspectives of a neurodevelopmental psychobiologist. In H. R. Lieberman, R. B. Kanarek, & C. Prasad (Eds.), *Nutrition, brain, and behavior* (pp. 163-186). Boca Raton, FL: CRC Press.

Wakschlag, L. S., Lahey, B. B., Loeber, R., et al. (1997). Maternal smoking during pregnancy and the risk of conduct disorder in boys. *Archives of General Psychiatry, 54*(7), 670-676.

Walker, G. C., Scott, P. S., & Koppersmith, G. (1998). Impact of child sexual abuse on addictions severity. *Journal of Psychosocial Nursing, 36,* 10-18.

Wallerstein, J., & Blakeslee, S. (1989). *Second chances: Men, women and children a decade after divorce.* New York: Tichnor & Fields.

Wallerstein, J., & Lewis, J. (2004). The unexpected legacy of divorce: Report of a 25-year study. *Psychoanalytic Psychology, 21*(3), 353-370.

Wang, X., Dow-Edwards, D., Anderson, V., et al. (2004). In utero marijuana exposure associated with abnormal amygdala dopamine D2 gene expression in the human fetus. *Biological Psychiatry, 56*(12), 909-915.

Watson, J. B., Mednick, S. A., Huttunen, M., et al. (1999). Prenatal teratogens and the development of adult mental illness. *Developmental Psychopathology, 11*(3), 457-466.

Watts, J. L., & Saigal, S. (2006). Outcome of extreme prematurity: As information increases so do the dilemmas. *Archives of Disease in Childhood. Fetal and Neonatal Edition, 91*(3), F221-225.

Webster, W. S. (1998). Teratogen update: Congenital rubella. *Teratology, 58*, 13-23.

Weiner, E., & Smith, R. S. (1992). *Overcoming the odds: High risk children from birth to adulthood.* Ithaca, NY: Cornell University Press.

Weinstrock, M. (2001). Alterations induced by gestational stress in brain morphology and behaviour of the offspring. *Progress in Neurobiology, 65*, 427-451.

Weiss, B. (1996). The deferred legacy of developmental neurotoxicity. *Neurotoxicology and Teratology, 18*(3), 327-343.

Welberg, L. A., & Seckl, J. R. (2001). Prenatal stress, glucocorticoids and the programming of the brain. *Journal of Neuroendocrinology, 13*(2), 113-128.

Werner, E. (1989). High-risk children in young adulthood: A longitudinal study from birth to 32 years. *American Journal of Orthopsychiatry, 59*(1), 72-81.

Werner, E. E., & Smith, R. S. (1982). *Vulnerable but invincible: A longitudinal study of resilient children and youth.* New York: Adams, Bannister and Cox.

Werner, E. E., & Smith, R. S. (1992). *Overcoming the odds: High risk children from birth to adulthood.* Ithaca, NY: Cornell University Press.

Whitaker, A., Van Rossem, R., Feldman, J., et al. (1997). Psychiatric outcomes in low-birth-weight children at age 6 years: Relation to neonatal cranial ultrasound abnormalities. *Archives of General Psychiatry, 54*, 785-789.

Whitfield, M., Grunau, R. V. E., & Holsti, L. (1997). Extremely premature (<800 g) schoolchildren: Multiple areas of hidden disability. *Archives of Diseases in Childhood, 77*, 83-90.

Widom, C. S. (2000). Understanding the consequences of childhood victimization. In R. M. Reece (Ed.), *Treatment of child abuse: Common ground for mental health medical and legal practitioners* (pp. 339-361). Baltimore: The Johns Hopkins University Press.

Williams, R. (2006). The psychosocial consequences for children and young people who are exposed to terrorism, war, conflict and natural disasters. *Current Opinion in Psychiatry, 19*(4), 337-349.

Willis, E., & Strasburger, V. (1998). Media violence. *The Pediatric Clinics of North America: Violence Among Children and Adolescents, 45*, 319-332.

Wilson, M., & Daly, M. (1987). The risk of maltreatment of children living with stepparents. In R. J. Gelles & J. B. Lancaster (Eds.), *Child abuse and neglect: Biosocial dimensions, foundations of human behavior* (p. 228). New York: Aldine de Gruyter.

Winneke, G., & Krämer, U. (1997). Neurobehavioral aspects of lead neurotoxicity in children. *Central European Journal of Public Health, 5*(2), 65-69.

Wolchik, S. A., Sandler, I. N., Millsap, R. E., et al. (2002). Six-year follow-up of preventive interventions for children of divorce: A randomized controlled trial. *Journal of the American Medical Association, 288*(5), 1874-1881.

Wolfe, D. A., Sas, L., & Wekerle, C. (1994). Factors associated with the development of posttraumatic stress disorder among child victims of sexual abuse. *Child Abuse and Neglect, 18*, 37-50.

Wolke, D. K. (1997). The preterm responses to the environment: Long term effects? In K. L. F. Cocburn (Ed.), *Advances in perinatal medicine* (pp. 305-314). Carnforth, UK: Parthenon Publishing.

Wood, N. L. S., Marlow, N., Costeloe, K., et al. (2000). Neurologic and developmental disability after extremely preterm birth. *The New England Journal of Medicine, 343*(6), 378-384.

Wooley, C., Gould, E., & McEwen, B. S. (1990). Exposure to excess glucocorticoids alters dendritic morphology of adult hippocampal pyramidal neurons. *Brain Research, 531*, 225-231.

Wright, M. O., & Masten, A. S. (2006). Resilience processes in development. In S. Goldstein & R. B. Brooks (Eds.), *Handbook of resilience in children* (pp. 17-37). New York: Springer Science & Business Media, Inc.

Wyszynski, D. F., Nambisan, M., Surve, T., et al. (2005). Antiepileptic Drug Pregnancy Registry. Increased rate of major malformations in offspring exposed to valproate during pregnancy. *Neurology, 64*(6), 961-965.

Yates, T. M., Egeland, B., & Sroufe, L. A. (2003). Rethinking resilience: A developmental perspective. In S. S. Luthar (Ed.), *Resilience and vulnerability: Adaptation in the context of childhood adversities* (pp. 243-266). New York: Cambridge University Press.

Yokota, F., & Thompson, K. M. (2000). Violence in G-rated animated films. *Journal of the American Medical Association, 283*, 2716-2720.

Ystgaard, M., Hestetun, I., Loeb, M., et al. (2004). Is there a specific relationship between childhood sexual and physical abuse and repeated suicidal behavior? *Child Abuse and Neglect, 28*(8), 863-875.

Zill, N., Morrison, D. R., & Coiro, M. J. (1993). Long-term effects of parental divorce on parent-child relationships, adjustment, and achievement in young adulthood. *Journal of Family Psychology, 7*(1), 91-103.

Zillmann, D., & Weaver, J. B. (1999). Effects of prolonged exposure to gratuitous media violence on provoked and unprovoked hostile behavior. *Journal of Applied Social Psychology, 29*, 145-165.

UNIT III

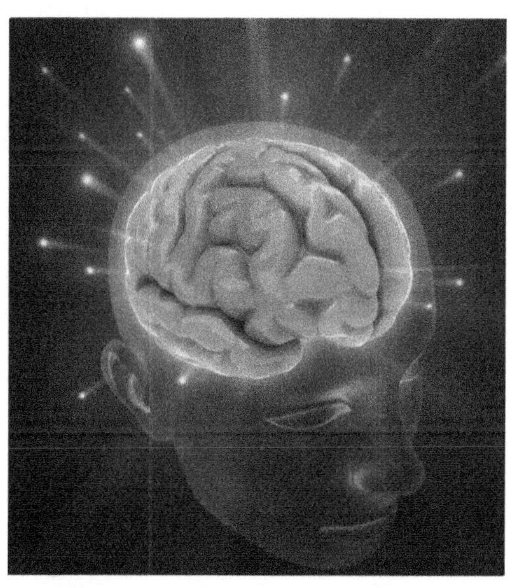

Levers of Change: Interventions Used by Psychiatric Advanced Practice Nurses

CHAPTER 4

Communicating, Interviewing, and Assessing

Ellen R. Portnoy, DNP, RN, PMHNP-BC

"One cannot not communicate" (Watzlawick, 1967, p. 49).

This chapter reviews the concept of communicating and the process of interviewing and assessing adult psychiatric patients. It is intended to provide clear explanations and guidelines for the practicing clinician in common hospital and outpatient settings. Experienced clinicians use their knowledge of all the basic components of communication and continually modify their approach to situations as interviews, assessments, and the relationship evolve.

Communication

In all aspects of nursing and health care, poor or ineffective communication is a major risk to patient safety. Nowhere is communication skill as important to the treatment process itself as in psychiatry. As the backbone of the therapeutic process, effective communication by both clinicians and patients is required in every setting, and it can be learned and improved. Communication skills are a key vehicle for promoting growth and healing. They influence the outcome of an encounter and set the tone for either the development of a working alliance and relationship or the derailment of the process (Schuster, 2002). Both the communication sender and the receiver are influenced by the environment, circumstance, history, and purpose for the encounter as well as by the ongoing interactions between them.

Communication Theory

Contributions to communication theory have come from many fields, including engineering, psychology, and the social and biological sciences, as well as nursing. Each field helps to explain some of the forces that operate between the clinician and patient during an encounter. Both the sender and the receiver of any piece of information are influenced by their own perceptions, history, and experience. In practical terms, the clinician's presentation and skill help mold and direct the content and process of the interactions.

Paul Watzlawick, an Austrian psychologist, is one of the early influences on modern communication theory and is notable for his axiom, "One cannot not communicate" (Watzlawick, Beavin, & Jackson, 1967, p. 49). The usefulness of this concept is clear: all behavioral presentations—both verbal and nonverbal, intended and unintended—are communication. Watzlawick et al. further defined additional communication axioms:

- "Every communication has a content and a relationship aspect such that the latter classifies the former and is therefore a metacommunication" (p. 54). This sentence means that, in addition to choosing certain words, the speaker indicates in other ways how she sees herself and how she wants to be understood. For example, a clinician who enters a room with a patient and sits behind a desk sends a different message than does a clinician who sits in a chair that is next to the patient.
- "Human beings communicate both digitally and analogically. Digital language has a highly complex and powerful logical syntax but lacks adequate semantics in the field of relationships, while analogic language possess the semantics but has no adequate syntax for the unambiguous definition of the nature of relationships" (p. 66). This axiom is referring to the nonverbal gestures and analog-verbal tones that are part of the verbal message. For example, a patient whose speech is barely audible is communicating a particular feeling in addition to the words being said.

It is important to know the potential meanings of all the aspects of communications of both the self and the patient. Whereas some messages have universal meanings, other messages may need to be clarified to avoid misunderstanding.

Another significant influence on communication theory came from Murray Bowen (1978), who applied general systems theory to communication in families. His use of the concept of triangles, in which a third individual is engaged to stabilize tension in a dyad, has wide applicability in understanding patterns of communication that can be influenced and corrected in order to understand and build healthy relationships.

Eric Berne's (Berne, 1961) use of transactional analysis is a classic application of use of the meaning and intention of a message in understanding its impact. He defined the content of a message as originating with the "parent," "adult," or "child" aspect of the individual sending the message. The message is then received by the "parent," "adult," or "child" aspect of the recipient, who reacts according to the tone of the message. Identifying the aspect and then changing the mode of the message to "adult" communication changes the dynamics of both the message and the relationship. Talking to an elderly adult as though she were a child is an example of initiating a communication with a diminishing message attached, i.e., as a parent to a child.

Classic sender-receiver models of communication are referred to most often in nursing literature (Fleischer, Berg, Zimmermann, et al., 2009). In Figure 4-1, a model illustrating factors that impact communication can be used to identify both controllable and uncontrollable aspects of the communication process.

Communications involve an environment, a sender, and a receiver:

- The ***environment*** where the interaction occurs can vary widely. The clinician should make any modification that will enhance the comfort of the patient and the clinician; these conditions should also enable a conversation to take place. For example, the clinician could minimize interruptions and noise, ensuring privacy and safety for all participants.
- The ***sender*** during a communication is the encoder, the one who initiates the message and "packages" it with both the digital and analog components. The skill or ability of the sender of the message will determine the accuracy of the content. A sender who is impaired for any reason may send a message that is confusing or that carries additional messages.
- The ***receiver*** during a communication is the decoder, the one who interprets the message and then responds. Impairment or inability of the receiver for any reason will distort or block the message.

Most of the factors in Figure 4-1 are self-explanatory, though two factors require a bit more description:

- ***Transference*** refers to an individual's tendency to apply his or her thoughts and feelings from past communications to the current communication. For example, a patient who has had negative experiences with clinicians in the past may initially go into a conversation with a current clinician feeling wary and closed-minded. Other experiences can set expectations and affect both the outcome and the process of the current interaction; thus, transference can clearly affect how a communication is interpreted.
- ***Perception and/or perceptual disturbance*** can affect the thought processes and senses, which may distort or completely transform the interaction. For example, a patient who has incorporated a clinician into his or her delusional system will respond as though the clinician had a different identity or intention. The patient or the clinician may also have such a high level of anxiety that information cannot be processed accurately.

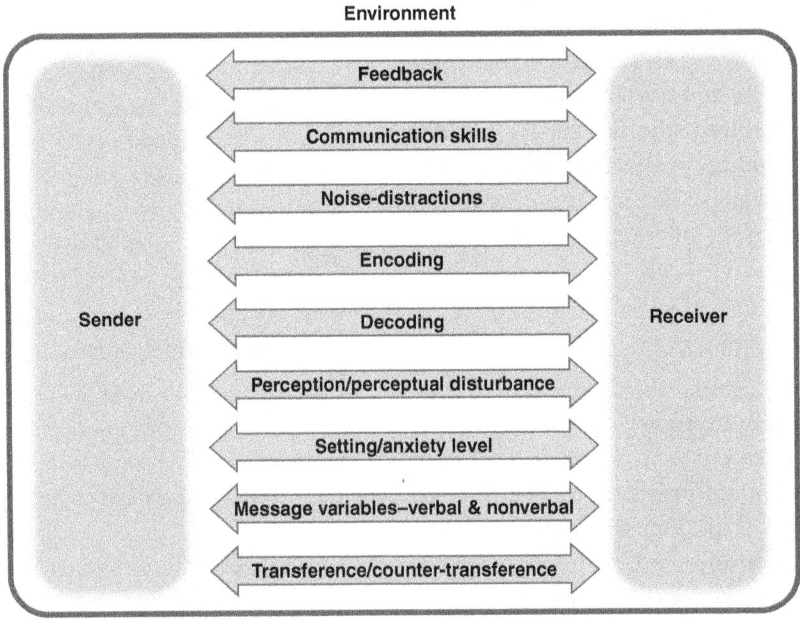

FIGURE 4-1: Factors that Influence Communication (Adapted from Wenburg, J., & Wilmot, W. [1973]. *The Personal Communication Process.* New York: John Wiley and Sons.)

Variation Within and Among Cultures

Differences in communication stemming from cultural preferences and practices can be profound. Even within a single culture, such as a religious or ethnic group, there can be wide variation due to regional differences, subgroups, or history. Clinicians working in an area where there is some diversity in demographics may want to clarify the meaning of verbal or nonverbal communications with the patient (if appropriate) or with a peer. Sensitivity to variation of expression and needs will enhance communication and the relationship and avoid misunderstandings and miscommunication (Ayonrinde, 2003).

Therapeutic Communication Strategies

Clinicians use many techniques to help patients describe concerns, conflicts, feelings, and thoughts. Clear communication should include

- An introduction
- The purpose of the interview
- The limits of the time available to help set the expectations for the interview

Sentences that are clear and that contain one idea at a time are most easily understood. For example, asking a patient in the same sentence if he or she is married and has children requires that the patient create a separation to answer both parts or give only a partial answer.

Clinicians use both verbal and nonverbal communication strategies when interacting with their patients. Additionally, clinicians' awareness of functional and dysfunctional communication helps them to respond to dysfunctional communication behaviors; it can also help them to recognize and correct any dysfunctional communication tendencies that they may have.

Verbal Communication Strategies

Verbal communication strategies include open-ended and closed-ended questions, focused listening, and responses.

Open-Ended Questions

Open-ended questions allow the patient to answer in any way that he or she chooses. Open-ended questions do not force the patient to follow one particular train of thought, and they do not define the focus of interest. They are useful to begin an interview, to open up new areas, or to learn what the patient is thinking or feeling. Examples are "How do you feel about... ?" or "What do you think would help you... ?"

Closed-Ended Questions

Closed-ended questions focus on one particular problem. The patient has limited options for response, e.g., "yes" or "no," a number, or a one-word response. An example of a closed-ended question is "Do you have trouble falling asleep?" Closed-ended questions are used to gather specific information. These can be followed with additional closed-ended questions such as "Once you fall asleep, how long do you stay asleep?" Open-ended questions can be used after closed-ended questions to obtain more information; for instance, "Describe what happens when you try to go to sleep" is an open-ended follow-up question.

Focused Listening

Letting the patient talk without interruption as much as possible lets the clinician listen to themes as well as content. Focused listening, sometimes referred to as "free speech," is particularly useful at the beginning of an initial interview or when difficult or emotionally laden material is being expressed. The clinician should encourage the patient to talk by using facilitating strategies such as nodding and making eye contact, perhaps leaning forward or subtly mirroring the patient's posture. The clinician should let the patient know that the clinician has heard the patient by using repetition, e.g., using one of the patient's key words, paraphrasing, or reflecting. Sometimes a simple sentence such as "That must have been tough" indicates listening and empathy and encourages the patient to continue.

Responses

The clinician must respond to what he or she has heard. Responses can include summarizing, asking further questions, providing factual information, offering reassurance, or displaying empathy, depending on the type of interview being conducted. Responses can also be nonverbal, as described below. Occasionally, the clinician's response will be an expression of doubt, particularly if the patient appears to be testing in some way. Reframing, or giving the situation an alternative context, may be helpful to the patient. Providing possible connections to the patient, such as noting similarities in the patient's experiences at different points in time or connecting a feeling to an event, may be useful. Sometimes, a patient may perceive the clinician's reassurance, which is designed to reduce the patient's anxiety, as a belittling of the problem. However, providing supportive comments to the patient as he or she communicates is often encouraging and will help the patient continue.

The response of empathy demonstrates understanding of the emotion that the patient is experiencing, shows that the clinician identifies the cause of the emotion, and indicates that he or she has made the connection between the emotion that the patient experienced and the cause. Often, a helpful response is to restate the identified emotion and the cause. Box 4-1 summarizes several interventions that are often used in both psychotherapy and interviewing to prompt the patient to describe emotions or more detail about interactions.

Nonverbal Communication Strategies

Nonverbal communications from the patient convey significant information not only on initial contact but also in

BOX 4-1 Interventions Used to Prompt the Patient for More Information

- **Clarification** is a technique in which the interviewer asks the patient for more information about a response. The interviewer seeks more information in order to have a clearer understanding of what the patient meant, such as *"Tell me what you mean when you say..."*
- **Reflection** involves repeating something or some of the words that a patient has used in response to the interviewer's question. The interviewer uses this technique to encourage the patient to give more information about the topic, such as *"You feel left out by your family?"*
- **Empathy statements** provide validation and let the patient know he was understood. A statement such as *"You must have felt very angry" (or hurt or frightened)* often facilitates a greater flow of feelings.
- **Interpretation** is a technique the interviewer uses to suggest a discrepancy between observed behaviors and expressed thoughts, such as *"You tell me you're relaxed, but you're picking your fingers."*
- **Summarizing** is used to let the patient know that the interviewer has heard what she has been saying; it is also used to clarify the interviewer's understanding of what was said or to close a topic, e.g., *"It sounds to me by what you have described that your many recent losses have contributed to your grief and depression."*
- **Probes** are used to gain information about a patient's understanding of his experiences, such as *"Describe more about what was said during that argument."*
- **Checks** are used to evaluate the presence or change of symptoms, such as *"Is there a difference in your appetite?"*
- **Validation** is a way of letting the patient know that his feeling or action is reasonable and what most people would feel or do in similar situations, such as *"Many people are anxious about their children in the city"* (Robinson, 2000).
- **Leads** prompt the patient to continue; examples include *"Go on" "What happened then?"* and *"Tell me more about..."*
- **Prompts** encourage the patient, e.g., *"You were telling me about..."* or *"You had mentioned..."*

subsequent sessions. The following are nonverbal factors of the patient to consider:

- General appearance, posture, facial expression, and eye contact; these will give instant information and indicate starting points that may require follow-up
- Where the patient sits; if he or she asks where to sit or just waits; if he or she is in a bed or gurney; the presence of restraints
- The presence of body movements, tremors, or indications of restlessness or agitation such as pacing and muscle tightness
- Hygiene, body odor, presence of makeup, and attention to dress
- The volume, tone, and rate of speech and if speech is goal directed or linear

While it is certainly not necessary to respond to everything that is noted, factors such as strong body odor or signs of agitation can alert the clinician to be mindful of safety, as the patient may be sending a message to maintain some distance. Other information gathered during this initial assessment can be used later during the interviewing and assessment process.

The following are nonverbal factors for the clinician to consider in his or her presentation:

- The clinician should consider his or her general appearance: professional dress, lab coats as appropriate in medical units, and grooming convey a message of competence to patients.
- The clinician should maintain good eye contact, with modifications as needed for suspicious, anxious, or agitated patients.
- The clinician should use affirmative head nods rather than an impassive poker face.
- The clinician should avoid tired, restless, or bored gestures, such as frequently looking at a watch or nervous hand gestures. These can be distracting and affect the patient's response (Preston, 2005).

Closeness, distance, and stance are nonverbal issues that greatly influence personal comfort and safety. If one party breaches the boundaries of personal space, the other may feel threatened. The exact distance to maintain varies with the situation, but approximately 4 to 6 feet all around is generally appropriate. If the patient is standing, the clinician should stand. If the patient is sitting, the clinician should avoid standing over him or her (Dubin & Jagarlamudi, 2010). It is important to be respectful, attentive, and nonthreatening. When patients come too close, it is certainly reasonable for the clinician to request or instruct them to move to a different location, or to move himself or herself. Remaining more than an arm's length from a patient in a bed or gurney is also wise, particularly when the patient is unknown to the clinician.

Depending on the setting and circumstance, obtaining additional safety resources, offering medication, or perhaps eliminating an audience by moving to a quieter location may be a useful beginning. An astute clinician will receive and decode the communication accurately and will provide the most appropriate approach.

Functional and Dysfunctional Communication Strategies

Sarcasm, minimizing, passive-aggressive communication, symbolic communication, and silence contain both verbal and nonverbal components with underlying intention.

Sarcasm

Sarcasm is communication intended to cut or criticize and can be displayed in both words and tone. The emotion attached to sarcasm is generally anger intended to disparage, and it is rarely useful in a therapeutic setting. When the patient uses sarcasm, it is important for the clinician to note and clarify or explore it. For example, if a patient says, "I just can't wait for the next visit," the clinician can follow up in several ways, such as, "I gather there is something about the upcoming visit that you really don't like," and then follow up with the feelings or content expressed.

Minimizing

Minimizing downplays the importance of a situation and can sound condescending, nonempathetic, or belittling, among other things. When used by the patient, it can indicate a lack of understanding of the significance of a situation or a reluctance to discuss it. It is best to clarify the meaning in a neutral manner. A patient's answering "Not really..." is a frequently used minimizing response. For example, if a clinician asks a question such as "Has anything significant happened in the last week?" and the patient says "Not really," the clinician could reply by saying "It sounds like you might not be sure," and see where that leads.

Passive-Aggressive Communication

Passive-aggressive communication delivers a negative message without seeming to do so. These messages are generally nonverbal and include such behaviors as chronic lateness, ignoring a promise, or doing something known to be disliked. Sometimes the behavior is simple avoidance, but over time and with repetition, the pattern generally becomes clear. These behaviors are often subtle and require exploration and occasional self-reflection. An example is as follows: A patient gives the clinician a form to complete for an employer, lawyer, or caseworker that is needed the next day. The clinician puts the form in the record without filling it out. The patient calls the next 2 days requesting the form, but it is continuing to fall to the bottom of the list. The same type of behavior can also be perpetrated by the patient; both situations require an honest investigation and often a discussion.

Symbolic Communication

Symbolic communication can be used to describe a situation in a way that is more easily understood. This type of communication may be particularly useful in talking with children, but it can also help in any situation when additional clarification is needed. Psychotic patients may describe events or experiences in symbolic terms, such as when describing physical symptoms. The clinician must take symbolic descriptions seriously and attempt to clarify and evaluate what is being expressed, because the symbolic references may be an attempt to communicate a serious problem. An example is the patient who relays that "voodoo is attacking my feet," which turns out to be a description of a diabetic neuropathy. Another example is the patient who describes his mother as a "helicopter" (hovering everywhere).

Silence

Silence can be both functional and nonfunctional. Some patients simply need time to gather their thoughts or sort through feelings. However, silence can also indicate resistance, hostility, or anger. Both patients and clinicians can become uncomfortably anxious when silence is protracted. Watching for nonverbal cues will help the clinician determine how long to wait for a response, or to determine if silence is the response. Potential meaning, signals, and direction can be clarified as the interview proceeds. The clinician should avoid allowing the patient's anxiety to become too uncomfortable initially because doing so will derail the communication.

Communicating in Special Situations

A number of challenging situations may require adaptations to the communication process. Communication can be affected when there is a difference in culture and vocabulary between the two communicating parties, when the patient is mute, when there is a language barrier, and when the patient is an involuntary participant.

Culture and Vocabulary Differences

Culture affects both verbal and nonverbal communication. Language of the "drug culture," "hip-hop" language, and use of culture-specific terminology in both diverse and mainstream cultures are common examples of situations that can present a need for clarification. The meaning of eye contact is an example of nonverbal communication that can easily be misinterpreted. In some age groups and cultures, maintaining eye contact may indicate that the speaker is being honest. In others, and frequently with young people, high level of eye contact when speaking indicates the opposite. In very paranoid patients, it can be interpreted as aggressive and hostile. Clinicians often have the opportunity to inquire about cultural norms and should take advantage when they present themselves. There are also many Web sites with definitions and explanations of various current word definitions and social norms. Clinicians who are working in localities or communities with diverse demographics should explore variations in meaning, behaviors, and norms in order to effectively understand and to communicate intelligently and respectfully.

Mute Patient

Having some history or prior information before meeting with a mute patient is useful. Because verbal information will not be obtained, the clinician will need to use cues from nonverbal behavior as well as information learned prior to the interview. Certainly, the presence of family or significant others can be helpful and informative. Statements should be short and clear. The same general practice of giving an introduction, stating the time that is available, and relaying the purpose of the meeting should be communicated. The behavior, responses, and reactions to the clinician's verbal statements should be noted. If possible the clinician should sit, but it is important to keep safety in mind because little may be known about the patient's potential behavior.

Language Barrier

It may be necessary to use a translator when verbal language cannot be understood or when the patient is deaf or significantly hard of hearing. The use of professional translators is clearly the best choice. When working with a translator, the expectation is that the clinician will look at and address not the translator but the patient. The translator will then give the identical message to the patient. The clinician should not expect or ask the translator to give opinions or information that the patient will not also be made aware of—the purpose is only to translate.

While clearly preferable, it is not always possible to arrange for a professional translator on short notice. In that case, the clinician should still attempt to avoid using minors, close relatives, or people who may know the patient personally so that the interview can remain confidential and objective. Of course, in an emergency situation, it is necessary to obtain basic facts. The clinician should clarify and record the source of the information and, when possible, identify whether it appears to be fact, opinion, or guess. This will help to indicate the reliability of the report. The information can be obtained in a supportive fashion to collect the most amount of information possible.

Involuntary Patient

The involuntary patient often (but not always) presents a challenge. Here again, having some prior information will be helpful. In some instances, owing to either the patient's internal "noise" or to distortion of thinking, the patient will be clearly psychotic and unable to either receive or send communication with any accuracy. The clinician will need to persistently clarify the message to understand the patient's situation or condition.

In some cases, involuntary patients will clearly state their belief that there is no reason for them to be there, that there is nothing wrong, and that there is nothing to discuss. They may say that there is no point in talking because nothing can help their situation. In these circumstances, it is important for the clinician to communicate to involuntary patients that he or she can help them get what they want or need by telling the clinician as much as they can.

Interviewing

There are several different types of interviews. The initial or consultation interview may be the only time the clinician and patient meet, or it may serve as the beginning of a treatment relationship. Morrison (2008) defined the hallmark of a good initial interview as one that collects the most accurate information in the shortest amount of time while maintaining an effective relationship and connection with the patient. While the first interview is focused on obtaining information to evaluate the nature, extent, and direction of treatment, all interviews share the need to develop and maintain a level of rapport to be effective. Content and process in an ongoing therapeutic relationship shifts the emphasis to the treatment aspects that have brought the patient for help.

Interviewing and the Therapeutic Alliance

The purposes of the psychiatric interview are to understand the patient's illness, to evaluate the effect of the illness on the patient's life, and to create a beginning diagnosis and treatment plan. This information is obtained most effectively within the context of a working alliance between the clinician and the patient (Havens, 1998). The clinician uses his or her therapeutic self—calm, warm, understanding, kind, respectful, concerned, and focused—to create a therapeutic alliance. Additional goals for the clinician are to elicit emotions, feelings, and attitudes; to reduce the patient's anxiety; to instill hope; to develop an assessment from which a tentative diagnosis can be made; and to develop hypotheses that will guide diagnosis and begin an initial plan of treatment (Meeks, Lanouette, Vahia, et al., 2009).

It is through the therapeutic alliance in the context of an ongoing relationship that the clinician is able to help the patient change. The patient has likely had questions in his or her mind since deciding to seek help, such as "Will I be safe or threatened, or will I be rejected?" and "Can this person help me?"

An important task in building a strong therapeutic relationship is to help the patient feel accepted. Regardless of the patient's actual presentation, the clinician should assume that the patient is anxious and seek to maintain the anxiety within workable limits. The clinician demonstrates empathy, which is the ability to understand what the patient feels, by using empathetic statements such as "It sounds to me as if you have been feeling some very painful emotions." Maintaining a professional manner and presentation reduces the threat of closeness that some patients may experience, particularly during an initial interview.

Patients want clinicians to have expertise that can be used to help them. The clinician's steadiness and responsiveness and the quality of the questions the clinician asks contribute to the patient's belief that the clinician knows what might help. For patients, knowledgeable questioning—such as fact-oriented questions that focus on concrete realities of patients' situations, symptoms, and problems—provides an impression of a strong knowledge base and experience with similar problems (Shea, 1998).

The Initial Clinical Interview

The initial clinical interview requires the most direction and focus in order to obtain an accurate and complete description of the problem. In medical inpatient and outpatient settings, in emergency settings, and in consult services, there is often only one opportunity to conduct the interview.

However, even in these situations the encounter can be therapeutic by focusing on specific issues, by helping the patient make connections, and by jointly working on an initial plan.

Many clinicians preface a consultation interview by stating how the interview will proceed. They may begin by telling the patient why the interview is occurring—for example, they were asked to see the patient by the emergency room physician because of the patient's high anxiety level. Then they tell the patient how much time is allotted, and they explain that the clinician will need to ask a lot of questions first and that the patient can talk a little more after that. Individual clinicians develop their own style over time, but the components are basically the same and help the clinician develop a partnership with the patient. An example of a basic form for recording an initial interview is shown in Box 4-2.

BOX 4-2 Psychiatry Intake (Compressed) for the Initial Interview

Name/ID # ______________________

Referral Source Name/Address ______________________

Reason for Referral ______________________

Telephone ______________________ Emergency Contact ______________________

(Obtain Release of Information if patient permits contact)

List primary language/culture/race: ______________________

Accommodations needed (translator, etc.): ______________________

List any vision/hearing barriers: ______________________

Accommodations needed: ______________________

I. **Chief complaint and history of present illness** (onset of illness, duration, precipitating factors, current symptoms):

____

II. **Past psychiatric history** (last treatment, date, and provider; include source of assessment information):

____

III. **Current substance abuse** (type, frequency, and date of onset, most recent use, and amount; include history of substance abuse and treatment): ______________________

IV. **Family psychiatric and substance abuse history:** ______________________

V. **Allergies:** ______________________

VI. **Current medications** (psych & physical medications; reactions/responses): ______________________

Current medical problems (indicate LMP, pregnancy/contraceptives): ______________________

Primary care physician: ______________________

Pain assessment: ______________________

VII. **Social History/Current Stressors**

A. Current living situation/relationships *(living arrangements, violence/abuse/neglect, divorce/loss, sexual issues, problems in environment, legal guardian, other pertinent information)*:

B. Educational/vocational/financial support *(financial problems, job stability [how long employed and longest job held], school/learning problems, worker's compensation, dates of military service, branch, how long, type of discharge)*:

C. Medical/legal issues *(serious illness [self or family], legal problems, accident/trauma, other information)*:

D. Family of origin *(childhood caregiver[s], violence/abuse/neglect, separation/loss[es], traumatic experiences, other childhood adversity)*:

E. Other immediate problems:

F. Current resources/strengths *(available support person/telephone numbers, current/previous therapist available, stable living arrangement, insight/motivation, community support[s], other information)*:

G. Environmental safety assessment:

PATIENT/SIGNIFICANT OTHER GENERAL APPRAISAL OF ENVIRONMENTAL SAFETY

In the home:	*Good*	*Fair*	*Poor*	Comments:
In the workplace:	*Good*	*Fair*	*Poor*	Comments:
In the neighborhood:	*Good*	*Fair*	*Poor*	Comments:

Continued

BOX 4-2 Psychiatry Intake (Compressed) for the Initial Interview—continued

VIII. Mental Status Examination

A. General appearance, attitude, and behavior:

B. Stream of mental activity *(speech pattern, reaction time, etc.)*:

C. Mental trends and thought content *(major theme, thought process)*:

D. Emotional reaction *(affect, mood)*:

E. Sensorium *(orientation, memory, attention, concentration)*:

F. Insight and judgment:

IX. Risk Assessment/Justification for Level of Service (Deterrents, access to weapons, plan, family history of suicide, plans for future, etc.)

A. Suicidal ideation *(plan, capability, access, intent, deterrents)*

B. Homicidal ideation *(plan, capability, access, intent, deterrents)*

C. Assaultive behaviors *(history of harm to others, property, animals, fire-setting, etc.)*

D. Other harm to self *(self-mutilation, risky behaviors, etc.)*

CLINICIAN FINDINGS/SUMMARY

Check all that apply, add specifics as needed

Appetite/sleep disturbance (specify)	Mania/hypomania
Assaultive/destructive ideation/behavior past or present	Medical/surgical factors complicating illness
Bizarre behavior/delusional thinking	Paranoia
Body rigidity/immobility	Positive drug/alcohol screen
Depressed mood, psychomotor depression	Severe agitation, anxiety, panic (specify)
Domestic violence/abuse	Severe eating disorder
Failed outpatient treatment	Severe impairment in familial, vocational or educational functioning
Hallucinations: specify	Social withdrawal
History of nonadherence to treatment	Somatic preoccupation
Homicidal threat/plan/ideation	Substance abuse
Hostility/poor impulse control	Suicide attempt/plan/ideation
Impaired judgment/memory	Toxic medication reaction
Impaired memory/orientation	Other (specify)

Diagnosis

Axis I ______________________ Code ______________

Axis II ______________________ Code ______________

Axis III ______________________ Code ______________

Axis IV ______________________ Code ______________

Axis V *Current* ____________ *Highest level past year* ______________

R/O ______________________ Code ______________

X. Treatment given/teaching/instructions

XI. Indirect collateral contacts made (family, physician, clinical, other)

XII. Initial treatment plan—include name and phone numbers of referrals, date of appointments made, e.g., support groups, AA, clinics, etc.)

Vital signs (if required): B/P ________ P ________ R ________ T ________

Time: Start ____________ End ____________ Date ____________

Signature ______________________

Print ______________ Pager #__________

Preparation for the Initial Clinical Interview

Patients and clinicians prepare differently for the initial clinical interview.

Patient's Preparation

The patient may have been having symptoms of a disorder for a long time, but something has changed to the extent that the patient, a family member, the primary care physician, or someone in the community has determined that the patient needs mental health care for the problems that he or she is no longer able to manage. The patient often feels shamed because he or she thinks that others view him or her as weak, and unable to cope. The patient feels the stigma of being considered mentally ill. He or she fears what being labeled "a mental patient" will mean to him or her and the roles in which the patient functions—partner, parent, worker, and community member. The patient worries about taking time off from work or turning the care of the family over to someone else. If the patient has never received mental health care, he or she is worried about what will be involved, how the patient will be received, and what will be expected of him or her. The patient may never have heard of the clinic or practice to which he or she has been referred and may wonder if he or she will be helped. In some cases, the patient has had a bad experience and brings feelings about it.

Interviewer's Preparation

The interviewer's preparation depends on the setting in which the interview will take place, his or her readiness to conduct the interview, and safety concerns. Providing for safety with attention to personal space is a necessary part of preparation. Decreasing distractions, such as noise from televisions and interruptions from cell phones or other electronic devices, will assist the exchange of information. If the patient has the devices, the clinician should request that they be turned off. Ideally, in an office setting, the room should be a quiet, peaceful space with sufficient seating. Chairs for the interviewer and patient should be arranged at an angle so that the interviewer does not directly face the patient. If there are to be others in the room, such as students or preceptors, their chairs should be at the back of the room and out of the patient's direct line of vision; doing so will lessen the likelihood of the patient's responding to them instead of to the interviewer. The interviewer should be able to see the wall clock or should use a small desk clock so that it is not necessary to check his or her wristwatch. All equipment—pens, forms, folders—should be assembled before the interview. The equipment should be neat and not carry the logo of a drug company. In providing for safety, the interviewer should know how the patient was brought for the evaluation—by family or friends or by the police—and if the patient is under the influence of alcohol or drugs. If the interviewer decides that there may be a risk of violence, he or she should ask other staff to be there for the interview or close by the office. To ensure safety, all heavy objects—e.g., books, vases, art objects—that can be used as weapons should be removed from the room. There should be plenty of space around the patient. More on interview settings can be found later in this chapter.

Privacy and confidentiality may be difficult to secure in some settings. Stating to the patient the nature and limits of confidentiality will give the patient additional information about how the content may be used. A clinician cannot withhold any information from the team that will affect treatment or safety, and the patient should be made aware of this. However, other information, experience, and feelings will be confidential and not released without permission or court order.

Process of the Psychiatric Interview

In some settings, the clinician will meet the patient at the door and accompany the patient to the interview room. While social comments about weather or directions may help the patient become more comfortable, it is best to avoid asking "How are you?" while walking in because the patient may begin to tell about his or her condition before there is an opportunity for privacy.

At the beginning of the interview, the clinician should introduce herself or himself by full name and identify his or her professional status. For example, "I am Lauren McCall. I am a Psychiatric Nurse Practitioner and I am a member of the practice group here." The clinician should also identify any other persons in the room and why they are there, e.g., students there for observation.

The next step is to find out what the patient understands about the reason for the interview. Robinson (2000) has suggested that the interviewer ask, "What is your understanding of why we are meeting?" The interviewer then tells the patient how long the interview will last and whether he or she will be seeing the patient again; for example, the clinician should say if it is a one-time interview that has been requested for evaluation of the patient. The clinician then explains that he or she will be asking questions about the patient's personal history and family history.

The process of the psychiatric interview involves the interaction between clinician and patient as the clinician asks questions and the patient responds with answers that will lead to the appropriate treatment of the patient's problems. Patients are often unfamiliar with this type of questioning, especially questions that they consider to be personal or that require sensitive information. To facilitate the process of obtaining information, the interviewer maintains a courteous, objective, nonjudgmental approach and makes sure that the patient is comfortable and understands what will take place in the interview.

All techniques that encourage patients to speak freely are effective. The interviewer may also use the techniques discussed earlier in this chapter, including

- Asking directly about emotional reactions
- Expressing sympathy
- Using open-ended questions
- Using interpretation
- Reflecting emotional cues

One of the clinician's goals early in the interview is to establish a therapeutic relationship. A strong therapeutic alliance provides the trust that patients need to be able to accept treatment—medications, psychotherapy, or psychosocial interventions—that will bring about change.

Transitioning From Topic to Topic

In order to include all the questions that must be covered in a psychiatric assessment, the interviewer must ask questions in many areas. Sometimes the interviewer can use a cause-and-effect transition, linking something that happened—such as being moved from home to an assisted living facility—with the development of difficulties, such as abnormal sleep patterns and reduced interest in doing things. Sometimes the interviewer uses the framework of time, such as linking the time after the patient retired with changes in behaviors, such as increased use of alcohol. Interviewers often use the strategy of summarizing what has just been discussed and then moving to another area, saying, "and now I want to find out about your work history." A simple preparation, such as saying "Now I'd like to ask you about..." also helps the interview flow.

During the interview, the clinician begins to develop a hypothesis of what the diagnosis might be. Robinson (2000) has suggested that the clinician use the cues that are presented as links to possible diagnoses. For example, for patients in an older age group, the clinician might consider medical disorders that cause psychiatric symptoms, trauma, substance abuse, and interactions of multiple medications. For adult patients with disruptive behaviors, the clinician might consider the possibility of a psychotic disorder, a psychiatric disorder due to a medical condition, or a substance-related disorder. For a patient who presents with poor grooming and hygiene, agitated behavior, and impaired judgment and insight, the clinician might consider a psychotic disorder or substance-related delirium or withdrawal. Obtaining time frames and clearly identifying symptoms is necessary to begin provisional diagnoses. As the interview progresses, the clinician formulates a clinical assessment including a tentative differential diagnosis.

The Motivational Interview

Motivational interviewing is an approach that helps patients to identify, explore, and resolve ambivalence about making behavioral changes. It was first used with patients with substance abuse and other addictive behaviors, but it can be applied in other situations in which a health-related behavioral change is necessary. An increasing amount of evidence-based literature demonstrates the effectiveness of the general principles and technique in improving patient adherence to medication, diet and exercise changes, and other health-related situations (Levensky, Forcehimes, O'Donohue, et al., 2007; Rosengren, 2009).

Several basic principles are involved in a motivational interview:

- Acknowledging the difficulty of the problem that the patient relates, and expressing empathy
- Identifying the discrepancy that exists between what the patient would like to happen and the difficulty he or she states about changing behavior
- Allowing and sympathizing with expressions of resistance
- Supporting self-efficacy and the patient's solutions (Levensky et al., 2007).

These principles are difficult for many health-care providers, who are often most willing to provide the solutions to the patient. It is a type of interviewing that actively involves both the patient and the clinician, and it begins with the patient's identifying readiness to make a change.

To use the principles of motivational interviewing, the clinician must apply several communication skills. The first skill is *reflective listening*, which involves repeating back to the patient the essence of what he has said. As an example, if a patient reports that he just cannot remember to take medication every day because he is too busy, the clinician might nod and agree that his life is busy and that it is hard to remember everything. The second skill is *asking open-ended questions*. In this situation, the clinician could ask, "What do you think would be the worst thing that would happen if you don't take the medicine?" (or stop the alcohol use, or lose some weight). The clinician should encourage as much description as possible and affirm and support the patient's description. The last skill involves *summarizing*, which is putting together what the patient has identified as the problem and the difficulty, acknowledging the predicament, and supporting the patient's ideas for a solution.

In some ways motivational interviewing is simple, but mastering the application takes practice in order to avoid the pitfalls, such as identifying a problem too quickly, having difficulty working with resistance and ambivalence, and becoming less directive with people who are making lifestyle changes. The clinician interested in this approach should consider bringing situations to a group or seasoned coach for practice and additional teaching (Rosengren, 2009).

Additional Types of Interviews

In addition to interviewing patients, there are times when clinicians must interview family members and other informants, such as the police, clergy, or other physicians. In any instance, patient confidentiality must be maintained.

Interviewing Family Members

There are a number of situations in which family or significant others are involved in the interview process. Sometimes it is the family that brings the patient into the clinic or emergency department. Sometimes the clinician will request that a family member come with the patient to provide additional history and to determine resources and level of support. Often, family members' input, judgment, and requests are very significant, and they should seldom be discounted. The clinician should investigate if there is a legal guardian status or if there is a social security relationship, such as a "payee" status; the clinician should also ask family members what they view as the problem.

If possible, the clinician should interview the patient alone first, letting the patient and the family member(s) know that the clinician will speak to them next in the presence of the patient, if possible. It is best to present this information as part of the process instead of as an option. The clinician should let the patient know what information about him or her will and will not be divulged. The clinician can ask which family member the patient feels closest to or trusts the most, and then honor that request if possible. It is often useful to quickly draw a family genogram (Fig. 4-2) to capture the names, relationships, and significant family events.

It is important to maintain loyalty to the patient while developing a relationship with each member of the family who is present. To build relationships with family members, the clinician can thank each member for contributions of information, comment on the significance of the information that they have provided, and offer appreciation for their assistance. Family members should be aware of the confidentiality requirements and exceptions, as well as what may be required in the future, depending on the setting and nature of the patient's situation. Family interviews usually end with a general communication of the plan or future appointments.

Interviewing Other Informants: The Police, Clergy, and Other Clinicians

In some situations, it is the police, clergy, or another clinician who accompanies a patient to the treatment setting. While it is important to maintain confidentiality, the clinician should be as cooperative as the situation will allow. While these professionals generally understand that a court order is required to obtain records, they can be excellent sources of information—particularly when safety is an issue—and they may have a good relationship with the patient. When the patient is an involuntary admission, these informants may have the first-hand knowledge

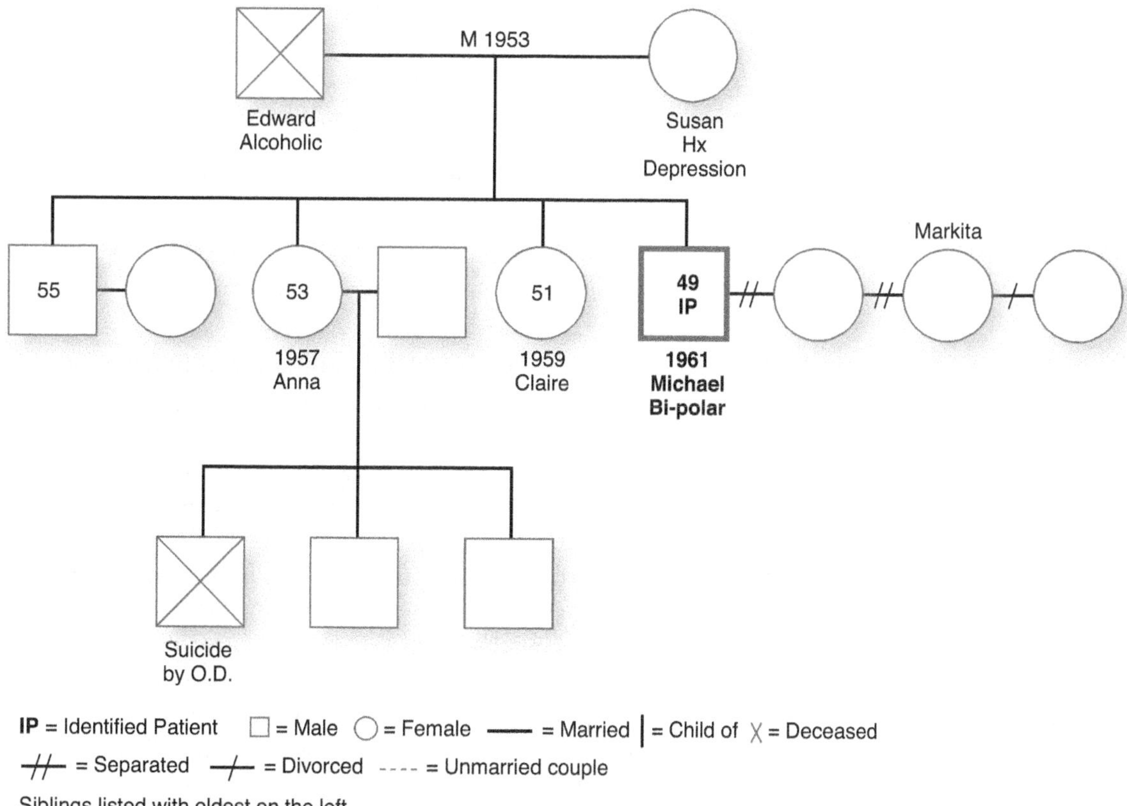

FIGURE 4-2: Sample Genogram. In this genogram, the Identified Patient is Michael, a 49-year-old male with a diagnosis of bipolar disorder. His father was an alcoholic, now deceased, and his mother has a history of depression. He has been married twice and is currently separated from his third wife. He is the youngest of four siblings: he has two older sisters and one older brother. His sister Anna's son committed suicide by an overdose. Genograms can be expanded to include additional detail about psychiatric, medical, and social history and will allow the clinician to refer to family members with accuracy.

required for a Petition for Hospitalization. Although state processes vary, direct and specific information taken on the appropriate forms provides the strongest documentation to proceed with an admission; this documentation will stand up in court if it becomes necessary.

Interviewing informants before they leave is the most efficient way to save time over the course of a hospitalization, and it can shorten the hospital admission. Other clinicians and clergy may have contact information or may be able to provide support services necessary for discharge planning. A request to plan aftercare by a clinician who had a previous treatment relationship with the patient should be honored if possible. If there are additional recommendations from the treatment team, they should be communicated with the permission of the patient.

The Difficult Interview

There are multiple circumstances that can make an interview difficult and can challenge even the most experienced clinician. Below are some examples of patient personalities, special situations, and interviewer tendencies that can make the interview less productive or derail it; also included are some possible approaches that the interviewer can make during the interview to accommodate the difficulties.

The Hostile Patient

The hostile patient is an angry individual who is determined not to cooperate. It may help to acknowledge the patient's feelings and advise that it is in the patient's best interest to tell his or her side of the story; otherwise, the clinician will have to assume the worst and make recommendations accordingly. If it is possible, then the clinician can offer to return later after the patient has had a chance to settle down.

The Overinclusive, Rambling Patient

The clinician should acknowledge that the overinclusive, rambling patient has a lot to say and should be prepared to explain the goals of the interview to the patient several times. It is useful if the clinician offers to talk more with the patient after they have finished communicating the required information. The overinclusive patient will require a great deal of direction and redirection. Taking notes will help the clinician to stay on track so that there is enough information to write the interview report when the interview has concluded.

The Suspicious Patient

There are many reasons for patients to be suspicious about a clinician. Suspiciousness may be part of the patient's psychopathology and can range from a personality disorder to a psychosis or to a dementing or organic process. Suspicion could be related to a general cultural belief based on factual historical experience or belief pattern, or it could also reflect previous experience. In any case, it is best for the clinician to be clear about the purpose of the interview, keep movements calm and open, and answer questions as honestly as possible. It is often wise to reduce direct eye contact to an intermittent level, as too much eye contact can be interpreted as aggressive or invasive. With some patients, an offer of water or juice will be helpful in clearing the tension; others will decline.

The Confused, Unreliable Patient

If the patient is confused or unreliable, obtaining names of contact people or family as soon as possible is essential. If there is history from another source, such as a previous encounter, it should be reviewed. The interview and assessment will focus on the possible sources for the confusion, including substances, seizures, and other medical or metabolic sources. Depending on the location of the initial interview, a medical work-up may need to be completed before the clinician can continue. Piecing together an evaluation will take time and teamwork. Maintaining updated communication in the medical record and in person is necessary to help the team stay on track.

The Vague, Evasive, or Manipulative Patient

The vague, evasive, or manipulative patient purposefully corrupts communication to provide minimal, distorted, or completely manufactured information, generally to obtain a primary or secondary gain. A patient may act evasively in an attempt to avoid a legal consequence, to seek drugs or shelter, to provide work excuses, or to explain away relationship issues. The patient may also want to minimize the extent of an illness, attract attention, or create a sense of disorder that mirrors his or her own internal state. The focus in the initial interview will be on the current situation. The patient's description of what she believes she needs will help the clinician determine the first level of dynamics that are operating. In subsequent interviews, focusing on the developmental history will provide the direction that treatment interventions will take.

The Patient Who Is a Victim of Abuse

This is often a very difficult situation, as abuse can involve patients of all ages. Abused and battered children, adults, and elders create many feelings in the staff at all levels. Whereas the medical issues are generally clear, the psychosocial issues are complicated. In many states, there is a legal requirement for Protective Services to be contacted for children and vulnerable adults; the contact can be made by any professional member of the team in a process that varies by state.

Rape assessment, while not significantly different from the management of any patient in an acute situation, can be particularly stressful for both the clinician and patient because it is a highly charged issue with preconceptions attached to the perpetrator and victim. Rape kits, police reports, or both may be appropriate. The psychiatric interview, if ordered, may be conducted by specifically trained nurses or by the psychiatric clinician. When a suspected domestic abuser is present in the evaluation setting, he or she should not be present during the interview; otherwise, the patient may not say anything (although that may happen anyway). The clinician's role in this interview is to obtain as much fact as possible and to provide as much support, anticipatory guidance, and resources as will be accepted. Often, small cards that can be tucked away with resource numbers are useful for patients in the future, as it often takes a number of episodes before a woman leaves an abusing partner. For rape victims, referrals or an appointment with specialized programs are the most preferable follow-up.

The Agitated Patient

In some instances, the clinician will be called to interview a patient who is clearly agitated. The purpose of the visit may be solely to help the patient calm down, or it may be the initial focus of an evaluation. If the patient is willing to talk, even if the communication is loud, it is acceptable to proceed provided that other staff members are nearby and the situation or setting is determined to be safe. Establishing violence potential is particularly important with patients who have comorbid antisocial and psychopathic traits because there is an increased risk of danger (Antonius, Fuchs, Herbert, et al., 2010). If there is reason to believe that the patient is intoxicated, the clinician should defer completing the interview until the level of intoxication is within legal limits. The clinician must be mindful of changes in the patient's presentation, content, and affect and should make sure that the patient's anxiety level is within tolerable limits.

Other reasons for patient agitation are psychosis, depression, physical illness, delirium due to an organic condition, or dementia; the setting of the interview may also agitate the patient. In many cases, the clinician's efforts to calm the agitated patient by (1) offering medication, juice, or water, (2) moving the interview to a quieter location if possible, and (3) verbalizing and displaying a willingness to listen to the patient will be sufficient to calm the patient so that the interview can proceed.

Interviewer Attitude or Transference

Some patients trigger an internal reaction in the clinician. It may be a particular personality type, such as a histrionic individual; a patient behavior, such as abuse; or a bias related to a particular subculture. In the same way, a patient can come to an interview with preconceived ideas about clinicians. Clearly, for the clinician, acknowledging the presence of a preconceived attitude is the first step, and remaining respectful and professional is absolute. If there are verbal or nonverbal indications from the patient that there is a problem, it is often useful for the clinician to ask directly if there is a concern about interviewing with the clinician and to make an attempt to resolve the issue if possible.

Delivering Bad News

While somewhat less of a catastrophic issue in mental health, delivering bad news to patients or family members may be necessary. For patients with psychiatric disorders, bad news may be the diagnosis of a major mental disorder, losses such as the death or departure of a trusted clinician, or disappointments such as being denied desired placements or other treatment options. The clinician should proceed first from where the patient is or what is already known, and then move on to what the patient would like to know. The clinician should inquire about how the patient believes the news will affect his or her future and ask what feelings the patient has. Lastly, the clinician should discuss ways to cope, what sources of support exist, and what the patient believes would be helpful in his or her own adaptation to the change.

Interview Settings

Psychiatric encounters with patients can occur in many different types of settings, including the crisis center/emergency room, an inpatient unit, an outpatient clinic, the patient's home, jail, a retail setting, a school, a mobile unit, and, increasingly, via telephone and the Internet. Each setting may require different approaches.

In practical terms, the clinician must consider the type of interaction that will be taking place and plan ahead by reviewing records, progress notes, and reports from other staff (Bowers, Brennan, Winship, et al., 2010). Having some knowledge of the patient history is particularly important before an interview so that the clinician comes prepared and with the appropriate resources. Knowing in advance whether a translator is needed, whether a supportive family member will be available, and whether it is necessary to obtain supplies such as paper and pencil or toys will allow the most efficient use of the interview time. In addition, the forms and equipment needed for taking notes, reviewing records, and generating reports may vary widely from all paper records to electronic health records, so it is important to know what methods the interview setting requires.

The following discussion focuses on common interview settings for clinicians, including the emergency room/crisis clinic, the office, impatient units, and via the telephone and Internet.

The Emergency Room/Crisis Clinic

Psychiatric services in hospital emergency settings benefit from having an interdisciplinary team available. Clinician roles may vary widely, but they often include having responsibility for the initial interview, which includes interviewing family, collateral informants, or both; arranging additional consultation; and performing the patient disposition. The information obtained during the initial interview is of key importance, as the clinician may be involved in a decision about using restraints and the level of risk related to discharge planning. Review of medical tests is also important. Some conditions, such as pregnancy, intoxication, and suicide attempts by cuts, hanging, gunshot, or poison, will require medical intervention first, delaying the patient's transfer to inpatient psychiatric services. Complete, clear, and timely communication to the team will keep the emergency management process as efficient as possible.

The Office

Outpatient psychiatric and mental health clinics are the traditional settings for initial and ongoing psychiatric evaluation, psychotherapy, and medication management. Interviews are generally scheduled in advance for specific periods of time. Procedures for case discussion and review are part of the process.

Many office settings built for this purpose are well equipped with the required space, office flow, and supports (such as reception staff and "panic alarms"). Other office settings have less ideal design that may be unalterable. Some examples of possible solutions are leaving the office door partly open, having another individual working nearby, changing offices or interview rooms, having a code word for the receptionist, or using portable alarms, which are readily available if there is not a built-in panic-alarm system. In both scenarios, it is important to have a plan to handle potentially dangerous situations, to be consistently conscious of safety precautions, and to keep in mind that even very well-known patients can be unpredictable and unsafe. Interviews can include very intense, ongoing work, and they can involve difficult decisions about treatment. Repeated interviews in the same location can create an illusion of safety and a sense of complacency, against which the clinician must guard, knowing that clinicians have been seriously harmed in repeat sessions.

The clinician should attempt to reduce the patient's anxiety near the end of the session.

Conventional wisdom for clinician safety is to place himself or herself nearest to the door without any barriers so that the clinician can leave without passing the patient if behavior escalates. However, another school of thought recommends easier egress for the patient, because a patient who feels trapped can be especially dangerous (Dubin & Jagarlamundi, 2010).

Inpatient Units

The psychiatric advanced practice nurse who functions on an inpatient unit often is responsible for interview assessments, initiating medical orders, and following up in a collaborative relationship with a physician. Generally, the team includes other professionals with defined roles, such as social workers, occupational/recreational therapists, resident or attending physicians, and pharmacy support. The clinician may have interviewed the patient first in the emergency setting and then continues to assess, note progress, and continue educational or interventional components in subsequent interviews. The clinician must arrange for privacy and safety, making use of designated consultation space where possible to minimize distractions.

The Telephone and the Internet

Psychiatry has used telephone consultations and interviews for some time, but the use of the Internet will likely become more frequent in the future. While there are clear attractions for some clinicians and patients, there are also risks. Some advantages to using the phone and Internet are accessibility for patients living in remote or underserved areas and for those with disabilities; ease of reaching distant family members; and perhaps ease of reaching patients with some types of phobias, such as social phobia or agoraphobia. Risks of using the Internet and telephone include potential security issues with information; a potential lack of nonverbal cues or tonal cues; and having patients living in states where the clinician may not be licensed to practice. A clinician choosing to work in these media should seek advice and proceed carefully (Dever Fitzgerald, Hunter, Hadjistavropoulos, et al., 2010).

Assessment

The purposes of a psychiatric assessment interview are to gather information that will enable the formulation of a diagnosis and differential diagnoses; to establish a therapeutic relationship with the patient; to reassure the patient that help will be provided; to begin to develop a treatment plan based on the information obtained; and to produce a written document for the patient's record that is organized in a standard format.

Interview Format

This interview proceeds in a standardized format:

A. Introduction

1. State whether patient was the sole informant, whether history was obtained from previous psychiatric records, or whether other persons provided the information.
2. State who referred patient for evaluation; whether the patient was self-referred or brought in by a family member, friend, or other individual.
3. Indicate how reliable you think the information is.

B. Reason for Referral for Evaluation/Chief Complaint

The interviewer may have information from the emergency room or from a family doctor that states the reason for referral. If not, the interviewer should ask the patient what problems he or she is having at this time or should ask the patient to tell why he or she is being referred. State the reason why the patient has come for treatment in the patient's own words. Add a sentence with information to expand on the patient's statement. The reason for referral and how the patient provides the information is a starting point for the clinician to begin to hypothesize about the diagnosis.

C. Identification of Patient

Identification of the patient includes the patient's full name, the name of those accompanying the patient, and the following information about the patient: age, gender, marital status, primary language and culture, and religion.

1. **Age.** The patient's age helps in narrowing the possible diagnoses to those disorders that have an age of onset in specific age ranges—late teens, early adulthood, middle to late adulthood, and old age. Among older patients, the interviewer would consider that the psychiatric symptoms might be due to existing medical disorders or drug interactions, alcohol, or depression. Age also influences acceptance of a diagnosis and treatment, response to treatment, and ability to make changes. Younger patients may be reluctant to accept the diagnosis of a psychiatric disorder and may refuse to take medication or to participate in psychotherapy. Older adults may have more medical disorders, may be taking multiple prescribed medications, may have limited finances and problems with transportation that may affect adherence to treatment, and may have suffered multiple losses such as loss of a partner, home, and role in life.
2. **Gender.** Gender differences are seen in the prevalence of psychiatric disorders. For example, women have higher rates of eating disorders, somatization disorder, panic disorder, dysthymia, major depression, and borderline personality disorder, and men have higher rates of alcoholism, other substance use disorders, paraphilias, and antisocial personality disorder (Robinson, 2000). Female gender raises concern about pregnancy because of the potential for increased stress and because some of the psychotropic medications have teratogenic effects. Female gender also is an issue with medications that cause hyperprolactinemia with resulting disruption of menses, along with possible links with future breast cancer. Male gender raises the concern of priapism when certain antipsychotics or antidepressants are used (see Chapter 6).
3. **Marital status.** A patient's marital status is an indication of the patient's social support and home environment. Many patients with psychiatric disorders are not married or never married. Therefore, marital status may suggest that the patient had a high level of functioning before his or her present illness. The presence of a spouse or partner suggests to the clinician that the patient may have help in adhering to treatment and keeping appointments. It also is a flag for the clinician to think in terms of family education as well as patient education.
4. **Primary language and culture.** Acceptance of mental illness differs among cultures. Individuals from different cultures may have problems in providing information and in understanding explanations or interpretations complicated by language barriers. Nonprofessional interpreters or family members serving as interpreters may distort questions during the assessment process, may add information not provided by the patient, and may omit information. Therefore, it is preferable to use the services of a professional interpreter, as described earlier in this chapter.
5. **Religion.** Individuals often look to their religious leaders or their writings for guidance in coping with life problems such as psychiatric disorders. It is important for the clinician to know what the patient's religious beliefs and practices are so that they may be considered in assessing the patient, formulating a diagnosis, and planning treatment for the patient. The clinician should be aware of the wide variations within cultures to avoid making an assumption that may be offensive. Asking a direct question, such as "Will having your husband wait outside during an examination create a difficulty?" can help create an alternative plan ahead of time in a neutral manner.

D. History of Present Illness

The goal of the history of present illness is to provide a concise history of the current problem.

1. Describe onset of symptoms: time, frequency, duration, aggravating and relieving factors, treatments tried, severity, characteristics of symptoms, and associated factors or "triggers."
2. State if this is the first psychiatric evaluation or hospitalization or if there has been other treatment, and then state when the last visit occurred.
3. Describe when the current psychiatric symptoms began and if they were acute or had a gradual onset.
4. Ask if symptoms were precipitated by an event or problem. Also ask if anything significant has happened in the last several months, because the patient may not make a connection between an event and the onset of symptoms. If something significant did happen, describe the event or problem. Are the symptoms lessened by anything? How does the patient cope with the symptoms? How do the symptoms affect the patient's social and work functioning?
5. Ask about current medical conditions, recent surgeries, and current medications. Has the patient been taking the medication regularly? Has anything changed recently? Did any medical conditions precipitate the psychiatric symptoms? Identify any treatment for present illness and include dose, how long the patient has been taking the medication, and effectiveness of medication. Ask if the last appointment was kept and if the patient has been actively involved in treatment.
6. Describe the influence of symptoms on patient's life and on family life.

7. Did drug or alcohol abuse precipitate the psychiatric symptoms?

E. Psychiatric History

1. Give a summary of past illnesses, problems, and treatment.
2. Identify the number of past hospitalizations and episodes of the illnesses.
3. Ask when the patient was first seen for psychiatric evaluation or the age when symptoms began.
4. Describe subsequent episodes, symptoms, severity, and response to treatment. What has been tried—e.g., medications, psychotherapy, somatic interventions such as electroconvulsive therapy, psychosocial interventions—and what was the effectiveness?

F. Substance Use History

1. Determine consumption pattern of substances: first use; last use; how the patient uses it (e.g., daily, weekends); amount; effects; problems with family or others.
2. Substance dependence: name of substance, age/time of onset, amount used, last use.
3. Presence of withdrawal symptoms; unsuccessful attempts to cut down; desire to quit; increased amounts required to achieve same effect; withdrawal from social and occupational activities.

G. Medical History

1. All current medications
2. All diagnoses
3. Names and telephone numbers of primary care physician and relevant specialists.
4. Allergies to medication, food, or other items, including latex
5. History of hospitalizations and surgeries
6. Laboratory values (if available), including complete blood count (CBC) with differential, electrolytes, hemoglobin A1c (HbA1c), thyroid-stimulating hormone (TSH), kidney and liver function, as well as others, as indicated

H. Family History

The family history helps with generating hypotheses and provides information on psychosocial factors that shaped the patient's life. Because it is a shift in questioning, tell the patient that you want to ask some questions about their family background. Consider creating a genogram (see Fig. 4-2) to describe or map the family. Inquire about:

1. The presence of psychiatric symptoms or unusual behaviors in the family
2. The presence of known psychiatric disorders and treatment received
3. Medical and neurological illnesses
4. Substance dependence
5. Members who prefer to live in isolation or unusual circumstances, or who are considered eccentric
6. History of suicide or attempted suicide
7. Unexplained changes in residence

I. Social History

1. Where was patient born? At home, in a hospital, or in another country?
2. Did the patient have any childhood problems, e.g., tantrums, school phobia, delinquency?
3. Who were the patient's childhood best friends? What were the patient's childhood interests and hobbies?
4. Stability of family: What was the patient's childhood like?
5. Was there childhood adversity, such as poverty, parental illness, contentious divorce, other? Childhood adversity arising from problems in family functioning is associated with all types of mental and emotional illness (Pearson, 2010; Scott, Varghese, & McGrath, 2010)
6. Where did patient grow up? (Patients have reported that their neighborhood gives them a sense of identity) (Perese, Rohloff, & Ryan, 2008).
7. What was the patient's relationship with parents and siblings?
8. What are the family's religious or cultural attitudes and practices relevant to patient's illness?
9. Describe interpersonal relationships during adolescence and early adulthood.
10. Identify current social supports.

J. Sexual History

1. When was the first sexual experience?
2. When was the patient last sexually active?
3. Is the patient attracted to men, women, or both?
4. How many sexual partners has the patient had?
5. What kind of sexual protection does the patient use?
6. Has the patient been tested for HIV?
7. Does the patient have any difficulties with any aspect of sexual activity?
8. Are there any interactions between medication and libido?

K. Abuse

1. What kind of punishment was used in the patient's family?
2. Was the patient ever touched by someone in a way that he or she didn't like?
3. Was the patient ever forced to do something sexual?
4. Is there any present abuse?

L. Educational and Work History

1. Years of school completed and how well the patient did. Were there particular academic interests? Interest in extracurricular activities?
2. Reason for leaving school
3. Current employment/position, number of jobs held, descriptions of jobs, responsibilities, reasons for leaving

4. Recent changes in position, e.g., possibilities for promotion

M. Military History

1. Branch of service and type of discharge
2. Combat exposure
3. Disciplinary action
4. Psychiatric referral

N. Legal History

1. History of charges, e.g., for what crimes
2. History of convictions, suspended sentences, probation, or parole
3. Offenses related to operating a motor vehicle
4. Upcoming court dates

O. Mental Status Examination

A mental status examination uses observations and direct questioning to evaluate several domains of mental functioning, including speech, behavior, emotional expressions, thinking, and perception and cognitive functions. It summarizes what has been presented in the interview and often adds some specific tasks to determine functional cognitive ability.

1. *General appearance, attitude, and behavior* are described to determine the presence of unspoken clues to the underlying condition. The presenting appearance can help determine the patients' ability to take care of himself or herself and his or her inability or unwillingness to comply with social norms. The presence of body odor, ability to sit still, level of cooperativeness, and observations such as hand and body gestures reflect underlying feelings.
2. *Speech* is assessed by noting spontaneity, syntax, rate, and volume. Abnormalities of speech should be noted, such as dysarthrias and aphasias, which may indicate a physical cause of the mental state.
3. *Emotional expression* can be assessed by asking the patient to describe his or her feelings. The patient's tone, posture, and facial expressions are all considered. Note the *mood*, which is the patient's subjective report of how he or she is feeling. Note *affect*, which is the clinician's observation of the range and depth of emotional responses. Some typical words to describe affect are as follows:
   a. *Full*, meaning that the patient is expressing a wide range of feelings.
   b. *Flat*, which means that the patient has minimal responses that reflect little or no emotion.
   c. *Constricted*, when the patient has limited expressiveness and is able to describe some feelings but stays in a restricted range.
   d. *Blunted*, which is very little emotional response.
   e. *Labile*, which is very changeable and may vary from laughter to tears.
   f. *Euphoric*, or elated.
   g. *Euthymic*, which is neutral and consistent with the circumstances.

An important aspect when looking at affect is whether what is being expressed is congruent with the content of the information described, e.g., the patient describes witnessing a motor vehicle accident in which there is great bodily injury, and his or her expression is smiling. The clinician can describe this incongruence as the affect's being inappropriate to the content expressed.

4. *Thought process* is an expression of the patient's stream of thought using quotes from the patient as examples. Words used to explain thought process include logical, tangential, circumstantial, impoverished. It may include the belief of thought broadcasting or insertion.
5. *Thought content* is the primary content expressed. This includes the patient's information and description related to symptoms or circumstances of depression, anxiety, compulsions, phobias, delusions, or the presence of self-injurious, suicidal, or homicidal ideation. It is the general description of what the patient talked about.
6. *Perception* describes whether the patient is in good contact with the environment or if there is a distortion of perceptions of reality, such as auditory or other hallucinations.
7. *Cognitive function* includes the information following:
   a. Orientation to person, place, time, and circumstance
   b. Ability to abstract: explain proverbs
   c. Memory and concentration
   d. An estimate of intellectual functioning
   e. Judgment, the ability to weigh consequences of doing or not doing something

P. Risk Assessment

One of the most important aspects of assessment is to identify the potential for violence toward self or others and the presence or history of assaultive or destructive behavior. This includes the risk of violence to the clinician or other staff and patients (Antonius et al., 2010). Information obtained throughout the interview will alert the clinician if there is an increased risk of suicidal, homicide, or other risk of violence. It may also include exploration of other risk behaviors such as self-cutting or burning, sexual acting out, or provoking others to retaliate. Factors such as age, gender, substance abuse, recent history, and mental status provide clues that may need further investigation. The clinician must use specific questions to elicit the information necessary to determine the relative risk involved, unless the risk is very obvious.

1. **Suicidal ideation:** Questioning about suicidal ideation can be difficult for the clinician. Feelings about the sanctity of life, religious beliefs, and judgments about right and wrong should be part of the

clinician's self-awareness. Patients who feel that they cannot continue to live are in significant pain and require sensitivity to complete a thorough assessment. The following is a suggested order of questioning:

a. *Are you having any thoughts of harming yourself or ending your life?* If there is any hesitation (or a "not really" response), then the clinician specifically asks:
b. *Can you tell me what you are thinking about? What is your plan? Do you intend to carry it out? Do you have weapons of any sort in your house that you have considered using? Do you have access to them?* The clinician then has to consider whether the patient's response to these questions are ideas, thoughts, or an active plan. If it is an active plan, is the plan realistic and potentially lethal, and is the individual capable of carrying it out? Is there any evidence of psychotic thinking? If so, the clinician must proceed carefully because patients with thought disorders may have very dangerous notions of how to solve their problems and may not communicate it clearly without support.
   (1) *Case example:* Robert, a 22-year-old single Caucasian male was referred to a partial hospital program for further evaluation due to psychotic undercurrents in his thought process. He admitted to hearing voices that were "not nice," but he was guarded about specifics. After further discussion, the nurse returned to the voices, asking specifically where he thought they were coming from. With little hesitation, he stated his belief that a receiver that had been implanted in this brain was transmitting messages to him from the outside. When asked if he thought anything could stop it, he produced a long, double-edged, curved knife that he planned to use to remove the transmitter through his ear. The voices were commanding him to take action.
c. *Have you ever attempted suicide or harmed yourself? If so, what did you do and when?* If there is a history, risk increases. Evaluate the attempt considering the patient's judgment of what happened, why it didn't work, if the patient would do it the same way again, or what he or she would change. Consider the possibility of the patient's acting seriously enough to accidently cause death.
   (1) *Case example:* Mark, a 42-year-old single African American male, had come to an emergency department stating that he planned to kill himself as he had "no place to go." He was well known to the staff for being positive for various drugs and alcohol, episodic homelessness, and a prison history. He was judged to be "manipulating" for an admission and was discharged from the ER. He went out of the hospital, into the street, and threw himself in front of a police car, not killing himself but sustaining significant injury.
d. *Has anyone in your immediate family attempted or committed suicide? Has anyone close died suddenly or violently recently?* Positive history increases risk. As part of history-taking, responses related to the impact of any trauma, particularly if relatively recent, warrant further scrutiny.
e. *What would stop you from harming yourself?* Are there deterrents, such as religious beliefs or concern about children or family that the patient states? Fear of jail? (Do not rely on a "no-suicide" contract.)
f. *Do you think anything or anyone can help you?*
g. *When you feel overwhelmed or out of control, how have you handled it in the past?*

2. **Homicidal ideation**

If the patient states he has no plan to harm himself, but does state that he wants to harm someone else, then ask:

a. *Is there a specific, identifiable individual?*
b. *Have you ever harmed anyone else?*
c. *Is there a specific plan? (or is it a wish?)*
d. *Is there anything that would stop you?*

Clearly, the presence of active suicidal or homicidal intent necessitates a psychiatric inpatient hospitalization. However, there are some patients, often with personality disorder or borderline disorder, with chronic suicidal thoughts that can be appropriately managed in an outpatient setting. The clinician should become familiar with the obligations under the Tarasoff Act, which requires that an identifiable intended victim, as well as the local police, be notified if hospitalization of a potentially dangerous individual does not occur. If the patient is hospitalized, the necessity for warning should be reevaluated prior to discharge.

Q. Case Formulation

Case formulation involves a brief description of primary factors operating in the patient's illness or presenting problem, the major dynamics, and the suggested treatment. It is most often used in the context of dynamic therapy and can be used to offer a brief explanation to the patient. For example, the clinician might say, *"You become very anxious when anyone in your workplace displays anger, and this may be related to the experiences you had with your father when you were young."* While this is a simplistic example, the formulation can become the starting place for treatment. The formulation is discussed further in Chapter 5.

R. Summary

The summary should include the identification of problem(s), provisional diagnosis, level of risk, and treatment plan, which should include follow-up appointments and medications, if prescribed. In some situations, it is also useful to indicate the patient's motivation for treatment or change as well as his or her resources. If appropriate, the patient's and family's response to the plan as well as options discussed should also be indicated.

Rating Scales and Their Use

There are a number of rating scales that clinicians may want to consider as part of their assessment or for initial benchmarking (Sajatovic & Ramirez, 2003). Some rating scales—such as the Abnormal Involuntary Movement Scale (AIMS) or Dyskinesia Identification System (DISCUS) for the evaluation of movement disorders, the Mini-Mental Status Exam (MMSE) for organicity, or screening for substance abuse—may be part of the evaluation process. Many scales and validated assessment tools are in the public domain so they can be used freely. Some examples of rating scales are

- Diagnostic: the Structured Clinical Interview for Axis-I *DSM-IV* Disorders (SCID)
- Symptom-Based: the Brief Psychiatric Rating Scale (BPRS)
- Diagnostic-specific scales: the Positive and Negative Symptom Scale for Schizophrenia (PANSS)
- Basic screening: PHQ-2, PHQ-4, PHQ-9, and various Dartmouth COOP charts can be used for general screening and are adaptable to various medical settings to detect possible depression and/or anxiety quickly. See Sajatovic and Ramirez (2003) for many sample tools.

Some scales can be done by self-rating, whereas others can be completed only by the clinician. There are also nonspecific, informal types of self-ratings that the clinician can ask the patient to do, such as asking, *"On a scale of 1 to 10 where 10 is the best, how do you feel?"* Any of these tools can help both the clinician and the patient to recognize progress or movement toward goals. The more formal tools can help narrow down areas of difficulty and aid with diagnosis. Formal testing, such as neuropsychological testing for intelligence or organicity, may be necessary for some placements.

Taking Notes: Issues Involved

Ideally, the clinician would be able to interview the patient and concentrate solely on the content and process. However, there is a great amount of information that needs to be collected and recorded accurately, making it necessary to take notes in some form (Morrison, 2008). In some settings, there is no choice: the history is recorded directly into a computer database as the interview takes place. In other settings, forms, formats, outlines, or the clinician's handwritten notes are used or become the basis for dictation.

One way for the clinician to record family information is to create a genogram while inquiring about the family composition and history. A genogram is a format for drawing a family tree that records information about family members and their relationships graphically. This provides a quick reference to family relationships and can clearly depict the way in which the current symptoms are related to family patterns (McGoldrich & Gerson, 1995). As shown in Figure 4-2, genograms can make a complicated amount of information clear and serve as a reference in future discussions.

The clinician should let the patient know that notes will be taken and give a brief explanation. He or she should make every attempt to make eye contact and listen as the interview proceeds.

Key Points

- All behavior, both intended and unintended, is communication. Communication techniques can be learned by both clinicians and patients and can be improved with practice and experience.
- Communication is influenced by many factors, including the setting, the relationship, perceptual interference, and verbal and nonverbal messages from both the sender and receiver. Variation within cultures, age group differences, and the impact of illness directly affect the process. Patterns of functional and dysfunctional communication are recognizable and can be influenced by the clinician.
- There are both consultative/diagnostic and interventional interviews. In both cases, the initial interview requires the clinician to obtain a great deal of information in a relatively short time while establishing a working rapport and alliance with the patient. Both types of interviews can be therapeutic to the patient and family.
- Psychiatric interviews can occur in diverse settings. Each setting requires some specific modifications that should be addressed in advance of the interview. In all settings, attention must be given to safety considerations for the clinician, other staff, and patients.
- A formal assessment followed by a written report is required. The evaluation content occurs in a specific order, although the format may differ according to the treatment setting. The process of the interview involves communication, interviewing, and assessment skill, as well as empathy and working alliance.

References

Antonius, D., Fuchs, L., Herbert, F., et al. (2010). Psychiatric assessment of aggressive patients: A violent attack on a resident. *American Journal of Psychiatry, 167*(3), 253-258.

Ayonrinde, O. (2003). Importance of cultural sensitivity in therapeutic transactions: Considerations for healthcare providers. *Disease Management Health Outcomes. 11*(4), 233-248.

Berne, E. (1961). *Transactional analysis in psychotherapy.* New York: Grove.

Bowen, M. (1978). *Family therapy in clinical practice.* New York: Jason Aronson, Inc.

Bowers, L., Brennan, G., Winship, G., et al. (2010). How expert nurses communicate with acutely psychotic patients. *Mental Health Practice, 12*(7), 24-26.

Dever Fitzgerald, T., Hunter, P., Hadjistavropoulos, T., et al. (2010). Ethical and legal considerations for internet-based psychotherapy. *Cognitive Behavior Therapy, 39*(3), 173-187. doi 10.1080/16506071003636046

Dubin, W., & Jagarlamundi, K. (2010). Safety in the evaluation of potentially violent patients: Decreasing the clinician's risk, *Psychiatric Times, 27*(7).

Fleisher, S., Berg, A., Zimmermann, M., et al. (2009). Nurse-patient interaction and communication: A systematic literature review. *Journal of Public Health, 17*, 339-353.

Havens, L. (1998). Forward. In S. C. Shea (Ed.), *Psychiatric interviewing: The art of understanding* (pp. vii-viii). Philadelphia: Saunders.

Levensky, E. R., Forcehimes, A., O'Donohue, W. T., et al. (2007). Motivational interviewing. *American Journal of Nursing, 107*(10), 50-58.

McGoldrich, M., & Gerson, R. (1995). *Genograms in family assessment*. New York: W. W. Norton & Company.

Meeks, T., Lanouette, N., Vahia, I., et al. (2009). Psychiatric assessment and diagnosis in older adults. *FOCUS: The Journal of Lifelong Learning in Psychiatry. Winter, VII*(1), 3-15.

Morrison, J. (2008). *The first interview* (3rd ed.). New York: Guilford Press.

Pearson, G. (2010). The past defines the present. *Perspectives in Psychiatric Care, 46*(3), 169-170.

Perese, E., Rohloff, M., & Ryan, E. (2008). Promoting positive clinical experiences with older adults through students' use of a therapeutic intervention—group reminiscence therapy. *Journal of Gerontological Nursing, 34*(12), 46-51.

Preston, P. (2005). Non-verbal communication: Do you really say what you mean? *Journal of Healthcare Management, 50*(2), 83-86.

Robinson, D. J. (2000). *Three spheres: A psychiatric interviewing primer.* Port Huron, MI: Rapid Psychler Press.

Rosengren, D. B. (2009). *Building motivational interviewing skills: A practitioner workbook*. New York: Guilford Press.

Sajatovic, M., & Ramirez, L. (2003). *Rating scales in mental health* (2nd ed.). Hudson, Ohio: Lexi-Comp. Inc.

Schuster, P. M. (2002). *Communication: The key to the therapeutic relationship.* Philadelphia: F. A. Davis.

Scott, J., Varghese, D., & McGrath, J. (2010). As the twig is bent, the tree inclines: Adult mental health consequences of childhood adversity. *Archives of General Psychiatry, 67*(2), 111-112.

Shea, S. C. (1998). *Psychiatric interviewing: The art of understanding* (pp. vii-viii). Philadelphia: Saunders.

Watzlawick, P., Beavin, J., & Jackson, J. (1967). *Pragmatics of human communication*. New York: W. W. Norton & Company.

Wenburg, J., & Wilmot, W. (1973). *The personal communication process.* New York: John Wiley and Sons.

CHAPTER 5

Case Formulation, Diagnosis, and Plan of Care

Dessye Dee Clark, PhD, APRN, PMHCNS-BC

This chapter provides guidance in how to develop a case formulation, make a provisional primary diagnosis, consider differential diagnoses, and create a preliminary treatment plan. There are different approaches to developing a case formulation, but as stated by Privitera and Lyness (2009) "Every psychiatric workup ends with some kind of summation" (p. 69). They describe a commonly used format that includes three sections: "a diagnostic impression, a formulation, and plan" (p. 69). The case formulation is derived from the information that the psychiatric advanced practice nurse (PAPN) compiles during the clinical interview and from data collected from other assessment sources, such as psychological assessments, neuroimaging studies, laboratory findings, academic records, legal records, and prior treatment providers. As to be expected, the more detailed the collection process, the better the case formulation. For example, the PAPN may be asked to evaluate an individual's mental capacity during a family law process in which parties are developing a parenting plan. Obtaining information about whether the individual was a registered sex offender, had obtained an honorable discharge from military service, or has had recent citations for DUI (Driving Under the Influence) might be relevant.

The extent of the formulation and the length of written documentation of diagnostic impressions vary greatly and depend on the clinical setting. In an academic medical center where children or young adults may present with early-onset or first-episode events of major psychiatric disorders such as schizophrenia and bipolar disorder, work-ups will be extensive and the duration of evaluation may cover days to weeks. Initial admission diagnoses selected at the time of first admission to a psychiatric unit may change substantially by the time of discharge to the community.

Often the term "provisional" is used to acknowledge the limitations of a preliminary diagnosis when there are time constraints. For example, when a patient with newly developing symptoms of psychosis meets some of the criteria for schizophrenia, that patient may be diagnosed with "schizophreniform disorder (provisional)." The use of the term "provisional" is recommended in the *Diagnostic and Statistical Manual of Mental Disorders,* 4th Edition Text Revision *(DSM-IV-TR)* quick-reference guide: "...when the diagnosis must be made without waiting for recovery, it should be qualified as provisional" (American Psychiatric Association, 2000, p. 158). Likewise, children referred early for mental health consultation or presenting with early-onset psychiatric mental health disorders will prompt the PAPN to conduct a careful evaluation of related factors, such as the presence of environmental toxins (e.g., lead poisoning), child maltreatment, neurodevelopmental dysregulation of biological origin, and other pathophysiological conditions that may provoke or present with psychiatric or behavioral symptoms. It is expected that children or young adults with a first psychotic presentation or major suicide attempt will require extensive treatment planning and community discharge resources. Patients with adult-onset psychiatric conditions who are already established with an outpatient psychiatric provider may have shorter, more abbreviated work-ups in the emergency room and very focused treatment plans that target specific aspects of the current crisis.

This chapter discusses both the formal structure and the mechanics of the diagnostic process using *DSM-IV-TR* procedures and illustrates the creative aspects of case formulation that reflect the "art" of diagnosis and treatment planning. Several case studies will illustrate how the PAPN may develop case formulations for patients across the life span and at specific intervention time points, primarily upon initial contact. However, it should be noted that *the diagnostic process is not static.* It is continuously employed when the PAPN has ongoing contact with a patient, and it is possible that the patient will no longer meet full criteria for a previous diagnosis at midtreatment or at the conclusion of therapy.

This chapter also provides information on the utility of screening tools, symptom rating scales, diagnostic decision trees, and specialized assessments that the PAPN may employ for comprehensive diagnostic work-up and differential diagnosis. These assessment tools provide an evidence base for diagnosis and may assist the patient to access additional care resources or receive financial or educational benefits necessary to cope with and recover from a specific mental health problem or psychiatric disorder. The chapter concludes with a discussion of case formulation strategies commonly used when the PAPN receives a previously treated patient from another provider or agency or is asked to provide a second opinion or an explanatory web of causation for some forensic purpose. In these situations, a patient with a chronic mental health condition may get a "fresh look." The PAPN has the opportunity to reframe the disease process and reorient the patient, perhaps emphasizing symptom self-management strategies and new community resources using a recovery model type of intervention plan.

Case Formulation: Making Sense of the Data

An important product of the clinical assessment is the case formulation. Case formulation has been defined as "a hypothesis about the causes, precipitants, and maintaining influences of a person's psychological, interpersonal, and behavioral problems" (Eells, Kendjelic, & Lucas, 1998, p. 146). It describes a process that organizes, explains, and makes sense of the data. It explains the patient's symptoms, prompts the PAPN to engage in critical thinking about etiology, and provides a working rationale for the treatment plan (Ingram, 2006).

When engaging in case formulation, the PAPN endeavors to differentially compare and contrast information in order to include or exclude clinical data and thus justify that sufficient criteria are met for a formal psychiatric diagnosis. For example, a woman in young adulthood might be late to work, have difficulty staying on task at her job as an office assistant, fail to socialize with coworkers, and spend excessive amounts of unapproved time on the Internet during her work hours. How the woman responds to her supervisor's confrontation would provide important insight into her understanding of the problem, her likelihood of improving her work performance, and the stability of her occupational functioning:

- One hypothesis that the PAPN might entertain is that the woman has an adjustment disorder related to maturational difficulties and developmental immaturity. The PAPN might also consider that the woman is unmotivated and using diversion to cope with feelings of boredom and disinterest. The PAPN might further assess for signs of depression or consider social factors contributing to relationship difficulties. For example, perhaps the woman has a hidden disappointment that she was not given financial support from her parents for college and is now acting out her anger by behaving poorly at a job she believes is "beneath her."
- Another hypothesis might have the PAPN focus on potential frontal lobe dysfunction as manifested in difficulties of attention, or consider impairment of executive functioning, with investigation of possible attention deficit disorder.
- With a third hypothesis, the PAPN would further explore the woman's impaired social interactions to determine if social phobia is contributing to avoidance and escape behaviors.
- A fourth hypothesis that the PAPN might entertain is the presence of a neurobehavioral disorder, such as Asperger's or high-functioning autism. In such cases, the woman may have an obsessive interest in certain Internet sites and compulsively engage in these activities, even with the obvious threat of being fired. If the PAPN inquires about sleep routines and daytime fatigue, she might discover that this young woman was up many nights on the computer, surfing Internet sites related to a special interest. The employer's computer might also show that the young woman went exclusively to certain Web sites. The PAPN would need to consider whether the quality of repetitive activity involved a checking ritual related to obsessive-compulsive disorder (OCD). Clarification would come from exploring the woman's thoughts about computer usage and assessing for obsessive ideas, repetitive thoughts, and compulsive behaviors and from the use of screening tools for OCD or more formal assessments such as the Yale-Brown Obsessive-Compulsive Scale (Y-BOCS) (Goodman, Price, Rasmussen, et al., 1989).

Role of Case Formulation in Diagnosing and Planning Treatment

Case formulation is an important step in finalizing the diagnostic process and providing a foundation for planning treatment. It can be thought of as the bridge between diagnosis and treatment (Horowitz, Wilner, & Alvarez, 1997). Case formulation is a method of describing that organizes, explains, and makes sense out of the data across time. It offers explanations for the patient's symptoms in the past and present. It provides a rationale for the treatment plan (Ingram, 2006). Like a puzzle strategy, the process of thinking through the information obtained from the clinical interview, laboratory work, imaging studies, patient self-report, and history from family and other referral sources to develop a case formulation is creative and recursive. It helps the PAPN to make sense of the data and allows for sequential consideration of alternative explanations for psychopathology until a precise endpoint is reached. This endpoint should not only satisfy the diagnostic requirements to meet "essential criteria" of the *DSM-IV-TR* manual

(American Psychiatric Association, 2000), but also reflect interrelationships of causality, etiology, historical development, maturation, and trajectory of the illness or disorder and predict the patient's potential recovery process.

A dynamic case formulation positions the PAPN's professional understanding of the patient's presenting concerns in relation to standardized criteria (e.g., laboratory work, psychological testing, structured interview responses) and provides the basis for the determination of diagnoses. As part of the process of developing the case formulation, the PAPN assesses the patient and evaluates the content of the clinical assessment through one or more theoretical schemas and at a variety of conceptual levels. On a practical level, the written case formulation is often used in treatment planning to justify a level of care, specify treatment needs, provide rationale for clinical urgency, identify rationale for legal adjudication and immediate safety measures, and ensure reasonable cost containment. Case formulation can also be useful as a clinical "road map" for future clinicians who will be assuming care for a patient.

Process, Purposes, and Features of Case Formulation

Case formulation is a creative endeavor that can be time-consuming but does not need to be. PAPNs who make a habit of conceptualizing their cases, whether in written or verbal form, will develop a stronger foundation for clinical practice. Developing a skill in case formulation prevents the negative consequences of "cookbook" diagnosis, which is sometimes observed in novice providers who are too dependent on DSM typology.

Process

To work up a case requires accurate clinical understanding. The PAPN must establish genuine rapport, engage in therapeutic communication, respect the patient's personal viewpoint, and assess the variables pertinent to cultural diversity. For example, are ghosts or visits from ancestral spirits essential beliefs in the patient's family? Without this understanding, the PAPN might easily misdiagnose reports of ghostly visions as hallucinations or delusions and formulate a plan for treating psychotic disorders, when the individual could be experiencing a culture-bound experience of normal grief.

Purposes

The purposes of the case formulation are:

1. Organize all of the key facts of a patient's situation around a single cause that integrates all the information obtained in the assessment process and explains the source of the problem
2. Frame the source of the problem in terms of factors that are amenable to direct intervention
3. Explain the source of the problem and its effects to the patient so that the patient can participate in identifying the focus of treatment, the interventions that will be used, and the desired goals of treatment (Bergner, 1998).

In brief, a case formulation is a concise description of the chief features of the case as well as an integration of diagnosis, etiology, treatment options, and prognosis for the patient's problem (Sim, Gwee, & Bateman, 2005).

Features

Five broad categories of information are contained in a case formulation: symptoms and problems, precipitating events or stressors, predisposing life events or stressors, mechanisms or causes, and other contributing factors (Eells et al., 1998).

Symptoms and Problems

This category includes the patient's presenting symptoms, the patient's chief complaints and problems, and problems such as unmet needs that may be noticed by the PAPN but not mentioned by the patient.

Precipitating Events or Stressors

Precipitating stressors or events are occurrences or situations that directly lead to the current problem or increase the level of existing problems. Examples of precipitating stressors include financial losses; death of a spouse, child, parent, or close friend; loss of housing; physical illness; and victimization.

Predisposing Life Events or Stressors

These are events that have occurred in the patient's past and are believed to have produced an increased vulnerability or risk for developing symptoms of a psychiatric disorder:

- *Events in childhood.* Events such as separation from the mother, neglect, physical or sexual abuse, insecure attachment, having been born "unwanted," bullying, illnesses or injuries, conflict in the family, and parental psychiatric disorders are associated with risk for later development of psychiatric disorders.
- *Past events in adulthood.* Certain life events are associated with increased risk of developing symptoms of psychiatric disorders. Head injuries, exposure to trauma, and neurological illnesses such as Parkinson's disease and multiple sclerosis are associated with increased risk.
- *Recent events in adulthood.* Recent events include military service, unemployment, retirement, divorce, exposure to trauma, legal problems, relocation, and death of loved ones.

Mechanism

The mechanism is the PAPN's hypothesis of what is the cause of the patient's present problem; it is what links symptoms, stressors, predisposing influences, and factors maintaining the patient's problems. According to Eells et al.

(1998), "There are three major categories under inferred mechanism: biological, psychological, and sociocultural" (p. 147). *Biological causes* include genetic influences, neurodevelopmental abnormalities (abnormalities of brain development), neurochemical abnormalities, and abnormalities of brain circuitry and functioning. *Psychological causes* include interpersonal conflicts; dysfunctional thoughts or perceptions; problems with regulation of emotions; deficits of social skills, problem-solving skills, and skills in maintaining friendships; use of inappropriate defense mechanisms; and dysfunctional coping strategies in response to stressors. *Sociocultural causes* are factors such as ethnicity, socioeconomic status, religion, social isolation, lack of social support, and victimization.

Other Contributing Factors

Other factors that are encompassed in the case formulation include developmental history, educational achievement, work history, treatments for medical and psychiatric illnesses and responses to treatments, deficits in functioning, and lack of social support.

Biopsychosocial Case Formulation

Although diagnoses are based on case formulations, it is the total case formulation—not merely the diagnosis—that guides selection of specific interventions. One part of the biopsychosocial case formulation involves conceptualizing the patient and his or her world. During the interviewing and assessment process, PAPNs form a mental model of the biopsychosocial health of the patient and the world in which the patient lives, the people in that world, the roles that the patient plays, patterns of coping, and the patient's internal and external resources. Another part of the biopsychosocial case formulation involves planning how to improve the patient's biopsychosocial health, the world in which he or she lives, and his or her functioning. The biopsychosocial case formulation includes key points of the psychiatric history, mental status examination, key developmental issues, and relevant stressors. It links the patient's past and present problems. Based on the biopsychosocial case formulation, PAPNs develop a working diagnosis using the five-axis classification system of the *DSM-IV-TR*, which is discussed in the diagnosis section of this chapter.

A biopsychosocial case formulation incorporates the information obtained in the psychiatric interview and mental status examination into a concise description of the patient and his or her world; this formulation will guide treatment (Engel, 1980; Privitera & Lyness, 2009). The *biological* part of the formulation will include a brief account of the patient's physical status, health problems, and functioning. The *psychological* part will include information about the patient's developmental history, themes that are associated with past and present problems, and current stressors that may have triggered the present problems. The *social* part will include information such as availability of social support and problems with living situation and financial situation. Kassaw and Gabbard (2002) suggested the following considerations in developing the biopsychosocial case formulation:

1. Focus on identifying one or two key psychodynamic themes that are the core of the patient's subjective view of the problem.
2. Identify, if possible, developmental experiences that may contribute to the current problem.
3. Identify current stressors that trigger symptoms or prompt the patient to seek help.
4. Predict how present relationships may be linked to childhood developmental experiences. For example, a basic premise of psychodynamic thinking is that relationships that are etched in neural networks from early childhood development tend to repeat themselves in adult relationships (Kassaw & Gabbard, 2002).
5. Keep in mind that a case formulation is a hypothesis or a set of hypotheses and may have to be changed as new information is obtained.

The case formulation links (1) *DSM-IV-TR* criteria, (2) information about patients' problems, their thoughts, and why the problem emerged at this time, and (3) course and proposed treatment. From the biopsychosocial case formulation, the clinician proposes a diagnosis using the five axes of the *DSM-IV-TR* (American Psychiatric Association, 2000) and decides where the patient should receive treatment—in a hospital, as an outpatient, or in an assertive community treatment program.

Other Approaches to Case Formulation

Other approaches that the clinician may use in case formulation include the problem-oriented method; the structural approach, which focuses on the characteristics of the patient's personality within a functional context; and the genetic approach, which focuses on exploration of early development and life events.

Problem-Oriented Method

In the problem-oriented method, a problem title is generated from the current, real-life difficulties, complaints, and problems for which the patient seeks treatment. It is a brief descriptive phase and often begins with words such as "difficulty," "inability to," "lack of," or "excessive." Examples of frequently encountered problems include depressed mood, excessive anxiety in public-speaking situations, auditory hallucinations, substance abuse, or difficulty getting along with others. Descriptive words may be added to the problem, such as "with depressed mood following relocation." Explanatory phrases such as "due to" or "because of" should not be used (Ingram, 2006).

The problem is defined as a solvable target of treatment. An outcome goal that is directly related to the problem title is also generated. The outcome goal is realistic, related to real-life functioning, and stated as a positive—for example, "stress symptoms will be reduced." The data that were obtained from the assessment are organized according to subjective data, objective data, assessment, and plan of treatment (SOAP) (Ingram, 2006).

- Subjective data include information that is learned from the patient and family members, such as age and number of years of school achieved. Direct quotations are helpful.
- Objective data include the PAPN's observations, test results, reports from professionals, and information obtained from review of records.
- The assessment is a written explanatory discussion of the PAPN's analysis of the patient's problem, hypotheses, and theoretical speculations. The assessment is based on the data and is designed to lead to treatment plans that will resolve the problem, with each treatment intervention supported by data in the assessment. It is expected that resolution of the problem will result in achievement of the outcome goal.
- The treatment plan should be appropriate for the treatment setting and should address the use of community resources and referrals, if needed (Ingram, 2006).

Structural Approach

The structural approach uses the concept of *ego strengths* to refer to the inner life of patients. One ego strength is a sense of reality or ability to distinguish self from others and to know what is real and what is not real, such as hallucinations and delusions. Another ego strength is the ability to relate in a meaningful way to significant others and to maintain a stable sense of self-identity. Ability to experience and tolerate a wide range of emotions—love, anger, joy, sadness, and humiliation—is an ego strength. Use of mature defense mechanism—altruism, anticipation, suppression, sublimation, and humor—in response to perceived danger, challenges, or painful emotions is an ego strength. Other ego strengths include ability to think clearly, logically, and abstractly; ability to organize oneself to be able to function in an integrated way; and presence of morals, ideals, and a conscience.

Genetic Approach

Certain neuropsychiatric disorders have strong familial-genetic inheritance. Tolerance and risk for dependence on alcohol is one example (Wolff, 1972; Yoshida, 1993). According to LeDoux (2002), "The essence of who we are is encoded in our brains and brain changes account for the alterations of thought, mood and behavior that occur in mental illness" (p. 260). Also according to LeDoux (p. 261), the "soup model" of understanding the biology of psychiatric disorders—which proposed that mental disorders are due to chemical imbalances in the brain—has been replaced by the circuit model. The circuit model is based on evidence that mental states are created by patterns of information processing within and between synaptic connected neural circuits. LeDoux said that neurochemicals (neurotransmitters) participate in the transmission of information from synapse to synapse, but it is the pattern of transmission in circuits—not the neurotransmitters—that determines the mental state. For example, both life events and psychotherapy are experiences of learning, and they leave lasting effects as stored memories in synaptic circuits. Both bring about changes in synaptic connections; that is, they alter the brain and thus its functioning.

Case Formulation and Culture-Bound Syndromes

Simons and Hughes (1993) described culture-bound syndromes as "recurrent, locality-specific patterns of aberrant behavior and experience that appear to fall outside of conventional Western psychiatric diagnostic categories" (p. 75). Because culture-bound syndromes occur within the context of culturally determined perceptions of autonomy, illness, transgressions, and supernatural forces, PAPNs need to be aware of the patient's way of understanding emotional reactions, functioning, and behaviors. Examples of culture-bound syndromes include

- **Amok:** This is a dissociative episode, marked by outbursts of violent and aggressive or homicidal behavior directed at people and objects; persecutory ideas; amnesia; and finally a return to consciousness. It is found in Malaysia and Indonesia.
- **Koro:** An intense and sudden anxiety that the penis (or, for females, the vulva and breasts) will recede into the body. The penis is held by the victim or someone else, or devices are attached to prevent its receding. It is found in Chinese and Malaysian populations.
- **Latah:** Hypersensitivity to sudden fright or startle, hypersuggestibility, echopraxia, echolalia, or dissociative or trance-like behavior. It is found in Malaysia and Indonesia.
- **Susto or Espanto:** A folk diagnosis made in Latin American countries. It describes tiredness and inability to function that is due to a fright that may be recent or very old.
- **Ataque de nervios:** An out-of-consciousness state in which the individual is unable to cope with overwhelming stressors. It is found among Puerto Ricans in New York City, who seek help from *espiritistas* (experts in mental health problems).
- **Brain fag:** Problems in concentration, remembering, and thinking. There may be fatigue and anxiety. Patients may complain of worms crawling in the head. It is found among people from Africa.
- **Falling-out:** This is a seizure-like affliction with a sudden collapse. There is no convulsive behavior, but individuals

say that they cannot see or move. Falling-out often occurs in response to crises such as accidents, robberies, and assaults. It is found primarily in the southeastern United States among African Americans and Afro-Caribbeans.

- **Ghost-sickness:** Weakness, loss of appetite, dizziness, bad dreams, and a feeling of suffocation. It is attributed to witches and other bad spirits and is found among Navajo populations. Traditional treatment proposes that the strength of the bad spirit must be countered by the spirit of the healer, who uses smoking, emetics, and other cleansing procedures.
- **Hwa-Byung:** A Korean disorder, whose main symptom is epigastric pain that the patient thinks will lead to death. It is associated with lack of harmony and anger.
- **Taijin kyofusho:** This is found in Japan and is similar to social anxiety disorder, but patients are afraid of embarrassing others with their behavior, or they may fear that their body order is offensive. Traditional therapy includes a variety of physiological interventions: sweating and massage, diet, and social support.
- **Voodoo death:** An individual's belief that someone has put the spell of death on him or her. Patients may believe that if someone has access to their fingernail clippings or hair, they can put a spell on them.
- **Wacinko:** It is a reaction to interpersonal problems. The symptoms are anger, withdrawal, mutism, and immobility. It has been said to lead to suicide. It is found among the Sioux population.
- **Wind illness:** A disorder found in Chinese populations, it is based on the balance of elements, yin and yang. The symptoms include a fear of the cold and of the wind. It is believed that cold is associated with becoming weak and susceptible to illness.
- **Boufee delirante:** It is a syndrome found in West Africa and Haiti. It is a French term that describes outbursts of aggressive and agitated behavior, confusion, agitation, and sometimes visual and auditory hallucinations or paranoid ideation.
- **Angst:** It describes anxiety, dread, anguish. The term comes from German and Danish languages.
- **Colera:** It is a Spanish word describing episodes of symptoms such as nausea, vomiting, fever, severe temper tantrums, and dissociative behaviors (adapted from Simons and Hughes, 1993).

Case Formulation for Patients With a Prior Evaluation, Diagnosis, and Treatment

A case formulation will continue to be useful to the PAPN, with utility even for established patients with an extensive history of prior evaluations. As summarized by Blatner in his Internet blog, "The art of case formulation" (2006), "So, case formulation is the psychodynamic equivalent of a physician understanding the pathophysiology of a patient's medical problem. Formulating a case means constructing a meaningful story, that is, placing the patient's present illness within the context of his or her life. Formulation is also the foundation for rational treatment planning and as such constitutes the key process in clinical practice! All diagnostic inquiries, examinations, and tests are oriented towards this end" (p. 1).

Case formulation is frequently underrated by both faculty and students. As Sim et al. (2005) commented, "some of the issues faced in the development of a case formulation include that of immediacy versus comprehensiveness, complexity versus simplicity, observation versus organization, and the need for cultural sensitivity toward each individual patient" (p. 289). In the ideal world, case formulation is an integrative, reiterative process that the PAPN uses to rebuild the assessment database into a manageable configuration that can guide treatment. While the basic diagnostic steps outlined in the *DSM-IV-TR* may identify required behaviors or "essential characteristics," this current format is primarily descriptive and atheoretical, and therefore it does not adequately explain patient motivation, environmental influences, or the contingencies the PAPN may modify to enhance the patient's recovery process. Case formulation is the essential step to developing a working diagnosis. The novice will find this process to be difficult, but worthwhile.

"Pathogenesis" is a much broader concept in psychiatric nursing than in traditional medicine. As noted by Blazer (2008) in his discussion of the etiology of mental illness and the evolution of the *DSM-IV-TR* (American Psychiatric Association, 2000), "psychiatric diagnostic systems disaggregate psychiatric disorders into discrete cases...an individual meets criteria for diagnosis...or he or she does not" (p. 7). Blazer noted that this strategy serves the purposes of epidemiological research but compromises the clinician's need to holistically comprehend the patient's experience. He emphasized that in actual clinical practice it is important to avoid unitary explanations of disease. He believed that it is essential to use a dynamic "biopsychosocial model" and explore the "web of causation" (p. 7). Privitera and Lyness (2009, p. 11) noted that treatment modalities derive from multiple levels of conceptual organization simultaneously. Thus, the PAPN may develop a plan of care that considers the patient at several levels—e.g., the neurochemical milieu of iron-deficiency anemia, history of precocious puberty secondary to childhood sexual abuse, and adjustment difficulties with features of depression and anxiety emerging after a patient drops out of high school—and the plan of care will also consider the patient's prior response to treatment. The astute PAPN may also factor in cognitive deficits related to neurotoxic effects, drug and alcohol abuse, and the potential for multigenerational learning disabilities. For example, some patients may need a wraparound community-based plan that accommodates their learning disabilities and those of immediate relatives who are expected to help the patient self-manage their mental illness. Some patients may need protection from those who have chemical dependency problems, leading to a recommendation for alternative housing or lock boxes at home and case management for medication monitoring. The treatment plan may require prescription of noncontrolled medications because of a family history of drug dealing or drug diversion.

Creating the Case Formulation

Each PAPN aggregates information in a unique manner, for we are all governed by personal learning styles and modes of sensing and perceiving the world. Some PAPNs tend to collect bits of information and then see how they "match up" with diagnostic criteria. Others tend to memorize diagnostic criteria and then observe the patient for evidence that will fulfill the criteria. According to Sim et al. (2005, p. 289), the quality of case formulation is determined by five case elements:

1. Integrative aspects of case formulation
2. Explanatory aspects of case formulation
3. Prescriptive aspects of case formulation
4. Predictive values of case formulation
5. Therapist variables of case formulation

First, the PAPN should identify major issues quickly and *integrate* salient features to reduce case complexity and organize key first steps. Second, the *explanatory* aspect of case formulation compares and contrasts dynamic and nondynamic factors that produce the current set of signs and symptoms and postulate the historic evolution of the illness. The third *prescriptive* aspect of case formulation identifies goals and proposes strategies that the PAPN can use to hold a particular course of action, even when the patient or significant others swing on an emotional pendulum.

A fourth important aspect is the *predictive* value of case formulation. While an initial rating scale or assessment protocol may suggest a poor prognosis, the iterative process of case formulation allows for new understanding as treatment proceeds. As new information surfaces and new technologies emerge, the PAPN and patient may be able to reconceptualize the problem and redefine treatment endpoints. Over time, the prognosis may become much more favorable. For example, a child presumed to have reactive attachment disorder might have been removed from the home on the grounds of possible abuse and neglect, then later reunited with family after revision of the diagnosis and identification of an autism spectrum disorder with nonverbal learning deficits. In another example, an adolescent with Tourette's disorder may have severe motor tics only moderately responsive to medications and hence may require homeschooling. However, this patient may have a dramatic response to psychosurgery when he receives an implant for deep brain stimulation, and the plan would be revised to allow for mainstream education.

Sim et al. (2005) identified *therapist* variables as the fifth important aspect of case formulation. Experienced therapists have a strong capacity for empathy and will inquire about a patient's personal explanatory model, even if it appears peculiar or vexing to them. In a healthy therapeutic alliance, the PAPN and patient will experience a reciprocal feedback loop and develop a working partnership. Over time, this mutual case formulation process helps to identify emerging skills or regained competencies. It also helps identify therapy-interfering behaviors, such as regressive dependencies and acting-out, and other defensive modes that may impede the recovery process. For example, a patient may resist switching antipsychotic agents, even when the PAPN believes a newer atypical agent may have less risk for dyslipidemia. This form of resistance may arise from learned helplessness and a sense of despair over medication-induced weight gain, or it may represent an idiosyncratic preference for tablets over capsules or a concrete wish to take less medication, equated with total number of pills or magical thoughts about milligram dosage. Reformulating the case to achieve greater medication adherence is an important aspect of psychiatric nursing care.

Case Formulation and Psychotherapy

Sim et al. (2005) viewed case formulation as a useful clinical tool in psychotherapy because they believed that diagnosis does not provide an adequate focus on causality. They noted that "case formulation can fill the gap between diagnosis and treatment, with the potential to provide insights into the integrative, explanatory, prescriptive, predictive, and therapist aspects of a case" (p. 289). Each provider executes case formulation in a slightly different manner, depending on the theoretical model used. For example, a depressed and anxious man with apparently good work skills may have a pattern of job hunting, proceeding with successful interviews, accepting the job, and then abruptly leaving a short time later. Different providers may formulate this case in different ways:

- In the cognitive behavioral therapy model, case formulation would consider that he may have performance-based social anxiety, and avoidance relieves his distress. Treatment would involve isolating the situational triggers for this anxiety, developing positive affirmations for himself as a worker, and systematically exposing him to the various stages of job orientation and work-role acquisition. During these stages, he would try out exercises to tolerate his distress without walking off the job. Imagining and rehearsing job tasks and instruction in deep-breathing and other relaxation strategies might be part of the care plan.
- In dynamic psychotherapy, the case will be formulated to consider relational dynamics that might be triggering performance anxiety, perceived feelings of inadequacy, and unrealistic fear of failure. There would be less treatment

focus on trying out new behaviors on the job and more treatment focus on discovering past relationships in which social approval was important, especially family-of-origin experiences, and the therapist might explore failed vocational events in the past. Or the dynamic psychotherapist might pursue the patient's needs for perfection and the affront to his narcissism if he could not instantly perform the new job "perfectly."

- A psychopharmacologist might make sure the patient slept well during the first few weeks of employment and might prescribe a benzodiazepine as a sleep aid and antianxiety medication.

According to Sim et al. (2005), "Therapists must evaluate patient suitability for specific types of psychotherapy and information such as demographic features, and symptom presentation are often inadequate; hence something more is needed. Case formulation can fill this gap between diagnosis and treatment and can be seen to lie at the intersection of etiology and description, theory and practice, and science and art" (p. 289).

Keep in mind that a case formulation is a hypothesis or a set of hypotheses. The hypothesis may have to be changed as new information is obtained. Embrace this fact. A PAPN's patients are on journeys of self-discovery, and the PAPN is a coach for their recovery. The patient may have tolerated some medical or psychological event for much of his or her life, not recognizing that it had symptomatic significance and not realizing that this information may be important to disclose for the sake of diagnostic clarity. Many times I have heard, "I didn't think to tell them that" or "Nobody has asked me about that before." Over time, with rapport and sincerity, these critical bits of information may surface and help the PAPN aggregate data in more meaningful ways. The best plans of care evolve from an iterative discovery process in which the PAPN and patient engage in mutual, successive exchanges over time. This can perfect the diagnosis and ensure the most accurate pathway to recovery.

Diagnosing Psychiatric Disorders

A diagnosis provides an important part of the foundation for the PAPN's plan of care (Ingram, 2006) and it can provide relief, hope, and a sense of direction for the patient. However, most comprehensive treatment plans will also be shaped by assessment data provided by others on the interdisciplinary team, such as educators, speech and language pathologists, and occupational specialists, and by others such as clergy, employers, spouses, other family members, and patient advocates.

Patient Considerations

When giving a diagnosis, the PAPN must take into consideration the feelings of the patient, the patient's eligibility for entitlements and insurance coverage, and the patient's credibility.

The Patient's Feelings

The medical model has been criticized for what some patients say is a "box" that makes them feel stigmatized, and some patients may respond to a diagnosis in a negative way, feeling "labeled" in a manner that makes them feel demoralized, marginalized, or defective. Informing a patient of a psychiatric diagnosis can have a profound impact on his or her personal identity and can have a ripple effect on family members, friends, and coworkers. Mental illness still holds stigma in many realms of our society. Some subcultures may be defensive or very reactive to the process of psychiatric diagnosis, especially if the process of diagnosis has been associated with efforts to control a group of individuals (e.g., political dissidents or people of color) or used to justify some secondary motive (loss of parental guardianship of a child or reason for attributing blame for criminal activity and subsequent incarceration).

Tremendous empathy is required when presenting a psychiatric diagnosis to a patient and to his or her family. The PAPN should also be vigilant for the patient's attitude about disclosure of the diagnosis. Some patients are so relieved, even excited to learn the "name" for the symptoms they have been suffering with that they blurt out this information impulsively in social forums where others may not yet be receptive. Part of the plan of care should include helping the patient to decide this process of self-disclosure and preparing him or her psychologically and politically for this process. This approach advocates for the patient's rights as a protected person under the Americans with Disabilities Act (ADA) and considers the fact that learning about a diagnosis is a life-changing event with stages of ambivalence, acceptance, and change. It is helpful to view the diagnostic process as part of a shared journey that involves mutual participation between the patient and the PAPN in promoting illness recovery and restoration of quality of life.

The Patient's Eligibility for Entitlements and Insurance Coverage

While diagnoses may identify therapies and educational strategies, the PAPN should keep in mind that diagnoses are also part of the criteria for inclusion and exclusion in various entitlement programs and may affect insurance coverage. For example, sleep disorders are treated by pulmonologists, neurologists, and psychiatric mental health professionals, among other specialties. The patient's same symptom might have different diagnoses depending on whether it was coded through *International Classification of Diseases, Ninth Revision (ICD-9)* or *DSM-IV-TR* manuals, and this could affect health insurance reimbursement, especially when there is a behavioral health carve-out plan. Autism is another example of a condition with a broad continuum. Neurodevelopmental pediatric specialists have often treated severe conditions, and some mental health centers have denied services to patients in the past on the rationale that autism was a "developmental or neurological condition" and not a traditional psychiatric mental health disorder. Milder conditions of pervasive developmental disorder (PDD), especially people diagnosed with Asperger's disorder, are now commonly treated in mental health settings. Cassels (2010) reported that the *DSM-V* Neurodevelopmental Work Group has recommended that a new category of autism spectrum disorders be created that will incorporate the current *DSM-IV-TR* diagnoses of Autistic disorder, Asperger's disorder, Childhood disintegrative disorder, and Pervasive developmental disorder not otherwise specified (PDD-NOS). This diagnostic evolution will remove Asperger's as a distinct disorder and place it wholly within the broader descriptive category as a mild form of autism. Cassels (2010) pointed out that it remains to be seen how insurance companies, schools, and mental health centers will respond to these changes.

In addition, depending on state and federal laws, economics, and political climate, some diagnoses may alter a patient's ability to serve in the armed forces, possess firearms, adopt a child, hold an elected office, have a driver's license, and work with vulnerable populations like children or the elderly.

The Patient's Credibility

The PAPN must also consider the possibility of a secondary gain of obtaining a particular diagnosis and the occasional circumstance in which an individual may intentionally exaggerate or fabricate symptom information in order to persuade a provider that it meets the criteria for a specific disorder. For example, during times of war, soldiers may feign psychosis to return home from battle zones; patients with addictions may fabricate symptoms of anxiety or pain to obtain controlled substances; and college students may exaggerate problems of inattention, hyperactivity, and poor concentration to obtain stimulants or other cognition-enhancing medications.

With regard to childhood victimization that can have lifetime health effects (Kendall-Tackett, 2003), both adults and children can make false allegations during the psychiatric interview or can be unreliable in their self-report (Bernet, 2008). These actions can occur for a multitude of reasons. Sometimes a parent is delusional and convinces family members of a false reality. In other circumstances, the child may have revenge fantasies or feel under pressure to live with one parent during a custody hearing (Bernet, 2002; Bernet & Corwin, 2006). The patient's credibility must be evaluated in a systematic, respectful manner that considers psychodynamic factors that might motivate false report. The PAPN should include an estimate of the patient's veracity in the case formulation, e.g., "the patient appears to be a reliable self-historian" or "the patient's recollection of events appears vague and contradictory." In a forensic case, the PAPN might state that the patient's "self-report is questionable, given the dramatic and implausible description of the events and the rigorous efforts of discovery made by law enforcement personnel at the crime scene."

Diagnostic Insights for the Novice PAPN

The novice PAPN should begin by understanding the organizational and hierarchical structure of the *DSM-IV-TR* classification scheme. It will help to have a firm grounding in the diagnostic features of each major diagnostic group and the associated features and comorbid disorders, which are discussed in the next section. Associated laboratory findings, general medical conditions, and physical examination findings are also essential areas to assess prior to establishing or confirming a diagnosis. For example, the onset of confusion and manic-like symptoms in a woman previously treated with citalopram (Celexa) for unipolar clinical depression may actually have been due to hyponatremia, not to a bipolar spectrum disorder. Thus, ordering blood work with a test for electrolytes would be critical for differential diagnosis.

Medical findings may also be critical to creating a viable treatment plan. For example, dysphagia and dysgraphia may be associated with attentional deficits and impulsivity in individuals who have a history of premature birth, perinatal difficulties, or a subtype of PDD. Some of these patients may have difficulty swallowing pills, especially halved (irregular) tablets or capsules. The PAPN may help the patient to be more adherent to treatment by selecting quick-dissolve tablets or by educating the patient to coat the pill with soft margarine or olive oil before swallowing. A subset of these patients may have a genetic-linked basis for their neurobehavioral presentation, such as social anxiety in fragile X syndrome and prosopagnosia (facial blindness) in autistic spectrum disorders. The treatment plan for someone with PDD should anticipate swallowing difficulties and be concerned about adherence if medications will be prescribed. As an example, one child with PDD had an eccentric preference for "squishy" pills and an obsession with the color blue, so she refused to swallow tablets and loved taking blue capsules.

The PAPN will find that the *DSM-IV-TR* decision trees for differential diagnosis (American Psychiatric Association, 2000, Appendix A, p. 745) will provide a useful method for streamlining the diagnostic process by focusing on the most relevant inclusion and exclusion criteria. However, these decision trees are often not mutually exclusive, so the PAPN must consider dynamic interactions across symptom clusters when doing differential diagnosis and case formulation. Privitera and Lyness (2009) have provided a helpful resource for this process (see their Table 6.3, "Symptom-Driven Guide to Differential Diagnosis," p. 73). Over time, the PAPN should develop the skill to consider how unique features of the patient may influence subtle variation in the manifestations of the diagnostic criteria. Age, gender, culture, and environmental exposure will create diversity in symptom formation and expression.

Generating a diagnosis is a way to organize information that makes it easier to understand the clinician's observations of the patient and the patient's report of experiences. Diagnosis helps with understanding the patients' situation, guiding treatment, and predicting response to treatment. As described earlier, diagnoses are also used for reimbursement purposes and to define length of treatment for a specific disorder; they are also used in litigation and in health-care epidemiology to determine prevalence and population changes (Andreasen & Black, 2006).

Mechanics of Diagnosis

Diagnoses help to predict course (episodic or chronic) and outcome, and they are also used to decide appropriate treatment. Evidence-based research has identified specific treatments that are effective in treating specific disorders. Diagnoses are also used for nonclinical purposes. For example, they are used to determine reimbursement by insurance companies and to define length of treatment for specific disorders; in litigation; and in epidemiology to determine prevalence and incidence of disorders in the population (Andreasen & Black, 2006).

Diagnoses are derived from the case formulation. That is, they are derived from the patient's information, clinical observations of signs and symptoms, history of course, and response to treatment that have been integrated into a case formulation. Psychiatric diagnoses accomplish several tasks: they provide a structured way of thinking and planning treatment, and they provide a way to divide symptoms—such as emotional, cognitive, and behavioral symptoms—into broad categories that include psychosis, substance abuse, dementia, anxiety, depression, and responses to traumatic events; these broad categories can be subdivided into specific disorders, such as specific anxiety disorders.

According to Andreasen and Black (2006, p. 4), in the ideal world, all diseases in medicine would be defined in terms of etiology, such as a disease that follows exposure to an agent that causes an infection. However, at this time, psychiatric diagnoses are syndrome based; that is, they are based on a syndrome or cluster of symptoms that occur together, have a characteristic course and outcome, and have a similar response to treatment. In most instances, psychiatric diagnoses are determined by the presence of the criteria listed for each disorder in the *DSM-IV-TR* (American Psychiatric Association, 2000). The criteria are characteristics or features that must be present to make a specific diagnosis. However, data are not always available to determine if the presentation and history of symptoms meet the criteria.

DSM-IV-TR

Classification Approach

The *DSM-IV-TR* (American Psychiatric Association, 2000) is the most commonly used system for classifying psychiatric disorders. The *DSM-IV-TR* uses a descriptive approach rather than an etiological approach. It relies on clinical descriptions and symptoms. It is organized on the syndrome principle; i.e., groups or patterns of symptoms appear together in the same time frame in many individuals with the same disorder. The developers of the *DSM-IV-TR* assumed that symptoms clustered together because they were associated with the same etiology. However, studies suggest that syndromes do not represent distinct etiologies. Although it would be ideal if all disorders could be defined in terms of their etiology, at this time, etiology is clear with infectious diseases but not with psychiatric disorders (Andreasen & Black, 2006).

The *DSM-IV-TR* uses a categorical system rather than a dimensional system, listing more than 250 categories of diagnosis. In using the categorical system, a patient's clinical presentation either meets the diagnostic criteria for a specific disorder or does not. This approach is similar to the one used in diagnosing medical disorders, such as colon cancer.

The multiaxial system of the *DSM-IV-TR* requires clinicians to examine all aspects of the individual's health and social background:

- Axis I is where the major psychiatric disorders are organized, which Panksepp (2004, p. 18) has described as the "broken parts" approach to diagnosis.
- Axis II lists patients' personality disorders or developmental conditions.
- Axis III is used to list general medical condition and any medical illnesses.
- Axis IV is used to list any psychosocial or environmental problems that may interact with the patient's psychiatric and medical illnesses, such as housing or economic problems, support network, social activities, educational or work problems, problems with accessing health care, and legal problems.
- Axis V is used to list global assessment of the patient's psychological, social, and vocational functioning.

In assessing patients for mental disorders, Zimmerman and Mattia (2000) emphasized that clinicians must be alert to the high rates of comorbidity of both medical disorders—some of which may mimic the symptoms of psychiatric disorders—and psychiatric disorders.

Limitations of DSM-IV-TR

One criticism of the *DSM-IV-TR* is that it does not adequately include psychodynamic or developmental data. Another criticism is that it functions like a categorical checklist and does not fully address the concept of "spectrum disorders" wherein symptoms present on a continuum (Seligman & Reichenberg, 2007, p. 529). The *DSM-V* committee is seeking to better integrate new knowledge from molecular genetics, and studies are underway to identify salient nonpathological markers for diagnosis. For example, in the early childhood identification of autism, a preference for geometric shapes may be predictive (Pierce, Conant, Hazin, et al., 2011). However, data may not be available to determine if all criteria are met or not, and some psychiatric disorders appear to be dimensional or on a continuum from "normal" behavior to psychiatric disorder. In addition, the *DSM-IV-TR* does not identify other factors that must be considered in creating a plan of care for the patient, such as the patient's adaptive or maladaptive characteristics, capacity for relationships, coping patterns, interpretation of life events, or life history (Winston, Rosenthal, & Pinsker, 2004); nor does it identify patients' unmet needs, attachments or loss of attachments, internal resources such as hope and hardiness, or external resources such as social support and helpful neighbors (see Chapter 1).

Although some researchers believe that a dimensional system should be used in diagnosing psychiatric disorders, at this time, academic and clinical presentations, etiology, epidemiology, course, prognosis, and treatment are based on the categorical system (First & Tasman, 2004).

Provisional Diagnosis

The initial or provisional diagnosis is typically generated through a tandem, bidirectional process. Initially, the novice PAPN will consult the *DSM-IV-TR* for relevant approved diagnostic categories (e.g., mood disorders, somatoform disorders) and pursue inquiry through established diagnostic decision trees, then carefully review criteria for inclusion and exclusion to select a provisional psychiatric diagnosis. However, the PAPN should also learn to work "backward" from the patient's presenting condition and give due consideration to all relevant clinical assessment data, such as symptoms and behaviors, presenting problems, precipitating stressors, past history, and predisposing life events (Eells et al., 1998). Consideration is also given to age at onset of exposure to stressors and predisposing neurodevelopmental features that relate to familial inheritance—for example, in utero Rh blood incompatibilities or variable-penetrance genetic expressions in neurofibromatosis. It is even possible that a particular diagnosis may never have arisen if not for the particular timing of a traumatic event. Genetic vulnerability and social mores that may play a part in the ultimate expression of psychopathology are also considered.

It is common for the novice provider to hesitate when being asked to make a rapid diagnosis for disposition planning, e.g., when he or she is in an emergency room setting. The PAPN must find an expeditious route through the minefield of data collection, neither obsessing on minor details nor engaging in premature closure of the assessment process. At the end of the interview, the PAPN will be expected to render some type of diagnosis, and this may feel uncomfortable for the new clinician.

Commonly, especially on first visits and in emergency room settings, the PAPN will select an Axis I diagnosis and then put "provisional" next to it. However, hedging conclusions by calling everything a "rule out" may prevent medical billers from submitting viable claims to insurance companies. On occasion, selecting one of the "NOS" (not otherwise specified) categories will be useful, implying either that the patient does not meet full criteria for a more specific diagnosis at this time or that relevant information necessary for the patient to meet full criteria for this diagnosis is not available at this time. The reader is referred to p. 26 in the *DSM-IV-TR* manual (American Psychiatric Association, 2000) for "additional codes" that can be used when codes are needed for reimbursement. Codes 300.9 Unspecified Mental Disorder (nonpsychotic), V71.09 No diagnosis or condition on Axis I, and 799.9 Diagnosis or Condition deferred on Axis I may be selected appropriately when there is only partial information (e.g., when working with a nonverbal individual or when an interpreter is not available). However, many insurance companies may not reimburse for these codes because they are so noncommittal, even if they best describe the patient's situation. Occasions when these codes might be relevant would be for patients seeking screening psychiatric evaluations as a required condition for employment, such as people entering the military, job corps, or the FBI. It is wise for the PAPN to develop some confidence in making a decision with partial data. Many patients do not happen to mention important symptoms until they deem certain details "relevant," until they acquire some understanding of their disease process, or until they feel a true sense of trust.

At all times, the PAPN must make an effort to be thorough and conscientious in the collection of relevant data. This effort should not be intrusive or invasive or in other means "objectify" the patient. For example, a patient coming to the emergency room for treatment following a suicide attempt may meet criteria for both major depression and post-traumatic stress disorder (PTSD) secondary to childhood abuse. On this first contact, the PAPN might be comfortable recording 296.23 for Major Depressive Episode, severe on Axis I for the *DSM-IV-TR* multiaxial system. However, due to the crisis nature of this first contact and the vulnerability of the individual's suicidal state, the PAPN might defer asking detailed questions about childhood abuse that might confirm a diagnosis of PTSD.

The next few paragraphs will show how case formulation aids initial patient diagnosis and provides a working foundation to revise the diagnostic process. Screening tools save precious time and help speed the diagnostic process. Decision trees may also be helpful. Later sections of the chapter will examine strategies for differential diagnosis and address the concepts of comorbidity and iatrogenic responses to diagnosis and treatment.

Screening Tools as a Preliminary Step to Diagnosis

Screening tools can improve initial diagnostic accuracy by quantifying patients' presenting problems, and screening tools often prompt a therapeutic dialogue with patients about their perception of the problem. Sajatovic and Ramirez (2003) have summarized an excellent resource for rating scales in mental health, and many of these scales are available free, in the public domain, or can be obtained by mental health professionals at low cost.

Common examples of general symptom screening tools can be found in Table 5-1. Using an array of written self-report or family observation screening tools can also help the PAPN understand the natural environment of the patient, habits of daily living activities, level of functionality, and personal/family beliefs and cultural strengths.

More formal diagnostic evaluation tools may also be used by the PAPN in clinical practice. Tools like the Y-BOCS (Goodman et al., 1989), its pediatric version, the Children's Yale-Brown Obsessive Compulsive Scale (CY-BOCS), and the Positive and Negative Syndrome Scale (PANSS) (Kay, Opler, & Fizbein, 1994) for psychotic disorders are semistructured interviews that help provide more extensive objective evidence for the PAPN to use in making a differential diagnosis.

Evidence-based practice recognizes the diversity of persons and the likelihood that some symptoms may be present in people who still fall within the normal standards of a given population. For example, normative sexual behavior inventories have been developed and tested to evaluate deviancy in both adult and pediatric populations. These inventories help to identify a substantial amount of sexual behavior as developmentally normal in pediatric populations, thus preventing the diagnostician from leaping to the assumption that a child has experienced sexual abuse (DiPietro, Runyan, & Fredrickson, 1997). Many individuals with depression or other mental illness also suffer from fibromyalgia or other neuropathic pain disorders. It is appropriate for PAPNs to use a neuropathic pain screening

TABLE 5-1 FREQUENTLY USED SCREENING TOOLS

Screening Tool	Description and Purpose
Adult ADHD Rating Scale (Conners, Erhardt, & Sparrow, 1998)	Assessment of symptoms of ADHD in adults
Asperger Syndrome Diagnostic Scale (ASDS) (Smith-Myles, Jones-Bock, Stacey, et al., 2001)	Assessment of individuals ages 5 through 18 who manifest the characteristics of Asperger's syndrome
Autism Quotient Scale (AQ) (Baron-Cohen, Wheelwright, Skinner, et al., 2001)	A self-rating scale of symptoms of autism or one of the autism spectrum disorders
Beck Anxiety Inventory (Beck, Epstein, Brown, et al., 1988)	An evaluation for generalized anxiety
Behavior Assessment System for Children, Second Edition (BASC-2) (Reynolds & Kamphaus, 1992)	A comprehensive, multidimensional measure designed to differentiate between children who potentially have a psychiatric disorder such as depression or a behavior problem and children who do not
Behavior Rating Inventory of Executive Function (BRIEF) (Gioia, Isquith, Guy, et al., 2000)	An assessment for cognitive executive function in children
CAGE Questionnaire (Ewing, 1984)	A screening tool for alcohol abuse
Child Behavior Check List (CBCL) (Achenbach, 1991)	A tool for determining developmental deviations in a variety of emotional, psychological, and behavioral domains in children
Childhood Depression Inventory (CDI) (Kovacs, 1981)	A screening tool for depression in prepubertal children
Hamilton Rating Scale for Anxiety (HAM) (Hamilton, 1959)	An evaluation for generalized anxiety
Hare Psychopathy Checklist-revised (2nd ed.) (Hare, 2003)	A tool for rating psychopathic personality characteristics and socially deviant behaviors
Impact of Event Scale (IES) (Horowitz, Wilner, & Alvarez, 1979)	An assessment of response to traumatic stressors or stressful life events
Michigan Alcohol Screening Test (MAST) (Selzer, 1971)	A screening tool for alcohol dependence
Mini-SPIN (Connor, Kobak, Churchill, et al., 2001)	A screening tool for social phobia or social anxiety disorder (SAD)
Mood Disorder Questionnaire (MDQ) (Hirschfeld, Williams, Spitzer, et al., 2000)	A screening tool for bipolar disorder
Patient Health Care Questionnaire-Nine Symptom Checklist (PHQ-9) (Spitzer, Kroenke, & Williams, 1999)	A screening tool for depression and mania in adults
Suicide Intent Scale (SIS) (Beck, Schuyler, & Herman, 1974)	A tool for determining suicide risk
Suicide Probability Scale (Cull & Gill, 1982)	An assessment for suicide risk in adolescents and adults
The 17-Item SPIN (Davidson, Hughes, George, et al., 1993)	A screening tool for social phobia in an individual presenting with major depression and panic symptoms
The 6-question Adult Self-Report Scale-V1.1 (ASRS-V1.1) Screener (World Health Organization, 2003)	An evaluation for adult ADHD
Zohar-Fineberg Obsessive Compulsive Screen (ZF-OCS) (Fineberg, O'Dougherty, Rajagopal, et al., 2003)	A tool to determine whether more extensive assessment of OCD is needed

questionnaire (Portenoy, 2006) as part of the differential diagnosis and case formulation. Children also experience pain, and this can contribute to depression, anxiety, and behavioral difficulties that may prompt referral to the PAPN. The OUCHER and the Wong-Baker FACES pain rating scales (2005) are two examples of clinical assessment tools used in pediatric mental health.

For pediatric assessment of autistic spectrum disorders and early childhood psychiatric disorders, students are referred to the review by Greenspan and Wieder (2008) of *The Interdisciplinary Council on Developmental and Learning Disorders Diagnostic Manual for Infants and Young Children (ICDL-DMIC)*. Pediatric bipolar disorder is an emerging diagnosis that is also inadequately delineated in the *DSM-IV-TR*. Clinicians may find on the Internet many useful self-report rating scales that are subject to professional review. The Online Asperger Syndrome Information and Support (OASIS) Web site (http://www.aspergersyndrome.org/), the Depression and Bipolar Support Alliance (DBSA) Web site (http://www.dbsalliance.org/site/PageServer?pagename=home), and the Child Adolescent Bipolar Foundation (CABF) Web site (www.cabf.org/) all offer tools designed by specialists that are accessible to the public. Asking families to participate in these online assessments may speed the process and open up dialogue with relatives, making the acceptance of diagnosis more comfortable.

The PAPN will find the following assessment tools helpful in the diagnosis of conversion disorder: Dissociative Experiences Scale, Somatoform Dissociation Questionnaire, Childhood Trauma Questionnaire, Spielberger Trait Anxiety Inventory, Clinician-Administered Dissociative State Scale, and Dissociative Disorders Interview Schedule (Japanese Society of Psychiatry and Neurology, 2009).

Other Screening Methods

Neuroimaging studies can help confirm or rule out psychopathology, but the extent of use of neuroimaging varies greatly across practice settings and is affected by access to services. In addition, there are some conditions that are detected only by serial studies, but cost and lack of patient follow-through may prevent reimaging efforts. There is also some controversy over which diagnoses require neuroimaging studies for either diagnosis or treatment. For example, functional magnetic resonance imaging (MRI) and single-photon emission computed tomography (SPECT) scans are used actively in research settings but may not be paid for by a patient's insurance. PAPNs must keep pace with the changing landscape of neuroimaging services, as certain imaging studies may become obsolete or may become useful (after a period of being inadequate, confusing, or cost prohibitive).

Furthermore, many psychiatric disorders can be determined almost exclusively by clinical interview; review of medical, academic, vocational, and military records; and careful history and physical examination. For example, current practice for diagnosing attention deficit-hyperactivity disorder (ADHD) does not require MRI or SPECT neuroimaging studies, and a computerized continuous-performance task would not be considered sufficient on its own to diagnose the condition. Sometimes the patient will already have had neuroimaging studies completed for a different purpose (a fall during the toddler period or motor vehicle accidents). In such circumstances, it may be useful for the PAPN to review these studies, even if they are now being used to ascertain a new psychiatric disorder.

New research findings appear all the time that can become useful for application in the practice setting. For example, it has been found that the growing brain naturally develops cortical asymmetries (Shaw, Lalonde, Lepage, et al., 2009), but this process may be disrupted owing to pathophysiology or as a result of genetic influences in neurodevelopmental disorders such as ADHD. It is important for PAPNs to track neurocognitive research because biological markers, including functional neural correlates, are being identified as aids in the identification of impaired cognitive control and social dysfunction in a variety of disorders, such as in autism spectrum disorders (Dichter, Felder, & Bodfish, 2009).

One challenging evaluation that requires careful differential diagnosis involves the assessment of somatoform disorders. A patient may be experiencing a physical or mental disorder, fabricating one or both of these, or denying any disorder in the presence of scientifically verified or "founded" pathophysiology. Conversion disorder is a case in point, one of the most puzzling presentations for the psychiatric professional. These cases are typically evaluated on medical units by consultation liaison psychiatrists and are not commonly seen in traditional outpatient community mental health settings. For somatoform disorder and conversion disorder, past or present predisposing life events or stressors may be major factors contributing to the severity of symptoms or to the way the patient presents to the provider. Sometimes the individual's body "shows the feelings" and there is a metaphoric presentation of symptoms. For example, a young woman who has been raped "can't stand" what happened to her and may present to the emergency room with a complaint of difficulty or inability to walk, as an unconscious communication of her psychological distress. As another example, a child may witness a parent's seizure and then acquire a similar affliction (e.g., pseudo-seizures) or another conversion symptom like dizziness or cyclic vomiting. In one study that measured the relationship between reported childhood trauma and dissociation in patients who have a conversion symptom, it was found that dissociative disorder was diagnosed in 46.9% of the patients with conversion disorder (Sar, Islam, & Ozturk, 2009). Conversion patients with a dissociative disorder had borderline personality disorder more frequently than those without a dissociative disorder. Among childhood trauma types, emotional abuse was the only significant predictor of dissociation in regression analysis. None of the childhood trauma types predicted borderline personality disorder criteria. Sar et al. concluded that borderline personality disorder, dissociation, and reports of childhood emotional abuse are associated with a subgroup of patients with conversion symptom. Dissociation seems to be a mediator between childhood trauma and borderline phenomena among these patients (Sar et al.).

Decision Trees

Similar to the structured interview methods and patient self-report screening tools, diagnostic decision trees can help the PAPN narrow down the complexity of data and focus on pivotal data needed for diagnosis. Decision trees aid decision making, but they should not be used blindly. The American Psychiatric Association has published several manuals that use flowcharts of decision rules that can take the PAPN through the basics of the diagnostic process. However, these flowcharts do not replace the creative, intuitive, gestalt assessment process involved in case formulation.

Differential Diagnosis

When making a provisional diagnosis or reviewing an established prior diagnosis, the PAPN must also consider the tandem process of differential diagnosis. Under time constraints, it is tempting to maintain prior diagnoses with little deliberation; however, premature closure on the process may result. The PAPN must tolerate uncertainty and enter into an inner dialogue, perhaps even dialectical, about opposing diagnostic viewpoints. Is the diagnosis consistent with one viewpoint, or another viewpoint, or is it consistent with both? In some instances, the chicken-or-the-egg theory comes to mind. The PAPN must get comfortable with this internal debate process.

Many psychiatric disorders share common symptoms, such as anxiety. The clinician must determine which one of two or more disorders with similar symptoms is the patient experiencing. The tasks incurred in making a differential diagnosis are to consider all possible diagnoses that could cause the symptoms; to collect and evaluate additional information, such as personal history and family history; and to consider the results of the mental status examination and the laboratory investigations (First & Tasman, 2004).

In addition, many medical disorders have symptoms that are similar to those of psychiatric disorders. To help in identifying medical mimics of mental disorders, Hedaya (1996) offered a mnemonic, "Thinc Med" (p. 189), to help with differential diagnoses. It stands for **t**umors; **h**ormones, such as thyroid; **i**nfectious and immune disease, such as syphilis, AIDS, or lupus; **n**utrition such as vitamin deficiencies; **c**entral nervous system disorders, such as head trauma, epilepsy, or Parkinson's disease; **m**iscellaneous (anemia, sleep disorders); **e**lectrolyte abnormalities (abnormal levels of potassium, sodium, chloride, or magnesium) and environmental toxins (insecticides, solvents); and **d**rugs (illegal, over-the-counter, herbs).

Comorbid Psychiatric Disorders

There are several mental disorders in the *DSM-IV-TR* that have extensive subtypes (e.g., bipolar spectrum disorders and anxiety disorders), and then there are a few unique and discrete diagnoses (e.g., circadian rhythm disorder or anorexia nervosa) that can either stand alone or be present with comorbid conditions. For example, people with Tourette's disorder may also meet criteria for OCD or ADHD. In one study, among patients with a primary diagnosis of major depression, 10% had a comorbid mental disorder diagnosis. A higher rate was found among patients with a primary diagnosis of social anxiety disorder, who had a 28% rate of comorbid mental disorders. In fact, all the anxiety disorders have high rates of comorbid mental disorders (Zimmerman & Mattia, 2000). Patients seek treatment for symptoms of disorders other than those of their primary psychiatric diagnosis. They want relief from the symptoms of the comorbid disorders as well as from the symptoms of the primary disorder, and sometimes they consider the comorbid disorder symptoms to be more distressing. Because patients with multiple disorders tend to have a poorer response to treatment and less favorable long-term outcomes, it is important that PAPNs identify and treat the comorbid disorders as well as the primary disorder.

Medical Mimics of Psychiatric Disorders

Medical mimics are physical disorders manifesting as psychiatric symptoms as the primary initial expression (e.g., systemic lupus erythematosus), during a later stage of the illness (e.g., psychosis in Huntington's disease), or as a result of some medical side effect (e.g., sexual dysfunction or depression in patients taking antihypertensive agents). Some common medical mimics that may be erroneously diagnosed as bipolar spectrum disorders include tuberous sclerosis, multiple sclerosis, complex-partial temporal lobe seizures, thyrotoxicosis, and frontal-temporal dementia.

Medication-Induced Psychiatric Symptoms

Certain medications may induce a short-term exacerbation of the very symptoms they are targeted to treat (e.g., selective serotonin reuptake inhibitors [SSRIs] or serotonergic atypical medications can be activating, causing physical anxiety), or the patient may experience an adverse drug reaction in the presence of a pre-existing disorder (e.g., a child with PDD-NOS and severe behavior problems becomes even more aggressive on antiepileptic drugs).

Behavioral Manifestations of Psychiatric Symptoms

The surface behavior displayed by a patient rarely has a one-to-one correspondence with one particular psychiatric disorder. For example, behavioral activities directed at the skin, such as picking, rubbing, marking, cutting, or tattooing, may have great diagnostic diversity. Skin picking is commonly seen in a variety of anxiety disorders but may be seen during opiate drug withdrawal. Rubbing or picking the skin is sometimes a self-soothing activity but may represent a symptom of drug abuse, a toxidrome from accidental poisoning, or a neurobehavioral symptom of dementia, or it may be part of a mental ritual or obsession, as seen with OCD or Tourette's disorder. Marking, cutting, burning, or tattooing the skin may represent personal coping responses to dissociative experience in PTSD; adjustment difficulties in someone with borderline personality disorder; or cultural markers for a rite of passage, social inclusion in gangs, or inmate cliques within prison settings.

Some presenting behaviors, like impulsivity, may be symptomatic of ADHD, mental retardation, or an undetected head injury. When present on a cyclical basis, the impulsivity may be part of mania. Other cases of presumed impulsivity may actually represent a form of childhood neglect in which children have access to dangerous materials and lack adult supervision. Environmental assessment, developmental context, and corroborating data are crucial.

In summary, for the PAPN to substantiate that differential diagnosis has been entertained, it is important to document the rationale for "the roads not taken." As noted by Eells et al. (1998), case formulation informs others about the "inferred mechanism," the therapist's hypothesis about causality. One case in point is the phenomena of fire-setting. There is not just "one reason" that people set fires, and this behavior may or may not be related to mental illness. For example, Williams and Clements (2005) identified six subtypes for fire setters: (1) Curiosity/Accidental Fire Setting, (2) Thought Disordered Fire Setting, (3) Delinquent Fire Setting, (4) Thrill Seeker Fire Setting, (5) Revenge Based Fire Setters, and (6) Compulsive Fire Setters. The PAPN will best understand the underlying motivation by careful clinical interview and sampling feedback from informed others surrounding the patient.

Treatment Plan: Biopsychosocial Plan of Care

The treatment plan is embedded in a developmental matrix that considers growth and aging factors across the life span. In the United States, mental disorders are the chronic illnesses of young people (Demyttenaere, Bruffaerts, Posada-villa, et al., 2004). Unlike most physical illnesses, mental disorders begin very early in life, with half of all lifetime cases of mental disorders beginning by 14 years of age (Kim-Cohen, Caspi, Moffitt, et al., 2003). For example, anxiety disorders often begin in late childhood, mood disorders in late adolescence, and substance abuse in early 20s (Kessler, Berglund, Demler, et al., 2005a). Thus, adolescents and young adults experience disability during the period of their lives when they would be expected to be most productive.

The prevalence of mental disorders is higher than that of any other class of chronic disorders (Murray & Lopez, 1996). Kessler et al. (2005a) report that among the general population in the United States, 46.4% had a lifetime history of a mental disorder; of these, 27.7% had two or more lifetime disorders, and 17.3% had three or more. The 1-year prevalence rate for mental disorders is 26.2% of the general population; however, the prevalence rate may be higher because the survey on which this estimate was based did not include people with schizophrenia or autism, people in nursing homes or other institutions, people who were homeless (Kessler, Chiu, Demler, et al., 2005b). Kessler et al. report lifetime prevalence estimates of 28.8% for anxiety disorders; 20.8% for mood disorders; 24.8% for impulse-control disorders; and 14.6% for substance-use disorders. Lifetime prevalence rates are high among the younger cohort of American adults (ages 18 to 29 years), and this higher rate among the younger cohort remains stable over time. Mental disorders vary in intensity and need for treatment but represent a significant cost to society (Olin & Rhoades, 2005).

Distribution of Treatment

Approximately 40% of mental disorders in a 12-month period are mild or transient and may not require treatment (Narrow, Rae, Robins, et al., 2002; Kessler et al., 2005a). Of the remaining 60%, among patients who have serious mental disorders—schizophrenia, bipolar disorder, drug dependence, OCD, oppositional defiant disorder, and mood disorders—35.5% to 50.3% do not receive any treatment (Demyttenaere et al., 2004). People with mental disorders are more likely to receive treatment from primary care physician/nurses (22.8%) or from a nonpsychiatrist mental health care provider such as a psychologist, counselor, or social worker (16%) than from a psychiatrist (12%). People with mental disorders also seek treatment from a counselor or spiritual advisor outside of the mental health setting (9.75%) and from alternative sources such as from a chiropractor or self-help group (6.9%). Demyttenaer et al. found that adequacy of treatment was best when it was provided by mental health practitioners.

Among those who do receive treatment, only one-third reported treatment that meets criteria for minimal adequacy; for instance, one-third of patients with serious mental disorders are receiving minimally adequate treatment (Wang, Lane, Olfson, et al., 2005). Among patients receiving treatment from specialty mental health providers, less than half (48%) received care that was minimally adequate. Among patients receiving treatment from general medical care providers, 12.8% received minimally adequate care; among those receiving care from non-health care providers, 13.1% received minimally adequate treatment (Wang et al.). Not only is treatment often inadequate, but there are long delays between onset of mental disorders and being evaluated, receiving a diagnosis, and beginning treatment (Insel & Fenton, 2005). The median delay across all mental disorders in getting treatment is 10 years (Wang, Berglund, Olfson, et al., 2004).

The majority of people who receive treatment for mental disorders are those with subthreshold disorders, whereas those with serious disorders are less likely to receive treatment. In the United States, this mental health care distribution pattern may be due to a decentralized and fragmented system of mental health care; a lack of perceived need for treatment; lack of access to insurance coverage; and lack of financial resources. Underserved groups such as the elderly, racial and ethnic minorities, and those with low income or no insurance had the greatest unmet need for treatment (Wang et al., 2005).

Untreated early-onset mental disorders are associated with school failure (50% for untreated social anxiety disorder), teenage childbearing, unstable employment, early marriage, marital instability, and violence (Kessler, Berglund, Foster, et al., 1997; Kessler, Foster, Saunders, et al., 1995; Kessler, Walters, & Forthofer, 1998). Untreated early-onset mental disorders can also lead to more severe, more difficult-to-treat disorders and to the development of concurrent mental disorders such as substance-related disorders (Kessler, 1997; Kessler & Price, 1993).

America's PAPNs are well prepared to help people move toward achieving Healthy People 2010's (2000) goals: improved mental health and provision of appropriate, quality treatment for patients with mental disorders. Choice of intervention or interventions is based on the issues emerging from the assessment and case formulation, the clinician's explanation of the patient's symptoms, and the clinician's assessment of the patient's biopsychosocial functioning.

Biopsychosocial Plan of Treatment

From the case formulation, the first step in planning treatment is to determine where the patient should receive treatment, e.g., hospital setting or outpatient setting. Within the biopsychosocial model of treatment, the biological domain of treatment includes a physical examination; appropriate laboratory tests; history of the medications currently being taken and whether they will be maintained, modified, or discontinued; and existing medical conditions and their treatment. The psychological domain includes possible referral for neuropsychiatric testing. It also includes discussion of psychotherapeutic interventions, such as cognitive behavioral therapy. In considering psychotherapy, the PAPN must decide if the patient's symptoms are likely to respond to psychotherapy and to which modality of psychotherapy. If the therapy is to be one of the psychodynamic therapies, the PAPN must decide if the patient has the psychological characteristics needed for psychodynamic therapy (Andrews, 2008). With regard to the social domain, the PAPN plans interventions to improve the patient's living, employment, financial, and social situations and the role that the patient plays in those situations.

The treatment plan is carefully written to meet the patient's needs and ensure that goals, interventions, and resources are culturally relevant, realistic, attainable, socially acceptable, and accessible.

Modifications to the Plan of Care: Ongoing Process

The PAPN will encounter some common difficulties when developing a patient's plan of care. For example, genetics, neurobiology, and psychodynamic theories about the origin and vector of dysfunctional behavior can provide insight about psychopathology, but they do not always illuminate effective treatments (Privitera & Lyness, 2009). The ultimate plan of care may be initiated, reviewed, modified, or discontinued based on the clinical frame of reference of one provider or through the interdisciplinary process of a team of providers in conjunction with the patient's choice of direction and that of the patient's advocates or proxy partners (e.g., parents or temporary guardian).

Many PAPNs will work in independent practices or with multiple agencies across a variety of community settings, so differences in theoretical orientation are common. Sometimes this leads to conflict, which can be very healthy and constructive; conflict resolution is a natural part of a PAPN's practice experience. Even within the confines of one agency, where all providers are coworkers, the providers will not always share the same theoretical frame of reference. As a result, the PAPN may sometimes find that the treatment team is divided on approaches to care. For example, some therapists with attachment-based theoretical orientation may not believe that medications will be helpful for children with autistic spectrum disorders and may even exclude this set of diagnoses in favor of a reactive attachment disorder diagnosis. However, there is ample opportunity to reformulate a patient's case and resolve the differences in theoretical orientations. As Privitera & Lyness (2009) rightly observed, "More than one theory may be invoked simultaneously to understand a patient's disorder" (p. 11). The PAPN should be prepared to take the initiative in offering additional biopsychosocial theories that can explain patient behavior or provide evidence for treatment plan modifications. For example, in the past, some parents of children with Asperger's disorder have been told that they were overanxious and "hovering" over their child and that poor parenting caused the delays in observed social skills and emotional maturity. The PAPN may disagree with this viewpoint and have conflict with a provider's descriptive label of "helicopter mother" but should be discreet when facing such conflict and sharing alternative biological information about brain development and executive function deficits. It is essential that the PAPN retain respect for the viewpoints of non-medical providers when engaging in interdisciplinary treatment planning.

CASE STUDY PRACTICE

The following case examples provide hypothetical patients with various backgrounds and symptoms. All of the cases are a composite of patients with identifiers removed, and all names are pseudonyms. While reading the case, consider possible differential diagnoses and the provisional psychiatric diagnoses. At the end of the case example, diagnosis is presented using the five-axis classification system of the *DSM-IV-TR* (American Psychiatric Association, 2000).

CASE STUDY 5-1

Emergency Room Triage: Initial Psychotic Break

Clinical Presentation

Jarred was diagnosed with social phobia when he was in high school 10 years ago. Guidance counselors wondered at the time about his obsessive and ruminative thinking because he was fascinated with alien worlds and drew repetitive pictures of exploding monsters and robotic creatures with magical abilities. Jarred appeared distracted in class, "off in another world," and often skipped entire days. His grades declined from B's and C's to D's and F's. For a while he hung out with "potheads," but then they seemed to just leave him alone. After urging from his parents, Jarred's primary care physician tried a brief trial of an SSRI medication, but that did not seem to help. Jarred has never been hospitalized or received counseling since that diagnosis.

Jarred dropped out of high school and has never really held down a job. His family saw him become more distant and withdrawn. When he was 19, his father had a huge argument with him over a missing set of tools in the garage and threatened to kick him out. His mother wondered if he had been wanting to make a bomb. Both parents were concerned, but Jarred just laughed it off and retreated to his bedroom for two weeks. They thought he was getting high every day, but they could not find any marijuana when they did a room search. His hygiene was poor and he needed to be pushed to pick up after himself.

Since dropping out, Jarred had not been able to work or manage his finances, so his parents finally set him up in a small apartment and asked his older brother to keep an eye out. When his older brother had to go overseas for business 2 months ago, Jarred put towels over the windows and would not go out to buy groceries. He lost 15 lbs. Now in his early 20s, Jarred avoids leaving the apartment because of paranoia. Jarred collects newspapers and has stacks of them in his apartment. It is difficult for others to make it down the hallway because of this accumulation. He asked his landlord if the other tenants could read his thoughts. One of the tenants told the landlord that he had seen Jarred standing on the roof of the apartment complex with a long stick last weekend when he came home from a bar at 1 a.m. Although Jarred did not say anything, the neighbor was worried because he was holding it "like a gun." Because Jarred went back down into his apartment immediately after this, the neighbor did not call the police. This week, Jarred's brother offered to give him a cell phone for emergencies, but Jarred declined, claiming that the phone would transmit magnetic waves from an alien world and take over his body. This alarmed his brother, who then called the local mental health center and set up a psychiatric evaluation.

During the initial intake Jarred admits to feeling afraid and thinks that somebody might be controlling his thoughts. He says that he feels anxious but denies feeling depressed. He denies thoughts of harming himself or others. However, he fears that others may harm him. He looks suspicious when asked about auditory hallucinations and denies hearing any specific voices or noises. Jarred believes that there may be alien beings living in the apartment next door to him. Jarred seems to have a hard time tracking conversations and needs to have questions restated in different ways to comprehend some of the history questions. His responses are slow, as though it takes great effort to think or speak. On occasions his eyes dart off to a corner of the office and he laughs, out of context with the conversation. Jarred makes only brief eye contact and tends to have an avoidant gaze. During the interview, he often seems perplexed or confused. Affect is blunted. Body movements are slowed but adequately coordinated. Speech is clear and soft, with some mumbled phrases. No gesturing or odd motor movements are seen. Jarred is unable to maintain a conversation about any topic. He often answers with "I dunno."

Differential Diagnosis

Psychotic disorder, NOS; delusional disorder; obsessive-compulsive disorder; dementia

Primary Diagnosis

I. Schizophreniform disorder, rule out paranoid schizophrenia subtype; social phobia (by history); rule out psychotic disorder due to a substance and/or medical condition; rule out cannabis dependence and polysubstance abuse

II. Rule out avoidant personality disorder; rule out schizotypal personality disorder

III. Dental caries

IV. Difficulties with immediate family, unemployment, conflicts with neighbors, recent absence of primary caretaker, financial difficulties

V. Global Assessment of Functioning (GAF): 35

Plan of Care

- Admit to inpatient psychiatric unit for further evaluation; provide 1:1 supervision for safety of self and others; obtain neuroimaging studies (e.g., MRI, EEG); complete lab work.
- Fully assess psychotic symptoms, using the PANSS.
- Begin trial of antipsychotic medication.
- Provide patient and family education concerning the recovery process following a psychotic episode and refer them to the National Alliance for the Mentally Ill (NAMI) for additional peer support.
- Develop a discharge plan for community aftercare that provides medication monitoring, case management, and a support program to improve Jarred's personal care and develop social and vocational skills. Refer patient for vocational assessment and consider SSI for major psychiatric disability.

Continued

CASE STUDY 5-1—continued

Clinical Pearls

Family members may try to shelter a loved one rather than seek psychiatric consultation in a timely manner. Neighbors in the community may discount a neighbor's behavior as simply "odd" if he keeps to himself, and they may not appreciate the safety risks. The need for extreme family support in early adulthood in response to declining self-care and occupational difficulties is a common pattern for the prodromal period during the onset of schizophrenia. It is common for patients with psychotic symptoms to use alcohol or marijuana to calm their anxiety or "self-medicate" auditory hallucinations.

Reflection Questions

When Jarred appears distracted, what is making him inattentive? Is he responding to internal stimuli? What would be possible safety concerns when he returns to the community? Would he need a less restrictive order for community commitment, to ensure participation in outpatient therapies? Many substances, including cannabis and alcohol, can also induce psychosis. What are some other common street drugs or prescribed drugs that are associated with psychotic symptoms? How would the PAPN begin to cluster symptoms into recognizable patterns that could fit a syndrome?

CASE STUDY 5-2

Outpatient Department Evaluation of Recently Incarcerated Individual

Clinical Presentation

Lone Bear is a young man in his twenties who grew up on the local Reservation. He has recently been released from jail after having served time for reportedly bizarre behavior and misdemeanor charges that he was intentionally scaring children in his neighborhood. He denies recollection of these events and states he would "never hurt a child." His release from the county jail is conditional with the expectation that he be evaluated by the local mental health clinic. Detention staff reports that he "seemed fine" while incarcerated and "did not cause any problems."

His probation officer believes that Lone Bear may have a major mental illness because he is reporting having "visions" and admits to seeing the ghost of his dead grandfather. There is a history of early childhood abuse, and Lone Bear spent many years in out-of-home placement, both in a foster home and in a group home residential facility. Lone Bear reports that he was "brainwashed" while in the group home: "I had to ask permission for everything, even to go to the bathroom." He is annoyed that his mother and probation officer think he is "crazy" and explains that he has "fallen in love" and "got religion." He believes his girlfriend may be carrying his baby, a child born to fulfill biblical prophecy, a boy child that will help save the world. He says his girlfriend also believes him and has seen visions too, "she's native tribal."

His uncle, who lives on the Reservation, reports that he has not seen any girlfriend and thinks she does not exist. When the PAPN asked Lone Bear if the girlfriend was real or someone he had wished for, Lone Bear explains, "Well I know it sounds strange to be having sex with a dead person, but she exists for me because I have been specially chosen. It all came to me in a vision. Her spirit and my spirit are one." Old medical records reveal that he was previously diagnosed with a psychotic disorder and given antipsychotic medication. Lone Bear says, "I was medicated against my will." He recently got a medical marijuana card to treat his "psychic pain" and believes he suffers from "post-traumatic stress disorder." Recent medical notes state that Lone Bear was also sent by ambulance to the emergency room for evaluation under the presumption of alcohol intoxication on two separate occasions over the past 4 months. On both occasions, his blood alcohol level was very low on lab study.

Lone Bear has not slept more than 2 to 4 hours a night over the last 2 weeks. He says that he is keeping a "vigil" to honor the dead girlfriend's spirit. "Because I believe in her, she has come to me and will have my baby, it will be a beautiful thing, I know I have a special purpose in this life now." Lone Bear is very excited when he talks. He jumps up and gestures widely about how he will be able to help the world. His speech is rapid and dramatic. Lone Bear tells the PAPN that he really does not want any drugs: "They might harm my visions, I need to be clearheaded to help the world...all they did was drug me when I was in the group home."

Differential Diagnosis

Included in the diagnostic differential would be the possibility of a manic episode in the presence of a bipolar spectrum disorder. The PAPN should also consider the possibility of a psychotic disorder, such as schizophrenia or schizoaffective disorder, and the more remote possibility of a cultural explanation for his symptoms. According to Beyerstein (1996), Western culture is uncomfortable with hallucinations, and providers may reflexively choose medications when there may be a cultural basis to the patient's visions. Tribal cultures often consider visions to be a privilege or a loving, protective message from the ancestors. Hallucinations are not always the result of drug intoxication or some neuropsychiatric pathology; in fact, they may present in the normal population. The PAPN should look at factors such as the coherence of themes, flow of thought, and logic of the patient's associations when considering psychotic symptoms. Do others in the patient's subculture perceive a change in personality or thinking process? How adequate is the patient's attendance to hygiene, food and drink, and other activities of daily living?

Primary Diagnosis

I. Psychotic disorder, NOS; rule out bipolar I disorder, most recent episode mania with psychotic features; rule out cannabis abuse and polysubstance abuse; rule out PTSD

II. Deferred (for personality disorders); rule out learning disability, NOS

III. Dental caries

CASE STUDY 5-2—continued

IV. History of severe child maltreatment, unemployment, poverty, recent incarceration; being on probation; unstable housing
V. GAF: 35

Plan of Care

- Establish rapport and trust with patient, who is very guarded about medications and mental health providers due to his years in the "system."
- Provide patient/family education about psychotropic medications (mood stabilizers and antipsychotic agents).
- Invite the patient to a depression and bipolar recovery support group.
- Provide a less restrictive alternative to hospitalization, but still provide a setting that offers more structure and supervision; e.g., the patient could be enrolled in an intensive case management program in the community and receive supported living in a halfway house.
- Work with the public defender and probation officer as a "team" with the patient to evaluate the extent of his chemical dependency issues; provide education about how cannabis and other substances may be harmful, even if "natural."
- Arrange safety surveillance and random drug urine analyses.

Clinical Pearls

The PAPN must become competent in discovering the subcultural beliefs of the patient, and it helps to have the patient and relatives "consult" with the provider to help distinguish actual symptoms of psychopathology.

Reflection Questions

What are the long-term sequelae for children "raised in the system," i.e., out of home care with multiple foster placements or institutional group care? What are some culturally relevant questions to ask Lone Bear's tribe?

CASE STUDY 5-3

Urgent Presentation of Established Patient in Outpatient Setting

Clinical Presentation

Margi is a woman in her early 40s who presented to a community psychologist with a history of depressed mood after being fired from her job as a bank loan officer due to declining work performance. Margi had been a very high functioning executive with meticulous attention to detail. Her husband first noticed changes 3 years ago, when he realized she made errors with family finances and was becoming distant from the children. The psychologist diagnosed Margi with a severe major depressive episode. Margi was tearful and had obsessive, ruminative thoughts, but she had no direct suicidal or homicidal ideation. After 6 months of insight-oriented psychotherapy that was ineffective, the psychologist referred Margi to a psychiatrist at the local hospital. This psychiatrist recommended baseline laboratory studies, a neurology consultation, and neuroimaging studies. The EEG was within normal limits (she was on Paxil 20 mg/day at the time). A brain MRI showed mild-to-moderate loss of parenchymal volume, but these findings were not considered to be significant at the time, and the neurologist could not determine any specific organic etiology for her depression. The psychiatrist suspected a psychotic break and probable bipolar spectrum disorder. Margi was uncooperative with seeing him in a hospital-like setting. He started her on Lamictal. The family did not see much improvement at a dosage of 200 mg/day, so this medication was discontinued after 4 months.

Since Margi had refused psychiatric evaluation in a hospital-like setting, a homebound program was initiated with the psychologist. The family decided to discontinue this treatment because the patient seemed to be getting "worse, not better." Margi's depression had deteriorated to the point of mutism and disorganized and noncompliant behavior, and she had periods of excessive sleep and wakefulness. Behavioral strategies did not seem to help with improving activities of daily living. The family thought the hospital-like environment they saw the psychiatrist in was making her anxious, so they stopped making her go. They compensated by providing increased supervision in the home, and Margi's children were often sent to stay with grandparents. The family physician strongly recommended that they get a secondary psychiatric consultation.

Margi's husband has now contacted the PAPN's outpatient office because both the former psychiatrist and psychologist have recommended the PAPN as a provider in the community. The family has agreed to see the PAPN, especially since the office looked "homey" and nonclinical when they made a preliminary visit. By this time, Margi has developed periods of high energy, compulsive eating, and mutism. She can go for days without sleep. Her family reports that she has darted out in front of cars, left the house in the middle of the night, and grabbed food off the counters of convenience stores without paying. Last week, she walked into a neighbor's house unannounced while they were not home and ate food from their kitchen, leaving a mess.

The PAPN notices that Margi has trouble staying seated. She gets up often and touches things without asking. Margi displays echopraxia and echolalia. She occasionally screeches and pounds her chest; some stereotypies are reminiscent of an autistic individual. Her family has brought small food packets to keep her occupied and to stay in the interview room. Eye contact is good and she does not appear fearful. There is very little reciprocal speech and no functional conversation. Margi is able to sign her name for consent to treatment but refuses to complete any intake paperwork. Family members help her to do this. Margi will answer questions with a "yes" or "no," but it is unclear if she has full comprehension of the interview questions. While it is presumed that she has psychotic features, she has disturbed attention, speech, and language processing, which makes this hard to

Continued

CASE STUDY 5-3—continued

assess. Her husband looks exhausted and very anxious. His wife's illness has begun to cause a burden for the family. They are ready to reconsider medication but do not feel comfortable "forcing her" against her will. There is no history of her wanting to harm herself or others, by family report.

Differential Diagnosis

Schizophrenia, catatonic subtype; psychotic disorder secondary to a medical condition (underlying illness, epilepsy, surreptitious poisoning, infectious disease; parasite infestation in the brain, brain tumor or cyst, etc.); psychosis secondary to occult drug abuse; major depression with psychotic features; schizoaffective disorder; delirium and various types of dementia

Primary Diagnosis

Bipolar disorder, catatonic subtype (primarily disorganized excited phase) with a plan to rule out catatonic schizophrenia.

Plan of Care

Margi originally experienced a major depressive episode several years ago, followed by a cognitive decline and probable psychotic process. She has presented with a cyclical pattern of sustained hyperactivity and insomnia (1- to 4-week periods) that appear to be features of mania with catatonic features resembling the excitatory phase. The PAPN considers that Margi may be gravely disabled and may need to be involuntarily detained and admitted to a psychiatric unit. The family does not like this plan and would like to try medication first on an outpatient basis. The PAPN agrees to do some medication trials first but recommends that the family simultaneously work with her to gain cooperation and confidence for admitting Margi to a hospital unit for additional work-ups.

The PAPN provides family education about the severity of Margi's condition. Her cognitive decline and prolonged confusional state warrant a comprehensive medical work-up. Although the family thinks that neurological disorders were ruled out 2 years ago, the PAPN reminds them that repeat imaging studies were recommended and should be done, even if the patient is uncooperative. The PAPN recommends an inpatient psychiatric evaluation in a hospital setting for 24-hour observation of her behavior and for repeat lab work and neuroimaging studies (MRI, CT scan, and EEG).

The PAPN starts Margi on a medication plan that will address symptoms of psychosis, mood swings, and catatonia. Margi's medications include Invega 9 mg/day; Lamictal 400 mg/day; Lorazepam 1 mg tid; and Provigil 200 mg/day. On this regimen, she made only minor improvement over the next 6 months. There is a modest increase in functional communication with the PAPN and with a receptionist. At home, she plays a simple card game with her children, washes her hair with supervision, and can be taken to the mall without impulsively grabbing things or darting off. But she is not "getting better."

The PAPN provides family education on medical-legal aspects of Margi's case. There is currently no health-care proxy in place, yet the severity of her mental illness warrants having a third party advocate for her basic needs. Her persisting altered mentation, dysfunctional behavior, and loss of self-care and parenting capacities have been a significant burden to the family. She needs 24-hour supervision, and her parents have been providing support while her husband is at work. The PAPN recommends that the husband become her legal guardian and conservator. Margi's husband and her parents are initially alarmed at this suggestion, though Margi's mental status is markedly changed from the person they knew 3 years ago. The PAPN supports their grieving process, facilitates family discussions, and helps them to look realistically at the circumstances.

The PAPN again advises that it is necessary to more completely assess for other sources of psychosis and catatonia, including dementia, and clarify whether an organic condition is present. The family is embarrassed to bring her to a hospital and are fearful of how others will handle her disruptive behavior there. They expect that she will refuse all lab work and testing and may become combative and get hurt. The PAPN provides emotional support to help the family make difficult decisions. The PAPN also offers hope, by providing education about the options for advanced therapies like electroconvulsive treatment (ECT). The family eventually agrees that it would be helpful to try ECT and likes the fact that a secondary review will be done by a judge to determine her eligibility for this treatment, as it lifts their own burden of guilt. Unfortunately, ECT is not available to Margi in her rural home state. The PAPN advises the family about how to access services out of state and advocates for them with the patient's insurance company and the state insurance commissioner.

The PAPN then consults with ECT psychiatrists in three states about Margi's case and makes a formal referral for inpatient care. The PAPN develops a patient transport plan for family members to escort Margi to the hospital, as Margi would be incapable of tolerating an airplane flight, and the cost of ambulance services out of state are prohibitive. A detailed map marking stops with access to medical services and cell phone reception is constructed. The family is provided with a notarized letter concerning Margi's medical condition to show innkeepers and to protect them legally in case she acts impulsively at a road stop and police are asked to intervene.

Margi is then admitted to an out-of-state psychiatric hospital where she is evaluated as a candidate for ECT, which includes doing baseline medical work-ups and neuroimaging studies. At this time, it becomes clear that Margi does not have bipolar disorder with catatonia; she is actually suffering from frontal-temporal dementia. This devastating diagnosis rarely occurs in a young woman of her age. The medical staff at the hospital provides anticipatory counseling regarding coping with progressive dementia. They recommended that Margi continue on the medications that the PAPN initiated, but also informed the family that this would simply slow her decline and make her behavior manageable. The family began the slow acceptance process and realized that "there is no cure." The family is now engaged in an extensive home-based supportive-rehabilitation program with strong nursing support and case management. The children are receiving counseling about the loss of their mother's parenting availability, and the family is moving on in a positive direction.

Clinical Pearls

- Patients like Margi would have been treated on an inpatient basis and institutionalized 30 years ago. Now, factors such

CASE STUDY 5-3—continued

as cost containment, declining psychiatric inpatient services, and emphasis on least-restrictive levels of care sometimes impede the full evaluation and treatment of severe neuropsychiatric disorders.

- Sometimes medications are used to treat symptom clusters, without confirmation of a specific diagnosis.
- There are many medical disorders that mimic psychiatric disorders or have behavioral and neurocognitive manifestations.
- Medical work-ups need to be monitored: sometimes certain tests are overlooked or the repeat testing is not followed up.
- Families may resist hospitalization because of stigma or fear of harm to their loved one; supportive counseling is necessary to give them confidence, to gain their trust, and to help them follow through with difficult medical decisions.
- Children may need counseling when a parent develops a medical condition that has an insidious onset, as they may misinterpret the parent's behavior as disinterest and feel neglected or rejected.
- It is difficult to access some medical services when the patient is demonstrating no threat to self or others. Being "gravely disabled" is no longer a sufficient reason for psychiatric admission in some areas.
- ECT is an effective treatment for catatonia in patients with bipolar spectrum disorders, but there are few treatment facilities providing this care.

Reflection Questions

What is the process for developing a health-care proxy for psychiatric patients? What are the PAPN's state's laws about conservatorship? How accessible is ECT in the PAPN's state?

CASE STUDY 5-4

Referral of a Child by Primary Care Physician for Psychiatric Evaluation

Clinical Presentation

Fonzy is an 8-year-old boy who has been treated for ADHD by his family physician for the past 4 years with psychostimulant medication. Currently, he is taking 10 mg of mixed amphetamine salts once each morning. Fonzy's mother, who was a teenager when he was born, is living in an institution. Her history is sketchy, but she is reported to have manic depression and was a drug addict. Fonzy's father was never identified. Fonzy has been raised by his maternal uncle (recently deceased) and grandparents. The school psychologist noted, "Fonzy shows some socially atypical behaviors that are not severe enough to qualify him for a PDD but are likely to set him apart from others and interfere with his social and perhaps academic progress. His social behavior is more immature than most 8-year-olds and makes him a target for peer bullying. He is likely to have Asperger's or high-functioning autism, particularly since he also shows advanced intellect in multiple cognitive domains and normal speech and language development, apart from some nasality and odd 'professor-like' word usage." Fonzy's uncle, his legal guardian, died 1 month ago by suicide. The grandparents have taken him into their home temporarily. Fonzy has not shown much of a grief reaction, but he has been hitting children on the playground and threw a stapler at the substitute teacher this week. He has been talking about "killing aliens."

Fonzy dislikes loud noises and any changes in routine. His teacher reports that he takes things very literally sometimes. The other children reject him from their games and he is the last picked for sports. Fonzy does not endear himself to others, as he will only talk about his favorite themes and picks his nose compulsively in class. Now, at the end of the school year, Fonzy's grades are poor and he is likely to be held back. He has not been sleeping much, and he sneaks onto the computer late at night. The primary care physician refers him to the PAPN for further psychiatric evaluation and medication consultation. There is a family history of depression, bipolar disorder, learning disorders, and ADHD.

In the initial intake, the PAPN observes that Fonzy has some mild motor stereotypies, such as flapping his hands when excited and tapping things. He has mild gaze aversion and prefers not to make eye contact. He hums to himself when playing. The PAPN notices that Fonzy repeatedly raises his eyebrows in a tic-like manner. Fonzy also frequently sniffs, but without trying to smell anything. There is also a brief throat clearing. He has narrow special interests, a fascination with dinosaurs and rocks. In some ways he appears very bright, like a dictionary when discussing science facts. Fonzy is idiosyncratic and perseverative with his play, not showing much interest in having the PAPN participate. His grandmother tells the PAPN that Fonzy will only wear red and orange and prefers toys and other objects with these colors; Fonzy pipes up, "they are my fire colors!" He does not cry or verbalize any sadness when the PAPN asks about his uncle. He does draw a picture of an alien with tears coming down from the enlarged eyeballs.

Differential Diagnosis

Attention deficit-hyperactivity disorder, combined type (ADHD); mood disorder related to a medical condition; complex partial seizures; myoclonus; obsessive-compulsive disorder; autistic spectrum disorder, such as Asperger's disorder, high-functioning autism, or pervasive developmental disorder, NOS; pediatric bipolar spectrum disorder; simple motor tics; Tourette's disorder; adjustment disorder with disturbance of emotions and conduct

Primary Diagnosis

1. Attention deficit-hyperactivity disorder, combined type; adjustment disorder with mixed emotions and conduct; rule out Asperger's disorder; rule out Tourrette's disorder; rule out early-onset pediatric bipolar spectrum disorder

Continued

CASE STUDY 5-4—continued

II. Rule out learning disorder; auditory processing disorder
III. Rule out allergic rhinitis, nasal polyps, hearing and vision difficulties, and neurological problems
IV. Peer rejection/bullying; inadequate school accommodations; loss of primary support figure due to suicide; unstable housing; academic difficulties; transition to summer; inadequate parenting; social isolation
V. GAF: 48

Plan of Care

Provide grief counseling for the family to help provide stability for this child. Fonzy may also be suffering a mild adjustment reaction to his uncle's death, which could possibly explain his recent repetitive talk of death. Individual therapy may be helpful. He will need assistance to comprehend these issues, and increased family support and family mourning practices may help. The family history of depression and suicide attempts suggests that Fonzy's mood and behavior should be closely monitored for depression, especially if the family relocates to new housing. However, Fonzy does not show an intent to harm himself and appears to be at low risk for suicide at this time.

ADHD does not fully explain some of his disturbed social relatedness and compulsive, ritualistic behaviors. The PAPN should conduct additional clinical assessments to confirm the presence of an autistic spectrum disorder or related condition, such as nonverbal learning disorder. Referral to a neuropsychologist is appropriate. The PAPN who has received additional training and experience with developmental disabilities may conduct some assessments for autistic spectrum disorders.

In terms of psychotropic medication, Fonzy's level of impulsivity and hyperactivity are excessive and he is responding to psychostimulant medications, although the dose may be too low. However, at this time of transition, it may not be advisable to do a new medication trial because school observations are not possible, steady parental supervision is lacking, and psychostimulants can sometimes induce mania or other adverse reaction as dose increases. The lack of close medical follow-up during this interim time of moving to his grandparents' home also contraindicates the use of clonidine. However, this fall, when the school year begins, trying an alternative to stimulants, such as guanfacine, may be of interest. Because summer has just started, an alternative medication to consider is sertraline (Zoloft), an SSRI that has been shown to be helpful for improving socialization and some obsessional behaviors associated with autism spectrum disorders. This medication is relatively safe and will not require frequent blood draws or blood pressure monitoring. Of course, any antidepressant must be monitored closely initially for risk of activation and induction of suicidal tendencies.

The PAPN should consider referral to a local community mental health center that provides child case management and in-home family-based services. If Fonzy's behavior deteriorates further, a "wraparound" plan to maintain him in the community with crisis respite services may be needed. The PAPN should also participate with school staff and the mental health center staff to develop a school Individualized Education Plan (IEP) that best meets his social and emotional accommodation needs. Social skills training and lunchtime 'friendship groups' would be helpful.

Clinical Pearls

- There is a higher likelihood of early-onset mood disorders in families in which many members have depression or bipolar disorder.
- There may also be a slight increased incidence of PDDs in the children of parents who have bipolar disorder.
- Children with complex behavioral difficulties may later present with comorbid major psychiatric disorders.
- Polypharmacy strategies may be needed to treat symptoms of mood difficulty, tics, obsessive anxiety, and executive function problems of ADHD.
- Children with complex behavioral difficulties often will eventually need inpatient psychiatric treatment for containment and medication adjustments.
- With strong family support and intensive wraparound services, these children can avoid being institutionalized and become contributing members of the community.

Reflection Questions

What should the PAPN do for medication adjustments when a child treated with psychostimulant medications begins to present with severe insomnia, mood swings, tics, or psychotic symptoms? What are wraparound services? Are there any national programs or models for this service? What is the current understanding of autism spectrum disorders? Should children be told about a family member's suicide? What resources are available to help families cope with suicide of a loved one?

Summary

The primary purpose of a case formulation is to integrate descriptive information about a patient obtained during the assessment process in order to generate a hypothesis about the causes, precipitants, and mechanisms that are involved in a patient's psychological, interpersonal, and behavioral problems. The mechanisms are the causes of patient's problems, and thus understanding the mechanisms that underlie the patient's symptoms and distress is key to planning treatment. A case formulation can serve as a structure for the clinician's understanding of the patient, a guide for treatment, and a way to measure change. Case formulation skills are fundamental to providing effective treatment.

Key Points

- The PAPN compiles information from (1) the clinical interview and (2) data collected from other assessment sources, such as psychological assessments, neuroimaging studies, laboratory findings, academic records, legal records, and prior treatment providers.

- Case formulation includes symptoms, precipitating stressors, predisposing life events, mechanisms or causes, patient's strengths and deficits, and support and resources.
- Symptoms include the symptoms and problems that the patient has identified and also biopsychosocial health problems that the clinician identifies.
- Precipitating stressors are events, situations, or perceptions that induce or exacerbate the patient's symptoms and behaviors.
- Predisposing life events include adverse events that happened in early life, childhood, adolescence, and adulthood and also recent or current events.
- Mechanisms that induce and maintain symptoms and behaviors can be biological, psychological, or social.
- Diagnoses are derived from case formulations.
- Diagnoses provide a basis for understanding the patient's situation, for determining treatment and place of treatment, for predicting course, and for reimbursement.
- At this time, psychiatric diagnoses are based on the *DSM-IV-TR* (American Psychiatric Association, 2000), which uses five axes to identify patients' psychiatric disorder, personality or developmental disorders, medical health problems, social problems, and functioning.
- Psychiatric diagnosis must also take into consideration the patient's adaptive characteristics, coping patterns, capacity for social relationships, and ability to interpret life events.
- PAPNs use a biopsychosocial plan of treatment.
- Within the biopsychosocial plan of treatment, the *biological* domain includes a physical examination, appropriate laboratory tests, and obtaining information about existing medical conditions and their treatment and about medications currently being taken. The *psychological* domain includes possible referral for neuropsychiatric testing and psychotherapeutic interventions. The *social* domain includes identification of interventions to improve the patient's living, employment, financial, and social situations and the role that the patient plays in those situations.
- The treatment plan meets the patient's needs and goals.
- Treatment interventions are culturally relevant, realistic, attainable, socially acceptable, and accessible.

References

Achenbach, T. M. (1991). *Manual for the child behavior checklist/4-18 and 1991 Profile.* Burlington, VT: University of Vermont.

American Psychiatric Association (2000). *Diagnostic and statistical manual of mental disorders* (4th ed., text rev.). Washington, DC: American Psychiatric Publishing, Inc.

Andreasen, N. C., & Black, D. W. (2006). *Introductory textbook of psychiatry* (4th ed.). Washington, DC: American Psychiatric Publishing, Inc.

Baron-Cohen, S., Wheelwright, I., Skinner, R., et al. (2001). The Autism-Spectrum Quotient (AQ) evidence from Asperger syndrome/high functioning autism, males and females, scientists and mathematicians. *Journal of Autism and Developmental Disorders, 31*(1), 5-17.

Beck, A. T., Epstein, N., Brown, G., et al. (1988). An inventory for measuring clinical anxiety: Psychometric properties. *Journal of Consulting Clinical Psychology, 56*, 893-897.

Beck, A., Schuyler, D., & Herman, I. (1974). Development of suicidal intent scales. In A. T. Beck, H. P. Resnik, D. J. Lettieri, et al. (Eds.), *Prevention of suicide.* Philadelphia: Charles Press.

Bergner, R. M. (1998). Characteristics of optimal clinical case formulations: The linchpin concept. *American Journal of Psychotherapy, 52*(3), 287-300.

Bernet, W. (2002). Child custody evaluations. *Child and Adolescent Psychiatric Clinics of North America, 11*, 781-804.

Bernet, W. (2008). Parental alienation syndrome and DSM-V. *Family Therapy, 36*(5), 349-366.

Beyerstein, B. L. (1996). Believing is seeing: Organic and psychological reasons for hallucinations and other anomalous psychiatric symptoms, Posted: 04/10/2002; *Medscape Psychiatry & Mental Health eJournal* 1(6) © 1996 Medscape. www.medscape.com/viewarticle/431517.

Blatner, A. (September 15, 2006). The art of case formulation [Internet blog] (email adam@blatner.com). This article is a complement to and/or extension of another paper on this Web site: The Art of Case Presentation. http://www.blatner.com/adam/papers.html#other originally published as: Blatner, A. (1993). The art of case presentation. *Resident & Staff Physician, 39*(2), 97-103.

Blazer, D. G. (2008). Psychiatric epidemiology. In M. Ebert, J. Leckman, P. Loosen, & B. Nurcombe (Eds.), *Current diagnosis & treatment psychiatry* (2nd ed.) (pp. 7-14). New York: McGraw-Hill/Lange Medical book.

Cassels, C. (2010). Medscape perspectives on the American Psychiatric Association Annual 2010 meeting: Proposed DSM-5 receives unprecedented public response. *Medscape Medical News*, June 15, 2010. Retrieved from www.medscape.com/viewarticle/723526

Conners, C. K., Erhardt, D., & Sparrow, E. (1998). *Adult ADHD rating scale.* Toronto: Multi-Health Systems.

Connor, K. M., Kobak, K. A., & Churchill, L. E., et al. (2001). Mini-SPIN: A brief screening assessment for generalized social anxiety disorder. *Depression and Anxiety*, 14, 137-140.

Cull, J. G., & Gill, W. W. (1982). *The suicide probability scale.* Los Angeles: Western Psychological Services.

Davidson, J. R. T., Hughes, D. L., George, L. K., et al. (1993). The epidemiology of social phobia: Findings from the Duke Epidemiological Catchment Area Study. *Psychological Medicine, 23*, 709-718.

Demyttenaere, K., Bruffaerts, R., Posada-villa, J., et al. (2004). The WHO World Mental Health Survey Consortium. Prevalence, severity and unmet need for treatment of mental disorders in the World Health Organization World Mental Health Surveys. *Journal of the American Medical Association, 291*(21), 2581-2590.

Dichter, G. S., Felder, J. N., & Bodfish, J. W. (2009). Autism is characterized by dorsal anterior cingulated hyperactivation during social target detection. *Social Cognitive and Affective Neuroscience, 4*(3), 215-226.

DiPietro, E. K., Runyan, D. K., & Fredrickson, D. D. (1997). Predictors of disclosure during medical evaluation for suspected sexual abuse. *Journal of Child Sexual Abuse, 6*(1), 133-142.

Eells, T. D., Kendjelic, E. M., & Lucas, C. P. (1998). What's in a case formulation? Development and use of a content coding manual. *The Journal of Psychotherapy Practice and Research, 7*, 144-153.

Engel, G. (1980). The clinical application of the biopsychosocial model. *American Journal of Psychiatry, 137*(3), 535-544.

Ewing, J. A. (1984). Detecting alcoholism: The CAGE Questionnaire. *Journal of the American Medical Association, 252*(14), 1905-1907.

Fineberg, N. A., O'Dougherty, C., Rajagopal, S., et al. (2003). How common is obsessive-compulsive disorder in a dermatology outpatient clinic? *Journal of Clinical Psychiatry, 64*, 152-155.

First, N. A., & Tasman, A. (2004). *DSM-IV-TR mental disorders: Diagnosis, etiology & treatment.* West Sussex, England: John Wiley & Sons, Ltd.

Gioia, G. A., Isquith, P. K., Guy, S. C., et al. (2000). *BRIEF Behavior Rating Inventory of Executive Function professional manual.* Lutz, FL: Psychological Assessment Resources, Inc.

Goodman, W. K., Price, L. H., Rasmussen, S. A., et al. (1989). The Yale-Brown Obsessive-Compulsive Scale I: Development, use and reliability. *Archives of General Psychiatry, 46*, 1012-1016.

Greenspan, S., & Wieder, S. (2008). The Interdisciplinary Council on Developmental and Learning Disorders diagnostic manual for infants and children. *Journal of Canadian Academy of Child and Adolescent Psychiatry, 17*(2), 76-89.

Hamilton, M. (1959). The assessment of anxiety states by rating. *British Journal of Medical Psychology, 32*, 50-55.

Hare, R. D. (2003). Hare psychopathy checklist-revised (2nd ed.). Toronto: Multi-Health Systems, Inc.

Healthy People 2010 (Conference Edition, in Two Volumes). (2000). Washington, DC: U.S. Department of Health and Human Services.

Hedaya, R. J. (1996). *Understanding biological psychiatry*. New York: W. W. Norton & Company.

Hirschfeld, R. M. A., Williams, J. B., Spitzer, R. L., et al. (2000). Development and validation of a screening instrument for bipolar spectrum disorder: The Mood Disorder Questionnaire. *American Journal of Psychiatry, 157*, 1873-1875.

Horowitz, M., Wilner, N., & Alvarez, W. (1979). Impact of Event Scale: A measure of subjective distress. *Psychosomatic Medicine, 41*, 209-218.

Ingram, B. L. (2006). *Clinical case formulations: Matching the integrative treatment plan to the patient*. Hoboken, NJ: John Wiley & Sons, Inc.

Insel, T. R., & Fenton, W. S. (2005). Psychiatric epidemiology: It's not just about counting anymore. *Archives of General Psychiatry, 62*(6), 590-592.

Kassaw, K., & Gabbard, G. (2002). Creating a psychodynamic formulation from a clinical evaluation. *The American Journal of Psychiatry, 159*(5), 721-726.

Kay, S. R., Opler, L. A., & Fizbein, A. (1994). *Positive and negative syndrome scale manual*. North Tonawanda, NY: Multi-Health Systems.

Kendall-Tackett, K. (2003). *Treating the lifetime health effects of childhood victimization*. Kingston, NJ: Civic Research Institute.

Kessler, R. C. (1997). The prevalence of psychiatric comorbidity. In S. Wetzler & W. C. Sanderson (Eds.), *Treatment strategies for patients with psychiatric comorbidity*. New York: John Wiley & Sons.

Kessler, R. C., Berglund, P., Demler, O., et al. (2005a). Lifetime prevalence and age-of-onset distributions of DSM-IV disorders in the national comorbidity survey replication. *Archives of General Psychiatry, 62*(6), 593-602.

Kessler, R. C., Berglund, P. A., Foster, C. L., et al. (1997). Social consequences of psychiatric disorders, II: Teenage parenthood. *American Journal of Psychiatry, 154*, 1405-1411.

Kessler, R. C., Chiu, W. T., Demler, O., et al. (2005b). Prevalence, severity, and comorbidity of 12-month DSM-IV disorders in the national comorbidity survey replication. *Archives of General Psychiatry, 62*(6), 617-627.

Kessler, R. C., Foster, C. L., Saunders, W. B., et al. (1995). Social consequences of psychiatric disorders, I: Educational attainment. *American Journal of Psychiatry, 152*, 1026-1032.

Kessler, R. C., & Price, R. H. (1993). Primary prevention of secondary disorders: A proposal and agenda. *American Journal of Community Psychology, 21*, 607-633.

Kessler, R. C., Walters, E. E., & Forthofer, M. S. (1998). The social consequences of psychiatric disorders, III: Probability of marital stability. *American Journal of Psychiatry, 155*, 1092-1096.

Kim-Cohen, J., Caspi, A., Moffitt, T. E., et al. (2003). Prior juvenile diagnoses in adults with mental disorder: Developmental follow-back of a prospective longitudinal cohort. *Archives of General Psychiatry, 60*(7), 709-717.

Kovacs, M. (1981). Rating scales to assess depression in school-aged children. *Acta Paedopsychiatrica, 46*, 305-315.

LeDoux, J. (2002). *Synaptic self: How our brains become who we are*. New York: Viking.

Murray, C. J. L., & Lopez, A. D. (1996). *The global burden of disease*. Geneva: World Health Organization, Harvard School of Public Health, World Bank.

Narrow, W. E., Rae, D. S., Robins, L. N., et al. (2002). Revised prevalence estimates of mental disorders in the United States using a clinical significance criterion to reconcile 2 surveys' estimates. *Archives of General Psychiatry, 59*, 115-123.

Olin, G. L., & Rhoades, J. A. (2005). The five most costly medical conditions, 1997-2002: Estimates for the U.S. civilian non-institutionalized population. Medical Expenditure Panel survey. *Agency for Healthcare Research and Quality, Statistical Brief # 80*.

Panksepp, J. (2004). Biological psychiatry sketched: Past, present & future. In J. Panksepp (Ed.), *Textbook of biological psychiatry* (pp. 3-32). Hoboken, NJ: Wiley-Liss.

Pierce, K., Conant, D., Hazin, R., et al. (2011). Preference for geometric patterns early in life as a risk factor for autism. *Archives of General Psychiatry, 68*(1), 101-109.

Portenoy, R. (2006). Development and testing of neuropathic pain screening questionnaire. *Current Medical Research and Opinion, 22*, 1555-1565.

Privitera, M. R., & Lyness, J. M. (2009). *Psychiatry mentor clerkship and shelf exam companion* (2nd ed.). Philadelphia: F. A. Davis.

Reynolds, C. R., & Kamphaus, R. W. (1992). *The behavior assessment system for children*. Circle Pines, MN: AGS Publishing.

Sajatovic, M., & Ramirez, L. F. (2003). *Rating scales in mental health* (2nd ed.). Hudson, OH: Lexi-Comp.

Sar, V., Islam, S., & Ozturk, E. (2009). Childhood emotional abuse and dissociation in patients with conversion symptoms. *Psychiatry and Clinical Neuroscience, 63*(5), 670-677.

Seligman, L., & Reichenberg, L. W. (2007). *Selecting effective treatments: A comprehensive systematic guide to treating mental disorders*. San Francisco: John Wiley & Sons, Inc.

Selzer, M. L. (1971). The Michigan Alcoholism Screening Test: The quest for a new diagnostic instrument. *American Journal of Psychiatry, 127*, 1653-1658.

Shaw P., Lalonde F., Lepage C., et al. (2009). Development of cortical asymmetry in typically developing children and its disruption in attention-deficit hyperactivity disorder. *Archives of General Psychiatry*, 66, 888-896.

Sim, K., Gwee, K. P., & Bateman, A. (2005). Case formulation in psychotherapy: Revitalizing its usefulness as a clinical tool. *Academic Psychiatry, 29*(3), 289-292.

Simons, R. D., & Hughes, C. C. (1993). Culture-bound syndromes. In A. C. Gaw (Ed.), *Culture, ethnicity and mental illness* (pp. 75-99). Washington, DC: American Psychiatric Publishing, Inc.

Smith-Myles, B., Jones-Bock, S., & Simpson, R. L. (2001). *Asperger syndrome diagnostic scale: Examiner's manual*. Austin, TX: PRO-ED, Inc.

Spitzer, R. L., Kroenke, K., & Williams, J. B. (1999). Validation and utility of a self-report version of PRIME-MD: The PHQ primary care study—Primary Care Evaluation of Mental Disorders, Patient Health Questionnaire. *Journal of the American Medical Association, 282*, 1737-1744.

Wang, P. S., Berglund, P. A., Olfson, M., et al. (2004). Delays in initial treatment contact after first onset of a mental disorder. *Health Services Research, 39*(2), 393-415.

Wang, P. S., Lane, M., Olfson, M., et al. (2005). Twelve-month use of mental health services in the U.S. Results from the National Co-morbidity Survey Replication (N CS-R). *Archives of General Psychiatry, 62*, 629-640.

Williams, D., & Clements, P. T. (2005). Intrapsychic dynamics, behavioral manifestations, and related interventions with youthful fire setters. *Journal of Forensic Nursing, 3*(1), 67-72.

Winston, H. A., Rosenthal, R. N., & Pinsker, H. (2004). *Introduction to supportive psychotherapy*. Washington, DC: American Psychiatric Publishing, Inc.

Wolff, P. H. (1972). Ethnic differences in alcohol sensitivity. *Science, 175*, 449-450.

Wong, D. L., & Baker, C. M. (2005). Pain rating scale. In M. J. Hockenberry, D. Wilson, & M. L. Winkelstein (Eds.), *Wong's essential of pediatric nursing* (7th ed.). St. Louis: Mosby.

World Health Organization (WHO) (2003). *Adult Self-Report Scale-V1.1 (ASRS-V1.1) Screener*. Geneva, Switzerland: World Health Organization.

Yoshida, A. (1993). Genetic polymorphisms of alcohol-metabolizing enzymes related to alcohol sensitivity and alcoholic diseases. In K. M. Lin, R. E. Poland, & G. Nakasaki (Eds.), *Psychopharmacology and psychobiology of ethnicity* (pp. 169-186). Washington, DC: American Psychiatric Publishing, Inc.

Zimmerman, M., & Mattia, J. I. (2000). Principal and additional DSM-IV disorders for which outpatients seek treatment. *Psychiatric Services, 51*(10), 1299-1304.

CHAPTER 6

Psychopharmacotherapy

Norman L. Keltner, EdD, CRNP, and Joan S. Grant, DNS, RN, CS

This chapter reviews basic information about psychopharmacology with the intent of providing readers with foundational concepts they can adapt to individualized patient care. The chapter also reviews the core psychotropic drugs: antipsychotic, antidepressant, antimanic, and antianxiety drugs. Specific applications of pharmacotherapy can be found in the chapters dealing with specific disorders.

Basics of Psychopharmacotherapy

The brain and its neurotransmitters are key components in understanding the basics of psychopharmacotherapy.

Brain

An individual is born with about 100 billion neurons. The fetal brain actually develops many more neurons, but the extra neurons are eliminated before birth (Sugerman, 2011).

At times during the gestational period, over 100,000 neurons are produced per minute. A road map of where the neurons will eventually go (or should go) is also developed. With such extensive neuronal activity taking place, the wonder is not how something "went wrong" in some individuals during these highly sensitive times, causing later mental problems, physical problems, or both; rather, the wonder is how so many people *survive* this intense neuronal generation period without apparent damage. More information about brain development can be found in Chapter 2.

Neurotransmitters

Neurotransmitters consist of monoamines, cholinergics, and amino acids. While there are many neurotransmitters, six are most commonly affected by psychotropic medications: dopamine (DA), norepinephrine (NE), serotonin (5-HT), acetylcholine (Ach), gamma-aminobutryic acid (GABA), and glutamate (Glu). An understanding of these transmitters will enable the clinician to meaningfully engage the psychopharmacology literature. Classifications of neurotransmitters and their locations and major pathways are summarized in Table 6-1 and described in more detail below. Psychotropic medications affect neuron activity typically by modulating neurotransmitters.

Monoamines

Dopamine, norepinephrine, and serotonin are referred to as monoamines because they have one amine (NH_2) group. They are all derived from amino acids, but an enzyme (a decarboxylase) removes the carboxylic acid (COOH) from their makeup. Because they still have the "amino" but not the "acid," they become monoamines.

Dopamine and norepinephrine are molecules in the catecholamine synthesis chain, with norepinephrine being a metabolite of dopamine. Brain dopamine is synthesized in the substantia nigra, ventral tegmental area (VTA), and hypothalamus. Brain norepinephrine is synthesized in the locus ceruleus located in the pons.

Serotonin is derived from the amino acid tryptophan. Serotonin is synthesized in the raphe nuclei of the brainstem, with rostral serotonin neurons projecting to the cerebrum and caudal serotonin neurons projecting to the cerebellum and down the spine (see Table 6-1 for serotonin's major pathways). Interestingly, most serotonin is synthesized not in the brain, but in the gut wall.

Cholinergics

Acetylcholine is the lone cholinergic. It is widely distributed in the peripheral nervous system and plays a key role in learning and memory in the central nervous system. Brain acetylcholine (~90%) is synthesized in the cerebrum in an area referred to as the basal nucleus of Meynert. Interestingly, drugs with anticholinergic effects can temporarily affect memory and learning; hence, cholinergic blocking drugs should be used cautiously in older individuals because they are at risk for memory and learning problems.

TABLE 6-1 CLASSIFICATION OF NEUROTRANSMITTERS AND PATHWAYS

Category	Neurotransmitter	Location in the Central Nervous System	Major Pathways
Cholinergic	Acetylcholine	Basal nucleus of Meynert and in pons	Basal nucleus of Meynert to cerebral cortex; septal area to hippocampus
Monoamines	Dopamine	Substantia nigra	Nigrostriatal
		Ventral tegmental area	Mesolimbic
		Ventral tegmental area	Mesocortical
		Hypothalamus	Tuberoinfundibular
	Norepinephrine	Locus ceruleus	Locus ceruleus (in pons) to thalamus, cerebral cortex, cerebellum, and spinal cord
	Serotonin	Raphe nuclei	Rostral raphe nuclei to thalamus, striatum, hypothalamus, hippocampus, nucleus accumbens, prefrontal cortex Caudal raphe nuclei to cerebellum and spinal cord
Amino acids	GABA	Most common inhibitory transmitter in brain	Purkinje cells to deep cerebellar nuclei; striatal
	Glutamate	Most common excitatory transmitter in brain	Widely distributed in central nervous system

Adapted from Keltner, N. L., & Folks, D. G. (2005). Psychotropic drugs *(4th ed.). St. Louis: Mosby.*

Amino Acids

GABA is the most common inhibitory neurotransmitter in the brain. GABA receptors control chloride channels that, when stimulated, allow more chloride into the neuron. Chloride influx can cause hyperpolarization, making it more difficult for the neuron to depolarize. Therefore, drugs such as the benzodiazepines slow neuronal firing and thus are effective medications for "slowing down" overexcited neurons.

Glutamate is the most common excitatory neurotransmitter. Two psychiatrically significant glutamate receptors exist: the *N*-methyl-D-aspartate (NMDA) receptor and the non-NMDA receptor (also referred to as the aminomethylisoxazole proprionate [AMPA] receptor). The NMDA receptor is of special interest because as it becomes activated, calcium enters the neuron, causing neuronal firing. When glutamate overstimulation occurs, neuron death (i.e., excitotoxicity) develops, which may be a major source for the damage occurring in Parkinson's disease, Alzheimer's disease, Huntington's disease, and neuronal loss after strokes. Interestingly, as NDMA receptors are blocked, schizophrenia-like symptoms may develop. For instance, phencyclidine and ketamine may cause a sense of depersonalization, delusions, and hallucinations. Though the exact mechanism is unclear, it is postulated that an underfunctioning glutamatergic system may be an etiologic factor in schizophrenia.

Neurotransmitters and Psychopharmacology

Basic premises about these neurotransmitters, though perhaps simplistic, continue to drive current psychopharmacology. For example: elevated dopamine is associated with positive symptoms of schizophrenia, hyperkinesias, and sexual enhancement. Hence, enhancing dopamine (e.g., amphetamines, levodopa, and bupropion) can produce hallucinations, dyskinesias, and hypersexuality. Reduced dopamine levels, on the other hand, are associated with improvement in positive symptoms of schizophrenia, temperature dysregulation, hypokinesias, and impaired sexuality. Thus, blocking dopamine (e.g., with antipsychotics) can relieve symptoms of schizophrenia, but it can also elevate temperature, cause extrapyramidal side effects (EPSEs), and reduce interest in sex. Tables 6-2 through 6-5 provide greater detail of the results of receptor activation (agonist) or antagonism for dopamine, norepinephrine, serotonin, and acetylcholine receptors, respectively.

TABLE 6-2 DOPAMINE ACTIVATION AND ANTAGONISM

Activation (Agonists)	Antagonism
Positive symptoms of schizophrenia: hallucinations, delusions	Negative symptoms Antipsychotic effect (i.e., improves positive symptoms)
Nausea, vomiting	Antiemetic effect
Dyskinesias	Parkinsonism and other EPSEs
Sexual function enhancement	Sexual dysfunction
Other problems: addictive behaviors	Other problems: negative symptoms, temperature dysregulation, cognitive problems, prolactin elevation, depression and/or anhedonia, lack of energy and/or motivation

EPSEs, extrapyramidal side effects.
Adapted from Keltner, N. L. (2000). Neuroreceptor function and psychopharmacologic response. Issues in Mental Health Nursing, 21, *31-50.*

TABLE 6-3 NOREPINEPHRINE ACTIVATION AND ANTAGONISM

Activation (Agonist)	Antagonism
Antidepressant effect	Depressive effect
Vasoconstriction (α_1)	Vasodilation (α_1 antagonism)
Increased heart rate (β_1)	Decreased heart rate (beta blocker)
Bronchial dilation	Sexual dysfunction
Other physical effects	Other physical effects

Adapted from Keltner, N. L. (2000). Neuroreceptor function and psychopharmacologic response. Issues in Mental Health Nursing, 21, *31-50.*

TABLE 6-4 SEROTONIN ACTIVATION AND ANTAGONISM

Activation (Agonist)	Antagonism
Antidepressant effect	Depression
Anxiety	Anxiety
Migraine headaches	Migraine headaches
Insomnia	Sleep-wake cycle disruption
Other problems: nausea, vomiting, and other gastrointestinal disturbances; sexual dysfunction and decrease in penile erection capability; reduced appetite and weight loss; movement disorders; temperature dysregulation; psychotic thinking	Other problems: dysthymia and suicidality; aggressiveness; obsessive thinking; pain; compulsive behavior; panic

Adapted from Keltner, N. L. (2000). Neuroreceptor function and psychopharmacologic response. Issues in Mental Health Nursing, 21, *31-50.*

TABLE 6-5 ACETYLCHOLINE ACTIVATION AND ANTAGONISM

Activation (Agonist)	Antagonism
Pupil constriction	Pupil dilation
Decreased heart rate	Increased heart rate
Constriction of bronchi	Dilation of bronchi
Increased respiratory secretions	Decreased respiratory secretions
Increased voiding	Decreased voiding
Salivation	Dry mouth
Increased gastric secretions	Decreased gastric secretions
Increased defecation	Constipation
Sweating	Decreased sweating
Enhancement of cognitive processes	Cognitive slowing

Adapted from Keltner, N. L. (2000). Neuroreceptor function and psychopharmacologic response. Issues in Mental Health Nursing, 21, *31-50.*

Pharmacokinetics of Psychopharmacology

The two major objectives for psychopharmacotherapy are to prevent and to cure mental disorders. Because these goals are often not feasible, less ambitious goals must be developed, such as symptom relief, reduction of disabling features, and slowing of disease progression. To best achieve these goals, the clinician must prescribe an appropriate psychotropic drug. Prerequisite properties are drug efficacy and safety. Preferably, the medication chosen will selectively attack the problem without undue side effects; unfortunately, such precision is often lacking. The clinician should command a basic understanding of pharmacokinetics so that he or she can prescribe medications that are safe and effective for patients.

In order for drugs to have an effect, they must be *absorbed* into the bloodstream, *distributed* into extracellular spaces and tissues, *metabolized* (typically into inactive and water-soluble forms), and *excreted* from the body. A brief review of the cytochrome P-450 enzymes, including their induction or inhibition (which interferes with "normal" metabolism), will be used to illustrate the metabolic process.

Absorption

Drugs taken by mouth must be absorbed into the general circulation. Drug molecules pass through the cell membrane (1) by slipping through pores and channels, (2) by a special transport system, or (3) by their lipid solubility. Most drugs are too large to pass through pores and channels and do not have a special transport system; therefore, an overwhelming amount of psychotropic drugs rely on lipid solubility.

While drugs' lipid solubility gets them into circulation, this property is also needed to get them into their site of action: the brain. This transport can be a problem, because drugs taken by mouth are ferried directly to the liver via the hepatic portal system. As a result, many drugs have a high extraction factor, meaning that a great proportion of the drug is metabolized by the liver's enzymes before entering systemic circulation. This high extraction factor is referred to as *the first-pass phenomenon*. The amount of the drug that reaches the general circulation is the drug's *bioavailability*. Bioavailability can be high (over 90%) or low (e.g., donepezil has 100% bioavailability, whereas buspirone's bioavailability is between 1% and 4%).

Distribution

Distribution is the body's ability to move the drug from the bloodstream to the extracellular fluids and to tissues. Lipid-soluble drug molecules pass through the cell membrane of the capillaries or go between the endothelial cells. Water-soluble drugs can only pass through the gaps between the cells; however, capillaries in the brain do not have gaps between the cells, as these gaps are closed (referred to as tight junctions). This barrier—the blood-brain barrier—helps maintain the brain's homeostasis, which is required for survival. Basically, only lipid-soluble drugs can penetrate the brain.

Another concept of keen interest to the advanced practitioner is volume of distribution. Volume of distribution can be roughly defined as the amount of drug that sequesters in fat tissue. The more fat an individual has (women and the elderly have a higher percentage of fat by weight than do nonelderly men), the greater the volume of distribution. Likewise, the more lipid soluble the drug, the greater the volume of distribution. Thus, highly lipid soluble drugs tend to have a high volume of distribution. In women, this pharmacokinetic variable accounts for a longer half-life for many psychotropic medications.

A third aspect of distribution is the level of protein binding. Because serum proteins are significantly larger than drug molecules, a drug is "stuck" in the bloodstream once it attaches to a serum protein. While attached to protein, the drug is said to be "protein bound." When not attached, the drug is free. Protein binding is referred to as a percentage or ratio. For example, sertraline has a protein binding of 99%, whereas venlafaxine has a much lower binding ratio of 23%. Only 1% of a dose of sertraline is free, and it is only the free drug that can have a pharmacologic effect. A bound drug cannot leave the bloodstream and thus cannot have a pharmacologic effect, cannot be metabolized in the liver, and cannot be excreted.

Metabolism

Metabolism is that part of the pharmacokinetic process that we are most familiar with. Drugs are changed metabolically by enzymes that are typically from the liver (but not always). The metabolic process is categorized as either phase I metabolism or phase II metabolism. Phase I is the type of metabolism that most nurses are aware of: during phase I, an enzyme attaches to a drug to cause a molecular change, e.g., it may oxidize or take away a chemical group such as a methyl group or hydroxyl group. In phase II, an endogenous water-soluble molecule is combined with the drug molecule (typically after a phase I action), rendering the molecule water soluble. Glucuronic acid, glutathione, and amino acids are typical molecules that accomplish this metabolic activity.

Another important aspect of metabolism is half-life. Half-life is the amount of time required to reduce serum levels by half. A drug with a 4-hour half-life will have half of the dosage gone from circulation in 4 hours; in 8 hours, only a quarter of the dosage will remain; and so on. The concept of "steady-state" is a dimension of half-life. When a drug is given consistently—that is, the same dosage at the same time interval (i.e., an interval shorter than the half-life)—then a steady-state or plasma plateau will be achieved after four half-lives. A drug with a long half-life—such as fluoxetine—can take several weeks to reach a plateau. Some antibiotics have half-lives of such short duration that they must be given by intravenous drip.

Metabolism and Cytochrome P-450

The cytochrome P-450 (CYP) enzymes metabolize 80% to 90% of drugs in the human body. There are 12 families of CYP enzymes with over 40 individual enzymes (Lehne, 2007). Six of these enzymes account for almost 90% of CYP enzymes in humans: 1A2, 3A4, 2C9, 2C19, 2D6, and 2E1 (Cozza, Armstrong, & Oesterheld, 2003). They are sometimes referred to as *isoenzymes* or *isozymes*, but they produce true enzymatic activity and thus are referred to here simply as "enzymes."

The CYP enzymes are found in the liver and in the bowel wall. The ability to produce these enzymes varies by ethnic group: for instance, 5% to 14% of Caucasians are genetically deficient in 2D6 and thus experience greater side effects at "normal" doses. Genetic polymorphism is the term used to describe the variance in genetic codes for producing these enzymes. Even the alteration of a single nucleotide in the DNA sequencing can affect the "potency" of enzymatic action. Some individuals metabolize extensively and others (about 30% of the population) are poor metabolizers. Extensive metabolizers will need a larger dose of a drug, whereas poor metabolizers will need a smaller dose of the same drug.

Cytochrome P-450 enzymes can also be induced or inhibited by other drugs. If induced, then drug substrates will be metabolized more rapidly; if inhibited, then substrates will develop increased serum levels. Lin, Smith, and Lin (2003) and Cozza et al. (2003) provided information on polymorphism consequences for specific ethnic groups. Although these variances do not necessarily hold true for all psychotropic substrates for a particular enzyme, they provided an interesting snapshot of what could happen:

- CYP 1A2: Reduced activity in 23% of Japanese; increased activity in 32% of Caucasians.
- CYP 2C19: Reduced activity in 2% to 6% of Caucasians, 5% to 20% of Japanese, 10% to 20% of Africans, and 20% of East Asians.
- CYP 2D6: Poor metabolism in 5% to 14% of Caucasians and 40% to 50% of Asians, Pacific Islanders, Africans, and African Americans.
- CYP 3A4: Polymorphisms of this enzyme have not been known to cause significant problems.

Excretion

Excretion is the body's action to rid the body of the drug molecule. Typically the kidneys perform excretion, but some excretion occurs in bile, feces, lungs, breast milk, and sweat. Excretion occurs because lipid-soluble molecules have been changed to water-soluble molecules by the metabolic process. Some drugs are so highly lipid soluble that if not for this process, it would take many years to rid the body of the drug.

Psychotropic Drugs

The information in this chapter provides a foundation for understanding the use and prescription of psychotropic drugs. Its broad information covers widely recognized basic concepts of these medications. New and unique applications of these agents are addressed in the chapters discussing specific disorders.

Antipsychotic Drugs

Antipsychotic drugs are the platform from which treatment of schizophrenia and other psychoses is launched. These drugs are so fundamental to psychiatric care that a thorough grounding in the information covered will help the clinician better understand other psychotropic agents as well.

Antipsychotic drugs are used to treat psychosis in schizophrenia, acute mania, depression, drug abuse intoxication, medication intoxication, dementia, delirium, some general medical conditions (e.g., seizures), and traumatic head injury. All of these disorders can be treated with antipsychotic drugs, but schizophrenia is the disorder most likely to be encountered by psychiatric advanced practice nurses.

Antipsychotic Drugs and Schizophrenia

Schizophrenia is a psychotic disorder that disrupts an individual's mental state and thus disrupts his or her life. It also disrupts the lives of those who are around them. These individuals struggle to distinguish the external world from their internal perceptions, and this distortion of thought is manifested in several related ways. Common symptoms of psychosis include hallucinations, delusions, and difficulty with thought organization.

Schizophrenia tends to be a lifelong illness. Keltner (2010) summarized the effects of schizophrenia as follows:

1. Schizophrenia devastates people.
2. Schizophrenia is an enormous health burden on the economy.
3. It overwhelms patients and families.
4. Its rate is not in decline.
5. More than $10 billion is spent on antipsychotic drugs each year.
6. People with schizophrenia have high rates of comorbid medical disorders, substance abuse, and unemployment, and they die younger than the general population.

The basic neurochemical theory of schizophrenia that has stood the test of time is simply this: too much dopamine causes the prominent symptoms of schizophrenia, i.e., hallucinations, delusions, and paranoid thinking. To be effective in treating schizophrenia, a drug must block dopamine receptors.

A good approach for understanding the biochemical changes associated with schizophrenia and its treatment is to look at Parkinson's disease (PD). PD is a neurodegenerative disease resulting from the premature dying of dopamine-producing neurons in an area of the midbrain called the substantia nigra (which is Latin for "black substance"). The substantia nigra projects neuronal axons to the basal ganglia or striatum. As these neurons die, less and less dopamine is synthesized, and dopamine is absolutely essential for normal movements and support for normal movements. The tipping point for the emergence of PD symptoms occurs when about 80% of these neurons die off (Agid, 1991). Because a balance between dopamine and acetylcholine is required for normal movement, the decline in dopamine levels leads to an unevenness or imbalance between the two neurotransmitters. Because both modulate striatal GABA (dopamine is inhibitory and acetylcholine is excitatory), this imbalance leads to motor difficulties. Treatment of PD often centers on increasing brain dopamine levels. Drugs such as levodopa, a precursor to dopamine in the catecholamine synthesis chain, are given in order to overcome the loss of dopamine. As seen in Table 6-2, it is apparent that dopamine elevations can cause schizophrenia-like symptoms, such as hallucinations and delusions, whereas dopamine depletions can lead to hypokinetic disorders. PD is a good model for understanding drug treatment for schizophrenia because, in treating PD with a dopaminergic agent, the clinician can inadvertently cause a schizophrenia-like problem. Similarly, in treating schizophrenia, the clinician can cause a PD-like problem.

Perhaps the most useful approach for thinking about schizophrenia in relation to pharmacotherapy is to use the approach described by Andreasen, Crowe, and others almost 30 years ago (Andreasen & Olsen, 1982; Crowe, 1982) that looks at schizophrenia as "positive" or "negative." Positive schizophrenia symptoms tend to be florid, whereas negative schizophrenia symptoms suggest a subtraction from the personality. The positive symptoms are thought to be related to elevations of dopamine, whereas the opposite may be true for the negative symptoms. Hence, blocking dopamine receptors is ideal for positive symptoms, but it may compound the negative symptoms. Table 6-6 outlines some distinctions between positive and negative symptoms of schizophrenia.

Traditional Antipsychotic Drugs

Antipsychotics can be viewed from the perspective of traditional agents (roughly those developed between 1950 and 1990) and the newer, atypical antipsychotic drugs (developed 1990 to present). The traditional drugs can be further subtyped based on potency. *Potency* refers to drug activity: if a drug has high potency, a smaller dose is needed to alleviate symptoms; if a drug has low potency, a larger dose is needed to alleviate symptoms. For example, 2 mg of haloperidol is as effective as 100 mg of chlorpromazine in treating the symptoms of schizophrenia,

TABLE 6-6 COMPARISON OF POSITIVE AND NEGATIVE SYMPTOMS OF SCHIZOPHRENIA

Parameter	Positive Symptoms	Negative Symptoms
Prognosis	Better	Poorer
Onset	Typically acute	Chronic
Intellect	More intact	Less intact
Pathophysiology	D_2 hyperactivity (limbic)	D_2 hypoactivity? (cortical)
Pathoanatomy	Unknown	Increased ventricular brain ratios, other atrophy

Adapted from Andreasen, N. C. (1985). Positive vs. negative schizophrenia: A critical evaluation. Schizophrenia Bulletin, 11, *380.*

BOX 6-1 Thresholds of Dopamine D_2 Receptor Antagonism Triggering Desired or Unwanted Effects

- When about 60% to 70% of dopamine D_2 receptors are blocked in the mesolimbic tract, a therapeutic effect occurs.
- When about 70% of dopamine D_2 receptors are blocked in the tuberoinfundibular tract, prolactin levels increase.
- When about 80% of dopamine D_2 receptors are blocked in the nigrostriatal tract, extrapyramidal side effects develop.

From Sedvall, G. (1995). PET studies on the neuroreceptor effects of antipsychotic drugs. Current Approaches to Psychosis, 4, 1; and Seeman, P., & Van Tol, H. H. (1994). Dopamine receptor pharmacology. Trends in Pharmacologic Science, 15*(7), 264.*

and thus haloperidol is more potent than chlorpromazine. A few drugs are somewhere between the polar designations of "high potency" and "low potency"; examples of these "moderate-potency" antipsychotics can be found in Table 6-7.

Depending on the symptoms that the clinician wishes to alleviate, a drug can be high potency for one symptom and low potency for another. For example, haloperidol is certainly not more potent at causing dry mouth or blurred vision, so in what way is it more potent than chlorpromazine? Haloperidol is more potent than chlorpromazine at blocking or antagonizing dopamine receptors; 2 mg of haloperidol will block as many dopamine receptors as 100 mg of chlorpromazine. Yet here we must become even more specific: there are five dopamine receptors, so is haloperidol more potent in blocking all of these five receptors? The answer is no. Of these five dopamine receptors, only the dopamine D_2 receptor is considered when describing a traditional antipsychotic as high potency or low potency. To reiterate, 2 mg of haloperidol blocks as many dopamine D_2 receptors as 100 mg of chlorpromazine. Box 6-1 outlines the thresholds of dopamine D_2 blockade triggering specific effects.

On the other hand, chlorpromazine and other low-potency traditional drugs would be described as having high potency if the object of discussion were cholinergic muscarinic or α_1-adrenergic receptors. The low-potency drugs cause a much higher incidence of dry mouth, blurred vision, constipation, and orthostatic hypotension. The high-potency antipsychotics have a higher incidence of extrapyramidal side effects (EPSEs). The conclusion to be drawn is simply this: dry mouth, blurred vision, and so forth are products of cholinergic muscarinic blockade, orthostatic hypotension results from antagonism of α_1 receptors, and blocking dopamine D_2 receptors (only in the nigrostriatal tract) leads to EPSEs. In looking at the latter side effect, an anticholinergic such as benztropine (Cogentin) is often given with a high-potency drug in order to prevent or treat EPSEs. Why? The benztropine rebalances the dopamine/acetylcholine equation: high-potency antipsychotics block dopamine, and the anticholinergic benztropine blocks acetylcholine, thus reestablishing the balance.

TABLE 6-7 RELATIVELY COMMON TRADITIONAL ANTIPSYCHOTICS

Low-Potency Antipsychotics	Moderate-Potency Antipsychotics	High-Potency Antipsychotics
Chlorpromazine (Thorazine)	Loxapine (Loxitane)	Haloperidol (Haldol)
Thioridazine (Mellaril)	Perphenazine (Trilafon)	Fluphenazine (Prolixin)

Among the side effects caused by traditional antipsychotics, three stand out:

1. EPSEs
2. Hyperprolactinemia
3. Increased negative/cognitive symptoms

An interesting matter of speculation is why the low-potency drugs do not cause as many EPSEs as the high-potency drugs. The answer probably resides in the non-dopamine receptors that low-potency agents block, i.e., cholinergic receptors. In other words, one could say that chlorpromazine does not cause as many EPSEs because chlorpromazine contains anticholinergic properties: the clinician need not add benztropine to the treatment plan because chlorpromazine is already anticholinergic. Table 6-8 outlines the common EPSEs.

Another major problem associated with traditional antipsychotic drugs is the issue of elevated prolactin levels, known as hyperprolactinemia. Elevated prolactin levels occur because dopamine D_2 receptors are blocked in the anterior pituitary by traditional antipsychotics. Consequences of hyperprolactinemia include impotence, decreased libido, amenorrhea, galactorrhea, gynecomastia, lowered sperm count, and feminization (Box 6-2). Prolactin elevation is a major drawback to traditional medications

TABLE 6-8 EXTRAPYRAMIDAL SIDE EFFECTS

Side Effect	Description
Drug-induced parkinsonism	Resting tremor, bradykinesia, rigidity, postural instability
Akathisia	Moderate to severe inner restlessness; inability to sit still
Akinesia	Inability to initiate movement
Dystonia	Sustained muscle contractions; muscle freezing
Dyskinesia	Diminished voluntary movement with increased involuntary movements such as tics and chorea
Tardive dyskinesia	Type of dyskinesia in which involuntary movements tend to occur in tongue and mouth muscles, e.g., tongue protrusion, lip smacking, teeth grinding
Neuroleptic malignant syndrome	Potentially life-threatening effect of antipsychotics typically expressed as high temperature and significant rigidity and rhabdomyolysis

BOX 6-2 Side Effects Associated With Elevated Prolactin

Side Effects in Women

- Amenorrhea
- Loss of libido
- Galactorrhea

Side Effects in Men

- Impotence
- Loss of libido
- Gynecomastia
- Lowered sperm count
- Feminization

and also a key obstacle to adherence to the drug regimen. Hyperprolactinemia will be reintroduced in the later discussion of atypical antipsychotics.

The third major concern is the increase in negative/cognitive symptoms. Traditional antipsychotics can increase negative/cognitive symptoms by dopamine antagonism and also by blocking cholinergic receptors. As noted above, acetylcholine has a key role in learning and memory. When acetylcholine receptors are blocked, learning and memory are compromised.

Atypical Antipsychotic Drugs

The search for new antischizophrenia drugs was propelled by the many problems associated with the traditional agents. EPSEs (including the potentially lethal neuroleptic malignant syndrome), elevated prolactin, and increased negative/cognitive symptoms caused many patients to choose between being miserable with side effects or being miserable with schizophrenia (i.e., nonadherence). Into this no-win situation, a number of laboratories began pursuing medicines that would continue to reduce positive symptoms while not causing the problems just mentioned. The question was simple, but the answer complex:

The Question: How do you manufacture a drug that will block hallucinations and delusions but not cause EPSEs, hyperprolactinemia, or increase negative/cognitive symptoms?

The Answer: You develop a drug that can decrease dopamine in one specific area while not decreasing dopamine in other areas.

The key to answering this simple question was based on the arduous task of uncovering four different dopamine tracts in the brain. If you review the question above and the discussion of major side effects in the traditional antipsychotics section, you will note that one positive event and three overarching negative events developed from taking traditional antipsychotic drugs:

1. Decreased positive symptoms (positive event)
2. EPSEs (negative event)
3. Elevated prolactin (negative event)
4. Increased negative/cognitive symptoms (negative event)

The total of these "events" is four, and there are four dopaminergic pathways in the brain that are directly related to these events:

1. Positive symptoms are linked to the mesolimbic dopamine tract.
2. EPSEs are linked to the nigrostriatal dopamine tract.
3. Elevated prolactin is linked to the tuberoinfundibular tract.
4. Increased negative/cognitive symptoms are linked to the mesocortical tract.

All of these "events" are caused by blockade of dopamine D_2 receptors. If one could find a drug that would continue to block dopamine in the mesolimbic tract but not decrease and perhaps even increase dopamine in the nigrostriatal, tuberoinfundibular, and mesocortical tracts, one could treat positive symptoms (mesolimbic tract) without causing EPSEs (nigrostriatal tract), hyperprolactinemia (tuberoinfundibular tract), or increased negative/cognitive symptoms (mesocortical tract).

Atypical antipsychotics are purported to do this very thing. It is said that they are effective in treating positive symptoms, do not cause EPSEs, do not elevate prolactin, and do not increase negative/cognitive symptoms (and may improve these symptoms). Actual practice with these drugs does not support a total agreement with these claims, but certainly these side effects are reduced when atypicals are prescribed (Asenjo Lobos, Komossa, Rummel-Kluge, et al., 2010; Komossa, Rummel-Kluge, Hunger, et al., 2009a; Komossa, Rummel-Kluge, Schmid, et al., 2009b; Komossa, Rummel-Kluge, Hunger, et al., 2010a; Komossa, Rummel-Kluge, Schmid, 2010b).

Mechanism of Action

The mechanism of action by which atypical drugs achieve this seemingly highly selective approach to treatment is the antagonism of a specific serotonin receptor, 5-HT_{2A}. This receptor can be found on the axon terminal of neurons that produce dopamine. When serotonin activates these receptors, the release of dopamine decreases. By building into the atypical antipsychotics a mechanism to block the 5-HT_{2A} receptors from serotonin, dopamine release is increased. Interestingly, this seems to affect the three tracts that have a negative impact on treatment: the nigrostriatal, tuberoinfundibular, and mesocortical tracts. For reasons not fully elucidated in the literature, dopamine blockade in the mesolimbic tracts continues to occur, thus diminishing hallucinations, delusions, and other positive symptoms. This recognition led to these drugs' being initially referred to as D_2/5-HT_{2A} receptor antagonists.

Atypical Antipsychotic Drugs

There are six atypical antipsychotic agents: clozapine, risperidone, olanzapine, quetiapine, ziprasidone, and aripiprazole.

Clozapine

Clozapine (Clozaril) was introduced in 1990 in the United States and was the first of the atypical antipsychotics to be marketed there. It had been in use in Europe and China for some time, but its debut in America was delayed due to a serious side effect: agranulocytosis. Aganulocytosis is a condition in which white blood cell counts (WBCs) drop so dramatically that there is a high possibility that the individual will be overwhelmed by an infection. Because this drug caused a number of deaths within the first years of its release, clinicians and agencies became very cautious about prescribing it. However, because clozapine is a very effective antipsychotic and has helped people seemingly out of the reach of other medications, clinicians persisted until they could develop protocols to make this drug safe.

The first line of defense in keeping patients safe when taking clozapine is a thorough work-up before therapy is initiated. If patients are deemed suitable for clozapine therapy, the next step is taken: frequent and regular analysis of WBCs. Typically, patients must submit to laboratory testing once per week; if no concerns are noted after 6 months, some patients are permitted to move to a biweekly schedule for blood draws. Box 6-3 outlines protocols for clozapine therapy.

BOX 6-3 Parameters for Clozapine Therapy Related to Agranulocytosis

1. To initiate clozapine therapy, WBC must be over 3500/mm³ and the ANC above 2000/mm³.
2. These parameters must be monitored weekly for 6 months and then biweekly if no problems arise.
3. If WBC drops below 3000/mm³ or the ANC drops below 1500/mm³, then stop clozapine.
4. If no infection develops, once the original parameters are reached again, clozapine can be restarted.
5. If WBC drops below 2000/mm³ and ANC drops below 1000/mm³, permanently discontinue clozapine.

ANC, absolute neutrophil count; WBC, white blood cell count.

Risperidone

Risperidone (Risperdal) was approved in 1994 and, while an atypical drug, is different from clozapine in that it does not cause agranulocytosis and has some variance in its mechanism of action. For instance, risperidone appears to have a greater affinity for dopamine D_2 receptors than does clozapine. At higher doses, risperidone is known to cause both EPSEs and hyperprolactinemia. Because *not* causing these two side effects is part of the rationale for an antipsychotic's being labeled "atypical," risperidone has detractors who question this designation. Nonetheless, it is an effective antipsychotic and one of the most prescribed. An injectable, long-acting version is also available, Risperdal Consta.

Paliperidone (Invega) is a relatively new drug. Paliperidone is a metabolite of risperidone and is thought to have a similar side-effect profile and mechanism of action. The formulation available as Invega comes in an extended-release form.

Olanzapine

Olanzapine (Zyprexa) is perhaps the most popular of the atypical antipsychotics among clinicians. Olanzapine is effective in the treatment of both schizophrenia and bipolar disorder. Unfortunately, olanzapine can cause significant weight gain and consequent diabetes. Fast-dissolving and intramuscular formulations are available.

Quetiapine

Quetiapine (Seroquel) was brought to market in 1997. It is similar in action to the drugs just mentioned. However, one dimension of quetiapine does stand out from the other drugs: it is being abused for its anxiolytic and sedative effects. Of course, these same qualities can be exploited clinically. Quetiapine abuse in jail and prison settings is a phenomenon creating a wave of attention (Keltner & Vance, 2008). Inmates are known to feign mental illness in order to obtain this medication, while others who legitimately need the drug are often coerced to turn it over to more powerful prisoners.

Ziprasidone

Ziprasidone (Geodon) is also recognized as an effective antipsychotic. It has been linked to heart problems brought on by a lengthening of the QTc interval, and thus careful pretreatment screening is indicated. An intramuscular version is available. Absorption of ziprasidone is increased with food. In contrast to the other atypical antipsychotics, ziprasidone has significant activation (is an agonist) of 5-HT_{1A} receptors. An agonist of this receptor can precipitate (1) decreased anxiety, (2) a decrease in depressive symptoms, and (3) an improvement in negative symptoms via a nondopamine avenue. Because of these "extra" actions, ziprasidone is favored by many clinicians.

Aripiprazole

Aripiprazole (Abilify) is the last atypical antipsychotic to be mentioned. Its mechanism of action is significantly different from the other agents: aripiprazole is described as a dopamine partial agonist. Although perhaps overly simplistic, a good way to conceptualize this feature is to think of aripiprazole as bringing all dopamine levels to some mid-level of availability. In areas of the brain in which overactivity of dopamine causes symptoms, aripiprazole reduces dopamine levels; in areas of the brain in which underactivity of dopamine causes symptoms, aripiprazole increases dopamine availability. It modulates dopamine downward in the mesolimbic tract while modulating dopamine upward in the nigrostriatal, tuberoinfundibular, and mesocortical tracts. Thus, through the unique action of being a partial agonist, aripiprazole theoretically brings dopamine availability to a consistent level within the four dopaminergic pathways.

Problems With Atypical Antipsychotics

Atypical antipsychotics can be sedating and, more importantly, may cause significant weight gain. Weight gain may lead to what is called metabolic syndrome (or insulin resistance syndrome) and type 2 diabetes. When metabolic syndrome develops, the body begins to struggle to metabolize glucose, and the body's insulin is resisted by insulin receptors on cells. This leaves the individual with elevated blood glucose levels and the concomitant problems of obesity, elevated lipids, and hypertension. Drug manufacturers are required to include a warning about these problems. Table 6-9 captures the dosages and incidence for EPSEs, anticholinergic effects, orthostasis, sedation, and weight gain in both the typical and atypical antipsychotics. The cost for a month's supply for a few selected drugs is also included in the table. As will be readily apparent, the atypical antipsychotics are significantly more expensive than the traditional drugs.

Antidepressant Drugs

Antidepressant drugs are widely prescribed. In fact, three of the top 15 brand name drugs sold in America are antidepressants: #3 Lexapro, #9 Effexor XR, and #13 Cymbalta (Drug Topics Staff, 2009). Antidepressants are used to treat depression, anxiety, panic disorder, obsessive-compulsive disorder, eating disorders, chronic pain, and post-traumatic stress disorder.

As will be discussed in Chapter 13, biochemical explanations for depression stress the importance of serotonin, norepinephrine, and dopamine deficiencies. All of the drugs and categories of drugs that are discussed in this chapter increase neuronal availability of one, two, or all three of these neurotransmitters (see Table 6-10 for neurotransmitter reuptake potency of the antidepressants). There are several categories of antidepressants. All but the last two of these categories (numbers 6 and 7, below) increase serotonin, norepinephrine, dopamine levels, or any combination of these by blocking the reuptake of the neurotransmitter after it is released into the synaptic cleft. The categories of antidepressants are

1. Tricyclic antidepressants (TCAs)
2. Selective serotonin reuptake inhibitors (SSRIs)
3. Serotonin-norepinephrine reuptake inhibitors (SNRIs)
4. Norepinephrine reuptake inhibitors (NRIs)
5. Norepinephrine dopamine reuptake inhibitors (NDRIs)
6. Noradrenergic and specific serotonergic antidepressants (NaSSAs)
7. Monoamine oxidase inhibitors (MAOIs)

With this large selection of antidepressant categories to choose from, it can be intimidating for the clinician to attempt to understand mechanisms of action and significant differences that help in providing the best medication for the patient. However, though each of these drugs may report a different lag time to clinical effectiveness, it is appropriate to tell patients that, in most cases, this effect will be achieved within 2 to 4 weeks. Not only is there a delayed response to contend with, but many patients must take these agents for several months to several years in order to overcome depressive symptoms.

Tricyclic Antidepressants

TRICYCLIC ANTIDEPRESSANTS

Serotonergic TCAs	Adrenergic TCAs
Amitriptyline (Elavil, Endep)	Desipramine (Norpramin)
Clomipramine (Anafranil)	Nortriptyline (Pamelor, Aventyl)
Imipramine (Tofranil)	Protriptyline (Vivactil)

TCAs were discovered early in the pursuit to fight depression with chemicals. These drugs are the standards by which succeeding generations of antidepressants have been compared. Truthfully, newer antidepressants, such as the SSRIs, are not *better* antidepressants (particularly for severe depression), but they do cause fewer side effects (Agius, Gardner, Liu, et al., 2010; Anderson, 2000; Bruce, Macgillivray, Ogston, et al., 2005; Chen, Gao, & Kemp, 2011; Cipriani, Furukawa, Salanti, et al., 2009; Parikh, 2009).

TCA side effects include anticholinergic, antihistaminic, and antiadrenergic effects. Anticholinergic effects are

TABLE 6-9 TRADITIONAL AND ATYPICAL ANTIPSYCHOTICS

Drug	Usual Adult Maintenance Range (mg/day)	Rate of Extrapyramidal Side Effects	Rate of Anticholinergic Effects	Rate of Orthostasis	Rate of Sedation	Rate of Weight Gain	Monthly Cost
Traditional (First Generation)							
HIGH-POTENCY DRUGS							
Fluphenazine (Prolixin)	0.5–40	High	Low	Low	Low	Low	$10-$30
Haloperidol (Haldol)	1–15	High	Low	Low	Low	Low	$14-$21
MODERATE-POTENCY DRUG							
Perphenazine (Etrafon, Trilafon)	12–64	High	Low	Low	Moderate	Low	$102
LOW-POTENCY DRUGS							
Chlorpromazine (Thorazine)	200–1000	Moderate	Moderate	High	Moderate	High	$23
Thioridazine (Mellaril)	200–800	Low	High	High	High	High	$12-$30
Atypical (Second Generation)							
Aripiprazole (Abilify)	10–30	Low	Low	Low	Low	Low	$589
Clozapine (Clozaril)	75–900	Low	High	High	High	High	$690
Olanzapine (Zyprexa)	5–20	Low	Moderate	Low	High	High	$546
Paliperidone (Invega)	3–12	Low	Low	Moderate	Moderate	Moderate	$532
Quetiapine (Seroquel)	200–800	Low	Low	Moderate	Moderate	Moderate	$549
Risperidone (Risperdal)	0.5–6.0	Low*	Low	Moderate	Moderate	Moderate	$450
Ziprasidone (Geodon)	40–160	Low	Low	Low	Low	Low	$622

Costs obtained from Consumer Reports Best Buy Drugs (2009) and Keltner and Vance (2008). Prices based on brand name for atypical agents.

*At higher doses risperidone causes extrapyramidal side effects.

TABLE 6-10 ANTIDEPRESSANTS: DAILY DOSAGE AND NEUROTRANSMITTER REUPTAKE POTENCY

Antidepressant	Daily Dosage Range (mg)	Neurotransmitter Reuptake Potency: 1 (Low) to 5 (High)		
		NE	5-HT	DA
Tricyclic Antidepressants				
Amitriptyline (Elavil)	75–300	1	3	1
Clomipramine (Anafranil)	75–300	1	4	1
Desipramine (Norpramin)	75–300	5	1	1
Imipramine (Tofranil)	75–300	2	3	1
Nortriptyline (Pamelor, Aventyl)	50–150	4	2	1
Selective Serotonin Reuptake Inhibitors				
Citalopram (Celexa)	10–60	1	4	1
Escitalopram (Lexapro)	10–20	1	4	1
Fluoxetine (Prozac)	10–80	1	3	1
Fluvoxamine (Luvox)	50–300	1	4	1
Paroxetine (Paxil)	10–60	1	5	1
Sertraline (Zoloft)	25–200	1	4	2
Other Antidepressants				
Bupropion (Wellbutrin)	150–450	1	0/1	2
Duloxetine (Cymbalta)	20–60	3	2	1
Mirtazapine (Remeron)	7.5–45	1	1	0
Trazodone (Desyrel)	150–600	0	2	1
Venlafaxine (Effexor)	75–225	2	4	1
Desvenlafaxine (Pristiq)	50	2	4	1
Monoamine Oxidase Inhibitors				
Phenelzine (Nardil)	30–90			
Tranylcypromine (Parnate)	20–60			
Moclobemide (Manerix)	300–600			
Selegiline (Emsam)	6–12			

DA, dopamine; 5-HT, serotonin; NE, norepinephrine.

the classic effects caused when muscarinic acetylcholine receptors are blocked in certain cranial nerves. Box 6-4 outlines the anticholinergic effect on cranial nerves of muscarinic acetylcholine receptor blockage. The histamine antagonism leads to drowsiness and weight gain. When α_1-adrenergic receptors are blocked by these agents, blood vessels lose their ability to constrict, leading to hypotension and dizziness.

A more concerning adverse effect of TCAs is the threat of deadly cardiac arrhythmias and seizures. These serious outcomes are primarily related to the disruption of sodium channels when TCAs are taken in very high doses (Stahl, 1998). For this reason, TCAs can be potentially hazardous to patients who are suicidal. Accordingly, the prescriber must be judicious when first ordering these for a depressed patient because as little as a 7-day supply can be fatal, because suicidal overdose can cause cardiac arrhythmias and seizures.

TCAs increase serotonin and norepinephrine by blocking the reuptake of these neurotransmitters back into the presynaptic neuron. Some TCAs are more efficient at blocking the reuptake of serotonin, and some are more efficient at blocking the reupake of norepinephrine. This property is typically expressed as a ratio. For example, amitriptyline preferentially blocks the reuptake of serotonin to norepinephrine at a 3:1 ratio. As opposed to some antidepressants, which will be discussed later, this preferential ratio is not affected by dosage. Drugs that are more serotonergic are referred to as tertiary amine TCAs, and those that preferentially boost norepinephrine are called secondary amine TCAs.

BOX 6-4 Anticholinergic Effects of Blocking Muscarinic Cholinergic Receptors on Four Cranial Nerves

- Cranial nerve III (oculomotor): mydriasis and blurred vision
- Cranial nerve IV (facial): dry mouth, decreased respiratory secretions, and decreased tearing
- Cranial nerve IX (glossopharyngeal): dry mouth and decreased respiratory secretions
- Cranial nerve X (vagus): constipation, urinary hesitancy, and increased heart rate

Selective Serotonin Reuptake Inhibitors

SELECTIVE SEROTONIN REUPTAKE INHIBITORS
Citalopram (Celexa)
Fluoxetine (Prozac)
Paroxetine (Paxil)
Escitalopram (Lexapro)
Fluvoxamine (Luvox)
Sertraline (Zoloft)

SSRIs are commonly prescribed antidepressants and work by increasing the availability of serotonin. Selection of SSRIs is typically driven by clinician experience and avoidance of side effects. These drugs are not better antidepressants than TCAs (Rush, Trivedi, Wisniewski, et al., 2006; Sachs, Nierenberg, Calabrese, et al., 2007), but they do provide a better side-effect profile overall (Cipriani et al., 2009; Parikh, 2009), particularly the absence of fatal cardiac effects (Sicouri & Antzelevitch, 2008). However, though the side-effect profile is less potentially lethal, adverse effects can become troubling to the point of nonadherence (Cooke & Keltner, 2008). Specifically, sexual dysfunction is very common, with anecdotal reports suggesting that 80% of patients taking these drugs have a significant change in their sexual life. Gastrointestinal disturbances are also major untoward effects of SSRIs.

SSRIs can affect all three stages of sexual intercourse: desire, arousal (lubrication or erection), and orgasm. The decrease in libido is related to the mesolimbic pathway (see Table 6-1); thus, it is most likely the inhibition of dopamine (the pleasure neurotransmitter) by serotonin in the mesolimbic pathway that causes this drop in sexual interest (Damsa, Bumb, Bianchi-Demicheli, et al., 2004). Serotonin axons that move caudally from the brainstem affect other neurotransmitters that facilitate lubrication/erection and orgasm. Though decline in all three stages is reported in the literature, first-hand experience (NLK) with male patients suggests that anorgasmia is the most common and most troubling sexual side effect. In the treatment of deficiency of stages 1 (desire) and 3 (orgasm), dopamine-enhancing agents such as bupropion are particularly helpful. Erection difficulties are treatable with sildenafil (Viagra) or a similar drug. Unfortunately, when sexual dysfunction occurs, discontinuing the SSRI may not restore normal sexual functioning. Some patients report continued sexual problems months and years later (Csoka, Bahrick, & Mehtonen, 2008).

As noted previously, the majority (90%) of serotonin is synthesized in the gut wall (Mason, Morris, & Balcezak, 2000). Elevations of serotonin, as caused by SSRIs, increase serotonin activation of 5-HT$_3$ receptors. These receptors are in the gastrointestinal tract and in the vomiting center of the medulla. Drugs that block 5-HT$_3$ receptors such as ondansetron (Zofran) can decrease gastrointestinal upset (cramps, diarrhea, nausea) and vomiting.

Mechanism of Action

In a classic treatise on antidepressants, Stahl (1998) moved the discussion of SSRIs beyond the simplistic notion of a drug blocking a return "tunnel" back into the presynaptic neuron. He pointed out that, initially, the reuptake transporter blockade occurs in the raphe nuclei. After serotonin levels rise around the soma of the neuron, the autoreceptors (5-HT$_{1A}$) in that area become desensitized to serotonin and cease functioning normally. This allows serotonin to increase because the feedback system is turned off. Serotonin release at the axon terminal into the synaptic cleft then increases as well. The blockade of these presynaptic reuptake transporters enhances the buildup of serotonin. The final piece of the antidepressant effect may be the desensitization of postsynaptic serotonin receptors. Stahl suggested that this sequential process may explain the delay observed in the therapeutic response to SSRIs.

Serotonin-Norepinephrine Reuptake Inhibitors

SEROTONIN-NOREPINEPHRINE REUPTAKE INHIBITORS
Desvenlafaxine (Pristiq)
Duloxetine (Cymbalta)
Venlafaxine (Effexor, Effexor XR)

Serotonin-norepinephrine reuptake inhibitors (SNRIs) have found wide acceptance by clinicians and patients and are two of the top 15 brand name drugs sold in America: venlafaxine (Effexor XR) at #9 and duloxetine (Cymbalta) at #13 (Drug Topics Staff, 2009). The SNRI venlafaxine increases serotonin at lower dosages and increases norepinephrine at mid-range doses; at higher dosages, it increases levels of dopamine (Lee & Keltner, 2006). Venlafaxine does not cause the same degree of side effects as the TCAs and SSRIs owing to lower affinity for muscarinic, histaminic, and adrenergic receptors. Common side effects include drowsiness, dry mouth, dizziness, constipation, nervousness, sweating, and anorexia. A few patients have experienced elevated blood pressure related to venlafaxine, and thus certain patients should be monitored for this effect.

Venlafaxine is not a potent inhibitor of CYP enzymes and, coupled with its low protein binding (23%), produces relatively few drug interactions. Desvenlafaxine (Pristiq) is a metabolite of venlafaxine and has similar levels of efficacy and a similar side-effect profile. Duloxetine also increases intrasynaptic serotonin and norepinephrine, although the exact mechanism remains to be fully elucidated. It is an effective antidepressant and has a similar side-effect profile to that of venlafaxine, though it has not been observed to elevate blood pressure. Duloxetine is used with relatively high frequency to treat diabetic neuropathy.

Norepinephrine Reuptake Inhibitors

NOREPINEPHRINE REUPTAKE INHIBITORS
Atomoxetine (Strattera)

Norepinephrine reuptake inhibitors (NRIs) are not as commonly prescribed or as well recognized by the lay public. Because norepinephrine deficiency is consistently mentioned as a factor in depression, one would expect elevation of this neurotransmitter to be therapeutic. Unfortunately, this does not appear to be the case. This ineffectiveness explains NRIs' lack of prescriptive endorsement. Atomoxetine is used to treat attention deficit-hyperactivity disorders. Side effects include dry mouth, insomnia, dizziness, elevations in heart rate and blood pressure, and constipation.

Norepinephrine Dopamine Reuptake Inhibitors

NOREPINEPHRINE DOPAMINE REUPTAKE INHIBITORS
Bupropion (Wellbutrin, Zyban)

Norepinephrine dopamine reuptake inhibitors (NDRIs) are the only antidepressants with dopamine reuptake inhibition as a major mechanism of action, and they do not affect serotonin systems. Bupropion is only one of these drugs with any kind of wide usage. Because bupropion does affect dopaminergic systems, it offers a true change in treatment strategy for patients not responding to the serotonin-enhancing agents. As noted above, dopamine suppression plays a role in antidepressant-induced sexual dysfunction. Bupropion is often used to augment other antidepressants in hopes of relieving these sexual problems; at other times, a switch is made to bupropion in order to alleviate sexual problems. Bupropion has a narrow therapeutic index, but it is far less lethal than the TCAs. Owing to its impact on the adrenergic system, overstimulation, insomnia, and agitation can develop. The short-acting formulation has been associated with seizures, but not the extended-release form. The Zyban trade name is marketed as a smoking cessation agent. Theoretically, Zyban's ability to increase dopamine overcomes the craving associated with withdrawal from nicotine (Keltner & Grant, 2006, 2008).

Noradrenergic and Specific Serotonergic Antidepressants

NONADRENERGIC AND SPECIFIC SEROTONERGIC ANTIDEPRESSANTS
Mirtazapine (Remeron, Remeron Sol Tabs)

Noradrenergic and specific serotonergic antidepressants (NaSSAs) are drugs that elevate serotonin and norepinephrine in a unique way. Mirtazapine owns perhaps the most interesting mechanisms of action:

1. First, it is an antagonist at the α_2 autoreceptor. This autoreceptor provides feedback to both the serotonergic and the adrenergic systems. When α_2 is blocked, it "tells" the neuron to synthesize and release more serotonin and more norepinephrine.
2. Second, mirtazapine is an antagonist at the 5-HT_{2a} receptor and the 5-HT_3 receptor. Remember that when 5-HT_{2A} is exposed to serotonin, dopamine release is reduced, causing sexual problems. When 5-HT_3 is activated by serotonin, gastrointestinal symptoms and vomiting can develop. Mirtazapine blocks both 5-HT_{2A} and 5-HT_3, thus avoiding or at least minimizing sexual dysfunction and gastrointestinal upset. Further, the elevation in serotonin can, in turn, desensitize the 5-HT_{1A} autoreceptor and disinhibit the synthesis and release of serotonin even further.

Mirtazapine is an effective antidepressant, and it is thought to have a more rapid clinical effect (Croom, Perry, & Plosker, 2009). Common side effects include somnolence, increased appetite, weight gain, and dizziness. At lower dosages (<15 mg), sedation is common because of mirtazapine's antihistaminic profile; paradoxically, at higher dosages, drowsiness decreases. This seeming contradiction is thought to result from a greater activation by norepinephrine, which counteracts antihistaminic-caused sedation. Beyond its antidepressive effects, mirtazapine has been useful in treating people with SSRI-induced sexual dysfunction, in treating depressed patients who have poor appetites, and in treating individuals who are struggling to sleep (at lower dosages). The orally dissolvable formulation is particularly attractive for patients with swallowing difficulties; it dissolves on the tongue in about 30 seconds.

Monoamine Oxidase Inhibitors

MONOAMINE OXIDASE INHIBITORS
Moclobemide (Manerix)
Phenelzine (Nardil)
Selegiline (Emsam)
Tranylcypromine (Parnate)

Monoamine oxidase inhibitors (MAOIs) are seldom prescribed. These drugs, though effective antidepressants, can and have caused serious and deadly reactions. Because they are so rarely prescribed, only a short mention will be made.

MAOIs work by blocking the metabolism of monoamines. As discussed previously, the monoamine neurotransmitters are dopamine, norepinephrine, and serotonin. When the degradation of these molecules is blocked, they build up in the axon terminal and are increasingly released into the synapse. Because deficiency in these molecules has been repeatedly postulated to cause depressive symptoms, one would surmise that by sharply reducing their metabolic demise, depression would be decreased. While this assumption is true, the buildup of these neurotransmitters can also cause a profound effect if, for some reason, the axonal supply is released all at once. Severe hypertension, central nervous system excitability, and death have occurred when agents that have the ability to release monoamine stores are ingested. These interactants include both drugs and foods. (See a pharmacology textbook for a list of substances that must be avoided.) In summary, however, drugs that are sympathomimetics (i.e., stimulate adrenergic receptors), drugs that increase serotonin levels (e.g., SSRIs), and some central nervous system drugs (such as meperidine, which should be absolutely avoided) can cause a lethal interaction. Foods that contain tyramine (an amine) should also be avoided.

Phenelzine (Nardil) and tranylcypromine (Parnate) are traditional MAOIs in that they inhibit both MAO-A (which metabolizes norepinephrine and 5-HT) and MAO-B (which metabolizes dopamine). They are referred to as nonselective. Moclobemide, on the other hand, is a selective inhibitor of just MAO-A and thus is dubbed a reversible inhibitor of monoamine oxidase A (RIMA). It increases the availability of serotonin and norepinephrine. Selegiline is selective for MAO-B and increases the availability of just dopamine. Selegiline is formulated as a transdermal patch, Emsam, that releases the medication slowly over the course of the day. Because it bypasses the stomach, there is less need for dietary control except when higher dosages are given (Bristol-Meyers Squibb, 2006).

Other Important Issues Related to Antidepressants

Five important issues should be briefly discussed in order to provide a more complete review of antidepressants: serotonin syndrome, antidepressant apathy syndrome, antidepressant withdrawal, antidepressant loss of effectiveness, and antidepressant-induced suicide.

Serotonin Syndrome

Serotonin syndrome is almost identical to neuroleptic malignant syndrome in terms of signs and symptoms: hyperthermia, rigidity, altered mental status, and autonomic changes. These physical expressions of dysfunction are precipitated by elevations of serotonin. Serotonin syndrome can develop from SSRI monotherapy, but most often it is the result of drug interactions. Elevations can develop due to interference with CYP metabolism, inhibition of monoamine oxidase, metabolism of serotonin, or prevention of serotonin reuptake (Wren, Frizzell, & Keltner, 2003). Drug combinations necessitating caution include SSRIs combined with serotonin agonists, MAOIs, lithium, levodopa, meperidine, or TCAs (Weitzel & Jiwanlal, 2001). Non-SSRI combinations have been lethal as well, including MAOIs, TCAs, amphetamine, venlafaxine, mirtazapine, and tramadol. Street drugs, such as Ecstasy and LSD, have also been reported to cause serotonin syndrome. It has been suggested that excessive stimulation of 5-HT_{1A} and perhaps 5-HT_2 receptors cause serotonin syndrome (Wren et al., 2003).

Antidepressant Apathy Syndrome

A relatively new concern that has surfaced in regard to antidepressants in general and SSRIs in particular is antidepressant apathy syndrome (Lee & Keltner, 2005). Many patients find the effect to be not so much a lack of depression but rather an overwhelming lack of interest. Some have referred to this phenomenon as mood anesthesia. Of course, indifference most likely "feels" better than depression, but it is not the goal of therapy and has been speculated to be related to some of the headline-making events linked to SSRIs.

Antidepressant Withdrawal

There is a withdrawal or discontinuation syndrome associated with antidepressants (Lader, 2007). It is perhaps most pronounced with the SSRIs, but it can occur with other agents. Physical symptoms include dizziness, lethargy, diarrhea, flu-like symptoms, insomnia, and vivid dreams. Psychological symptoms are anxiety, agitation, irritability, confusion, and slowed thinking. Most clinicians titrate the dosage downward to prevent antidepressant withdrawal. Without chemical assistance, this antidepressant withdrawal will last a couple of weeks (Howland, 2010; Inott, 2009).

Antidepressant Loss of Effectiveness

Antidepressant loss of effectiveness, or drug "poop-out," is another issue prescribers must address. Some patients stop responding to the antidepressant (Keltner, 2011). This is perhaps most common with SSRIs.

Antidepressant-Induced Suicide

The Food and Drug Administration (FDA) requires a black box warning on antidepressant packaging inserts alerting patients to the increased risk of suicide. Specifically, the FDA warns that increased suicidal thinking and behavior can occur in patients up to age 24 during the initial treatment period (generally within the first 1 to 2 months) (Reeves & Ladner, 2010).

Antimanic Drugs

Antimanic drugs or mood stabilizers are very important in the nurse practitioner's therapeutic arsenal. Antimanic drugs include lithium, divalproex and other anticonvulsants, and antipsychotics.

During the manic phase of bipolar disorder, the brain is "firing" too rapidly. Most clinicians have worked with patients who were talking too much and too fast, whose minds were racing, and who exhibited or reported an elevated mood, grandiosity, irritability, anger, insomnia, distractibility, and so on. During the depressive phase, withdrawal, passivity, sluggishness, difficulty thinking, and apathy are apparent. The antimanic drugs mentioned above are prescribed to stabilize the individual between these two emotional extremes.

Lithium

Lithium is a naturally occurring element found in the same column as other salts on the periodic table. Lithium is still considered the gold standard for bipolar disorder, though it is not the drug most frequently prescribed (Hirschowitz, Kolevzon, & Garakani, 2010; Ventimiglia, Kalali, & McIntyre, 2009). Lithium is effective in approximately half of the patients for whom it is prescribed. The exact mechanism of how lithium works has not been clearly identified. A number of interesting hypotheses exist, however:

1. Lithium substitutes for sodium.
2. Lithium inhibits the release of and facilitates the reuptake of norepinephrine and serotonin.
3. Lithium regulates the Na^+, K^+-ATPase pump.
4. Lithium stabilizes the second-messenger system, thus regulating intracellular signaling (El-Mallakh, 1996; Nestler, Hyman, & Malenka, 2009).

The typical dosage of lithium is 600 mg three times a day with the goal of achieving a serum level of 0.6 to 1.2 mEq/L. This serum level can usually be maintained at a slightly lower dosage (900 to 1200 mg/day). Because lithium has a narrow therapeutic index, seemingly slight changes in doses can yield a toxic reaction. For instance, though 1.2 mEq/L is a therapeutic level for lithium, blood levels above 1.5 mEq/L can be toxic and should be avoided. Interestingly and perhaps unfortunately, common side effects overlap with the beginning symptoms of toxicity. The unfortunate aspect is that neither patient nor clinician may know if diarrhea, for instance, is just an annoying side effect or the manifestation of mild toxicity. Keltner and Grant (2008) detailed cases of two men who appear to have irreversible neuropathy (to the point of losing the ability to ambulate) related to toxic levels of lithium. Clinicians should also prescribe lower doses for older adults and monitor for lower serum levels. For instance, in most older patients, a serum level of 0.4 to 0.8 mEq/L is desirable. Box 6-5 lists signs and symptoms associated with therapeutic to very high serum lithium levels. Table 6-11 shows the dosage of lithium and other antimanic drugs.

BOX 6-5 Adverse Effects of Lithium at Therapeutic and at Mild, Moderate, and Severe Levels of Toxicity

Therapeutic Serum Levels (0.6 to 1.2 mEq/L)
- Hand tremor (mild)
- Memory problems
- Goiter
- Hypothyroidism
- Mild diarrhea
- Anorexia
- Nausea
- Edema
- Weight gain
- Polydipsia, polyuria

Mild to Moderate Toxicity (1.5 to 2.0 mEq/L)
- Diarrhea
- Vomiting
- Drowsiness
- Dizziness
- Hand tremor (coarse)
- Muscular weakness
- Lack of coordination
- Dry mouth

Moderate to Severe Toxicity (2 to 3 mEq/L)
Previous symptoms and
- Ataxia
- Giddiness
- Tinnitus
- Blurred vision
- Large output of dilute urine
- Delirium
- Nystagmus

Severe Toxicity (greater than 3 mEq/L)
Previous symptoms and
- Seizures
- Organ failure
- Renal failure
- Coma
- Death

Anticonvulsants

The drug most commonly prescribed for bipolar disorder is the anticonvulsant divalproex (Depakote). This drug has a more rapid onset action than lithium, can be used without attempting to use lithium, and is better tolerated than lithium. Disadvantages include transient hair loss, weight gain, tremors, gastrointestinal problems, and a dose-related thrombocytopenia. It is highly protein bound and can be "knocked off" the protein sites by other highly bound drugs. When this occurs, toxic levels can develop (Chateauvieux, Morceau, Dicato, et al., 2010; Hirschowitz et al., 2010). Serum levels for treating bipolar disorder are slightly higher than accepted levels when this drug is used to address a seizure disorder (50 to 115 mcg/mL).

Other anticonvulsants used to treat bipolar disorder include carbamazepine (Tegretol), lamotrigine (Lamictal), oxcarbazepine (Trileptal), gabapentin (Neurontin), and topiramate (Topamax) (Grunze, 2010). All of these drugs work by decreasing the firing rate of the overly excited neurons. Carbamazepine normalizes sodium channels; lamotrigine modulates the GABA system while blocking sodium and calcium channels; oxcarbazepine normalizes sodium channels; gabapentin fortifies GABA neurotransmission; and topiramate increases GABA while blocking sodium and calcium channels (Lehne, 2007).

Antipsychotics

Most antipsychotics have a role in treating bipolar disorder. Of particular note, the following antipsychotics are prescribed

TABLE 6-11 LITHIUM AND SELECTED ANTICONVULSANTS USED IN THE TREATMENT OF BIPOLAR DISORDER

Antimanic Drug	Usual Adult Daily Dosage	Half-life (hr)	Therapeutic Serum Level	Monthly Cost	Common Side Effects	Warnings
Lithium	Acute: 600–1800 mg Maintenance: 900–1200 mg	~24	0.6–1.2 mEq/L	$12–$24	N/V, diarrhea, polyuria, polydipsia, weight gain, tremor, fatigue	Lithium toxicity; teratogenicity
Carbamazepine	800–1000 mg and titrated upward until side effects of serum level reached	12–17; induces own metabolism	4–12 mcg/mL	$6–$15 (generic)	N/V, dizziness, sedation, rash, HA	Blood dyscrasias; teratogenicity
Divalproex	1000–1500 mg	6–16	50-115 mcg/mL	$57–$228 (Depakote)	N/V, sedation, weight gain, hair loss	Hepatoxicity, teratogenicity, pancreatitis
Lamotrigine	Begin at 25–50 mg and increase by 12.5-25 mg/wk, up to 250 mg bid	~24 with chronic use	N/A	$123–$486 (Lamictal)	HA, sedation, cognitive dulling, insomnia, ataxia, N/V, dizziness, diplopia	Serious rash, e.g., Stevens-Johnson; breastfeeding?
Oxcarbazepine	600–2400 mg in two or three divided doses	7–20 with active metabolites	15–35 mcg/mL	$222–$555 (Trileptal)	Fatigue, N/V, dizziness, sedation, diplopia, hyponatremia	Teratogenicity; breast-feeding?; cognitive dulling

HA, headache; N/V, nausea and vomiting; ?, safety has not been established.

Modified from Bezchlibnyk-Butler, K. Z., & Jeffries, J. J. (2007). Clinical handbook of psychotropic drugs. *Seattle: Hogrefe & Huber; Keltner, N. L., & Folks, D. G. (2005). Psychotropic drugs. St. Louis: Mosby; Keltner, N. L., Bostrom, C. E., & McGuinness, T. M. (2011).* Psychiatric nursing *(6th ed.). St. Louis: Mosby; and Consumer Reports Best Buy Drugs, 2009.*

relatively frequently for this condition: olanzapine, risperidone, quetiapine, ziprasidone, clozapine, and aripiprazole (El-Mallakh, Elmaadawi, Loganathan, et al., 2010). Refer to the Atypical Antipsychotics section above that discusses these drugs.

Antianxiety Drugs

Antianxiety drugs include benzodiazepines, SSRIs, and buspirone. The benzodiazepines are the agents most commonly thought of as anxiolytic.

Benzodiazepines

Most clinicians are reluctant to prescribe benzodiazepines for any length of time because of potential abuse of these drugs. Nonetheless, because anxiety can be almost unbearable, medications that can quickly subdue the symptoms are valued. Thus, many prescribers do use benzodiazepines, particularly in the early stages of anxiety treatment. Table 6-12 features the more commonly prescribed benzodiazepines and also nonbenzodiazepines.

Benzodiazepines cause an anxiolytic response by enhancing GABA receptor reaction to GABA. As will be remembered, GABA receptors are the most common inhibitory neurotransmitter in the brain, with a full 40% of neurons possessing these receptors (Martin & Dunn, 2002). The GABA receptor is actually composed of five subunits that encircle a chloride channel. These subunits are identified as α, β, and γ. There are also variations among these subunits, such as α_1, α_2, α_3, β_2, γ_1, and γ_2. These subunits can be arranged in several different configurations to form the chloride channel. Some configurations have an *allosteric site* for benzodiazepines and some do not. An allosteric site is one that is not in the traditional active neurotransmitter place on the receptor. By attaching to this allosteric site, benzodiazepines make the "regular" GABA binding sites more sensitive to GABA. Simply put, benzodiazepines make GABA receptors more responsive to GABA (Atack, 2010; Henry, Jensen, Licata, et al., 2010; Juergens, 2010).

Similar allosteric sites exist for alcohol and for barbiturates. With GABA enhancement, more chloride is drawn into the neuron, thus increasing the negativity of the membrane potential. In other words, the neuron becomes hyperpolarized, thus slowing the depolarization event. Benzodiazepines slow neuronal firing, and this slowdown causes depression of cognitive functions in the frontal lobe and emotional blunting that no doubt arises from inhibition of mesolimbic function. A benzodiazepine-induced apathy can develop in long-term users of these drugs (Atack, 2010; Henry et al., 2010; Juergens, 2010). As is evident, such effects reduce anxiety, but at a high cost.

An important consideration for clinicians is the pharmacokinetic process of metabolism. While most benzodiazepines are metabolized by liver CYP enzymes or by phase I metabolism, a few rely on phase II or conjugation entirely (oxazepam and lorazepam, for instance) or primarily (alprazolam). Because phase I metabolism capability declines with age or in hepatically compromised individuals whereas phase II metabolism does not, some of these agents should not be prescribed in individuals with liver disease or ordered routinely in older individuals. Agents most appropriate for people with declining liver function are oxazepam and lorazepam. These two drugs and alprazolam do not have pharmacologically active metabolites, thus adding to their value in this population. Benzodiazepines are almost completely absorbed, highly bound to serum proteins (80% to 90%), and most have active metabolites (Greenblatt, Shader, Divoll, et al., 1981). They are also very lipophilic, entering the brain easily. As can be discerned

TABLE 6-12 COMMONLY PRESCRIBED BENZODIAZEPINES AND NONBENZODIAZEPINES: DOSAGE, EQUIVALENCE TO LORAZEPAM, HALF-LIFE, AND ANXIOLYTIC AND SEDATIVE EFFECTS

	Usual Daily Dose (mg/day)	Lorazepam-Equivalent Dose (mg)	Half-life (hr)	Anxiolytic Effect	Sedative Effect
Benzodiazepines					
Short-acting	Triazolam (Halcion) 0.125–0.5	0.25	1.5–5	Weak	Strong
Intermediate	Alprazolam (Xanax) 0.75–4*	0.5	12–15	Moderate	Weak
Intermediate	Lorazepam (Ativan) 2–6*	1	10–20	Strong	Moderate
Intermediate	Oxazepam (Serax) 30–60*	15	5–20	Moderate	Weak
Intermediate	Temazepam (Restoril) 10–60	10	10–15	Weak	Strong
Long-acting	Chlordiazepoxide (Librium) 15–100*	25	5–30†	Moderate	—
Long-acting	Clonazepam (Klonopin) 0.5–10*	0.25	18–60†	Moderate	Weak
Long-acting	Diazepam (Valium) 4–40*	5	20–80†	Strong	Moderate
Nonbenzodiazepines					
	Buspirone (Buspar) 15–40*	—	2–11†	Strong	—

*Given in divided doses.
†With active metabolite.
Adapted from Keltner, N. L., & Folks, D. G. (2005). Psychotropic drugs. *St. Louis: Mosby;* and Consumer Report Best Buy Drugs (2009).

from Table 6-12, variance in half-life is considerable. Triazolam has a short half-life of 5 hours or less, whereas diazepam can stay in the system for up to 80 hours before being reduced in half (therefore, in once per day dosing, diazepam can accumulate in some individuals). Tolerance—another key pharmacokinetic issue—develops quickly in benzodiazepine use. Tolerance simply means that the individual no longer experiences the same effect at the same dosage; more is required to achieve the same effects. Tolerance to sedation occurs within weeks, whereas tolerance to anxiolytic properties takes months (Ashton, 2000; Juergens, 2010).

Important side effects of benzodiazepines include sedation, decreased cognitive functioning such as memory impairment, and reduced coordination. Such impairments can lead to difficulties at work, at home, and in the environment (mishandling of automobiles). On the other hand, poor memory of a colonoscopy (due to the effect of midazolam [Versed] used for sedation) can be considered to be a therapeutic side effect (Lee & Kim, 2009).

Benzodiazepines are also very disinhibiting, creating many social and legal problems. The list of inappropriate benzodiazepine-induced words and deeds that individuals wish they could recall is almost endless (Rothschild, 1992; Rothschild, Bessette, Carter-Campbell, et al., 1993). Further, some people have a paradoxical reaction and actually develop anxiety, insomnia, hyperactivity, and aggressive behavior related to benzodiazepines. Aggressive behavior—whether verbal or physical—may be the result of disinhibition, a paradoxical reaction, or both. Common side effects of benzodiazepines are

- Drowsiness
- Light-headedness
- Lassitude
- Increased reaction time
- Dysarthria
- Ataxia
- Motor incoordination
- Impairment of mental functions
- Sexual dysfunction
- Weight gain
- Skin reactions
- Headache
- Confusion
- Depression
- Anterograde amnesia (Charlson, Degenhardt, McLaren, et al., 2009; Keltner & Folks, 2005)

Benzodiazepines have a wide therapeutic index, and serious overdose of these drugs most often is in combination with other central nervous system depressants (e.g., with alcohol). After chronic use of benzodiazepines, individuals can become addicted to them. Like other addictions, "coming off" these drugs can be both painful and deadly. The painfulness comes from the withdrawal syndrome (Ashton, 2004), with both physical and psychological symptoms:

- Physical: headache, pain/stiffness, tingling/numbness, weakness, muscle twitches, tremor, dizziness, blurred vision, tinnitus, overbreathing
- Psychological: excitability, insomnia, increased anxiety, agoraphobia, perceptual distortions, depersonalization, hallucinations, depression, rage, aggression, irritability, poor memory and concentration

Because unassisted withdrawal can cause convulsions, abrupt cessation of these drugs in dependent individuals should be guarded against. People addicted to benzodiazepines should become drug free if possible, but only under the care of a trained professional.

Selective Serotonin Reuptake Inhibitors

Whereas benzodiazepines are often prescribed for anxiety, it is the SSRIs that are the predominant drugs used for long-term benefit. SSRIs, because of their effect on second-messenger systems, alter neuronal physiology and output (Keltner & Gorman, 2007). Often, an SSRI and a benzodiazepine will be prescribed initially with the objective to wean the patient off the benzodiazepine but have him or her remain on the SSRI. Many clinicians are so averse to the use of benzodiazepines that they do not use them even in this limited way (Lader, Tylee, & Donoghue, 2009). Nonetheless, many prescribers do so, however reluctantly. See the antidepressant section above and Unit IV: Anxiety Disorders for further comments on the use of SSRIs.

Buspirone

Buspirone (Buspar) differs substantially from the benzodiazepines and can be used successfully for anxiety. It is dosed at 15 to 40 mg/day and has an anxiolytic effect equivalent to lorazepam's. It is nonsedating and does not interact with central nervous system depressants, though interactions with haloperidol and MAOIs have been observed (Keltner & Folks, 2005). On the other hand, for individuals who are miserable from their anxiousness, buspirone does not offer "a quick fix." Time to a full clinical effect can range from 3 to 6 weeks, though some target symptoms begin to improve within days. Its mechanism of action is thought to be related to partial agonist effects at the 5-HT_{1A} receptor (Blier, Bergeron, & de Montigny, 1997). Buspirone has a very low bioavailability (1% to 4%) and is almost completely bound to serum proteins (~95%).

Summary

This chapter has reviewed the classic categories of psychotropic drugs. The discussion emphasis focused on disorder pathology and elaboration of drug mechanisms aimed at chemically confronting those deficits. These foci were prefaced by an overview of the brain, neurotransmitters, receptors, and pharmacokinetics. Particularly, metabolism and the induction or inhibition of enzymes was emphasized as important considerations.

Psychiatric advanced practice nurses must be aware of these concepts in order to provide the care psychiatric patients require. For example, many psychiatric drug interactions are caused by disruptions in enzymatic breakdown of pharmaceuticals. A review of the pharmacokinetic processes discussed in this chapter affords the clinician a basis for understanding those interactions. Further, by understanding each drug category's mechanism of action, the clinician is prepared to understand psychotropic drugs more thoroughly, including better prediction of drug performance, its side effects, and potential interactions. In adopting this approach, the authors attempt to provide information that is both fundamental to care and state-of-the-art. With this information, the practitioner should be able to incorporate the ever-expanding knowledge more seamlessly into his or her understanding of psychopharmacology.

Key Points

- Psychiatric disorders are brain disorders.
- Many psychiatric disorders are treated with medications that work in the brain.
- Most psychiatric drugs affect one or more of six neurotransmitters.
- In order to understand psychiatric drugs, the clinician must have a firm grasp of pharmacokinetics.
- There are four major psychotropic drug categories: antipsychotic, antidepressant, antimanic, and antianxiety drugs.
- Antipsychotic agents have wide utility, but most use is targeted at the treatment of psychoses.
- Antipsychotic drugs can be roughly divided into traditional and atypical categories.
- Antidepressant drugs are used chiefly for treatment of depression and anxiety.
- Antimanic agents are used to stabilize mood. Lithium is the gold standard, while divalproex is most often prescribed.
- Antianxiety agents are used to treat anxiety disorders and include SSRIs, benzodiazepines, and the nonbenzodiazepine buspirone.

References

Agid, Y. (1991). Parkinson's disease: Pathophysiology. *Lancet, 337,* 1321-1323.

Agius, M., Gardner, J., Liu, K., et al. (2010). An audit to compare discharge rates and suicidality between antidepressant monotherapies prescribed for unipolar depression. *Psychiatria Danubina, 22,* 350-353.

Anderson, I. M. (2000). Selective serotonin reuptake inhibitors versus tricyclic antidepressants: A meta-analysis of efficacy and tolerability. *Journal of Affective Disorders, 58*(1), 19-36.

Andreasen, N. C. (1985). Positive vs. negative schizophrenia: A critical evaluation. *Schizophrenia Bulletin, 11,* 380.

Andreasen, N. C., & Olsen, S. (1982). Negative vs. positive schizophrenia. *Archives of General Psychiatry, 139,* 789.

Asenjo Lobos, C., Komossa, K., Rummel-Kluge, C., et al. (2010). Clozapine versus other atypical antipsychotics for schizophrenia. *The Cochrane Database of Systematic Reviews,* (11). CD006633.

Ashton, C. H. (2000). *Benzodiazepines: How they work & how to withdraw.* New Castle, UK: University of Newcastle.

Ashton, H. (2004). Benzodiazepine dependence. In P. Haddad, S. Dursun, and B. Deakin (Eds.), *Adverse syndromes and psychiatric drugs: A clinical guide* (pp. 239–260). New York: Oxford University Press.

Atack, J. R. (2010). GABA(A) receptor subtype-selective modulators. I. $\alpha2/\alpha3$-selective agonists as non-sedating anxiolytics. *Current Topics in Medicinal Chemistry, 11*(9), 1176-1202.

Bezchlibnyk-Butler, K. Z., & Jeffries, J. J. (2007). *Clinical handbook of psychotropic drugs.* Seattle: Hogrefe & Huber.

Blier, P., Bergeron, R., & de Montigny, C. (1997). Selective activation of postsynaptic $5HT_{1A}$ receptors induces rapid antidepressant response. *Neuropsychopharmacology, 16,* 333-338.

Bristol-Meyers Squibb. (2006). Emsam Package Insert. New York: Bristol-Meyers Squibb.

Bruce, A., Macgillivray, S., Ogston, S., et al. (2005). Efficacy and tolerability of tricyclic antidepressants and SSRIs compared with placebo for treatment of depression in primary care: A meta-analysis. *Annals of Family Medicine, 3,* 449-456.

Charlson, F., Degenhardt, L., McLaren, J., et al. (2009). A systematic review of research examining benzodiazepine-related mortality. *Pharmacoepidemiology and Drug Safety, 18,* 93-103.

Chateauvieux, S., Morceau, F., Dicato, M., et al. (2010). Molecular and therapeutic potential and toxicity of valproic acid. *Journal of Biomedicine & Biotechnology,* pii: 479364. Retrieved from http://www.ncbi.nlm.nih.gov/pmc/articles/PMC2926634/?tool=pmcentrez

Chen, J., Gao, K., & Kemp, D. E. (2011). Second-generation antipsychotics in major depressive disorder: Update and clinical perspective. *Current Opinion in Psychiatry, 24*(1), 10-17.

Cipriani, A., Furukawa, T. A., Salanti, G., et al. (2009). Comparative efficacy and acceptability of 12 new-generation antidepressants: A multiple-treatments meta-analysis. *Lancet, 373,* 746-758.

Consumer Reports Best Buy Drugs (2009). *Treating schizophrenia and bipolar disorder: The antipsychotics—Comparing effectiveness, safety, and price.* Yonkers, NY: Consumer Reports Best Buy Drugs. Retrieved from http://www.consumerreports.org/health/resources/pdf/best-buy-drugs/Antipsychs-2pager-FINAL.pdf

Cooke, B. B., & Keltner, N. L. (2008). Traumatic brain injury-war related: Part II. *Perspectives in Psychiatric Care, 44*(1), 54-57.

Cozza, K. L., Armstrong, S. C., & Oesterheld, J. R. (2003). *Drug interaction principles for medical practice.* Washington, DC: American Psychiatric Publishing, Inc.

Croom, K. F., Perry, C. M., & Plosker, G. L. (2009). Mirtazapine: A review of its use in major depression and other psychiatric disorders. *CNS Drugs, 23(5),* 427-452.

Crowe, T. J. (1982). Two dimensions of pathology in schizophrenia: Dopaminergic and nondopaminergic. *Psychopharmacology Bulletin, 18,* 22.

Csoka, A. B., Bahrick, A., & Mehtonen, O. P. (2008). Persistent sexual dysfunction after discontinuation of selective serotonin reuptake inhibitors. *The Journal of Sexual Medicine, 5,* 227-233.

Damsa, C., Bumb, A., Bianchi-Demicheli, F., et al. (2004). "Dopamine-dependent" side effects of selective serotonin reuptake inhibitors: A clinical review. *Journal of Clinical Psychiatry, 65,* 1064-1068.

Drug Topics Staff (2009). Pharmacy facts and figures. Retrieved January 8, 2010 from http://drugtopics.modernmedicine.com/Pharmacy+Facts+&+Figures

El-Mallakh, R. S. (1996). *Lithium: Actions and mechanisms.* Washington, DC: American Psychiatric Publishing, Inc.

El-Mallakh, R. S., Elmaadawi, A. Z., Loganathan, M., et al. (2010). Bipolar disorder: An update. *Postgraduate Medicine, 122*(4), 24-31.

Greenblatt, D. J., Shader, R. I., Divoll, M., et al. (1981). Benzodiazepines: A summary of pharmacokinetic properties. *British Journal of Clinical Pharmacology, 11*(Suppl 1), 11S-16S.

Grunze, H. C. (2010). Anticonvulsants in bipolar disorder. *Journal of Mental Health, 19*(2), 127-141.

Henry, M. E., Jensen, J. E., Licata, S. C., et al. (2010). The acute and late CNS glutamine response to benzodiazepine challenge: A pilot pharmacokinetic study using proton magnetic resonance spectroscopy. *Psychiatry Research, 184,* 171-176.

Hirschowitz, J., Kolevzon, A., & Garakani, A. (2010). The pharmacological treatment of bipolar disorder: The question of modern advances. *Harvard Review of Psychiatry, 18,* 266-278.

Howland, R. H. (2010). Potential adverse effects of discontinuing psychotropic drugs: Part 2: Antidepressant drugs. *Journal of Psychosocial Nursing and Mental Health Services, 48*(7), 9-12.

Inott, T. J. (2009). The dark side of SSRIs: Selective serotonin reuptake inhibitors. *Nursing, 39*(8), 31–33.

Juergens, S. M. (2010). Understanding benzodiazepines. Retrieved from http://www.csam-asam.org/pdf/misc/Juergens.pdf

Keltner, N. L. (2000). Neuroreceptor function and psychopharmacologic response. *Issues in Mental Health Nursing, 21,* 31-50.

Keltner, N. L. (2010). Schizophrenia: What do we know and how do we know it? *Journal of the American Psychiatric Nurses Association. 16*(1), 5-6.

Keltner, N. L. (2011). Antidepressants. In N. L. Keltner, C. E. Bostrom, & T. M. McGuinness (Eds.), *Psychiatric nursing* (6th ed.) (pp. 178-193). St. Louis: Elsevier.

Keltner, N. L., & Folks, D. G. (2005). *Psychotropic drugs* (4th ed.). St. Louis: Mosby.

Keltner, N. L., & Gorman, A. G. (2007). Second messengers. *Perspectives in Psychiatric Care, 43*(1), 60-64.

Keltner, N. L., & Grant, J. S. (2006). Smoke, smoke, smoke that cigarette. *Perspectives in Psychiatric Care, 42*(4), 256-260.

Keltner, N. L., & Grant, J. S. (2008). Irreversible lithium-induced neuropathy: Two cases. *Perspectives in Psychiatric Care, 44*(4), 290-293.

Keltner, N. L., & Vance, D. E. (2008). Incarcerated care and quetiapine abuse. *Perspectives in Psychiatric Care, 44*(3), 202-206.

Komossa, K., Rummel-Kluge, C., Hunger, H., et al. (2009a). Ziprasidone versus other atypical antipsychotics for schizophrenia. *The Cochrane Database of Systematic Reviews,* (4). CD006627.

Komossa, K., Rummel-Kluge, C., Hunger, H., et al. (2010a). Olanzapine versus other atypical antipsychotics for schizophrenia. *The Cochrane Database of Systematic Reviews,* (3). CD006654.

Komossa, K., Rummel-Kluge, C., Schmid, F., et al. (2009b). Aripiprazole versus other atypical antipsychotics for schizophrenia. *The Cochrane Database of Systematic Reviews,* (4). CD006569.

Komossa, K., Rummel-Kluge, C., Schmid, F., et al. (2010b). Quetiapine versus other atypical antipsychotics for schizophrenia. *The Cochrane Database of Systematic Reviews,* (1). CD006625.

Lader, M. (2007). Pharmacotherapy of mood disorders and treatment discontinuation. *Drugs, 67,* 1657-1663.

Lader, M., Tylee, A., & Donoghue, J. (2009). Withdrawing benzodiazepines in primary care. *CNS Drugs, 23*(1), 19-34.

Lee, S. I., & Keltner, N. L. (2005). Antidepressant apathy syndrome. *Perspectives in Psychiatric Care, 41*(4), 188-192.

Lee, S. I., & Keltner, N. L. (2006). Serotonin and norepinephrine reuptake inhibitors (SNRIs): Venlafaxine and duloxetine. *Perspectives in Psychiatric Care, 42*(2), 144-148.

Lee, H., & Kim, J. H. (2009). Superiority of split dose midazolam as conscious sedation for outpatient colonoscopy. *World Journal of Gastroenterology, 15,* 3783-3787.

Lehne, R. A. (2007). *Pharmacology for nursing care.* St. Louis: Elsevier.

Lin, K. M., Smith, M., & Lin, M. T. (2003). Psychopharmacology: Ethnic and cultural perspectives. In A. Tasman, J. Kay, & J. A. Lieberman (Eds.), *Psychiatry* (2nd ed.) (pp. 1915-1927). West Essex, UK: John Wiley & Sons.

Martin, I. L., & Dunn, S. M. J. (2002). GABA receptors. *Tacris Review, 20,* 1.

Mason, P. J., Morris, V. A., & Balcezak, T. J. (2000). Serotonin syndrome: Presentation of 2 cases and review of the literature. *Medicine, 79,* 201-209.

Nestler, E. J., Hyman, S. E., & Malenka, R. C. (2009). *Molecular neuropharmacology: A foundation for clinical science* (2nd ed.). New York: McGraw Medical.

Parikh, S. V. (2009). Antidepressants are not all created equal. *Lancet, 373,* 700-701.

Reeves, R. R., & Ladner, M. E. (2010). Antidepressant-induced suicidality: An update. *CNS Neuroscience & Therapeutics, 16,* 227-234.

Rothschild, A. J. (1992). Disinhibition, amnestic reactions, and other adverse reactions secondary to triazolam: A review of the literature. *Journal of Clinical Psychiatry, 53*(Suppl), 69-79.

Rothschild, A. J., Bessette, M. P., Carter-Campbell, J., et al. (1993). Triazolam and disinhibition. *Lancet, 341,* 186.

Rush, A. J., Trivedi, M. H., Wisniewski, S. R., et al. (2006). Bupropion-SR, sertraline, or venlafaxine-XR after failure of SSRIs for depression. *The New England Journal of Medicine, 354,* 1231-1242.

Sachs, G. S., Nierenberg, A. A., Calabrese, J. R., et al. (2007). Effectiveness of adjunctive antidepressant treatment for bipolar depression. *The New England Journal of Medicine, 356,* 1711-1722.

Sedvall, G. (1995). PET studies on the neuroreceptor effects of antipsychotic drugs. *Current Approaches to Psychosis, 4,* 1.

Seeman, P., & Van Tol, H. H. (1994). Dopamine receptor pharmacology. *Trends in Pharmacologic Science, 15*(7), 264.

Sicouri, S., & Antzelevitch, C. (2008). Sudden cardiac death secondary to antidepressant and antipsychotic drugs. *Expert Opinion on Drug Safety, 7*(2), 181-194.

Stahl, S. M. (1998). Basic psychopharmacology of antidepressants, Part 1: Antidepressants have several distinct mechanisms of action. *Journal of Clinical Psychiatry, 59*(Suppl 4), 5-14.

Sugerman, R. A. (2011). Psychobiologic basis for behavior. In N. L. Keltner, C. E. Bostrom, & T. M. McGuinness (Eds.), *Psychiatric nursing* (6th ed.) (pp. 44-59). St. Louis: Elsevier.

Ventimiglia, J., Kalali, A. H., & McIntyre, R. (2009). Treatment of bipolar disorder. *Psychiatry, 6*(10), 12-14.

Weitzel, C., & Jiwanlal, S. (2001). The darker side of SSRIs. *RN, 64*(8), 43-47.

Wren, P., Frizzell, L. A., & Keltner, N. L. (2003). Three potentially fatal adverse effects of psychotropic medications. *Perspectives in Psychiatric Care, 39*(2), 75-81.

CHAPTER 7

Psychotherapies

Diane M. Wieland, PhD, MSN, RN, PMHCNS-BC, and Sharon R. Katz, PMH-APRN, BC

Psychotherapy is a powerful healing method that engages a patient at a vulnerable point and enables change. It is a living and adaptable art based on the establishment of a psychotherapeutic confidential relationship between the individual patient and a qualified mental health practitioner; it provides attention to issues and complex relationships and addresses and alters perspectives that are inhibiting the patient's growth and development.

Psychotherapy is the bedrock of treatment for patients with psychiatric disorders, and it is the foundation of psychiatric advanced practice nurses' clinical work. It requires specialized knowledge, an understanding of the psychotherapeutic relationship and psychotherapeutic modalities, expertise in generating diagnoses and identifying patients' goals, and provision of evidence-based practice. This chapter illuminates the techniques that need to be developed to (1) facilitate the psychiatric advanced practice nurse's role as a psychotherapist, (2) adhere to the standards that mental health third-party payers require for assessment and documentation of psychotherapy practice, and (3) facilitate the evolution of psychiatric mental health care and the role of the psychiatric advanced practice nurse, which has shifted recently to the unified role of nurse, psychotherapist, and prescriber of psychotropic medications. With this unification, psychiatric advanced practice nurses work with the whole patient's mental health process, complementing his or her care in integrated health settings, community outpatient practices, or psychiatric crisis or acute settings (Cozolino, 2002).

Psychotherapy has a long-term impact. Even after the treatment is terminated, the insight, adaptation, and healing may continue for many years without further intervention. Change requires (1) addressing the central core of factors (psychological, physiological, and neurobiological) that contributed to the development of the brain and to behavior, using a systematic process to engage healing, and (2) understanding the psychotherapeutic process, which includes attending sessions, managing discomfort from exploring issues, and adaptation.

Learning to be a nurse psychotherapist involves understanding and implementing a wide range of skills and theories that are practiced by all mental health providers (psychiatrists, psychologists, social workers, licensed professional counselors, and marriage and family therapists) as well as specifically psychiatric nursing skills and theories. As mental health providers, nurses have a common bond with other practitioners in the mental health profession through the shared standards of treatment and documentation and use of clinical modalities. Psychiatric advanced practice nurses follow medical documentation standards: establishing a diagnosis using clinical criteria that reflect mental and medical symptoms, using evidence-based interventions, maintaining records that track progress and safety, developing treatment plans that reflect symptom reduction, and evaluating patient progress. Psychiatric mental health nursing also brings a strong nursing theoretical base to the psychotherapeutic relationship, which is central to healing. While psychiatric nurses incorporate medical and psychological clinical models to treat patients, they also incorporate nursing's comprehensive scope of practice. Psychiatric advanced practice nurses have a duty to apply theories that integrate the mind and body in assessment and treatment planning, to engage the patient's view of self, and to prescribe evidence-based interventions that facilitate patients' adaptation. To reframe and treat mental illness and substance abuse, the psychiatric advanced practice nurse incorporates into psychotherapy principles of empathetic communication, psychopathology, psychopharmacology, family systems, and growth and development. The psychiatric advanced practice nurse's goal for treatment is to return the patient to his or her highest level of wellness or recovery.

No other area of health care has undergone as many significant changes over the last few decades as has psychiatric mental health care (Rice, 2008). Psychiatric advanced practice nurses are continuing to evolve and to define clinical science through evidence-based practices and evolution of models of care that reflect nursing's scope of practice.

Psychiatric advanced practice nurses' scope of practice is comprehensive and complex, combining many skills of other mental health professionals. Working alongside psychologists, psychiatrists, social workers, and other licensed mental health providers, psychiatric advanced practice nurses extend their mental health skills to offer a comprehensive scope of practice to patients that combines psychopharmacology, psychiatric diagnosis, developmental assessment and treatment, teaching of coping skills, understanding of family adaptation, and monitoring of health. Through the psychotherapeutic session, psychiatric advanced practice nurses provide a healing environment that promotes the development of an empathetic relationship with patients and their families.

Because the practice of psychiatric nursing is multimodal and flexible, it allows integration of various modalities based on the patient's needs and the setting of the therapeutic process. For example, psychiatric advanced practice nurses may be referred a patient with a significant medical illness who has comorbid mental health illnesses that have created a shift in functioning in relationships or family dynamics. Psychiatric advanced practice nurses assess and treat individuals and their families. They address significant unconscious and multigenerational patterns that affect coping, and they identify supports within the family and extended community. As clinicians, psychiatric advanced practice nurses have the duty to demonstrate clear boundaries in relationships, follow the psychological theories that give structure to the psychotherapy sessions, and use theoretical models as tools to define the change process. Patients look for competency in their therapists and for comprehensive psychotherapy that can heal individual and family functioning, but they have little understanding about the differences among professional approaches or disciplines. Patients build relationships with psychotherapists, and many patients may be challenged by knowing who to trust and how to work within boundaries in a relationship.

This chapter introduces nursing students in psychiatric advanced practice nursing programs to the process of the nurse psychotherapist that reflects six decades of development and adaptation of nursing and psychological theories. The nurse psychotherapist's clinical preparation must align with standards of mental health treatment and documentation reflected universally with *Psychiatric Mental-Health Nursing: Scope and Standards of Practice* (American Nurses Association, 2007) as well as the standards of the mental health industry.

This chapter begins by presenting a historical perspective of psychotherapy and nursing and then discusses the nurse as a psychotherapist and the core principles of psychotherapy. A new model for psychiatric nursing, MINDFUL CARE—which is an acronym for a plan of psychotherapeutic intervention that will be described later—helps unify the skills of clinical nurse specialists and psychiatric nurse practitioners, allowing for a theoretical framework to guide psychotherapy and select a traditional clinical modality. Models of brief psychotherapies—relational, learning, and contextual—and supportive psychotherapy are important to master as evidence-based therapeutic strategies and are included in the chapters discussing individual disorders (Chapters 9 to 18).

Historical Perspective of Psychotherapy and Psychiatric Nursing

After World War II, concern for the mental health treatment of American veterans led to the National Mental Health Act of 1946. This act established psychiatric nursing as one of the original four disciplines authorized to treat patients with mental illnesses and receive payment for services (American Nurses Association, 2007). The earliest modern nursing theory is attributed to Hildegard Peplau's (1952) *Interpersonal Relations in Nursing*, which detailed the psychotherapeutic role of nursing as an interpersonal process that assesses and develops a course of action to solve problems that affect healing. This process was noted as a life span process that incorporated the whole family structure, developmental assessment and theories, and the "biological-psychological-spiritual-sociological" aspects of the individual in relation to the health-care issue (Peplau, 1988). Peplau's theory prescribed ways to challenge patients' perceptions, structured nursing interventions to address issues assessed by nurses, and taught communication techniques that decrease crisis and stress response. The theory still stands as the first nursing theory leading to long-term healing and change resulting from a nursing psychotherapeutic approach. Peplau's theory enabled nursing to establish the groundwork for advanced practice roles. (The first role to be developed was the clinical nurse specialist in psychiatric nursing.) Peplau's contribution supported the inclusion of the nursing profession as one of the four recognized professional designations licensed to work with the mentally ill. Psychotherapy became more mainstream with the advent of psychotropic medications and the use of medications in combination with talk therapy.

The surge of second generation antidepressants and antipsychotic medications has had a significant impact on public perception of treatment of mental illnesses. In the past, psychotherapy lacked an empirical research base that demonstrated its effectiveness. With the development of selective serotonin reuptake inhibitors (SSRIs) and serotonin-norepinephrine reuptake inhibitors (SNRIs), patients have been prescribed significant amounts of psychotropic medications. Extensive side-effect panels, tainted pharmaceutical industry studies, and lack of effect with mild and moderate symptoms, such as mild and moderate symptoms of depression, have led to a reexamination of reported efficacy of pharmacology research (Fournier, DeRubeis, Hollon, et al., 2010). It is now widely accepted that patients with moderate and severe symptom profiles benefit from a combination of psychotherapy and medication (Hellerstin, 2009).

Over the past five decades, psychiatric clinical nurse specialists continued the original work of Peplau's commitment to the therapeutic relationship as independent practitioners of psychotherapy. Many states extended prescription-writing privileges—previously granted only to nurse practitioners—to psychiatric clinical nurse specialists; however, this privilege was not universal, and there was a rapid growth of psychiatric nurse practitioner programs (see Chapter 1). Psychiatric nurse practitioners' education and clinical experiences overlapped significantly with the psychiatric clinical nurse specialists' scope of practice; however, the psychiatric nurse practitioner's preparation focused more on pharmacotherapy and prescriptive practice, and less on provision of psychotherapy. Recent changes in nursing led to the discussion of a future role for psychiatric advanced practice nurses based on the Consensus Model for APRN Regulation: Licensure, Accreditation, Certification, and Education (American Nurses Association, 2010; APRN Consensus Work Group & National Council of State Boards of Nursing APRN Advisory Committee, 2008). The psychiatric advanced practice nurse role would include psychotherapy as a clinical modality for all psychiatric advanced practice nurses and a life span approach to care. In keeping with these proposed changes, many of the psychotherapeutic approaches discussed in this chapter are beneficial at all stages of life.

The Nurse as Psychotherapist

Mental health problems, which are unique to the individual and to his or her family structure and functioning, need to be understood in the context of the individual's life; the nurse psychotherapist needs to be able to hear the process of illness as well as provide the right interventions. It takes years for nurse psychotherapists to develop to their full ability and expertise. Because the process of becoming effective nurse psychotherapists is intimidating to most new psychotherapists, we will break down the process by presenting core psychotherapy principles, introducing a nursing model for psychiatric assessment and psychotherapy, and discussing traditional clinical psychological modalities that are useful tools for evidence-based psychotherapy.

Psychotherapy is a holistic treatment that relies on the nurse's processing of what the patient is experiencing. Similar to pharmacotherapy, psychotherapy is a powerful treatment that results in a shift in functioning. Psychiatric advanced practice nurses need to develop skills to therapeutically pace psychological interventions that enhance the patient's ability to cope. Developing the ability to attune to patient's needs, to pace assessment and hence prevent premature judgment, and to direct the patient toward adaptation requires learning through supervision, detailed investigation of options that have worked in the past or with others with similar issues, and extensive continuing education that extends beyond the traditional coursework.

Peplau's theory of interpersonal relationships, integrated with psychological theories of interpersonal relations and communication theories, is the foundation of many of the psychological theories that nurse psychotherapists use in providing psychotherapy. During the psychotherapy process, the psychiatric advanced practice nurse does the following:

- With the patient, addresses the individual and family processes
- Assesses the identified problems during the orientation phase of the therapeutic relationship
- Determines, together with the patient, the underlying health-care issues
- Collects psychiatric data
- Establishes a trusting relationship

According to Peplau (1988), by working in a family systems context to understand multigenerational transmission and genetic influences, nurses are able to keep the focus balanced between the present situation and the individual's relationship to others in the family system and patterns of emotional dysfunction.

Regardless of the setting, psychiatric advanced practice nurses are able to apply core principles of psychotherapy as well as nursing theory to promote recovery through adaptation. By structuring the consultation and focusing on the nurse-patient relationship, nurse psychotherapists transcend the limits of the four walls of the treatment setting and can reach patients. This transformative experience might take place in a private session, at a bedside consultation, in a primary care clinic, or in a prison setting.

Being present as a psychotherapist begins with taking care of oneself—one's own psychological issues and one's personal and professional balance. Without the psychotherapist's having a good sense of how he or she is functioning in relationships, projection can occur and emotional boundaries can be blurred, with the risk of causing harm to those who are most vulnerable and those who are determining whom to trust (Duncan, Miller, Wampold, et al., 2010). As with anything nurses do, it is important to know one's own issues and limits as a person. The psychiatric advanced practice nurse needs to have a strong sense of self to responsibly engage a patient in psychotherapy. Nurses must be able to both acknowledge their own pathologies and put those personal pathologies aside when working with and giving messages to patients. Psychiatric advanced practice nurses should resolve their own issues or avoid taking patients with similar problems. For example, if the nurse psychotherapist is going through a life transition, having legal issues, or abusing substances, then it is the nurse's responsibility to receive appropriate psychotherapy or supervision to prevent projection, violation of boundaries, or other licensure compromises.

Through clinical supervision, ongoing continuing education, and professional interaction, nurse psychotherapists continue to build an understanding of the evolving science of relationships and to attain further skills that can be used in implementing the healing process. The American Nursing Credentialing Center (ANCC) and states require continuing education credits, but participating in a professional organization such as the American Psychiatric Nurses Association (APNA) or the International Society of Psychiatric Nurses (ISPN) helps to perpetuate the development of the profession through networking and presenting advances in the science of psychiatric nursing.

Core Principles of Psychotherapy

Psychotherapy is a healing process that mutually engages the nurse psychotherapist and the patient and provides for developing a trusting alliance and enabling history to be collected, problematic behavior to be assessed, diagnostic process to be revealed, and a mutually agreed upon treatment plan to be formulated. The interpersonal clinical relationship that develops follows a structured approach that enforces professional boundaries and enables clinical interventions to focus on adaptation. Although the focus in a nurse-patient relationship might be on the patient, it also encompasses a life span and family systems approach, which may bring into focus more than just the patient in any given session.

There are principles and activities that are followed by all psychotherapists:

- Psychotherapists must understand how to conduct themselves professionally.
- Psychotherapists' documentation must be complete, and it must reflect the patient's diagnosis, the symptom progression, and a clear plan of action.
- Psychotherapists' approaches to symptom reduction and interventions should reflect adaptation of a clinical modality (individual, couple, family, or group psychotherapy) to address a patient's individual needs.
- Psychotherapists' review of progress and collaboration with other health-care professionals who also see the patient is important in providing safe, quality care.

The major components of psychotherapy are confidentiality, counter-transference and therapeutic use of self, empathy, and safety.

Confidentiality

A major element in developing a trusting relationship is maintaining privacy. Patients come into psychotherapeutic sessions with multiple issues, complex histories, and significant fears. Their shame, guilt, and struggles are sensitive information that should be treated with respect (Gabbard, 2009).

The nurse psychotherapist must obtain consistent clinical data, which includes the patient's history, issues, suicidality/homicidality, history of abuse, and other clinical information. Information obtained in a session should not be discussed or used in any way. Even in clinical supervision, it is necessary to protect the patient's identity. State statutes and professional ethics, which are enforceable by law, protect information. However, there are exceptions, which the nurse should discuss with the patient during the initial session. For example, licensed mental health providers are required to break confidentiality in situations in which the patient is endangered or could endanger another. The nurse psychotherapist should consult state statutes regarding confidentiality laws, as they vary by state. Transferring of confidential mental health information (whether verbally or in written documents) is also protected. Patients need to request in writing that their records be transferred to another practitioner or communicated to another health-care provider.

To receive reimbursement from federal, state, and commercial insurances, the psychiatric advanced practice nurse needs to be aware of requirements for credentialing, supervision, insurance company contract requirements, and billing codes. Documentation should reflect a clinical record of services and levels of treatment for each date of service, ensuring that treatment was done in an ethically appropriate and safe manner. Insurance companies have the right to audit patients' charts to ensure that proper documentation and treatment plans are followed, as per their contract with the patient.

The psychotherapeutic relationship is different from the medical relationship. As mental health professionals, psychiatric advanced practice nurses are trusted with a rich and personal history of the patient and their family life, and keeping this trusting relationship is essential. Mental health providers have debated for years about privacy of mental health records and documentation. There is a great deal of personal information that does not need to be in an accessible mental health document that is open to insurance audits. Documentation should always reflect the following:

- The patient's subjective symptoms
- Behavioral issues that are triggering the psychotherapeutic interaction
- Intervention(s) prescribed
- Medical or behavioral health changes or challenges to substantiate the level of care billed

The psychiatric advanced practice nurse should consult federal, state, and consumer insurance contracts for specific information regarding contracting, expected reimbursement levels, and state regulations regarding billing for psychiatric advanced practice nurse services. The functions of "certified nursing specialist" and "nurse practitioner" are frequently assigned to different levels of treatment and reimbursement.

Counter-Transference and Therapeutic Use of Self

Nurse psychotherapists are human beings and experience common situations and events just like anyone else. However, accepting patients' confidence is a serious commitment to maintaining their safety. If the nurse psychotherapist is experiencing anxiety, obsessive thoughts, or a need to process a case or something a patient revealed in a session, it is important to consult with a supervisor or colleague, in a confidential manner, to examine what is making the therapist uncomfortable. In the rare occasions when there are intimate emotions, it is essential to seek supervision and terminate the therapeutic relationship.

Sometimes it is therapeutic to share common experiences, but sharing should be focused on enhancing trust or used to show interest. Excessive self-disclosure is not therapeutic. It is unprofessional to share any intimate information or unresolved emotional crises that illuminate the therapist's inability to manage personal affairs or family matters. Frequently a patient will ask if the nurse psychotherapist has children, is married, or has been through similar experiences as a way of relieving his or her anxiety or a way of testing if the therapeutic relationship would be reliable. The nurse psychotherapist needs to assess if requests for information are part of the broader nature of the patient's symptomatology or are being made to develop trust in the therapeutic alliance. One's shared history should be devoid of as many details as possible so as not to compromise one's family or sexual boundaries. Establishing a therapeutic relationship with friends or offering to house or host a patient for a meal opens the relationship to blurred boundaries of the therapeutic alliance and is professionally inappropriate.

Empathy

Psychotherapy relies on the clinician's ability to understand the issues that patients bring into the relationship. Patients are looking for someone who understands them and the psychological processes that they are experiencing. Patients are revealing their most difficult issues, a history that overwhelms them, and deep relationship issues for the psychotherapist to help them through. Establishing a trusting relationship begins with *empathy*, which is the psychotherapist's ability to understand the emotional process of the patient. Fostering empathy involves reflective listening, cognitive processing, and tracking while processing what the patient is conveying verbally and nonverbally through body language (see Chapter 4 for more information on communication). An empathetic relationship reflects sensitivity, or the understanding of thoughts, feelings, and struggles. Psychiatric advanced practice nurses track the narrative while observing areas of distress and brain functioning.

Not every patient is able to develop an empathetic link in psychotherapy, especially if they have a developmental disorder or post-traumatic stress disorder. Awareness of the patient's level of distress regarding information revealed in sessions is important because psychotherapy might activate suicidal or homicidal thoughts. If suicidal or homicidal thoughts result from the discussions, the psychotherapist assesses the patient for safety and suicidality and offers additional sessions or emergency support options.

Remaining "mindful" of the emotional struggle exhibited by the patient engages the patient and the therapist in "paying attention" to the evolution of thoughts, feelings, choices, and levels of self-understanding that contribute to the balance of the patient in the environment. Being mindful triggers attunement and insight that crosses the cultural barriers respectfully and allows the therapeutic bond to be established. Mindfulness allows people of all cultural backgrounds to pay attention to the messages that are being transmitted to themselves and others, and to develop self-understanding and self-inquiry (Kabat-Zinn, 2003, 2005).

Safety

Mental illness significantly impacts mortality (Parks, Radke, & Mazade, 2008). Documenting assessment of safety and treatment is important to protect the psychiatric advanced practice nurse from adverse professional actions. Mental illness can create deep negative thoughts, which can erode both perspective and the will to live. In addition, psychotherapy can reveal areas of insecurity, abuse, and unsafe behaviors that patients have not been able to deal with by themselves. Patients become fragile and impulsive due to a variety of circumstances; hence, patient safety must be assessed and reflected in treatment goals, and patients need to be informed of how to access emergency treatment. Understanding and documenting risk for suicide is lifesaving, and it opens opportunities for valuable interventions. Previous suicide attempts, family history of suicide, and current obsessions or messages indicate the emotional level of vulnerability. Assessment tools, such as the SAD PERSONS scale, will assist in documentation and assessment of suicide risk (Patterson, Duhn, Bird, et al., 1983):

S Sex
A Age
D Depression
P Previous attempts
E Ethanol abuse
R Relational loss
S Social supports lacking
O Organized plan
N No spouse
S Sickness

Psychiatric advanced practice nurses working in psychotherapy must use an organized clinical process that incorporates an ongoing comprehensive assessment and tracking of complex mental health and family dynamics. Psychiatric advanced practice nurses' scope of practice shifts focus among core principals of psychiatry, psychology, and psychotherapy. Using a clinical model such as MINDFUL CARE, the nurse psychotherapist can balance listening to the individual's processing of emotional distress with the process of assessment and the identification of goal-focused interventions.

The MINDFUL CARE Model

The MINDFUL CARE model is a nurse psychotherapy model that provides a framework for psychotherapy. It integrates scope of practice, assessment, treatment, clinical models, and evidence-based practice. It reflects recent developments in understanding (1) changes in gene expression (see Chapter 1), (2) changes related to developmental stress, and (3) how to work to change patterns of adaptation. By understanding stress responses and maladaptive patterns of communication and behavior, nurse psychotherapists can help patients change behavior to more adaptive patterns and more effective transmission of messages. For example, psychotherapy has been demonstrated to decrease the activation and reshape the perceptions, thus decreasing the neural firing of synapses that trigger the hypothalamic-pituitary-adrenal axis. The role of the nurse psychotherapist is not just to listen empathically, but also to direct the process toward growth and wellness, with the ultimate goal of recovery.

Psychiatric advanced practice nurses have a comprehensive preparation that enables them to assess and treat the whole person who presents with mental health issues. The MINDFUL CARE model addresses the whole person by organizing a comprehensive assessment and treatment process (Katz, 2008), and it works regardless of the patient's age and stage of life or the setting of the therapeutic process (discussed later in this chapter).

MINDFUL CARE does the following:

- It relies on emotional presence and attunement during ongoing assessment and therapeutic process, as well as insight into the patterns of the patient's mental, physical, and family process. When the practitioner works through a MINDFUL CARE assessment process, the areas of classical nursing—psychiatry and psychology—and epidemiological factors can be integrated into the psychotherapy model chosen for the treatment of mental illness.
- It focuses on assessment of potential levels of functioning, establishment of hope, and identification of potential availability of peer support and community resources, thus using a recovery model for mental health and substance abuse (Katz, 2008).
- It reflects the whole treatment team's role as well as that of the psychiatric advanced practice nurse and places priority on the patient's adaptation, with evidence-based practice as the center of the recovery plan.

The MINDFUL CARE diagram (Fig. 7-1) is useful as a visual tool. It illustrates and gives perspective to the whole person's baseline strengths and their functioning, and it qualifies treatment planning, treatment focus, and realistic goals of patient care. The main areas of the MINDFUL CARE diagram are as follows:

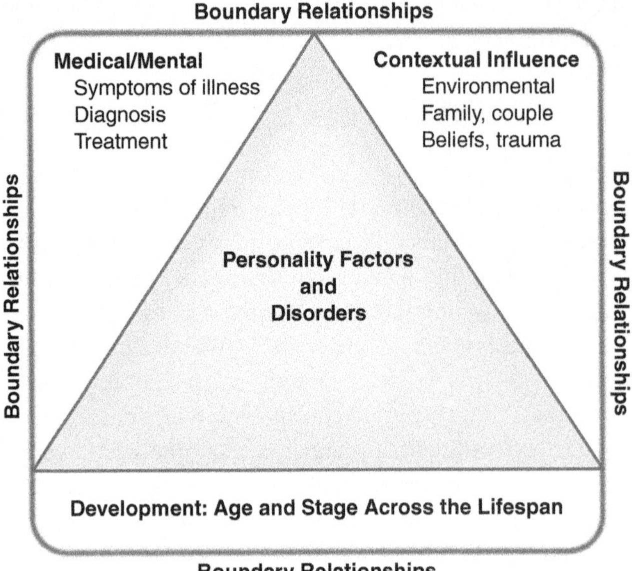

FIGURE 7-1: The MINDFUL CARE model provides a way to assess patients' baseline strengths and functioning, personality traits, medical and mental disorders, and contextual influences across the life span within the boundary of relationships. This model of assessment provides the basis for setting realistic patient goals and planning appropriate treatment interventions.

- *Medical/mental illness/substance abuse* history and comorbidities (mental illness or medical diagnosis, adverse behaviors, pharmacology, medical risks, and genetics)
- *Contextual influences* (environmental circumstances, key family/relationships, occupational or educational stability, and home life)
- *Developmental obstacles* (actual age verses stage of life demonstrated) and underlying influence of *personality disorders*

Personality factors, addictions, defense mechanisms, and unconscious response to crisis need to be considered in the assessment, and the therapist must take care to select appropriate patient-centered clinical treatment modalities. Goals of patient care depend on the patient's overall functioning. Although the nurse psychotherapist assesses a large scope of issues, the MINDFUL CARE diagram assists in understanding and organizing diagnosis and treatment goals, just like a genogram illuminates the family dynamics.

The MINDFUL CARE model puts into context the professional role and boundaries of patient education and nursing insight in the delivery of psychotherapy. The assessment process frames the clinical process by addressing areas of the brain, of behavior, and of the mind/body continuum that have been altered by imbalances in brain chemistry, physical illness, or neurobiological or developmental dysfunctions. It also addresses areas of family, individual, and social dysfunction that interfere with physical or mental health recovery.

For the new psychiatric advanced practice nurse, it can be intimidating to "see" the therapeutic process and understand the balance of issues that need to be altered to heal the patient systematically. To simplify the nursing process in psychiatric nursing, the acronym MINDFUL consolidates assessment areas, with CARE focusing on the process of intervention, coordination, and resources to develop a plan of psychotherapeutic intervention:

- **M** Medical and mental health review of systems, mental status examination, data collection, and review of physical, mental and substance-abuse history
- **I** Identity of the patient in the family and environment
- **N** Nutrition and nurturing of self
- **D** Developmental age and stage
- **F** Family system
- **U** Unconscious mental process: personality, defense mechanisms
- **L** Level of life functioning

—

- **C** Collaborative care
- **A** Adaptation
- **R** Recovery and instillation of hope
- **E** Evidence-based practice and patient education

The rest of this section will further explain the steps in the MINDFUL CARE model.

M: Medical and Mental Health History and Review of Systems

While the structure of the initial interview varies, it is essential to focus on the patient's current, past, and family history of illnesses (medical illnesses, mental health problems including suicidality, and substance abuse). Accuracy of the information obtained reflects effective engagement, clear communication of goals, and maintenance of the boundaries of the confidential relationship. Depending on the situation, the maturity of the patient and therapist, and previous therapeutic experiences, the first interview can either be very intimidating or progress with ease. Although psychological assessment forms provide an excellent guide for the interview, the nursing process needs to address the integration of systems that influence healing the whole person in his or her environment.

Psychiatric Mental Health History, Medications, and Survey of Psychiatric Symptoms

The psychiatric issues presented have a history or trigger that needs to be documented. Using the assessment format, the mental health history can be helpful to document family history, genetic history, substance abuse, or stressors that have triggered the psychiatric mental health process. While the bulk of the initial interview is based on the patient's subjective story, to the trained practitioner, engagement in the story opens the unconscious process of the psychotherapeutic relationship. Mental status examination is documentation of the clinician's perception of the patient's behavioral and cognitive functioning. Tracking the symptoms, assessing communication, and testing perception or memory enables the clinician to understand thoughts, impulses, and how the brain is functioning. It is difficult to assess defense mechanisms and projective patterns during the initial interview, but thoughts regarding their unconscious processing should be noted for further investigation in later sessions, as they might be inhibiting mental wellness and adaptation.

Medical History, Medications, and Symptoms

Comorbidity of mental health problems and medical disorders creates higher acuity and mortality. Documentation through noting detailed history and the age of initiation of a chronic medical condition can give details of how the patient's life has been affected by medical issues and interventions. When multigenerational transmission of illness is viewed in the MINDFUL CARE or holistic perspective, psychotherapy can work to resolve somatic transmission of behavioral patterns. Assessment of the patient's reaction to physical and emotional stress will open up an understanding of how the mind and body tolerate distress, will identify defense mechanisms or personality traits, and will determine the presence of protective factors, such as spirituality. Documentation of prescribed medications is essential in considering the effectiveness of treatment as well as adherence factors. Medical symptoms illuminate ongoing disease state management, need for collaboration with other healthcare providers, and integration of treatment for mental health problems and for medical pathology.

Psychotherapy can be instrumental in connecting the mind and body reactions. For example, when examining the interaction of the hypothalamic-pituitary-adrenal axis and the stress reaction, the clinician can select a therapeutic modality that will decrease the trigger stressor on both the mental illness and the medical issue. Physical, emotional, and sexual abuse or traumas have been noted to trigger emotional or physical symptoms that can interrupt coping or developmental stages or can even trigger automatic nervous system patterns.

I: Identity of the Patient in the Family and Environment

In psychotherapy, it is easy to focus on symptoms or on the story that the patient tells, however, to empower patients to alter health patterns requires an understanding of their identity. The patient's identity encompasses the patient's functioning in the context of his or her environment, occupation, expectations, relationships, losses, life choices, addictions, and legal or military history. The individual's sense of self reflects his past in the context of his current life circumstances. The human experience in developing identity incorporates sense of belonging and sense of being different

(Minuchin, 1974). Family and individuation are central to patient perception, function, personality, and choices, and they account for many poor health behaviors and mental health issues. Having a clear picture of who a person is, how he or she functions, and what his or her personal obstacles are will make it easier to identify and address issues.

As the psychotherapeutic relationship develops, goals for incorporation of positive traits and strengthening techniques that can enhance mental health and functioning are identified. Patients need to accept themselves for who they are and understand areas that they can change. They may demonstrate problems with this acceptance and understanding by resisting treatment or being nonadherent with medications. The nurse therapist may focus on understanding the patients' perception of engaging in an appropriate trial of treatment or on developing an alternative holistic treatment plan.

Ethnic and cultural identity integration creates a sense of self and mental health, regardless of the outward cultural or religious practice. Family history of mental illness and how the mental illness was treated or adapted to as a multigenerational problem may impact patient recovery. Addressing cultural and ethnic identity integration could be an effective method in developing the patient's ego strength that will be needed for changing emotional and physical processes.

Addictions are core behaviors central to a patient's identity, with socializing and coping directly linked to substance use or addictive behaviors. In addition, patients with addictions have difficulty seeing the impact of their substance abuse problem or addiction (such as gambling, sex, eating, or computer addiction) on themselves, their family, and their functioning. In working to address addictions or dual diagnosis (in which the patient has both a mental illness and a substance use disorder), it is necessary for patients to understand how their identity will change if they adopt a sober or addiction-free lifestyle. (See Chapter 17 for information on Co-occurring Substance Use and Psychiatric Disorders.)

N: Nutrition and Nurturing

What and how patients eat and nurture themselves is essential to mental health and overall healing. Nutrition and nurturing create emotional connections that begin in early childhood and last a lifetime, and they engage internal unconscious messages about self-worth. Developmental interruption of maternal-child nurturing and nutrition can create painful feelings of deprivation and abandonment, increasing the potential for mental illness later in life (Bowlby, 1988; Briere, 2002).

Medical issues can have underlying nutritional deficiencies, requiring augmentation or special diet. Thyroid function impacts body weight and mental health; thus, it is a primary concern in patients' assessment and diagnosis. Inability to adhere to primary care providers' recommendations for proper nutrition can indicate symptoms of depression, obsessive-compulsive eating, and other eating disorders. Baseline data collection of weight, height, and blood chemistry in combination with a discussion of daily dietary intake will be helpful in selecting a psychotropic medication, monitoring for side effects, and providing a baseline of psychological functioning. Patients will frequently return to normal metabolic weight when they are in optimal mental balance.

Eating disorders can be life threatening, with severe implications for all body systems, especially cardiac, digestive, and metabolic systems. The underlying issue of eating disorders is not food, but the inability to nurture self, construct identity, communicate, and tolerate stress independently; the patient often experiences faulty perceptions and a faulty sense of self-worth (Sobel, 2008). Morbid obesity, which has increased significantly in recent years, has a significant link to brain functioning and depression. Even with good diet and weight supervision, oral defenses (the need to use or refuse food to decrease anxiety), mental health problems, and addictions draw patients back to a disease state. Depression and other psychiatric symptoms increase with body mass index (Vogelzangs, Kritchevsky, Beekman, et al., 2008). Treating morbid obesity without mental health treatment will not allow for full recovery.

D: Developmental Age and Stage

The sequence of normal development involves learning specific tasks that link neural development, mastery of psychological stages, evolving personality, psychopathology, and communication skills that enable adaptation through life. Erik Erikson created a theory of identified stages and developed stages of development throughout the life span (see Chapter 1). Erikson theorized that without appropriate developmental mastery, subsequent stages, if stagnated or never mastered, could create physical, cognitive, social, and emotional maladjustment (Erikson, 1980). Regardless of chronological age, maturity through developmental stages sets reaction formation patterns that might be inhibiting the development of ego states needed to tolerate distress (Siegel, 1999; Watkins & Watkins, 1997). Adaptation might follow predictable patterns, but if out of sequence the patterns can trigger psychopathology or personality issues. Sexual development and emotional security enable ego development and object relations that lead to mastery of steps toward emotional independence/dependence, subsequently impacting patterns in brain functioning (Amen, 1998; Cozolino, 2010). Traumatic events, especially physical or sexual abuse, trigger developmental scarring that is evident many years after the traumatic event (see Chapter 3).

Maladaptive developmental milestones can be healed through psychotherapy as long as the patient can engage in a trusting relationship and work through unconscious defenses that have developed through years of maladaptive reaction formation and regression. For example, treating post-traumatic stress disorder close to the time of the trauma will help prevent trauma reenactment, defense formation, and other maladaptive reactions (Briere, 2002).

Psychotherapists can choose from a number of directions how to identify the impact of development on psychopathology. This impact is identified by taking a thorough history of patients' growth and development, by defining their relationship to parents and siblings, and by recording their history of trauma, abuse, losses, and obstacles during the growth process in the overall family experience. Many people cannot recall their childhood, and the trust found in a therapeutic relationship can provide a safe place to remember traumatic experiences, but these recollections need to occur without suggestion and be kept safe to explore and to live with after disclosure. Many therapists use a family genogram and timeline, filled out by patients at home. Unconscious messages are introjected into one's personality by parents and others during childhood, so positive or negative messages regarding their growth are important to note.

Developmental disabilities are becoming more prevalent, treatable, and hopefully curable, and many psychiatric advanced practice nurses will work in developmental disabilities centers or pediatric practices. Developmental issues of a sibling affect the whole family system, and this needs to be addressed at some time during the psychotherapeutic relationship, as it might be the underlying cause of the psychiatric diagnosis.

F: Family Systems

The family system is a transactional system that provides direct messages regarding roles, expectations, genetics, support systems, and coping skills. The family establishes cultural and individual expectations that follow the individual through the life span.

A detailed family history includes a family genogram or a timeline of family or developmental history, which illuminates various factors that impact emotional growth and adaptation. This important therapeutic tool is a way for the psychotherapist to keep the case clear in his or her mind and for the patient to demonstrate connections within the family of origin (Carter and McGoldrick, 1999). A genogram tracks the multigenerational transmission of patterns and provides necessary data to enhance the therapist's insight. Life stressors and birth order affect development, communication, relationship modeling, and functioning in group settings. Assessment of sibling order and patterns can illuminate mental health disorders, substance abuse, and suicide potential. Information about birth order, pregnancies, miscarriages, adoptions, and divorces will enhance understanding of developmental obstacles and sources of distress. Family triggers are identified by understanding parental relationships and influences, both in the current context and in the past. Traumatic family events, military experiences, and other issues might have had an impact on the patient's growth and development of self and on the family unit. Household moves as well as job loss and the economic distress of parents might have had a lasting impact on development and security.

Family Systems Core Concepts

Family systems work begins with understanding the impact that family birth order, family issues, addictions, projection process, conditions of birth, relocations, deaths, economic issues, and family diseases had on the individual. Through understanding the family process and factors that created patterns in personality, defense mechanisms, and psychiatric illnesses, patients can be empowered to make changes within themselves that encourage healthy relationships and decisions. Underlying every family system are the core family organizational patterns:

- Adaptability
- Connectedness
- Family boundaries
- Triangulation
- The family projection process

Consider the family as the psychological equivalent to the womb. While the baby is in the womb, the mother may do everything possible to ensure that it is healthy; or, as in the case of a mother who has an addiction, she may abuse the fetus through neglect such as lack of prenatal care and good nutrition and exposure to alcohol and drugs. The family can be seen in the same way as a womb, in that parents and other family members can either nurture and protect other family members, or neglect or abuse them. Psychotherapy works to treat maladaptive coping that was established by families, thus altering the multigenerational transmission of dysfunction and messages that trigger mental illnesses. Through identifying maladaptive responses to family circumstances, the psychotherapist can provide adaptive models of boundaries and responses.

Adaptability

Family systems communicate adaptability through systems of rules, modeling of coping styles, and values. Change is constant within each individual's stages of growth and development; flexibility within the family structure contributes to nurturing and attachment, whereas reactivity or rigidity will contribute to fight-or-flight reactions. Family leadership, organization, and roles within the family need to be assessed for a counterbalance of flexibility and stability as they contribute to adaptation during the various life stages. For instance, the way a family adapts to the diagnosis of a significant illness can illuminate elements of family adaptation that might inhibit wellness (Rolland, 1994).

Connectedness or Attachment

John Bowlby and Mary Ainsworth's landmark research into attachment of infants to their parents established the value of family attachments during early development as the major contributor to resilience and ego strength in dealing with illness or trauma (Bowlby, 1988; Bretherton, 1992; Siegel,

1999). Establishing attachment in the family engages a balance between closeness and mutual support, giving reinforcement to emotional brain development throughout the life span. Extremes of family disengagement or enmeshment alter responsiveness, leading to dysfunctional reaction formation (Siegel) (see Chapter 1 for discussion of attachment).

Through a psychotherapeutic relationship, patient attachment and connectedness can be mirrored through transference and reinforcement of emotional connectedness by processing the loss and consistency of a relationship. This process increases neuroplasticity and adaptation, resulting in more appropriate adaptation to internal messages (Cozolino, 2010).

Family Boundaries

Family systems have natural boundaries that vary in terms of rules of closeness and clarity of roles between individuals (Bowen, 1978; Minuchin, 1974). Defining appropriateness of boundaries during childhood is critical to personality formation, and it involves organization of emotional security that promotes differentiation and independence in responsibility for thoughts and actions. Psychotherapy is an active mechanism to address the inappropriate formation of boundaries, as it offers opportunities to mimic boundary formation.

Triangulation

All families and relationships have a triangulation process that can be either *functional* and demonstrate appropriate boundaries or *dysfunctional* and scapegoat a third person into a role that deflects tension (Bowen, 1978; Minuchin, 1974). Understanding the role of triangulation of patients in their family of origin may reveal the origin of imbalances and pathology. Early response to triangulation can stimulate parentification (taking on a parental role that is inappropriate for the age of the child) or regression. When seen in family illness, parentification can lead to premature emotional entitlement that interrupts normal boundaries of relationships. Regression from the stress of the triangulation can be seen in lack of differentiation, continued regression, or dependence when stress or illness is present.

Family Projection Process

All families have projections or expectations within reason. When families transmit their emotional problems onto their offspring, the process can impair the child to the extent that he or she has an increased vulnerability to symptoms of illness (Bowen, 1978). Understanding the messages that might have led to dependency or reactivity will enhance healing in the therapeutic relationship.

U: Unconscious

During the psychotherapeutic process, it is important to notice not only what is being said and observed, but also what is being unconsciously blocked. Patients naturally transfer or project deep unconscious patterns or emotions onto the therapeutic process and act out in subsequent relationships. Being unconscious of this emotional reactivity and process and lacking the depth of insight to see where their reaction might be coming from, they subsequently lack the insight to alter their own automatic or instinctual process to make effective changes. As seen in family systems, the capacity of forming satisfying relationships is related to internal messages that have origins within early family relationship development. The unconscious process is a complex concept involving the struggle between id, ego, and superego to suppress thoughts and actions that compromise the integrity of the individual's ability to exert control or avoid mental pain or uncontrollable impulses (Freud, 1938). Carl Jung's study of the unconscious helps the nurse psychotherapist to understand the role of the unconscious process, and it illuminates the elements of the unconscious mind that trigger roles, behaviors, and illnesses (Stein, 1998).

Jung's clinical instinct and insight provided him with the basis for creating a map of the unconscious, detailing elements that underlie behavior and insight into patterns. The psychotherapist makes connections regarding the conscious and unconscious patterns by understanding instincts, archetypes, and the psyche's ability to control emotional energy. Our minds have intangible symbolic representations and emotional characteristics that are universal, regardless of age, stage, or society. These unconscious thoughts trigger both physical and psychological responses in the form of hormone excretion and generational or occupational tendencies. Patients gain insight into their patterns and behaviors by working with a psychotherapist to bring the unconscious to consciousness through disclosure in a safe psychotherapeutic relationship. Psychotherapists use direct investigation of unconscious tendencies to diffuse maladaptive reactions, transference, and resistance that trigger psychopathology (Rosenthal, 2010). Assessing and encountering unconscious patterns are key features of many clinical modalities and are evident in all psychotherapeutic relationships.

When a patient presents with emotionally disabling issues, psychic energy needs to be assessed and understood to prescribe a modality that will enable change. Looking for history or "constellations" of behaviors and schemas that predated reactions may lead to an understanding of the unconscious patterns of character or reactivity. Jung attempted to scientifically categorize and make concrete the unconscious, which is a spectrum of the psyche processing. Psychotherapists can identify both instincts and the archetypes the patient displays, giving conscious illumination to the unconscious constellation of complexes that initiate behaviors and impulsivity.

Patients display the unconscious traits through the symbolism, schemas, dreams, and fantasies that they bring to sessions (Jung, 1938). The therapist analyzes the unconscious through understanding the instincts and archetypes that dictate the schemas. Instincts are the physiologic responses to psychic impulses, producing instinctual memory, automatic physical response ("knee-jerk reactions"), fantasy, dreams, and emotions (Stein, 1998). Stimulation of hormones and emotional reactions (tears) are an indication that instinctual information converts from the unconscious psyche to the somatic/physiologic response. Hunger and sexuality are examples of instincts that are unconscious processes. Archetypes are described as "permanent covert structures within the collective and radical unconscious" that can be seen as typical images in personality, roles, reactions, desires, life events, and defenses (Watkins & Watkins, 1997, p. 5).

Unconscious processes in psychotherapy are also seen in the transference and defense mechanisms exhibited by patients toward significant people in their lives and their psychotherapists. Patients displace emotions onto the psychotherapist or significant others, opening the psychotherapist to the deeper emotional process that underlies their dysfunctional process or illness (Sadock & Sadock, 2008). Defense mechanisms are seen as distortions of the psychodynamic unconscious that help us regulate negative emotions by reducing or minimizing anxiety, shame, or guilt and by decreasing awareness of depressing and demoralizing realities (Cozolino, 2010).

L: Life Functioning

Psychiatric advanced practice nurses are consulted not only regarding mental illnesses, but also when quality of life is being weighed in medical treatment and when life transitions affect coping. The overall composition of dysfunction and its impact greatly influence patients' prognosis and ability to progress past the illness as seen in a present state. Knowledge of impairment of functioning and its impact on the patient's life enables psychiatric advanced practice nurses to consistently assess patient safety and independence through the psychotherapeutic process.

Psychiatric advanced practice nurses are clinically competent to assist patients and their families in confronting serious medical decisions that affect the family functioning and coping. These coping decisions span the life cycle, including fertility and pregnancy, developmental disabilities, chronic medical conditions, and hospice care. Much unconscious processing is associated with decisions regarding life and death, and an individual needs to assess and understand it in order to make decisions. The psychiatric advanced practice nurse uses a patient-centered approach to assist patients in identifying core beliefs about their inner self with regard to their feelings about the disease process, their needs, and what the collaborative team can do to facilitate meeting their needs (Green, 2006).

In dealing with life issues, patients need to understand

1. Their own situation through self-actualization
2. What they need to do to accommodate to changes in their concept of self
3. How they are going to communicate their feelings or their decision to enlist a family or support system to assist in achieving adaptation

This process of understanding life issues is universal, applicable to situations from adaptation to raising a child with developmental differences to facing end of life. Psychotherapy might be enlisted in the individual process, or it may be used in family work.

Alterations in life functioning can also occur with natural or manmade disasters, such as the 9/11 tragedy, earthquakes, fires, mud slides, or catastrophic oil spills, or with situational traumatic events such as divorce or death of spouse (see Chapter 11). In addition to alterations in functioning, the individual's sense of safety and trust are unpredictably disrupted. Working with contextual loss brings to consciousness the lack of control of environment and life projection. Spirituality and relationships come into awareness and are used as concrete means to deal with the loss of control, to engage in healing, and to promote security. Family relationships are revisited and emotional support systems are reassessed.

As patients strive to be responsible in life, there are shifts in life functioning that greatly add to the complexity of significant psychiatric disorders and character disorders. Divorce, separation, loss, and other changes can compromise ability to respond to normal stress, with resulting distress. Acute distress can compromise sleep cycles and is associated with the development of anxiety, depression, addictions, and other psychiatric issues. Addressing sleep issues can give a clearer perspective of the depth of psychiatric issues. Interventions to diffuse reactivity include a short course of psychotropic medications, crisis debriefing, eye movement desensitization and reprocessing, and psychotherapy that focuses on diffusing crisis response and developing a new life focus.

Tracking life functioning is essential to evidence-based practice, with the Global Assessment of Functioning (GAF) scale used as the fifth axis of *Diagnostic and Statistical Manual of Mental Disorders (DSM-IV-TR)* diagnosis. The GAF scale is a compilation of social, occupational, and psychological factors. Psychiatric treatment must take into consideration a patient's ability to be responsible for his or her actions and to perform functions independently. The GAF scale reflects the severity of the patient's symptoms, functioning, safety, and ability to be responsible for his or her decisions and actions. While the assessment tool is universally used, the clinician determines its application, based on evaluation of information obtained during the patient assessment. The scale is instrumental in determining hospitalization, progress in treatment, and treatment planning (American Psychiatric Association, 2000).

C: Collaboration and Integrated Care

The Institute of Medicine (2006) report, *Improving the Quality of Health Care for Mental Health and Substance Use Conditions*, stated that "healthcare for general, mental, and substance use problems and illnesses must be delivered with the understanding of the inherent interactions between the mind/brain and the rest of the body" (pp. 71-72). General health, mental health, and substance use conditions are highly related. For example, one in five patients hospitalized for a heart attack suffers from major depression for up to 1 to 4 months after the heart attack, and the presence of major depression increases the risk of dying from heart-related illness. Depression may also result in a delay of returning to work, poorer quality of life, and a worsening of both physical and mental health (Bush, Ziegeldtein, Patel, et al., 2005).

The importance of collaboration and communication about treatment among health-care providers has been supported by countless studies over the past decade. For example, there are significant advantages in overall health of patients with mental and substance use disorders and in health-care delivery when the patient's physical and mental care are integrated into the same office, are co-located, or benefit from distant collaboration (Mauer & Druss, 2007). The rationale and data related to the advantages of collaboration have been incorporated into health-care reform legislation, shifting mental health and substance use disorder treatment to a collaborative or integrated approach. Regardless of whether the psychiatric advanced practice nurse is located in an independent office away from a medical system, is co-located with that medical system, is integrated with it, or is on a collaborative health-care team, communication and collaboration are needed to ensure safety and health of patients. Communication should include information about overall patient health issues, health-care data and treatment, clinical goals, accountability of health-care roles, and outcome measurement.

Psychotherapists who routinely collaborate in providing care for patients have found that doing so enhances patient health and referrals. As the psychiatric advanced practice nurses' role shifts to an enhanced presence in primary care environments, their ability to work collaboratively is even more valued. Collaborating and communicating are valued parts of the therapeutic relationship, especially when patients are prescribed medications by multiple health-care professionals, have chronic medical problems or substance-abuse issues, or have acute changes in health that affect both medical and mental health of the individual within the family.

Collaboration begins with the patient-psychotherapist relationship and can involve multiple other reciprocal professional relationships, depending on the needs of the patient. Lack of collaboration between medical and mental-health professionals reduces the effectiveness of both the medical and the psychotherapeutic treatments (Riba & Balon, 2008; Ruddy, Borresen, & Gunn, 2008). It is important to consistently document treatment's influences on behavioral health challenges and changes in mental and physical health throughout treatment. Through collaboration, therapeutic modalities of medical care, psychotherapy, pharmacotherapy, and psychosocial interventions such as case management or vocational rehabilitation are evaluated and balanced.

During the collaboration process, the nurse needs to document clinical assessment data and coordinate with other involved health-care professionals, then gain the patient's permission to release information to collaborate with these providers. It is important to obtain a list of all medications and their dosages, medical rationales, and prescribers. If the psychiatric advanced practice nurse is prescribing medications, it is important to communicate medication changes to the other providers who are prescribing. Patients need to be active members in their health-care coordination and understand their role in their mental health, substance use, or medical treatment. Obstacles to treatment need to be discussed and explored in psychotherapy sessions.

One obstacle to collaboration includes the confidential nature of this discipline. The importance of collaboration and adherence to care recommendations needs to be discussed during psychotherapy to address misconceptions and to ensure that a high level of confidentiality is maintained while exchanging essential information. Patients routinely allow collaboration or communication with primary care providers because it is imperative that other disciplines involved in their care have knowledge of prescription and safety issues that might compromise patients' lives. Communicating treatment goals, issues, and progress can be done verbally through consultation reports or through a short summary of recommended interventions and medications prescribed. Documentation of this communication is an important part of the medical record.

Psychiatric advanced practice nurses are well prepared to make a difference with patients who have such complex needs. Addressing medical treatment and adherence to recommendations, smoking cessation, addictions, and poor sexual or other health practices in psychotherapy sessions allows the intervention to be congruent with preventive strategies. Adapting psychotherapy modalities to medical issues is an important component of psychiatric advanced practice nurses' practice, and it can be accomplished by setting goals, providing affirmations, and challenging the cognitive process and distortions in context with the behavior. Box 7-1 shows the psychiatric advanced practice nurse's clinical toolbox of psychiatric nursing interventions.

A: Adaptation

Work on enhancing adaptation to mental disorders, physical illnesses, and recovery must be adjusted to the patient's needs; it also must address issues on the patient's agenda as they are presented in psychotherapeutic sessions. The timing of these issues depends on exposure during life experiences and is applied to a theoretical adaptation process. In addition to psychology-based clinical modalities, psychiatric

BOX 7-1 Clinical Toolbox

Recovery is the ultimate goal of all psychiatric nursing interventions, and the process of psychotherapy, which enhances patients' adaption to stress or change, plays a crucial role in moving them toward recovery. The psychiatric advanced practice nurse's toolbox for clinical practice may include

- Patient education materials
- Traditional psychotherapy models
- Holistic modalities (hypnosis, guided imagery, Reiki, emotional freedom technique, etc.)
- Involvement of significant family members or others in patients' lives

Deciding which modality to use in a session is influenced by the psychiatric advanced practice nurse's mastery of the type of psychotherapy and supervision, as well as the patient's philosophy of care.

nursing models can be especially useful tools to guide the thought process of adaptation.

R: Recovery and Establishing Hope

Research into brain development and changes that occur throughout life have demonstrated that therapeutic relationships can promote a shift in brain chemistry and a change in emotional dynamics that can result in long-term adaptation (Cozolino, 2002, 2010). Knowledge of this shift of brain chemistry supports the validity of many psychotherapeutic clinical modalities that are employed in clinical settings (Wampold, 2010). Research studies have established that patients can recover from mental illness if given the right support and treatment. Psychotherapists now can identify what works to shift the brain chemistry and thus can modify multigenerational transmission of mental health traits. Short-term cognitive therapies challenge beliefs and perceptions, provide opportunities for patients to learn alternative strategies, explore roots to reactions, and employ new skills. Nurse psychotherapists can enhance the cognitive therapeutic session through health education and medication management of symptoms, and they can combine clinical modalities with holistic tools that decrease reactivity and perception of stress.

Recent consumer-based research and evolution in mental health treatment has led to adopting the Recovery and Resilience Model to move treatment from patient dependence to patient independence. The recovery model empowers patients with the freedom to understand their abilities, deal with challenges, and connect with others. The principal values of the recovery model reframe and support significant mental illness by instilling hope, establishing peer support, cultivating respect by identifying strengths, providing patient education and choices, instilling personal responsibility, and empowering the patient. These principles of the recovery model should be addressed with the patient as treatment goals in individual or group psychotherapy sessions (Substance Abuse and Mental Health Services Administration, 2009).

E: Evidence-Based Practice and Patient Education

Mental health care is an evolving science that incorporates a wide scope of practice and research from psychiatry, psychology, nursing, human development, neurology, neuroscience, and primary care medicine into clinical practices with real patient problems. Psychiatric advanced practice nurses have the responsibility (1) to provide research-based clinical care that reflects professional research and supporting literature and (2) to develop care plans that are acceptable for patients' needs while providing cost-effective outcomes (Rice, 2008). The history of psychiatry illustrates how, before evidence-based practice, patients received less than optimal care that compromised patient health, inhibited human rights, and created dependence. As a profession, we are obligated to continue to update our knowledge base on patient problem presentations and to adapt research and professional standards of care to clinically proven methods (Mundy & Stein, 2008).

Evidence-Based Practice

Documenting evidence-based practice demonstrates consistent treatment approaches and outcomes. While reimbursement is not currently linked to evidence-based practice outcomes, there has been a movement to have patients complete mental health surveys, either through direct contact with their insurance carriers or at the clinician's initiation in the office for later review. The most commonly used clinical scale in clinical outpatient practices is the Patient Health Questionaire-9 (PHQ-9). This scale is a nine-item depression scale based directly on the *DSM-IV-TR* that can be used to track symptom changes, overall level of distress, and suicide potential and to evaluate treatment outcomes. Greater use of clinical scales will be helpful in establishing measurable goals of treatment.

Evidence-based practice in mental health treatment is dependent on the patient-psychotherapist relationship, most notably the establishment of empathy and trust. Using clinical scales or other strategies to quantify care objectively allows for a problem-oriented approach that also factors in the adaptation and human variables that patients bring to the psychotherapy session. According to Melnyk and Fineout-Overholt (2005), evidence-based practice in psychotherapy involves a five-step process:

1. Ask a clinical question regarding the best approach to patient care.
2. Search and appraise the existing evidence.
3. Combine the research evidence with clinical expertise and experience and patient preferences and values.
4. Plan and carry out the intervention.
5. Evaluate the outcomes.

Evidence-based practice provides insight not only into the patients' progress, but also into what works in psychotherapy. With documentation of psychotherapy with evidence-based practice guidelines in mind, we can illustrate the impact of psychiatric nursing's scope of practice and can develop research-based treatment guidelines.

Patient Education

The stigma of mental illness has been perpetuated by lack of knowledge of mental health disorders and common treatments and by lack of patient empowerment to change. Patients sometimes do not understand the facts about their mental health condition, creating a self-stigma that can inhibit treatment. Working with a patient and his or her family to understand basic facts about the patient's illness can empower everyone to take an active role in the patient's recovery (The Substance Abuse and Mental Health Services Administration, 2009). Patients receive information from a variety of media, especially commercials for psychotropic medications and television programs. While most of this information enhances understanding of common conditions, the information frequently does not present a balanced perspective, allowing projection and personalization by patients and their families. The patient's perspective of his or her mental health can inhibit appropriate treatment adherence. Patients' perceptions and understanding of their diagnosis, medications, treatment options, community options, and course of illness are important topics to address in individual or group psychotherapy sessions.

Summary of MINDFUL CARE in the Context of Mental Health Treatment

Psychiatric advanced practice nurses have been valued as psychotherapists in clinical settings for over 60 years. Learning the process of psychotherapy is different for psychiatric advanced practice nurses than for other types of psychotherapists, as the psychiatric advanced practice nursing profession is based on clinical theories reflecting the biopsychosocial foundation of nursing as well as on theories of psychology and psychiatry. Defining their skills and using them in diverse clinical settings involves speaking the same language as their mental health colleagues. The nursing model, MINDFUL CARE, consolidates the assessment areas and focuses on the process of identifying interventions, coordination, communication, and resources that are incorporated into a plan of psychotherapeutic intervention for the patient. The psychotherapy models presented in the later part of the chapter are clinical modalities used by all licensed mental health professionals.

An Introduction to Brief Psychotherapies

Psychotherapy is an integral part of psychiatric treatment. In a time when psychopharmacology may appear to "be the answer," consider the following metaphor: "Tranquilizers and psychotropic drugs serve as a life jacket—they keep you afloat, but they do not show you the way back to shore" (Van Pelt, 2009, in Carlat, 2010, p. 10). Psychotherapy gets patients back to shore.

Psychotherapeutic approaches to treatment have various focuses, goals, and lengths of treatment. The following presentation includes the major types of psychotherapies but does not exhaust the approaches available to nurse psychotherapists. Of the many tools available to them in their "psychotherapy tool chest," nurse psychotherapists will most frequently use brief (or short-term) psychotherapies, which are divided into three models:

- Relational therapies (psychodynamic psychotherapy and interpersonal psychotherapy)
- Learning therapies (cognitive therapy, behavioral therapy, and dialectical behavioral therapy)
- Contextual therapies (strategic psychotherapy and solution-focused psychotherapy)

Brief therapy refers to a class of psychotherapies that seek patient behavioral change through active patient involvement via the use of therapist-initiated focused interventions (Dewan, Steenbarger, & Greenberg, 2010). Brief psychotherapy sessions can range from a single session to 20 or more psychodynamic therapy sessions. The popularity of brief therapies increased with the advent of behavioral therapy, cognitive therapy, and strategic therapy.

Behavioral therapy started to gain prominence during the 1970s, and it contributed to the increased use of brief therapies. In lieu of self-exploration and acquisition of insight by the patient, behavioral treatments focused on the role of the therapist as teacher and the role of the patient as learner. The focus of treatment sessions was on obtaining more adaptive coping skills and behaviors, with supplementation of work done outside the formal sessions through use of homework assignments.

From the behavioral paradigm, other models of therapy evolved, such as *cognitive therapy* (Beck, 1976) and *rational-emotive therapy* (Ellis & Dryden, 1997). Both cognitive therapy and rational-emotive therapy addressed dysfunctional thinking patterns, which, when challenged with thoughts that were more reality based, changed the patient's thoughts, perceptions, and mood.

Jay Haley's works, *Strategies of Psychotherapy* (1963) and *Problem-solving Therapy: New Strategies for Effective Family Therapy* (1976) (which drew from work of Milton Erickson), addressed patients' difficulties with solving problems of daily living via *strategic therapy*. For example, if the patient consistently takes the same or a similar approach to solving problems and is unsuccessful, a downward spiral of coping results. In the strategic or problem-solving model of psychotherapy, the therapist is more directive and is a problem solver. Added to the work done in the 1970s on the change process (Watzlawick, Weakland, & Fish, 1974), Haley's strategic approach was adopted and frequently used as a family therapy model.

With the advent of managed care and cost containment that began in the 1980s, brief therapy became more widespread and was seen as economically efficient. Steenbarger (1992) supported brief therapy in managed care organizations, and with the prevalence of evidence-based practice, such brief therapies have tended to become manualized, highly structured, and time restricted (Huppert, Fabbro, & Barlow, 2006). The challenge of time limitations of brief therapies are under discussion. In particular, brief therapies may have their greatest challenges in treating patients with severe and persistent mental illness, who tend to experience higher relapse rates and who respond better to supportive psychotherapy (Reed & Eisman, 2006). Because it is commonly used by nurses for many psychiatric populations, supportive psychotherapy—which is not a brief therapy—is also introduced in this chapter. Table 7-1 provides an overview of the various psychotherapies, including their therapeutic focus, the role of the therapist, their targeted behavioral change, and their structure.

Relational Therapies

Relational therapies (Dewan et al., 2010) include psychodynamic psychotherapy and interpersonal psychotherapy (IPT). The core feature that categorizes these therapies as relational therapies is that the presenting problems reflect difficulties in the relationships that the patient has with others. There are differences between the two psychotherapies, most notably the focus on the therapeutic relationship as a means of patient change in behavior.

Psychodynamic Psychotherapy

In psychodynamic psychotherapy, the presenting problem results from an internalization of conflicts from earlier relationships; anxiety related to these conflicts is controlled through the use of ego defenses. Defense mechanisms help the patient cope with conflicts in the short term, but the same mechanisms delay the resolution of the core relationship conflict. Some people do not enjoy conflict, and resolution of conflict is "swept under the rug" or ignored, which results in resurfacing of the conflict in similar situations. Anxiety results from the triggering of conflicts and the overuse of defenses that do not work in the long term. It is the ongoing conflicts with others that bring a patient into therapy.

Goals

The goal of psychodynamic psychotherapy is to focus on the effect of past experiences on present behaviors, thoughts, emotions, and actions; thus, focus is not on the past but on how past patterns and conflicts continue to affect relationships in the present. The psychotherapist must see the patient's symptoms as more than diagnostic criteria—for instance, to see the use of repeated, maladaptive defenses as a way to deal with conflict, which may be

TABLE 7-1 PSYCHOTHERAPIES

Type of Psychotherapy	Therapeutic Focus	Role of the Therapist	Goal/Targeted Behavioral Change	Structure
Relational Therapies				
Psychodynamic psychotherapy	Internalization of past interpersonal conflicts emerges in current relationships. Transference issues dealt with within therapeutic relationship.	Active role by assessing patient's history with significant others; interpretation and assisting patient to develop insight. Transference used within actual relationship between nurse and patient, and therapist is seen as significant other.	Corrective emotional experience for patient within the therapeutic relationship. Challenge and confront resistance.	Brief, 20 or more sessions may be needed.
Interpersonal psychotherapy	Current interpersonal relationships are found to be difficult to deal with for the patient.	Active role of problem-solver. Therapeutic relationship is not used in the same way as in psychodynamic psychotherapy.	Communication patterns, attachments, and expectations of current interpersonal relationships are discussed.	Brief, 12-20 sessions; patients may need to return to therapy to maintain self and to prevent relapse.
Learning Theories				
Cognitive behavioral therapy (CBT)	Result of use of dysfunctional schemas due to information processing distortions.	Collaborative empiricist.	Challenge negative distorted thoughts and replace them with realistic constructive thoughts.	Usual number of CBT sessions is 16. CBT is highly instructive, and patients are assigned homework between sessions.
Behavioral therapy	Conditioned patterns of emotions and behaviors are triggered by internal and environmental cues.	Directive teacher.	Decondition patterns through skill enactment during exposure to symptom triggers.	Exposure may be gradual or rapid and intensive.

Continued

TABLE 7-1 **PSYCHOTHERAPIES—continued**

Type of Psychotherapy	Therapeutic Focus	Role of the Therapist	Goal/Targeted Behavioral Change	Structure
Dialectical behavioral therapy (DBT)	A therapy approach based on learning theory that is most effective in patients with borderline personality disorder and patterns of suicide attempts and non-suicidal self-injury such as cutting or burning of oneself; however, it has been used with other populations. Integrated and comprehensive strategies of acceptance and change are used in aspects of individual and group therapy sessions. Patients are validated for their feelings while supported in the change process to deal more effectively with behavioral and emotional dysregulation and hypersensitivity to others. The dialectical approach takes the middle road between universalistic and relativistic modes of thought (i.e., there are gray areas of life, and not everything is black and white). Dialectical thinking is the overarching dimension to treatment. Reduction of blaming the victim is emphasized through patient problem-solving.	Therapist is an active participant in both individual and group skills training of patients as well as gaining support and understanding of self through group meetings with other therapists.	Patients may not have been the cause of their emotional hypersensitivity and resulting behaviors, but they are motivated to solve their own problems. Validation is stressed due to patients' being in invalidating environments during development. Seeing both sides of issues, as part of learning dialectical thinking, helps modify extremes in emotions and behaviors, seeing the world differently than in past dichotomous thinking patterns. Skills training in groups offers highly structured format. Telephone consultation may occur for patients when coaching is needed. Change occurs when addressing four levels: (1) severe behavioral dyscontrol; (2) quiet desperation; (3) problematic patterns of living; and (4) incompleteness.	Highly structured and manualized therapy.
Contextual Therapies				
Strategic therapy	Attempting solutions to problems are only reinforcing the problem.	Therapist is a facilitator to change through structured tasks and experiences.	To reframe problems and interrupt current problem-solving cycle, and to initiate novel actions to solve problems.	Highly abbreviated, but not highly structured.
Solution-focused therapy	Emphasis on exceptions to problem patterns and de-emphasis on problem.	Therapist is a facilitator to change through constructing of solution patterns.	Creating and enactment of solution patterns.	Highly abbreviated; often manualized; highly structured.
Supportive Psychotherapy	A dyadic treatment approach that is implemented with a conversational style by the therapist and characterized by the use of techniques to ameliorate symptoms and to maintain, restore, or improve self-esteem, adaptive skills, and psychological functioning. It can be used in a broad continuum of patient diagnoses and levels of functioning.	Therapist helps patient cope with symptoms; prevent relapse of serious mental illnesses; help patient deal with crisis or transient problems; the extent of supportive vs. expressive psychotherapy depends on patient's diagnosis and level of functioning; psychoanalytical approaches (ego psychology, object relations and attachment, self-psychology, interpersonal and relational approach) as well as cognitive behavioral therapy and learning theory/teaching are all used in supportive psychotherapy.	Use of praise, advice, reassurance, and encouragement, exhortation, inspiration, anxiety-reducing interventions, clarification, humor, confrontation, skills building, teaching, redirecting, promoting autonomy, and modeling of adaptive behavior to restore and improve self-esteem, ego functions, and adaptive skills.	Flexible, based on the patient's diagnosis and level of functioning. It is not a brief therapy.

experienced as anxiety or depressed mood. In psychodynamic psychotherapy, the nurse explores the patient's problems of living and brings about behavioral change through interpretation and insight in an effort to reduce a patient's suffering. Acquiring insight into repetitive patterns and their consequences is done in the safety of the therapist's office. If insight is not achievable (because it may take a longer time to acquire), change can be promoted by corrective experiences with the therapist. Reworking ways to handle new situations, relationships, and threats is achieved in therapy sessions.

Indications

Psychodynamic psychotherapy is indicated for depression, dysthymic disorders, anxiety disorders (panic disorder, social phobia, generalized anxiety disorder, post-traumatic stress disorder), somatoform disorders, eating disorders, substance-related disorders, and personality disorders (Leichsenring, 2009). Psychodynamic therapists focus on the psychodynamic features presented by a patient such as conflicts, defenses, and personality organization. Psychodynamic psychotherapy is described as being short term, with a range of 7 to 24 sessions, or long term, with a range of 25 to 46 sessions.

Assessment and Case Formulation

The therapist "works backward" not only to assess the symptoms presented in an intake interview, but also to interpret the presenting complaints within the psychodynamic framework, such as having meaningful ties to past experiences and conflicts that have not been resolved. Certain patient features have a positive impact on the outcome of short-term treatment. These patient features include high motivation, realistic expectations, circumscribed focus, high-quality object relations, and absence of personality disorder (Heglend, 1993; Messer, 2001; Piper, Azim, Joyce, et al., 2001). Case Study 7-1 presents a scenario in which the patient may benefit from psychodynamic therapy. After reading the case, try to describe the issues, conflicts, and defenses the psychiatric advanced practice nurse would discuss with the patient when using psychodynamic psychotherapy.

Strategies

The use of interpretation and the resulting insight gained by the patient is the therapist's strategy in psychodynamic psychotherapy. A patient history will need to include a developmental history and events leading up to the current therapy session to assess for (1) past patterns of conflict that the patient had with significant others, (2) the lack of resolution of such conflicts, and (3) the relationship of those events to current relationship difficulties. The therapist engages the real relationship between the patient and the therapist to assist the patient to see what is happening in the present.

Interventions

Interventions focus on identifying recurring conflictual relationship themes and on the present-day situations in which such themes are acted out. The therapist's aim is to create a positive emotional corrective experience with the therapy itself; thus, change is catalyzed by active involvement in the therapy. Counter-transference is used to provide feedback to the patient. Heightened emotional contexts (Davanloo, 1980; Sifneos, 1972) may assist the patient in a breakthrough within the therapeutic relationship occurring in the here and now. The anxiety may resurrect past memories and feelings about the original conflictual relationship with parents and significant others (Black & Andreasen, 2011). Solving interpersonal problems builds social skills and relieves symptoms.

Efficacy Research

Fisher and Greenberg (1985) and Wallerstein (1989) stated that an abbreviated form of psychoanalytical psychotherapy can achieve positive results, and research suggests that relationship factors, persuasion, suggestion, catharsis, and therapist-as-a-model are more pivotal to the change process than was previously recognized. For example, in the treatment of depression with psychodynamic psychotherapy, the therapist will focus on ego functions and conflicts

CASE STUDY 7-1

Patient Who May Benefit From Psychodynamic Therapy

Jackie is a 48-year-old married woman with three grown children. She is currently on Social Security Disability (SSD) and comes in for her first visit in almost a year. She has a reputation in the clinic for being manipulative and noncompliant. During the last episode of therapy, she was abusing the psychiatric prescribed medications lorazepam and Adderall, and she was not consistent with keeping appointments. She now reports she has been sober for 10 months and is coming back into the clinic "to really work" on her issues. She admits to polysubstance abuse (alcohol and oxycodone) since she was a teen and significant self-medication with over-the-counter drugs. She has been diagnosed with bipolar affective disorder II, borderline personality disorder, and polysubstance abuse. She is currently disabled due to her mental health issues. She has been going to Narcotics Anonymous (NA) meetings and reports that she has a sponsor and is working on her third step. In addition to her history of substance abuse, her father and brother had sexually abused her from ages 12 to 16. Jackie has never dealt with the abuse in previous therapeutic alliances with therapists, but she is determined to deal with it now because she has been told that it might have something to do with her sobriety. However, she states that talking about the abuse makes her feel numb. She demonstrates a monotone voice, a distant gaze, and eventually an overwhelming level of anxiety that is evident in her shaking of her legs and feet, which then moves up her body.

experienced by the patient. Efficacy studies are represented by randomized controlled trials, which are the highest level of research evidence in quantitative research; a meta-analysis of four randomized controlled trial studies comparing cognitive behavioral therapy (CBT) with short-term psychodynamic psychotherapy found that they were equally efficacious in reducing depressive symptoms and improving social functioning (Leichsenring, 2001). The findings of Gowers, Norton, Halek, et al. (1994) showed that short-term psychodynamic psychotherapy combined with four sessions of nutritional counseling demonstrated improvement in patients with anorexia nervosa. In treatment of patients with borderline personality disorder, randomized controlled trials conducted by Munroe-Blum and Marziali (1995) showed improvement of depressive, borderline, and general psychiatric symptoms and found that short-term psychodynamic psychotherapy was as efficacious as interpersonal therapy.

Interpersonal Psychotherapy

IPT began in 1984 as a brief manualized treatment to sustain and focus on the patient's interpersonal relationship with others, but IPT does not focus on the interpersonal relationship with the therapist, as in psychodynamic psychotherapy. Instead, IPT focuses on life events that occurred after early childhood that influence the development of psychopathology. For example, social losses serve as triggers to mental distress, whereas social supports help to protect the patient from distress.

Goals

The goal of IPT is to focus on the difficulties and changes that patients are experiencing in current relationships and on the ways those relationships can be handled. Lengthy review of past relationships is not the goal, as it is in psychodynamic psychotherapy. Rather, overall goals are

1. To change patterns of communication
2. To alter expectations within relationships
3. To use social supports to help patients deal with stress and improve the patient's environment
4. To relieve symptoms
5. To build social skills (Markowitz, 2008; Stuart, 2004; Weissman, Markowitz, & Klerman, 2000)

Indications

The American Psychiatric Association practice guidelines for adults with major depression include IPT among the recommended therapies (Markowitz, 2008). It is useful for patients with depression related to life events or interpersonal conflicts. IPT is considered effective in the treatment of nonpsychotic mild to moderate depression. The Agency for Health Care Policy and Research (1993) lists IPT along with CBT and behavioral therapy as effective in reducing symptoms of major depression. Support for IPT is found for depressive episodes related to

- Complicated bereavement/grief
- Marital and other interpersonal conflicts, such as role disputes
- Life events, such as role transitions
- Isolation, lack of support, and interpersonal deficits (Markowitz, 2008)

Assessment and Case Formulation

Case Study 7-2 presents a complicated patient with depressive symptoms. What would be your psychotherapeutic treatment plan to get her to a calmer state? What is the neuropsychiatric process that was achieved in psychotherapy?

CASE STUDY 7-2

Patient Who May Benefit From Interpersonal Therapy

Rachel, a 68-year-old widow, was referred to you by a colleague. She has a diagnosis of bipolar affective disorder II and borderline personality disorder. The colleague reports that the patient is needy and histrionic during sessions and has been difficult to keep on track. The psychiatrist is also concerned that she is prescribing too much medication, and she is fearful for her license that the patient will overdose.

During the initial session, it is noted that Rachel had good stable mental health and worked as a school nurse until she was 40 years old. That was the year her beloved husband was diagnosed with a brain tumor, and he died the following year. She has two grown children, both married, but her daughter lives in Israel. She now has eight grandchildren whom she had enjoyed visiting twice a year. Her son is married with no children, and he has a very poor relationship with her. He is in charge of her finances, and she has difficulty having a conversation with him without his putting her down or controlling her. She reports having had a very close relationship with her father, who also recently died, leaving a large inheritance. Though her father's death was traumatic, she appears to have tolerated it well. Her psychiatric history includes multiple hospitalizations during the last 20 years and a long relationship with a previous psychiatrist. When her previous psychiatrist wanted to do electroconvulsive therapy, she refused, feeling that it would ruin her memory of her husband. She left the psychiatrist about a year ago because she no longer felt that the medication was helping her and because she no longer trusted the psychiatrist's judgment after a recent hospitalization. She states that she never attempted suicide, but sometimes she gets angry and says that she would be better off dead. She has had no psychotherapy between leaving her previous psychiatrist and coming to the clinic. She is currently taking a laundry list of medications, mostly psychotropic medications. Her only medical problems are hypertension and high cholesterol.

Rachel's current stressor is her loneliness and depression. She lives alone in the house where she and her husband raised their children, and she has been isolating herself from

CASE STUDY 7-2—continued

her relatives and friends by not attending events. She explains that it doesn't bother her if her family members don't check on her if she misses or doesn't attend family social events.

She remarks that she has learned from psychotherapy, but she does not feel that she ever was "heard" with the other therapists. She wishes she could just die, and then her head won't hurt anymore. On assessment for bipolar affective disorder, she reports one significant buying binge of jewelry when her husband gave her money to pay bills. She frequently is depressed, spending days in bed, not answering the phone, or taking a shower. She hates how she looks, her hair is brittle, and she has gained weight since her former psychiatrist put her on Synthroid.

A year later: Rachel is now in an apartment that gets lots of sunshine. Her son, still in control of her finances, is talking to her when needed. She has visited her daughter, and they noted that she is a different person: much calmer, energetic, and able to tolerate distress in a large family. She is now on a minimal dose of medication, has no suicidal thoughts, and is even thinking about dating and having a sex life.

How would you apply interpersonal psychotherapy as a treatment modality in this case?

Strategies

IPT does not focus on transference issues within the relationship with the therapist. Instead, the strategy includes addressing patterns of communication and attachment. The therapist has an active role in the treatment but sustains the focus on the relationship issues experienced by the patient. The therapist is a collaborative problem solver, confronting any patient resistance in a straightforward manner. Future sessions may be necessary after termination of prescribed therapy to maintain gains made and to prevent relapse of symptoms.

Interventions

Interventions include (1) developing a therapeutic contract, (2) exploring interpersonal concerns and brainstorming ways to handle the concerns, (3) providing a means for the patient to be actively involved between sessions based on issues discussed, and (4) refining and reviewing problem-solving efforts. Three phases of interpersonal psychotherapy are early phase, middle phase, and termination phase.

In the *early phase* of therapy, the therapist identifies the depressive symptoms, evaluates the patient, and generates a formal diagnosis. The patient will receive psychoeducation and support to be in the "sick role." Patient's symptoms will be evaluated for the use of medications to treat the depression. The patient's history of depressive symptoms related to interpersonal issues is completed through an interpersonal inventory. The interpersonal inventory involves five areas of assessment:

1. The nature of the interactions the patient has with significant others
2. Identification of reciprocal relationships with significant others and if needs were satisfied
3. Discussion of both satisfying and dissatisfying aspects of the relationship
4. Recent changes in key relationships the patient has with others
5. Changes the patient desires in relationships

The therapist determines the problem area and sets treatment goals. The therapist then explains the IPT process and asks the patient to sign a contract that outlines the problem areas and the treatment goals. Brief therapy and a timeline are developed by the therapist. The target of IPT in this stage is to address the depression related to interpersonal issues and to do so in the here and now (Markowitz, 2008).

During the *middle phase* of therapy, the patient and therapist derive more specific strategies to deal with role transitions, grief, disputes within interpersonal relationships, and the need to improve social skills. In response to grief, the therapist encourages the process of mourning and assists the patient to find other relationships and activities to compensate for the loss. In the case of role transitions, such as transitioning to a new residence, job, role, or developmental stage in life, the patient learns to adapt to the change by mourning the old role and is challenged to transition to the new role. In cases of conflict or role disputes with significant others, the therapist engages the patient to explore the relationship and the nature of the dispute and alternatives to negotiate a resolution. When interpersonal deficits exist or when patients do not report recent life events (such as those described in the previous three problem areas of grief, role transitions, and conflict/role disputes), the therapist focuses on patient symptoms such as loneliness, lack of friends, and poor social skills and on behaviors in beginning and sustaining satisfying relationships with others. Because the sessions focus on the here and now, an opening statement made by the therapist may be, "How have things been since we last met?" (Markowitz, 2008).

During the *termination phase* of therapy, the following are set as goals: (1) to consolidate gains; (2) to foster independence in the patient; (3) to address feelings of guilt; (4) to review the risk of relapse and recurrence of depressive symptoms; and (5) to contract again for continuation and maintenance treatment as needed (Markowitz, 2008). The therapist discusses success in therapy and the fact that the patient was actively involved in making the changes in interpersonal relationships, which directly affected the depressed mood.

Efficacy Research

A pilot matched-control study compared 16 depressed women who received 8 IPT sessions to a control group of 16 depressed women who received the SSRI sertraline

(Zoloft). The findings showed that both groups had significant improvement in symptoms and functional abilities; however, the women who received the IPT improved more quickly than the women treated with sertraline (Swartz, Frank, Shear, et al., 2004).

In a second study created to treat antepartum depression, a 16-week bilingual controlled clinical trial of IPT was compared with subjects in a control group who received a didactic parental education intervention. Fifty women with a *DSM-IV-TR*–b—based diagnosis of major depressive disorder were randomly assigned to the two groups. Depressed mood was measured with several instruments including the Edinburgh Postnatal Depression Scale, the Beck Depression Inventory, and the Hamilton Depression Rating Scale. Recovery was measured using the Clinical Global Impression and the Hamilton Depression Scale. The results demonstrated that IPT is an effective form of treatment for depression during pregnancy, and it is recommended that it be the first-line treatment in the hierarchy of treatment in women during their pregnancy (Spinelli & Endicott, 2003).

In a third study, a randomized trial of weekly, twice-monthly, and monthly IPT as maintenance treatment for women with recurrent depression was carried out to compare the effect of increased frequency of therapy to the traditional monthly IPT. A total of 233 women between the ages of 20 and 60 who were experiencing recurrent unipolar depression were the subjects. After these women had achieved remission with weekly IPT plus antidepressant drug therapy, they were randomly assigned to weekly, twice-weekly, or monthly maintenance IPT. Results indicated that women who did not need an antidepressant could be maintained on once-a-month IPT, as compared to the women who needed the addition of an antidepressant, in whom IPT alone was less significantly efficacious in maintaining their recovery (Frank, Kupfer, Buysse, et al., 2007).

Learning Therapies

Learning therapies include cognitive therapy, behavioral therapy, and dialectical behavioral therapy.

Cognitive Therapy

Cognitive therapy is a form of psychotherapy based on the theory that pathological information processing is linked to emotional reactions and dysfunctional behavioral patterns. Treatment is focused on changing dysfunctional thoughts and mental schemas by asking the patient to be an active participant in critically analyzing the evidence for and against the cognitions that increase the patient's anxious and depressive symptoms.

According to Beck, Rush, Shaw, et al. (1979), depressed patients can have three areas of cognitive distortions, called the negative cognitive triad: negative feelings about the self, about the world, and about the future. Patients with anxiety habitually overestimate the danger or risk in situations and become risk averse and afraid. A vicious cycle results, with negative thoughts affecting mood, thus confirming and amplifying the patient's negative distorted cognitions to such a point that the patient may call himself "a loser" or claim to "give up trying" or state that "I will be alone the rest of my life because no one will want me." It is assumed that cognition has its basis in neuroscience and the biology of mental illness; thus, cognitive therapy is often supplemented with pharmacotherapy to enhance the positive outcome (Wright, Thase, & Beck, 2008).

Cognitive therapy interventions are focused and problem oriented. Although there are specific techniques, the therapy must focus on the therapeutic relationship, a thorough history and case formulation, and aspects of cognitive therapy that are centered on the issues important to the patient. Beck et al. (1979) said that cognitive therapy includes theories and treatment methods of behavioral therapy through use of techniques such as activity scheduling, graded task assignments, exposure, and social skills training. Psychoeducation is also used (Box 7-2). Ellis' rational emotive therapy (Ellis & Dryden, 1997) has helped to advance cognitive therapy. Cognitive therapy techniques, however, are built first upon a solid therapeutic relationship.

The therapeutic relationship in cognitive therapy is characterized by collaboration between the patient and therapist. It takes on an empirical tone because the goal is to work together as an investigative team to discern the nature of the cognitive errors and to empirically analyze the validity of the distorted thoughts and overall mental schemas that patients use in their daily lives. Beck et al. (1979) called this form of a relationship *collaborative empiricism*. There are several methods of enhancing this type of relationship, which are noted in Box 7-3.

Goals

The goals of cognitive therapy are to

1. Establish a nurse-patient therapeutic relationship
2. Complete a full assessment of the patient (via intake interview)
3. Set an agenda for therapy sessions
4. Give constructive feedback to direct the course of the therapy

BOX 7-2 Psychoeducation as an Aspect of Cognitive Therapy

Psychoeducation is a routine part of cognitive therapy. The patient first is socialized to the process of therapy and then is introduced to concepts inherent in cognitive therapy and the format of cognitive therapy sessions. Expectations of both therapist and patient in the therapeutic process of cognitive therapy are reviewed. The therapist introduces the patient to reading and computer-assisted materials and minilectures, and the therapist assigns homework. The cognitive therapy process enhances learning and self-awareness through these assignments. Table 7-2 provides a sample of commonly used resources for psychoeducation for cognitive therapy.

TABLE 7-2 EXAMPLES OF PSYCHOEDUCATIONAL MATERIALS AND COMPUTER ASSISTED PROGRAM FOR COGNITIVE BEHAVIORAL THERAPY

Title of Pamphlet, Book, or Computer-Assisted Program	Authors	Type of Psychoeducational Material
Coping with Depression	Beck & Greenberg, 1974	Pamphlet/flyer
Feeling Good: The New Mood Therapy	Burns, 1999	Book with self-help program
Getting Your Life Back: The Complete Guide to Recovery from Depression	Wright & Basco, 2002	Book with self-help program; integration of cognitive therapy and the biological perspective
Good Days Ahead: The Interactive Program for Depression and Anxiety	Wright, Wright, & Beck, 2003	Computer-assisted therapy and self-help program; information: http://www.mindstreet.com
Mastery of Your Anxiety and Panic	Craske and Barlow, 2006	Self-help for anxiety
Mind Over Mood: Change How You Feel by Changing the Way You Think	Greenberger and Padesky, 1995	Self-help workbook
Never Good Enough: How to Use Perfectionism to Your Advantage Without Letting It Ruin Your Life	Basco, 2000	Book on perfectionism
Stop Obsessing: How to Overcome Your Obsessions and Compulsions	Foa and Wilson, 2001	Self-help for obsessive-compulsive disorder
The Worry Cure: Seven Steps to Stop Worry From Stopping You	Leahy, 2006	Book with self-help for anxiety and worry
The Bipolar Workbook: Tools for Controlling Your Mood Swings	Basco, 2005	Self-help workbook
The Depression Workbook: A Guide for Living with Depression and Manic Depression	Copeland and McKay, 2002	Self-help book for depression and manic-depression
The Cognitive-behavioral Workbook for Depression: A Step-by-step Program	Knaus, 2006	CBT self-help workbook
The Depression Solutions Workbook: A Strength and Skill-Based Approach	Corcoran, 2009	Self-help book; focus on cultivating resiliency

BOX 7-3 The Therapeutic Relationship in Cognitive Therapy: Enhancing Collaborative Empiricism

In cognitive therapy, the patient and therapist work together to form an investigative team. The therapist should

- Establish a therapeutic relationship based on trust, warmth, and rapport
- Encourage the patient to use self-help and self-monitoring in the process of therapy
- Assess and establish the validity of cognitions and the efficacy of the patient's behavior
- Encourage the patient to develop coping strategies for real losses or deficits experienced
- Provide and request feedback from the patient during each visit
- Be sensitive to social or cultural differences in the therapy
- Use gentle humor
- Provide customized patient-centered interventions

5. Use cognitive therapy techniques at each session
6. Assign homework outside of the session
7. Encourage active self-help by the patient
8. Ultimately alter the distorted cognitions and schemas, which will then improve mood or decrease anxiety

In the process of implementing cognitive therapy, the therapist sets the scene for the treatment by accomplishing four things at the beginning of the therapy: (1) setting an agenda for therapy sessions; (2) giving constructive feedback in an effort to direct the therapy; (3) using common cognitive therapy techniques; and (4) assigning homework to the patient between sessions.

The therapist creates the agenda after collaborating with the patient, and the schedule should be flexible. The agenda combats the helplessness often felt by patients who experience depression. Encouraging remarks set the tone for the feedback by the therapist. Directives such as scheduling activities, recording thoughts, and completing homework assignments help patients feel more empowered and in control as opposed to feeling incompetent and helpless. In using the activities in the book *Getting Your Life Back* (Wright & Basco, 2001), for example, a patient would become actively engaged in recovery from depression through assessments and activities related to the "5 keys": (1) the thinking key; (2) the action key; (3) the biological key; (4) the relationships key; and (5) the spiritual key (Table 7-3). Self-help materials assist the patient to focus on goals as part of the therapeutic process and also play a role in the psychoeducation that occurs in the process of reading and discussing mental health concepts with the therapist.

Indications

Cognitive therapy is indicated for the treatment of depression, panic disorder, obsessive-compulsive disorder, personality disorders, and somatoform disorders. Treatment is provided on an individual level (Sadock & Sadock, 2008).

TABLE 7-3 **THE FIVE KEYS TO RECOVERY FROM DEPRESSION**

Keys to Recovery from Depression	Problems	Things You Can Do to Counter Depressed Feelings and Thoughts
1. The Thinking Key	Negative thoughts; hopelessness; poor self-esteem.	Challenge and control automatic negative thoughts. Build self-esteem. Improve problem-solving abilities.
2. The Action Key	Withdrawal from other people and usual activities; procrastination; helplessness.	Plan and implement activities. Set goals. Change negative behavioral patterns.
3. The Biology Key	Depressive symptoms; poor sleep; change in appetite or weight; lack of exercise.	Learn about the biological causes of depression. Take prescribed antidepressant medications. Eat healthy, nutritious foods. Practice sleep hygiene to improve the quality and amount of sleep. Increase exercise/movement per physical abilities.
4. The Relationship Key	Difficulty communicating with others; strained or poor relationships; unable to get or use support.	Attempt to reach out to others and let them know what your needs and feelings are. Ask others to be supportive versus isolating self from others.
5. The Spirituality Key	Lack of sense of purpose or meaning in life; questioning of one's values.	Practice spiritual activities. Deepen or grow a sense of meaning or purpose.

Source: Modified from Wright, J., & Basco, M. (2002). **Getting your life back. The complete guide to recovery from depression** *(p. 8). New York: Simon & Schuster.*

Assessment and Case Formulation

In this cognitive therapy process, the nurse assesses patient symptoms; notes the influences of the formative years and of biological, genetic, and medical factors; assesses patient strengths; and identifies automatic negative thoughts, emotions, behaviors, and schemas that the patient has developed. This thorough assessment is the basis for a *DSM-IV-TR* diagnosis and working hypotheses, with the outcome being an individualized treatment plan. Case Study 7-3 includes a scenario in which a particular patient may benefit from cognitive therapy. The therapist decides to use cognitive therapy to address Lisa's perfectionism and poor self-esteem. Explain how the nurse psychotherapist would set up the first session and what activities and homework the nurse could use in subsequent sessions. Why would cognitive therapy be useful in this case?

Strategies

The therapist who uses cognitive therapy addresses two types of cognitive errors that result in stress to the patient: (1) identifying and modifying automatic negative, anxious, or illogical thoughts and (2) identifying and modifying schemas. When behavioral procedures are used in addition to cognitive procedures, the technique is called cognitive behavioral therapy.

Identifying Automatic Negative, Anxious, or Illogical Thoughts or Cognitive Errors

The premise of cognitive therapy is that negative, anxious, and illogical thoughts that seem to automatically jump to the foreground of a patient's thinking result in a change in mood—one filled with anxiety, sadness, depression, or anger. The therapist is able to perceive the change in mood during the interview. For example, say a 30-year-old man with computer skills who works for an electric company says that his company did not get a desired contract. He states that the focus is on him because he was part of a team and he is afraid that he will be fired from his job. He is anxious and depressed because he knows he will be asked to leave, so he works 80 hours a week and takes work home every night so that he can prove he is worthy of his job. His poor concentration skills did create a few instances in

CASE STUDY 7-3

Patient Who May Benefit From Cognitive Therapy

Lisa is a 29-year-old Caucasian woman who presents with anxiety and depression after having difficulties in her marriage and self-esteem issues about her need for perfection at work. She had a history of anxiety and eating disorders as a teenager, and she tends to run 5 miles a day to keep her weight under control and to reduce stress. Even when she has a bad head cold and fever, she does not "give herself any slack" and has to complete the total 5 miles to make her feel that she has accomplished this goal.

Lisa is married to Ed, age 30, who, upon interview, is noted to have a flat affect and has a family history of depression (his father had depression). Ed has been depressed also and cannot make decisions, but he gets angry if Lisa prods him to make a decision, such as where to go for dinner or what household project needs attention. Lisa had been an excellent student in college and has excelled in her job as a beginning scientist. She decided to get a graduate degree and has a negative emotional reaction if she earns less than a grade of A. She is getting only 4 to 5 hours of sleep, does not eat well-rounded meals, and is unable to be frank with her husband about their poor marital relationship. Instead, she avoids discussing difficult issues and has purposely used hard liquor to numb her feelings. On one occasion she had too much to drink and was concerned later that she might overdose accidentally by drinking too much. Her husband is disgusted with her drinking and sees it as a personal flaw in Lisa and takes no responsibility for their relationship and poor communication.

which he made some programming mistakes, but they were quickly rectified. He feels totally responsible for the company's not getting the contract, although he is not in a management position. He calls himself stupid, saying that he is "making stupid mistakes." He states that he "is a loser because he cannot count on providing for his new baby and his wife."

The therapist can use several techniques to identify and modify automatic thoughts, such as (1) assessing for mood shifts; (2) use of Socratic questioning in an effort to guide the patient to explore the rationality of the thoughts; (3) role play; (4) examining the evidence; and (5) thought recording. Often the automatic thoughts are illogical, overblown, catastrophic, or personalized. Table 7-4 has examples of automatic negative thoughts (cognitive errors).

In an effort to make the thoughts more understandable and to examine the evidence for or against the thoughts, a written tool called a Thought Recording can be used (Table 7-5). With Thought Recording, the patient identifies his situation and the automatic thoughts that result from the situation. In the example, the patient feels pressured at work to "do beyond what everyone else is doing" in terms of work effort and hours in an attempt to "stay below the radar and be prepared so administration cannot blame him." He feels over-responsible, not only for his own work, but for the company as a whole and other productive coworkers.

Once some of the situations are understood or made clearer and the automatic thoughts are noted and discussed, the therapist helps the patient to challenge the automatic negative, anxious, or illogical thoughts so that the

TABLE 7-4 EXAMPLES OF AUTOMATIC NEGATIVE OR ANXIOUS THOUGHTS/COGNITIVE ERRORS

Automatic Thoughts	Definition of Automatic Negative or Anxious Thoughts	Example
Selective abstraction (or mental filter)	Drawing a conclusion on a small portion of data. Ignoring the positive things that occur to and around self, focusing instead on the negative	A teacher receives course evaluations from 50 students, two of which demean her teaching ability. The teacher feels like a failure and wants to find another profession because of the way such negative comments make her feel about herself.
Arbitrary inference	Coming to a conclusion without adequate supporting evidence or despite evidence that is contradictory	An employee works 80 hours instead of the typical 60 because he knows there will be employees let go and he suspects he may be one of them if he doesn't show his boss how much harder he is working compared to others.
Absolutistic thinking, "all or nothing thinking," or " black and white thinking"	Dichotomous thinking, i.e., right vs. wrong; black vs. white; all good or all bad, perfect vs. completely flawed; being successful or being a total failure	A teenager's dream date does not ask her to the prom. Because this person asks another girl, she states that she knows she is unattractive and a loser and that she will not do anything right in life.
Magnification and minimization	Overvaluing or undervaluing the significance of personal attributes, life situations, or a future possibility	A woman receives a yearly evaluation from her boss and magnifies any low score on the form, but minimizes the positive comments on the evaluation.
Personification	Taking blame, assuming responsibility, critical of self by linking external events to the self. This happens when there is little or no evidence for making these associations.	A woman feels that the failure of her marriage is totally her fault, and that if she had not gone back to school, her husband would not have left her for another woman.
Catastrophic thinking	Predicting the worst possible outcome while ignoring at the same time more likely outcomes	"I can't go up for a promotion because, if I do, my job responsibilities will increase and no one will take care of my children in the same way I do. They will not do as well in school if I take the promotion."
Exaggerating	Making self-critical or other-critical statements that include terms such as never, nothing, everything, or always.	"I earned the grade of B in biochemistry. I am a failure. I will never be a doctor now. Everything I dreamed of is lost."
Discounting	Rejecting positive experiences as not being important or meaningful.	"I really did not deserve the award."
Judging	Being critical of self or others, with a heavy emphasis on the use of "should have," "ought to," "must," "have to," and "should not have"	"I should have been there for my mother when she was dying despite the fact that I am single mother of 3 school-age children and could not move across country to be with her."
Mind reading	Making negative assumptions regarding other people's thoughts and motives	"I know my boss does not like me and therefore sabotages my successes."
Feelings are facts	Because you feel a certain way, reality is seen as fitting that feeling.	A woman is sad over the loss of a business contract and is pessimistic that her company will ever be really financially stable.
Labeling	Calling self or others a bad name when displeased with a behavior	"I am a stupid idiot for hiring John for the job as project manager."

Source: Modified from Beck, A., Rush, A., Shaw, B., et al. (1979). Cognitive therapy of depression *(p. 14). New York: Guilford Press.*

TABLE 7-5 AN EXAMPLE OF A TWO-COLUMN THOUGHT RECORDING

Situation	Automatic Thoughts
Pressure at work to do extra work above and beyond the 8-hour day.	If I don't do the extra work or projects, no one will do them; but also I have to do more than others or I will be picked out as the person to fire.
I found out that I made a mistake on a report, but the people who I sent it to realized the error, corrected it, and let me know.	I am stupid. I make stupid mistakes.
I work on things on my laptop at home because I don't have enough time in the day. I know my wife wants more of my attention.	I am a bad husband because I cannot relax and give my wife the love and attention she needs.
My thoughts are slowed down and I cannot concentrate as well as I used to before the recession and the increased stress at work.	I will never feel back to normal. My depression is too much and at times I can't deal with it. I never used to be this way and I wonder if there is a way out of this. I don't know if there is.

patient can begin to do this on his own. A tool that can be used for homework assignments, The Thought Change Record, is a 5-column record that includes the situation, automatic thoughts, the emotions that result from the automatic thoughts, a rational response, and an outcome (Table 7-6). The patient initially rates his belief in his autonomic thoughts and his degree of emotional/mood changes (on a scale from 0% to 100%), then does so again after identifying and challenging the irrational thoughts. A patient is able to modify his automatic thoughts when he is able to (1) generate alternatives; (2) critically evaluate the evidence for or against the thought; (3) identify when he is catastrophizing the situation; (4) use reattribution; and (5) practice cognitive rehearsals.

In our case example, to replace the patient's automatically thinking he would be fired, the therapist promoted healthy means of coping and problem-solving. In using reattribution, the nurse therapist assists the depressed patient to address negatively based attributions—e.g., global versus specific; internal versus external; and fixed versus variable attributions—which are more prominent in depressed individuals (Wright et al., 2008). In the case study above, the patient was threatened by the thoughts that the company would "fold due to the lost contract," that "the lost contract was his fault," and that "he had no way to get another job in this poor economy."

In modifying the automatic negative thoughts, the patient was able to see that he was catastrophizing the situation and personalizing the failed contract to himself and not others who were also involved. To combat his idea about not getting another job, he realized that, given the stress in the work environment, it was best to have an updated resume and to post it online. He had discussed this with his wife, who volunteered to help him type and post his resume as a way to be supportive.

Identifying and Modifying Schemas

Schemas are a person's core beliefs or basic assumptions about the self or life in general that have been developing for a long time. Schemas may not be in the patient's awareness. However, these larger patterns of behaviors and thoughts used in life may become evident when patterns of behavior and thinking are revealed by identifying automatic negative thoughts.

TABLE 7-6 THOUGHT CHANGE RECORD

Situation	Automatic Thoughts	Emotion(s)	Rational Response	Outcome
1. Describe the actual event leading to the unpleasant emotion; or 2. Describe stream of thoughts, daydreams, or recollection leading to the unpleasant emotion; or 3. Describe unpleasant physiological sensations	1. Write the automatic thought(s) that preceded the emotion(s) 2. Rate belief in automatic thought(s) (0%-100%)	1. Specify sad, anxious, angry, or other feelings 2. Rate degree of emotions (0%-100%)	1. Identify cognitive errors 2. Write a rational response to automatic thought(s) 3. Rate belief in rational response (0%-100%)	1. Once again, rate belief in automatic thought(s) (0%-100%) 2. Specify and rate subsequent emotion(s) (0%-100%)
Day #1 Date:				
Day #2 Date:				

While the process of identifying and modifying schemas is more difficult than that of challenging negative automatic thoughts, the techniques are the same. For example, a young woman may have the schema, "I must be perfect or I won't be accepted." The therapist can ask the patient to evaluate the evidence for and against being perfect and also the advantages and disadvantages of being perfect. Finally, to alter the schema, alternatives could be developed that assist the patient to realize that perfection is impossible and that life is not an "all or nothing situation"; that is, life does not follow the formula that to be perfect is to be loved and that, if not perfect, one will not be loved. Psychoeducation using the book *Never Good Enough* (Basco, 1999) would help the patient work through this life schema. Table 7-7 provides an example of the schema of perfectionism.

Interventions

Behavioral interventions are used along with cognitive therapy for the following three reasons: (1) to change dysfunctional patterns of behavior such as helplessness, isolation, lack of energy; (2) to reduce symptoms such as tension, anxiety, and intrusive thinking; and (3) to assist in identifying and changing maladaptive thoughts. The cognitive model of therapy incorporates an interactive relationship between cognition and behavior: if behavioral interventions influence cognition, then cognition can influence behavior. Behavioral techniques include activity scheduling, graded task assignments, coping cards, and exposure therapy.

In an *activity schedule*, the patient identifies the activities that he or she is involved with on a daily basis and records the activities on a log. Often a depressed person will say, "I don't enjoy anything anymore." Activities are first graded for pleasure and mastery, then discussed with the therapist in a future session. Activities that provide either pleasure or a sense of efficacy could be added. The actual record of activities and level of pleasure and mastery may reveal that the patient's perceptions of enjoyment and mastery conflict with the actual activities that are accomplished.

Depressed or anxious patients may feel overwhelmed by the thought of accomplishing a large project. The use of the *graded task assignment* can help the patient break down the task into small pieces, thus reducing the feeling of helplessness and increasing self-esteem and empowerment. Such a situation may occur in a patient who wishes to write the perfect term paper, only to procrastinate due to perfectionism, and then feel overwhelmed by the assignment.

Coping cards, which include cognitive and behavioral interventions, are used to help a patient cope with an anticipatory problem. The cognitive and behavioral interventions are written on a small card and carried with the patient as a reminder of how to facilitate problem-solving.

Exposure therapy is a core feature of the CBT approach to treating anxiety disorders. For example, a patient may have an unrealistic fear and use avoidance as a conditional pattern to the fear. The therapist would help the patient develop a hierarchy of feared stimuli, ranking them from 0 to 100. Gradual exposure beginning at the lowest-ranked items would occur. Use of relaxation techniques, deep breathing, and other methods would be used to enhance the patient's coping abilities and to carry out the exposure protocol.

In some cases, virtual images are used to simulate feared experiences. An example is the use of virtual combat exposure in servicemen and servicewomen in the Iraq and Afghanistan Wars who suffer from post-traumatic stress disorder. The virtual combat exposure may depict being in the Middle East and driving in a Humvee, and then having an improvised explosive device detonate (a common occurrence in the combat zone).

Efficacy Research

Epp, Dobson, & Cottraux (2009) have provided an overview of the efficacy studies of cognitive therapy for mood disorders, anxiety disorders, schizophrenia, bulimia nervosa, and personality disorders. CBT has been shown to be efficacious across this range of psychiatric disorders. In the United Kingdom, use of cognitive therapy in addition to an antipsychotic medication regimen is the standard of care for patients with schizophrenia (Turkington, Kingdon, & Weiden, 2006). In an RTC study on treatment of acute post-traumatic stress disorder with brief CBT, it was found

TABLE 7-7 MANAGING SCHEMAS: COMPARING ADVANTAGES AND DISADVANTAGES

Example: "I must be perfect in what I do at work."

Advantages of Schema	Disadvantages of Schema
I earned my MBA in an Executive-Weekend Program Pharmaceuticals in 18 months while working full time. I was disappointed in myself if I did not earn As in the courses, but I learned a lot and hopefully this will advance my career.	I cannot relax. I am on the computer at 3AM; I read email and instant messenger all day long. I cannot put my computer down once I get home—I cannot turn work off. I feel overwhelmed. I must be on my toes and not make any mistakes.
My company can rely on me. I have several teams reporting to me. They know I am meticulous in my work and will follow through.	I feel everyone overly depends on me and some of my team members do not do their share of the work.
Life can be predictable and controllable.	Everything is planned. Even my running every day is planned. Nothing in my life is spontaneous. My partner plans out every activity and I go along with this because I know what to expect.
I can count on myself to get things done.	This enables me to count on myself to get things done versus having to count on others.

that brief early CBT accelerated recovery from acute post-traumatic stress disorder symptoms; however, it did not influence effects in the long term (Sijbrandij, Olff, Reitsma, et al., 2007). Cognitive therapy in conjunction with pharmacotherapy can reduce relapse in the short term and improve social functioning in the long term in patients with bipolar disorder. In unipolar depression, cognitive therapy can be very efficacious (Friedman & Thase, 2009). Cognitive therapy and pharmacotherapy are seen to be equally efficacious in the acute treatment of depression, but there may also be an additional benefit beyond one treatment alone; that is, there is a synergy between cognitive therapy and psychopharmacology (Friedman & Thase). According to Sijbrandij et al., meta-analyses of the use of cognitive therapy in patients who are experiencing schizophrenia found that the focus was on cognitive restructuring and on decreasing hallucinations and delusions. Cognitive therapy is more efficacious than medication in patients with bulimia, but a combination of cognitive therapy with medications may be more effective than only cognitive therapy. There is evidence of the effectiveness of cognitive therapy in reducing symptoms of patients with borderline personality disorder (Epp et al.). In a study that compared short-term psychodynamic psychotherapy and CBT in generalized anxiety disorder in a randomized controlled trial design (Leichsenring, Salzer, Jaeger, et al., 2009), the results suggested that both CBT and short-term psychodynamic psychotherapy were beneficial for patients with generalized anxiety disorder, noting no significant differences between the treatments. However, in measures of trait anxiety, worry, and depression, CBT was found to be superior. Research has also been completed on computer-assisted cognitive therapy (Box 7-4).

Behavioral Therapy

Behavioral therapy is a type of learning therapy in which exposure to the source of fear is the core component. This work is well known to be useful in anxiety disorders, especially phobias and post-traumatic stress disorder, and has been well documented by Foa, Keane, & Friedman (2000) and others. Treatment begins with an assessment and some patient teaching to explain the therapy and how participating with the therapy will enhance patient mastery over fears. In one example of exposure therapy in which a patient with obsessive-compulsive disorder fears germs and thus washes the hands frequently, the therapist may purposely place dirty materials on the patient's hands (exposure), with the goal of preventing the patient from immediately washing his or her hands (response prevention). Shapiro (2001) notes that exposure therapy is effective because the patient learns to reprocess environmental cues associated with distress. Exposure therapy is used in the treatment of post-traumatic stress disorder in combat veterans and in other individuals exposed to trauma.

Behavioral therapy is used in child and adolescent settings, where points are earned or privilege levels are increased for positive behaviors and taken away for negative behaviors. Time out on a bench or in one's room is a type of behavioral therapy for the child or adolescent to reflect on behavior away from any stimulus in the environment. It is based on operative conditioning under the school of behaviorism.

Dialectical Behavioral Therapy

Dialectical behavioral therapy (DBT) was introduced by Linehan (1993a). She developed a skills training manual to implement DBT therapy (1993b). The unique focus of DBT

BOX 7-4 Computer-Assisted Cognitive Therapy

Selmi, Klein, Greist, et al. (1990) developed an early prototype of computerized therapy: a text-based program that taught patients how to use cognitive therapy to cope with their depression. Today, there are computer programs that have multimedia, virtual reality, and palm-top technology that produce therapy experiences that are effective and appealing to patients. One example is the DVD-ROM "Good Days Ahead," an interactive program for depression. It has interactive exercises that can be used on a computer or printed out to use in daily life. The DVD shows examples of how to solve problems, increase self-esteem, and make positive changes in one's life. It also includes exercises to increase skills to fight depression and anxiety. The program has a modest cost, under $100.00, and is user-friendly, especially in our computer-oriented world. Each computer session could last 20 to 60 minutes.

Efficacy Research of Computer-Assisted Cognitive Therapy

A randomized controlled trial of computer-assisted cognitive therapy for depression was conducted by Wright, Wright, Albano, et al. (2005). They found that computer-assisted cognitive therapy was equivalent to standard cognitive therapy, despite a reduction of total therapist time in computer-assisted cognitive therapy to 4 hours. Research subjects were drug free. Both computer-assisted therapy and standard cognitive therapy were highly effective in reducing depressive symptoms, and both were superior to delayed treatment control conditions.

Proudfoot, Ryden, Everitt, et al. (2004) studied the use of the computer-assisted program "Beating the Blues." Computer-assisted cognitive therapy was found to be effective in a controlled trial with subjects who were primary care patients. Patients who received the computer-assisted program had a greater improvement of depression than those who received treatment as usual.

Cognitive therapy has been used primarily to treat the target symptoms of depressed mood and anxiety; however, it has also been used for the following conditions: schizophrenia, eating disorders, bipolar disorder, substance abuse, personality disorders, chronic pain, irritable bowel syndrome, and fibromyalgia. It has been used in groups and families as well as in child-adolescent populations (Sadock & Sadock, 2008).

is to develop comprehensive strategies of acceptance with change in both the patient and therapist through a dialectical approach to thinking and problem-solving. For example, DBT is used for patients with borderline personality disorder who (1) experience severe emotional dysregulation, (2) are sensitive to environmental cues, (3) often feel slighted by others and as though they are not getting their needs met, and (4) may feel that they exist in an environment that invalidates their experiences. They act impulsively on these feelings with cutting behaviors, substance abuse, and suicidal ideation, intent, plan, and follow-through.

DBT is based in learning theory. Similar to CBT, DBT focuses on evaluating precipitating events, actions, and environmental cues that are present before and after a response by the patient. DBT uses traditional cognitive-behavioral tools, such as psychoeducation, challenging of automatic negative thoughts, skills training, and problem-solving. Other techniques are also used in DBT to unlearn dysfunctional responses, such as exposure, systematic desensitization, and cognitive restructuring (Wheelis, 2009). One goal of DBT is to create a dialectic, or tension, in thinking so that all-or-nothing thinking prevails less in the way the person sees and responds to the world. For example, if a nurse does not give a totally friendly response, it is not because the nurse is "mean and doesn't like me," but perhaps because he or she is stressed or not feeling well. In addition, patients are given validation as support for their experiences. A combination of individual and group therapy is offered to patients to promote the healing process.

Contextual Therapies

The contextual therapy approaches—strategic psychotherapy and solution-focused psychotherapy—are different from relational or learning therapies in that contextual brief therapies do not view problems as intrinsic to the person, but view them within a person-situation interaction (Dewan et al., 2008).

Strategic Psychotherapy

Strategic therapy attempts to help patients try different ways of solving their problems because the way the person currently perceives his or her problem is actually creating a situation in which the problem does not get solved. Reframing the situation may open options to approach the problem in a different manner.

In strategic therapy, the therapist listens to patients' current complaints and their current solutions while keeping in mind the question: What current situational factors continue to maintain the patient's presenting issues? The therapist listens to the problem, the people involved, the patient's view of the situation, the specific context of the concerns, and the patient's responses. The therapist can understand after the intake interview why the patient "feels stuck." The goal of the therapy (Rosenbaum, 1990) is not to find a solution to the patient's problem. Instead, the therapist helps the patient not to be "stuck" anymore by focusing on the patient's strengths, thus allowing the change process to take its course. For example, shy people can be less shy if they see themselves as nice, compassionate people who want to help others. By focusing on their strength in helping others, they will naturally become less shy, and they will receive positive feedback from the therapist in the process. The problems the patient brings to therapy are usually self-reinforcing problem-solving cycles, and the goal of the therapist is to change the pattern. Strategic therapy can include single-session therapy sessions or short-term therapy sessions.

Solution-Focused Therapy

Solution-focused therapy is a type of strategic therapy whereby the approach is to focus on a solution to a problem rather than on the problem itself. People face problems every day, and they either solve the problems to their satisfaction or they do not. The more that patients focus on their problems, the more they feel downtrodden. Sometimes this perspective negates situations in which the person actually satisfactorily solves his or her problems. In solution-focused therapy, then, the therapist listens to the patient and tries to help the patient find the answer to the question, "What have I done that is already helping me to fix the problem?"

Solution-focused therapy builds on the patients' current thoughts and behaviors; it does not initiate new behaviors. It is highly targeted and brief, and it frames problems in a positive way and focuses on actions to be accomplished. There is often a "miracle question" in solution-focused therapy, e.g., if you woke up tomorrow and solved your problem, what would your solution be? Solution-focused therapy de-emphasizes problems and emphasizes exceptions to problems in an effort to facilitate change through enactment of solutions (Dewan et al., 2008). As Walter & Peller (1992) advised, "Focusing on the positive, the solution, and the future facilitates change in the desired direction. Therefore, focus on the solution-oriented talk rather than the problem-oriented talk" (p. 37).

Supportive Psychotherapy

It is important for psychiatric advanced practice nurses to have a working knowledge of supportive psychotherapy because it has wide applicability to many populations of patients.

Supportive psychotherapy is a broadly defined approach that uses direct measures to reduce symptoms and maintain, restore, or improve self-esteem, ego function, and adaptive skills (Pinsker, 1997; Pinsker & Rosenthal, 1988; Pinsker, Rosenthal, & McCullough, 1991; Winston, Rosenthal, & Pinsker, 2004). *Direct measures* means that "the patient's response of symptom reduction or adoption of more adaptive behavioral patterns is not the result of insight into unconscious conflict and its working through, but rather because the patient has greater self-esteem, ego functions, and adaptive skills as a result of therapist interventions" (Rosenthal, 2010, p. 417). *Self-esteem* is addressed to improve the patient's sense of self-regard, confidence, hope, and self-efficacy. *Ego functions*—such as relation to reality, object relations, affect, impulse control, defenses, thought processes, autonomous functions, synthetic functions, and conscience, morals, and ideals—are identified and strengthened through supportive psychotherapy (Bellak & Goldsmith, 1984; Winston et al., 2004). *Adaptive functioning skills* are strengthened to help the patient with effective functioning in multiple spheres. The objective is not to change personality, but to assist healthy patients in their ability to cope with crises or transient problems and to assist patients with more serious mental illnesses to cope with and ameliorate psychiatric symptoms.

In supportive psychotherapy, the therapist is responsive to the patient's goals for therapy, and goals are based on specific developmental or reparative tasks that the clinician has identified. Three theoretical approaches are applied in supportive psychotherapy:

- Psychoanalytical approaches (ego psychology and development, object relations and attachment, self-psychology, and interpersonal and relational approach)
- CBT techniques
- Patient education (Winston & Goldstein, 2010)

Treatment may involve examination of relationships, both real and transferential (past and present), and current patterns of emotional response or behavior. The therapist must be able to use these approaches in an integrative manner to meet the needs of the patient within the therapeutic nurse-patient relationship. There are several supportive psychotherapy techniques under three categories: contextual techniques, tactical techniques, and skills building. Integration of these approaches by the therapist provides a cohesive and well-organized psychotherapy for the patient in which the therapist is active in treatment and is cognizant to provide a caring, therapeutic relationship.

Treatment also involves the examination of patient symptoms, relationships, daily functioning, emotional responses, and behavioral patterns. The treatment approach is determined by the extent of patient functioning on a health-illness continuum, from most impaired to least impaired. Level of patient impairment determines the need for increased support (for most-impaired patients) versus use of more expressive therapy and less support (for least-impaired patients). Expressive therapies use an interpersonal/conflict model. *Expressive therapy* is a collective term for a variety of approaches that seek personality change through analysis of the relationship between the therapist and patient, and through development of insight into previously unrecognized feelings, thoughts, needs, and conflicts (Dewald, 1994; Winston & Goldstein, 2010).

Goals

The goals of supportive psychotherapy are to (1) help patients cope with symptoms, (2) prevent relapse of serious mental illnesses, and (3) help individuals deal with a crisis or life transition by improving coping skills. As a result, the outcome for the patient is that there is a reduction in symptoms and improvement in adaptation, self-esteem, and overall functioning.

Theoretical Approaches

Theoretical approaches include psychoanalytical theories, CBT techniques, and learning theory.

Psychoanalytical Theories

Psychoanalytical theories used in supportive psychotherapy include ego psychology and development, object relations and attachment, self-psychology, and the interpersonal and relational approach.

Ego Psychology and Development

Ego psychology—which encompasses developmental theory and is based on Freud's (1923) structural approach of the ego, id, and superego—offers insight to patients with serious mental illnesses and serves as the foundation for therapists to evaluate ego function in patients. The more disturbance seen in a patient's ego function, the more support is needed within supportive psychotherapy. The patient's ego function is compared to functionally normal behavior. Table 7-8 provides the definitions of ego function and areas of assessment. Ego assessment can be used for patient case formulation, with ego strengths and limitations noted. For more information on ego function, see sources by Vaillant (1977, 1992, 1997, 2002, & 2008).

Object Relations and Attachment

Fairbairn (1952, 1994), Winnicott (1965, 1971), and Bowlby (1969, 1988), British psychoanalysts, developed the field of object relations. They viewed children as attempting to seek satisfactory relationships with parents and, through this, developing a sense of self in relation to others. Certain psychopathologies develop in children in their attempts to get their needs met from parents who may be rejecting, invalidating, or lacking the ability to be responsive to children's needs. The internal object relations in child-parent relationships are acted out in the therapeutic nurse-patient relationship; therapy is focused on being a "good enough mother/parent" and providing a "holding environment." The patient experiences a new type of relationship with the therapist, which causes a change in the patient's ability to relate to others in a more healthy way.

Bowlby (1988) discussed how infants and children develop either a secure or insecure attachment to parental figures (see Chapter 1 for discussion of attachment theory). Among patients with insecure attachments, those who experience a rupture in a relationship often cannot repair such

TABLE 7-8 EGO FUNCTION ASSESSMENT

Ego Function	Definition	Assessment
Reality testing	The ability to reach a logical conclusion from data or events that can be observed	Assess for 1. Ability to distinguish between ideas and perceptions 2. Accuracy of perceptions 3. Testing internal reality (orientation, illusions, delusions, hallucinations)
Judgment	The relationship between events; consists of connections between action and resulting consequences	Assess for 1. Anticipation of consequences of behavior 2. Appropriateness of behavior 3. Whether patient is aware of possible consequences combined with repetition of maladaptive actions
Sense of reality	Sense that phenomena going on around and within are real	Assess for 1. Body image 2. Ego boundaries 3. Self-identity
Regulation of drives, affects, and impulses	Ability to regulate feelings and drives, particularly sexual and aggressive feelings	Assess for 1. The ability to endure delay in gratification, frustration, and disappointment 2. Toleration of feelings of anxiety and depression 3. Impulses requiring action are controlled by thinking prior to taking action on an impulse. Impulses to assess: aggressive drive and anger; frustration; sexuality; affect
Object relations	Interpersonal relationships between human beings are warm and loving relationships	Assess relationships 1. With family members 2. With friends 3. With other relationships (work)
Thought processes	Involves the abilities to concentrate, form concepts, and think clearly and logically, using abstract thought, and expressing of thoughts through use of language and to store those thoughts in memory	Assess for 1. The ability to concentrate and pay attention 2. Short-term and long-term memory. 3. Logical thoughts and use of abstract thinking
ARISE (Adaptive regression in service to the ego)	The ability to let go, to relax control, and to permit fantasy and primary process thinking to take place. It involves imagination and creativity, capacity to problem-solve, to find new or original solutions; use of wit and humor; experience love, mothering, orgasm.	Assess levels of 1. Imagination 2. Creativity 3. Spontaneity 4. Pleasure in art, music, poetry, etc.
Defensive functioning	All processes that protect the ego against instinctual demands and dysphoric affects, such as anxiety, fear, anger, and depression	Assess for 1. Defense mechanisms used, which are immature versus mature; adaptive versus maladaptive 2. Success or failure of defenses to reduce anxiety
Stimulus barrier	A protective shield against overwhelming stimuli of all five senses	Assess for 1. Sensitivity to light, sound temperature, and odor 2. Sleep inhibited due to light and sound 3. Pain or discomfort as noxious stimuli
Autonomous functioning	The competence in psychomotor skills. Primary autonomous functioning is concerned with the degree of freedom from impairment of sight, hearing, language, learning, motor functions, and intellect. Secondary autonomous functioning is concerned with the degree of freedom from impairment of habits, skills, hobbies, and interests.	Assess for 1. Degree of difficulty with which work or self-care is performed 2. The patient's level of energy (Does patient express the need to exert more energy to accomplish usual tasks?) 3. How much the patient procrastinates in getting work done; putting off responsibilities
Synthetic integrative functioning	A coordinating function concerned with planning and organization; working in a coherent manner and reconciling contradictory experience or points of view	Assess for 1. The ability to balance different roles in life, e.g., wife/mother/worker; leader/follower; daughter/student 2. The ability to cope with more than one task at a time 3. The organization of daily life and the ability to carry out planned activities 4. The ability to adapt to change; ability to accommodate shifts in plans; ability to meet changing demands in work or school

Continued

TABLE 7-8 EGO FUNCTION ASSESSMENT—continued

Ego Function	Definition	Assessment
Mastery competence	The drive to master or control the external world. The urge to learn to do things and to do them. Striving or trying to achieve a goal and working up to one's ability. Difficulties result if patient does not interact with the environment, has feelings of powerlessness, and low self-esteem.	Assess for 1. The function of the patient to trust his/her own judgment; ability to cope with difficult tasks 2. Functional ability and if patient gives a positive evaluation of his/her own competence. 3. Whether the patient is in charge of his/her own life or whether events control him/her 4. The level of self-esteem. Is the patient able to state feelings of self-worth that is realistic in nature?
Conscience, morals, and ideals	These functions of the superego derive from the internalization of aspects of parental figures and mores in society. Impairment may interfere with the nurse-patient relationship, such as if the patient cannot be truthful. This affects psychotherapy success.	Assess for 1. Truth-telling (or lying) 2. Stealing 3. Damage to other people or their property 4. Lack of conscience or remorse

Source: Adapted from Bellak, L., & Goldsmith, L. (1984). The broad scope of ego function assessment. *New York: John Wiley; Winston, A., & Goldsmith, M. (2010). Theory of supportive psychotherapy. In G. O. Gabbard (Ed.),* Textbook of psychotherapeutic treatments. *Washington, DC: American Psychiatric Publishing, Inc.*

relationships. When therapists are aware of ruptures in the relationship and repair the relationship, this is a new type of experience for the patient. This repair of the rupture within the relationship is what Alexander and French (1946) called the corrective emotional experience. The patient learns to change his or her response to the therapist in a healthy manner because the therapist actively seeks to repair any rifts that occur and increase security and support for the patient. Such modeling of supportive behavior has an impact on the patient and the patient's future relationships with others.

Self-Psychology

Kohut (1971, 1977) is the theorist of self-psychology who, like other psychoanalysts, believed that early object relations are crucial in the development of the self. When the therapist offers a supportive relationship that is notably different from what the parents offer, the therapist has an "empathetic/introspective" stance, which offers a type of caring and empathetic relationship that the patient has not experienced before. If the therapist fails to meet the needs of the patient, there is negative energy generated from the patient toward the therapist because the therapeutic alliance is not as strong as it could be. The patient may feel dismissed or rejected. If the therapist understands this and reestablishes the relationship, it is called a repair of the therapeutic alliance. This repair of the therapeutic alliance leads to strengthening of the patient's self-system and internalization of the good qualities inherent in the therapist by the patient.

Interpersonal and Relational Approach

Hildegard Peplau (1952) built her nursing theory on the therapeutic nurse-patient relationship, trust building, and the stages of the relationship over time, and according to Gaston (1990) and Horvath and Symonds (1991), the therapeutic relationship may be the most important and positive therapeutic outcome. Supportive psychotherapy and CBTs focus more on the real relationship, whereas psychodynamic psychotherapy emphasizes more heavily the issue of transference. If negative transference issues do arise in supportive psychotherapy, however, they must be dealt with within the relationship, because not to address them may result in the patient's dropping out of therapy early. The real relationship exists in the here and now. It addresses the needs of the patient, focusing on "where the patient is," and is patient centered, not therapist centered. The therapeutic alliance is part of the real relationship and is necessary if the work of psychotherapy is to be successful. A positive therapeutic alliance early in the therapy should be established because it is predictive of a positive outcome (Hellerstein, Rosenthal, Pinsker, et al., 1998; Luborsky, McLellan, Woody, et al., 1984). The therapist and patient work collaboratively to create therapeutic change through an affectionate bond, agreement on goals of therapy, the therapist's ability to be empathetic and involved in therapy, and the ability of the patient to do the work of therapy. All of these components of a therapeutic alliance are elements of supportive psychotherapy (Bordin, 1979; Gaston, 1990; Greenson, 1967). Alliance "ruptures" occur less often in supportive psychotherapy than in expressive psychotherapy, and when they do occur, the therapist makes an active attempt to "repair the rupture" and address the misunderstanding in a practical way (for instance, if a therapist was late to a session) before addressing transference issues.

Cognitive Behavioral Therapy Techniques

CBT techniques are an important aspect of supportive psychotherapy and can be used with patients who have anxiety and depressive symptoms, in which dysfunctional thinking influences the patient's mood, responses, and actions. Within the supportive psychotherapy model, dysfunctional or negative thoughts are recognized, and the therapist helps the patient to challenge the reality of such thoughts and assists the patient to come up with alternatives. Reframing situations also are part of CBT. Such activities are done within the therapeutic relationship.

Learning Theory (Patient Education)

One of the interventions therapists use within the supportive psychotherapy is patient teaching. Therapists provide information, principles, and skills in order to empower the patient to care for self and to make adaptive decisions and actions. Theories of adult education are useful because adults want to learn things that solve immediate problems or concerns (Brookfield, 1995; Knowles, Holton, & Swanson, 1998); however, patients who have neural impairments related to mental illnesses may have difficulty learning, such as encoding and processing information. In psychotherapy, which is considered a "controlled form of learning" (Etkin, Phil, Pittenger, et al., 2005), the therapist asks the patient to participate in "active learning" so that information can be stored through the process of relating the material to meanings, associations, and relationships of previously learned knowledge.

Indications

Supportive psychotherapy is the most extensively practiced form of psychotherapy and can be used in a variety of patient populations. Case Study 7-4 presents a scenario in which a patient may benefit from supportive psychotherapy. In the scenario, how would the therapist use supportive psychotherapy as a modality? Is she safe? What would need to be established before medication is suggested for this patient? What mind/body interaction would the nurse find in this case? What interventions would the nurse pursue to change the pattern seen in this case?

Assessment and Case Formulation

Case formulation is based on the assessment of the patient through the intake interview, which assesses psychopathology, strengths, and functioning. The patient's presenting problems or issues are discussed with the therapist, who should respond in an empathetic manner. The *DSM-IV-TR* diagnosis is important, but how a person interprets relationships and adapts to life issues are also important. The approaches used in supportive psychotherapy often overlap during treatment (Winston et al., 2004).

Interventions/Techniques

There are two levels of technique used when conducting supportive psychotherapy: contextual and tactical. The contextual techniques are used with all patients to form a foundation of treatment, whereas the tactical techniques are based on content of current communication, characteristics of the patient, and goals established by the patient and therapist (Rosenthal, 2010). Table 7-9 provides an overview of contextual and tactical techniques used in supportive psychotherapy.

Efficacy Research

Supportive psychotherapy is effective in a broad range of disorders, including schizophrenia, anxiety disorders, personality disorders, and anorexia nervosa. It has not been sufficiently defined or tested in controlled clinical trials to be considered evidence based. In a National Institute of Mental Health study of patients with schizophrenia, insight-oriented psychotherapy was compared with reality-adaptive supportive psychotherapy. Results reported a better outcome for supportive psychotherapy, especially with gains in patients' coping abilities. The supportive psychotherapy was once per week. Supportive psychotherapy combined with psychopharmacology was the treatment of choice for patients with chronic schizophrenia (Gunderson, Frank, Katz, et al., 1984). Supportive psychotherapy is useful across several patient populations and incorporates cognitive therapy and psychodynamic therapy, which are psychotherapies with demonstrated efficacy. Supportive psychotherapy's premise is that the foundation of a therapeutic nurse-patient alliance is the basis for psychotherapy's success and should not be underestimated. For a primer on this type of therapy, the reader is referred to the text by Winston et al. (2004).

CASE STUDY 7-4

Patient Who May Benefit From Supportive Psychotherapy

Audrey is a 72-year-old married woman referred by her cardiologist because she has been calling 2 or 3 times a week, reporting heart palpitations that are unsubstantiated in the medical tests. She was diagnosed with supraventricular tachycardia (SVT) when she was 45 years old but likely has been symptomatic since high school. She had worked as a private child care provider and has three grown children. The eldest is her only daughter, who was adopted when Audrey thought she would never be able to conceive. After the adoption, Audrey had two natural conceptions. She still does not understand how that happened.

Recent heart symptoms make her fearful of sudden vascular collapse or a heart attack when she is alone. She reports that she has been unable to leave her apartment complex without someone with her, and she does not feel comfortable walking even across the parking lot or in separate aisles of the supermarket without her cell phone in hand in case she collapses. Her husband still works but has a significant cardiovascular history, including aortic aneurysm and myocardial infarction. He also has diabetes. When medication was discussed in the session, Audrey became increasingly agitated, stating that her brother is a professor of pharmacy and she is resistant to medication unless absolutely necessary. She states she is fearful of a reaction of another drug with her cardiac medication.

TABLE 7-9 SUPPORTIVE PSYCHOTHERAPY TECHNIQUES

Technique	Examples
Contextual Techniques Adopting a conversational style	Provides a familiar nonchallenging interaction that reduces anxiety.
Maintaining the frame of treatment	Includes office setting, therapist's role, expectations, setting fees, and handling missed appointments. Providing a "holding environment" that is structured, predictable, and reliable provides security and support.
Being like a good parent	Therapist encourages patient autonomy but, like a good parent, balances protection and age-appropriate expectations. Therapist can confront the patient without the patient's having a sense of being punished.
Focusing on the real relationship	Uses the here and now relationship versus focusing on transference-focused treatment. Negative transference is addressed when it threatens the nurse-patient alliance.
Tactical Techniques Alliance building	Expression of interest: Noting information from the previous session relays that the therapist sees the patient as important. Expression of empathy: Empathy helps the patient feel that he/she has been understood. Expressing understanding: Giving feedback to the patient to be sure the therapist clearly understands the patient's communication Repairing a rupture in the therapeutic alliance with the patient: Handling misunderstandings and repairing issues in the relationship. Self-disclosure: Therapist discloses information about self that is therapeutic to the issue experienced by the patient and models appropriate behavior. Sustaining comments: Making bridging statements or refocusing the patient in a supportive way.
Self-esteem building	Praise: Used proactively and liberally to raise self-esteem through patient awareness of strengths or goals that have been met. Reassurance: Best when based on data or principles, such as normalizing a person's situation, for example, that grief is an expected reaction to losses. Encouragement: When patients feels demoralized, they need encouragement to address feelings of powerlessness; to instill hope; and to see that small changes add up and spur patients to reach a goal. Exhortation: An insistent form of encouragement, such as "I see what you are capable of...you can do this." Inspiration: Words by the therapist that go beyond inspiration to increase motivation and promote self-actualizing behaviors.
Enhancement of ego functioning and anxiety-reducing interventions	Structuring the environment: In some cases, case managers and family members may be added to increase structure in the patient's environment. Maintaining a protected environment: Within the outpatient office setting, but also in inpatient settings where a secure, contained unit is needed when the patient needs to be safe from self-harm. Setting limits: Rules of therapy are explained and enforced, i.e., length of time in session; coming to therapy session on time. Naming the problem: Identifying the problem helps patient to conceptualize and cope with the problem more effectively. Modulating affect: Helping the patient regulate emotional responses to things that occur in the environment. Supporting defense mechanisms: Defenses are supportive unless they are maladaptive. Universalizing experiences: Not personalizing remarks, but explaining a comment in an impersonal way, for example, "Sometimes people hear what they want to hear." Rationalizing: Patient is allowed to explain unacceptable attitudes or behaviors so as to make them bearable through use of this defense mechanism. Reframing: Discusses the situation using a different perspective. Minimization: A form of rationalization in which therapist substitutes minimization for the patient's denial of affect in order to make the affect more palatable to accept it.
Awareness-expanding interventions	Clarification: Pointing out patterns, paraphrasing, summarizing, and organizing the patient's statements. Using humor: Using humor to put things into perspective or clarify an issue. Confrontation: Bringing to the patient's awareness things that might be avoiding; gives a clear rationale. Interpretation: Although used infrequently, interpretation focuses patient's awareness on a thought, behavior, affect, defense, or symptom by connecting it to an unconscious source or meaning.
Skill Building Teaching	Imparting to the patient information and principles to assist with life skills and coping.
Modeling adaptive behavior	Demonstrating appropriate and healthy behavior the patient can emulate.
Providing anticipatory guidance	Discussing concerns that the patient needs to consider in advance of the situation; for example, coping with the impending death of a critically ill family member.
Redirecting	Directing the patient to do other activities (such as relaxation techniques) to distract the patient temporarily or to reduce anxiety.
Promoting autonomy	Promoting self-efficacy and independence.

Source: Modified from Rosenthal, R. (2010). Techniques of individual supportive psychotherapy. In G. O. Gabbard (Ed.), The textbook of psychotherapeutic treatments. *Washington, DC: American Psychiatric Publishing, Inc.*

Summary

In summary, the psychiatric advanced practice nurse must evaluate the patient and decide—in agreement with the patient—which psychotherapy would be the most beneficial to the patient. More than one mode of psychotherapy may be used. For example, some patients may not be motivated to undergo cognitive therapy, and thus the nurse psychotherapist must be creative, compassionate, and flexible to find a therapy that works best for the patient and family; for instance, a female patient with depression may benefit from cognitive therapy, interpersonal therapy, and family therapy to address all of the issues presented. From their tool chest of psychotherapy modalities, psychiatric advanced practice nurses select a model of psychotherapy based on (1) the patient's perspective, needs, and capabilities, and (2) the potential of the model to facilitate the patient's movement toward recovery.

Key Points

- Psychotherapy is the bedrock of treatment for patients with psychiatric disorders, and it is foundational in the education of nurse psychotherapists. Psychotherapy incorporates an understanding of the nurse-patient relationship, professional boundaries, and evidence-based psychotherapy modalities that are individualized to the patient's needs and codified for billing and reimbursement purposes.
- The scope of psychiatric advanced practice nurses continues to evolve. It includes psychiatric assessment and diagnosis, developmental assessment and treatment, psychopharmacotherapy, teaching of coping skills, understanding family processes and psychopathology, and monitoring health, wellness, and recovery.
- Hildegard Peplau emphasized the therapeutic nurse-patient relationship and the establishment of the psychiatric clinical nurse specialist role. Two roles exist currently—the psychiatric nurse practitioner and the psychiatric clinical nurse specialist. There have been recommendations that the roles be combined into one role, the psychiatric advanced practice nurse, and that there be a life span approach.
- The MINDFUL CARE model is a nurse psychotherapy model that integrates scope of practice, assessment, treatment, clinical models, and evidence-based practice.
- The nurse psychotherapist understands family systems as a transactional system that provides direct messages regarding role, expectations, genetics, support systems, and coping skills. Nurse therapists complete family genograms. They understand the core concepts of family systems such as adaptability, connectedness, family boundaries, triangulation, and family projection process.
- Brief or short-term therapy refers to a class of psychotherapies that seek behavioral change in patients through active patient involvement via the use of therapist-initiated focused interventions. Behavioral change can occur through this emotionally corrective experience.
- Psychodynamic psychotherapy addresses internal conflicts and anxiety and the resultant use of defense mechanisms. The goal is to focus on the effects of past experiences on the patient's present behaviors, thoughts, emotions, and actions that occur in the here and now.
- Interpersonal psychotherapy focuses on the patient's interpersonal relationships and on life events that occurred after early childhood that continue to influence the patient's psychopathology. Loss serves as triggers to mental illness. The therapist focuses on social support networks, communication, expectations within relationships, relief of symptoms, and building of social skills.
- Cognitive therapy is a form of psychotherapy based on the theory that negative or anxious thoughts are linking with depressed and anxious mood states, and if the thoughts are challenged for their merit, they may be seen as overexaggerated. If thoughts were more in line with reality, rather than exaggerated or global, the patient's mood would change to being less depressed or anxious. Life schemas about core beliefs about self are also challenged.
- Cognitive behavioral procedures are used to change behavior through actions and activities, and the positive changes are rewarded. Behavioral techniques include activity scheduling, graded task assignments, coping cards, and exposure therapy.
- Behavioral therapy uses exposure as a therapeutic component in which the fear that triggers the presenting symptoms is deliberately introduced in imagery or in vivo exercises. This results in response prevention and mastery to handle the stressor and thus symptom reduction by reprocessing of environmental cures associated with the distressful situation.
- Dialectical behavioral therapy (DBT) was developed by Linehan to address the chaotic life course and suicidal and nonsuicidal self-injury patterns (such as cutting, burning, and substance abuse) in patients who primarily are diagnosed with borderline personality disorder. Patients use individual and group therapy, and therapists themselves have interactions with each other to process the work they do with patients with this complex diagnosis. DBT is based on learning theory. Dialectic thinking represents the opposite of all-or-nothing dichotomous thinking, as it provides a discourse about the limitations of such thinking and enhances the outcome of different views in a process with the patient that is transactional.
- Contextual brief therapies do not view problems as coming from the patient, but as coming from the person-situation context. Strategic therapy and solution-focused therapy are two types of contextual therapy. Strategic therapy views the patient's presenting concerns as the result of attempts at finding successful solutions to life's

problems, but the solutions chosen by the patient, unbeknownst to the patient, reinforce the very problems they are attempting to solve. Solution-focused therapy, an offshoot of strategic therapy, looks to address patient strengths that can be built upon to solve problems, thus not focusing on the problem-based thinking that allows patients to get stuck in their usual way of solving problems.

- Supportive psychotherapy is not a short-term or brief psychotherapy, but one that is used by nurse therapists with many types of patients, especially those with chronic and persistent mental illnesses. The goals of supportive psychotherapy are to help the patient cope with symptoms, prevent relapse, and improve coping skills, self-esteem, and overall functioning.

References

Agency for Health Care Policy and Research. (1993). *Depression in primary care* (Vol 4. Depression is a treatable illness: A patient's guide). Consumer Guideline Number 5, AHCRQPubl No 93-0553. Rockville, MD: Agency for Health Care Policy and Research.

Alexander, F., & Freinch, T. (1946). *Psychoanalytic therapy: Principles and applications.* New York: Ronald Press.

Amen, D. (1998). *Change your brain, change your life: The breakthrough program for conquering anxiety, depression, obsessiveness, anger and impulsiveness.* New York: Three Rivers Press.

American Nurses Association. (2007). *Psychiatric-mental health nursing: Scope and standards of practice.* Silver Spring, MD: American Nurses Association.

American Nurses Association. (2010). *Nursing: Scope and standards of practice* (2nd ed.). Silver Spring, MD: American Nurses Association.

American Psychiatric Association. (2000). *The diagnostic and statistical manual of mental disorders* (4th ed., text rev.). Washington, DC: American Psychiatric Publishing, Inc.

APRN Consensus Work Group & National Council of State Boards of Nursing APRN Advisory Committee. (2008). *Consensus model for APRN regulation: Licensure, Accreditation, Certification and Education.* Retrieved from www.aacn.nche.edu/Education/pdf/APRNReport.pdf

Basco, M. (2000). *Never good enough: How to use perfectionism to your advantage without letting it ruin your life.* New York: Free Press.

Basco, M. (2005). *The bipolar workbook: Tools for controlling your mood swings.* New York: Guilford Press.

Beck, A. (1976). *Cognitive therapy and the emotional disorders.* New York: International Universities Press.

Beck, A., & Greenberg, R. (1974). *Coping with depression.* Philadelphia: Beck Institute for Cognitive Therapy and Research. Retrieved from http://www.anapsys.co.uk/Disorders/depression_article.htm

Beck, A., Rush, A., Shaw, B., et al. (1979). *Cognitive therapy of depression.* New York: Guilford Press.

Bellak, L., & Goldsmith, L. (1984). *The broad scope of ego function assessment.* New York: John Wiley.

Black, D., & Andreasen, N. (2011). *Introductory textbook of psychiatry.* Washington, DC: American Psychiatric Publishing, Inc.

Bordin, E. (1979). The generalizability of the psycho-analytic concept of the working alliance. *Psychotherapy: Theory, Research and Practice, 16,* 252-260.

Bowen, M. (1978). *Family therapy in clinical practice.* New York: Jason Aronson, Inc.

Bowlby, J. (1969). *Attachment and loss* (Vol. 1. Attachment). New York: Basic Books.

Bowlby, J. (1988). *A secure base: Parent-child attachment and healthy human development.* New York: Basic Books.

Bretherton, I. (1992). *Origins of attachment theory: John Bowlby and Mary Ainsworth. Developmental Psychology, 28,* 759-775.

Briere, J. (2002). Treating adult survivors of severe childhood abuse and neglect: Further development of an integrated model. In J. E. B. Myers, L. Berliner, J. Briere, et al. (Eds.), *The APSAC handbook on child maltreatment* (2nd ed.). Newbury Park, CA: Sage Publications.

Brookfield, S. (1995). *Becoming a critically reflective teacher.* San Francisco: Jossey Bass.

Burns, D. (1999). *Feeling good: The new therapy* (revised). New York: Avon.

Bush, D., Ziegeldtein, R., Patel, U., et al. (2005). *Post-myocardial infarction depression. Summary.* AHRQ Publication Number 05-E018-1. Evidence Report/Technology Assessment Number 123, Rockville, MD: Agency for Healthcare Research and Quality.

Carlat, D. (2010). *Unhinged.* New York: Free Press.

Carter, B., & McGoldrick, M. (1999). *The expanded family life cycle: Individual, family, and social perspectives* (3rd ed.). New York: Allyn & Bacon.

Copeland, M., & McKay, M. (2002). *The depression workbook: A guide for living with depression and manic depression* (2nd ed.). Oakland, CA: New Harbinger Publications.

Corcoran, J. (2009). *The depression solutions workbook: A strength and skill-based approach.* Oakland, CA: New Harbinger Publications.

Cozolino, L. (2002). *The neuroscience of psychotherapy: Building and rebuilding the human brain.* New York: W. W. Norton & Company.

Cozolino, L. (2010). *The neuroscience of psychotherapy* (2nd ed.). New York: W. W. Norton & Company.

Craske, M., & Barlow, D. (2006). *Mastery of your anxiety and panic* (4th ed.). London: Oxford University Press.

Davanloo, H. (1980). *Short-term psychotherapy.* New York: Jason Aronson, Inc.

Dewald, P. (1994). Principles of supportive psychotherapy. *American Journal of Psychotherapy, 48,* 505-518.

Dewan, M., Steenbarger, B., & Greenberg, R. (2010). Brief psychotherapies. In R. E. Hales, S. C. Yudofsky, & G. O. Gabbard (Eds.), *The American psychiatric publishing textbook of clinical psychiatry* (5th ed.). Washington, DC: American Psychiatric Publishing, Inc. Retrieved from www.psychiatryonline.com

Duncan, B., Miller, S., Wampold, B., et al. (2010). The heart and soul of change. Washington, DC: American Psychological Association.

Ellis, A., & Dryden, W. (1997). *The practice of rational emotive behavior therapy* (2nd ed.). New York: Springer.

Epp, A., Dobson, K., & Cottraux, J. (2009). Applications of individual cognitive-behavioral therapy to specific disorders: Efficacy and indications. In G. O. Gabbard (Ed.), *Textbook of psychotherapeutic treatments* (pp. 239-262). Washington, DC: American Psychiatric Publishing, Inc.

Erikson, E. (1963). *Childhood and society.* New York: W. W. Norton & Company.

Erickson, E. (1980). *Identity and the life cycle* (Vol. 1). New York: W. W. Norton & Company.

Etkin, A., Phil, M., Pittenger, C., et al. (2005). Toward a neurobiology of psychotherapy: Basic science and clinical applications. *Journal of Neuropsychiatry Clinical Neuroscience, 17,* 145-158.

Fairbairn, W. (1952). *An object-relations theory of the personality.* New York: Basic Books.

Fairbairn, W. (1994). *From instinct to self: Selected papers of WRD Fairbairn* (Vols. 1-2.). E. Birtles and D. Sharff (Eds.), Northvale, NJ: Jason Aronson Publishers Inc.

Fisher, S., & Greenberg, R. (1985). *The scientific credibility of Freud's theories and therapy.* New York: Columbia University Press.

Foa, E., Keane, T., & Friedman, M. (2000). *Effective treatment for PTSD.* New York: Guilford Press.

Foa, E., & Wilson, R. (2001). *Stop obsessing! How to overcome your obsessions and compulsions* (revised edition). New York: Bantam.

Fournier, J., DeRubeis, R., Hollon, S., et al. (2010). Antidepressant drug effects and depression severity. A patient meta-analysis. *Journal of the American Medical Association, 303*(1), 47-53.

Frank, E., Kupfer, D., Buysse, D., et al. (2007). Randomized trial of weekly, twice-monthly, and monthly interpersonal psychotherapy as maintenance treatment for women with recurrent depression. *American Journal of Psychiatry, 164*(5), 761-767.

Freud, S. (1923). The ego and the id. In J. Strachey (Ed.), *The standard edition of the complete psychological works of Sigmund Freud,* Vol. 19. London, England: Hogarth Press, 1961, 12-66.

Freud, S. (1938). *The basic writings of Sigmund Freud.* New York: The Modern Library.

Friedman, E., & Thase, M. (2009). Combining cognitive-behavioral therapy with medications. In G. O. Gabbard (Ed.), *Textbook of psychotherapeutic treatments* (pp. 263-285). Washington, DC: American Psychiatric Publishing, Inc.

Gabbard, G. (2009). Professional boundaries in psychotherapy. In G. O. Gabbard (Ed.), *Textbook of psychotherapeutic treatments* (pp. 809-827). Washington, DC: American Psychiatric Publishing, Inc.

Gaston, L. (1990). The concept of the alliance and its role in psychotherapy: Theoretical and empirical considerations. *Psychotherapy, 27,* 143-153.

Gowers, D., Norton, K., Halek, C., et al. (1994). Outcomes of outpatient psychotherapy in a random allocation treatment study of anorexia nervosa. *International Journal of Eating Disorders, 15,* 165-177.

Green, A. (2006). Patient centered approach to palliative nursing. *Journal of Hospice and Palliative Nursing, 8*(5), 294-301.

Greenberger, D., & Padesky, C. (1995). *Mind over mood: Change how you feel by changing the way you think.* New York: Guilford Press.

Greenson, R. (1967). *The technique and practice of psychoanalysis.* New York: International Universities Press.

Gunderson, J., Frank, A., Katz, M., et al. (1984). Effects of psychotherapy in schizophrenia. Comparative outcomes of 2 forms of treatment. *Schizophrenia Bulletin, 10*(4), 564-598.

Haley, J. (1963). *Strategies of psychotherapy* (2nd ed.). New York: Grune & Stratton.

Haley, J. (1976). *Problem-solving therapy: New strategies for effective family therapy.* New York: Harper & Row.

Heglend, P. (1993). Suitability for brief dynamic psychotherapy: Psychodynamic variables as predictors of outcome. *Acta Psychiatric Scandinavia, 88,* 104-110.

Hellerstein, D. (2009). Combining supportive psychotherapy with medication. In G. O. Gabbard (Ed.), *Textbook of psychotherapeutic treatments* (pp. 465-496). Washington, DC: American Psychiatric Publishing, Inc.

Hellerstein, D., Rosenthal R., Pinsker, H., et al. (1998). A randomized prospective study comparing supportive and dynamic therapies: Outcome and alliance. *Journal of Psychotherapeutic Practice and Research, 7,* 261-271.

Horvath, A., & Symonds, B. (1991). Relation between working alliance and outcome in psychotherapy: A meta-analysis. *Journal of Counseling Psychology, 38,* 139-149.

Huppert, J., Fabbro, A., & Barlow, D. (2006). Evidence-based practice and psychological treatments. In G. Goodheart, A. Kazdin, & R. Sternberg (Eds.), *Evidence-based psychotherapy: Where practice and research meet.* Washington, DC: American Psychological Association, 131-152.

Institute of Medicine. (2006). *Improving the quality of health care for mental and substance-use disorders.* Washington, DC: National Academies Press.

Jung, C. (1938). *Psychology and religion.* New Haven: Yale Press.

Jung, C. (1983). *Essential Jung.* Selected and introduced by Anthony Storr. Princeton, NJ: Princeton University Press.

Kabat-Zinn, J. (2003). Mindfulness-based interventions in context: Past, present and future. *Clinical Psychology: Science and Practice, 10,* 144-156.

Kabat-Zinn, J. (2005). Bringing mindfulness to medicine: An interview with Jon Kabat-Zinn: Interview by Karolyn Gazella. *Advances in Mind-Body Medicine, 21*(2), 22.

Katz, S. (2008). MINDFUL CARE: An integrated tool to guide holistic treatment in enhancing fertility. *Perspectives of Psychiatric Care, 44*(3), 207-210.

Knaus, W. (2006). *The cognitive-behavioral workbook for depression: A step-by-step program.* Oakland, CA: New Harbinger Publications.

Knowles, M., Holton, E., & Swanson, R. (1998). *The adult learner: The definitive classic in adult education and human resource development.* Burlington, MA: Gulf Professional Publishing.

Kohut, H. (1971). *The analysis of the self.* New York: International Universities Press.

Kohut, H. (1997). *The restoration of the self.* New York: International Universities Press.

Leahy, R. (2006). *The worry cure: Seven steps to stop worry from stopping you.* New York: Harmony Press.

Leichsenring, F. (2001). Comparative effects of short-term psychodynamic psychotherapy and cognitive-behavioral therapy in depression: A meta-analytic approach. *Clinical Psychological Review, 21,* 401-419.

Leichsenring, F. (2009). Application of psychodynamic psychotherapy to specific disorders: Efficacy and indications. In G. O. Gabbard (Ed.), *Textbook of psychotherapeutic treatments* (pp. 97-132). Washington, DC: American Psychiatric Publishing, Inc.

Leichsenring, F., Salzer, S., Jaeger, U., et al. (2009). Short-term psychodynamic psychotherapy and cognitive-behavioral therapy in generalized anxiety disorder: A randomized, controlled trial. *American Journal of Psychiatry, 166*(8), 875-881.

Linehan, M. (1993a). *Cognitive behavioral therapy for borderline personality disorder.* New York: Guilford Press.

Linehan, M. (1993b). *Skills training manual for treating borderline personality disorder.* New York: Guilford Press.

Luborsky, L., McLellan, A., Woody, G., et al. (1985). Therapist success and its determinants. *Archives of General Psychiatry, 82,* 602-611.

Markowitz, J. (2008). Interpersonal psychotherapy. In R. E. Hales, S. C. Yudofsky, & G. O. Gabbard (Eds.), *The American psychiatric publishing textbook of clinical psychiatry* (5th ed.) (pp. 1191-1210). Washington, DC: American Psychiatric Publishing, Inc.

Mauer, B., & Druss, B. (2007). *Mind and body reunited: Improving care at behavioral and primary care interface.* American College of Mental Health Administration Summit, March, 2008.

Melnyk, B. M., & Fineout-Overholt, E. (2005). Rapid critical appraisal of randomized controlled trials (RCTs): An essential skill for evidence-based practice (EBP). *Pediatric Nursing, 31*(1), 50-52.

Messer, S. (2001). What makes brief psychodynamic therapy time efficient. *Clinical Psychology: Science and Practice, 8,* 5-22.

Minuchin, S. (1974). *Families and family therapy.* Cambridge, MA: Harvard University Press.

Mundy, K., & Stein, K. (2008). Meta-analysis as basis for evidence-based practice: The question is, why not? *Journal of the American Psychiatric Nurses Association, 14*(4), 326-328.

Munroe-Blum, H., & Marziali, E. (1995). A controlled trial of short-term group treatment for borderline personality disorder. *Journal of Personality Disorders, 9,* 190-198.

Parks, J., Radke, A., & Mazade, N. (2008). *Behavioral health and primary care collaboration.* Retrieved from https://www.thenationalcouncil.org

Patterson, W. M., Duhn, H. H., Bird, J., et al. (1983). Evaluating of suicidal patients: The SAD PERSONS scale. *Psychosomatics 24,* 343-349.

Peplau, H. (1952). *Interpersonal relations in nursing: A conceptual frame of reference for psychodynamic nursing.* New York: Putnam.

Peplau, H. (1988). *Interpersonal relations in nursing.* New York: Springer. (Original work published in 1952, New York: G.P. Putnam's Sons.)

Pinsker, H. (1997). *A primer of supportive psychotherapy.* Hillsdale, NJ: Analytic Press.

Pinsker, H., & Rosenthal, R. (1988). *Beth Israel Medical Center supportive psychotherapy manual.* Social and Behavioral Sciences Documents, 18, #2886. Washington, DC: American Psychological Association.

Pinsker, H., Rosenthal, R., & McCullough, L. (1991). Dynamic supportive psychotherapy. In P. Crits-Christoph & J. Barber (Eds.), *Handbook of short term dynamic psychotherapy.* New York: Basic Books.

Piper, W., Azim, H., Joyce, A., et al. (2001). Patient personality and time-limited group psychotherapy for complicated grief. *International Journal of Group Psychotherapy, 51,* 525-552.

Proudfoot, J., Ryden, C., Everitt, B., et al. (2004). Clinical efficacy of computerized cognitive-behavioral therapy for anxiety and depression in primary care: Randomized controlled trial. *British Journal of Psychiatry, 185,* 46-53.

Reed, G., & Eisman, D. (2006). Uses and misuses of evidence: Managed care, treatment guidelines and outcomes measurement in professional practice. In C. Goodheart, A. Kazdin, & R. Sternberg (Eds.), *Evidence-based psychotherapy: Where practice and research meet* (pp. 13-36). Washington, DC: American Psychological Association.

Riba, M., & Balon, R. (2008). Combining psychotherapy and pharmacology. In R. E. Hales, S. C. Yudofsky, & G. O. Gabbard (Eds.), *American psychiatric publishing textbook of clinical psychiatry* (5th ed.) (pp. 1279-1301). Washington, DC: American Psychiatric Publishing, Inc.

Rice, M. J. (2008). Psychiatric mental health evidence-based practice. *Journal of the American Psychiatric Nurses Association, 14*(2), 107-111.

Rolland, J. (1994). *Families, illness and disability: An integrated approach.* New York: Basic Books.

Rosenbaum, R. (1990). Strategic psychotherapy. In R. Wells & V. Giannetti (Eds.), *Handbook of the brief psychotherapies* (pp. 351-404). New York: Plenum Press.

Rosenthal, R. (2010). Techniques of individual supportive psychotherapy. In G. O. Gabbard (Ed.), *Textbook of psychotherapeutic treatments* (pp. 417-464). Washington, DC: American Psychiatric Publishing, Inc.

Ruddy, N., Borresen, D., & Gunn, W. (2008). *The collaborative psychotherapist: Creating reciprocal relationships with medical professionals.* Washington, DC: American Psychological Association.

Sadock, B., & Sadock, V. (2008). *Kaplan and Sadock's concise textbook of clinical psychiatry* (3rd ed.). Philadelphia: Wolters, Kluwer/Lippincott Williams, & Wilkins.

Selmi, P., Klein, M., Greist, J., et al. (1990). Computer-administered therapy for depression. *American Journal of Psychiatry, 147,* 51-56.

Shapiro, R. (2001). *Eye movement desensitization and reprocessing: Basic principles, protocols, and procedures* (2nd ed.). New York: Guilford Press.

Sifneos, P. (1972). *Short-term psychotherapy and emotional crisis.* Cambridge, MA: Harvard University Press.

Sijbrandij, M., Olff, M., Reitsma, J., et al. (2007). Treatment of acute posttraumatic stress disorder with brief cognitive behavioral therapy: A randomized controlled trial. *American Journal of Psychiatry, 164*(1), 82-90.

Sobel, S. (2008). *Hunger for health: The successful treatment of bulimia.* San Diego, CA: U.S. Psychiatric and Mental Health Congress. Retrieved from http://www.cmell.compsychcongress/images/08/pdg/32-3%20Sobel.pdf

Spinelli, M., & Endicott, J. (2003). Controlled clinical trial of interpersonal psychotherapy versus parenting education program for depressed pregnant women. *American Journal of Psychiatry, 160*(3), 555-562.

Stanton, A., Gunderson, J., Knapp, P., et al. (1984). Effects of psychotherapy in schizophrenia, I: Design and implementation of a controlled study. *Schizophrenia Bulletin, 10,* 520-563.

Steenbarger, B. (1992). Toward science practice integration in brief counseling and therapy. *Counseling Psychology, 20,* 403-450.

Stein, M. (1998). *Jung's map of the soul.* Chicago: Open Court Publishers.

Stuart, S. (2004). Interpersonal psychotherapy. In M. Dewan, B. Steenberger, & R. Greenberg (Eds.), *The art and science of brief psychotherapies: A practitioner's guide* (pp. 119-156). Washington, DC: American Psychiatric Publishing, Inc.

Stuart, S., & Robertson, M. (2003). *Interpersonal psychotherapy: A clinical guide.* London: Edward Arnold.

Substance Abuse and Mental Health Services Administration. (2009). Recovery. A philosophy of hope and resilience. *SAMHSA News, 17*(5), 1-2.

Swartz, H., Frank, E., Shear, M., et al. (2004). A pilot study of brief interpersonal psychotherapy for depression among women. *Psychiatric Services, 55*(4), 448-450.

Thompson, L., & Gallagher, D. (1985). Depression and its treatment. *Aging, 348,* 14-18.

Turkington, D., Kingdon, D., & Weiden, P. J. (2006). Cognitive behavior therapy for schizophrenia. *American Journal of Psychiatry, 163*(3), 365-373.

Vaillant, G. (1977). *Adaptation to life.* Boston: Little, Brown.

Vaillant, G. (1997). *Wisdom of the ego.* Cambridge, MA: Harvard University Press.

Vaillant, G. (1992). *Ego mechanisms of defense: A guide for clinicians and researchers.* Washington, DC: American Psychiatric Press.

Vaillant, G. (2002). *Aging well: Surprising guideposts to a happier life from the landmark Harvard study of adult development.* Boston: Little Brown and Company.

Vaillant, G. (2008). *Spiritual evolution: How we are wired for faith, hope, and love.* Three Rivers, MI: Three Rivers Press.

Van Pelt, I. (2009). Where is the hurt? How do we help? *Clinical Psychiatry News,* 37(6), 10.

Vogelzangs, N., Kritchevsky, S. B., Beekman, A. T., et al. (2008). Depressive symptoms and change in abdominal obesity in older persons. *Archives of General Psychiatry, 65*(12), 1386-1393.

Wallerstein, R. (1989). The psychotherapy research project of the Menninger Foundation: An overview. *Journal of Consulting Clinical Psychology, 57,* 195-205.

Walter, J., & Peller, J. (1992). *Becoming solution-focused in brief therapy.* New York: Brunner-Mazel.

Wampold, B. (2001). *The great psychotherapy debate.* New York: Routledge.

Wampold, B. (2010). *The basics of psychotherapy.* Washington, DC: American Psychological Association.

Watkins, J., & Watkins, H. (1997). *Ego states: Theory and therapy.* New York: W. W. Norton & Company.

Watzlawick, P., Weakland, H., & Fish, R. (1974). *Change: Principles of problem formulation and problem resolution.* New York: W. W. Norton & Company.

Weissman, M., Markowitz, J., & Klerman, G. (2000). *Comprehensive guide to interpersonal psychotherapy.* New York: Basic Books.

Wheelis, J. (2009). Theory and practice of dialectical behavioral therapy. In G. O. Gabbard (Ed.), *Textbook of psychotherapeutic treatment* (pp. 727-756). Washington, DC: American Psychiatric Publishing, Inc.

Winnicott, D. (1965). *The maturational process and the facilitating environment: Studies in the theory of emotional development.* London: Hogarth Press.

Winnicott, D. (1971). *Playing and reality.* New York: Basic Books.

Winston, A., & Goldstein, M. (2010). Theory of supportive psychotherapy. In G. O. Gabbard (Ed.), *Textbook of psychotherapeutic treatments* (pp. 393-416). Washington, DC: American Psychiatric Publishing, Inc.

Winston, A., Pinsker, H., & McCullough, L. (1986). A review of supportive psychotherapy. *Hospital and Community Psychiatry, 37,* 1105-1114.

Winston, A., Rosenthal, R., & Pinsker, H. (2004). *Introduction to supportive psychotherapy (Core competencies in psychotherapy series).* Washington, DC: American Psychiatric Publishing, Inc.

Wright, J., & Basco, M. (2002). *Getting your life back: The complete guide to recovery from depression.* New York: Free Press.

Wright, J., Basco, M., & Thase, M. (2006). *Learning cognitive-behavior therapy: An illustrated guide (Core competencies in psychotherapy series).* Washington, DC: American Psychiatric Publishing, Inc.

Wright, J., Salmon, P., Wright, A., et al. (1995). *Cognitive therapy: A multimedia learning program.* Louisville, KY: Mindstreet.

Wright, J., Salmon, P., Wright, A., et al. (2002). Development and initial testing of a multimedia program for computer-assisted cognitive therapy. *American Journal of Psychotherapy. 56,* 76-87.

Wright, J., Thase, M., & Beck, A. (2008). Cognitive therapy. In R. E. Hales, S. C. Yudofsky, & G. O. Gabbard (Eds.), *The American psychiatric publishing textbook of clinical psychiatry* (5th ed.) (pp. 1211-1256). Washington, DC: American Psychiatric Publishing, Inc.

Wright, J., Wright, A., Albano, A., et al. (2005). Computer-assisted cognitive therapy for depression: Maintaining efficacy while reducing therapist time. *American Journal of Psychiatry, 162,* 1158-1164.

Wright, J., Wright, A., & Beck, A. (2003). *Good days ahead: The interactive program for depression and anxiety.* Louisville, KY: Mindstreet.

Wright, J., Wright, A., Salmon, P., et al. (2002). Development and initial testing of a multi-media program for computer-assisted cognitive therapy. *American Journal of Psychotherapy. 56,* 76-86.

CHAPTER 8

Psychosocial Interventions

Eris F. Perese, APRN-PMH

Psychosocial interventions are nonpharmacological interventions that are designed to (1) relieve symptoms of distress, such as loneliness, anxiety, and depression; (2) reduce the severity of symptoms and the need for hospitalizations; and (3) improve psychosocial functioning and quality of life (Addington, Piskulic, & Marshal, 2010; Beebe, 2007, 2010; Mueser, Bond, & Drake, 2001). Psychosocial interventions include components such as effective communication, cognitive restructuring, problem-solving, management of stigma, teaching of coping skills, and ongoing support. Psychosocial interventions have the potential to promote resilience (McEwen, 2009) and to help patients to change negative thinking, dysfunctional emotional and behavioral responses, and unhealthy lifestyle practices. They help patients move toward recovery by increasing knowledge, hope, sense of self-identity and self-efficacy, skills for community connectedness, and resilience (International Federation Reference Centre for Psychosocial Support, 2009). According to the President's New Freedom Commission, in addition to pharmacotherapy and psychotherapy, psychosocial interventions are crucial to promoting recovery for patients with psychiatric disorders (Hogan, 2003). (See Chapter 1 for discussion of resilience and recovery.)

Individuals who participate in psychosocial interventions expect that they will change and that their situation will change. They expect to improve their physical, emotional, and social functioning and their sense of self-confidence (Hasson-Ohayon, Roe, & Kravetz, 2006). Psychosocial interventions have been found to be effective adjuncts in the treatment of psychiatric disorders such as bipolar disorder (Miklowitz, Goodwin, Bauer, et al., 2008), acute stress disorder, post-traumatic stress disorder (Marmar & Spiegel, 2007), schizophrenia, co-occurring mental illness and substance use disorders (Drake, O'Neal, & Wallach, 2008), and somatization disorder (Phillips, 2007). Psychosocial interventions have also been found to help in facilitating adjustment following exposure to traumatic events (Horowitz, 2003).

Overall, integrated approaches that combine psychotherapy, pharmacotherapy, and psychosocial interventions have been found to produce the optimum control of symptoms and highest levels of community functioning in patients with psychiatric disorders (Kopelowicz, Wallace, & Liberman, 2007). Integrated approaches are viewed as the most effective way of helping patients move toward recovery (Corrigan, 2006). Corrigan stated that the interaction of combined pharmacotherapy and psychosocial interventions is circulatory: medications help to decrease symptoms and improve cognition, and these changes enable patients to participate in psychosocial interventions that help them to understand the role of medications in recovery.

Families, patients, mental health care providers, and administrators of health-care organizations believe that psychosocial interventions must be evidence based and selected to meet the specific needs of each patient (Lehman, Kreyenbuhl, Buchanan, et al., 2004). Psychosocial interventions can be

- Preventive, as with psychological first aid and parish nursing
- Supplementary, as with psychoeducational programs, sleep management programs, social rhythms therapy, and socializing interventions
- Compensatory, as with coping enhancement programs, support programs, and care management programs
- Remedial, as with cognitive restructuring, cognitive adaptation training, cognitive remediation, and vocational rehabilitation

The categories listed above are fluid; one intervention may fulfill many purposes. For instance, stress management is a coping enhancement technique that can be both compensatory and preventive. Thus, having knowledge about evidence-based psychosocial interventions enables psychiatric advanced practice nurses to select the appropriate intervention for implementation or referral.

Preventive Psychosocial Interventions

The purpose of preventive psychosocial interventions is to help individuals to adapt positively to the effects of a traumatic event or situation as soon as possible in order to prevent the development of maladaptive responses or psychopathology. Examples of preventive psychosocial interventions include psychological first aid and parish nursing.

Psychological First Aid (PFA)

An individual's response to a crisis, trauma, or disaster is unique to that individual. Losses usually result from a tragic event: an individual may experience the loss of loved ones, of property, of his or her livelihood, of his or her status in a community, and of his or her sense of dignity, control, and security. Following the crisis, victims may experience shock from the actual event, grief for what has been lost, and feelings of distress such as fear, anxiety, depression, and anger. They often have a sense of "loss of place," which is a loss of confidence in the norms and networks of society that are supposed to protect them (International Federation Reference Centre for Psychosocial Support, 2009; McFarlane, 2010). Preschool children often experience separation anxiety, nightmares, and regressive behaviors. School-age children may experience somatic symptoms, arousal, and reexperiencing of the trauma. Adolescents often experience anxiety, depression, and fear of a foreshortened future (Shibley, 2010). Crisis-intervention specialists recommend the use of an approach known as psychological first aid (PFA) for individuals who have experienced a crisis such as a traumatic event or disaster (Gard & Ruzek, 2006). PFA is used to help victims—children, adults, families, and groups of people—come to terms with the event, reduce distress, increase resilience, and move toward recovery.

PFA is not a plan for delivery of mental health services; rather, it is a set of principles that can be used in diverse situations to guide care in response to crises and disasters. The primary principles of PFA are (1) meeting individuals' crisis-related biopsychosocial needs in a practical manner and (2) developing a plan for their recovery (Rodriguez & Kohn, 2008). The objectives of PFA are to

- Establish a helping relationship with individuals in crisis in a compassionate manner
- Provide for individuals' safety and physical and emotional comfort
- Calm and orient individuals who may feel overwhelmed and are experiencing intense grief
- Offer practical assistance and information to help individuals meet their needs and concerns
- Connect individuals with their family members, friends, neighbors, and community helping resources
- Support individuals' adaptive coping and encourage them in taking an active role in their recovery (adapted from Rodriguez & Kohn, 2008, pp. 375-376)

Activities taken to carry out the goals of PFA include

- Creating a safe, sheltering place where the victims can stay, and treating temporary living arrangements as villages
- Reuniting families, and keeping children with relatives or neighbors if they have lost their parents
- Providing clean water, sanitation, nutrition, and medical care (Ursano, Bell, Friedman, et al., 2006; Yule, 2006)
- Comforting and consoling victims who are grieving for what they have lost
- Providing information about what is being done to help them and when to expect the help
- Protecting victims from further threat and from exposure to media as far as possible
- Allowing victims to tell their story of the trauma if they wish to do so and to express their emotions after the danger/threat has subsided
- Helping victims—including children—to accept death and to understand grief and bereavement
- Encouraging a return to normal routines, such as children going to school
- Linking victims with systems of support by providing names of agencies and institutions and how to contact them
- Facilitating a sense of hope, mastery, and belief in recovery (Marmar & Spiegel, 2007; Yule).

In short, PFA involves providing information, basic survival supplies, resources, and support to individuals who have been affected by a traumatic event. Providing information about the trauma helps individuals to recognize and accept the details of what happened, though information needs to be given in a way that conveys hope and, at the same time, realistic expectations of what may happen in the future. Basic survival resources—including shelter, food, water, clothing, sanitation, and medical care—create a sense of safety. Support involves both strengthening the coping strategies that the individuals have used successfully in the past and promoting the use of new, adaptive coping strategies. For example, it is known that individuals do better after exposure to a traumatic event if they recognize the need to take responsibility for a successful outcome, are actively involved in overcoming the problems associated with the traumatic event, and are involved in helping others (LeDoux & Gorman, 2001).

Outcomes

In discussing outcomes of PFA, it is helpful to remember that PFA is based on the study of survivors of traumatic events who coped well after the event. The simple actions that helped them to recover their ability to function were identified and incorporated into the principles of PFA (Leach, 1995). Thus, PFA is built on a track record of successful functioning after a crisis. For example, in a study of the 9/11 terror attacks on the World Trade Center, Boscarino and Adams (2008) concluded that early, brief interventions at the site of the disaster were the most effective form of post-disaster treatment.

Parish Nursing

Faith-based providers are the only source of care for some individuals with mental disorders. They are often the primary source of care for those who are impoverished, recent immigrants, members of minority groups, older adults, and caregivers providing home care to a loved one (Anderson, 2004; Dossett, Fuentes, Klap, et al., 2005). For example, in a survey of 42 religious organizations that provide care to low-income, uninsured residents of Los Angeles County, more than half of the organizations reported that the parishioners receiving care tended to be Hispanic, Asian American, Pacific Islanders, and African Americans (Dossett et al.).

Parish nursing is a model of nursing provided by registered nurses with a minimum of 2 years of experience that focuses on health promotion and disease prevention within a faith community (Brudenell, 2003). The first parish nursing program was started in 1987 in Chicago by Dr. Granger Westberg and was an interdenominational endeavor by Catholic and Protestant churches. Now, in addition to Christian Parish Nurses, there are Jewish Congregational Nurses and Muslim Crescent Nurses. There are parish nurses in 15 countries, with approximately 12,000 parish nurses in the United States (Parish Nursing Fact Sheet, 2009).

In 1998, the American Nursing Association (ANA) recognized parish nursing as a specialty area of practice and published its scope and standards of practice (American Nursing Association, 1998). The ANA identified seven role functions for the parish nurse: the parish nurse is an integrator of faith and health, a provider of health education, a health counselor, a referral agent, a trainer of volunteers, an organizer of support groups, and an advocate for health.

Parish nursing is based on Engle's (1977) biopsychosocial approach to health care. The goals of parish nursing are to promote health, prevent illnesses, and provide the initiative for individuals to take care of themselves. Parish nurses help members of the faith community to be "good stewards of the gift of life" (Anderson, 2004, p. 119).

Faith communities often develop parish nurse programs to meet the needs of medically underserved members of their congregations. In most programs, parish nurses do not provide hands-on nursing care; they serve as educators, counselors, and support-group organizers. They are expected to serve as liaisons to community agencies, be knowledgeable about accessing community resources, and make referrals when needed for medical and psychiatric care (Anderson, 2004; Brudenell, 2003).

Parish nurses have developed and provided educational programs on self-esteem, depression, breast cancer, sexual education, healthy diets, stress reduction, immunizations, diabetic care, newborn care, medications, financial planning, and lightening the load of caregivers. They have organized blood pressure screening groups and written articles about health promotion and disease prevention for the organizations' newsletters. Some parish nursing programs provide case management. Other programs provide telephone access to the parish nurse so that parishioners can seek health advice, emotional support, or help in an emergency. Many programs provide mental health services, such as information about available mental health care, education about mental illnesses, individual counseling, and family counseling (Dossett et al., 2005).

Outcomes

The groups that parish nurses organize to provide health education have been found to provide opportunities for parishioners to build new relationships, increase social support, and reduce social isolation (Anderson, 2004). When parish nurses were involved in helping elderly parishioners with their health problems and providing emotional support for caregivers of elderly family members, there was improvement of the parishioners' quality of life and reduction of caregivers' feelings of isolation and being overwhelmed. Parish nurses' assistance to caregivers has been found to enable elderly patients to remain in their homes, thus reducing the cost of nursing home placements (Biddix & Brown, 1999; Rydholm, 1997).

Supplementary Psychosocial Interventions

Supplementary psychosocial interventions are used in combination with other interventions to increase patients' understanding of their illnesses, to facilitate self-care management of symptoms (such as with sleep disruptions), to reduce social isolation, and to increase connectedness to the community. Common supplemental interventions include psychoeducation, sleep management, social rhythms therapy, and socializing interventions.

Psychoeducational Programs

Patients with severe mental illness are no longer viewed as being passive recipients of care but rather as being actively involved in managing their illnesses. One intervention that has been developed to facilitate self-management of psychiatric disorders is psychoeducation for patients. Because the majority of patients with severe mental illness stay in close contact with their families, psychoeducation for families was also developed to help families in their role in managing patients' day-to-day care and in managing crises.

Patient Psychoeducation

Psychoeducation involves teaching patients about psychiatric disorders, treatment, coping strategies for managing stress and symptoms, and how to recognize and respond to early warning signs of relapse. Psychoeducation for patients also includes teaching skills for adhering to treatment, which is a key component of illness self-management. Approaches to improving medication adherence include social skills training, motivational enhancement, and behavioral tailoring.

Social skills training improves medication adherence by increasing protective factors, e.g., lessening the adverse effects of cognitive deficits, stressful events, daily hassles, and problems with social interactions by strengthening communication and coping skills, problem-solving ability, and resilience. Protective factors of reduced stress and increased involvement in managing their illness help patients to improve their adherence to treatment (Kopelowicz, Liberman, & Zarate, 2006).

Motivational enhancement increases patients' awareness of the obstacles that stand between them and their goals. In addition, identification of behavioral changes that must occur to achieve their goals often leads to increased medication adherence.

Behavioral tailoring is the patient's process of developing a routine for taking medications that fits into his or her daily habits. It includes natural prompts, such as placing medications beside the coffee cup. Because education about psychiatric disorders, their course, and their treatment may make patients more aware of lost dreams and stigma, psychiatric advanced practice nurses should monitor patients receiving psychoeducation for signs of depression and thoughts of suicide (Lysaker & Buck, 2006).

Outcomes

In a meta-analysis of ten randomized controlled studies, Pekkala and Merinder (2002) found that psychoeducation for patients improved adherence to medications and significantly decreased relapse and hospital readmission rates. However, some researchers believe that education that increases patients' awareness of illnesses such as schizophrenia may increase depression. Lysaker and Buck (2006) stated that it is the meaning of the illness, the stigma, and the lost dreams that generate adverse responses such as depression and suicidality.

Family Psychoeducation

In the past, family educational programs focused on families who had a member in the chronic phase of illness; the emphasis of these programs was frequently on preventing rehospitalization. The current approach to family psychoeducation is to involve families at the start of the illness in order to minimize the impact of the illness on the entire family, to facilitate the family's adaptation to the illness, and to reduce the family's grief, stress, and burden (Addington et al., 2010). Programs developed to help families often include both educational and supportive components; they focus on teaching about the nature of serious mental illness and the need for adherence to treatment. Specific content should include information about the illness, course, and treatment options; crisis intervention; use of community resources; methods for decreasing stress for the entire family; use of effective skills to cope with symptoms associated with the patient's illness, such as communication and problem-solving skills; and emotional support for the family (Dixon, Adams, & Luckstead, 2000; Lehman et al., 2004).

Families are also provided with information about how to help the patient manage his or her illness. For example, they are given information about the effect that the patient's illness-related symptoms—e.g., irritability, lack of energy, and fatigue—may have on the patient's ability to work and get along with people. Information is also provided about the relationship between stressful events in the patient's life—such as his or her inability to get a job, a change in living situation, or arguments with spouse, partner, or family members—and the patient's development of depression or an increase in severity of the symptoms of schizophrenia.

In addition, families are taught specific strategies for lowering their own anxiety, for reducing conflict with the patient, and for decreasing their expression of negative, hostile emotions or criticism (Skarsater, Agren, & Dencker, 2001). Most of these strategies are simple, such as the advice to go slow, give the patient space, set limits, keep directions simple, lower expectations, pick your battles, and solve problems step by step.

Families are also taught to develop a crisis plan that includes recognizing cues that warn of an approaching crisis and knowing what options there are if a crisis develops.

Outcomes

Adding family intervention programs to pharmacotherapy or case management produces better results than either of the two alone (Pilling, Bebbington, Kuipers, et al., 2002a, 2002b). Family intervention programs reduce symptoms and rates of relapse and rehospitalization among patients with schizophrenia and improve the outcome of patients with bipolar disorder (Mueser et al., 2001). Family educational programs have been found to reduce families' distress (Addington, McCleery, & Addington, 2005). To be effective, the family intervention program should be provided for at least 9 months (Lehman et al., 2004).

Sleep Management Programs

Sleep plays a role in physical and mental health, and disruptions of sleep have long been associated with both medical disorders and psychiatric disorders (Reite, 2009). Sleep disruptions occur frequently in medical disorders, such as with cardiovascular diseases, diabetes, asthma, arthritis, gastrointestinal reflux disorder, and obesity (Epstein & Mardon, 2007). Sleep deprivation that is often accompanied by feelings of being "stressed out" is associated with these medical disorders and also with impairment of cognitive functioning and memory (McEwen, 2007, p. 881). Psychiatric disorders characterized by sleep disturbances include anxiety disorders, depression, bipolar disorder, schizophrenia, and Alzheimer's disease. For example, the symptom of sleep disturbance is a red flag for depression. In the past, the assumption has been that depression causes sleep disturbances (Hassed, 2003). More recently, it has been proposed that poor sleep plays a role in the etiology of depression (Holsboer-Trachsler & Seifritz, 2000). For example, Morawetz (2001) found that 70% of individuals with depression who used sleep improvement strategies experienced a decrease in their symptoms of depression.

Thus, research has established that lack of sleep—defined as less than 7 or 7.5 hours for most people—affects alertness, memory, cognition, creativity, and quality of life; it is also linked to the risk of developing obesity, diabetes, heart disease, depression, and a shorter life span (Epstein & Mardon, 2007). Getting enough sleep is as essential for health as a healthy diet, exercise, or socialization. In order to get enough sleep each night, patients must modify lifestyle practices that sabotage sleep, set time aside for it consistently, follow sleep hygiene practices, prepare the environment for optimal sleep, and occasionally, use supplemental approaches to promote sleep.

Modification of Lifestyle Practices

A healthy diet that prevents obesity and other medical problems plays a role in promoting optimal sleep. Substances in the diet that contain caffeine such as coffee, tea, and caffeinated sodas block the production of adenosine, which is a neurotransmitter that promotes sleep. Therefore, caffeinated drinks should be limited to two or three drinks a day, preferably none after noon. Foods that cause heartburn, such as fatty foods or spicy foods, should be avoided for several hours before bedtime.

Exercise also plays a role in setting the circadian rhythm of sleep and wakefulness: it reduces stress and anxiety; increases serotonin, which promotes sleep; and affects the body's biological clock (Epstein & Mardon, 2007). Exercise is also linked with falling asleep faster, having a deeper sleep, and waking less during the night, so exercises such as walking, bicycling, swimming, and aerobics can be used to improve sleep.

Nicotine, a central nervous system stimulant, increases brain activity and thus interferes with sleep. Individuals who stopped smoking have found that they fall asleep more quickly and do not wake up as often during the night.

Sleep Plans and Preparation

Sleep planning includes setting aside a block of time for sleep that will enable the individual to feel rested and able to carry out required work, studying, parenting, homemaking, or other activities when he or she gets up in the morning. The time for sleep must be adhered to consistently, and other activities such as eating, exercising, and engaging in leisure activities should also be carried out at the same time each day.

Sleep preparation includes establishing a pre-sleep routine that is designed to reduce stress and mental activity. The pre-sleep routine may include tasks related to preparing for the next day, e.g., unloading the dishwasher, picking up clutter, setting the coffee maker, and making notes of what must be done the next day. The pre-sleep routine should include relaxing activities such as reading, listening to music, or watching nonstimulating television programs. It should produce a sense of relaxation and readiness for sleep.

Sleep Hygiene

Sleep hygiene refers to both routines associated with preparing to go to sleep and sleep habits. Good sleep hygiene activities include going to bed when sleepy; using the bedroom for only two purposes, sleep and sex; not taking daytime naps; getting up and doing something else if unable to fall asleep within 20 minutes of going to bed; and getting up at the same time each day. Poor sleep hygiene activities include napping during the day, drinking caffeinated beverages within 10 hours of bedtime, drinking alcohol 3 hours before bedtime, exercising within 4 hours of bedtime, worrying about important matters at bedtime, reading or watching television in bed, and sleeping in a room that is too hot, too noisy, or too bright (Gellis & Lichstein, 2008).

The Optimal Sleep Environment

Everything in the bedroom should encourage sleep. It should be cool and airy. Colors should be soothing and decorations should convey peace. The bed and pillows should be comfortable, the linens clean and crisp. There should be shades or curtains to block out light. Noise should be reduced by muting the phones and doorbells and by the use of earplugs if necessary. Finally, clocks should be turned so that it is not possible to see the time while falling asleep or waking during the night (Epstein & Mardon, 2007).

Supplemental Approaches to Sleep

Approximately half of adults in the United States experience sleep problems. Sleep-inducing medications (such as synthetic melatonin) are the most commonly used approach, but herbal supplements and hot baths are also used.

Medications

In the United States, 10% of adults use prescription medications or over-the-counter medications to promote sleep (National Sleep Foundation, 2008). However, sleep medications have many adverse effects that must be considered.

First, there are safety issues associated with the use of sleep medications, such as impairment of coordination and judgment, risk for falls, and increased death rates (Reite, 2009). Some sleep medications produce psychological dependency, which is the patients' belief that they cannot sleep without the medication, and some medications have a rebound effect, e.g., patients experience worse insomnia when they stop taking the medication. Reite suggested that if medications are to be used for short-term treatment of insomnia, the newer *hypnotic medications* should be used rather than benzodiazepines because they are less likely to cause habituation, tolerance, and altered sleep patterns. Newer hypnotic medications include zolpidem (Ambien, Ambien CR), zaleplon (Sonata), and eszopiclone (Lunesta). Zolpidem is sometimes used for short-term insomnias, such as stress-related insomnia due to an event that generates excitement or worry that interferes with sleep. Side effects include feeling groggy in the morning, dizziness, and upset stomach.

Many over-the-counter sleep medications have an *antihistamine* as a primary ingredient. Antihistamines block the release of histamine and thus cause drowsiness. However, tolerance to the sleepiness effect develops in just a few days (Schatzberg, Cole, & DeBattista, 2007).

Melatonin, a hormone secreted by the pineal gland at night, is involved in controlling the sleep-wake cycle. The body produces melatonin from the precursor tryptophan, which is found in foods such as meats, grains, fruits, and vegetables. Tryptophan is converted to serotonin and then to melatonin. The production of melatonin is controlled by the body's major internal clock, which is located in the suprachiasmatic nucleus of the hypothalamus and regulates the body's circadian rhythms. The internal clock is controlled by light. Based on the light information that it receives, the internal clock sends messages to the pineal gland that produces melatonin. Melatonin levels are highest at night, but bright light during normally dark times will block production of melatonin (Reite, 2009, p. 1245). Natural melatonin levels decline with age, and some older adults produce very little melatonin. It is estimated that 50% of older Americans have chronic sleep problems (Foley, Monjan, Brown, et al., 1995).

Synthetic melatonin, which is available as a food supplement, is sometimes used to treat sleep problems. It is used to reset the circadian cycle in those experiencing jet lag or doing shift work (Cardinali, Furio, Reyes, et al., 2006). It seems to be effective for individuals with delayed-sleep phase disorder (who do not feel sleepy until hours after their normal bedtime), but not for other types of insomnia. Synthetic melatonin has side effects that must be considered, including sleepiness, lower body temperature, stomach problems, headache, morning grogginess, and vivid dreams.

Ramelteon (Rozerem) is a melatonin receptor agonist that is used to treat sleep-onset insomnia. It mimics melatonin's sleep-promoting properties and shortens the time to sleep onset. Side effects include headache, sleepiness, fatigue, nausea, dizziness, diarrhea, and sometimes sleep driving, which is a condition similar to sleepwalking in which individuals may actually drive their cars and have serious auto accidents but not remember driving or the accident (Reite, 2009).

New medications under development for insomnia include the *orexin-modulating agents*. Orexin is a neuropeptide that acts on the sleep-wake cycle. Agents that act as orexin antagonists have been found to induce sleep, but they are not yet available for clinical use (Brisbare-Roch, Dingemanse, Koberstein, et al., 2007).

Herbal Supplements

Some individuals use herbal supplements for insomnia. Herbs that are proposed to alleviate insomnia include valerian, lavender, chamomile, and passionflower. Although some reports note that valerian is mildly sedating, other reports point out that valerian contains other substances and has several side effects. Lavender—in soaps, teas, and oils for massage—makes some individuals feel relaxed and may lead to a restful sleep. Chamomile, often used as a tea, has been reported to bring on drowsiness. Passionflower, either as tea or in a capsule, has been described as reducing anxiety and insomnia. All herbal supplements contain chemicals and have side effects or untoward effects. Like herbs, over-the-counter sleep medications and food supplements have many side effects, and the long-term effects of use are not known (Newall, Anderson, & Phillipson, 1996).

Hot Baths

The daily sleep-wake cycle is linked to daily body temperature. The initiation of nighttime sleep is normally preceded by a slight drop in body temperature. Taking a hot bath an hour or two before bedtime raises the core body temperature slightly and is thought to increase the normal nighttime drop of body temperature that triggers sleep induction. This artificially modified change in the body's core temperature may help some individuals to fall asleep (Epstein & Mardon, 2007).

Social Rhythms Therapy

Maintaining stable social rhythms includes establishing regular patterns of sleeping, eating, physical activity, social activities, emotional stimulation, and leisure activities (Kahn, Sachs, Printz, et al., 2000). Because studies have shown that keeping a record of their daily activities results in more stable daily routines, patients with disruptions of circadian rhythms are taught to track their mood, sleep, eating, activities, and interpersonal interactions daily (Frank, Swartz, & Kupfer, 2000).

Although social rhythms therapy has been studied most often among patients with bipolar disorder, it is now thought that it may be beneficial for other conditions in which disruption of circadian rhythms may be involved (Germain & Kupfer, 2008). Among patients with bipolar disorder, disruptions of sleep-wake cycles are more likely to trigger mania than depression (Malkoff-Schwartz, Frank, Anderson, et al., 1998), so establishing regular times for sleep and wakefulness is important. Patients with major depressive disorder also have alterations of circadian rhythms, and they have benefited from social rhythms therapy (Germain & Kupfer, 2008). Recent evidence suggests that alterations of circadian rhythms may contribute to the pathogenesis of metabolic syndrome and obesity and that social rhythms therapy may be helpful in augmenting treatment for these conditions (Maury, Ramsey, & Bass, 2010).

Socializing Interventions Designed to Reduce Social Isolation or Loneliness

Patients with severe mental illness tend to have much smaller social networks than people without mental illness (Cresswell, Kuipers, & Power, 1992). Their social networks begin to shrink around the time of the first psychotic episode and continue to deteriorate to the point of including only family members and mental health care providers. Having smaller social networks is associated with more frequent admissions to psychiatric hospitals and poorer outcomes (Bradshaw & Haddock, 1998). Interventions to help patients with severe mental illness increase their social network have included strategies to build new relationships, to improve the quality of existing relationships, and to provide patients with ready-made friends (Perese & Wolf, 2005). Some of these interventions include Compeer, Befriending, and Friendship Centers.

Compeer

Compeer is a nonprofit organization that matches trained community volunteers with children and adults receiving mental health treatment on a one-to-one basis. Compeer was started in 1973 in Rochester, New York. In 1982, the National Institute of Mental Health (NIMH) chose Compeer as a model program and funded the development of similar programs throughout the nation. Today, Compeer has over 100 affiliates in the United States, Canada, and Australia (National Compeer Website, 2003). Compeer recognizes that people with mental illness often experience loneliness, loss of self-esteem, fear, and failure. Compeer's philosophy is that these distressing feelings and experiences can be modified by the presence of a caring, supportive friend (National Compeer Website).

Compeer is regarded as an adjunct to therapy for which an individual with a mental illness is referred by a mental health professional. Mental health professionals provide initial consultation with the volunteer and are available for backup support. Volunteers receive 3 hours of training from a Compeer staff member before being assigned to an individual with a mental illness, and they provide mental health professionals with a copy of their monthly report. Volunteers commit to spending 1 hour a week with the patient in either face-to-face or telephone contact. Volunteers may provide socializing activities, rehabilitative social support, advocacy, educational and vocational mentoring, and access to community resources.

Outcomes

In a study evaluating the Compeer Model of providing volunteers who are trained to fill the role of friends, the individuals with severe mental illness receiving Compeer services had a greater increase in social support and sense of well-being and a greater reduction of psychiatric symptoms than individuals with severe mental illness who received community treatment as usual (McCorkle, Rogers, Dunn, et al., 2008).

Befriending

Cox (1993) has defined befriending as "an activity that aims to develop a relationship between individuals that is distinct from professional/client relationships" (p. 9). The relationship consists of the befriender, who is the volunteer friend, and the befriended, who is the individual receiving the friendship. While the original goal of befriending was to alleviate loneliness, the current expanded goals of befriending are to improve quality of life, reduce social isolation, help people meet emotional needs, promote and maintain mental health, and reduce the risk of developing mental illness (Andrews, Gavin, Begley, et al., 2003). Bradshaw and Haddock (1998) viewed befriending as a way of connecting people with severe mental illness with their communities, which is a primary goal of recovery (Davidson, Haglund, Stayner, et al., 2001).

Befriending aims to develop a relationship between individuals that incorporates the strengths of a day-to-day friendship. A befriending relationship is characterized by

- The befriender's commitment to the befriended individual
- The befriender's seeing the befriended individual as someone similar to him or her
- Mutual emotional attachment and self-disclosing
- The freely given friendship of the befriender

Because befrienders want to be friends, their involvement is highly valued by patients. That involvement has the power to change the befriendeds' view of themselves: they see themselves as worthy of another individual's interest (Cox, 1993). Befriending may be provided through a program or an organizational network. Befriending programs can be found in many countries, including Canada and the United States.

Befriending as a Programmatic Intervention

In response to research that revealed that programs that merely put lonely people together or offer structured activities—like discussion groups—did not reduce loneliness, a social service agency in the Netherlands developed a friendship program. The purpose of the friendship program is to help older women who are experiencing loneliness learn how to make friends. The program focuses on building skills such as listening, self-disclosure, expressing appreciation and empathy, and setting appropriate limits.

Participants experienced a decrease in loneliness and an increase in friendships (Stevens, 2001).

Befriending by an Organizational Network

An example of a larger organization of befriending is The Befriending Network, which is a charity based in London that was established in 1994. The original goals of the Befriending Network were (1) to provide help, support, and encouragement to people who were diagnosed with a terminal or life-threatening illness and (2) to improve their quality of life by offering the friendship of trained volunteers. The organization has since expanded to meet the needs of other groups of people, including those with mental illness and suicide ideation and those who are lonely and isolated or who have no close friends or nearby relatives (Befriending Network, UK, 2003).

People in need of befriending may contact a befriending network on their own, or their family, doctor, or nurse can refer them to the network. However, at some point, the individual's health care providers must be contacted and made aware of the befriending relationship (Befriending Network, UK, 2003). Befrienders are not meant to replace nurses or other medical staff; rather, they are viewed as augmenting treatment. Similar to Compeer, volunteers are matched with the individuals to be befriended on the basis of similar interests, if possible. Volunteers receive 4 days of training. Volunteers must offer a minimal 1-year commitment (in order to develop a trusting, deeper relationship) and spend at least 1 to 2 hours per week with the befriended individual. Shared activities include talking together, going out for coffee, sharing a meal at a restaurant, or shopping (Bradshaw & Haddock, 1998).

Although befriending is most often provided in face-to-face interactions in order to meet the needs of people in different situations, it may be offered in other ways, such as through Befriending Centers—which are drop-in centers that provide people to talk to, books, snacks, and resource information—and through telephone hotline services that enable callers to receive free help at home. For example, befriending by telephone was introduced into the Ukraine to compensate for lack of services and for the stigma experienced by individuals with mental illness that made them reluctant to seek help (Mokhovikov & Keir, 1999). Mokhovikov and Keir stated that the volunteer's emotional support and active listening decreases the befriended individual's sense of social isolation and brings about positive changes.

The Befriending Network of Scotland

The Befriending Network of Scotland's primary goal is to improve the mental health and well-being of individuals (Befriending Network, Scotland, 2002). The network trains volunteers to befriend individuals with mental illness who are isolated or lonely as a way of building their social networks. The aims of The Befriending Network of Scotland are to help people with mental illness to

- Take part in activities along with others in the community
- Develop positive friendships and relationships with people living in the local area
- Develop their skills
- Build self-confidence
- Gain respect as valued people living in the community

The activities that the volunteer and patient engage in include chatting and having a cup of tea, walking, cooking, reading the Bible, eating out, bowling, playing video games, shopping, and going to the movies.

Outcomes of Befriending

In a study of befriending of impoverished young mothers, many of whom were depressed and 40% of whom were single mothers, befriending was found to be effective in improving the young mothers' self-esteem, their control over their lives, and their interactions with their children (Cox, 1993). According to Andrews et al. (2003), befriended individuals appreciated the reliability of the befriender and valued the gift of the befriender's involvement and time. Bradshaw and Haddock's (1998) study of the effect of befriending for people with severe mental illness found that although only 44% said that there had been an increase in their social activities, all believed that they had benefited and that the primary benefit was having someone with whom to talk. The authors concluded that for people with severe mental illness who lived alone, befriending provided a link to the outside world.

In evaluating the outcomes of The Befriending Network of Scotland, slight improvement in overall social functioning was found among those receiving befriending. Approximately 44% reported an increase in social activity and 67% reported increased confidence in going out. About half reported increased energy. They valued having someone to talk to, having someone to support them as they increased their involvement in the community, and being helped to become aware of their own strengths (Bradshaw & Haddock, 1998).

Friendship Centers

Friendship Centers are social clubs for individuals recovering from mental illness. They provide an accepting, supportive environment where individuals can enjoy normal daily activities: they can talk with others about their problems; participate in music, arts, and crafts; exercise; play memory-stimulating games; celebrate holidays and birthdays; work on projects; and go on trips together.

Friendship Centers are sponsored by diverse organizations: Mental Health Associations, National Institute on Mental Illness, Veterans Administration, and mental health service providers such as Assertive Community Treatment programs. Psychosocial clubs can also serve as Friendship Centers. Friendship Centers can also be sponsored by community organizations and churches. An example of a Friendship Center that was developed by church congregations is described by Wheaton (1997). The churches provide social-recreation programs, and members of the congregations become one-on-one friends with the patients who are members of the Friendship Center. The Friendship

Center offers a place for the recovering individual to make friends, to develop relationships, and to receive peer support; friendship centers that are sponsored by churches also allow the recovering patient to have a friend who is not only a church member, but who also serves as an advocate and a community resource contact.

Outcomes

There is very little information about the outcomes of Friendship Centers.

Compensatory Psychosocial Interventions

Compensatory psychosocial interventions make up for patients' illness-related deficits in adapting to challenges or stressors, social functioning, and self-care management. Examples of compensatory interventions include building coping skills, increasing social support, and providing case management.

Coping Enhancement Programs

Coping involves the thoughts and behaviors that individuals use (1) when they believe that goals important to them have been threatened, harmed, or lost, or (2) when they encounter obstacles to attaining their goals; in other words, coping is how people respond to problems (Folkman & Moskowitz, 2004). Problems may arise from relationships with others, from actions of others that are hurtful or that keep patients from reaching their goal, or from events such as illnesses, losses, or traumas. Problems may also arise from individuals' unique attributes, such as fear, anxiety, or lack of self-esteem or self-confidence (Nezu, Nezu, & D'Zurilla, 2007). Effective coping is associated with gaining hope, optimism, greater self-esteem, improved self-confidence, better physical and mental health, and greater life satisfaction, all of which are the goals of psychiatric recovery (Nezu et al.). Unsuccessful coping often leads to health problems, impaired function, marital problems, depression, anxiety, substance use, and suicidal thoughts (Nezu et al.). Psychiatric advanced practice nurses can help patients to develop successful coping skills through the use of problem-solving therapy (PST), social skills training, stress management, and reminiscence therapy.

Problem-Solving Therapy (PST)

Problems are the obstacles between an individual's present situation and the goal that he or she wants to achieve. Solutions are attempts to overcome the obstacles so that the goal can be reached. If the obstacles cannot be changed, the solution is for the individual to learn to accept the problem or change his or her negative reaction to the problem. An effective solution is one that "(a) maximizes positive consequences, and (b) minimizes negative consequences" (Nezu et al., 2007, p. 5). Individuals who are effective problem-solvers see problems as challenges or opportunities, not as threats. In seeking a solution, they take time to gather information about the problem, to think carefully about it, to make plans, and to weigh the benefits and costs. These effective problem-solving skills can increase overall health and emotional well-being.

Effective problem-solving skills are the basis of PST, which was developed in the 1960s and 1970s as a way to increase social competence. *Social competence* is the ability to use a variety of pathways to reach goals, to use resources available within society (employment, schools, neighborhoods, social services, and health care) to facilitate movement toward goals, and to understand the world and how it works (Gladwin, 1967; Kopelowicz et al., 2006). Phillips and Zigler (1961) observed that patients with psychiatric disorders who had greater social competence before they were hospitalized did better after discharge than patients who did not have social competence before hospitalization. Thus, they concluded that increasing social competence through interventions such as PST should be included in treatment plans for patients with psychiatric disorders who are discharged from hospitals to the community.

PST is based on the theory that problem-solving moderates the effects of stress by reducing or eliminating the obstacles to goal attainment or by changing how the stressors are perceived (D'Zurilla & Nezu, 2009). Frequently occurring obstacles include not knowing what to do; seeing the problem as being very complicated; having conflicting goals; lacking skills to overcome the obstacles; lacking resources such as time, money, supplies, or services; uncertainty; and emotions such as fear of failure or rejection (Nezu et al., 2007).

Steps in Problem-Solving Therapy

Nezu et al. (2007) revealed that, ideally, an individual who is problem-solving must

1. Have a positive problem-solving attitude
2. Define the problem
3. Generate alternative solutions
4. Predict the consequences of the alternative solutions
5. Select one solution and try it

By completing each of these steps, the individual directs his or her energy toward finding a solution rather than dwelling on the problem.

Having a Positive Attitude

Problem-solving attitude can be positive or negative. Individuals with a positive problem-solving attitude see the problems as challenges; they believe that problems are a normal part of life and are solvable. People with positive problem-solving attitudes have confidence that they can be successful in solving the problem. They know that it may take time, but they choose to commit themselves to solving the problem rather than ignoring it. A positive problem-solving attitude is associated with higher levels of hope, optimism, and emotional health than a negative problem-solving attitude.

Individuals with a negative problem-solving attitude view the problem as a threat to their well-being. They believe that the problem is due to a defect in themselves, e.g., their incompetence. They doubt their ability to solve it, and they respond to problems with emotional distress, impulsive behaviors, or avoidance. They would prefer to have someone else solve the problem for them (D'Zurilla & Nezu, 1999). Negative problem-solving attitude is associated with high levels of depression, anxiety, anger, and hopelessness and low levels of self-esteem (Nezu et al., 2007).

Psychiatric advanced practice nurses can help patients to have a positive problem-solving attitude by teaching them that problems are a normal part of life and that how they think about a problem affects how they feel about the problem and their ability to solve it.

Defining the Problem

The first step in the process of defining the problem is to identify the desired goals. The next step is to clearly define the obstacles between the present state and the desired goals, that is, the problem itself. Lastly, information about the causes of the obstacles must be gathered. Questions to ask include the following: What keeps the obstacles in place? Is it lack of resources, knowledge, or self-confidence, or is it conflict over which goal to pursue? What is needed to overcome the obstacles? Are the benefits of achieving the goals greater than the cost/efforts that are required to achieve the goal? Defining the problem clearly and precisely is the first step toward finding a solution, a way to achieve the desired goals.

Generating Alternative Solutions

Individuals experience higher levels of hopelessness and helplessness when they can see only one solution to a problem than when they can see alternative solutions (Nezu et al., 2007). When they believe that they have several options or solutions to choose from, they feel safe, hopeful, and in control. Helping patients to generate a list of possible solutions to the problem increases hope and flexibility and reduces the tendency for impulsive actions.

One of the primary obstacles to generating alternative solutions to a problem is habit: what was used before feels right (D'Zurilla & Nezu, 1999). To overcome this obstacle, patients can be encouraged to think of many possible solutions (brainstorming approach) and then select relevant goal-oriented solutions, such as taking small steps to accomplish a task in comparison to approaching the task as an overwhelming demand. For example, when feeling overwhelmed by a stress-producing event or situation, patients can be encouraged to think of solutions that lead to reduction of stress, e.g., exercise, talking to a friend, reading, getting more information about the stressor, writing in a journal, identifying someone who is in a similar situation but handling it better and copying their behavior, and visualizing themselves as coping effectively and achieving their goals. These steps are likely to lead to the generation of more problem-solving solutions.

Predicting the Consequences of the Alternative Solutions

Each solution that appears to have potential for resolving the problem is evaluated (1) by thinking through the positive and negative consequences that are likely to follow if the solution is implemented and (2) by estimating the amount of time and effort required to implement each solution. The consequences should be evaluated in relation to the effect that they will have on the individual's physical and emotional well-being, relationships, finances, present and future employment, and social status. The choice of a solution is determined by its ability to solve the problem, the individual's capacity to carry out the solution, and the odds that the solution will maximize positive consequences and minimize negative consequences.

Trying a Solution

An individual must be motivated in order to try out a solution. Motivation is mobilized through knowledge of what will happen after the problem is resolved, immediate and long-term cost-benefit ratios, and the consequences if no action is taken.

Once the individual is motivated, he or she must plan how the solution will be carried out and obtain the resources or supplies that will be needed. After the solution is tried, the individual should evaluate the solution to determine if the problem was solved and if the effect was more positive than negative.

Outcomes of Problem-Solving Therapy

PST has been found to be an effective treatment for depression (Bell & D'Zurilla, 2009; Cuijpers, van Straten, & Warmerdam, 2007), and among older adults, PST has been found to be more effective than supportive therapy in reducing depressive symptoms and disability and in improving executive functioning (Alexopoulos, Raue, & Aredin, 2003). The action within PST that seems to be involved in improving depression, disabilities, and functioning is the increased ability of the patients to identify alternatives and to make decisions. In addition to depression, PST has been found to be beneficial for patients with other psychiatric disorders, for instance, with social phobia (DiGiuseppe, Simon, McGowan, et al., 1990), schizophrenia (Bradshaw, 1993), and suicidal ideation in adults and adolescents (Lerner & Clum, 1990). Among older adults, PST has been found to reduce symptoms of depression and anxiety (Kant, D'Zurilla, & Maydeu-Olivares, 1997). Other health problems that have been found to improve with effective problem-solving include stress, obesity, substance abuse, and suicidality (Nezu et al., 2007).

Social Skills Training

The purpose of social skills training is to improve patients' social competence by helping them learn how to manage problems with activities of daily living, leisure time activities, relationships, employment, and community integration

(Bustillo, Lauriello, Horan, et al., 2001; Horsfall, Cleary, Hunt, et al., 2009).

Social Competence

Social competence is made up of skills—which are learned ways to perform—that are acquired through life experiences (Bellack, Meuser, Gingerich, et al., 1998). The social skills that are the basis of social competence include social perception, social cognition, and behavioral response (Meier & Hope, 1998). *Social perception* is the ability to read others' moods and social cues, such as facial expressions, tone of voice, gestures, and posture. *Social cognition* is the process of analyzing the social situation, integrating previously acquired information or experiences, and planning an appropriate response. *Behavioral response* includes the ability to produce appropriate verbal responses; to use appropriate facial expressions, gestures, and body movements; and to respond in a social situation with appropriate actions. It is an individual's social competence that is involved in getting positive reinforcement, rewards, or good feelings in response to efforts made in social situations, such as interacting with partners, friends, or coworkers and participating in leisure or community activities. Low levels of social competence may result in lack of positive reinforcement and the experiencing of anxiety, frustration, and social isolation (Bellack et al.).

Many of the social skills that make up social competence are learned in early childhood, such as sharing, waiting one's turn, and saying "please" and "thank you." Other social skills—such as the skills involved in intimacy, marriage, getting and keeping a job, being a neighbor, and contributing to the community—are mastered when individuals meet the challenges of adolescence and early adulthood (Pratt & Mueser, 2002). Psychiatric disorders such as schizophrenia, major depressive disorder, bipolar disorder, anxiety disorders, and personality disorders that have an early onset may prevent individuals from mastering the skills needed for social competence; psychiatric symptoms may also prevent individuals from using the social skills that they have acquired (Kurtz & Mueser, 2008). Social skills training closes the gap between the patient's present skills and the skills that he or she needs to improve functioning.

Areas in which individuals with psychiatric disorders often need skills training include communication, assertiveness, friendship and dating, money management, getting a job and maintaining employment, coping with symptoms of mental illness, managing conflict or anger, safe sex practices, and living in the community (Bellack, Mueser, Gingerich, et al., 2004; Liberman, Wallace, Blackwell, et al., 1998).

Steps in Social Skills Training

Social skills training is based on principles of social learning theory (Bandura, 1969) and operant conditioning theory (Skinner, 1953). To teach social skills to an individual, the instructor must

1. Create motivation to learn a new behavioral skill by providing a reason for the change. For example, the instructor can explain to the patient that learning how to start a conversation is helpful in making friends.
2. Break down the social behavior into small elements and then teach the individual to perform each element. The material to be learned should be presented in brief units and repeated. Visual aids are useful, such as a video of someone approaching a stranger, introducing himself, shaking hands, exchanging a few words, and saying goodbye.
3. Combine the individual elements into one social behavior, and then model the new behavior for the patient to see. The patients practice the behaviors by role-playing; the instructors provide feedback to shape their behavior.

Social skills training programs for patients with psychiatric disorders often target specific skills within broad areas of functioning, such as self-care, money management, shopping, and preparing meals (Horsfall et al., 2009); because patients with psychiatric disorders often have cognitive impairment, social skills training programs minimize reliance on cognitive functioning and use direct strategies to teach new skills (Heinssen, Liberman, & Kopelowicz, 2000).

Outcomes

Social skills training has been found to improve patients' knowledge, behaviors, and skills (Nathan & Gorman, 1998). It has also been found to have a positive effect on self-confidence, self-efficacy, social or vocational role functioning, medication adherence, and reducing exposure to HIV (Bellack et al., 2004).

Recent outcome studies have shown that social skills training is associated with increased assertiveness and social interactions and with decreased symptoms of psychopathology and relapse (Kurtz & Mueser, 2008). Tsang (2001) found that social skills training was useful in helping individuals with severe mental illness to get a job and keep it. There is less evidence of patients' ability to transfer the skills learned in the office or clinic to the real-life environment of the community (Bellack et al., 2004); however, patients who receive skills training and additional support or help in using their new skills in their living situations have greater ability to transfer the skills learned (Lieberman et al., 1998; Tauber, Wallace, & LeComte. 2000).

Social skills training is most effective when used in conjunction with pharmacotherapy, case management, substance-abuse treatment for patients with dual diagnosis, and an appropriate housing environment (Bellack et al., 2004). Social skills training can provide the basic skills needed to develop competence (Kopelowicz et al., 2006).

Stress Management

The most common sources of stress are related to work; problems with people in the workplace; lifestyle; environment; life crises; and demanding living, academic, or work situations (Duhault, 2002). Each individual's unique response to these stressors is influenced by his or her brain's vulnerability to stress and by the presence of supportive or buffering factors.

Repeated or ongoing exposure to stress across the life span has been found to be associated with lasting adverse effects on the brain. Prenatal exposure to maternal stress, adverse events, or glucocorticoids is associated with lower birth weight; increased activity of the hypothalamic-pituitary-adrenal axis; abnormalities of development of the hippocampus, frontal cortex, and amygdala; and later, disturbances of neurological, cognitive, and behavioral functioning (Lupien, McEwen, Gunnar, et al., 2009). Exposure to stress during the preschool years is thought to be associated with abnormal functioning of the hypothalamic-pituitary-adrenal axis, alterations in frontal lobe functioning, and changes in the cortisol receptors (Lupien et al.). In adolescents, the effects of early exposure to stress are manifested in elevated levels of cortisol and reduced volume of the frontal cortex and anterior cingulate cortex. In older adults, stress has an adverse effect on brain structures (hippocampus, neurons, and dendrites) that are undergoing age-related changes. The long-term effects of early exposure to stress, which may have resulted in reorganization of synaptic connections, increase vulnerability for later development of psychiatric disorders, such as anxiety and depressive disorders (Lupien et al.). Synaptic connections can also be reorganized through the promotion of resilience—which is the ability to overcome an adverse situation and bounce back. In those who have been exposed to stressful situations, resilience may remediate the effect of stress on the brain and may also foster the development of new synaptic connections. Psychosocial interventions for reducing stress and increasing resilience include exercise or activity, relaxation, stress management education, use of leisure time, use of mood charts, and writing/journaling therapy.

Exercise

Exercise—such as using a stationary bicycle, walking, or jogging—has been found to reduce emotional distress and depressive symptoms (Barbour, Edenfield, & Blumenthal, 2007). Among patients with major depression, the benefit of exercise has been found to be similar to that of cognitive therapy (Lawlor & Hopker, 2001) and to that of pharmacotherapy with sertraline (Zoloft), which is a selective serotonin reuptake inhibiting antidepressant medication (Blumenthal, Babyak, Moore, et al., 1999). Among patients with bipolar disorder, exercise consisting of walking 30 minutes a day had a moderating effect on their response to stressful situations (Barbour et al.). Exercise has also been found to reduce symptoms of anxiety and panic (Strohle, Feller, Onken, et al., 2005).

Outcomes

Some studies of older adults have shown that exercise improves cognitive functioning—working memory, ability to plan, and ability to multitask (Colcombe & Kramer, 2003). Other studies have found that engaging in physical activity—long walks, participating in sports, and swimming—is associated with a lower rate of developing depression among older adults (Strawbridge, Deleger, Roberts, et al., 2002). In addition, some studies have found that exercise is associated with lower rates of developing dementia (Larson, Wang, Bowen, et al., 2006).

Leisure Time

A new approach to stress management is the use of leisure time for coping with stress (Iwasaki, Mactavish, & Mackay, 2005). It involves changing behavior—for instance, taking a time-out from the stress-causing situation—and creating a new or different situation in which the patient can experience a sense of rejuvenation and renewal. The effects of the leisure time-out approach include a rebalancing of life, increased ability to cope with stressors, and the acquisition of resilience.

Outcomes

There is no information about the outcomes of the use of leisure time as an intervention to reduce stress.

Mood Charts

Mood charts are a strategy for helping patients to understand how their mood fluctuates over the course of the day and over time. Mood charts can be expanded to include major stressors and daily hassles, medications, interpersonal conflicts, hours of sleep, and leisure-time activities. Information from the mood chart helps patients to gain insight into their illness and to identify both triggers and early warning signs (Torrey & Knable, 2002). Mood charts can be very complex, such as the *Life Chart Manual for Recurrent Affective Illness* (National Depressive and Manic-Depressive Association, www.ndmda.org) (Torrey & Knable), or they can be simple, as shown in Figure 8-1.

Outcomes

Mood charts have been found to help patients understand their illness, to help parents of children with mood disorders to identify triggers for changes in moods, and to help clinicians in treating the mood disorder (Torrey & Knable, 2002). It is generally accepted by patients and clinicians that mood charts are helpful as a nonmedication form of treatment for mood disorders (Torrey & Knable).

Writing/Journaling Therapy

Writing therapy involves building resilience to stress by managing negative emotions and finding a meaning to distressful situations or traumatic events through writing (Smyth, Hockemeyer, & Tulloch, 2008; Smyth, Stone, Hurewitz, et al., 1999). Writing therapy has some of the same components as cognitive behavioral therapy; for instance, they both use imaginal exposure and cognitive restructuring. In writing therapy, patients write detailed accounts of the traumatic event, including sensory experiences, painful facts related to the trauma, and emotions experienced. Then, they write to an imaginary close associate who experienced the same event with advice on how to deal with the event and its consequences. Finally, they write

Date	Mood rated from 1, very depressed, to 10, manic	Medications taken	Major stressors or daily hassles	Hours of sleep	Leisure time activities: sports, socializing, walking, etc.

FIGURE 8-1: Weekly Mood Chart. Mood charts are a strategy for helping patients to understand how their mood fluctuates over the course of the day and over time. Information from the mood chart helps patients to gain insight into their illness and to identify both triggers and early warning signs.

about the traumatic event, its impact, and their coping efforts as part of their life experiences (van Emmerik, Kamphuis, & Emmelkamp, 2008). Writing therapy has been linked to an increase of positive emotions and movement toward recovery (Smyth et al., 2008)

Outcomes

In a study that measured the outcome of structured writing therapy, it was found that patients with acute stress disorder and post-traumatic stress disorder had improvement of intrusive symptoms and symptoms of anxiety and depression (Bugg, Turpin, Mason, et al., 2008; van Emmerik et al., 2008).

Reminiscence Therapy

Reminiscence therapy has been defined by Dochterman & Bulechek (2004) as "using the recall of past events, feelings, and thoughts to facilitate pleasure, quality of life, or adaptation to present circumstances" (p. 602). More specifically, reminiscence therapy is a psychosocial intervention that is used to

- Provide a pleasant social experience
- Prevent or reduce depression
- Promote an individual's sense of self-identity and self-esteem
- Reduce social isolation
- Increase communication skills
- Help individuals adjust to the losses of life associated with aging
- Promote a sense of well-being (Harrand & Bollstetter, 2000; Miller, 2009)

The theoretical basis for reminiscence therapy is the theory of continuity (Parker, 1995), which proposes that individuals who experience changes in their lives try to make sense of the changes by recalling people, events, and experiences from their past. The process of recalling past changes or challenges and the knowledge, skills, and strategies they used to cope with the changes produces a sense of continuity in their lives and the ability to use familiar coping methods to adapt to present changes (Atchley, 1989).

In using reminiscence therapy, individuals are encouraged to talk about pleasant memories from an earlier time in their lives. Sometimes, photographs, music, or objects from the past are used to stimulate memories; in fact, reminiscence therapy that includes the use of objects and photographs has been found to be more effective in improving well-being than crafts, games, or socializing groups with no structured activity (Brooker & Duce, 2000; Woods, Bruce, Edwards, et al., 2009). As they recall positive experiences from the past, older adults are able to use familiar knowledge, skills, and strategies to adapt to the stressors of aging: that is, engaging in reminiscence facilitates their adaptation (Parker, 1995). In addition, when memories are shared with others, they provide evidence of past successful coping and establish the individual's identity as a competent individual (Perese, Rohloff, & Ryan, 2008; Watt & Cappeliez, 2000).

Outcomes

Reminiscence therapy can be done with groups of patients or with individual patients. Outcome studies are limited to group reminiscence therapy. Group reminiscence therapy has been found to reduce social isolation; to improve cognitive functioning and depression; and to increase self-esteem, sense of self-worth, social skills, and life satisfaction (Chao, Liu, Wu, et al., 2006; Lin, Dai, & Hwang, 2003). Group reminiscence therapy appears to be most effective when provided for six to twelve sessions of 30 to 45 minutes (Ashton, 1990; Hamilton, 1992); group therapy is also more effective when the group members have similar interests (Jones, 2003).

Based on a review of the literature, Jones (2003) said that reminiscence therapy appears to be effective "in preventing or reducing depression, increasing life satisfaction, improving self-care, improving self-esteem and helping older adults deal with crises, losses and life transitions" (p. 27). Reminiscence therapy has been used in many settings—such as in adult day-care centers, senior centers, and long-term care facilities—and has been observed to benefit older adults by improving their mood, coping abilities, and functioning (Cook, 1998; Youssef, 1990). Older adults who participate in reminiscence therapy have been found to be more optimistic about the future (Miller, 2009). In studies that compared group reminiscence therapy to other group interventions—such as talking about current problems, friendly visit groups, or structured life review—no difference in outcomes was found between reminiscence therapy and the other interventions; reminiscence therapy was found to be equally effective (Burnside, 1990; Hewett, 1989).

Social Support

Although "social support" and "social networks" are often used interchangeably, the term *social networks* refers to all the people with whom an individual has ongoing relationships, and the term *social support* refers to supportive exchanges that take place in social network relationships. Hawkins and Abrams (2007) defined supportive exchanges as "emotional encouragement, advice, information, guidance, and concrete aid, etc" (p. 2032).

Fingeld-Connett (2005) described social support as having two types: emotional and instrumental. Emotional support can include comforting gestures, such as listening, that are designed to reduce anxiety or stress; praying for the distressed individual; being physically present, if desired; normalizing the situation by focusing on other things; or engaging the individual in enjoyable activities. Instrumental support includes providing goods, supplies, money, childcare, or services such as transportation and housekeeping.

Social support and a social support network are associated with health and recovery and have been found to have a beneficial effect on mental health (Fingeld-Connett, 2005). For example, among patients with psychiatric disorders, higher levels of interactions with social networks and increased levels of social support have been found to be associated with reduced use of psychiatric services (Maulik, Eaton, & Bradshaw, 2009). For patients with deficits in social support or small support networks, ready-made social support interventions—such as support groups, self-help groups, and mutual help groups—have been found to compensate for lack of support.

Individuals with severe mental illness often have difficulty in making and keeping friends (Steinwachs, Kasper, & Skinner, 1992), and many have very small social networks that often are limited to family, mental health care providers, and others with mental illnesses (Angell, 2003). Among individuals with severe mental illness, the most frequently identified unmet need is for a friend (Perese, 1997). More than half of individuals with severe mental illness identify problems with social isolation and loneliness (Beebe, 2010; Clinton, Lunney, Edwards, et al., 1998).

Social isolation—a situation in which the number of relationships or closeness of relationships is less than desired—is often experienced as loneliness (Lauder, Sharkey, & Mummery, 2004). However, loneliness is a taboo subject. People are embarrassed or ashamed to say that they are lonely or that they have no friends (Killeen, 1997). Loneliness has a negative effect on self-esteem, depression, anxiety, self-evaluation, and physical health (Killeen; Lauder et al.). In addition to their direct effects on mental and physical health, functioning, and well-being, social isolation and loneliness are barriers to recovery (Deegan, 1990).

Causes of loneliness are most often situational, such as loss or disruption of relationships and friendships, but they may also be due to poverty, inadequate transportation, undesirable housing, and lack of opportunities for social interactions (Killeen, 1997). Individuals with severe mental illness are often unmarried and unemployed. They frequently live in housing situations that may not promote the development of friendships (Padgett, Henwood, & Abrams, 2008). They lack the financial resources needed to pursue recreational activities, and they do not know how to connect socially.

Most friendships are developed where an individual lives or through school, work, religious institutions, hobbies, sports, or recreation. It is common interests that usually attract people to each other (Cope: The Family Guide, 1999). Individuals with severe mental illness often must learn the basics of friendship building: how to ask people their names, how to introduce themselves, how to be friendly without being intrusive, and how to carry on a conversation; they also need an opportunity to practice these skills in a safe setting, such as in support groups, self-help groups, and mutual-help groups.

Support Groups

Support groups are often used by people in stressful circumstances or by people who lack contact with others. Support groups bridge the models of self-help groups and therapy groups. In comparison to therapy groups, which focus on specific problems or symptoms, and self-help groups, which stress empowerment (see next section on Self-Help groups), support groups strengthen "the central core" of individuals who consider themselves marginal or stigmatized (Rosenberg, 1984, p. 180). The goals of support groups are to increase members' coping ability in the face of stress, to give advice and feedback, to share information, and to build interpersonal skills (Rosenberg). Support groups use professional leaders to guide the group process, but like self-help groups, they expect that members will self-disclose, heal each other, and develop a sense of belonging. Support groups for patients with severe mental illness should be flexible and must feel safe (Stone, 1996).

Outcomes

There are several early, descriptive studies of supportive therapy groups with goals similar to those of support groups. Outcomes were described as expanding social networks, developing caring relationships with group members, providing advice with problems (Ely, 1985), and improving quality of life (Profita, Carrey, & Klein, 1989). More recently, in a study of psychosocial club members with severe mental illness, it was found that participation in a support group was associated with participants' increased ability to talk about the daily hassles and stressful events in their lives and an increased perception of having friends. Seventy-five percent of the participants rated the support group as helpful or very helpful (Getty, Perese, & Wooldridge, unpublished).

Self-Help Groups

Self-help is now a recognized service in the mental health care system (Hodges & Segal, 2002). According to Brown, Shepherd, Wituk, et al. (2008), "Mental health self-help refers to any mutual support oriented initiative directed by people with mental illness or their family members" (p. 105). Many individuals with psychiatric disorders participate in self-help groups because self-help groups provide a safe setting where they can gather, cultivate friendships, give mutual support, and develop a feeling of empowerment. Self-help participants make the decision to attend or not; there is no requirement that they attend (Swarbrick, 2007).

Self-help is characterized by the reliance on peers rather than professionals for help (Hardiman & Segal, 2003). Self-help groups are consumer-run, and their theoretical foundation is the belief that people who are empowered—i.e., those who have access to information, are able to make decisions, and have options—are better able to thrive and recover (Chamberlin, 1997). Group members support each other in meeting daily challenges, and they exchange information and expertise. Self-help groups use an approach based on individuals' strengths rather than on their disabilities. They promote empowerment, control over one's life situation, and independent social functioning, such as friendships and supportive relationships (Hardiman & Segal; Hodges & Segal, 2002).

In contrast to mental health care settings, where goals for patients often include increasing treatment adherence and independent living skills, self-help group settings allow participants to identify concrete goals that are important to them, such as having a better place to live or having more income (Hodges & Segal, 2002). Hodges and Segal suggested that these concrete goals are the precursors to more distal goals of successful community functioning.

There are many different types of programs under the umbrella of self-help: mutual-help groups, mutual support groups, self-help organizations, consumer-run organizations, consumer/survivor initiatives, consumer drop-in centers, self-help agencies, and peer-run organizations (Brown et al., 2008). They vary by organizational structure, with mutual support groups having less formal structure and consumer-run services having a more formal structure. Some of the self-help groups for individuals with psychiatric disorders are called "consumer-operated self-help centers" (Swarbrick, 2007), and some are called "psychosocial clubs." Both groups emphasize providing a place where individuals with psychiatric disorders can be with peers and get help from each other. They promote wellness, advocacy, and recovery (Swarbrick, Schmidt, & Pratt, 2009). Activities include providing recreational and educational opportunities, drop-in-centers, and support groups; arranging field trips; providing information and advocacy for participants; and volunteering in the community (Brown, 2009). Some self-help groups offer services such as counseling, housing, and work opportunities.

Consumer-Operated Self-Help Center

Consumer-operated services were developed in response to the mental health consumer movement that was based on consumers' belief that they had limited choices of services and limited participation in the mental health care system (Swarbrick, 2007). One model of a consumer-operated self-help center is the Consumer-Operated Self-Help Center program, developed by the New Jersey Department of Human Services, that shifts treatment from institutional settings to community settings. Consumer-operated self-help centers have been implemented in every county in the state of New Jersey (Swarbrick). Management of the program is shared by participants, and the centers are open weekends, evenings, and holidays. In an evaluation of the program, it was found that the participants ranged in age from 18 to 75, that more than half were single and never married, and that 25% had not completed high school. The most frequently occurring diagnosis was schizophrenia. Patients' satisfaction with the program was related to feeling connected to peers, to relationships at the center being positive and helpful, and to an environment that was orderly and predictable (Swarbrick et al., 2009).

Outcomes

Participation in consumer-operated services has been found to be associated with an increase in the factors involved in empowerment—a sense of self-esteem, self efficacy, power, autonomy, and optimism about the future—and with factors associated with recovery, such as "personal confidence and hope, willingness to ask for help, being goal and success oriented, reliance on others, and not being dominated by symptoms" (Corrigan, 2006, p. 1493). In a study of 194 mutual-help-group participants who were asked what personal change they noticed after participating, 20% reported an increase in self-esteem and self-confidence; 19% reported an increase in social skills such as talking and listening; 14% reported being better able to get along with people; and 11% reported better coping and problem-solving skills and less stress (Brown, 2009). In a review of empirical studies of outcomes of participation in mutual-help groups, Pistrang, Barker, and Humphreys (2008) found that mutual-help groups were beneficial for participants with chronic mental illness, depression, anxiety, and bereavement.

Psychosocial Clubs

Psychosocial clubs are modeled on the first psychosocial club, Fountain House, which is a self-help group founded by former psychiatric patients and social work volunteers (Beard, Propst, & Malamud, 1982; Sweet, 1999). Psychosocial clubs are based on a philosophy of empowerment, and their goal is to improve the lives of people with mental illness so that they can reach their potential and be coworkers, neighbors, and friends in their communities ("Gold Award", 1999). Early psychosocial clubs provided social support and a safe haven for patients with severe mental illness who, after long hospitalizations, were discharged to live in the community. The goal of psychosocial clubs was to provide an opportunity for members to interact socially (Macias & Rodican, 1997). Later, psychosocial clubs focused on providing vocational, educational, social, and recreational programs. Currently, there is interest in psychosocial clubs as cost-effective rehabilitative interventions for individuals with severe mental illness (Plotnick & Salzer, 2008).

In a study of psychosocial club members, it was found that there were more male members, that more than half (55.9%) were young adults 39 years of age or younger, that 80% were not married, and that most (79.4%) had completed high school. In spite of relatively high levels of educational preparation, no club members were competitively employed. They identified their greatest unmet needs as needs for self-identity, a role in life, and a friend (Perese, Getty, & Wooldridge, 2003). As previously noted by Ireland and Morgan (1997), Macias and Robican (1997), and Stone (1991), psychosocial clubs do not directly address the impaired ability of individuals with severe mental illness to make and keep friends. Outcome studies of psychosocial clubs have demonstrated benefits of club membership as being primarily a decrease in hospital readmissions and an increase in employment (Barton, 1999; Ireland & Morgan, 1997).

Self-help groups for individuals with mental illness include Recovery International (formerly Recovery, Inc.) (McFadden, Seidman, & Rappaport, 1992), Emotions Anonymous (Kurtz & Chambon, 1987), Schizophrenics Anonymous (Snowdon, 1980), and the National Alliance on Mental Illness (NAMI) (Howe & Howe, 1987). Recovery International is known as one of the first self-help groups for individuals with mental illness, and NAMI is a group that helps both mentally ill individuals and their families.

Recovery International

Recovery International was founded as Recovery, Inc., in 1937 by a psychiatrist, Dr. Abraham Low, and now has 800 groups worldwide (McFadden et al., 1992). It is now often known as "Recovery." The focus of Recovery is helping people with affective problems, such as depression or anxiety, to change from using negative or fearful thinking to self-supportive thinking and health-promoting behaviors (Murray, 1996). The meetings are structured around readings from Dr. Low's book, *Mental Health Through Will Training* (Low, 1971), which focus on problem behaviors. In Recovery meetings, a leader moderates discussions about the specific problems that members want to address; the leader also suggests a range of coping techniques.

National Alliance on Mental Illness

NAMI is an example of a self-help group for mentally ill people and their families (Howe & Howe, 1987). It was started in 1979 to help families by offering education, informational resources, social support, and advocacy activities. Families who join NAMI tend to have smaller social networks and higher functioning mentally ill relatives than those who do not choose to join (Mannion, Meisel, & Draine, et al., 1996). Those who participated report an improvement in their relationships with their mentally ill family members (Heller, Roccoforte, Hsieh, et al., 1997).

Outcomes

Early measured outcomes of self-help interventions for people with severe mental illness included reduction of severity of symptoms (Overall & Gorham, 1962), reduction of hospital readmissions, and shorter hospitalizations (Bond & Resnick, 2000). Later, emphasis shifted from measuring the reduction of severity of symptoms to measuring improvement of social relationships and employment (Carpenter & Strauss, 1991). Now, with the acceptance of recovery as the goal for individuals with psychiatric disorders, there is a need to identify outcomes that reflect both the process of recovery and recovery as an outcome (Hasson-Ohayon et al., 2006).

For example, Hodges and Segal (2002) studied how goals are advanced in self-help groups. They found that 91% of the participants in a self-help group were able to identify goals important to them, e.g., improvement of health, better job/income, a better place to live, and education/training. After 6 months, 19% of the participants had accomplished their most important goal and 55% were still interested in pursuing their goal. The researchers believed that obstacles such as a high rate of homelessness (46%), low levels of academic achievement and social support, limited finances, and severity of psychiatric disorders had a strong negative influence on goal attainment. Interestingly, among participants who were in a self-help group that emphasizes peer support and help, 64% responded that the best help comes from professional psychiatric care providers rather than from a peer, and 49% believed that a psychiatrist should be responsible for treatment decisions (Hodges & Segal, 2002). In a study of 255 participants in self-help agencies, there was an increase in empowerment that was measured as control over certain life domains such as housing, income, homelessness, and personal danger. However, there was no improvement in independent social functioning—social contacts in the community, use of community resources, contact with family and friends—and no change in involvement in academic or work activities (Hodges & Segal). Overall, evidence about the effectiveness of self-help groups or consumer-provided help is not consistent, and Solomon and Draine (2001) suggested that although they seem to be beneficial, no conclusions can be drawn at this time.

Mutual-Help Groups

Mutual-help groups are generally less structured than consumer-run organizations (Brown, 2009). In mutual-help groups, people voluntarily come together to help each other by sharing common problems or experiences (Davidson, Chinman, Kloos, et al., 1999). The goal of mutual-help groups is recovery: helping individuals to heal and to overcome their problems (Corrigan, Slopen, Gracia, et al., 2005). This process may increase the individual's understanding of his or her situation and decrease social isolation.

Mutual-help groups create social roles for the participants—such as team leaders, coordinators of activities, and representatives to policy-making organizations—so that the members have opportunities to gain a role identity as they help each other (Davidson et al., 1999). Mutual-support groups often include structured procedures and routines for addressing problems. They emphasize learning new information, developing new coping strategies, and using problem-solving techniques. They provide both emotional and instrumental support. One example of a mutual-help group is GROW (McFadden et al., 1992).

GROW

Recovering mental-hospital patients founded GROW in Australia in 1957, and there are now 500 GROW groups worldwide. One of GROW's beliefs is that members should strive to be all that they can be. The group encourages members to use their own experiences to help others and emphasizes the importance of friendship among members. GROW uses a pamphlet of short statements and phrases that are designed to help people with mental illness deal with daily life stressors and take steps toward recovery (McFadden et al., 1992). Members have identified self-reliance, industriousness, and self-esteem as key ingredients of recovery. They believed that GROW helped them in recovery through the program's philosophy, spirituality in the group, and sense of community and through the promotion of hope and power, self-acceptance, and healthy decision making (Corrigan et al., 2005).

Outcomes

There are very few studies of the outcomes of mutual-help groups. What information is available suggests that group participants have reduced psychiatric symptoms, hospitalizations, and social isolation (Galanter, 1988); improved self-concept and well-being (Carpinello, Knight, & Jatulis, 1992); and larger support networks (Carpinello, Knight, & Janis, 1991).

Care Management Programs: Case Management and Assertive Community Treatment

Case management includes the assessment, coordination, and provision of different components of care for an individual with severe mental illness (Mueser et al., 2001). People with a severe mental illness such as schizophrenia often have residual disabilities that hinder their accessing and using the community services that they need. Case managers are the mental health care providers who help in securing services and in managing the patients' use of these services, either individually through intensive case management or through the team approach of Assertive Community Treatment (ACT) (Bustillo et al., 2001).

Intensive Case Management

In intensive case management, the emphasis is on continuous, anticipatory patient-centered care rather than reactive, crisis-oriented care. Intensive case management has a wellness and recovery orientation and includes patient education, teaching self-management skills, and setting goals that are relevant for the patient. In intensive case management, provider decision making is supported by expert guidance, e.g., with practice guidelines. Information passes between the provider and patient, and care is reorganized both to support an effective partnership between clinicians and patients and to improve outcomes that are relevant to patients (Bodenheimer, Lorig, Holman, et al., 2002). Interventions include patient education about early warning signs and appropriate coping responses; scheduled care, such as regularly scheduled appointments; demand-responsive services, such as those requested by the patients related to issues in their lives that cannot wait for the next scheduled appointment; and outreach as a follow-up for missed appointments and to monitor response to recommendations from other providers.

Outcomes

Intensive case management has been found to be associated with reduction of hospitalizations, improved housing stability, reduced time in jail, and reduction of symptoms (Muesser, Bond, Drake, et al., 1998; Preston & Fazio, 2000).

Assertive Community Treatment (ACT)

ACT was developed in response to the needs of patients with severe mental illness who were (1) noncompliant with treatment and (2) high users of psychiatric services, such as inpatient hospitalization and emergency department treatment. In contrast to mental health programs that refer patients to other agencies for housing, food, clothing, case management, health care, and care for comorbid substance-related disorders, ACT provides comprehensive services, which includes facilitating access to the supplies, services, and resources that patients need for living and functioning in the community (Stein & Test, 1980). ACT is characterized by shared caseloads among clinicians; direct provision of services (health care, housing, and financial management); 24-hour coverage 7 days a week, including emergencies; close management of illnesses; provision of services in the community; assistance with problems of daily living; frequent contact; and outreach to maintain continuity of care.

Outcomes

ACT programs have been found to improve patients' psychiatric symptoms and substance abuse; increase adherence to medications; and decrease hospitalizations, homelessness, and incarcerations (Bond, Drake, Mueser, et al., 2001; Mueser et al., 2001). The ACT approach is effective in reducing hospitalizations and improving housing stability (Nelson, Aubry, & Lafrance, 2007; Stein, Barry, Van Dien, et al., 1999), but it is less effective in improving social connectedness, employment, and victimization (Mueser, Bond, Drake, et al., 1998; Perese, Wu, & Ram, 2005; Perese & Wu, 2010).

Remedial Psychosocial Interventions

Remedial psychosocial interventions are designed to correct faulty perceptions and cognitions, repair deficits in the processes of cognitive functioning, and build/rebuild skills. They include cognitive restructuring, cognitive adaptation training (CAT), cognitive remediation, and vocational rehabilitation, such as supported employment.

Modification of Cognitive Responses

Cognitive responses can be restructured, adapted, or remediated.

Cognitive Restructuring

Cognitive restructuring is a process by which patients' unrealistic views of themselves, of others, and of the world are challenged in order to replace those inaccurate views with more realistic views (Dochterman & Bulechek, 2004). Cognitive restructuring is used to help patients (1) to change negative thinking about themselves, (2) to overcome the fear of negative evaluation by others, and (3) to decrease their tendency to think that good outcomes happen by chance and that poor outcomes are due to their inadequacies.

The process of cognitive restructuring includes identifying negative thoughts, testing them for accuracy, and reframing them in a positive light. Cognitive restructuring helps patients learn that unhealthy thinking produces negative thoughts that can result in behavior problems, disturbances of interpersonal relationships, and maladaptive coping. They are taught how to change their thinking with the expectation that changes in thinking will result in reduced stress and improved health and functioning (Hollander & Simeon, 2008).

Outcomes

Cognitive restructuring has been found to be effective in preventing post-traumatic stress disorder among patients with acute stress disorder; however, it is less effective than therapies that use prolonged exposure to the stressor with prevention of response (Bryant, Mastrodomenico, Felmingham, et al., 2008). (See Chapter 11 for more information on acute stress disorder and post-traumatic stress disorder and exposure therapies.)

Cognitive Adaptation Training (CAT)

CAT is a psychosocial intervention that uses strategies designed to compensate for cognitive impairments and for impaired cognitive functioning (Velligan, Mueller, Wang, et al., 2006). The strategies are designed for each individual patient and are based on three observations:

1. An assessment of the patient's cognitive functioning, e.g., his or her executive functioning, problem-solving skills, ability to pay attention to a task over time, memory, learning, judgment, and ability to organize information.
2. Observation of the patient's self-care functioning, such as grooming, shopping, caring for belongings, and avoiding hazards.
3. Observation of the patient's performance of daily activities in the home.

Specific CAT strategies include step-by-step structuring of activities; prompting and cueing; checklists, signs, or pictures of the steps required to complete each activity; daily calendars and medication boxes; reminder notes for hygiene; anticipatory activities, such as placing a complete outfit together in one box with the day to wear it written in big letters; and lists of things to do in leisure time.

Outcomes

Patients with schizophrenia receiving CAT had fewer symptoms, better community functioning, more motivation, and fewer rehospitalizations than patients receiving standard care (Velligan, Bow-Thomas, Huntzinger, et al., 2000).

Cognitive Remediation

Cognitive impairment is a frequent symptom among individuals with schizophrenia, and the impairments of attention, memory, and abstract thinking interfere with their functioning and movement toward recovery. Cognitive remediation, which is a new approach to correcting malfunctioning cognitive processes and to building new ones, is being used to improve the cognitive deficits of individuals with schizophrenia (McGurk, Twamley, Sitzer, et al., 2007). The goal of cognitive remediative interventions is to improve cognitive processes, not to compensate for cognitive deficits. Cognitive remediation involves the use of training approaches that target specific cognitive skills, such as learning, attention, memory, planning, organization, and abstract thinking. Interventions include written tests, group activities, and computerized exercises.

Outcomes

Studies have found that cognitive remediation in individuals with schizophrenia has resulted in improvement of cognitive processes (Hodge, Siciliano, Withey, et al., 2010; Kurzban, Davis, & Brekke, 2010). Cognitive improvement of memory has been found to be associated with improvement of social functioning (Wykes, Reeder, Landau, et al., 2009). Younger patients—those 40 years of age or younger—achieved greater overall improvement of cognitive functioning than older patients, defined as those patients who were over 40 years of age (Wykes et al.).

Vocational Rehabilitation: Supported Employment

Although many patients with severe mental illness would like to be employed, the rate of competitive employment for this population is very low (Anthony & Blanch, 1987). Competitive employment, or holding a regular community job, is achieved by less than 20% of individuals with severe mental illness; the rate is even lower among individuals with schizophrenia (Lehman, 1995). Among the different programs designed to improve competitive employment, supported employment is more effective than the traditional vocational-rehabilitation approaches (Drake, McHugo, Becker, et al., 1996; Drake, McHugo, Bebout, et al., 1999).

Traditionally, patients received extensive skills training or work experience in sheltered workshops before they were placed in competitive work situations. Evaluation of this approach has shown that it is ineffective, with very low rates of eventual placement in competitive employment. Under the supported employment approach, patients are placed in a competitive job and then receive training and ongoing support; this method is also referred to as the "place, then train" model of supported employment (Addington et al., 2010, p. 262). This model follows six principles:

1. Participation is based on the patient's choice.
2. Supported employment is part of the overall treatment plan.
3. Competitive employment is the end goal.
4. Search for a job based on the patient's interest starts as soon as the patient indicates an interest in employment.
5. Support for the patient is continuous.
6. Preferences of the patient are essential.

One model of supported employment is the clubhouse model, in which members—psychiatric patients—provide support for each other and work together in the community. Other models of supported employment are ACT programs that help patients to achieve their goal of employment using a model called choose-get-keep. In the choose-get-keep model, patients identify the work and career areas that are of interest to them; then, they are helped to get and keep the job (Danley & Anthony, 1987).

Outcomes

Studies of supported employment have shown that it improves employment outcomes of patients with severe mental illness (Addington et al., 2010). For example, patients receiving supported employment treatment had higher rates of competitive employment (58%) than patients receiving usual services (19%). Patients receiving supported employment treatment also worked more hours and received higher wages (Bond, Drake, Mueser, et al., 1997).

Outcomes of Psychosocial Interventions

Because recovery is the desired outcome of psychosocial interventions and because it is unique to each individual with mental illness, Hasson-Ohayon et al. (2006) believed that measurement of outcomes of psychosocial interventions should reflect the individual's evaluation of the effectiveness of an intervention in moving them toward recovery. They developed a 16-item interview that asks questions such as "What change, if any, took place during participation in the intervention?" and "Did you benefit from the intervention?" (p. 266). In a study of 64 individuals receiving psychosocial interventions, the researchers found that the participants identified outcomes of the interventions as follows:

- Increased sense of mastery over their body despite their illnesses
- Improvement of emotional status
- Increase in leisure activities
- Greater social involvement, e.g., learning how to give and receive help from a peer
- Learning how to be a friend

Key Points

- Psychosocial interventions are a key component of comprehensive psychiatric care.
- Psychosocial interventions are nonpharmacological interventions.
- Psychosocial interventions can be preventive, supplemental, compensatory, or remedial.
- Psychosocial interventions decrease symptom severity; relieve symptoms of distress, such as loneliness, anxiety, and depression; reduce the need for hospitalizations; and improve psychosocial functioning and quality of life.
- Psychosocial interventions have the potential to reduce the effects of stress on the brain and body, to protect

the brain and improve brain functioning, and to promote resilience.

- Evidence-based psychosocial interventions have the potential to move patients toward recovery.

Resources

Toolkits

Psychosocial intervention toolkits that contain guidelines for the application of the evidence-based treatments, workbooks, training materials, and procedures have been developed (Drake, Goldman, Leff, et al., 2001). Toolkits such as Illness Management and Recovery, Family Psychoeducation, Supported Employment, and Co-occurring Disorders are available from the Substance Abuse and Mental Health Services Administration on their Web site: http://mentalhealth.samhsa.gov/cmhs/communitysupport/toolkits/.

Organizations

Recovery International
www.lowselfhelpsystems.org/
National Alliance on Mental Illness
http://www.nami.org
Compeer, Inc.
259 Monroe Avenue
Rochester, NY 14607
1-800-836-0475
Befriending
www.befrienders.org/
Assertive Community Treatment
www.actassociation.org/
Parish Nursing, International Parish Nurse Resource Center
214-918-2527
www.parishnurses.org
The National Center for School Crisis and Bereavement
1-513-803-2222
The Family Resource Center
140 Old Orangeburg Road
Orangeburg, NY 10962

Books

Resources also include books by and about individuals with serious mental illness; videotapes; reference guides; and staff who are willing to assist family members.

Medalia, A., Revheim, N., & Herlands, T. (2002). *Remediation of cognitive deficits in psychiatric patients: A clinician's manual.* New York: Montefiore Medical Center.

Adamec, C. (1996). *How to live with a mentally ill person: A handbook of day-to-day strategies.* New York: John Wiley & Sons.

References

Addington, J., McCleery, A., & Addington, D. (2005). Three-year outcome of family work in an early psychosis program. *Schizophrenia Research, 79,* 107-116.

Addington, J., Piskulic, D., & Marshall, C. (2010). Psychosocial treatments for schizophrenia. *Current Directions in Psychological Science, 19,* 260-263.

Ahern, L., & Fisher, D. (2001). Recovery at your own pace: Personal Assistance in Community Existence. *Journal of Psychosocial Nursing and Mental Health Services, 39*(4), 22-32.

Alexopoulos, G. S., Raue, P., & Aredin, P. (2003). Problem-solving therapy versus supportive therapy in geriatric major depression with executive dysfunction. *American Journal of Geriatric Psychiatry, 11*(1), 46-52.

American Nursing Association. (1998). *Scope and standards of parish nursing practice.* Washington, DC: American Nurses Association.

Anderson, C. M. (2004). The delivery of health care in faith-based organizations: Parish nurses and promoters of health. *Health Communication, 16*(1), 117-128.

Andrews, G. J., Gavin, N., Begley, S., & Brodie, D. (2003). Assisting friendships, combating loneliness: Users' views on a "befriending" scheme. *Ageing & Society, 23*(3), 349-362.

Angell, B. (2003). Contexts of social relationship development among assertive community treatment clients. *Mental Health Services Research, 5*(1), 13-25.

Anthony, W. A., & Blanch, A. (1987). Supported employment for persons who are psychiatrically disabled: An historical and conceptual perspective. *Psychosocial Rehabilitation Journal, 11,* 5-23.

Ashton, D. (1990). Therapeutic use of reminiscence with the elderly. *British Journal of Nursing, 2,* 1993-1997.

Atchley, R. (1989). A continuity theory of normal aging. *Gerontologist, 29*(2), 183-190.

Bandura, A. (1969). *Principles of behavior modification.* New York: Holt, Rinehart and Winston.

Barbour, K. A., Edenfield, T. M., & Blumenthal, J. A. (2007). Exercise as a treatment for depression and other psychiatric disorders: A review. *Journal of Cardiopulmonary Rehabilitation and Prevention, 27,* 359-367.

Barton, R. (1999). Psychosocial rehabilitation services in Community Support Systems: A review of outcomes and policy recommendations. *Psychiatric Services, 50*(4), 525-534.

Beard, J., Propst, R., & Malamud, T. (1982). The Fountain House: Model of psychiatric rehabilitation. *Psychosocial Rehabilitation Journal, 5*(1), 47-53.

Beebe, L. H. (2007). Beyond the prescription pad. *Journal of Psychosocial Nursing, 45*(3), 35-43.

Beebe, L. H. (2010). What community living problems do persons with schizophrenia report during periods of stability. *Perspective in Psychiatric Care, 46*(1), 48-55.

Befriending Network, Scotland. (2002). Retrieved from www.befriending.co.uk

Befriending Network, UK. (2003). Retrieved from www.befriending.net

Bell, A. C., & D'Zurilla, T. J. (2009). Problem-solving therapy for depression: A meta-analysis. *Clinical Psychology Review, 29,* 348-353.

Bellack, A. S., Meuser, K. T., Gingerich, S., et al. (1998). *Social skills training for schizophrenia: A step-by-step guide.* New York: Guilford Press.

Bellack, A. S., Mueser, K. T., Gingerich, S., et al. (2004). *Social skills training for schizophrenia: A step by step guide* (2nd ed.). New York: Guilford Press.

Biddix, V., & Brown, H. (1999). Establishing a parish nursing program. *Nursing and Health Care Perspectives, 20*(2), 72-90.

Blumenthal, J. A., Babyak, M. A., Moore, K. A., et al. (1999). Effects of exercise training on older patients with major depression. *Archives of Internal Medicine, 150,* 2349-2356.

Bodenheimer, T., Lorig, K., Holman, H., et al. (2002). Patient self-management of chronic disease in primary care. *Journal of the American Medical Association, 288*(19), 2469-2475.

Bond, G. R., Drake, R. E., Mueser, K. T., et al. (1997). An update on supported employment for people with severe mental illness. *Psychiatric Services, 48,* 335-346.

Bond, G. R., Drake, R. E., Mueser, K. T., et al. (2001). Assertive community treatment for people with severe mental illness: Critical ingredients and impact on clients. *Disease Management and Health Outcomes, 9,* 141-159.

Bond, G. R., & Resnick, S. G. (2000). Psychiatric rehabilitation. In R. G. Frank & T. R. Elliot (Eds.), *The handbook of rehabilitation psychology* (pp. 235-258). Washington, DC: American Psychological Association.

Boscarino, J. A., & Adams, R. E. (2008). Overview of findings from the World Trade Center disaster outcome study: Recommendations for future research after exposure to psychological trauma. *International Journal of Emergency Mental Health, 10*(4), 275-290.

Bradshaw, W. H. (1993). Coping-skills training versus a problem-solving approach with schizophrenic patients. *Hospital and Community Psychiatry, 44,* 1102-1104.

Bradshaw, R., & Haddock, G. (1998). Is befriending by trained volunteers of value to people suffering from long-term mental illness? *Journal of Advanced Nursing, 27*(4), 713-720.

Brisbare-Roch, C., Dingemanse, J., Koberstein, R., et al. (2007). Promotion of sleep by targeting the orexin system in rats, dogs, and humans. *Nature Medicine, 13*(2), 150-155.

Brooker, D., & Duce, L. (2000). Wellbeing and activity in dementia: A comparison of group reminiscence therapy, structured goal-directed group activity and unstructured time. *Aging & Mental Health, 4*(4), 354-358.

Brown, L. D. (2009). How people can benefit from mental health consumer-run organizations. *American Journal of Community Psychology, 43,* 177-188.

Brown, L. D., Shepherd, M. D., Wituk, S. A., et al. (2008). Introduction to the special issue on mental health self-help. *American Journal of Community Psychology, 42,* 105-109.

Brudenell, I. (2003). Parish nursing: Nurturing body, mind, spirit, and community. *Public Health Nursing, 20*(2), 85-94.

Bryant, R. A., Mastrodomenico, J., Felmingham, K. L., et al. (2008). Treatment of acute stress disorder. *Archives of General Psychiatry, 65*(6), 659-667.

Bugg, A., Turpin, G., Mason, S., et al. (2008). A randomized controlled trial of the effectiveness of writing as a self-help intervention for traumatic injury patients at risk of developing post-traumatic stress disorder. *Behaviour Research and Therapy, 311,* 7-12.

Burnside, I. M. (1990). *The effect of reminiscence groups on fatigue, affect, and life satisfaction in older women.* Unpublished doctoral dissertation, University of Texas at Austin, Austin, TX.

Bustillo, J. R., Lauriello, J., Horan, W. P., et al. (2001). The psychosocial treatment of schizophrenia: An update. *American Journal of Psychiatry, 158,* 163-175.

Cardinali, D. P., Furio, A. M., Reyes, M. P., et al. (2006). The use of chronobiotics in the resynchronization of the sleep-wake cycle. *Cancer Causes & Control, 17,* 601-609.

Carpenter, W. T., & Strauss, J. S. (1991). The prediction of outcome in schizophrenia IV: Eleven year follow-up of the Washington IPSS cohort. *Journal of Nervous and Mental Diseases, 179,* 517-525.

Carpinello, S., Knight, E., & Janis, L. (1991). *A qualitative study of the perceptions of the meaning of self-help, self-help group processes and outcomes.* Albany, New York: New York State Office of Mental Health.

Carpinello, S., Knight, E., & Jatulis, L. (1992). *A study of the meaning of self-help, self help group process, and outcomes* (pp. 37-44). Proceedings: 1992 NASMHPD Research Conference, Alexandria, VA.

Chamberlin, J. (1997). A working definition of empowerment. *Psychiatric Rehabilitation Journal, 20*(4), 43-46.

Chao, S., Liu, H-Y, Wu, C-Y, et al. (2006). The effects of group reminiscence therapy on depression, self esteem, and life satisfaction of elderly nursing home residents. *Journal of Nursing Research, 14*(1), 36-45.

Clinton, M., Lunney, P., Edward, H., et al. (1998). Perceived social support and community adaptation in schizophrenia. *Journal of Advanced Nursing, 27,* 955-965.

Colcombe, S., & Kramer, A. F. (2003). Fitness effects on the cognitive function of older adults: A meta-analytic study. *Psychological Science, 14,* 125-130.

Cook, E. A. (1998). Effects of reminiscence on life satisfaction of elderly female nursing home residents. *Health Care for Women International, 19,* 109-118.

Cope: The Family Guide. (1999). DE: AstraZeneca: A resource program from a Business Unit of Zeneca, Inc.

Corrigan, P. W. (2006). Recovery from schizophrenia and the role of evidence-based psychosocial interventions. *Expert Review of Neurotherapeutics, 6*(7), 993-1004.

Corrigan, P. W., Slopen, N., Gracia, G., et al. (2005). Some recovery processes in mutual-help groups for persons with mental illness; II: Qualitative analysis of participant interviews. *Community Mental Health Journal, 4*(6), 721-735.

Cox, A. D. (1993). Befriending young mothers. *British Journal of Psychiatry, 163,* 6-18.

Cresswell, C. M., Kuipers, L., & Power, M. J. (1992). Social networks and support in long-term psychiatric patients. *Psychological Medicine, 22,* 1019-1026.

Cuijpers, P., van Straten, A., & Warmerdam, L. (2007). Problem solving therapies for depression: A meta-analysis. *European Psychiatry, 22,* 9-15.

Danley, M. S., & Anthony, W. A. (1987). The choose-get-keep model: Serving severely psychiatrically disabled people. *American Rehabilitation, 13*(4), 27-29.

Davidson, L., Chinman, M., Kloos, B., et al. (1999). Peer support among individuals with severe mental illness: A review of the evidence. *Clinical Psychology: Science and Practice, 6*(2), 165-187.

Davidson, L., Haglund, K., Stayner, D., et al. (2001). "It was just realizing . . .that life isn't one big horror": A qualitative study of supported socialization. *Psychiatric Rehabilitation Journal, 24*(3), 275-292.

Deegan, P. (1990). Spirit breaking: When the helping professions hurt. *Humanistic Psychologist, 18*(3), 301-313.

DiGiuseppe, R., Simon, K. S., McGowan, L., et al. (1990). A comparative outcome study of four cognitive therapies in the treatment of social anxiety. *Journal of Rational-emotive & Cognitive-Behavior Therapy, 8,* 129-146.

Dixon, L., Adams, C., & Luckstead, A. (2000). Update on family psychoeducation for schizophrenia. *Schizophrenia Bulletin, 26,* 5-20.

Dochterman, J. M., & Bulechek, G. M. (Eds.). (2004). *Nursing interventions classification (NIC)* (4th ed.). St. Louis: Mosby.

Dossett, E., Fuentes, S., Klap, R., et al. (2005). Obstacles and opportunities in providing mental health services through a Faith-Based Network in Los Angeles. *Psychiatric Services, 56,* 206-208.

Drake, R. E., Goldman, H. H., Leff, S., et al. (2001). Implementing evidence-based practices in routine mental health settings. *Psychiatric Services, 52,* 179-182.

Drake, R. E., McHugo, G. J., Bebout, R. R., et al. (1999). A randomized clinical trial of supported employment for inner-city patients with severe mental disorders. *Archives of General Psychiatry, 56*(7), 627-633.

Drake, R. E., McHugo, G. J., Becker, D. R., et al. (1996). The New Hampshire study of supported employment for people with severe mental illness. *Journal of Consulting and Clinical Psychology, 64*(2), 391-399.

Drake, R. E., O'Neal, E. L., & Wallach, M. A. (2008). A systematic review of psychosocial research on psychosocial interventions for people with co-occurring severe mental and substance use disorders. *Journal of Substance Abuse Treatment, 34,* 123-138.

Duhault, J. L. (2002). Stress prevention and management: A challenge for patients and physicians. *Metabolism, 51*(6), 46-49.

D'Zurilla, T. J., & Nezu, A. M. (1999). *Problem-solving therapy: A social competence approach to clinical intervention* (2nd ed.). New York: Springer Publishing Company.

D'Zurilla, T. J., & Nezu, A. M. (2009). Problem-solving therapy. In K. S. Dobson (Ed.), *Handbook of cognitive-behavioral therapies* (3rd ed.). New York: Guilford Press.

Ely, A. (1985). Long-term group treatment for young male schizopaths. *Social Work, Jan.-Feb.,* 5-10.

Engle, G. L. (1977). The need for a new medical model: A challenge for biomedicine. *Science, 196,* 129-136.

Epstein, L. J., & Mardon, S. (2007). *The Harvard Medical School guide to a good night's sleep.* New York: McGraw Hill.

Fingeld-Connett, D. (2005). Clarification of social support. *Journal of Nursing Scholarship, 37*(1), 4-9.

Foley, D. J., Monjan, A. A., Brown, S. L., et al. (1995). Sleep complaints among elderly persons: An epidemiologic study for three communities. *Sleep, 18,* 425-432.

Folkman, S., & Moskowitz, T. (2004). Coping: Pitfalls and promise. *Annual Review of Psychology, 55,* 745-774.

Frank, E. I., Swartz, H. A., & Kupfer, K. J. (2000). Interpersonal and social rhythm therapy: Managing the chaos of bipolar disorder. *Biological Psychiatry, 48,* 593-604.

Galanter, M. (1988). Zealous self-help groups as adjuncts to psychiatric treatment: A study of Recovery, Inc. *American Journal of Psychiatry, 145,* 1248-1253.

Gard, B. A., & Ruzek, J. I. (2006). Community mental health response to crisis. *Journal of Clinical Psychology, 62*(8), 1029-1041.

Gellis, L. A., & Lichstein, K. L. (2009). Sleep hygiene practices of good and poor sleepers in the United States: An internet-based study. *Behavior Therapy, 40*(1), 1-9.

Germain, A., & Kupfer, D. J. (2008). Circadian rhythm disturbances in depression. *Human Psychopharmacology: Clinical and Experimental, 23*(7), 571-585.

Getty, C., Perese, E., & Wooldridge, P. (unpublished). Nurse facilitated support groups for individuals with severe mental illness: Participation, therapeutic factors, content, and satisfaction.

Gladwin, T. (1967). Social competence and clinical practice. *Psychiatry: Journal for the Study of Interpersonal Processes, 3,* 30-43.

Gold Award: The Wellspring of the clubhouse model for social and vocational adjustment of persons with serious mental illness. (1999). *Psychiatric Services, 50*(1), 1473-1476.

Hamilton, D. (1992). Reminiscence therapy. In G. Bulechek & J. McCloskey (Eds.), *Nursing interventions: Essential nursing treatments* (pp. 292-303). Philadelphia: W. B. Saunders.

Hardiman, E. R., & Segal, S. P. (2003). Community membership and social networks in mental health self-help agencies. *Psychiatric Rehabilitation Journal, 27*(1), 25-33.

Harrand, A. G., & Bollstetter, J. (2000). Developing a community-based reminiscence group for the elderly. *Clinical Nurse Specialist, 14*(1), 17-22.

Hassed, C. (2003). Sleep that knits the raveled sleeve of care. *Australian Family Physician, 32*(11), 945-946.

Hasson-Ohayon, H., Roe, D., & Kravetz, S. (2006). A qualitative approach to the evaluation of psychosocial interventions for persons with severe mental illness. *Psychological Services, 3*(4), 262-273.

Hawkins, R. L., & Abrams, C. (2007). Disappearing acts: The social networks of formerly homeless individuals with co-occurring disorders. *Social Science & Medicine, 65,* 2031-2042.

Heinssen, R. K., Liberman, R. P., & Kopelowicz, A. (2000). Psychosocial skills training for schizophrenia: Lessons from the laboratory. *Schizophrenia Bulletin, 26,* 21-46.

Heller, T., Roccoforte, J. A., Hsieh, K., et al. (1997). Benefits of support groups for families of adults with severe mental illness. *American Journal of Orthopsychiatry, 67*(2), 187-198.

Hewett, L. J. (1989). *Group reminiscence/life review with cognitively and/or affectively impaired nursing home residents—"Does it make a difference?"* Unpublished dissertation. Pepperdine University: Malibu, CA.

Hodge, M. A., Siciliano, D., Withey, P., et al. (2010). A randomized controlled trial of cognitive remediation in schizophrenia. *Schizophrenia Bulletin, 36*(2), 419-427.

Hodges, J. Q., & Segal, S. P. (2002). Goal advancement among mental health self-help agency members. *Psychiatric Rehabilitation Journal, 26*(1), 78-85.

Hogan, M. F. (2003). The President's New Freedom Commission: Recommendations to transform mental health care in America. *Psychiatric Services, 54*(11), 1467-1474.

Hollander, E., & Simeon, D. (2008). Anxiety disorders. In R. E. Hales, S. C. Yudofsky, & G. O. Gabbard (Eds.), *The American psychiatric publishing textbook of psychiatry* (5th ed.) (pp. 505-607). Washington, DC: American Psychiatric Publishing, Inc.

Holsboer-Trachsler, E., & Seifritz, E. (2000). Sleep in depression and sleep deprivation: A brief conceptual review. *World Journal of Biological Psychiatry, 1*(4), 180-186.

Horowitz, M. J. (2003). *Treatment of stress response syndromes.* Washington, DC: American Psychiatric Publishing, Inc.

Horsfall, J., Cleary, M., Hunt, G. E., et al. (2009). Psychosocial treatments for people with co-occurring severe mental illnesses and substance use disorders (Dual diagnosis): A review of empirical evidence. *Harvard Review of Psychiatry, 17,* 24-34.

Howe, C., & Howe, J. (1987). The National Alliance for the Mentally Ill: History and ideology. *New Directions for Mental Health Services, Summer* (34), 23-33.

International Federation Reference Centre for Psychosocial Support. (2009). *Psychosocial interventions: A handbook.* Copenhagen, Denmark: International Federation Reference Centre for Psychosocial Support.

Ireland, G., & Morgan, P. (1997). The club house effect. *Living with Schizophrenia, 2*(1), 6, 12.

Iwasaki, Y., Mactavish, H., & Mackay, K. (2005). Building strengths and resilience: Leisure as a stress survival strategy. *British Journal of Guidance Counseling, 33*(1), 81-100.

Jones, E. D. (2003). Reminiscence therapy for older women with depression: Effects of nursing intervention classification in assisted-living long term care. *Journal of Gerontological Nursing, 29,* 26-33.

Kahn, D. A., Sachs, G. S., Printz, D. J., et al. (2000). Medication treatment of bipolar disorder: A summary of the expert consensus guidelines. *Journal of Psychiatric Practice, 6*(4), 197-211.

Kant, G. L., D'Zurilla, T. J., & Maydeu-Olivares, A. (1997). Social problem-solving as a mediator of stress-related depression and anxiety in middle-aged and elderly community residents. *Cognitive Therapy and Research, 21,* 73-96.

Killeen, C. (1997). Loneliness: An epidemic in modern society. *Journal of Advanced Nursing, 28*(4), 762-770.

Kopelowicz, A., Liberman, R. P., & Zarate, R. (2006). Recent advances in social skills training for schizophrenia. *Schizophrenia Bulletin, 30,* S12-S23.

Kopelowicz, A., Wallace, C. J., & Liberman, R. P. (2007). In G. O. Gabbard (Ed.), *Gabbard's treatments of psychiatric disorders* (4th ed.) (pp. 361-384). Washington, DC: American Psychiatric Publishing, Inc.

Kurtz, L. F., & Chambon, A. (1988). Comparison of self-help groups for mental health. *Health & Social Work, 12*(4), 275-283.

Kurtz, M. M., & Mueser, K. T. (2007). A meta-analysis of controlled research on social skills training for schizophrenia. *Journal of Counseling and Clinical Psychology, 76*(3), 491-504.

Kurzban, S., Davis, L., & Brekke, J. S. (2010). Vocational, social, and cognitive rehabilitation for individuals diagnosed with schizophrenia: A review of recent research and trends. *Current Psychiatry Reports, 12*(4), 345.

Larson, E. B., Wang, L., Bowen, J. D., et al. (2006). Exercise is associated with reduced risk for incident dementia among persons 65 years of age and older. *Annals of Internal Medicine, 144,* 73-81.

Lauder, W., Sharkey, S., & Mummery, K. (2004). A community survey of loneliness. *Journal of Advanced Nursing, 46*(1), 88-94.

Lawlor, D. A., & Hopker, S. W. (2001). The effectiveness of exercise as an intervention in the management of depression: Systematic review and meta-regression analysis of randomized controlled trials. *British Medical Journal, 322*(7289), 763-767.

Leach, J. (1995). Psychological first aid: a practical aide-memoire. *Aviation, Space, and Environmental Medicine, 66*(7), 608.

LeDoux, J. E., & Gorman, J. M. (2001). A call to action: Overcoming anxiety through active coping. *American Journal of Psychiatry, 158*(12), 1953-1995.

Lehman, A. F. (1995). Vocational rehabilitation in schizophrenia. *Schizophrenia Bulletin, 21*(4), 645-656.

Lehman, A. F., Kreyenbuhl, J., Buchanan, R. W., et al. (2004). The Schizophrenia Patient Outcomes Research Team (PORT) updated treatment recommendations 2003. *Schizophrenia Bulletin, 30,* 193-217.

Lerner, M. S., & Clum, G. A. (1990). Treatment of suicide ideators: A problem-solving approach. *Behavior Therapy, 21,* 403-411.

Lieberman, R. P., Wallace, C. J., Blackwell, G., et al. (1998). Skills training versus psychosocial occupational therapy for persons with persistent schizophrenia. *American Journal of Psychiatry, 155,* 1087-1091.

Lin, Y-C, Dai, Y-T, & Hwang, S-L. (2003). The effect of reminiscence on the elderly population: A systematic review. *Public Health Nursing, 20*(4), 297-306.

Low, A. (1971). *Mental health through will training.* Boston: Christopher Publishing.

Lupien, S. J., McEwen, B. S., Gunnar, M. R., et al. (2009). Effects of stress throughout the lifespan on the brain, behaviour and cognition. *Nature Reviews. Neuroscience, 10,* 434-445.

Lysaker, P., & Buck, K. (2006). Moving toward recovery within clients' personal narratives: Directions for a recovery-focused therapy. *Journal of Psychosocial Nursing and Mental Health Services, 44*(1), 28-35.

Macias, C., & Rodican, C. (1997). Coping with recurrent loss in mental illness: Unique aspects of Clubhouse Communities. *Journal of Personal and Interpersonal Loss,* 205-221.

Malkoff-Schwartz, S., Frank, E., Anderson, B., et al. (1998). Stressful life events and social rhythm disruption in the onset of manic and depressive bipolar episodes: A preliminary investigation. *Archives of General Psychiatry, 55*(8), 702-707.

Mannion, E., Meisel, P. M., Draine, S., et al. (1996). A comparative analysis of families with mentally ill adult relatives: Support group members vs. non-members. *Psychiatric Rehabilitation Journal, 20*(1), 43-50.

Marmar, C. R., & Spiegel, D. (2007). Posttraumatic stress disorder and acute stress disorder. In G. O. Gabbard (Ed.), *Gabbard's treatments of psychiatric disorders* (4th ed.) (pp. 517-536). Washington, DC: American Psychiatric Publishing, Inc.

Maulik, P. K., Eaton, W. W., & Bradshaw, C. P. (2009). The role of social network and support in mental health service use: Findings from the Baltimore ECA Study. *Psychiatric Services, 60*(9), 1222-1229.

Maury, E., Ramsey, K., & Bass, J. (2010). Circadian rhythms and metabolic syndrome: From experimental genetics to human disease. *Circulation Research, 106*(3), 447-462.

McCorkle, B. H., Rogers, E. S., Dunn, E. C., et al. (2008). Increasing social support for individuals with serious mental illness: Evaluating the Compeer mode of intentional friendship. *Community Mental Health Journal, 45*(5), 359-366.

McEwen, B. S. (2007). Physiology and neurobiology of stress and adaptation: Central role of the brain. *Physiology Review, 87,* 873-904.

McEwen, B. S. (2009). The brain is the central organ of stress and adaptation. *NeuroImage, 47*(3), 911-913.

McFadden, L., Seidman, E., & Rappaport, J. (1992). A comparison of espoused theories of self- and mutual help: Implications for mental health professionals. *Professional Psychology: Research and Practice, 23*(6), 515-520.

McFarlane, A. C. (2010). Phenomenology of posttraumatic stress disorder. In D. J. Stein, E. Hollander, & B. O. Rothbaum (Eds.), *Textbook of anxiety disorders* (2nd ed.) (pp. 547-565). Washington, DC: American Psychiatric Publishing, Inc.

McGurk, S. R., Twamley, E. W., Sitzer, D. I., et al. (2007). A meta-analysis of cognitive remediation in schizophrenia. *American Journal of Psychiatry, 164*, 1791-1802.

Meier, V. J., & Hope, D. A. (1998). Assessment of social skills. In A. S. Bellack & M. Hersen (Eds.), *Behavioral assessment* (4th ed.) (pp. 232-255). Needham Heights, MA: Allyn & Bacon.

Miklowitz, D. J., Goodwin, G. M., Bauer, M. S., et al. (2008). Common and specific elements of psychosocial treatments for bipolar disorder: A survey of clinicians participating in randomized trials. *Journal of Psychiatric Practice, 14*(2), 77-85.

Miller, M. C. (2009). What is reminiscence therapy. *Harvard Mental Health Letter, 25*(10), 8.

Mokhovikov, A., & Keir, N. (1999). Befriending mental patients: Experience in the Ukraine. *Crisis: Journal of Crisis Intervention & Suicide, 20*(4), 150-154.

Morawetz, D. (2001). Sleep better without drugs! Depression and insomnia: Which comes first? *Australian Journal of Counselling Psychology, 3*(1), 19-24.

Murray, P. (1996). Recovery, Inc., as an adjunct to treatment in an era of managed care. *Psychiatric Services, 47*(12), 1378-1381.

Mueser, K. T., Bond, G. R., & Drake, R. E. (2001). Community-based treatment of schizophrenia and other severe mental disorders: Treatment outcomes. *Medscape General Medicine, 3*(1). Retrieved from http://www.medscape.com/viewarticle/430529_print

Mueser, K. T., Bond, G. R., Drake, R. E., et al. (1998). Models of community care for severe mental illness: A review of research on case management. *Schizophrenia Bulletin, 24*(1), 37-74.

Nathan, P. E., & Gorman, J. M. (1998). Treatments that work and what convinces us they do. In P. E. Nathan & J. M. Gorman (Eds.), *A guide to treatments that work* (pp. 2-25). New York: Oxford University Press.

National Compeer Website. (2003). Retrieved from http://Compeer.org/

National Sleep Foundation. (2008). Longer work days leave Americans nodding. *National Sleep Foundation, March 3, 2008*. Retrieved from http://www.sleepfoundation.org

Nelson, G., Aubry, T., & Lafrance, A. (2007). A review of the literature on the effectiveness of housing and support, Assertive Community Treatment and intensive case management interventions for persons with mental illness who have been homeless. *American Journal of Orthopsychiatry, 77*(3), 35. Retieved from http://www.nami.o0-364

Newall, C. A., Anderson, L. A., & Phillipson, J. D. (1996). *Herbal medicines: A guide for health-care professionals.* London: The Pharmaceutical Press.

Nezu, A. M., Nezu, C. M., & D'Zurilla, T. J. (2007). *Solving life's problems: A 5-step guide to enhanced well-being.* New York: Spring Publishing Company.

Overall, J. E., & Gorham, D. R. (1962). The brief psychiatric rating scale. *Psychological Reports, 10*, 799-812.

Padgett, D. K., Henwood, B., Abrams, C., et al. (2008). Social relationships among persons who have experienced serious mental illness, substance abuse, and homelessness: Implications for recovery. *American Journal of Orthopsychiatry, 78*(3), 333-339.

Parish Nursing Fact Sheet (2009). International Parish Nurse Resource Center. Retrieved from www.parishnurses.org

Parker, R. G. (1995). Reminiscence: A continuity theory frame work. *Gerontologist, 35*(4), 515-525.

Pekkala, E. T., & Merinder, L. B. (2002). Psychoeducation for schizophrenia. *The Cochrane Database of Systematic Reviews,* (2). doi:10.1002/14651858.CD002831.

Perese, E. (1997). Unmet needs of persons with chronic mental illness: Relationship to their adaptation to community living. *Issues in Mental Health Nursing, 18*(1), 18-34.

Perese, E., Getty, C., & Wooldridge, P. (2003). Characteristics of psychosocial club members and their readiness to use a support group. *Issues in Mental Health Nursing, 24*, 1-22.

Perese, E., Rohloff, M., & Ryan, E. (2008). Promoting positive clinical experiences with older adults through students' use of a therapeutic intervention-group reminiscence therapy. *Journal of Gerontological Nursing, 34*(12), 46-51.

Perese, E., & Wolf, M. (2005). Combating loneliness among persons with severe mental illness: Social network interventions' characteristics, effectiveness, and applicability. *Issues in Mental Health Nursing, 26*(6), 591-609.

Perese, E., & Wu, B. (2010). Shortfalls of treatment for patients with schizophrenia: Unmet needs, obstacles to recovery. *International Journal of Psychosocial Rehabilitation, 14*(2), 43-56.

Perese, E., Wu, B., & Ram, R. (2005). Effectiveness of assertive community treatment for patients referred under Kendra's Law: Proximal and distal outcomes. *The International Journal of Psychosocial Rehabilitation, 9*(1), 5-9.

Phillips, K. A. (2007). Somatoform and factitious disorders. In G. O. Gabbard (Ed.), *Gabbard's treatments of psychiatric disorders* (4th ed.) (pp. 517-536). Washington, DC: American Psychiatric Publishing, Inc.

Phillips, L., & Zigler, E. (1961). Social competence: The action-thought parameter and vicariousness in normal and pathological behaviors. *Journal of Abnormal and Social Psychology, 63*, 137-146.

Pilling, S., Bebbington, P., Kuipers, E., et al. (2002a). Psychological treatments in schizophrenia, I: Meta-analyses of randomized controlled trials of social skills training and cognitive remediation. *Psychological Medicine, 32*, 763-782.

Pilling, S., Bebbington, P., Kuipers, E., et al. (2002b). Psychological treatments in schizophrenia, II: Meta-analyses of randomized controlled trials of social skills training and cognitive remediation. *Psychological Medicine, 32*, 783-791.

Pistrang, N., Barker, C., & Humphreys, K. (2008). Mutual help groups for mental health problems: A review of effectiveness studies. *American Journal of Community Psychology, 42*, 110-121.

Plotnick, D. F., & Salzer, M. S. (2008). Clubhouse costs and implications for policy analysis in the context of system transformation initiatives. *Psychiatric Rehabilitation Journal, 32*(2), 128-131.

Pratt, S., & Mueser, K. T. (2002). Social skills training for schizophrenia. In S. G. Hofmann & M. C. Tompson (Eds.), *Treating chronic and severe mental disorders: A handbook of empirically supported interventions* (pp. 18-52). New York: Guilford Press.

Preston, N. J., & Fazio, S. (2000). Establishing the efficacy and cost effectiveness of community intensive case management of long-term mentally ill: A matched control group study. *Australian and New Zealand Journal of Psychiatry, 34*, 114-121.

Profita, J., Carrey, R., & Klein, F. (1989). Sustained multimodal outpatient group therapy for psychotic patients. *Hospital and Community Psychiatry, 40*(9), 943-946.

Reite, M. (2009). Treatment of insomnia. In A. F. Schatzberg & C. B. Nemeroff (Eds.), *The American psychiatric publishing textbook of psychopharmacology* (4th ed.) (pp. 1241-1266). Washington, DC: American Psychiatric Publishing, Inc.

Rodriguez, J. J., & Kohn, R. (2008). Use of mental health services among disaster survivors. *Current Opinion in Psychiatry, 21*, 370-378.

Rosenberg, P. (1984). Support groups: A special therapeutic entity. *Small Group Behavior, 15*(2), 173-186.

Rydholm, L. (1997). Patient focused care in parish nursing. *Holistic Nurse Practitioner, 11*(3), 47-60.

Schatzberg, A. F., Cole, J. O., & DeBattista, C. (2007). *Manual of clinical psychopharmacology* (6th ed.). Washington, DC: American Psychiatric Publishing, Inc.

Shibley, H. (2010). Psychological first aid: Helping children overcome disasters. *The Brown University Child and Adolescent Behavior Letter, 26*(4), 1059-1073.

Skarsater, I., Agren, H., & Dencker, K. (2001). Subjective lack of social support and presence of dependent stressful life events characterize patients suffering from major depression compared with healthy volunteers. *Journal of Psychiatric & Mental Health Nursing, 8*(2), 107-114.

Skinner, B. F. (1953). *Science and human behavior.* New York: Macmillan.

Smyth, J. M., Hockemeyer, J. R., & Tulloch, H. (2008). Expressive writing and post-traumatic stress disorder: Effects on trauma symptoms, mood states, and cortisol reactivity. *British Journal of Health Psychology, 13*(Pt. 1), 85-93.

Smyth, J. M., Stone, A. A., Hurewitz, A., et al. (1999). Effects of writing about stressful experiences on symptom reduction in patients with asthma or rheumatoid arthritis: A randomized trial. *Journal of the American Medical Association, 281*(14), 1304-1309.

Snowdon, J. (1980). Self-help groups and schizophrenia. *Australian and New Zealand Journal of Psychiatry, 14,* 265-268.

Solomon, P., & Draine, J. (2001). The state of knowledge of the effectiveness of consumer provided services. *Psychiatric Rehabilitation Journal, 25*(1), 20-27.

Spiegel, D. (1999). Healing words: Emotional expression and disease outcome. *Journal of the American Medical Association, 281*(14), 1328-1329.

Stein, L., Barry, K., Van Dien, G., et al. (1999). Work and social support: A comparison of consumers who have achieved stability in ACT and Clubhouse Programs. *Community Mental Health Journal, 35*(2), 193-204.

Stein, L. I., & Test, M. A. (1980). Alternatives to mental hospital treatment: Conceptual, model, treatment program and clinical evaluation. *Archives of General Psychiatry, 37,* 392-397.

Steinwachs, E., Kasper, J., & Skinner, E. (1992). Patterns of use and costs among severely mentally ill people. *Health Affairs, 11*(3), 178-185.

Stevens, N. (2001). Combating loneliness: A friendship enrichment programme for older women. *Ageing & Society, 21*(2), 183-202.

Stone, W. (1991). Treatment of the chronically mentally ill: An opportunity for the group therapist. *International Journal of Group Psychotherapy, 41*(1), 11-23.

Stone, W. (1996). *Group psychotherapy for people with chronic mental illness.* New York: Guilford Press.

Strawbridge, W. J., Deleger, S., Roberts, R. E., et al. (2002). Physical activity reduces the risk of subsequent depression for older adults. *American Journal of Epidemiology, 156*(4), 328-334.

Strohle, A., Feller, C., Onken, M., et al. (2005). The acute antipanic activity of aerobic exercise. *American Journal of Psychiatry, 162,* 2376-2378.

Swarbrick, M. (2007). Consumer-operated self-help centers. *Psychiatric Rehabilitation Journal, 31,* 76-79.

Swarbrick, M., Schmidt, L. T., & Pratt, C. P. (2009). Consumer-operated self-help centers: Environment, empowerment, and satisfaction. *Journal of Psychosocial Nursing, 47*(7), 40-47.

Sweet, T. (1999). The Wellspring of the Clubhouse Model for social and vocational adjustment of persons with serious mental illness: Fountain House, New York City. *Psychiatric Services, 50*(11), 1473-1480.

Tauber, R., Wallace, C. J., & LeComte, T. (2000). Enlisting indigenous community supporters in skills training programs for persons with severe mental illness. *Psychiatric Services, 51,* 1428-1432.

Torrey, E. F., & Knable, M. B. (2002). *Surviving manic depression: A manual on bipolar disorder for patients, families and providers.* New York: Basic Books.

Tsang, H. W. H. (2001). Rehab rounds: Social skills training to help mentally ill persons find and keep a job. *Psychiatric Services, 52,* 891-894.

Ursano, E. J., Bell, E. S., Friedman, M., et al. (2006). Practice guideline for the treatment of patients with acute stress disorder and posttraumatic stress disorder. In *American psychiatric association practice guidelines for the treatment of psychiatric disorders: Compendium 2006* (pp. 1003-1095). Washington, DC: American Psychiatric Publishing, Inc.

van Emmerik, A. A., Kamphuis, J. H., Emmelkamp P. M., et al. (2008). Treating acute stress disorder and posttraumatic stress disorder with cognitive behavioral therapy or structured writing therapy: A randomized controlled trial. *Psychotherapy and Psychosomatics, 77*(2), 93-100.

Velligan, D. I., Bow-Thomas, C., Huntzinger, C., et al. (2000). Randomized controlled trial of the use of compensatory strategies to enhance adaptive functioning in outpatients with schizophrenia. *The American Journal of Psychiatry, 157*(8), 1317-1323.

Velligan, D. I., Mueller, J., Wang, M., et al. (2006). Use of environmental supports among patients with schizophrenia. *Psychiatric Services, 57*(2), 219-224.

Watt, L. M., & Cappeliez, P. (2000). Integrative and instrumental reminiscence therapies for depression in older adults: Intervention strategies and treatment effectiveness. *Aging & Mental Health, 4*(2), 166-177.

Wheaton, P. (1997). Friendship centres: A treat, not a treatment. *The Journal of the California Alliance for the Mentally Ill,* 44-45.

Woods, R. T., Bruce, E., Edwards, R. T., et al. (2009). Reminiscence groups for people with dementia and their family careers: Pragmatic eight-centre randomized trial of joint reminiscence and maintenance versus usual treatment: A protocol. *Trials, 10,* 64.

Wykes, T., Reeder, C., Landau, S., et al. (2009). Does age matter: Effects of cognitive rehabilitation across the age span. *Schizophrenia Research, 113,* 252-258.

Youssef, F. A. (1990). The impact of group reminiscence counseling on a depressed elderly population. *Nurse Practitioner, 15*(4), 32-38.

Yule, W. (2006). Theory, training and timing: Psychosocial interventions in complex emergencies. *International Review of Psychiatry, 18*(3), 259-264.

UNIT IV

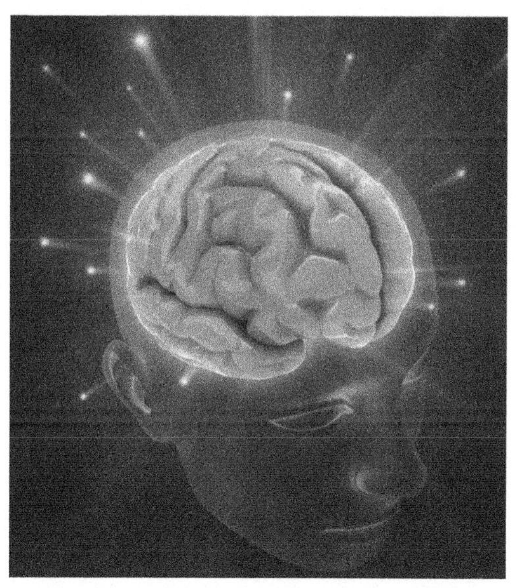

Psychiatric Disorders: Anxiety Disorders

CHAPTER 9

Stress-Related Responses: Adaptive Behaviors, Bereavement, and Adjustment Disorder

Eris F. Perese, APRN-PMH

Stressors can be thought of as negative events that threaten an individual's ability to self-regulate cognition, emotions, and behaviors and to attain desired goals (Brown, Westbrook, & Challagalla, 2005). All individuals face stressors on a daily basis, and most face significant stressors during their lifetime (Solomon, 1999). However, although stressors are known to have a strong influence on the development of stress-related disorders such as adjustment disorder, acute stress disorder, and post-traumatic stress disorder, not all individuals who are exposed to stressors develop psychopathology (Sgoifo, Coe, Parmigiani, et al., 2005). In fact, the majority of individuals exposed to traumatic events do not develop psychopathology (Galea, Vlahov, Resnick, et al., 2003).

Individuals' cognitive appraisal of the stressor and their style of coping have a greater influence on the consequences of exposure to a stressor than the physical aspects of the stressor itself (Sgoifo et al., 2005). The individual's appraisal of the threat results in emotions and coping strategies that may be adaptive—which are effective in helping the individual to overcome the stressor—or maladaptive—which are not effective in helping the individual to overcome the stressor. Whereas maladaptive coping strategies are associated with impairment of functioning, difficulties with interpersonal and vocational relationships, and diminished likelihood of accomplishing goals, adaptive coping strategies are associated with a reduction of feelings of distress, modification of the stressful situation, and movement toward achieving goals (see Box 9-1 for information on the four categories of coping strategies).

BOX 9-1 Coping Strategies

Coping strategies are the ways that people use to modify their situation and reduce feelings of distress. Coping strategies can be placed in four categories:

Category 1. Using direct methods to handle stressors, e.g., problem-solving, which is dealing with the problem by using activities directed toward solving the problem, or restraint, which is waiting for an appropriate opportunity to act.

Category 2. Using cognitive or internal strategies such as avoiding, minimizing, distancing, or seeking value in negative events.

Category 3: Using situational or environmental resources to reduce stress, such as seeking help and social support.

Category 4: Using personal attributes of hardiness, resilience, and sense of control.

Within the coping strategies, four factors have been found to be effective in maintaining health:

1. Factual knowledge about one's situation
2. Inner resources, such as optimism
3. Social support, with more support leading to better coping skills
4. Spirituality or the ability to find strength or obtain comfort from religion or beliefs (Ray, 2004)

Although most individuals learn to manage everyday stressful events, some feel overwhelmed and develop symptoms of distress, such as grief; anxiety; depression; impairment of academic, vocational, or self-care functioning; and problems with family and social interactions (Andreasen & Black, 2006). Some of these individuals may develop stress-related psychiatric disorders. Psychiatric disorders that have a stressful event as a direct cause include adjustment disorder, acute stress disorder, and post-traumatic stress disorder (Casey, Dowrick, & Wilkinson, 2001; Strain & Klipstein, 2007). Adjustment disorder, that develops in response to a variety of stressful events encountered in the course of everyday life, is characterized by a response that is judged to be in excess of a normal response in relation to the severity of the stressor (Black & Andreasen, 2011; Casey et al.). Acute stress disorder and post-traumatic stress disorder develop in response to exceptionally threatening experiences, such as sexual or physical assault; exposure to disasters, military combat, terrorist attacks, threats of death, or harm; witnessing death or injury; and being diagnosed with a life-threatening illness (Hollander & Simeon, 2011). Acute stress disorder and post-traumatic stress disorder will be discussed in detail in Chapter 11.

Normal Stress Response: Theories and Biological Basis for Adaptive Behaviors

Humans owe their survival to their ability to adapt to stressors and traumatic events.

It is fear that activates the stress response that supports survival by changing the functioning of the autonomic nervous system, neuroendocrine functioning, and the processing of information by the brain's emotional and cognitive systems (Rodrigues, LeDoux, & Sapolsky, 2009).

Early stress response theories—specifically, Selye's (1936) general adaptation syndrome—proposed that exposure to stress evoked the same pattern of response in all individuals: alarm with increased release of norepinephrine and cortisol to achieve homeostasis; adaptation; and, if the stressor persisted, exhaustion of individuals' defense mechanisms that could be used to achieve adaptation. Pathological processes begin to develop in the exhaustion stage (Deak & Panksepp, 2004).

Today, response to a stressor or traumatic event is no longer thought to be the same for all individuals. Instead, it is now accepted that the stress response is influenced by an individual's attributes, including genetic influences, experiences, and modifying or buffering factors (Strain, Klipstein, & Newcorn, 2011). For example, among individual attributes, gender has been found to influence response to stressors. In males, exposure to a stressor is likely to elicit a fight-or-flight response. Females are more likely to engage in caretaking activities, to use attachment-promoting behaviors, and to mobilize social support by creating a network of supporters—often other females—to protect them and their children from danger; i.e., females are likely to exhibit the "tend-and-befriend" response (Taylor, Klein, Lewis, et al., 2000).

Life situations such as low socioeconomic status or poverty and life experiences such as early childhood maltreatment have a negative influence on adaptive response to stressors in adulthood. External resources (e.g., social networks and social support) have been found to buffer the effects of stressors (McEwen, 2000). For example, having three or more regular social contacts has been found to be associated with lower stress scores (Seeman, Singer, Ryff, et al., 2002). Physical exercise has been found to have a buffering effect (Rovio, Kareholt, Helkala, et al., 2005), and the internal resources of self-esteem, a positive outlook on life, and a sense of mastery also modulate the effect of stressors (Strain et al., 2011).

Allostasis, Allostatic Load, and Allostatic Overload

Although it has long been accepted that there is a relationship between stress and disease, the ambiguous use of the terms "stress" and "being overstressed" or "burned out" has made it difficult to describe the processes by which the body copes with psychosocial, physical, and environmental challenges. Some researchers believed that a framework for understanding the processes of adaptation to stressors could guide interventions for helping individuals who are experiencing difficulties in adaptation (McEwen, 2008). A recent reconceptualization of the stress response has been within the framework of allostasis, allostatic load, and allostatic overload (Bartolomucci, Palanza, Sacerdote, et al., 2005). Allostasis, or alterations of the primary mediators of stress (neurochemicals), can be considered the primary or initial effect of response to stressors; allostatic load can be thought of as the secondary or proximal outcome; and allostatic overload can be considered the tertiary or distal outcome.

According to McEwen (2008), "Allostasis refers to the active processes by which the body responds to daily events and maintains homeostasis. Allostasis literally means achieving stability through change and is not intended to replace homeostasis" (p. 175). When an individual is exposed to a stressor, the changes that occur within the process of allostasis include

- Mobilization of energy for a behavioral response through the release of hormones, neurotransmitters, and cytokines (Bartolomucci et al., 2005)
- Activation of brain structures that integrate prior experiences, memories, anticipation, appraisal of the stressor, and the individual's reevaluation of needs and coping strategies (Korte, Koolhaas, Wingfield, et al., 2005)
- Changes in behaviors, e.g., increased aggression; smoking; consumption of food, alcohol, and drugs; engagement in more risk-taking behaviors; and decreased amounts of exercise and sleep (McEwen, 2000)

Allostatic States

The changes brought about by the process of allostasis produce "allostatic states," or altered and sustained activity levels of the primary mediators of stress. The primary mediators of stress are the neurochemicals involved in the stress response, which are glucocorticosteroids (cortisol), adrenaline (epinephrine), noradrenaline (norepinephrine), and dehydroepiandrosterone (DHEA) (McEwen, 2000; McEwen, 2005). These primary mediators of stress act as transcription factors and so regulate gene expression, which is involved in the body's response to stress (Lupien, McEwen, Gunnar, et al., 2009).

Allostatic states (alterations of neurochemicals) can be maintained for limited periods of time before they begin to produce wear and tear on the regulatory systems of the brain and body. Examples of the results of prolonged allostatic states include chronic hypertension and chronic fatigue syndrome (McEwen, 2005).

Allostatic Load

The accumulated effect of prolonged allostatic states is known as allostatic load. McEwen and Wingfield (2003) stated that allostatic load refers to the price the body pays for being challenged repeatedly by a variety of stressors. It replaces the vague term "the burden of chronic stress" (McEwen, 2008, p. 176), which does not take into account the contribution of changes of lifestyle practices to allostatic load. Measures of allostatic load that results from the processes of allostasis include blood pressure, weight, cortisol activity, cholesterol levels, glucose metabolism, serum dihydroepiandrosterone sulfate (DHEA-S) levels, and norepinephrine and epinephrine levels (McEwen, 2000, p. 112).

Allostatic Overload

Allostatic overload is the state in which serious pathophysiology occurs. Allostatic overload occurs with any of the following:

- Increased frequency of exposure to stressors
- Increased intensities of these stressors
- Decreased efficiency in coordinating the onset and termination of the physiological response

Allostatic overload is the mechanism through which acute physiological responses result in permanent tissue damage. Medical conditions and psychiatric disorders that result from allostatic overload include obesity, diabetes, atherosclerosis, bone demineralization, atrophy of structures of the brain, cognitive impairment, depression, and anxiety disorders (McEwen, 2004; McEwen & Wingfield, 2003; Reagan, Grillo, & Piroli, 2008). The effects of allostasis and the results of allostatic overload are different for various systems, as shown in Table 9-1.

Biological Basis of Stress Response

The biological basis of the stress response involves brain structures, brain circuitry, and neurochemical responses.

Brain Structures and Circuitry: The Fear/Anxiety Neural Circuit

Individuals experience the emotions of fear and anxiety if they feel threatened or if their welfare is endangered when they are engaged in meeting their survival needs, such as employment to generate financial resources, housing for shelter and safety, food and other sustenance supplies, an intimate relationship, affiliation, role in the community, and a respected status among their family, friends, and coworkers (Hofer, 2010).

Fear

Fear is a response to a known, definite, and external threat (Craig & Chamberlain, 2010; Panksepp, 2004). The response to fear is hardwired into the brain (Shelton, 2004). It protects humans from danger by preparing them to flee from the danger, to face the danger and fight, or to freeze (Amiel, Mathew, Garakani, et al., 2009).

Anxiety

In contrast to fear, anxiety is a response to a threat that is unknown, vague, or internal. Anxiety is also a response to an indirect threat, such as loss of people or things that represent security, e.g., loss of job, home, financial support, role in life, status, or relationships (Craig & Chamberlain, 2010; LeDoux, 2002).

Fear/Anxiety Circuit

Fear and anxiety use the same neural circuitry in promoting responses that are essential to survival. The concept of a neural circuit of fear and anxiety provides the basis for understanding the process through which threatening stimuli that enter through the primary senses—visual, auditory, vestibular (balance), gustatory, and somatosensory (touch, sensations pertaining to position in space and muscular activity, temperature, and pain)—are transformed into mental images that ultimately trigger appropriate mental and physical responses (Bremner & Charney, 2010). The structures of the fear/anxiety circuit are as follows:

- Amygdala, which serves as the brain's alarm center for responses to danger.
- Hypothalamus, which releases hormones that raise heart rate and blood pressure.

TABLE 9-1 EFFECTS OF ALLOSTASIS AND ALLOSTATIC OVERLOAD

System	Allostasis	Allostatic Overload
Immune	Promotion of immune function	Suppression of immune function
Cardiovascular	Maintenance of blood pressure according to need	Persistent elevation of blood pressure
Metabolic	Increases in appetite; replenishment of energy reserves after exposure to stressor	Insulin resistance; depositing of body fat in the abdominal area
Nervous	Improvement in memory	Death and atrophy of neurons; inhibition of new growth of neurons in the hippocampus; impairment of memory and enhancement of fear. Impaired ability to regulate emotions; development of depression and post-traumatic stress disorder

Adapted from McEwen, B. S. (2004). Protection and damage from acute and chronic stress: Allostasis and allostatic overload and relevance to the pathophysiology of psychiatric disorders. Annals of the New York Academy of Sciences, 1032, 1-7.

- Periaqueductal gray matter of the midbrain, which modulates brainstem involvement in behavioral and body responses such as fight, flight, or freeze.
- Tegmental fields (floor of the medulla) of the midbrain, which are involved in regulation of somatic and autonomic responses.
- Hippocampus, which records in memory the time and space dimensions of the stimuli and how they relate to previously stored information about similar stimuli; the hippocampus then relays that information to the amygdala (Bremner & Charney, 2010). However, if the emotional significance placed on an event by the amygdala is very high or if the event is terrifying, horrifying, or life threatening, processing of information by the hippocampus may be prevented and the sensory information remains as isolated bodily sensations, smells, and sounds (LeDoux, 2002; Verfaellie & Vasterling, 2009).
- Prefrontal and parietal cortexes, which are involved in cognitive appraisal of danger, in integrating information of previous experiences with present danger, and in planning responses to danger (Bonne, Crevets, Neumeister, et al., 2004; Bremner & Charney, 2010). The parietal cortex is also involved in locating a traumatic event in space (Debiec & LeDoux, 2009).

In normal functioning, the fear/anxiety circuit protects individuals from physical and psychological danger. Adaptive functioning of the fear/anxiety circuitry reduces distress and restores homeostasis, but dysregulation of the fear/anxiety circuitry may result in impaired functioning and the development of physical illness, such as hypertension, insulin-resistant diabetes and disorders of the immune system, and psychiatric disorders such as post-traumatic stress disorder (Amiel et al., 2009; Parsons & Rizzo, 2008; Rodrigues et al., 2009).

The first step of converting awareness of a threatening or dangerous stimulus into an appropriate response is activation of the fear/anxiety system (Fig. 9-1). Activation results from fear that may be generated by pain, noise, the presence of predators, open spaces, sudden movements, and information from all of an individual's senses. The thalamus starts the process of integrating information related to the stressor with previously stored information. From the thalamus, information is transmitted to the amygdala by way of two parallel loops: the short loop and the long loop. (The one exception to this process is sensory information from the olfactory system, which bypasses the thalamus and goes directly to the entorhinal cortex of the brain.)

The short loop, which LeDoux (2002) called "the quick and dirty low road" (p. 123), is a direct pathway from the thalamus to the amygdala; emotional evaluation of the stimulus by the amygdala is initially based on the fragments of information transmitted by the thalamus. The short loop "jump starts" the fear system, preparing it to process later-arriving integrated information from the cortex (LeDoux, 2002, p. 122). The short loop transmits the unprocessed information directly to the brainstem, which is involved in autonomic responses, neurohormonal responses, and behavioral responses such as fight, flight, or freeze (Debiec & LeDuox, 2009). The information that arrives at the amygdala via the short loop can be less accurate than the information that passes from the thalamus through the cerebral cortex via the long loop.

The longer, slower, regulatory loop that LeDoux (2002) called the "slow but accurate high road" (p. 122) is the cortical pathway that includes the following:

- Somatosensory cortexes
- Insula, which is an island of cortex located between the two hemispheres that is involved in generating, planning, and coordinating movements necessary for speech and in generating signals of present body state and predicted change
- Anterior cingulate cortex, which is involved in initiation of speech, memory, learning, emotions, and selecting responses for action
- Prefrontal cortex, which is involved in attention, emotion, planning, and feeling in control (Bremner & Charney, 2010; Higgins & George, 2007; Mathew, Price, & Charney, 2008) (see Chapter 2 for discussion of the function of brain structures).

In the long loop, sensory information about stimuli that produce fear and anxiety is first processed in the sensory cortexes of the brain before being transmitted as integrated information back to the amygdala and other subcortical structures—the hypothalamus and brainstem—that are involved in emotional, behavioral, and somatic responses. The long loop regulates the response of the amygdala: whether to continue or cease the response to the fear-producing stimulus. However, as previously described, the amygdala receives nonprocessed sensory information directly from the thalamus by way of the short loop before the processed and more accurate information from the cerebral cortex arrives by way of the long loop. Thus, the initial response to a stressor is activation of the amygdala, which immediately begins to transform the sensory information into emotional and hormonal responses (Debiec & LeDuox, 2009).

Some researchers believe that anxiety disorders reflect an imbalance of control of the long loop over the short loop (Bonne et al., 2004). Because altered functioning of one component of the long loop, the insula, has been found in patients with anxiety disorders (generalized anxiety disorder, panic disorder, obsessive-compulsive disorder, and post-traumatic stress disorder), it has been proposed that, in comparison to *fear*, which is primarily related to functioning of the amygdala, *anxiety* may be due to abnormalities of the insula. The insula integrates information from the amygdala, nucleus accumbens, and orbitofrontal cortex and generates signals that represent the difference between the present and the future. It is

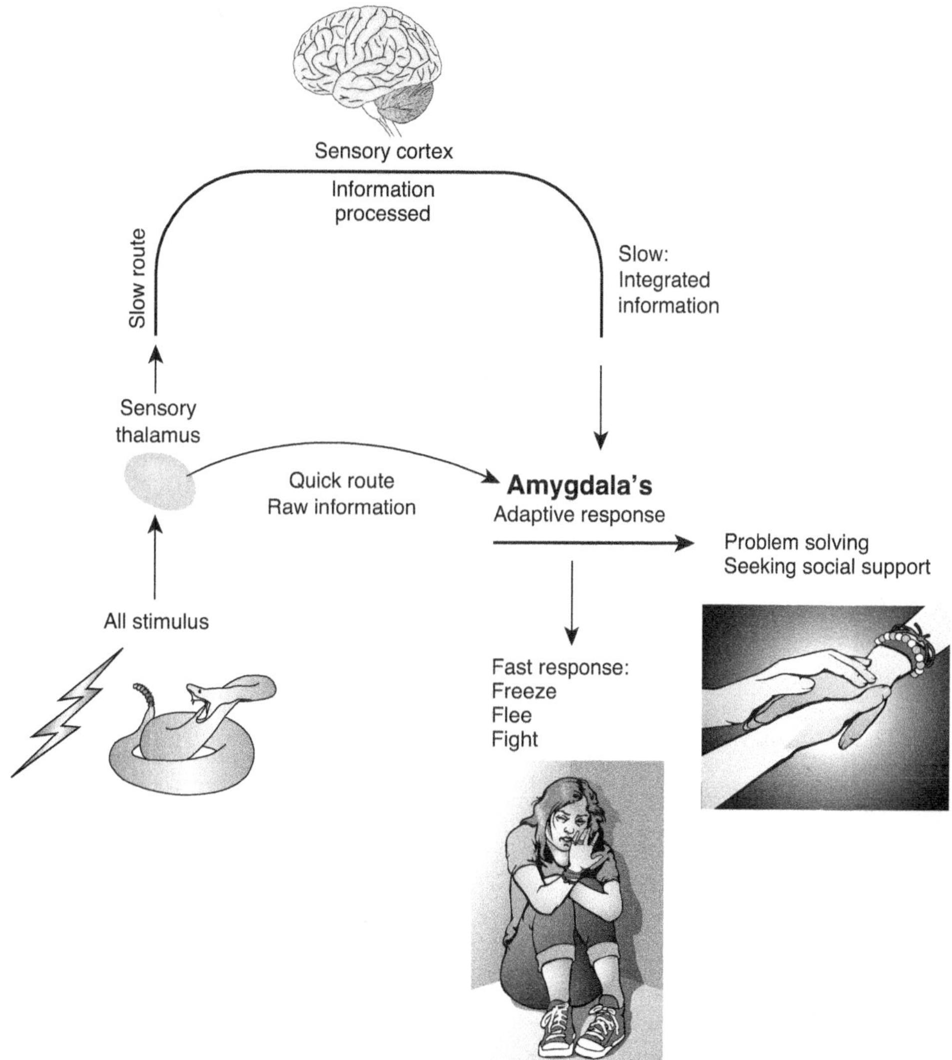

FIGURE 9-1: Fear/Anxiety Circuitry. The fear/anxiety circuit has two loops. In the short loop, emotional stimulus is received by the thalamus and then transmitted directly to the amygdala. In the long loop, the emotional stimulus is transmitted from the thalamus to the sensory cortex of the brain, where it is processed and integrated with other information and then transmitted to the amygdala. The short loop is faster but provides the amygdala with less information about the stimulus. The longer loop provides more complex information about the stimulus.

thought that the insula's signals of predicted change may be abnormal in individuals with anxiety disorders (Mathew et al., 2008).

Through these brain activities, individuals form associations that tell them what to fear. If the mechanism for forming these associations becomes hypersensitive as a result of early exposure to severe or chronic stress, individuals may anticipate danger inaccurately and experience anxiety in association with situations, thoughts, and memories that are not realistic sources of fear ("Generalized anxiety disorder: Toxic worry," 2003; Bremner & Charney, 2010). In time, an individual's thoughts—rather than external events or situations—create fears that activate the amygdala and initiate or maintain a response to danger.

Neurochemical Response

Experiencing stressors and traumatic events triggers the release of neurotransmitters and neuropeptides to defend against the present danger and to prevent it from happening again (Amiel et al., 2009). The neurochemicals released prepare the body to defend itself by

- Increasing oxygen
- Channeling more blood flow to the brain and muscles
- Making stored energy available

The amygdala stimulates the hypothalamus to produce corticotropin-releasing factor (CRF). CRF is associated with fear behaviors, increased arousal, and inhibition of neurovegetative functioning. That inhibition is manifested in disturbances of sleeping and eating and in fatigue and decreased sexual interest (Charney, 2004). CRF shuts down these functions so that resources can be devoted to *fighting* or *fleeing*. Release of CRF from the hypothalamus activates the hypothalamic-pituitary-adrenal (HPA) axis and stimulates the release of adrenocorticotropic hormone (ACTH) from the pituitary. ACTH stimulates the adrenal cortex to release adrenaline, norepinephrine, cortisol, and DHEA (Charney, 2004; Harvey & Byrant, 2002):

- Adrenaline increases cardiac output, raises blood pressure, constricts small blood vessels, releases glucose stored in the liver, and relaxes certain involuntary muscles while it contracts others.
- Norepinephrine raises blood pressure by constricting peripheral blood vessels. It inhibits gastrointestinal activity, and dilates the pupils of the eye. It is associated with symptoms of anxiety such as panic, insomnia, hyperarousal, increased startle response, and hypervigilance (Amiel et al., 2009).
- Cortisol mobilizes and replenishes energy stores and contributes to arousal, vigilance, focused attention, and memory formation (especially emotion-related memories); all of these actions are involved in an individual's ability to respond to stressors and traumatic events (Amiel et al., 2009; Charney, 2004). Cortisol is associated with alterations of the serotonin system that may result in increased anxiety and reduced ability to suppress memories of the traumatic event. Increased levels of cortisol are believed to cause atrophy and death of neurons in the hippocampus with resulting impairment of learning and memory (Amiel et al., 2009; Friedman, Charney, & Deutch, 1995). Stress-induced increase of cortisol is limited by feedback loops of the hippocampus. Without adequate feedback from the hippocampus, excessive and sustained cortisol secretion may occur (van der Kolk, 2006); this can have serious adverse effects including hypertension, osteoporosis, immunosuppression, insulin resistance, cardiovascular disease (Charney, 2004; Karlamangla, Singer, McEwen, et al., 2002), and increased amygdala activity, which increases the encoding of emotion-related memories such as memories of traumatic events.
- DHEA is an adrenal steroid that is released in response to a stressor. It is secreted with cortisol. In the brain, DHEA has antiglucocorticoid activity (Charney, 2004) that may reduce the uptake of cortisol by glucocortical receptors and provide protection for neurons (Kimonides, Khatibi, Svendsen, et al., 1998). Through these actions, DHEA may promote psychological resilience (Charney, 2004). More on psychological resilience can be found in Chapter 1.

Stress-Related Responses: Normal Distress and Bereavement

Experiencing stressors, which can range from daily hassles (e.g., family conflicts, money problems, disagreements at work, or relocation) to death of a loved one, is part of everyone's life. Stressors are stimuli or challenges that require behavioral, psychological and physiological changes in order for individuals to adapt and survive (Esch & Stefano, 2010). Knowing how the body normally responds to stressors provides an understanding of why distressed individuals react the way they do and how psychiatric advanced practice nurses can facilitate reduction of distress and grief and improvement of functioning.

Normal Distress

Normal response to a stressor may be evidenced as an unpleasant sense of arousal, restlessness, confusion, anxiety, and changes in emotions (Higgins & George, 2007). Individuals often experience difficulty concentrating and making decisions and have thoughts of failure. Behavioral responses include crying, acting impulsively, clenching the jaw, and increased smoking and use of alcohol or other drugs. Physical symptoms include tight muscles, headaches, back or neck pain, and sleep disturbances. Classic signs of distress include narrowing of focus of attention, increased use of attachment behaviors (seeking sources of attachment), diminished sense of self-identity and self-competence, impairment of social role functioning, and difficulty in making decisions (Hansell, 1976; Higgins & George, 2007; Panksepp, 2004; University of Texas at Austin Counseling and Mental Health Center, 2004).

Following exposure to a stressor, many individuals are able to use their coping skills to restore conditions to as close to normal as possible, but others may experience changes in their normal coping strategies; for instance, they may increase their smoking, alcohol, or substance use; they may experience sleep disturbances; and they may alter their eating patterns and patterns of activity (Shelby & McCance, 2002). These individuals may need help in developing new coping strategies. Because individuals who have experienced stressors often have an altered sense of self-identity and self-efficacy, interventions should emphasize empowerment and promotion of self-efficacy (LeDoux & Gorman, 2001). Psychiatric advanced practice nurses can foster return of functioning by supporting patients' new coping skills, by encouraging their sense of hope, and by demonstrating the expectation that they have the ability to gain mastery over the problems caused by the stressor.

Bereavement, Grief, and Complicated Grief

Normal grief associated with bereavement is a common stressor for individuals, and most individuals find ways to cope with their losses over time. Complicated grief, however, often requires treatment because it is longer lasting, is frequently comorbid with depression and post-traumatic stress disorder, and has greater negative consequences on health. Table 9-2 lists characteristics of bereavement and normal grieving and of complicated grieving.

TABLE 9-2 BEREAVEMENT AND NORMAL GRIEVING, AND COMPLICATED GRIEVING

Stage or Intervention	Description
Bereavement and Normal Grieving	
Initial response to loss	*Cognitive state:* shock, disbelief, a wish to deny the loss, a desire to reverse the event *Physical state:* shortness of breath, muscle weakness, lack of energy, dry mouth, chest and throat tightness *Behaviors:* sleep disturbances, appetite disturbances; absentminded behaviors; social withdrawal; dreams of the deceased; sighing and crying
Acceptance of loss	Sadness, reminiscing, regret for lost opportunities, search for meaning to the death
Encapsulation of loss	Views the relationship as a significant part of his or her life, addresses new challenges, develops new relationships
Complicated Grieving	
Complicated grieving symptoms	Despair over the loss Withdrawal from normal activities Bereavement becomes a way of life Insistence of keeping things exactly the way they were when the deceased was alive Symptoms of recurrent insomnia or loss of appetite Grieving is debilitating, e.g., patient is unable to resume usual work or activities Yearning for contact with the deceased Dissociative state (imagines deceased is still with him or her) Self-destructive behaviors
Complicated grieving interventions	Provide the individual the opportunity to express feelings of anger, hurt, guilt, and sense of personal loss. Help the individual to review the qualities of the persons. Help the individual to review the nature of the relationship, e.g., what has been lost. Discuss the individual's fears of the future without the loved one. Help the individual to shift to a forward focus, e.g., develop adaptive plans. Help the individual to develop plans for coping with the identified fears for the future without the loved one.

Sources: France, 2002; Parry, 1994; Roberts & Berry, 2002; Shear, 2005.

Bereavement and Grief

Bereavement, which is the loss of a loved one through death, can be anticipated, can occur unexpectedly, or can occur within a disaster that involves other losses (Stroebe, Schut, & Stroebe, 2005). Death of a spouse is a life occurrence that requires readjustment in many life domains, with nearly half (46%) of women older than 65 years experiencing widowhood (Stroebe et al., 2005). *Grief* includes the thoughts and feelings related to the individuals' perception of their loss. The emotions of grief include sadness, anxiety, guilt, anger, and shame (Shear, 2005). *Mourning* is the process that individuals go through following the loss; mourning consists of the behaviors and activities that are related to adjusting to death. Ways of mourning are influenced by gender, ethnicity, and culture (Stroebe, Stroebe, & Schut, 2001).

Bereavement may lead to a period of distress, impaired functioning, and health problems such as headaches, indigestion, chest pain, disability, and increased use of medications. There is an increased risk of death and suicide in the early months following the death of a loved one. There may be reduced ability to take in new information; impaired thinking, planning, and problem-solving; and a reduced sense of self-efficacy (Kowalski & Bondmass, 2008; Stroebe, Schut, & Stroebe, et al., 2007). A few individuals may experience symptoms of depression, anxiety, and post-traumatic stress disorder (Stroebe et al.).

Eventually, bereaved individuals adapt to the change by building a life without the loved one, creating new relationships, and restructuring their views of themselves, their goals in life, and their beliefs about the control that they have over their lives (Roberts & Berry, 2002). In the past, studies of bereavement in widows suggested that the highest levels of grief occur during the first 4 months after the death of a spouse and that it took 2 years for widows to recover from their grief (Hyrkas, Kaunonen, & Paunonen, 1997). However, some researchers found that it was 3 years before grief symptoms of depression, social isolation, bodily pains, and poor eating diminished (Wilcox, Evenson, Aragaki, et al., 2003), and others have found that it is 5 years before symptoms of grief diminish (Kowalski & Bondmass, 2008). More than half of widows report health-related problems and changes in lifestyle practices. For example, among those who smoked, 44% increased their smoking after the death of their spouse, and 21% of the total study population increased their alcohol consumption (Kowalski & Bondmass).

Treatment of Grief

In the past, it was thought that grief work was essential for adapting to bereavement. Grief work consists of sharing and disclosing feelings, accepting death, confronting the reality of loss, and giving up the bond to the deceased. Recent research has shown that individuals who do not engage in grief work recover as well as, if not better than, those who do (Bonanno, 2001; Wortman & Silver, 2001). Usually, families, friends, neighbors, and religious groups provide all the support that is necessary following bereavement (Parkes, 1998). Researchers have also investigated the benefits of psychotherapy, pharmacotherapy, and psychosocial interventions in helping an individual overcome grief.

- ***Psychotherapy.*** Studies of counseling for bereavement are inconclusive. Although bereavement counseling may serve as additional support to that provided by family and friends, there is no evidence for a selected preventive approach of referring everyone who is experiencing bereavement for counseling (Parkes, 1998) because individuals who receive bereavement interventions are not appreciably less distressed than those who do not receive any formalized help. However, preventive interventions are beneficial when targeted to bereaved individuals who are in need of help (Currier, Neimeyer, & Berman, 2008).
- ***Pharmacotherapy.*** Antidepressant medications may be helpful when depression is present during bereavement (Barraclough, Palmer, & Dombrowe, 1998). The antidepressant bupropion (Wellbutrin) has been found to relieve depressive symptoms, and a decrease in depressive symptoms is associated with a decrease in grief intensity (Zisook, Shuchter, Pedrelli, et al., 2001). During acute grief, which is grief at the level of a psychiatric emergency, interventions that may be used include a short course of sedative-hypnotic medications, a short course of benzodiazepines, and use of selective serotonin reuptake inhibitor antidepressant medications (Schatzberg & Nemeroff, 2006).
- ***Psychosocial interventions.*** Psychiatric advanced practice nurses can assist patients to find solutions to the problems that result from bereavement. Common problems for the patient include needing time off from work, needing to identify financial resources, and needing to provide care for family members. Psychiatric advanced practice nurses can encourage contact with friends outside of the family. They can also refer patients to support groups for bereavement (Berghuis & Jongsma, 2008). One psychosocial intervention found to be helpful is bibliotherapy that includes readings to help the patient understand the grieving process. Two books that have been found to be helpful are *The Grief Recovery Handbook: The Action Program for Moving Beyond Death, Divorce, and Other Losses* (James & Friedman, 1998) and *Getting to the Other Side of Grief* (Zonnebelt-Smeenge & DeVries, 1998).

Complicated Grief

Complicated grief differs from normal grieving in intensity, length of time, or both. It is characterized by

- Persistent longing or yearning for the deceased that lasts at least 6 months
- Sense of disbelief that the individual has died
- Anger and bitterness over the death
- Preoccupation with thoughts of the loved one
- Intrusive thoughts related to the death (Shear, Frank, Houck, et al., 2005)

Complicated grief can be identified by using the Inventory of Complicated Grief (Prigerson, Maciejewski, Reynolds, et al., 1995).

One hypothesis for failure to adapt to the death of a loved one involves the nucleus accumbens, which is the reward center of the brain that is activated by feelings of attachment. Bereaved individuals who do not have complicated grief respond to reminders of the deceased with pain-related neural activity, but not with activity in the reward center of the brain. In contrast, individuals with complicated grief respond to reminders of the deceased with both pain-related neural activity and reward-related activation in the nucleus accumbens. It is suggested that yearning is a form of attachment that activates the nucleus accumbens and produces a pleasurable sensation. Thus, among patients with complicated grief, yearning for the deceased is a form of attachment that activates the reward center of the brain and may interfere with the individual's adapting to the realities of the loss (O'Connor, Wellisch, Eisenberger, et al., 2008).

Risk factors associated with the development of complicated grief include death that is sudden, untimely, or traumatic; the presence of multiple stressors associated with the death; caregiver strain; the death of a child; and being isolated. Factors that seem to protect against the development of complicated grief include having secure attachment patterns with others; high self-esteem; sense of control over one's life; the presence of social support; and spirituality (Stroebe et al., 2007). Prigerson and Jacobs (2001) revealed that 9% to 20% of adults who experience bereavement have complicated grief; however, this statistic may be as high as 58% for parents whose child has died from sudden infant death syndrome and 78% for parents who have lost a child because of an accident or suicide (Dyregrov, Nordanger, & Dyregrov, 2003).

Treatment of Complicated Grief

Early studies suggested that antidepressant medications relieved symptoms of depression but did not change symptoms of complicated grief (Prigerson, Frank, Kasl, et al., 1995). Later studies found that selective serotonin reuptake inhibitor antidepressant medications and other antidepressants such as nortriptyline (Pamelor) improved both depressive symptoms and complicated grief symptoms (Zisook et al., 2001; Zygmont, Prigerson, Houch, et al., 1998). Complicated grief treatment that includes information about normal and complicated grief and that focuses on (1) restoration of a satisfying life, (2) adjustment to loss, (3) managing symptoms by retelling the story of the death with gradual emphasis on positive memories, and (4) confrontation with avoided situations has been found to be effective in improving complicated grief symptoms (Shear et al., 2005). Cognitive behavioral therapy that includes exposure therapy (where patients gradually confront reminders of their losses and discuss effects of the loss on their lives) was associated with greater improvement than supportive counseling in which patients discussed the emotional, social, and practical difficulties that were occurring in their everyday lives (Boelen, de Keijser, van den Hout, et al., 2007).

In conclusion, recovery from complicated grief involves restructuring life without the loved one. Interventions designed specifically for individuals experiencing complicated grief seem to be more effective than nonspecific interventions (Currier et al., 2008).

Adjustment Disorder

Before adjustment disorder was included in the *Diagnostic and Statistical Manual of Mental Disorders,* 2nd Edition *(DSM-II)* (American Psychiatric Association, 1968), it was described as "transient situational disturbance" (Casey et al., 2001, p. 479). Now, adjustment disorder is considered to be a stress-related occurrence in which experiencing a stressor has been followed by (1) maladaptation or difficulty adjusting to the event and (2) development of symptoms of distress (Black & Andreasen, 2011). Some researchers consider patients with adjustment disorder to be in a middle area between patients with specific mental disorders—such as major depressive disorder—and patients with good mental health; in other words, patients with adjustment disorders are individuals who do not develop major psychiatric disorders in response to exposure to stressors (Gur, Hermesh, Laufer, et al., 2005). Others believe that for some individuals, the signs and symptoms of adjustment disorder may be early signs of an emerging psychiatric disorder (Strain et al., 2011).

To meet the *Diagnostic and Statistical Manual of Mental Disorders, Fourth Edition, Text Revision (DSM-IV-TR)* (American Psychiatric Association, 2000) criteria for adjustment disorder, the symptoms must have developed within 3 months of the stressor, and the amount of distress must be in excess of what might be expected in relation to the stressor, or the individual must experience significant impairment in social, occupational, or other important functioning. The stressor may be a one-time event—such as finding out that a spouse has been unfaithful or that financial losses may result in foreclosure on a home—or a chronic condition—such as having parents who are constantly fighting or having a spouse who hoards things. Symptoms should resolve within 6 months of the end of the stressor or its consequences (Casey et al., 2001). Symptoms may persist longer if they are in response to a chronic stressor or if the consequences persist. The diagnosis of adjustment disorder is not used (1) if the symptoms meet the criteria for another Axis I psychiatric disorder, such as one of the anxiety disorders or mood disorders, (2) if the symptoms are an exacerbation of an existing Axis I or Axis II psychiatric disorder, or (3) if the symptoms represent bereavement.

Although adjustment disorder is often considered to be a minor psychiatric disorder with less severe symptoms in comparison to other psychiatric disorders (Greenberg, Rosenfield, & Ortega, 1995), it is frequently associated with lost time from work, which is costly to society. For example, in the Netherlands, half of work disabilities for chronic illnesses are stress-related disorders such as adjustment disorder (Van der Klink, Blank, Schene, et al., 2003). In addition to high levels of disability, adjustment disorder also carries a high risk for suicide (Goldston, Daniel, Reboussin, et al., 1998; Kryzhanovskaya & Canterbury, 2001; Schnyder & Valach, 1997), excessive substance use, somatic complaints, and poorer response to treatment among patients with medical illness (Strain et al., 2011).

Several researchers have challenged the validity of the diagnosis of adjustment disorder because (1) the disorder does not have a specific symptom profile or biological correlates and (2) the symptoms of adjustment disorder often overlap with the symptoms of major depressive disorder (Snyder & Strain, 1989) or with symptoms of some anxiety disorders (Casey et al., 2001). For example, adjustment disorder with depressed mood is frequently misdiagnosed as a mood disorder such as major depressive disorder that may need pharmacological treatment. Casey et al. stated that more careful application of the criteria for adjustment disorder for patients who may be experiencing an adjustment disorder with multiple symptoms could differentiate it from major depressive disorder, thus avoiding the use of pharmacotherapy, which is often associated with treatment of major depressive disorder. Others have pointed out that the explanation that temporary emotional symptoms have occurred in response to an identifiable stressful life event may be less stigmatizing and more acceptable for the patient than a diagnosis of a major psychiatric disorder (Takei & Sugihara, 2006). At this time, there appears to be support for the diagnosis of adjustment disorder (Strain, Klipstein, & Newcorn, 2008).

Epidemiology of Adjustment Disorder

The epidemiology of adjustment disorder includes prevalence, risk factors, and protective factors.

Prevalence

Prevalence varies depending on the population studied. According to *DSM-IV-TR*, adjustment disorder has been found in 12% of general hospital inpatients referred for mental health consultation; 10% to 30% of patients in outpatient mental health settings; and 50% of individuals who have experienced a specific stressor, such as cardiac surgery (American Psychiatric Association, 2000, p. 681). In a community sample, the prevalence of adjustment disorder among children, adolescents, and older adults has been found to be 2% to 8%. However, among older adults admitted to the hospital for an acute medical condition, the prevalence of adjustment disorder is 20% (Gonzalez-Jaimes & Turnbill-Plaza, 2003; Schatzberg, 1990).

Adjustment disorder is more common among women, unmarried individuals, and younger individuals (Black &

Andreasen, 2011). For example, women are diagnosed with adjustment disorder twice as often as men (American Psychiatric Association, 2000). Table 9-3 shows the prevalence of adjustment disorder among certain patient populations.

Risk Factors

Individuals from disadvantaged backgrounds, those who are indigent, and those who have a medical illness may be at increased risk for adjustment disorder (Strain et al., 2008). The presence of separation anxiety in childhood has been found to be associated with later development of adjustment disorder (Giotakos & Konstantakopoulos, 2002). Other risk factors include lack of social support, family disruptions or marital problems, frequent moves, recent losses, and prior history of mental illness (Casey et al., 2001; Jones, Yates, Williams, et al., 1999).

Protective Factors

Certain factors may mediate the likelihood of an individual's developing an adjustment disorder in response to a stressor (Mazure, 1998). These factors include individual attributes such as hardiness, effective coping skills, support systems, and prior mastery of stressful events (Strain et al., 2008). Healthy lifestyle practices, having a sense of humor, being resilient, and thinking positively about oneself are also protective factors (Mayo Clinic, 2011; McEwen, 2007).

Among adults, specific mediating factors include ability to bond with a group, altruism, and ability to participate in teamwork (Gur et al., 2005). Among children, individual attributes associated with successful adaptation include "good intellectual functioning, effective self-regulation of emotions and attachment behaviors, a positive self-concept, optimism, altruism, and a capacity to convert traumatic helplessness into learned helpfulness" (p. 727).

Etiology of Adjustment Disorder

Adjustment disorder is precipitated by exposure to one or more stressors. In determining the diagnosis, the clinician accepts that the identifiable stressor is the cause of the response and that the response to the stressor is time limited (a transitory response). The stressor may be a single event, such as loss of a job, or an event that has indirect effects or multiple effects, such as divorce, change of residence, retirement, severe illness, or the loss of an important source of social support (Weigel, Purselle, D'Orio, et al., 2009). The stressor may be recurrent (such as a seasonal difficulty) or continuous (such as poverty or the effects of chronic illness), or the stressor may be a recent minor event added to a previous major stressor that did not appear to have an effect (Strain et al., 2008). The effect of the stressor is influenced by the presence or absence of protective factors and by what the stressor means to the individual immediately and for the long term (McEwen, 2007; Strain & Klipstein, 2007).

Psychodynamic Factors

Throughout childhood, the development of defense mechanisms—which are techniques that reduce anxiety when one is dealing with stressful events—is influenced by the child's unique attributes as he or she interacts with people in his or her attachment networks and social support systems (Strain et al., 2008). Children and adolescents often develop immature defense mechanisms, such as denial, distortion, acting-out behaviors, and somatization. Retention and use of these immature defense mechanisms is maladaptive in managing stressful situations in adulthood. Development of more mature defense mechanisms, such as anticipation, humor, suppression, sublimation, and altruism, leads to the acquisition of resilience, which is the ability to bounce back from a stressful or adverse situation (Werner & Smith, 1982).

Biological Basis for Adjustment Disorder

Stress depletes glucose in the neurons of the hippocampus, making the neurons vulnerable to the action of excitatory neurotransmitters, such as glutamate; exposure to excessive glutamate can result in neuron shrinkage and cell death.

TABLE 9-3 PREVALENCE OF ADJUSTMENT DISORDER IN CERTAIN POPULATIONS

Population	Prevalence	Study
Individuals with severe burns	60%	Perez Jimenez, Gomez Bajo, Lopez Castillo, et al., 1994
Elderly individuals receiving elective surgery for coronary artery disease	50.7%	Oxman, Barrett, Freeman, et al., 1994
Individuals with cancer	50%	Spiegel, 1996
Individuals after stroke	40%	Shima, Kitagawa, Kitamura, et al., 1994
Children with new-onset of diabetes	35%	Kovacs et al., 1995
Elderly individuals with a cerebrovascular accident	27%	Kellerman, Jehete, Gesztelyi, et al., 1994
Individuals attempting suicide	22%	Schnyder & Valach, 1997
Individuals in early stages of multiple sclerosis	20%	Sullivan et al., 1995
Individuals receiving head and neck surgery	16.8%	Kugaya, Akechi, Okuyama, et al., 2000

Prolonged exposure to stress may prevent neurogenesis (the birth of new neurons) in the dentate gyrus of the hippocampus, which is one of the areas in the brain that has been found to have the ability to generate new neurons that could lead to increased learning and memory formation. In addition, the stress hormone cortisol affects the functioning of the prefrontal cortex, which is involved in judgment, decision making, and perception, and it affects the amygdala's ability to regulate fear (LeDoux, 2002; McEwen, 2007). Each of these activities plays a role in individuals' ability to respond to stressors and is believed to be involved in the development of adjustment disorder.

Clinical Presentation of Adjustment Disorder

Adjustment disorders are characterized by maladaptive psychological responses to an identifiable stressor or stressors or a change in life circumstances (Maercker, Forstmeier, Enzler, et al., 2008; Strain & Klipstein, 2007). The stressors are everyday events in an individual's life, such as divorce or separation, unemployment, accidents, financial problems, and retiring, rather than catastrophic events, such as earthquakes (Maercker). Maladaptive responses to such stressors are manifested in emotional, cognitive, or behavioral symptoms (American Psychiatric Association, 2000) (Box 9-2).

Suicidal behavior is common in patients with adjustment disorder (Tripodianakis, Markianos, Sarantidis, et al., 2000). In fact, according to Gur (2005), 30% of patients with adjustment disorder have suicidal thoughts.

BOX 9-2 Emotional, Cognitive, and Behavioral Symptoms of Adjustment Disorder

Emotional Symptoms

- Nervousness and anxiety
- Depressed mood
- Sadness and crying spells
- Hopelessness
- Lack of enjoyment in activities that were previously enjoyed
- Feelings of being overwhelmed
- Feelings of desperation

Cognitive Symptoms

- Worry
- Difficulty concentrating
- Thoughts of suicide

Behavioral Symptoms

- Sleep disturbances
- Changes in eating
- Avoiding family or friends
- Ignoring need to pay bills
- Poor work performance
- Fighting
- Reckless driving

Sources: Gur et al. (2005); Mayo Clinic (2011).

The *DSM-IV-TR* (American Psychiatric Association, 2000) lists six categories of adjustment disorder:

1. Adjustment disorder with depressed mood
2. Adjustment disorder with anxiety
3. Adjustment disorder with mixed anxiety and depressed mood
4. Adjustment disorder with disturbance of conduct
5. Adjustment disorder with mixed disturbance of emotions and conduct
6. Adjustment disorder unspecified (See Box 9-3 for a description of the categories.)

The adjustment disorder may be specified as *acute* if the disturbance lasts less than 6 months and *chronic* if the disturbance lasts longer than 6 months and is in response to a chronic stressor or to the lasting consequences of a stressor. The symptoms or behaviors are clinically significant, as indicated by distress in excess of what might be expected from the severity of the stressor or by significant impairment of social, occupational, or academic functioning (American Psychiatric Association, 2000). The symptoms may not be present for more than 6 months after the stressor or its consequences end.

Adjustment Disorder in Specific Populations

Adjustment disorder affects children and adolescents, adults, older adults, and military personnel.

Children and Adolescents

In children, adjustment disorder is most often related to the challenge of moving through Erikson's developmental stages, to school problems, to family conflicts, and to peer difficulties (Strain & Klipstein, 2007). Among children ages 8 to 13 years with adjustment disorder, the most frequent category is adjustment disorder with depressed mood (63%) (Kovacs, Gatsonis, Pollock, et al., 1994), and the most common symptoms are feeling sad, suicidal ideation, no pleasure, self-depreciation, and irritability. For children with other types of adjustment disorder, symptoms include disobedience, irritability, feeling sad, anger, fighting, and anxiety (Kovacs et al.). Poor school performance, skipping school, vandalism, substance use, and suicidal thoughts and behaviors may occur in children and adolescents with any type of adjustment disorder (Mayo Clinic, 2011). Among children, early problems in adjusting to the stress of a medical illness appear to predict vulnerability to later development of psychopathology (Kovacs, Ho, & Pollock, 1995).

The most common stressors among adolescents are family-related events, peer-related problems, school problems, parental alcohol and drug problems, parental separation or divorce, and parental rejection (Andreasen & Black, 2006). Symptoms include anxiety, depression, and disturbances of conduct such as aggressive behavior. There may be absences from school, alcohol misuse, and learning difficulties. Symptoms in males are more likely to be aggressive behavior, truancy, depression, restlessness, and problems

BOX 9-3 Description of Categories of Adjustment Disorder

Adjustment Disorder With Depressed Mood
Symptoms include hyposomnia, decreased appetite, weight loss, decreased motor activity, social withdrawal, depressed mood, low self-esteem, tearfulness, sense of hopelessness, alcohol use, and increased risk for suicide (Strain et al., 2008). Patients no longer find pleasure in things that they used to enjoy (Mayo Clinic, 2011).

Adjustment Disorder With Anxiety
Symptoms include generalized anxiety, increased motor activity, nervousness, worry, difficulty concentrating or remembering things, low self-esteem, hyposomnia, somatic complaints, and feeling overwhelmed (Mayo Clinic, 2011; Strain et al., 2008). There are often co-occurring generalized anxiety, situational anxiety, and panic attacks (Strain et al.). Children may fear being separated from their parents (Mayo Clinic).

Adjustment Disorder With Mixed Anxiety and Depressed Mood
There may be concurrent symptoms of anxiety and depression, impulsivity, hostility, excessive alcohol use, antisocial behaviors, lack of insight, self-centeredness, hostility, elated mood, and homicidal ideation (Strain et al., 2008).

Adjustment Disorder With Disturbance of Conduct
Symptoms include impulsive and violent behaviors and conduct in which the rights of others are violated or social norms are disregarded. These behaviors include truancy, vandalism, reckless driving, fighting, defaulting on legal responsibilities, withdrawal, vegetative signs, insomnia, and suicidal behavior. Children may skip school, vandalize property, and get into fights (Mayo Clinic, 2011; Strain et al., 2008).

Adjustment Disorder With Mixed Disturbance of Emotions and Conduct
There may be symptoms of depression and anxiety and behavioral problems (Mayo Clinic, 2011).

Adjustment Disorder Unspecified
There may be emotional or behavioral responses soon after a difficult event, but the symptoms do not meet the criteria for the other subtypes (Mayo Clinic, 2011).

with the law; in females, symptoms are more likely to be internalizing symptoms of anxiety, depression, and self-reproach (Pelkonen, Marttunen, Henriksson, et al., 2007).

Adjustment disorder with depressed mood has been found to be a frequent diagnosis among young people who make suicide attempts (Skopek & Perkins, 1998; Wai, Hong, & Heok, 1999). The duration between first communication of thoughts of suicide and suicide among adolescents with adjustment disorder is shorter (less than 1 month) than among individuals with major depressive disorder (less than 3 months) or individuals with schizophrenia (47 months) (Runeson, Beskow, & Waern, 1996). Based on information obtained from a psychological autopsy study, Portzky, Audenaert, and van Heeringen (2005) reported that the suicide process in adolescents with adjustment disorder moves very quickly from first communications of suicidal ideation to suicide, with an average duration of 3 months and mean duration of 2 months, and that the suicide process was triggered by experiencing an adverse event. They did not identify the adverse events, nor did they identify whether the adverse event occurred one time or was chronic. However, Black and Andreasen (2011) provided information about the type of stressors and the acuity or chronicity of stressors experienced by adolescents with adjustment disorder. Only 9% of adolescents with adjustment disorder had experienced a stressor within 3 months. For 60% of adolescents with adjustment disorder, the stressors were chronic, present for a year or more. The most frequently identified stressor was school problems (60%), followed by parental rejection (27%), alcohol and/or drug use (26%), parental separation or divorce (25%), and problems with girlfriends or boyfriends (20%). Less frequently identified stressors included parents' marital problems, moving, legal problems, work problems, and other problems (p. 363). The very short time between communicating ideas of suicide and completing suicide among adolescents with adjustment disorder is a red flag for psychiatric advanced practice nurses to assess suicide risk and to implement preventive interventions. There is a very small window of time for preventing suicide among adolescents with adjustment disorder.

Adults

Stressors frequently associated with the development of adjustment disorder in adults include adverse events—such as breakups, marital conflict, and divorce; accidents; layoffs, loss of a promotion, or retirement; new or unanticipated medical diagnoses; or relocation—and positive events, such as marriage, birth of a child, or a child's leaving home for college. In adults, the most common stressors associated with the development of adjustment disorder are marital problems, separation or divorce, relocation, and financial problems. Frequently, the stressors are multiple, recurrent, or continuous (Andreasen & Black, 2006). Case Study 9-1 presents adjustment disorder with disturbances of emotion and conduct in an adult.

Older Adults

Older adults face multiple stressors: death of loved ones, coping with chronic medical conditions and disabilities, and loss of roles, home, financial security, neighborhood friends, social support, and independence (Lantz, 2008). In

CASE STUDY 9-1

Adjustment Disorder With Disturbances of Emotion and Conduct in an Adult

Mr. W is a 30-year-old male who immigrated to the United States from Poland. He was sponsored to this country through a Catholic organization that initially helped him find a place to live in a Polish American neighborhood and provided minimal financial assistance. He was referred to the community mental health clinic by Social Services.

With the help of an interpreter, it was discovered that Mr. W had immigrated alone and had no immediate or distant family in the United States. He was never married. On interview, he complained of constant anxiety, insomnia, and sense of helplessness and hopelessness, but he denied suicidal ideation and attempts and was deeply affronted when asked. He expressed deep religious faith and beliefs and felt that his Catholic faith was his main source of comfort and support at this time. He was unable to find even a menial type of entry-level work owing to the language barrier. He was reluctant to leave his studio apartment for fear of having encounters where he would not know how to respond or how to react. He was spending more and more time at home, doubting his decision to immigrate, anxious and uncertain about his future, and feeling alone and alienated.

Questions

1. What are the clinical features of adjustment disorder?
2. Is there a difference between adjustment disorder and major depressive disorder with regard to suicidal ideation?
3. What issues and barriers do immigrants face that may make them susceptible to adjustment disorders?

Answers to these questions can be found at the end of this chapter.

Source: Sophie Knab, MSN-PMH

combination with impairments of functioning and loss of protective or buffering resources, these stressors place older adults at risk for developing adjustment disorders.

Among older adults, the most frequent subtype of adjustment disorder has mixed emotional features, but older adults frequently have adjustment disorder with disturbances of behavior that may be manifested in refusal of treatment (Lantz, 2008). In a recent study of older adults, among those 65 years of age to 96 years of age, 52.1% had experienced a stressor (severe illness, illness of a relative, family conflicts, and financial problems) that was considered to be the index stressor for making the diagnosis of adjustment disorder (Maercker et al., 2008). Adjustment disorder with anxiety occurs frequently among older adults who have experienced personal stressful events such as moving from one room to another in a nursing home, developing a new physical illness, or experiencing changes in the family or financial situation (Spar & La Rue, 2006).

Military Personnel

The U.S. military is involved in response and defense during times of conflict and disaster (Riddle, Smith, Smith, et al., 2007, p. 192), and it requires optimal mental and physical health of its members (Smith, Zamorski, Smith, et al., 2007). In fact, the overall mental and physical health of the military is better than that of the U.S. general population of the same age and sex (Smith et al.). However, certain subgroups within the military—including women, those with short-term service, enlisted personnel, those on active duty, members of the Army, and those who are younger, less educated, and single—have been found to be at greater risk for developing mental disorders (Riddle et al.).

Military service provides multiple stressors, such as being away from family, living closely with others, having contact with firearms, adjusting to military hierarchy, and experiencing military duty with the potential of war (Hageman, Pinborg, & Andersen, 2008). In the study by Hageman et al. of Danish conscripts, 52.9% of those referred to the Military Psychiatric Department for psychiatric complaints were diagnosed as having adjustment disorder. Although adjustment disorder is thought to be transient and it is assumed that individuals will return to normal life, a 10-year follow-up of conscripts with adjustment disorder challenges those assumptions.

At 10-year follow-up, among those initially diagnosed as having an adjustment disorder, 21.8% had had additional contact with psychiatric services. Among those diagnosed with adjustment disorder, 30.4% had nervous or stress-related disorders; 17.4% had personality disorders; 17.4% had affective disorders; 13% had schizophrenia; 8.7% had substance-related disorders; 6.5% had schizotypy, and others had behavioral disorders. In comparison to a control group consisting of conscripts who did not have any psychiatric complaints, the conscripts who did have psychiatric complaints had higher mortality rates, with death resulting most frequently from suicide and second most frequently from accidents. Hageman et al. (2008) suggested that because nearly one-fourth of the conscripts with adjustment disorder went on to develop major psychiatric disorders, the diagnosis of adjustment disorder should be considered to have a predictive value.

Among military personnel who were evacuated during the Afghanistan and Iraq military operations, 10.1% were evacuated for psychiatric reasons. These evacuated personnel had not responded to front-line mental health counseling by trained counselors and were considered dangerous to themselves or others at the time of evacuation. Among those evacuated, less than 5% were able to be return to active duty. Fourteen percent were sent to a U.S. military hospital for treatment, and 81% were returned as outpatients to their home base (Rundell, 2006, p. 354). The most common diagnosis among evacuated personnel was adjustment disorder (37.6%). Other psychiatric disorders were mood disorders (22.1%), personality disorders (15.7%), and anxiety disorders (15.4%) (Rundell).

Risk factors for developing adjustment disorder among young soldiers included a history of childhood exposure to abuse, childhood separation anxiety, adverse events in the family, or having overprotective parents (For-Wey, Fei-Yin, & Bih-Ching, 2002; Hansen-Schwartz, Kijne, Johnsen, et al., 2005). Risk factors for needing to be evacuated for psychiatric reasons were being female, being African American, and being in the reserve as opposed to serving in active duty military. The need for evacuation was greatest during the first 6 months of deployment. The stressors that were identified more frequently than combat exposure or being fired on were problematic day-to-day deployment environment and family problems back home. Problems in the day-to-day deployment environment included stressful living conditions, weather extremes, problems with peers or supervisors, sleep deprivation, and sexual or physical abuse. Female service members were ten times more likely than male service members to have experienced recent sexual abuse and four times more likely to have experienced recent physical abuse. Female service members were also twelve times as likely to have experienced sexual abuse in their lifetime and five times as likely to have experienced physical abuse in their lifetime (Tiet, Finney, & Moos, 2006).

Comorbidity

Approximately 70% of patients—children, adolescents, and adults—with adjustment disorder have at least one other Axis I diagnosis (Fabrega, Mezzich, & Mezzich, 1987; Kryzhanovskaya & Canterbury, 2001). Axis II personality disorders are frequently comorbid with adjustment disorder (Gur et al., 2005). Casey et al. (2001) suggested that personality traits—such as impulsivity, dramatization, and unstable relationships—play a role in the development of adjustment disorder.

Assessment

In the initial interview of the patient, the goal of the psychiatric advanced practice nurse is to establish rapport and a collaborative relationship with the patient. During the interview, the following information is elicited:

- Chief complaint
- History of present illness
- History of any previous psychiatric disorders
- History of past medical disorders
- Past social history
- Developmental history that includes any adverse prenatal events and accomplishment of developmental milestones
- Early childhood living situation
- Attachment pattern with parents
- History of childhood separations and verbal, physical, and sexual abuse
- How life transitions—such as going away to college or leaving home—were accomplished

Because treatment involves (1) eliminating or reducing the stressor, (2) changing the patient's perception of the stressor, or (3) promoting adaptation to the stressor, the assessment must include clarification of what the identified stressor means to the patient in relation to changes in functioning, loss of sense of self-identity and valued roles, acceptance in social networks, alterations of living situation, and the need to modify plans for the future. To determine the patient's capacity for eliminating, reducing, or adapting to the stressor, the patient's inner strengths, coping skills, hardiness, resilience, sense of mastery, attachment network, social support system, and spirituality should be assessed (Strain & Klipstein, 2007).

Psychiatric advanced practice nurses assimilate the data obtained into a biopsychosocial case formulation that includes key biological, psychological, and social elements of the history and mental status examination. Based on the case formulation, the psychiatric advanced practice nurse develops a biopsychosocial plan of treatment. The biological part of the plan contains a physical examination (often performed by the primary care clinician); laboratory tests; review of medications that the patient is taking; and referrals for treatment of medical, dental, and vision problems, if indicated. The psychological part of the treatment plan contains neuropsychological testing (if indicated) and psychotherapy. The social part of the treatment plan may contain approaches to improve housing, living situation, employment, finances, social support, and connectedness with religious or spiritual groups (Andrews, 2008).

Screeners for Adjustment Disorder

Screeners or assessment tools may be used as part of the assessment and treatment planning. Examples include the following:

- *The Perceived Stress Scale* (Cohen, Kamarck, & Mermelstein, 1983), a 10-item scale that measures the degrees to which situations in one's life are appraised as stressful. It measures global perception of stress.
- The *Life Events Questionnaire*, a 12-item instrument that measures common life events that tend to be threatening (Brugha & Cragg, 1990).
- The *Hospital Anxiety and Depression Scale*, a 14-item self-report questionnaire that measures anxiety and depressive symptoms during the previous week. It has been used for patients with medical illnesses. It does not screen for adjustment disorder specifically but has been found to be predictive for the development of

adjustment disorder in patients with cancer (Akechi, Okuyama, Sugawara, et al., 2004).

Brief one-item instruments have been developed to detect adjustment disorder in patients with cancer. For example:

- *The One-Question Interview* was recently developed to screen for adjustment disorder and depression. It consists of one question: "Please grade your mood during the past week by assigning it a score from 0 to 100, with a score of 100 representing your usual relaxed mood. A score of 60 is considered the passing grade" (Akizuki, Akechi, Nakanishi, et al., 2003, p. 2607).
- The *Distress Thermometer* (Roth, Kornblith, Batel-Copel, et al., 1998) is a one-item self-report analog scale of distress. Scores range from 0 (no distress) to 10 (extreme distress).

Brief questionnaires may be useful in identifying which patients need further evaluation, but they do not distinguish between adjustment disorder and other depressive disorders (Strain et al., 2008).

Differential Diagnosis

In considering the diagnosis of adjustment disorder, a stressor to which the patient is having difficulty adapting must be identified. The stressor cannot be bereavement. If the patient has experienced a stressor within the previous 3 months and the symptoms of anxiety or depression meet the criteria for an anxiety disorder or major depressive disorder, then the Axis I disorder takes precedence over the diagnosis of adjustment disorder (Black & Andreasen, 2011).

Psychiatric Disorders as Differential Diagnoses

Depressive disorders, anxiety disorders (acute stress disorder and post-traumatic stress disorder), substance-related disorders, disruptive behavior disorders, brief psychotic disorder, personality disorders, and bereavement must be considered as differential diagnoses:

- ***Depressive disorders.*** Although symptoms may overlap, the threshold of the symptoms and the duration of the symptoms of major depressive disorder are useful in distinguishing adjustment disorder from major depression.
- ***Anxiety disorders.*** To differentiate *generalized anxiety disorder* from adjustment disorder, three of six symptoms of anxiety must be present for more days than not for a period of 6 months. To diagnose *acute stress disorder*, the stressor must be extreme (not a common stressor) and there must be depersonalization and dissociation that resolves within 4 weeks. In *post-traumatic stress disorder*, the stressor must be extreme (life threatening) and the symptoms must include intense fear, helplessness, or horror. Other symptoms that may be present include increased arousal (hypervigilance and disruptions of sleep), reexperiencing of the trauma, and avoidance of stimuli associated with the trauma (American Psychiatric Association, 2000; Casey, 2001).
- ***Substance-related disorders.*** Individuals with substance-related disorders have a history of multiple symptoms that have occurred over time, including compulsive use, withdrawal, medical complications, problems with work and money, marital conflict, and legal problems.
- ***Disruptive disorders.*** According to the *DSM-IV-TR*, in disruptive behavior disorders, there must be a specific number of behaviors or pattern of behaviors that must have been present for at least 6 months (American Psychiatric Association, 2000).
- ***Brief psychotic disorder.*** In response to a stressor, individuals develop psychotic symptoms, delusions, hallucinations, disorganized speech, or disorganized or catatonic behavior that lasts at least 1 day but less than 1 month. They are often very confused or in emotional turmoil (American Psychiatric Association, 2000).
- ***Personality disorders.*** Individuals with personality disorders may show patterns of thinking and behavior that deviate from the usual cultural patterns, e.g., deviations in interpreting events, emotional responses (mood instability), interpersonal functioning, and impulse control. The deviations are long-standing and sometimes can be traced back to childhood (American Psychiatric Association, 2000).
- ***Other disorders: bereavement.*** In considering the differential diagnosis of bereavement, it is important for psychiatric advanced practice nurses to remember that grief comes in waves. There are moments of happy reminiscences. Although there may be expressions of guilt, the theme is that of not having done enough for the deceased. In bereavement, suicidal ideation is low, and depressive symptoms, although usually present soon after the loss, tend to resolve by 2 months. Psychiatric advanced practice nurses must be aware of abnormal or complicated grief that may be manifested as absent or delayed grief, excessively intense mourning, self-destructive behaviors, suicidal ideation, and psychotic symptoms, such as the bereaved's believing that he or she is the deceased individual or is dying from the same condition as the deceased (Roberts & Berry, 2002). There may be persistent auditory hallucinations, suicidal ideation, and psychotic symptoms (Hales, Yudofsky, & Gabbard, 2008).

In summary, differential psychiatric diagnoses that must be considered include generalized anxiety disorder (see Chapter 10); acute and post-traumatic stress disorders (see Chapter 11); major depressive disorder (see Chapter 13); substance-related disorder (see Chapter 17); personality disorders (see Chapter 18); and brief psychotic disorder and somatization disorder (see a textbook of psychiatry such as Black and Andreasen, 2011 or Hales, Yudofsky, & Gabbard, 2011).

Treatment of Adjustment Disorder

The overall goal of treatment for adjustment disorder is to return the patient to his or her previous level of functioning or better as soon as possible (Weigel et al., 2009). The focus is on reducing or eliminating the stressor that precipitated the adjustment disorder; increasing coping skills to manage the stressor; and increasing the patient's support system to help in achieving positive adaptation (Strain et al., 2008). When the symptoms of adjustment disorder are at low levels, the family often treats the symptoms with culturally approved approaches, which are a form of emotional first aid; however, if the symptoms are more severe, the family often sees them as a medical illness and requiring of outside help (Gur et al., 2005). Treatment for adjustment disorder should be provided as soon as possible to prevent a maladaptive response to the stressor or stressors that may result in impaired relationships and decreased functioning at work, school, or home.

Treatment interventions for adjustment disorder include immediate treatment or emotional first aid, psychotherapy, a multimodal approach, pharmacotherapy, psychosocial interventions, activating intervention, and alternative treatments. Group therapy is helpful for patients who are able to benefit from being with others who have experienced similar stressors, such as patients with the same medical illnesses. Individual therapy is helpful for some patients to explore the meaning of the trauma for them and to examine previous traumas in their lives with the goal of strengthening their coping in the face of future stressors (Strain et al., 2011).

Immediate Treatment

The principle of immediate treatment for patients with adjustment disorder is to use a direct approach and deal with the situation at hand that is troubling the individual (First & Tasman, 2004). The first step in immediate treatment includes practical support offered in a sympathetic manner that fits the patient's needs and complements the help being given by family and friends. For example, information about housing, financial problems, or medical problems may be needed (Bisson, Brayne, Ochberg, et al., 2007).

Emotional first aid is an example of a brief intervention. It is designed to help individuals accept the reality of the stressor, identify sources of help, and participate in resuming their lives (Bisson et al., 2007; First & Tasman, 2004). Principles of emotional first aid are based on the BICEPS approach (brevity, immediacy, centrality, expectancy, proximity, and simplicity). BICEPS is a military approach, but it has also been used for adjustment disorder (Lundin, 1994; Wise, 1988). The BICEPS approach embodies the following principles:

- Brevity: treatment is expected to be brief
- Immediacy: treatment is provided immediately after exposure to a stressor, e.g., after learning of diagnosis of cancer
- Centrality: treatment and needed services are coordinated
- Expectancy: it is expected that the individual will return to normal functioning
- Proximity: treatment is provided as close to the scene of the stressor as possible
- Simplicity: treatment is focused on maintaining a reintegrative approach

The BICEPS approach provides emotional first aid that gets the individual started in the process of active coping that is crucial for positive adaptation.

Psychotherapy

Psychotherapy is the treatment of choice for adjustment disorders (Weigel et al., 2009). Psychotherapy allows the patient to express feelings of fear, anxiety, anger, rage, and helplessness in relation to the stressor; psychotherapy also allows the patient to reframe the stressor, to learn new ways of coping, and to learn ways to develop alternative interests and relationships (Pollen & Holland, 1992). Psychotherapeutic interventions include therapies such as supportive psychotherapy, brief dynamic psychotherapy, cognitive behavioral therapy (CBT), interpersonal relationship therapy, and eye movement desensitization and reprocessing (EMDR) therapy (Strain et al., 2011).

Brief Psychotherapy

Brief psychotherapy refers to a class of psychotherapies that seek to bring about change through active, focused interventions that involve direct participation of therapist and patient. It proposes that change comes about through new experiences rather than through the fostering of insight. The therapist actively promotes corrective emotional experiences. The use of brief therapies is indicated when

1. The duration of the problem is brief
2. The patient has good interpersonal skills and can build a trusting relationship
3. The severity of the problem is mild to moderate
4. The problem is circumscribed
5. The patient understands the need for change
6. Social support is strong and accessible

The outcome of brief therapy depends on the therapist's skills in introducing new corrective emotional experiences and the patient's willingness and ability to participate (Dewan, Steenbarger, & Greenberg, 2008).

Brief psychotherapy interventions may not be sufficient for patients with ongoing stressors or for patients who have personality traits that make them more vulnerable to stress (Katzman & Tomori, 2005). Additional treatment is based on knowledge that adjustment disorder comes from a psychological response to a stressor. Therefore, the stressor must be identified and described to the patient so that the patient understands its properties; in other words, the meaning of the stressor for the patient must be clarified and interpreted (Strain & Klipstein,

2007). Longer-term treatment plans are developed to include interventions to reduce or eliminate the stressor or its consequences; to enhance coping skills in relation to the stressor; to help patients gain a different perspective on the stressful event; to foster willingness on the part of the patient to adapt to the changes that occurred as a consequence of the stressor; and to facilitate the establishment of support systems and engagement in support groups or self-help groups that can help with adaptation (Strain & Klipstein).

Supportive Psychotherapy

The goal of supportive psychotherapy is to help patients cope with symptoms or to help healthy people deal with a crisis or transient problems. It is indicated for patients experiencing overwhelming anxiety, for those responding to a stressful event or situation, and for patients with adjustment disorder (Winston, 2008). Supportive psychotherapy uses direct strategies to reduce symptoms, to increase adaptive coping skills, and to promote ego strengths, such as thinking/interpreting information and regulating affect and behaviors. It helps patients to review the stressor in terms of (1) their views on the stressor's significance in their life, (2) their ability to achieve their goals, and (3) their ability to self-regulate emotions and behaviors in relation to the problem (Brown et al., 2005).

Brief Dynamic Psychotherapy

Brief dynamic psychotherapy challenges maladaptive defense patterns and provides new corrective relationship experiences (Dewan et al., 2008). Among patients with adjustment disorder with depressed mood, with dysthymic disorder, and with depressive disorder not otherwise specified, both brief dynamic therapy and supportive psychotherapy were associated with greater improvement of symptoms immediately after treatment in comparison to a control group and to patients on the waiting list. Brief dynamic therapy was more effective than supportive psychotherapy at 6-month follow-up (Maina, Forner, & Bogetto, 2005).

Cognitive Behavioral Therapy (CBT)

There are no studies that specifically focus on the effects of CBT on adjustment disorder; however, some studies suggest that CBT benefits those with minor depressive disorder, which is a diagnosis sometimes used instead of "adjustment disorder with depressed mood" (Strain & Klipstein, 2007). Thus, in the future, treatment for adjustment disorder may include the use of technology that offers computerized cognitive behavioral therapy (CCBT) for patients with anxiety and depressive disorders using programs such as *Stresspac*, *Beating the Blues*, and *Restoring the Balance* (Andrews & Erskine, 2003; Whitfield, Hinshelwood, Pashley, et al., 2006).

These CCBT programs are based on the principles of therapist-delivered cognitive behavioral therapy, and they have the potential to make treatment more accessible. The *Kessler Self-Assessed Psychological Distress Scale* can be used to measure clinical response of patients with anxiety and depression (Andrews & Slade, 2001). Studies comparing therapist-led cognitive behavioral therapy and CCBT have had mixed results, with some indicating that CCBT may be most useful as an adjunctive intervention to CBT.

Interpersonal Relationship Therapy

The goal of interpersonal relationship therapy—originally designed to treat depression—is to help patients overcome problems in their role functioning or social environment. The usual areas of focus are problems with grief, marital conflict, life changes, isolation, lack of social support, and role transitions. Interpersonal relationship therapy seeks to relieve symptoms, to improve the patients' environment, to build social skills, and to foster a sense of mastery over the environment. It has been found to be useful in helping patients to interpret the meaning of stressors, to use a here-and-now approach to understanding the problem, to explore options for changing dysfunctional behavior patterns, and to identify interpersonal problem areas (Markowitz, 2008).

Eye Movement Desensitization and Reprocessing Therapy (EMDR)

EMDR is a form of psychotherapy that assists patients in processing information related to past traumatic experiences that may be the source of present dysfunctional beliefs and to distressing images, sensations, and emotions. In EMDR, patients focus on the disturbing image, thoughts, and sensations and on a preferred positive belief that they have identified while moving their eyes to follow the therapist's finger as it passes across their field of vision. Eye movements are the most commonly used external stimuli, but tapping or sounds are also used. There is evidence that supports the effectiveness of EMDR in treating patients with post-traumatic stress disorder (Wheeler, 2008). EMDR has also been used for patients with adjustment disorder. Patients with adjustment disorder with anxiety or with mixed features showed improvement, but those with adjustment disorder with depressed mood and those with ongoing stressors did not show improvement (Mihelich, 2000; Strain et al., 2011).

Multimodal Approach

Lazarus (1992) developed a multimodal approach to treating minor depression, which is a term sometimes used to describe adjustment disorder with depressed mood. Lazarus' multimodal approach was based on the assumption that most psychological problems result from an interaction of external stressors, internal conflicts, misinformation or lack of information about the stressor, maladaptive habits or behaviors, interpersonal difficulties, and biological disorders. He believed that treatment should address all of these factors.

In the multimodal model, patients are asked to identify behaviors, sensations, images, ideas, people, and places that they formerly found to be pleasing or rewarding; patients are then encouraged to engage in these pleasing activities or social interactions. To change affect that is depressed, gloomy, or sad, patients are taught to use relaxation exercises, meditation, and calming self-statements that have been found to have antidepressant effects. They are taught to use imagery to recall previous positive coping, and they are taught to use time projection in which they imagine themselves in a future time when they would be happier, coping adaptively, and engaging in pleasurable activities. Patients' cognitive distortions are challenged in multimodal therapy, and they are taught assertiveness skills. They are also taught lifestyle practices that are known to be effective for individuals with depression, e.g., exercise, sleep hygiene, and relaxation (Lazarus, 1992). Multimodal therapy has been found to be more effective than cognitive therapy alone, behavior modification alone, or no treatment (Taylor & Marshall, 1977).

Pharmacotherapy

Studies of the use of pharmacotherapy for adjustment disorder are inconclusive (Strain et al., 2008, p. 771). Medications may be used to treat specific symptoms for a brief time: for example, sleep disturbance may be treated with short-term use of diphenhydramine (Benadryl), trazadone (Desyrel), or zolpidem (Ambien) to reestablish sleep-wake cycles (Weigel et al., 2009). Selective serotonin reuptake inhibitors and venlafaxine (Effexor) have been found to be effective in relieving anxiety and depressive symptoms.

Pharmacotherapy for Adjustment Disorder With Anxiety

Patients with adjustment disorder with anxiety may benefit from a brief course (days to weeks) of a benzodiazepine such as lorazepam (Ativan) (Strain et al., 2008).

Pharmacotherapy for Adjustment Disorder With Depression

Patients with adjustment disorder with depressed mood were found to have an equally favorable response to citalopram (Celexa), paroxetine (Paxil), sertraline (Zoloft), and venlafaxine (Effexor) (Hameed, Schwartz, Malhotra, et al., 2005). Patients with adjustment disorder with depressed mood were twice as likely as patients diagnosed with major depressive disorder to respond to antidepressant medications, and their response to the medication was also sustained longer. Combining antidepressants did not improve response or remission rates. The addition of psychotherapy to pharmacotherapy did not improve response or remission rates over pharmacotherapy alone. Hameed et al. suggested that identification and treatment of patients with adjustment disorder with depressed mood in primary care settings has the potential to prevent progression to a more serious depressive disorder.

Psychosocial Interventions

Psychosocial interventions include activities described as part of the multimodal approach (education about the reality of the situation, assertiveness training, and time projection), role-playing, biofeedback, and support groups (Mayo Clinic, 2011) (see Chapter 8 for a description of support groups). Psychosocial interventions also include promotion of self-care activities.

Self-Care Interventions

Self-care interventions that patients can be taught include preventive strategies that can be used (1) before an anticipated stressful event and (2) after experiencing a stressful event. Preventive interventions include performing stress management strategies, such as exercise, yoga, and meditation; reviewing inner strengths; and remembering coping skills that have been used successfully in past stressful situations. Interventions that can be used after experiencing a stressful event include maintaining healthy lifestyle practices, talking with caring family or friends, working at a hobby, joining a support group of people experiencing a similar stressful event, and seeking support from a spiritual group (Mayo Clinic, 2011).

Patient Activities to Reduce Distress

Individuals who have been exposed to stressors often feel anxious, agitated, restless, or uneasy. They may avoid thoughts that lead to arousal of fear and anxiety. These feelings may be reduced by focusing the individual on problem-solving activities and also by encouraging engagement in less difficult tasks, such as activities that serve as distractions during which the patient is asked to turn away from distressing thoughts by doing something else. LeDoux and Gorman (2001) suggested that engaging in an active coping response rather than using avoidance reroutes the processing of thoughts and actions from passive fear responses to successful interactions with the environment. LeDoux and Gorman recommended that clinicians encourage patients who have been exposed to stressors to engage in activities that lead to pleasure. Box 9-4 provides examples of specific stress-reducing activities.

Activating Intervention

The activating intervention is a 12-month intervention designed to prevent the disabling long-term effects of adjustment disorders and thus reduce sickness duration and rates of failing to return to work. It is a three-stage intervention based on principles of time contingency in which "activities increase according to a pre-structured time scheme" (van der Klink et al., 2003, p. 429); it is also based on cognitive behavioral therapy. Instead of waiting for a reduction of distressful symptoms, the patient is encouraged to engage in work activities immediately.

In the first stage of the intervention, the emphasis is on information: the patient learns to understand the origin of the adjustment disorder. During this stage, patients are

BOX 9-4 Stress-Reducing Activities

Activities that patients could engage in to reduce stress levels or buffer the effect of stress include the following:

- Getting more sleep
- Developing a positive outlook
- Adopting a healthy diet
- Engaging in moderate physical activity, such as walking
- Participating in social activities
- Avoiding smoking and excessive alcohol use
- Making things, e.g., food, crafts, and gardens
- Making lists or plans
- Listening to music or making music.
- Using spiritual resources, such as meditating, praying, reading affirmations; participating in rituals and ceremonies; and listening to spiritual programs on the radio.

Sources: Copeland (2002) McEwen (2008); Rovio et al. (2005); Seeman et al. (2002).

encouraged to increase their participation in nondemanding daily activities. In the second stage, patients write a list of stressors and develop problem-solving strategies for these stressors. In the third stage, the patients put the strategies into practice and add more demanding activities to their daily activities. Throughout the intervention, the patient's responsibilities and role in promoting recovery are emphasized.

When the three-stage intervention was compared to usual care (counseling, instruction about stress, lifestyle advice, and discussion about work problems), significantly more patients in the intervention group returned to work at 3 months, showing that sick leave was shorter in the intervention group. Patients in both groups showed improvement of physical symptoms and of symptoms of distress, anxiety, and depression and an increase in sense of mastery. There was no difference between the groups in these changes. At 12 months, all patients had returned to work, with the intervention group having returned earlier.

Alternative Treatments

Bourin, Bougerol, Guitton, et al. (1997) described a multicenter, double-blind, placebo-controlled study that examined the use of plant extracts in the treatment of outpatients with adjustment disorder with anxious mood. Among patients taking Euphytose (EUP) for 28 days, repeat measures using the Hamilton Anxiety Scale showed a significant difference between the patients receiving EUP and those receiving placebo. It has been reported that Ginkgo biloba special extract EGb761 reduced symptoms of anxiety and somatic symptoms in patients with adjustment disorder with anxiety (Woelk, Arnoldt, Kieser, et al., 2007). Woelk et al. noted that EGb761 does not cause dependence or sedation and may improve cognitive functioning in older adults. Kava was also found to reduce symptoms in patients with adjustment disorder with anxiety (Volz & Kieser, 1997).

Course of Adjustment Disorder

The course of adjustment disorder for adults is usually favorable and brief. In a 5-year follow-up of patients diagnosed with adjustment disorder, 71% of adult patients were completely well; 8% had had an intervening psychiatric disorder; and 21% had developed a major depressive disorder or alcoholism. The course of adjustment disorder is less favorable for adolescents: among adolescents, in a 5-year follow-up, 44% were well and 13% had had an intervening psychiatric disorder; among those with an intervening psychiatric disorder, 43% had a major psychiatric disorder such as schizophrenia, major depression, alcohol and substance abuse, or antisocial personality disorder (Andreasen & Hoenk, 1982).

Summary

In managing the care of patients who have been exposed to stressors, psychiatric advanced practice nurses teach that feelings of distress in response to many of life stressors are natural and have a natural course (Weigel et al., 2009). Psychiatric advanced practice nurses provide interventions that will reduce the distress of the symptoms; limit adverse effects on relationships, work, study, and pursuit of goals; and promote adaptive coping.

Key Points

- Humans owe their survival to their ability to adapt to stressors.
- Individuals' stress response is influenced by their attributes, including genetic influences, their experiences, and the presence of modifying or buffering factors.
- Allostasis refers to the active processes by which the body responds to daily events and maintains homeostasis.
- A fear/anxiety brain circuit processes response to stressors.
- Major brain structures in the fear/anxiety circuit are the amygdala, hypothalamus, hippocampus, and prefrontal and parietal cortexes.
- Many individuals are able to use their coping skills to restore conditions to as close to normal as possible after experiencing a stressful event.
- Others use maladaptive coping: increased eating, smoking, alcohol, or substance use and decreased sleep and exercise.
- Normal grief results from experiencing bereavement and is expressed in mourning.
- Complicated grief includes a sense of disbelief that the individual has died, anger and bitterness over the death, preoccupation with thoughts of the loved one, and yearning for the deceased.
- Adjustment disorder is a stress-related disorder in which experiencing a stressor has been followed by problems in adjusting to the stressor and development of symptoms of distress.

- Children with adjustment disorders have symptoms of disobedience, irritability, sadness, anger, fighting, and anxiety, and suicidal thoughts.
- Adolescents with adjustment disorder have symptoms of anxiety, depression, and disturbances of conduct such as aggressive behavior and suicidality.
- Poor school performance, skipping school, vandalism, substance use, and suicidal thoughts and behaviors may occur in children and adolescents with any type of adjustment disorder.
- There is a very short duration between first communicating ideas of suicide and completion of suicide among adolescents and young adults with adjustment disorder.
- Adjustment disorder with anxiety occurs frequently among older adults who have experienced personal stressful events, such as relocation, illnesses, or changes in social support.
- Among those in the military with adjustment disorder, nearly one-fourth develop major psychiatric disorders.
- Treatment of adjustment disorder involves (1) eliminating or reducing the stressor, (2) changing the patient's perception of the stressor, or (3) promoting adaptation to the stressor.
- The course of adjustment disorder is usually favorable and brief for adults, but it is less favorable for adolescents.

Resources

Organizations

Anxiety Disorders Association of America
www.adaa.org
Center for the Neuroscience of Fear and Anxiety
http://www.cns.nyu.edu/CNFA/

References

Akechi, T., Okuyama, T., Sugawara, Y., et al. (2004). Major depression, adjustment disorders, and post-traumatic stress disorder in terminally ill cancer patients: Associated and predictive factors. *Journal of Clinical Oncology, 22*(10), 1957-1965.

Akizuki, N., Akechi, T., Nakanishi, T., et al. (2003). Development of a brief screen interview for adjustment disorders and major depression in patients with cancer. *Cancer, 97,* 2605-2613.

American Psychiatric Association. (1968). *Diagnostic and statistical manual of mental disorders* (2nd ed.). Prepared by the Committee on Nomenclature and Statistics of the American Psychiatric Association. Washington, DC: American Psychiatric Publishing, Inc.

American Psychiatric Association. (2000). *Diagnostic and statistical manual of mental disorders* (4th ed., Text Revision). Washington, DC: American Psychiatric Publishing, Inc.

Amiel, J. M., Mathew, S. J., Garakani, A., et al. (2009). Neurobiology of anxiety disorders. In A. F. Schatzberg & C. B. Nemeroff (Eds.), *The American psychiatric publishing textbook of psychopharmacology* (pp. 965-985). Washington, DC: American Psychiatric Publishing, Inc.

Andreasen, N. C., & Black, D. W. (2006). *Introductory textbook of psychiatry* (4th ed.). Washington, DC: American Psychiatric Publishing, Inc.

Andreasen, N. C., & Hoenk, P. R. (1982). The predictive value of adjustment disorders: A follow-up study. *American Journal of Psychiatry, 139,* 584-590.

Andrews, L. B. (2008). The psychiatric interview and mental status examination. In R. E. Hales, S. C. Yudofsky, & G. O. Gabbard (Eds.), *The American psychiatric publishing textbook of psychiatry* (5th ed.) (pp. 3-17). Washington, DC: American Psychiatric Publishing, Inc.

Andrews, G., & Erskine, A. (2003). Reducing the burden of anxiety and depression disorders: The role of computerized clinician assistance. *Current Opinion in Psychiatry, 16*(1), 41-44.

Andrews, G., & Slade, T. (2001). Interpreting scores on the Kessler psychological distress scale (K1). *Australian and New Zealand Journal of Public Health, 25,* 494-497.

Barraclough, J., Palmer, S., & Dombrowe, A. (1998). Bereavement in adult life: Psychotropic drugs may be appropriate treatment. *British Medical Journal, 317*(7157), 539.

Bartolomucci, A., Palanza, P., Sacerdote, P., et al. (2005). Social factors and individual vulnerability to chronic stress exposure. *Neuroscience and Biobehavioral Reviews, 29,* 67-81.

Berghuis, D. J., & Jongsma, A. C. (2008). *The severe and persistent mental illness treatment planner.* Hoboken, NJ: John Wiley & Sons, Inc.

Bisson, J., Brayne, M., Ochberg, F., et al. (2007). Early psychosocial intervention following traumatic events. *The American Journal of Psychiatry, 164*(7), 1016-1019.

Black, D. W., & Andreasen, N. C. (2011). *Introductory textbook of psychiatry* (5th ed.). Washington, DC: American Psychiatric Publishing, Inc.

Boelen, P., de Keijser, J., van den Hout, M., et al. (2007). Treatment of complicated grief: A comparison between cognitive-behavioral therapy and supportive counseling. *Journal of Counseling and Clinical Psychology, 75,* 277-284.

Bonanno, G. A. (2001). Grief and emotion: A social-functional perspective. In M. S. Stroebe, R. O. Hansson, W. Stroebe, et al. (Eds.), *Handbook of bereavement research: Consequences, coping, and care* (pp. 493-515). Washington, DC: American Psychological Association.

Bonne, O., Crevets, W. C., Neumeister, A., et al. (2004). Neurobiology of anxiety disorders. In A. Schatzberg & C. B. Nemeroff (Eds.), *The American psychiatric publishing textbook of psychopharmacology* (3rd ed.) (pp. 775-792). Washington, DC: American Psychiatric Publishing, Inc.

Bourin, M., Bougerol, T., Guitton, B., et al. (1997). A combination of plant extracts in the treatment of outpatients with adjustment disorder with anxious mood: Controlled study versus placebo. *Fundamental & Clinical Pharmacology, 11*(2), 127-132.

Bremner, J. D. (2003). Functional neuroanatomical correlates of traumatic stress revisited 7 years later, this time with data. *Psychopharmacology Bulletin, 37*(2), 6-25.

Bremner, J. D., & Charney, D. S. (2010). Neural circuits in fear and anxiety. In E. Hollander & B. O. Rothbaum (Eds.), *The American psychiatric publishing textbook of anxiety disorders* (2nd ed.) (pp. 55-67). Washington, DC: American Psychiatric Publishing, Inc.

Brown, S. P., Westbrook, R. A., & Challagalla, G. (2005). Good cope, bad cope: Adaptive and maladaptive coping strategies following a critical negative work event. *Journal of Applied Psychology, 90*(4), 792-798.

Brugha, T. S., & Cragg, D. (1990). The list of threatening experiences: The reliability and validity of a brief Life Events Questionnaire. *Acta Psychiatrica Scandinavica, 82,* 77-81.

Casey, P. (2001). Adult adjustment disorder: A review of its current diagnostic status. *Journal of Psychiatric Practice, 7*(1), 32-40.

Casey, P., Dowrick, C., & Wilkinson, G. (2001). Adjustment disorders: Fault line in the psychiatric glossary. *The British Journal of Psychiatry, 179,* 479-481.

Charney, D. S. (2004). Psychobiological mechanisms of resilience and vulnerability: Implications for successful adaptation to extreme stress. *The American Journal of Psychiatry, 161*(2), 195-216.

Cohen, S., Kamarck, T., & Mermelstein, R. (1983). A global measure of perceived stress. *Journal of Health and Social Behavior, 24,* 385-396.

Copeland, M. E. (2002). *Dealing with the effects of trauma: A self-help guide.* Rockville, MD: U.S. Department of Health and Human Services, Substance Abuse and Mental Health Services Administration, Center for Mental Health Services.

Craig, K. J., & Chamberlain, S. R. (2010). The neuropsychology of anxiety disorders. In D. J. Stein, E. Hollander, & B. O. Rothbaum (Eds.), *Textbook of anxiety disorders* (2nd ed.) (pp. 87-102). Washington, DC: American Psychiatric Publishing, Inc.

Currier, J. M., Neimeyer, R. A., & Berman, J. S. (2008). The effectiveness of psychotherapeutic interventions for bereaved persons: A comprehensive quantitative review. *Psychological Bulletin, 134*(5), 648-661.

Deak, T., & Panksepp, J. (2004). Stress, sleep & sexuality in psychiatric disorders. In J. Panksepp (Ed.), *Textbook of biological psychiatry* (pp. 111-143). Hoboken, NJ: John Wiley & Sons, Inc.

Debiec, J., & LeDoux, J. E. (2009). The amygdala and the neural pathways of fear. In P. J. Shiromani, R. M. Keane, & J. E. LeDoux (Eds.), *Post-traumatic stress disorder: Basic science and clinical practice* (pp. 23-38). New York: Humana Press.

Dewan, M. J., Steenbarger, B. N., & Greenberg, R. P. (2008). Brief psychotherapies. In R. E. Hales, S. C. Yudofsky, & G. O. Gabbard (Eds.), *The American psychiatric publishing textbook of psychiatry* (5th ed.) (pp. 1158-1170). Washington, DC: American Psychiatric Publishing, Inc.

Dyregrov, K., Nordanger, D., & Dyregrov, A. (2003). Predictors of psychosocial distress after suicide, SIDS and accidents. *Death Studies, 27,* 143-165.

Esch, T., & Stefano, G. B. (2010). The neurobiology of stress management. *Neuro Endocrinology Letters, 31*(1), 19-39.

Fabrega, H. Jr., Mezzich, J. E., & Mezzich, A. C. (1987). Adjustment disorder as a marginal or transitional illness category in DSM-III. *Archives of General Psychiatry, 44,* 567-572.

First, M. B., & Tasman, A. (2004). Adjustment disorders. In M. B. First & A. Tasman (Eds.), *DSM-IV-TR mental disorders: Diagnosis, etiology and treatment* (pp. 1216-1227). West Essex, UK: John Wiley & Sons, Ltd.

For-Wey, L., Fei-Yin, L., & Bih-Ching, S. (2002). The relationship between life adjustment and parental bonding in military personnel with adjustment disorder in Taiwan. *Military Medicine, 167,* 678-682.

France, K. (2002). *Crisis intervention: A handbook of immediate person-to-person help* (4th ed.). Springfield, IL: Charles C Thomas Publisher, Ltd.

Friedman, M., Charney, D., & Deutch, A. (Eds.). (1995). *Neurobiological and clinical consequences of stress.* Philadelphia: Lippincott-Raven.

Galea, S., Vlahov, D., Resnick, H., et al. (2003). Trends of probable post-traumatic stress disorder in New York City after the September 11 terrorist attacks. *American Journal of Epidemiology, 158,* 514-524.

Generalized anxiety disorder: Toxic worry. (2003). *Harvard Mental Health Letter, 19*(7), 1-5

Giotakos, O., & Konstantakopoulos, G. (2002). Parenting received in childhood and early separation anxiety in male conscripts with adjustment disorder. *Military Medicine 167,* 28-33.

Goldston, D., Daniel, S. S., Reboussin, B. A., et al. (1998). Psychiatric diagnoses of previous suicide attempters, first-time attempters, and repeat attempters on an adolescent inpatient psychiatry unit. *Journal of the American Academy of Child & Adolescent Psychiatry, 37,* 924-932.

Gonzalez-Jaimes, E. I., & Turnbill-Plaza, B. (2003). Selection of psychotherapeutic treatment for adjustment disorder with depressive mood due to acute myocardial infarction. *Archives of Medical Research, 34*(4), 298-304.

Greenberg, W. M., Rosenfield, D. M., & Ortega, E. A. (1995). Adjustment disorder as an admission diagnosis. *American Journal of Psychiatry, 152,* 459-461.

Gur, S., Hermesh, H., Laufer, N., et al. (2005). Adjustment disorders: A review of diagnostic pitfalls. *Journal of the American Medical Association, 7,* 726-731.

Hageman, I., Pinborg, A., & Andersen, H. S. (2008). Complaints of stress in young soldiers strongly predispose to psychiatric morbidity and mortality: Danish national cohort study with 10-year follow-up. *Acta Psychiatrica Scandinavica, 117,* 148-155.

Hales, R. E., Yudofsky, S. C., & Gabbard, G. O. (Eds.). (2008). *The American psychiatric publishing textbook of psychiatry* (5th ed.). Washington, DC: American Psychiatric Publishing, Inc.

Hales, R. E., Yudofsky, S. C., & Gabbard, G. O. (Eds.). (2011). *Essential of psychiatry* (3rd ed.). Washington, DC: American Psychiatric Publishing, Inc.

Hameed, U., Schwartz, T. L., Malhotra, K., et al. (2005). Antidepressant treatment in the primary care office: Outcomes for adjustment disorder versus major depression. *Annals of Clinical Psychiatry, 17*(2), 71-81.

Hansell, N. (1976). *The person-in-distress: On the biosocial dynamics of adaptation.* New York: Human Sciences Press.

Hansen-Schwartz, J., Kijne, B., Johnsen, A., et al. (2005). The course of adjustment disorder in Danish male conscripts. *Nordic Journal of Psychiatry, 59,* 193-196.

Harvey, A. G., & Bryant, R. A. (2002). Acute stress disorder: A synthesis and critique. *Psychological Bulletin, 128*(6), 886-902.

Higgins, E. S., & George, M. S. (2007). *The neuroscience of clinical psychiatry: The pathophysiology of behavior and mental illness.* Philadelphia: Wolters Kluwer-Lippincott Williams & Wilkins.

Hofer, M. A. (2010). Evolutionary concepts of anxiety. In D. J. Stein, E. Hollander, & B. O. Rothbaum (Eds.), *Textbook of anxiety disorders* (2nd ed.) (pp. 129-145). Washington, DC: American Psychiatric Publishing, Inc.

Hollander, E., & Simeon, D. (2011). Anxiety disorders. In R. E. Hales, S. C. Yudofsky, & G. O. Gabbard (Eds.), *Essential of psychiatry* (3rd ed.) (pp. 185-228). Washington, DC: American Psychiatric Publishing, Inc.

Hyrkas, K., Kaunonen, M., & Paunonen, M. (1997). Recovering from the death of a spouse. *Journal of Advanced Nursing, 25,* 775-779.

James, J., & Friedman, R. (1998). *The grief recovery handbook: The action program for moving beyond death, divorce, and other losses.* New York: Harper Collins.

Jones, R., Yates, W. R., Williams, S., et al. (1999). Outcome for adjustment disorder with depressed mood: Comparison with other mood disorders. *Journal of Affective Disorders, 55*(1), 55-61.

Karlamangla, A. S., Singer, B. H., McEwen, B. S., et al. (2002). Allostatic load as a predictor of functional decline: MacArthur studies of successful aging. *Journal of Clinical Epidemiology, 55,* 696-710.

Katzman, J. W., & Tomori, O. (2005). Adjustment disorders. In B. J. Sadock & V. A. Sadock (Eds.), *Kaplan & Sadock's comprehensive textbook of psychiatry* (8th ed.) (pp. 2055-2062). Philadelphia: Lippincott, Williams & Wilkins.

Kellerman, M., Jehete, I., Gesztelyi, R., et al. (1994). Screening for depressive symptoms in acute phase of a stroke. *General Hospital Psychiatry, 21,* 116-121.

Kimonides, V. G., Khatibi, N. H., Svendsen, C. N., et al. (1998). Dehydroepiandrosterone (DHEA) and DHEA-sulfate (DHEAS) protect hippocampal neurons against excitatory amine acid-induced neurotoxicity. *Proceedings of the National Academy of Science, USA, 95,* 1852-1857.

Korte, S. M., Koolhaas, J. M., Wingfield, J. C., et al. (2005). The Darwinian concept of stress: Benefits of allostasis and costs of allostatic load and the trade-offs in health and disease. *Neuroscience & Biobehavioral Reviews, 29*(1), 3-38.

Kovacs, M., Gatsonis, C., Pollock, M., et al. (1994). A controlled prospective study of DSM-III adjustment disorder in childhood: Short-term prognosis and long-term predictive validity. *Archives of General Psychiatry, 51,* 535-541.

Kovacs, M., Ho, V., & Pollock, M. H. (1995). Criterion and predictive validity of the diagnosis of adjustment disorder: A prospective study of youths with new-onset insulin-dependent diabetes mellitus. *American Journal Psychiatry, 152*(4), 523-528.

Kowalski, S. D., & Bondmass, M. D. (2008). Physiological and psychological symptoms of grief in widows. *Research in Nursing & Health, 31,* 23-30.

Kryzhanovskaya, L., & Canterbury, R. (2001). Suicidal behavior in patients with adjustment disorders. *Crisis: The Journal of Crisis Intervention and Suicide Prevention, 22*(3), 125-131.

Kugaya, A., Akechi, T., Okuyama, T., et al. (2000). Prevalence, predictive factors and screening for psychological distress in patients with newly diagnosed head and neck cancers. *Cancer, 88,* 2817-2823.

Lantz, M. S. (2008). Adjustment disorders in the older adult. *Clinical Geriatrics, 16*(5), 17-19.

Lazarus, A. A. (1992). The multimodal approach to the treatment of minor depression. *American Journal of Psychotherapy, 46*(1), 50-57.

LeDoux, J. (2002). *Synaptic self: How our brains become who we are.* New York: Viking Press.

LeDoux, J. E., & Gorman, J. M. (2001). A call to action: Overcoming anxiety through active coping. *American Journal of Psychiatry, 158*(12), 1953-1995.

Lundin, T. (1994). The treatment of acute trauma: Posttraumatic stress disorder prevention. *Psychiatric Clinics of North America, 17,* 385-391.

Lupien, S. J., McEwen, B. S., Gunnar, M. R., et al. (2009). Effects of stress throughout the lifespan on the brain, behaviour, and cognition. *Neuroscience, 10,* 434-445.

Maercker, A., Forstmeier, S., Enzler, A., et al. (2008). Adjustment disorders, posttraumatic stress disorder, and depressive disorders in old age: Findings from a community survey. *Comprehensive Psychiatry, 49*(2), 113-120.

Maina, G., Forner, F., & Bogetto, F. (2005). Randomized controlled trial comparing brief dynamic and supportive therapy with waiting list condition in minor depressive disorders. *Psychotherapy & Psychosomatics, 74*(1), 43-50.

Markowitz, J. C. (2008). Interpersonal psychotherapy. In R. E. Hales, S. C. Yudofsky, & G. O. Gabbard (Eds.), *The American psychiatric publishing textbook of psychiatry* (5th ed.). (pp. 1191-1210). Washington, DC: American Psychiatric Publishing, Inc.

Mathew, S. J., Price, R. B., & Charney, D. S. (2008). Recent advances in the neurobiology of anxiety disorders: Implications for novel therapeutics. *American Journal of Medical Genetics. Part C, Seminars in Medical Genetics 148C*(2), 89-98.

Mayo Clinic. (March 17, 2011). *Adjustment disorders.* Retrieved from http://www.mayoclinic.com/health/adjustment-disorders/DS00584.

Mazure, C. (1998). Life stressors as risk factors in depression. *Clinical Psychology: Science and Practice, 5,* 291-313.

McEwen, B. S. (2000). Allostasis and allostatic load: Implications for neuropsychopharmacology. *Neuropsychopharmacology, 22*(2), 108-124.

McEwen, B. S. (2004). Protection and damage from acute and chronic stress: Allostasis and allostatic overload and relevance to the pathophysiology of psychiatric disorders. *Annals of the New York Academy of Sciences, 1032,* 1-7.

McEwen, B. S. (2005). Stressed or stressed out: What is the difference? *Journal of Psychiatry and Neuroscience, 30*(5), 315-318.

McEwen, B. S. (2007). Physiology and neurobiology of stress and adaptation: Central role of the brain. *Psychological Review, 87,* 873-904.

McEwen, B. S. (2008). Central effects of stress hormones in health and disease: Understanding the protective and damaging effects of stress and stress mediators. *European Journal of Pharmacology, 583*(2-3), 174-185.

McEwen, B. S., & Wingfield, J. C. (2003). The concept of allostasis in biology and biomedicine. *Hormones & Behavior, 43*(1), 2-15.

Mihelich, M. L. (2000). Eye movement desensitization and reprocessing treatment of adjustment disorder: Dissertation. *Abstracts International, 61*(2B), 1091.

O'Connor, M-F, Wellisch, D. K., Eisenberger, A. L., et al. (2008). Craving love? Enduring grief activates brain's reward center. *NeuroImage, 42*(2), 969-972.

Oxman, T. E., Barrett, J. E., Freeman, D. H., et al. (1994). Frequency and correlates of adjustment disorder relates to cardiac surgery in older patients. *Psychosomatics, 35,* 557-568.

Panksepp, J. (2004). *Textbook of biological psychiatry.* Hoboken, NJ: Wiley-Liss.

Parkes, C. M. (1998). Editorial comments. *Bereavement Care,* 17, 18.

Parry, J. K. (1994). Death review: An important component of grief resolution. *Social Work in Health Care, 20*(2), 97-107.

Parsons, T. D., & Rizzo, A. A. (2008). Affective outcomes of virtual reality exposure therapy for anxiety and specific phobias: A meta-analysis. *Journal of Behavior Therapy and Experimental Psychiatry, 39,* 250-261

Pelkonen, M., Marttunen, M., Henriksson, M., et al. (2007). Adolescent adjustment disorder: Precipitant stressors and distress symptoms of 89 outpatients. *European Psychiatry, 22,* 288-295.

Perez Jimenez, J. P., Gomez Bajo, G. J., Lopez Castillo, J. J., et al. (1994). Psychiatric consultation and post-traumatic stress disorder in burned patients. *Burns, 20,* 532-536.

Pollen, I. S., & Holland, J. (1992). A model for counseling the medically ill: The Linda Pollin Foundation approach. *General Hospital Psychiatry, 14*(Suppl 6), 15-25.

Portzky, G., Audenaert, K., & van Heeringen, K. (2005). Adjustment disorder and the course of the suicidal process in adolescents. *Journal of Affective Disorders, 87,* 265-270.

Prigerson, H. G., Frank, E., Kasl, S. V., et al. (1995). Complicated grief and bereavement-related depression as distinct disorders: Preliminary empirical validation in elderly bereaved spouses. *American Journal of Psychiatry, 152*(1), 22-30.

Prigerson, H., & Jacobs, S. (2001). Traumatic grief as a distinct disorder: A rationale, consensus criteria, and a preliminary empirical test. In M. S. Stroebe, R. O. Hansson, W. Stroebe, et al. (Eds.), *Handbook of bereavement research: Consequences, coping, and care* (pp. 613-645). Washington, DC: American Psychological Association.

Prigerson, H., Maciejewski, P. K., Reynolds, C. F., et al. (1995). Inventory of complicated grief: A scale to measure maladaptive symptoms of loss. *Psychiatric Research, 59,* 65-79.

Ray, O. (2004). How the mind hurts and heals the body. *American Psychologist, 59*(1), 7-13.

Reagan, L. P., Grillo, C., & Piroli, G. G. (2008). The As and Ds of stress: Metabolic, morphological and behavioral consequences. *European Journal of Pharmacology, 585,* 64-75.

Riddle, J. R., Smith, T. C., Smith, B., et al., for the Millennium Cohort Study Team (2007). Millennium cohort: The 2001-2003 baseline prevalence of mental disorders in the U. S. Military. *Journal of Clinical Epidemiology, 60,* 192-201.

Roberts, K. F., & Berry, P. H. (2002). Grief and bereavement. In K. K. Kuebler, P. H. Berry, & D. E. Heidrich (Eds.), *End of life care* (pp. 53-63). Philadelphia: Saunders.

Rodrigues, S. M., LeDoux, J. E., & Sapolsky, R. M. (2009). The influence of stress hormones on fear circuitry. *Annual Review of Neuroscience, 32,* 289-293.

Roth, A. J., Kornblith, A. B., Batel-Copel, L., et al. (1998). Rapid screening for psychologic distress in men with prostate carcinoma: A pilot study. *Cancer, 82*(10), 1904-1908.

Rovio, S., Kareholt, I., Helkala, E. L., et al. (2005). Leisure-time physical activity at midlife and the risk of dementia and Alzheimer's disease. *Lancet Neurology, 4,* 705-711.

Rundell, J. R. (2006). Demographics of and diagnoses in Operation Enduring Freedom and Operation Iraqi Freedom personnel who were psychiatrically evacuated from the theater of operations. *General Hospital Psychiatry, 28,* 352-356.

Runeson, B. S., Beskow, J., & Waern, M. (1996). The suicidal process in suicides among young people. *Acta Psychiatrica Scandinavica, 93,* 35-42.

Schatzberg, A. F. (1990). Anxiety and adjustment disorder: A treatment approach. *Journal of Clinical Psychiatry, 51*(Suppl 1), 20-24.

Schatzberg, A. F., & Nemeroff, C. B. (Eds.). (2006). *Essentials of clinical psychopharmacology* (2nd ed.). Washington, DC: American Psychiatric Publishing, Inc.

Schnyder, R., & Valach, L. (1997). Suicide attempters in a psychiatric emergency room population. *General Hospital Psychiatry, 19,* 119-129.

Seeman, T. E., Singer, B. H., Ryff, C. D., et al. (2002). Social relationships, gender, and allostatic load across two age cohorts. *Psychosomatic Medicine, 64,* 395-406.

Selye, H. (1936). A syndrome produced by diverse nocuous agents. *Nature, 138,* 32.

Sgoifo, A., Coe, C., Parmigiani, S., et al. (2005). Individual differences in behavior and physiology: Causes and consequences. *Neuroscience and Biobehavioral Reviews, 29,* 1-2.

Shear, K. (2005). Bereavement-related depression in the elderly. *Primary Psychiatry, 12*(8 Suppl 7), 3-9.

Shear, K., Frank, E., Houck, P., et al. (2005). Treatment of complicated grief: A randomized controlled trial. *Journal of American Medical Association, 293*(21), 2601-2608.

Shelby, J., & McCance, K. L. (2002). Stress & disease. In K. L. McCance & S. E. Huether (Eds.), *Pathophysiology: The biologic basis for disease in adults & children* (4th ed.) (pp. 272-289). St. Louis: Mosby.

Shelton, C. J. (2004). Diagnosis and management of anxiety disorders. *The Journal of the American Orthopedic Association, 104*(3 Suppl 1), 2-5.

Shima, S., Kitagawa, W., Kitamura, T., et al. (1994). Post-stroke depression. *General Hospital Psychiatry, 16,* 286-289.

Skopek, M. A., & Perkins, R. (1998). Deliberate exposure to motor vehicle exhaust gas: The psychosocial profile of attempted suicide. *Australian and New Zealand Journal of Psychiatry, 32,* 830-838.

Smith, T. C., Zamorski, M., Smith, B., et al., for the Millennium Cohort Study Team. (2007). The physical and mental health of a large military cohort: Baseline functional health status of the Millennium Cohort. *BMC Public Health, 7,* 340.

Snyder, S., & Strain, J. J. (1989). Differentiation of major depression and adjustment disorder with depressed mood in the medical setting. *General Hospital Psychiatry, 12,* 159-165.

Solomon, S. D. (1999). Interventions for acute trauma response. *Current Opinions in Psychiatry, 12,* 175-180.

Spar, J. E., & La Rue, A. (2006). *Clinical manual of geriatric psychiatry.* Washington, DC: American Psychiatric Publishing, Inc.

Spiegel, D. (1996). Cancer and depression. *British Journal of Psychiatry, 168*(Suppl 30), 104-116.

Strain, J. J., & Klipstein, K. G. (2007). Adjustment disorder. In G. O. Gabbard (Ed.), *Gabbard's treatments of psychiatric disorders* (4th ed.) (pp. 573-579). Washington, DC: American Psychiatric Publishing, Inc.

Strain, J. J., Klipstein, K. G., & Newcorn, J. H. (2008). Adjustment disorder. In R. E. Hales, S. C. Yudofsky, & G. O. Gabbard (Eds.), *The American psychiatric publishing textbook of psychiatry* (5th ed.) (pp. 755-775). Washington, DC: American Psychiatric Publishing, Inc.

Strain, J. J., Klipstein, K. G., & Newcorn, J. H. (2011). Adjustment disorders. In R. E. Hales, S. C. Yudofsky, & G. O. Gabbard (Eds.), *Essentials of psychiatry* (3rd ed.) (pp. 255-269). Washington, DC: American Psychiatric Publishing, Inc.

Stroebe, W., Schut, H., & Stroebe, M. S. (2005). Grief work, disclosure and counseling: Do they help the bereaved. *Clinical Psychology Review, 25,* 395-414.

Stroebe, M., Schut, H., & Stroebe, W. (2007). Health outcomes of bereavement. *Lancet, 370,* 1960-1973.

Stroebe, M. S., Stroebe, W., & Schut, H. (2001). Gender differences in adjustment to bereavement: An empirical and theoretical review. *Review of General Psychology, 5,* 62-83.

Sullivan, M.J., Winshenker, B., Mikail, S., et al. (1995). Screening for major depression in the early stages of multiple sclerosis. *Canadian Journal of Neurological Sciences, 22*(3), 228-231.

Takei, N., & Sugihara, G. (2006). Diagnostic ambiguity of subthreshold depression: Minor depression vs. adjustment disorder with depressive mood. *Acta Psychiatrica Scandinavica, 114,* 144.

Taylor, S. E., Klein, L. C., Lewis, B. P., et al. (2000). Biobehavioral responses to stress in females: Tend-and-befriend, not fight-or-flight. *Psychological Reviews, 107*(3), 411-429.

Taylor, F. G., & Marshall, W. L. (1977). Experimental analysis of a cognitive-behavioral therapy for depression. *Cognitive Therapy & Research, 1,* 59-72.

Tiet, Q. Q., Finney, J. W., & Moos, R. H. (2006). Recent sexual abuse, physical abuse, and suicide attempts among male veterans seeking psychiatric treatment. *Psychiatric Services, 57*(1), 107-113.

Tripodianakis, J., Markianos, M., Sarantidis, D., et al. (2000). Neurochemical variables in subjects with adjustment disorder after suicide attempts. *European Psychiatry: The Journal of the Association of European Psychiatrists, 15*(3), 190-195.

University of Texas at Austin Counseling and Mental Health Center. (2004). *Stress signals.* Retrieved from http://www.utexas.edu/student/cmhac/booklets/stress/stress.html

Van der Klink, J. J. L., Blank, W. B., Schene, A. H., et al. (2003). Reducing long term sickness absence by an activating intervention in adjustment disorders: A cluster randomized controlled design. *Occupation Environmental Medicine, 60,* 429-437.

van der Kolk, B. A. (2006). The body keeps the score. Approaches to the psychobiology of posttraumatic stress disorder. In B. A. van der Kolk, A. C. McFarlane, & L. Weisaeth (Eds.), *Traumatic stress: The effects of overwhelming experience on mind, body and society* (pp. 214-241). New York: Guilford Press.

Verfaellie, M., & Vasterling, J. J. (2009). Memory in PTSD: A neurocognitive approach. In P. J. Shiromani, T. M. Keane, & J. E. LeDoux (Eds.), *Post-traumatic stress disorder: Basic science and clinical practice* (pp. 105-130). New York: Humana Press.

Volz, H. P., & Kieser, M. (1997). Kava-kava extract WS1490 versus placebo in anxiety disorders: A randomized placebo controlled 25 week outpatient trial. *Pharmacopsychiatry, 30,* 1-5.

Wai, B. H., Hong, C., & Heok, K. E. (1999). Suicidal behavior among young people in Singapore. *General Hospital Psychiatry, 21,* 128-133.

Weigel, M. B., Purselle, D. C., D'Orio, B., et al. (2009). Treatment of psychiatric emergencies. In A. F. Schatzberg & C. B. Nemeroff (Eds.), *American psychiatric publishing textbook of psychopharmacology* (4th ed.) (pp. 1287-1308). Washington, DC: American Psychiatric Publishing, Inc.

Werner, E. E., & Smith, R. S. (1982). *Vulnerable but invincible.* New York: McGraw-Hill.

Wheeler, K. (2008). Processing trauma. In K. Wheeler (Ed.), *Psychotherapy for the advanced practice psychiatric nurse* (pp. 310-329). St. Louis: Mosby Elsevier.

Whitfield, G., Hinshelwood, R., Pashley, A., et al. (2006). The impact of a novel computerized CBT CD rom (overcoming depression) offered to patients referred to clinical psychology. *Behavioural and Cognitive Psychotherapy, 34*(1), 1-11.

Wilcox, S., Evenson, K. R., Aragaki, A., et al. (2003). The effects of widowhood on physical and mental health, health behaviors and health outcomes. The Women's Health Initiative. *Health Psychology, 22,* 513-522.

Winston, A. (2008). Supportive psychotherapy. In R. E. Hales, S. C. Yudofsky, & G. O. Gabbard (Eds.), *The American psychiatric publishing textbook of psychiatry* (5th ed.) (pp. 1257-1277). Washington, DC: American Psychiatric Publishing, Inc.

Wise, M. G. (1988). Adjustment disorders and impulse control disorders not otherwise classified. In J. A. Talbot, R. Hales, & S. C. Yudofsky (Eds.), *Textbook of psychiatry.* Washington, DC: American Psychiatric Publishing, Inc.

Woelk, H., Arnoldt, K. H., Kieser, M., et al. (2007). Ginkgo biloba special extract EGv761 R in generalized anxiety disorder and adjustment disorder with anxious mood: A randomized, double-blind, placebo-controlled trial. *Journal of Psychiatric Research, 41,* 472-480.

Wortman, C., & Silver, R. (2001). The myths of coping with loss revisited. In M. S. Stroebe, R. O. Hansson, W. Stroebe, et al. (Eds.), *Handbook of bereavement research: Consequences, coping, and care* (pp. 405-429). Washington, DC: American Psychological Association.

Zisook, S., Shuchter, S. R., Pedrelli, P., et al. (2001). Bupropion sustained release bereavement: Results of an open trial. *Journal of Clinical Psychiatry, 62,* 227-230.

Zonnebelt-Smeenge, S. J., & DeVries, R. C. (1998). *Getting to the other side of grief.* Grand Rapids, MI: Baker Books.

Zygmont, M., Prigerson, H. G., Houch, P. R., et al. (1998). A post hoc comparison of paroxetine and nortriptyline for symptoms of traumatic grief. *Journal of Clinical Psychiatry, 59*(5), 241-245.

Answers to Case Study 9-1 Questions

1. Diagnosing adjustment disorder in clinical practice can be difficult because of overlapping of symptoms among the various subcategories of adjustment disorder and other psychiatric syndromes, such as generalized anxiety and major depression. The diagnosis is based on clinical judgment concerning the response to a stressful event and/or its consequences. The key requirement for diagnosing adjustment disorder is either a response to a stressful event that has occurred within the last 3 months that is in excess of what might be expected from exposure to the stressor, or significant impairment in social, academic, or occupational functioning.
2. Adjustment disorder carries the same risk factors for self-harm as do other psychiatric diagnoses. The studies to date indicate that suicide is more likely to be carried out under the influence of alcohol and to be unplanned.
3. There are a myriad of adjustments necessary when an individual enters a new culture. The inability to read or speak English provides the greatest barrier as it prevents the individual from obtaining even basic entry-level jobs. For many immigrants, any type of work provides feelings of self-respect and independence and the sense of fulfilling their American dream. Work also provides a source of possible social contacts and decreases feelings of alienation.

CHAPTER 10

Anxiety Disorders: Phobic Disorders, Generalized Anxiety Disorder, Social Anxiety Disorder, and Panic Disorder

Eris F. Perese, APRN-PMH

Anxiety disorders were once thought of as the psychiatric disorders closest to normal mental functioning: people with anxiety were normal but worried, or "the worried well" (DuPont, DuPont, & Rice, 2002, p. 475). Now, anxiety disorders are viewed as major psychiatric disorders that cause great distress and impairment of functioning and that are associated with increased morbidity and mortality. The most frequently occurring anxiety disorders are phobic disorders, generalized anxiety disorder (GAD); social anxiety disorder (SAD); panic disorder with and without agoraphobia; agoraphobia; acute stress disorder (ASD); posttraumatic stress disorder (PTSD); and obsessive-compulsive disorder (OCD) (Andreasen & Black, 2006). Anxiety disorders must be differentiated from anxiety due to other causes, such as medical conditions, medications, or illicit substances (Table 10-1).

Phobic disorders, GAD, SAD, and panic disorder are discussed in this chapter. ASD and PTSD are discussed in Chapter 11, and OCD is discussed in Chapter 12.

Phobic Disorders

Black and Andreasen (2011) described phobic disorders as "an irrational fear of specific objects, places, or situations or activities" (p. 183). Phobic disorders are characterized by a persistent, unreasonable fear that is triggered by the presence of an object or situation and by the desire to avoid the object or situation (Gamble, Harvey, & Rapee, 2010). Phobias have three components: (1) anticipatory anxiety, which is caused by thinking of the possibility of experiencing the feared stimulus; (2) fear that is not so much of the *object* or situation as it is of the *outcome* that might result from contact with the object or of being in the situation; and (3) avoidance behaviors that are used to prevent anxiety (Hales, Yudofsky, & Gabbard, 2011). Phobias can be classified as follows:

- Animal type (fear of animals)
- Environmental type (fear of heights, storms, thunder, fire, or water)
- Situational type (fear of enclosed places, flying, driving, elevators, tunnels)
- Blood-injection-injury type (fear of the sight of blood, injections, or any injury)
- Other type (choking or vomiting; and in children, fear of strangers or loud sounds) (Gamble et al., 2010)

The stimulus almost always causes an anxiety response. Individuals recognize that the response is excessive or unrealistic and they will avoid situations that are likely to put them in contact with the stimulus. However, continual avoidance of feared situations may compromise their personal, vocational, and social functioning. (See the *Diagnostic and Statistical Manual of Mental Disorders*, 4th edition, Text Revision *[DSM-IV-TR]* diagnostic criteria for specific phobias [American Psychiatric Association, 2000, pp. 449-450].)

Epidemiology

Among the general population, the prevalence of phobic disorders is 10% (Emmelkamp & Wittchen, 2009). They occur twice as often in women than in men, except for the blood-injection-injury phobia, which occurs equally in men and women (Becker, Rinck, Turke, et al., 2007; Gamble et al., 2010). Phobias pertaining to animals, blood, storms, and water tend to begin in early childhood or before age 12 years (Black & Andreasen, 2011). Phobias of heights tend

TABLE 10-1 MEDICAL CONDITIONS, MEDICATIONS, AND SUBSTANCES CAUSING ANXIETY

Medical Conditions Causing Anxiety	Medications Causing Anxiety	Substances Causing Anxiety
Neurological Disorders: Brain tumors, postconcussion syndrome, cerebrovascular disease, multiple sclerosis, epilepsy (especially temporal lobe epilepsy), cerebral syphilis, encephalopathies	Over-the-counter cold medications	Caffeine, monosodium glutamate, lysergic acid diethylamide (LSD)
Cardiovascular and Circulatory Disorders: Angina, arrhythmias, congestive heart failure, anemia, atrial fibrillation, myocardial infarction, coronary insufficiency, mitral valve prolapse	Antidepressants, e.g., tricyclic antidepressants and selective serotonin reuptake inhibitors (SSRIs) Antipsychotic medication Thyroid hormones	Methylenedioxymethamphetamine (MDMA)
Medical Disorders: Migraine headaches, severe pain, irritable bowel syndrome, peptic ulcer, thyrotoxicosis, hypoglycemia, and hyperglycemia Withdrawal from alcohol, benzodiazepines, and sedative-hypnotics	Corticosteroids Aminophylline and related compounds Sympathomimetics (agonists for norepinephrine) Also found in decongestants, bronchodilators, and diet pills	Hallucinogens, cocaine, amphetamine, marijuana
Endocrine Disorders: Pituitary dysfunction; thyroid (hyperthyroidism or hypothyroidism) or adrenal dysfunction; Addison's disease, Cushing's syndrome; pheochromocytoma (vascular tumor of adrenal medulla or sympathetic paraganglia with hypersecretion of epinephrine and norepinephrine)	Oral contraceptives	Inhalants
Inflammatory Disorders: Lupus erythematosus, rheumatoid arthritis	Anticonvulsants	Phencyclidine
Vitamin B_{12}	Antihypertensive agents; anti-inflammatory agents, anti-parkinsonian agents, and antihistamines; digitalis Caffeine Herbal medicines such as ginseng (Fricchione, 2004; Hansen, 2004)	Withdrawal syndromes; e.g., alcohol, narcotics, sedative-hypnotics

Sources: Black & Andreasen, 2011; First & Tasman, 2004; Sadock & Sadock, 2007.

to begin in the teens, and situational phobias tend to begin in late teens to middle twenties (First & Tasman, 2004; Hollander & Simeon, 2008). Phobias have been found to be less prevalent in older adults (Emmelkamp & Wittchen, 2009) and in Asian and Hispanic adults (Stinson, Dawson, Chou, et al., 2007).

Etiology

Specific phobias tend to run in families, although the same phobia may not be evidenced (First & Tasman, 2004). There seems to be a stronger genetic influence for blood-injection-injury phobia (Gamble et al., 2010). Maladaptive cognitive functioning, such as negative self-statements or unrealistic thoughts about the consequences of exposure to a feared object or situation, may play a role in the development of specific phobias (Gamble et al.). Development of specific phobias has also been found to be associated with trauma to the brain. Among individuals who experienced a traumatic brain injury, 6% developed specific phobias (Hibbard, Uysal, Kepler, et al., 1998), and among individuals with a history of a head injury in their lifetime, 11.2% had specific phobias (Silver, Kramer, Greenwald, et al., 2001).

Biological Basis

The biological basis of phobias is not well understood (Black & Andreasen, 2011). Research suggests that phobic responses are the result of dysfunction of the neural circuitry involved in attention (anterior cingulate cortex, prefrontal cortex, insula, amygdala, and thalamus) that is manifested in an overestimation of the danger of the phobic stimulus or deficient emotional regulation (Britton, Gold, Deckersbach, et al., 2009). For example, in a study of spider phobia, activity was increased in the amygdala (involved in fear responses), in the insula (involved in registering disgust), and in the dorsal anterior cerebral cortex (involved in expression of fear responses), and activity was decreased in the ventromedial prefrontal cortex, which is involved in automatic regulation of emotion (Hermann, Schafer, Walter, et al., 2009).

Clinical Presentation

Individuals with specific phobias do not usually seek treatment (Black & Andreasen, 2011). They accept their fear as part of their personality and avoid the feared object (Gamble et al., 2010). Individuals with specific phobias—with the exception of those with blood-injection-injury phobia—manifest two sets of symptoms following exposure or anticipation of exposure to a feared stimulus: (1) symptoms related to sympathetic nervous system activation, which include unsteadiness, dryness of the mouth, pounding heart, nausea, sweating, shortness of breath, feelings of choking or being smothered, chest pain, chest discomfort, faintness, trembling, fear of dying, fear of going crazy, feelings of unreality, and perception of impending doom; and (2) symptoms of avoidance behaviors; if unable to avoid the situation, the individual will tolerate it with increased anxiety and escape as quickly as possible (Gamble et al.).

Individuals with blood-injection-injury phobia may have one of two sets of symptoms: (1) sympathetic nervous system activation as described above, or (2) fainting. Fainting is due to a sharp drop of blood pressure after an initial rise on exposure to the feared situation. Individuals with blood-injection-injury phobia are more likely to describe disgust than fear on exposure to the feared object.

In clinical practice, there appears to be a considerable overlap of the subtypes (Gamble et al., 2010). Nearly three-fourths of individuals reporting one specific phobia subtype also reported symptoms of other specific phobia subtypes (Stinson et al., 2007).

Differential Diagnosis

Several psychiatric disorders are associated with fear and avoidance of stimuli or situations (Table 10-2). Differentiating specific phobia from other disorders depends on evaluating the individual's targeted fear, the reasons for avoidance, and the number or range of situations feared (First & Tasman, 2004; Gamble et al., 2010). The individual with a specific phobia does not usually complain of generalized anxiety and often has insight into the irrationality of the phobia.

Treatment

Although individuals with specific phobias are not usually impaired by their phobia and do not seek treatment (Davidson, Connor, & Zhang, 2009), they may do so if the phobia interferes with social or vocational activities, such as fear of water or fear of flying. The goal of treatment is to reduce distress and functional impairment by decreasing fear and avoidance. Interventions that help to reduce the distress that results from specific phobias include exposure therapy, pharmacotherapy, and psychosocial interventions.

Exposure Therapy

The first-line treatment choice is exposure therapy, which has the goal of extinguishing fear associated with a specific phobia (Davidson et al., 2009). Treatment interventions include in vivo exposure (live exposure to the phobic stimulus); virtual reality exposure, in which the patient is exposed to a virtual environment that arouses fear and anxiety, such as flying or heights; and computer-aided self-help exposure programs (Krijn, Emmelkamp, Olafsson, et al., 2004b). Virtual reality has been found to be as effective as in vivo exposure in the treatment of flying phobia (Rothbaum, Hodges, Anderson, et al., 2002) and height phobia (Krijn, Emmelkamp, Biemond, et al., 2004a). Treating blood-injection-injury phobias with muscle tension exercises—such as rapidly and frequently tensing various muscle groups during exposure—has been found to be more effective than exposure alone (Gamble et al., 2010; Swinson, Antony, Bleau, et al., 2006).

Pharmacotherapy

No drug has been approved by the U.S. Food and Drug Administration (FDA) for the treatment of specific phobias (Davidson et al., 2009). The antidepressants paroxetine (Paxil) and escitalopram (Lexapro) have been found to reduce the distress of patients with specific phobias (Davidson et al.), and selective serotonin reuptake inhibitors (SSRIs) have been found to reduce panic sensations for situational phobias that are similar to panic disorder, such as claustrophobia (First & Tasman, 2004). Recently, there has been interest in using medications that have been found to facilitate new learning, such as D-cycloserine (Seromycin), in combination with exposure therapy. Early results suggest that the combination treatment is associated with improvement and that the improvement is maintained (Ressler, Rothbaum, Tannenbaum, et al., 2004).

TABLE 10-2 DIFFERENTIAL DIAGNOSIS OF SPECIFIC PHOBIAS

Other Psychiatric Disorder	Differentiating Characteristics of Other Psychiatric Disorder
Panic disorder with agoraphobia	Avoidance of many different situations because of fear of having a panic attack
Social phobia	Avoidance of social situations because of fear of embarrassment or rejection
Avoidance in post-traumatic stress disorder	Avoidance of stimuli that trigger reminders of a previously experienced life-threatening event Presence of intrusive thoughts and nightmares
Avoidance in obsessive-compulsive disorder	Avoidance is associated with the content of obsessions (e.g., dirt) Presence of obsessions and compulsions
Avoidance in psychotic disorders	Avoidance is in response to a delusion (without the recognition that the fear is excessive or unreasonable) Lack of insight

Sources: First, Frances, & Pincus, 2002; Gamble, Harvey, & Rapee, 2010.

Psychosocial Interventions

Psychosocial interventions used for specific phobias that have been found to be effective include exposure-based treatments (real-life exposure and computer-based exposure) that involve repeatedly approaching fear-provoking situations until they no longer cause fear. Effectiveness is greater when the exposure sessions are spaced close together, when a longer duration of exposure is used, when there is limited use of avoidance strategies (such as distraction or being accompanied by a partner), when real-life exposure is used rather than exposure in imagination, and when there is some therapist involvement in the sessions. Computer-administered treatments have been used successfully for specific phobias, such as fear of spiders (Smith, Kirkby, Montgomery, et al., 1997).

Course

Some childhood phobias—mostly fear of animals—resolve without treatment. However, phobias that continue into adolescence are less likely to resolve. Complete spontaneous remission is rare, occurring in approximately 10% of those with phobias. Treatment with exposure therapy is beneficial. Pharmacotherapy has not been found to have a lasting benefit (Emmelkamp & Wittchen, 2009).

Key Points

- Phobic disorders are fear of specific objects, places, situations, or activities.
- Phobias have three components: (1) the anticipatory anxiety; (2) the fear; and (3) the avoidance behaviors.
- The first-line treatment choice for phobic disorders is exposure therapy.
- Although some childhood phobias resolve, other phobias tend to be chronic conditions.

Generalized Anxiety Disorder (GAD)

GAD is characterized by excessive anxiety and pervasive worry that have been present for at least 6 months (Allgulander, Bandelow, Hollander, et al., 2003). Some researchers believe that these criteria—6-month duration and excessive worry—should be reexamined because patients often have chronic symptoms and impairment of functioning (Ruscio, Lane, & Roy-Byrne, 2005) and because many patients have symptoms for 1 to 5 months (Kessler, Brandenburg, Lane, et al., 2005b). Additional criteria listed in the *DSM-IV-TR* (American Psychiatric Association, 2000) include restlessness, fatigue, poor concentration, irritability, muscle tension, and poor sleep. The hypervigilance and somatic symptoms that commonly occur in GAD are especially distressing to patients (Papp, 2010; Rynn, Russell, Erickson, et al., 2008).

GAD is associated with impaired cognitive functioning (Martin, Kubzansky, LeWinn, et al., 2007); with impairment of functioning in interpersonal, social, and vocational roles (Olfson, Fireman, Weissman, et al., 1997); and with diminished sense of good health, well-being, and quality of life (Allgulander, 2010; Ballenger, Davidson, Lecrubier, et al., 2001; Rynn et al., 2008). Patients with GAD worry about everyday things, such as work, finances, health, repairs, tardiness, being accepted in social situations, confronting others, their competence, the welfare of family members, and their marital relationship. Their degree of worrying is out of proportion both to the likelihood that something adverse will happen and to the impact if something does occur (Andreasen & Black, 2006). Individuals with GAD are more likely to think that negative things will happen than that positive things will happen, and they think that they do not have the coping skills to manage if something bad or dangerous happens (Huppert & Sanderson, 2010). They experience greater emotional dysregulation than individuals without GAD; for example, they experience greater intensity of emotions, poorer understanding of their emotions, more negative reactions to emotional experiences, less ability to self-soothe, and greater difficulty managing their emotional reactions (Mennin, Heimberg, Turk, et al., 2005).

Children worry about their ability to do things or about their level of performance on things such as homework. Their anxiety is often expressed in relation to schoolwork or sporting activities. They may also express anxiety about events such as earthquakes and terrorist attacks (see *DSM-IV-TR* for specific criteria for Generalized Anxiety Disorder [American Psychiatric Association, 2000]).

Epidemiology

Prevalence

The 1-year prevalence of GAD in adults is 6% to 8% (Fyer & Brown, 2009). The prevalence of GAD in school-age children is approximately 3% (Sadock & Sadock, 2007), but it has been reported to be as high as 10% in children and adolescents (Keeton, Kolos, & Walkup, 2009).

Onset

Onset in adults tends to be after the age of 20 years (American Psychiatric Association, 2000; Papp, 2010), and onset in children tends to be between 8 and 9 years (Keeton et al., 2009). Based on studies of continuity of anxiety disorders, some researchers believe that GAD is a continuation of childhood anxiety disorders. For example, 42% of 26-year-old patients with GAD had a history of childhood anxiety disorders—overanxious disorder, separation disorder, and phobias (Poulton, Pine, & Harrington, 2009). Onset of GAD may follow an episode of depression (Kandel, Schwartz, & Jessell, 2000) or a specific negative event that occurred in the year prior to the onset of GAD (First & Tasman, 2004). Other patients develop GAD after the birth of their first child, in which case the onset of GAD appears to be related to their sense of increased responsibility and their desire to be perfect in childrearing (Huppert & Sanderson, 2010).

There is also late onset of GAD, after age 50. Whereas early-onset GAD is associated with more psychiatric comorbidities and greater severity of worrying, late-onset GAD is associated with more functional impairment due to physical problems (Le Roux, Gatz, & Wetherell, 2005). Among older adults, GAD frequently co-occurs with other anxiety disorders. The rate of anxiety problems among older adults may be as high as 20% (Sheikh, 1992).

Gender

GAD is diagnosed twice as often in women as in men (Pollack, 2009). There is increased risk for development of GAD during pregnancy and the postpartum period; if GAD is already present before pregnancy or the postpartum period, its severity tends to increase (Cohen, Nonacs, & Viguera, 2004).

Culture

In some societies, anxiety is expressed through somatic symptoms (American Psychiatric Association, 2000). Patients of certain cultures may complain of feelings of heat in the head, while patients from other cultures may describe anxiety as tightness in the chest. In some cultures, males may ascribe anxiety to the presence of semen in their urine. In many cultures, anxiety is described as "nerves." In some cultures, anxiety may be stigmatized as a loss of emotional control, and the individual complaining of "nerves" or "nervousness" may be viewed as a less valued member of the community (Friedman, 1997).

Risk Factors

Factors associated with the development of GAD include family history of GAD; increase in the amount of stressors in an individual's life; onset of a serious medical illness; losses (financial, personal, or career); history of physical or emotional trauma (Fricchione, 2004); presence of a medical illness, such as diabetes; smoking (Brantley, Mehan, Ames, et al., 1999; Brown, Fulton, Wilkeson, et al., 2000; Johnson, Cohen, Pine, et al., 2000); and being separated, divorced, or widowed (Papp, 2010).

Risk factors also include factors attributable to the individual and to his or her experiences in life. Risk factors attributable to the individual include the trait of behavioral inhibition, which is the tendency to be shy or timid in new situations (Lightfoot, Seay, & Goddard, 2010); a low tolerance for uncertainty (Dugas, Savard, Gaudet, et al., 2007); lower levels of cognitive functioning in childhood; conduct problems; anxiety and depression; and a high-arousal coping style in response to minor stressors (Hettema, Prescott, & Kendler, 2004; Katzman, 2009; Martin et al., 2007). Risk factors attributable to experience include history of childhood physical or sexual abuse (Windle, Windle, Scheidt, et al., 1995) and parenting that is controlling and excessively protective (Rapee, 1997).

Etiology

The cause of GAD is unknown. Most models of GAD propose that worrying is the avoidance of internal affective experiences (thoughts, beliefs, and emotions) and that worrying is perpetuated by certain mechanisms, e.g., by intolerance of uncertainty, by positive beliefs about the importance or value of worrying, and by emotional dysregulation (Behar, DiMarco, Hekler, et al., 2009).

Theories of the etiology of GAD have continued to evolve from early psychoanalytical theory. Some of the recently proposed theories include genetic theory, attachment theory, avoidance theory, intolerance of uncertainty theory, and psychoanalytical theory.

Genetic Theory

There appears to be a genetic predisposition to the development of GAD with heritability of 22% to 37%, which means that 22% to 37% of the variance of developing GAD is due to genetic influence (Hettema, Neale, & Kendler, 2001). Stein (2009) described the heritability of GAD as moderate. However, some researchers believe that there is not sufficient evidence to support the role of genetics in the development of GAD (Mendlewicz, Papadimitriou, & Wimotte, 1993), and others believe that genetic influence combined with exposure to stress in the early periods of brain development creates a neurobiological vulnerability to stress with a resulting lower threshold for developing anxiety disorder following later exposure to stress (Jetty, Charney, & Goddard, 2001).

Attachment Theory

Attachment theory proposes that insecure attachment patterns that create early models of the world as a dangerous place may contribute to later development of anxiety (Cassidy, 1995; Cassidy, Lichtenstein-Phelps, Sibrava, et al., 2009). Bowlby (1973) proposed that an infant's feeling of distress at separation from his or her primary caregiver (usually the mother) created the prototype of anxiety. Under optimal circumstances, the mother relieves the child's anxiety and restores the child's sense of security. However, if the mother is unavailable owing to illness, depression, drug abuse, separation, or other causes and is not there to relieve the child's distress, anxiety develops. Thus, an insecure attachment pattern may cause anxiety problems in childhood that develop into GAD in adulthood (Cassidy et al.). This theory is supported by research findings that insecure attachment patterns are more common among individuals with GAD than in the general population (Eng & Heimberg, 2006).

Avoidance Theory

Borkovec, Alcaine, and Behar's (2004) avoidance theory of GAD builds on attachment theory. Borkovec et al. noted that insecure attachment patterns, early life traumas, and poor interpersonal skills underlie the development of GAD, and that patients with GAD perceive the world as a dangerous place. Worrying is the patient's attempt to avoid exposure to future negative experiences. While worrying inhibits distressing mental images of threats or danger, somatic responses, and emotional activation, it prevents the emotional processing of fear that is needed to extinguish it. Extinction of fear comes from (1) exposure to the feared object or situation and (2) exposure to the potential meaning behind the fear (Foa, Huppert, & Cahill, 2006). Therefore, although worrying provides short-term relief, it prevents effective problem-solving (Behar et al., 2009; Lightfoot et al., 2010).

Intolerance of Uncertainty Theory

Difficulty tolerating uncertainty can be viewed as a cognitive vulnerability that is specific to GAD (Behar et al., 2009). According to the theory of intolerance of uncertainty, individuals with GAD find situations that are uncertain to be stressful. They experience a state of chronic worry in uncertain situations. They believe that worrying helps them to cope and may prevent the feared event from happening. However, the chronic worrying is associated with lack of confidence in their problem-solving ability, with seeing all problems as threats, with becoming frustrated in dealing with problems, and with being pessimistic about the possibility that problem-solving can lead to positive results (Behar et al.).

Psychoanalytical Theory

According to psychoanalytical theory, anxiety is a symptom of unresolved unconscious conflicts (Josephs, 1994). Freud believed that conflict between the id (basic instincts or drives), the ego (the executive force that modulates the id and controls what we do, how we perceive things, and our contact with reality), and the superego (conscience, judge of performance) was the basis of anxiety (Sadock & Sadock, 2007). Psychoanalytical theory proposes that anxiety-causing conflict in adulthood is based on similar unresolved conflict in childhood.

Biological Basis

Individuals with GAD appear to have impairment of cognition. They view ambiguous information as threatening or negative and focus more attention on potentially threatening information than on positive information. Patients with GAD have also been found to have problems with memory and attention (Weisberg, 2009). There is evidence that patients with GAD have abnormalities of brain structures, of brain functioning, and of neurochemistry Abnormalities of brain structures include abnormalities of the occipital lobe, basal ganglia, limbic system, hippocampus, brainstem, and frontal cortex (Jetty et al., 2001). One abnormality of brain functioning is sustained activity in the medial prefrontal area after termination of the threatening stimulus. Worrying activates the medial regions of the frontal lobe, and whereas individuals who are low worriers could stop worrying after termination of the threatening stimuli, thus reducing activity in the medial prefrontal area, individuals who are high worriers could not (Paulesu, Sambugaro, Torti, et al., 2009). Figure 10-1 shows the increased activity in the temporal limbic area and in the prefrontal area of the brain of a patient with GAD.

The neurotransmitters that are involved in the fear/anxiety circuit include gamma-aminobutyric acid (GABA), norepinephrine, serotonin, glutamate, and cholecystokinin (Panksepp, 2004). (The fear/anxiety circuit is discussed in Chapter 9.) Increased levels of norepinephrine and abnormalities of serotonin activity have been found in patients with GAD (Lightfoot et al., 2010). Serotonin is involved in regulation of mood, impulse control, sleep, vigilance, memory, and the processing of anxiety and fear (Akimova, Lanzenberger, & Kasper, 2009). The serotonin receptor 5-HT_{1A} is thought to play a major role in the etiology of anxiety disorders: it has been found to have less binding capability in individuals with some anxiety disorders. Medications such as SSRIs change serotonin neurotransmission, including the binding of the 5-HT_{1A} receptor; thus, SSRIs may reduce anxiety by increasing binding of serotonin to 5-HT_{1A} receptors (Akimova et al.).

Decreased GABA functioning has been found in many patients with GAD (Jetty et al., 2001; Lightfoot et al., 2010); supporting this finding, pilot studies have found that pregabalin (Lyrica), which is an analog to GABA (has a similar structure to GABA's), is effective in improving the symptoms of GAD (Feltner, Crockatt, Dubovsky, et al., 2003).

Glutamate is thought to be involved in the "...danger processing functions of the amygdala..." (Amiel, Mathew,

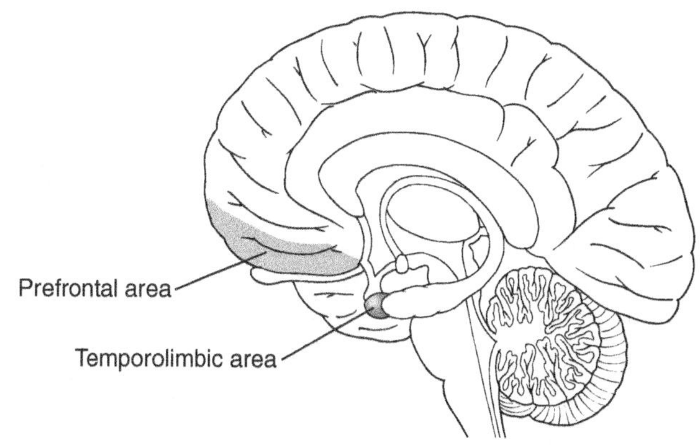

FIGURE 10-1: Neuroanatomical model of the brain in generalized anxiety disorder that shows increased activity in the temporal limbic area (Tiihonen, Kuikka, Räsänen, et al., 1997; Wu, Buchsbaum, Hershey, et al., 1991) and in the prefrontal area (Rauch, Savage, Alpert, et al., 1997; Wu et al.).
Reprinted from Stein, D. J. (2000). *False alarm! How to conquer the anxiety disorders.* Cape Town, South Africa: University of Stellenbosch. Used with permission.

Garakani, et al., 2009, p. 974). Treatment of GAD with riluzole (Rilutek), a glutamatergic agent that inhibits the release of glutamate and is used in the treatment of patients with amyotropic lateral sclerosis, has been found to reduce anxiety (Mathew, Amiel, Coplan, et al., 2005).

Neurohormones are also involved in GAD. For example, in response to threatening or dangerous situations, corticotropin-releasing hormone promotes an increase in the output of cortisol, which results in anxiety in the form of agitated arousal that leads to freezing behaviors that are evolutionary responses to danger (Panksepp, 2004). Freezing behaviors—such as keeping absolutely still or dropping to a crouching position—are automatic responses to fear. They are activated by the sympathetic nervous system and occur seconds before the fight-or-flight response to danger (LeDoux, 2002).

Clinical Presentation

The primary feature of GAD is excessive anxiety and worry that is difficult to control, causes serious distress, and interferes with the patient's daily activities (Huppert & Sanderson, 2010; Lightfoot et al., 2010). Patients with GAD often report physical symptoms, including muscle tension, headaches, and muscle pain in the neck, shoulders, and lower back (Papp, 2010); additionally, approximately two-thirds of patients with GAD complain of sleep disturbances (Allgulander, 2010). The majority of patients with GAD report being anxious at least half of each day. Although patients may describe worries about work, family, finances, health, and interpersonal relationships (Papp, 2010), the primary focus of their worrying is usually on interpersonal difficulties (Roemer, Molina, & Borkovec, 1997). They may describe themselves as being the nurturing partner in their relationships and often say that they are exploited (Salzer, Pincus, Hoyer, et al., 2008).

Patients may give a history of early anxiety, social isolation, academic difficulties, obsessions, and disturbed family situations (First & Tasman, 2004). They may have tried many treatments and may be ashamed of their failure to control their symptoms. They may display characteristics of perfectionism and need for control, and they may express the belief that they are responsible for negative events. Some patients believe that they have no control over their worrying, and some believe that worrying has value; e.g., by worrying, they prevent negative events from occurring (Huppert & Sanderson, 2010). They are often angry and think that people do not take their symptoms seriously. Clinical presentation usually includes biological, psychological, and social symptoms (Box 10-1).

BOX 10-1 Biological, Psychological, and Social Symptoms of Generalized Anxiety Disorder

Biological

- Gastrointestinal irritability
- Diarrhea
- Frequent urination
- Tachycardia
- Sweaty palms
- Dryness of the mouth
- Shallow respirations
- Muscle tenseness or spasms
- Irritable bowel syndrome

Psychological

- Apprehensive expectation of bad things happening
- Jumpiness
- Irritability
- Difficulty falling asleep
- Problems concentrating
- Fear of not being accepted by others
- Hypervigilance

Social

- Inability to relax with social activities
- Problems in work situation due to worry about possible problems
- Limited social and leisure activities due to worry about potential harm to family members

Sources: Lightfoot, Seay, Goddard, 2010; Panksepp, 2004; Shelton, 2004.

Comorbidity

About 90% of patients with GAD have at least one other psychiatric disorder (Pollack, 2009). For example, approximately two-thirds of patients with GAD have co-occurring major depressive disorder (Fricchione, 2004; Pollack), which increases the risk of suicide attempts (Pollack). One-fourth of patients with GAD have co-occurring panic disorder, and approximately one-third have co-occurring alcohol or drug abuse (Fricchione; Pollack). The Axis II personality disorders that belong to Cluster C (anxious and fearful)—such as avoidant personality disorder, dependent personality disorder, and obsessive-compulsive personality disorder—are often comorbid with GAD. Co-occurring medical conditions include migraine, rheumatoid arthritis, peptic ulcer disease, irritable bowel syndrome, coronary heart disease, hyperthyroidism, diabetes, asthma, and chronic obstructive pulmonary disease (Culpepper, 2009).

Differential Diagnosis

Differential diagnoses to be considered include high-level worrying, medical disorders, and psychiatric disorders. High-level worriers are individuals who experience a high level of worrying but do not meet the criteria for GAD. They are less impaired by their worrying than are patients with GAD. In comparison to high-level worriers, patients with GAD experience less control over negative, intrusive thoughts and experience higher levels of somatic hyperarousal (Ruscio & Borkovec, 2004).

In differentiating anxiety related to medical conditions from GAD, the following classes of medical conditions should be considered: cardiac, pulmonary, neurological, and endocrine disorders including hyperthyroidism. Individuals with anxiety related to medical conditions often include those who have

- An age of onset older than 35 years (whereas GAD is common for individuals in their early 20s)
- No family history of generalized anxiety disorder
- No presence of increased stressors in life
- No avoidance of situations that cause anxiety
- Poor response to antianxiety medications (Fricchione, 2004)

Table 10-3 shows psychiatric disorders that should be considered in the differential diagnoses for GAD.

Treatment

The immediate goal of treatment for patients with GAD is improvement of symptoms. The distal goal is remission of the disorder (Katzman, 2009). Patients with GAD need to be helped to understand that their symptoms are part of a health problem, not a character weakness; that treatment may relieve symptoms and reduce distress without curing the disorder; and that their response to treatment may be gradual. Assessment may include the use of screening instruments such as the 14-item *Hamilton Anxiety Rating Scale (HARS)* (Hamilton, 1959) or the seven-item *GAD-7 scale* that includes some of the *DSM-IV* symptoms for GAD (Kroenke, Spitzer, Williams, et al., 2007; Spitzer, Kroenke, Williams, et al., 2006).

Treatment for GAD includes psychotherapy, pharmacotherapy, and psychosocial interventions. Complementary and alternative interventions are also being investigated. Both cognitive behavioral therapy (CBT) and pharmacotherapy have been found to be effective in treating GAD (Anderson & Palm, 2006; Fisher, 2006). Medications appear to be effective in reducing symptoms of anxiety, but they do not appear to be effective in reducing the symptoms of worry (Anderson & Palm). CBT is effective in reducing both anxiety and worry (Covin, Quimet, Seeds, et al., 2008).

Psychotherapy

CBT, supportive psychotherapy, and insight-oriented therapy have been found to be beneficial for patients with GAD. CBT is considered to be the first line of treatment (Allgulander et al., 2003; Huppert & Sanderson, 2010; Milrod, 2009).

Because patients with GAD misperceive events, exaggerate difficulties, make pessimistic assumptions on little evidence, and have automatic thoughts, CBT that involves cognitive restructuring, relaxation, worry exposure, behavior modification, and problem-solving has been found to be effective for patients with this disorder (Lang, 2004). For example, it has been found that 50% of patients with GAD respond to CBT (Huppert & Sanderson, 2010). The greatest benefits are achieved after 6 months of weekly sessions. CBT has been found to be associated with a 30% to 60% reduction of anxiety symptoms (Huppert & Sanderson). Long-term benefits are maintained in approximately half

TABLE 10-3 DIFFERENTIAL DIAGNOSIS OF GENERALIZED ANXIETY DISORDER

Other Psychiatric Disorder	Differentiating Characteristics of Other Psychiatric Disorder
Obsessive-compulsive disorder	Obsessional thoughts are not excessive worries about everyday or real-life problems Obsessional thoughts are ego-dystonic intrusions Obsessional thoughts tend to be urges and impulses and are accompanied by compulsive acts that reduce the anxiety associated with the obsessions (American Psychiatric Association, 2000)
Panic disorder	Co-occurs in 25% of patients with GAD (Fricchione, 2004) Presence of symptoms of numbing, choking, trouble breathing, tingling, rapid heartbeat, panic attacks, and impairment of functioning (First & Tasman, 2004) Patients seek treatment (Papp, 2010)
Major depressive disorder	Co-occurs in two-thirds of patients with GAD (Fricchione, 2004); higher rates of dysphoric mood, psychomotor retardation, suicidal ideation, and feelings of guilt, hopelessness, and helplessness; more work impairment (First & Tasman, 2004); presence of vegetative signs of depression and early morning sleep disturbances (Papp, 2010).
Social phobia	Avoidance of specific social situations in which the individual's performance might be evaluated; focus is on avoiding embarrassment or rejection (Papp, 2010)
Phobias	Specific object or situation is avoided; focus is fear of the result of contact with object (e.g., spiders) or of being in the situation (e.g., flying) (Gamble, Harvey, & Rapee, 2010)
Adjustment disorder with anxiety	Anxiety occurs in response to a life stressor experienced within previous 3 months (e.g., retirement, marital problems, relocation) (American Psychiatric Association, 2000)
Social anxiety disorder	Social anxiety disorder has anticipatory anxiety related to social situations and avoidance behaviors; focus is fear of not performing well and being rejected (Hales, Yudofsky, & Gabbard, 2011)
Nonpathological anxiety	Everyday worries are seen as more controllable; they are not usually accompanied by physical symptoms such as excessive fatigue, restlessness, and irritability (American Psychiatric Association, 2000)
Substance-related disorders	Direct physiological effects of a substance including medications; co-occurs in one-third of patients with GAD (Fricchione, 2004)

GAD, generalized anxiety disorder.

of patients who received CBT (Durham, Chambers, MacDonald, et al., 2003), and there may be continued improvement over time (Huppert & Sanderson). Other interventions that are being studied include cognitive therapy with the addition of a mindfulness approach, meditation, acceptance-based techniques, or problem-solving. There is no evidence at this time that additions to CBT provide an additional benefit (Huppert & Sanderson).

Pharmacotherapy

Patients with GAD often need long-term medication management (Davidson et al., 2009; Rynn & Brawman-Mintzer, 2004) that includes the use of SSRIs, serotonin-norepinephrine reuptake inhibitors (SNRIs), benzodiazepines, azapirones such as buspirone, other antidepressant medications, anticonvulsants, and atypical antipsychotics. The SSRIs and SNRIs have become accepted as the first-line pharmacological intervention (Hoffman & Mathew, 2008; van Ameringen, Mancini, Patterson, et al., 2010). Patients usually respond to medications within 8 weeks (Friccione, 2004), and treatment is usually continued for 6 to 12 months, although some patients may need to be on medication longer.

Selective Serotonin Reuptake Inhibitors (SSRIs)

In comparison to the use of benzodiazepines, the use of SSRIs is safer and more effective for treating symptoms of anxiety, including worry, tension, irritability, and problems with concentration (Snyderman, Rynn, Bellew, et al., 2004).

Several of the SSRIs are effective in treating GAD. Floxetine (Prozac) may transiently increase anxiety, but paroxetine and sertraline (Zoloft) do not (Allgulander et al., 2003). Paroxetine has been found to reduce anxiety symptoms, with improvement evident after 1 week (Pollack, Zaninelli, Goddary, et al., 2001; Rickels, Zaninelli, McCafferty, et al., 2003; Rocca, Fonzo, Scotta, et al., 1997). It has also been found to improve social functioning (Pollack et al.).

Escitalopram has been found to be as effective for GAD as paroxetine (Bielski, Bose, & Chang, 2005). Among patients receiving escitalopram, 68% showed improvement after 8 weeks, in comparison to 41% of patients receiving placebo (Davidson, Bose, Korotzer, et al., 2004). Escitalopram has been found to be effective in treating older adults with GAD (Lenze, Rollman, Shear, et al., 2009).

In a comparison, both paroxetine and sertraline resulted in decreased anxiety while maintaining patients' remission rates and quality of life. Occurrence of undesired side effects was comparable (Ball, Kuhn, Wall, et al., 2005).

Serotonin Norepinephrine Reuptake Inhibitors (SNRIs)

The SNRIs venlafaxine (Effexor) and duloxetine (Cymbalta) are considered to be a first-line choice of treatment for GAD (Pollack, Kornstein, Spann, et al., 2008) and are approved for treatment by the FDA.

Venlafaxine has been found to be effective in treating patients with GAD and co-occurring major depressive disorder (Fricchione, 2004). Response rate is about 70%, with benefits evidenced within 2 weeks (Hollander & Simeon, 2008). It is effective in treating symptoms of insomnia, restlessness, poor concentration, irritability, and excessive muscle tension. Anxiety symptoms are reduced after 2 weeks, and somatic symptoms are improved after 4 to 8 weeks of treatment (Allgulander, Hackett, & Salinas, 2001). Adverse effects of venlafaxine ER include nausea, somnolence, dry mouth, sexual dysfunction, and blood pressure elevation in some patients. Discontinuation of treatment may be accompanied by dizziness, light-headedness, tinnitus, nausea, vomiting, and loss of appetite (Allgulander et al., 2001).

Duloxetine has been found to be effective in the treatment of GAD (Khan & Macaluso, 2009). When compared to a group receiving a placebo, patients with GAD who received duloxetine showed significant improvement in anxiety symptoms, fear, depressed mood, overall functioning, and quality of life (Pollack et al., 2008; Rynn et al., 2008). Improvement of anxiety symptoms was seen as early as 2 weeks, and early response to duloxetine has been found to be correlated with better outcome (Pollack et al.). Side effects of nausea and dizziness, which occurred in one-third of the patients, were associated with the patients' discontinuation of treatment (Carter & McCormack, 2009). In a study comparing venlafaxine XR, duloxetine, and placebo, there was significant decrease of anxiety symptoms for those receiving venlafaxine and duloxetine, with the percentage of patients achieving remission greater among those receiving venlafaxine (Hartford, Kornstein, Liebowitz, et al., 2007).

Benzodiazepines

Benzodiazepines were the traditional method of treating anxiety disorders; however, they have been replaced by newer medications such as the SSRIs, SNRIs, and buspirone (Buspar). Benzodiazepines such as lorazepam (Ativan), oxazepam (Serax), clonazepam (Klonopin), alprazolam (Xanax), and diazepam (Valium) are effective anxiolytics in the acute phase and for treatment of physical symptoms of anxiety. They act through potentiation of the inhibitory neurotransmitter GABA (Davidson et al., 2009). Their strongest effect is on hypervigilance and somatic symptoms, and they are less effective in relieving symptoms of irritability and worry (Davidson et al.).

Benzodiazepines provide immediate relief, but their side effects of dependence, cognitive impairment, drowsiness, unsteadiness of gait (risk for falls), and withdrawal symptoms (anxiety, delirium, and seizures) are of major concern (Davidson et al., 2009; Fricchione, 2004; Rynn & Brawman-Mintzer, 2004). To avoid these problems if benzodiazepines are used, treatment should start with a benzodiazepine that has an intermediate half-life, such as oxazepam or lorazepam, or with a long half-life such as clonazepam or chlordiazepoxide (Librium). Discontinuation of high-potency short-acting benzodiazepines such as alprazolam requires a long, slow taper and often the use of anxiolytic antidepressants (Rickels, DeMartinis, Garcia-Espana, et al., 2000). If benzodiazepines are to be withdrawn, the dose is decreased over 3 to 6 months (Dubovsky, 2005). To lessen the risk of dependency, benzodiazepines should be avoided in patients who have a history of alcohol or substance abuse (Pollack, 2009).

Azapirones: Buspirone

Buspirone is a serotonin partial agonist of serotonin 1A receptors that has been approved by the FDA for the treatment of GAD (van Ameringen et al., 2010). Early studies in research centers reported its effectiveness for GAD, but in clinical practice its effectiveness has been found to be inconsistent (Pollack, 2009). It is effective in 60% to 80% of patients with GAD. Buspirone causes little drowsiness, memory impairment, or sexual dysfunction and does not cause dependence or withdrawal symptoms. It is effective in treating the psychological components of GAD, but it may be less effective in decreasing somatic complaints (Davidson et al., 2009). It has no antidepressant effect, and response may take 2 to 4 weeks (Fricchione, 2004). Although buspirone has been found to be equal in efficacy to traditional benzodiazepines, the benzodiazepine alprazolam has a more rapid response; however, it also has more adverse events (van Ameringen et al.). Buspirone must be taken regularly and is the first choice for patients with a history of substance abuse or pulmonary disease and for patients who operate equipment such as trucks or airplanes (Dubovsky, 2005).

Other Antidepressants

Mirtazapine (Remeron) has been found to be effective in treating GAD (Goodnick, Puig, DeVane, et al., 1999). In one study, a 50% improvement of symptoms was noted in 80% of the patients receiving mirtazapine (Gambi, De-Berardis, Campanella, et al., 2005). If other antidepressants are not effective, tricyclic antidepressants (TCAs) such as imipramine (Tofranil) may be used to reduce symptoms of GAD (Fricchione, 2004). TCAs may also be useful in managing the discontinuation of benzodiazepines (Rickels et al., 2000). However, TCAs have many side effects that may limit their use. Some problematic side effects include weight gain, orthostatic hypotension, urinary retention, constipation, and sedation. There is also a serious problem of lethality associated with overdoses: a dose of 10 times the total daily dose can be fatal (Nelson, 2009).

Most antidepressants are effective for GAD. However, antidepressants can cause initial symptoms of agitation, tremor, sweating, insomnia, and increased anxiety (Dubovsky, 2005). To overcome antidepressant-caused jitteriness, a benzodiazepine may be used first and the antidepressant added while tapering off the benzodiazepine (Dubovsky).

Anticonvulsants

Some anticonvulsant medications have antianxiety properties and some modulate the GABA and glutamate systems, both of which are involved in GAD (van Ameringen et al., 2010). They are useful for patients with a history of substance abuse or for patients who cannot tolerate antidepressants. For example, gabapentin (Neurontin) has been found to be useful in patients who cannot tolerate antidepressants (Dubovsky, 2005). In addition, pregabalin, which is approved for use for patients with GAD in Europe but not in the United States (Pollack, 2009), modulates excitatory neurotransmitters—such as glutamate—and has been found to reduce symptoms of GAD. Onset of response is rapid, similar to that with benzodiazepines, and it has few withdrawal symptoms (Hoffman & Mathew, 2008; Pollack).

Atypical Antipsychotics

Although there is evidence of the effectiveness of quetiapine (Seroquel) for GAD, the FDA decided in April 2009 not to approve its use for GAD because of potential metabolic problems, the possibility of extrapyramidal side effects, and the risk of sudden death due to ventricular arrhythmias (Allgulander, 2010). For treatment of refractory GAD, augmentation with atypical antipsychotics, such as risperidone (Risperdal) and olanzapine (Zyprexa), may be helpful (van Ameringen et al., 2010).

Other Pharmacotherapeutic Approaches

Other treatment approaches include riluzole, eszopiclone, and herbal treatments:

- ***Riluzole (Rilutek).*** Based on the knowledge that there are abnormalities of regulation of the excitatory neurotransmitter glutamate in patients with anxiety, the use of riluzole, a presynaptic glutamate release inhibitor, has been studied in a small group of patients with GAD. Two-thirds of the patients experienced a reduction of anxiety symptoms within 8 weeks (Pollack, 2009).
- ***Eszopiclone (Lunesta).*** Sleep disturbance is a frequent problem for patients with GAD. Treating sleep problems by augmenting SSRI treatment with the hypnotic eszopiclone was found to improve anxiety symptoms, sleep, and functioning (Pollack, 2009).
- ***Herbal treatments.*** The use of herbal treatments such as kava, valerian, passionflower, and Ginkgo biloba has been tried by some individuals for the relief of anxiety, but they are not considered to be effective treatment for GAD (Davidson et al., 2009; van Ameringen et al., 2010).

Long-term Use of Pharmacotherapy

Long-term treatment with medications may be necessary to prevent GAD relapse and to achieve remission (Davidson, 2009). Venlafaxine XR and escitalopram have been found to be effective in long-term treatment of GAD (van Ameringen et al., 2010). Paroxetine, escitalopram, duloxetine, quetiapine XR, and pregabalin have been found to be effective in relapse-prevention studies (van Ameringen et al., 2010).

In summary, several categories of medications—SSRIs, SNRIs, benzodiazepines, azapirones, other antidepressants, anticonvulsants, and atypical antipsychotics—have been found to be effective in the treatment of GAD. However, many patients do not receive adequate treatment. For example, it has been found that 35.2% of patients with GAD who were treated in the primary care sector and 56.6% of patients who were treated in mental health care settings do not receive the care that is suggested by evidence-based guidelines (Davidson, 2009).

Psychosocial Interventions

Individuals with milder forms of GAD may respond to psychosocial interventions, such as altering lifestyle practices and relaxation strategies (First & Tasman, 2004).

Promoting Healthy Lifestyle Practices

Patients with GAD should be encouraged to practice good sleep habits; follow healthy eating habits; reduce or eliminate caffeine, nicotine, and alcohol; exercise regularly; use relaxation techniques; and seek treatment for co-occurring medical illnesses. Teaching patients to increase problem-solving skills and social skills if there is a deficit and teaching patients to use effective communication and stress management has been found to be helpful. Basic supportive techniques such as reassurance, clarification, direct suggestions, anticipatory guidance, and providing advice are also helpful (Fava, Ruini, Rafanelli, et al., 2005; First & Tasman, 2004).

Relaxation Therapy

Relaxation therapy is beneficial for some patients with GAD. In relaxation therapy, patients imagine calming situations to achieve muscular and mental relaxation. Applied relaxation therapy that involves using progressive relaxation, slowed breathing, relaxing imagery, and meditational relaxation throughout the day and in response to any anxiety cues has been shown to achieve benefits similar to those achieved with CBT (Borkovec, Newman, Pincus, et al., 2002; Fisher & Durham, 1999; Huppert & Sanderson, 2002).

Exercise

Lavie and Milani (2004) found that exercise training is associated with a 50% reduction in the prevalence of symptoms of anxiety among patients in cardiac rehabilitation, and based on this finding they suggest the use of exercise in the management of GAD. Other researchers have found that exercise is effective in reducing anxiety symptoms and the symptoms of panic disorder (Barbour, Edenfield, & Blumenthal, 2007).

Self-Help Interventions

Self-help interventions are also beneficial for patients with GAD. A computer-based self-help intervention, *Stresspac*, has been found to be helpful (White, 1998b). Other self-help computer programs that can be used for anxiety include *FearFighter* (http://www.FearFighter.com) and *Restoring the Balance* (http://www.mentalhealth.org.uk/publications/?entryid5=41591&char-R). *FearFighter* is designed for phobia, anxiety, and panic, and *Restoring the Balance* is designed for individuals experiencing anxiety and depression (Stuhlmiller & Tolchard, 2009).

Other self-help strategies for reducing anxiety include:

- Limiting time spent thinking, by doing physical activities (gardening, cooking, crafts)
- Spending time doing enjoyable activities (drawing, sewing, jigsaw puzzles, working with clay, or painting)
- Doing relaxation exercises
- Exercising: taking a walk, riding a bike, or dancing
- Reducing caffeine intake
- Finding something to laugh at
- Doing something relaxing: a hot bath, a video game, a book, a television show that explores another country, or listening to music

Complementary and Alternative Interventions for Reducing Anxiety

Individuals with GAD often use complementary or alternative interventions in addition to prescribed treatment (Antonacci, Davis, Bloch, et al., 2010). Among the few studies of the efficacy of alternative interventions, there are studies of the anxiety-reducing benefits of yoga (Sharma, Azmi, & Settiwar, 1991; Kirkwood, Rampes, Tuffrehy, et al., 2005), dietary supplements (Pittler & Ernst, 2003), and balneotherapy (mineral water therapy in a spa setting) (Dubois, Salamon, Germain, et al., 2010). The study of Dubois et al. was a controlled study that compared balneotherapy with paroxetine over an 8-week period. They found that balneotherapy was associated with a greater reduction of anxiety (Dubois et al.).

Course

Some patients with GAD report having been anxious all their lives. They may have been moderately anxious as children and they may have had a history of childhood fears and school problems (Papp, 2010). GAD often develops following exposure to stressors, such as leaving home to enter college or starting work (Papp). Although the symptoms of GAD may fluctuate, they often persist throughout an individual's life, with less than one-third of patients with GAD experiencing spontaneous remission (Rickels & Rynn, 2002) and with about 80% of patients continuing to have symptoms that interfere with their functioning, especially with work performance (Wittchen, Zhao, Kessler, et al., 1994). The negative effects of GAD on quality of life are primarily due to worrying about life circumstances, financial situations, and harm to family members. The worrying associated with GAD can also have a negative effect on relationships with family members, friends, and coworkers (Cramer, Torgersen, & Kringlen, 2005; Gabbard, 2005).

Key Points

- GAD is characterized by chronic anxiety, uncontrollable worry, expectation of negative outcomes, and impairment of functioning.

- Etiology includes genetic influences, biological abnormalities, behavioral inhibition, and exposure to adverse childhood experiences.
- Cognitive behavioral therapy is the first choice for psychotherapy.
- SSRIs and SNRIs are the first choice for pharmacotherapy.
- The course is chronic with fluctuating severity of symptoms that often require maintenance treatment (Allgulander, 2010).

Social Anxiety Disorder (SAD)

SAD can be viewed as a response to a perceived threat to social status or reputation (Crozier & Alden, 2005a); the core feature of the SAD response is the fear of being evaluated by others, judged to be inadequate, and rejected (Bogels & Stein, 2009). SAD is characterized by a fear of social or performance situations in which the individual may experience embarrassment, such as in meeting new people; dealing with people in authority; attending parties, meetings, or interviews; speaking in front of people; eating in front of people; and using public bathrooms (Hollander & Simeon, 2008). Approximately 25% of patients with SAD will have nongeneralized SAD, and the remaining 75% will have generalized SAD, in which nearly all social interactions are stressful (Lydiard, 2002). In nongeneralized SAD, the patient has a limited social fear that occurs in one situation (e.g., when speaking in public), whereas in generalized SAD, fears occur in many social situations. In comparison to individuals with nongeneralized SAD, individuals with generalized SAD have more symptoms of overall distress, anxiety, and depression; more impairment of functioning, such as in their ability to work; fewer social skills; and a greater degree of self-criticism and fear of negative evaluation (Carter & Wu, 2010; Ramsawh, Chavira, & Stein, 2010). They are also more likely to be unemployed (Heimberg, Hope, Dodge, et al., 1990).

When exposed to feared situations, individuals with SAD experience anxiety, somatic symptoms, distortions of cognition, and impairment of functioning. Somatic symptoms include tremors, sweating, blushing, and dry mouth. Blushing is the key physical symptom of SAD (Ramsawh et al., 2010; Black & Andreasen, 2011). Distortions of cognition include evaluating their social performances negatively and discounting their social competence in positive interactions (Ramsawh et al.). Fear of a situation interferes with the individual's life: it affects his or her daily routine, academic achievement, work, and social interactions. Patients are afraid that others will think they are weak, crazy, or stupid. In severe forms, SAD can lead to unemployment because of the individual's inability to participate in job interviews (Bonne, Grillon, Vythilingam, et al., 2004). Their social interactions are limited to the family, and they have a diminished quality of life (Cramer et al., 2005; Stein & Keane, 2000) and increased risk for suicide (American Psychiatric Association, 2000; Sareen, Cox, Afifi, et al., 2005). Among children, SAD is associated with failing a grade; among adolescents, it is associated with dropping out of school, not graduating from high school, and increased risk for alcohol abuse (van Ameringen, Mancini, & Farvolden, 2003).

Epidemiology

Prevalence

In the United States, the prevalence of SAD is 4% to 13% among adults and adolescents (Kessler, Berglund, Demler, et al., 2005a). Similar rates have been found in Canada, Sweden, and Switzerland, but lower rates have been found in non-Western countries (Ramsawh et al., 2010).

Onset and Gender

SAD begins in midadolescence and may follow childhood social inhibition or shyness, or it may develop following exposure to a stressful or embarrassing situation (Ollendick & Hirshfeld-Becker, 2002). Although the mean age of onset is 15 years, the mean age of first treatment is 12 years later, and 80% of individuals with SAD never received treatment (Black & Andreasen, 2011). SAD appears to occur more frequently in individuals who are female, single, and unemployed and who have lower incomes and less education (Ruscio, Brown, Chiu, et al. 2008). For example, two-thirds of patients with SAD are single, divorced, or widowed. A tragic finding is that more than half of patients with SAD never completed high school, and one-fifth are too disabled to work (Friedman, 1997; Stahl, 2000).

Culture

In some cultures, SAD is manifested as a fear of giving offense to others in social situations rather than as a fear of embarrassing oneself or experiencing humiliation, e.g., Taijin Kyofusho (Ramsawh et al., 2010, p. 441). Among other cultures, social anxiety may be manifested as a fear of evaluation or a fear of failing, e.g., fear of failing the extended family and the black race (Neal-Barnett & Smith, 1997). Lower rates of SAD have been found among Hispanics and non-Hispanic blacks (Breslau, Aguilar-Gaxiola, Kendler et al., 2006). Breslau et al. suggested that strong identification with an ethnic group or culture may be protective during childhood, reducing the risk of development of SAD.

Risk Factors

Retrospective information obtained from adults with SAD indicates that 40% to 60% of them could recall a specific traumatic incident that led to the development of their SAD (Morreale, Tancer, & Uhde, 2010). Other risk factors for the development of SAD include

- History of inhibited temperament (tendency to withdraw, cry, cling, or freeze in unfamiliar situations) (Hirshfeld-Becker, Biederman, Henin, et al., 2007)

- Ambivalent attachment patterns (Warren, Huston, Egeland, et al., 1997)
- Childhood separation anxiety
- Childhood language difficulties (16% of children with language problems developed SAD later) (Voci, Beitchman, Brownlie, et al., 2006)
- Shyness in childhood and adolescence
- Perfectionism; fear of making mistakes
- Problems with schoolwork
- Parents who used shame as a way of discipline
- Parental history of psychiatric disorders
- Parents having SAD (Ogliari, Citterio, Zanoni, et al., 2006)
- Parental conflict
- Childhood maltreatment
- Frequent relocations during childhood (Hollander & Simeon, 2008)

Etiology

The etiology of SAD is not known (Morreale et al., 2010). It is thought to develop from the interaction of the following factors:

- Genetic vulnerability
- Insecure attachment patterns
- Experienced factors (parental behaviors including parental modeling of social avoidance, exposure to humiliating social experiences, and experiencing peer rejection)
- Fear of social evaluation (Ollendick & Hirshfeld-Becker, 2002)

Individuals with nongeneralized SAD are more likely to have been exposed to traumatic experiences that conditioned their response to new situations, whereas individuals with generalized SAD are more likely to have a history of childhood shyness (Cox, MacPherson, & Enns, 2005).

Genetic Influence

There appears to be a familial pattern, with SAD occurring frequently among first-degree relatives (Bogels & Stein, 2009). The heritability of SAD is 28%, indicating that more than one-fourth of the variance is due to genetic influence (Hettema et al., 2001). Genetic influence is stronger for generalized SAD than for nongeneralized SAD (Morreale et al., 2010). Genetic influence may be through temperament—such as behavioral inhibition in response to unfamiliar stimuli that is seen in infants with slow-to-warm-up temperament—and, later, in shyness in preschool and early school years (Kagan & Snidman, 1991). Inhibited children have biological markers, such as electroencephalographic abnormalities, increased startle response, and increased cortisol levels (Schmidt, Polak, & Spooner, 2005). Thus, some children are born with a vulnerability to respond to new stimuli with anxiety. However, many children with a genetic or biological vulnerability to behavioral inhibition do not develop shyness or behavioral inhibition. They may be protected by buffering factors such as warm, supportive caregivers (Schmidt et al., 2005).

Experienced Factors

Toward the end of the third year of life, children are able to judge their behavior relative to standards that they have been taught. They develop shame, pride, guilt, and forms of embarrassment in response to others' evaluation of their performance or in response to their own evaluation of their performance (Crozier & Alden, 2005b). Studies have found that parents who provide sensitive, warm, and supportive family environments and who set clear expectations for behavior have socially competent and sociable children; parents who are distant and rejecting tend to have children who are shy and socially withdrawn (Schmidt et al., 2005). Maternal depression, nervousness, irritability, and shyness may also contribute to the development of a child's inhibited behaviors (Schmidt et al.). Children with insecure attachment patterns or inhibited temperament may not have had the opportunities and support to develop appropriate social skills and competencies. They are often aware of their deficiencies and judge themselves negatively (Morreale et al., 2010).

Biological Basis

Patients with SAD have some reactions that are similar to those of patients with panic disorder (discussed next). When exposed to high concentrations of substances—such as carbon dioxide, caffeine, or cholecystokinin—that stimulate release of adrenocorticotropic hormone and cortisol, patients with SAD and those with panic disorder have more intense reactions than controls. During anticipation of public speaking, patients with nongeneralized SAD have elevated heart rates that are similar to those of patients with panic disorder (Carter & Wu, 2010). When patients with SAD were exposed to threatening images during neuroimaging studies, their brains showed increased activity in the amygdala and insula (Shah, Klumpp, Angstadt, et al., 2009). These brain structures are involved in cognitive appraisal of environmental stimuli, in integrating emotional information, in responding to fear, in self-perception, and in evaluating others' intentions (Aquizerate, Martin-Guehl, & Tignol, 2004; Pietrini, Godini, Lazzeretti, et al., 2010; Shah et al., 2009). The neuroimaging studies showed less activity in the prefrontal cortex, which is involved in cognitive evaluation of situations, self-regulatory processes, and inhibition of the activity of the amygdala (Furmark, 2009). It is thought that patients with SAD become so anxious that they cannot think clearly (Lorberbaum, Kose, Johnson, et al., 2004), and instead they use the brain's more primitive system of responding to threats or danger (Morreale et al., 2010). Figure 10-2 shows increased temporal limbic activity, decreased basal ganglia dopaminergic activity, and some increase of prefrontal activity in a patient with SAD.

Abnormalities of neurotransmitter systems have also been found in patients with SAD. The two most studied

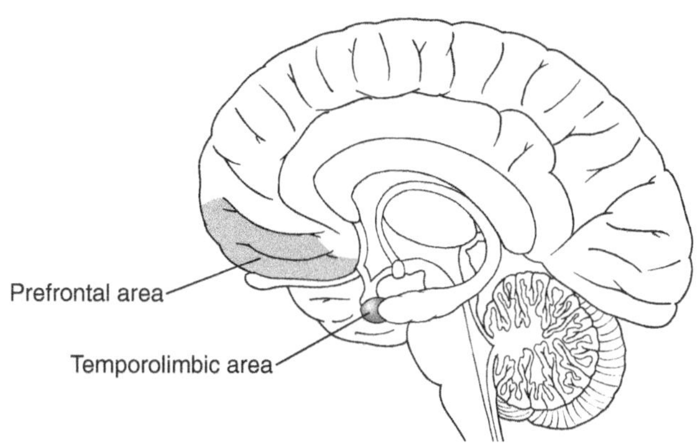

FIGURE 10-2: Neuroanatomical model of the brain in social anxiety disorder that shows increased temporal limbic activity (van der Linden, van Heerden, Warwick, et al., 2000), decreased basal ganglia dopaminergic activity (Tiihonen, Kuikka, Räsänen, et al., 1997), and some increased prefrontal activity (Rauch, Savage, Alpert, et al., 1997; van der Linden et al.).
Reprinted from Stein, D. J. (2000). *False alarm! How to conquer the anxiety disorders.* Cape Town, South Africa: University of Stellenbosch. Used with permission.

systems are the serotonin and dopamine systems. In the serotonin system, which is involved in modulating fear and anxiety, the serotonin 1A receptor has a diminished binding potential (hence the improvement seen with the use of SSRIs). In the dopamine system, which is involved in motivation and reward-seeking behaviors, reduced dopamine activity has been found in patients with SAD (Furmark, 2009). Furmark pointed out that increased knowledge about the neurochemistry of SAD is needed for the development of new treatment options.

Clinical Presentation

Patients with SAD often describe symptoms of anxiety, including palpitations, trembling, sweating, shaking of their hands, diarrhea, blushing, and confusion. They may describe anticipating and worrying about an event or situation weeks in advance (Antai-Otong, 2008). They may also describe being hypersensitive to criticism, negative evaluation, or rejection and to having problems with assertiveness and self-esteem. They often complain of sleep disturbances, difficulty falling asleep, and poor quality of sleep (Morreale et al., 2010). They may demonstrate poor social skills such as in making eye contact, initiating conversations, and responding to others. They may describe being afraid to talk to strangers and avoiding parties. If they are in academic settings, they may describe test anxiety and difficulties in participating in class. They may have dropped out of school. If employed, they may describe problems at work because of inability to speak in public, be assertive with others, eat in front of others, or use public bathrooms. They may describe their physical health as poor (Shields, 2004). Patients with SAD will often describe using "safety behaviors" (Clark, 2005, p. 196). For example, if they anticipate that they will blush or become red in a situation in which they may be observed, they avoid hot drinks, sit near a window, or wear cool clothing.

Children with SAD may present with a history of avoiding activities such as speaking in class, eating in the cafeteria, or changing their clothes in front of others. They may say that they are sick and stay home to avoid school days when they have to do things that are frightening to them (First & Tasman, 2004). They also have a high rate of sleep problems: 90% have at least one sleep-related problem (Alfano, Ginsberg, & Kingery, 2007).

Comorbidity

Although SAD frequently co-occurs with other psychiatric disorders—such as anxiety disorders, mood disorders, substance-related disorders, eating disorders, and avoidant personality disorder (Kessler, Stang, Wittchen, et al., 1999; Ramsawh et al., 2010)—it usually precedes the development of these disorders. Suicidal thoughts and suicide attempts have been reported among patients with SAD. The suicide attempts have been found to be associated with the presence of co-morbid conditions (Ramsawh et al.).

Differential Diagnoses

Before making the diagnosis of SAD, other disorders that cause irrational fear or avoidance of feared situations should be ruled out (Hollander & Simeon, 2008). Patients with some psychiatric disorders—such as schizophrenia, paranoid disorders, and avoidant personality disorder—fear that something will be done to them. In contrast, patients with SAD fear that they will do something wrong and will be humiliated (Hollander & Simeon).

SAD is also often mistaken for shyness (Keller, 2003). SAD and shyness have many of the same symptoms, including somatic arousal, increased heart rate, and fear of negative evaluation. However, SAD and shyness differ in prevalence and severity. SAD occurs in 4% to 13% of the population (Kessler et al., 2005a), but shyness has been reported by 40% to 50% of college students (Carducci & Zimbardo, 1995). Shyness and SAD differ in degree of severity of avoidance, impairment, and course, with SAD having greater severity of symptoms, more avoidance behaviors, greater impairment of functioning, and a more chronic course (Ramsawh et al., 2010). However, many extremely shy individuals meet the criteria for generalized SAD and for avoidant personality disorder. Ramsawh et al. suggest that shyness may be part of the continuum of SAD. Other researchers have found that among shy individuals, 53% of women and 40% of men develop an anxiety disorder during their lifetime, with SAD the most common (Morreale et al., 2010).

Medical and psychiatric disorders can also be mistaken for SAD. Medical disorders, medications, and substances causing anxiety were discussed in the introduction section of this chapter (see Table 10-1). Table 10-4 provides information about psychiatric disorders that should be considered as differential diagnoses for SAD.

TABLE 10-4 DIFFERENTIAL DIAGNOSIS OF SOCIAL ANXIETY DISORDER

Other Psychiatric Disorder	Differentiating Characteristics of Other Psychiatric Disorder
Panic disorder with agoraphobia	Characterized by the initial onset of unexpected panic attacks; avoidance is not limited to social situations; focus is on avoiding places or situations where it might not be possible to get help if a panic attack occurs (e.g., elevators, bridges, malls) (Pollack, Smoller, Otto, et al., 2010)
Agoraphobia without history of panic disorder, generalized anxiety disorder, specific phobia	Involves anxiety not limited to situations that involve scrutiny by others
Separation anxiety disorder	Characterized by fears of separation from home or caretakers; children may avoid being away from caregiver (e.g., sleepovers)
Pervasive developmental disorders, schizoid personality disorder	Characterized by avoidance of social situations due to lack of interest in relating to others
Avoidant personality disorder	May describe the same individuals as those with generalized social anxiety disorder; symptoms may be less severe; patients with avoidant personality disorder have more interpersonal sensitivity and fewer social skills (First & Tasman, 2004)
Social anxiety and avoidance associated with other mental disorders	Characterized by anxiety that occurs only during the course of the other mental disorders; if the anxiety is better accounted for by the other mental disorder, a diagnosis of social anxiety is not given
Nonpathological performance anxiety, stage fright, or shyness	Lacks clinically significant impairment or marked distress

Sources: Black & Andreasen, 2011; First, Frances, & Pincus, 2002; Hales, Yudofsky, & Gabbard, 2011.

Treatment

The goals of treatment for patients with SAD are to reduce or eliminate the symptoms of fear, avoidance behaviors, and physiological distress; to improve functioning; to treat comorbidities and disabilities; and to improve quality of life (Davidson et al., 2009). Treatment is based on an assessment that includes a comprehensive psychiatric evaluation. Screening instruments that may be useful in identifying SAD include the 17-item self-rated *Social Phobia Inventory (SPIN)* (Connor, Davidson, Churchill, et al., 2000) or the shorter three-question screening tool, *MINI-SPIN* (Connor, Kobak, Churchill, et al., 2001). Screening instruments for children include the *Revised Children's Manifest Anxiety Scale (MASC)* (Reynolds & Paget, 1981) and the *Screen for Child Anxiety Related Emotional Disorders (SCARED)* (Birmaher, Khetarpal, Brent, et al., 1997). Treatment includes psychotherapy, pharmacotherapy, and psychosocial interventions.

Psychotherapy

Individuals with SAD see social situations as dangerous because the thought that they will be scrutinized and evaluated causes anxiety. They develop a negative image of how they will appear to the audience and an exaggerated image of what the audience expects of them. With these negative images in mind, they become hypersensitive to any sign of disinterest, boredom, or lack of acceptance from the audience and are more aware of their internal sensations of distress. These images remain with them after the social event and become part of the memory of the event that influences their actions in future events. Treatment involves exposure to stressful social situations and cognitive restructuring that allows patients to reexamine their thoughts about themselves and others (Pontoski, Heimberg, Turk, et al., 2010). Examples of psychotherapy modalities include CBT, exposure therapy, virtual reality exposure therapy, self-help interventions, interpersonal therapy, and psychodynamic therapy.

Cognitive Behavioral Therapy

CBT, a form of exposure therapy, has been found to be effective for SAD (Rodebaugh, Holaway, & Heimberg, 2004; Rowa & Anthony, 2005). CBT is based on three core assumptions:

1. Cognitive activity affects behavior (e.g., an individual's thoughts about an event or situation influence his or her actions or behaviors).
2. Cognitive activity may be identified and changed.
3. Behavior may be changed by changing cognitive activity, e.g., by changing thoughts about an event or situation (Dobson & Dozois, 2010).

CBT changes an individual's view of self by decreasing negative thoughts and by increasing positive thoughts about his or her ability to do things (First & Tasman, 2004; Pontoski et al., 2010). The patient identifies stressful situations, and the therapy focuses on changing the patient's thinking about the stressful situations while being exposed to them. The response rate for CBT is 50% to 66% following completion of 12 to 16 sessions (Schneier, 2006).

CBT is the most effective of the psychotherapy interventions for SAD (Pontoski et al., 2010). It is comparable in effectiveness to pharmacotherapy for SAD, but the relapse rates after discontinuation of treatment are lower for CBT than they are for pharmacotherapy. Although the evidence is inconclusive, adding CBT to medications or medications to CBT does not appear to increase the benefits of either modality (Davidson et al., 2009; Pontoski et al.).

Exposure Therapy

Exposure therapy leads to the formation of new memories of a feared situation: the individual confronts the feared stimulus, which activates the fear network and causes the individual to acquire new information about the stimulus (Parsons & Rizzo, 2008). Exposure treatment provides an opportunity for the patient to experience correct information in a safe situation, which may help to modify dysfunctional beliefs (Pontoski et al., 2010). Exposure treatment has been found to be effective in reducing the symptoms of SAD, and it has been found to be more effective than progressive relaxation training (Al-Kubaisy, Marks, Logsdail, et al., 1992).

Virtual Reality Exposure Therapy

In studies of the use of virtual reality therapy, in which patients were exposed to virtual environments that re-created feared social situations and performance situations, improvement with virtual reality therapy was comparable to standard CBT (Klinger, Bouchard, Legeron, et al., 2005; Krijn et al., 2004a).

Self-Help Interventions

Andersson, Carlbring, Holmstrom, et al. (2006) described a combination intervention that uses an Internet-based self-help program that includes group exposure to real-life stressful situations and e-mail contact with a therapist. Patients experienced improvement of their symptoms of SAD and of their quality of life. The benefits were maintained at 1-year follow-up.

Interpersonal Therapy

Interpersonal therapy (IPT) has also been found to be effective for SAD (Borge, Hoffart, Sexton, et al., 2008; Lipsitz, Gur, Vermes, et al., 2008). The foundation of IPT is the assumption that psychiatric disorders result from and are maintained within a psychosocial and interpersonal context. This assumption is supported in part by the fact that patients with SAD are often unmarried, have difficulties with family and peer relationships, and often report early adverse parenting experiences, problems with peers, and multiple stressful life events (Lipsitz et al.). IPT aims to reduce symptoms by improving interpersonal functioning through the process of identifying interpersonal problems, exploring feelings and thoughts related to the problems, encouraging the expression of feelings, analyzing decisions, and role playing (Pontoski et al., 2010). IPT has been found to reduce the symptoms of SAD (fear and avoidance), to reduce symptoms of depression, and to improve social, work, and leisure-time functioning (Lipsitz et al.).

Psychodynamic Therapy

Psychodynamic therapy is also effective for SAD. According to a psychodynamic perspective, SAD is due (1) to feelings of shame because of the patients' belief that they can never measure up to others' expectations and (2) to separation anxiety related to earlier loss of a caregiver's love (Pontoski et al., 2010). In psychodynamic therapy, there is a focus on relationship problems, goal setting, developing insight, and understanding the role of shame and unrealistic expectations. With support, patients are encouraged to confront feared social situations.

Pharmacotherapy for Generalized Social Anxiety Disorder

The FDA-approved drugs for the treatment of SAD include the SSRIs—paroxetine, sertraline, and fluvoxamine CR (Luvox CR)—and the SNRI venlafaxine SR (Blanco, Schneier, Vesga-Lopez, et al., 2010).

Pharmacotherapy for generalized SAD includes first-line medications, second-line medications, and other approaches. The effectiveness of combination psychotherapy and pharmacotherapy has also been investigated in individuals with generalized SAD.

First-line Medications

The SSRIs paroxetine, sertraline, and fluvoxamine CR and the SNRI venlafaxine are considered to be the first line medications for generalized SAD (Antai-Otong, 2008; Davidson et al., 2009; Schneier, 2006). These medications are also effective for SAD with comorbid depression, panic disorder, generalized anxiety disorder, and OCD (Hollander & Simeon, 2008).

Response rates are 50% to 80% after 8 to 12 weeks of treatment. Treatment is often started at half the usual dose and increased after a week. Patients who respond by 12 weeks should receive maintenance treatment to reduce risk of relapse (Schneier, 2006).

Among the SSRIs, sertraline has been found to be effective in reducing symptoms of fear and avoidance and the physiological arousal symptoms of blushing and palpitations, but it is not effective in reducing the symptoms of trembling and sweating (Connor, Davidson, Chung, et al., 2006). Fluvoxamine has been found to be effective in reducing fear, avoidance, and physiological arousal (Davidson et al., 2009; Stein, Fyer, Davidson, et al., 1999; van Vliet, den Boer, & Westenberg, 1994) and in improving psychosocial functioning (Asakura, Tajima, & Koyama, 2007). In a small open-label trial, citalopram (Celexa) was found to be effective in reducing the symptoms of SAD and in improving work and social functioning (Simon, Korbly, Worthington, et al., 2002). Escitalopram has been found to reduce symptoms of SAD—such as the fears associated with social interactions, eating or drinking in public, and speaking in public—and to improve work and social functioning (Kasper, Stein, Loft, et al., 2005). Studies that included a longer follow-up time found that escitalopram was more effective than paroxetine at 24 weeks (Lader, Stender, Burger, et al., 2004).

The SNRI venlafaxine ER has been found to be effective in treating patients with SAD (Thase, 2006), with patients receiving it showing a reduction of anxiety symptoms and improvement of their social life at 4 to 12 weeks and better work functioning at 12 weeks (Rickels, Mangano, & Khan, 2004).

Second-line Medications

Second-line medications for generalized SAD include benzodiazepines and the antidepressant mirtazapine (Davidson et al., 2009). Benzodiazepines are used for patients with performance anxiety on an as-needed basis; they are also used for patients who do not respond to SSRIs or venlafaxine (Blanco, Schneier, Vesga-Lopez, et al., 2010). However, benzodiazepines do not relieve comorbid depression, and dependence can develop within 2 weeks of use. To reduce the risk of dependence, the long-acting benzodiazepine clonazepam may be used. When it is discontinued, it should be tapered by a reduction of 0.25 mg every 2 weeks. Mirtazapine has been found to improve symptoms of SAD and also to improve social functioning (Muehlbacher, Nickel, Nickel, et al., 2005).

Other Pharmacotherapeutic Approaches

Other medications that have been reported to be effective for generalized SAD include antidepressants, anticonvulsants, and atypical antipsychotics.

Among antidepressant medications, the monoamine oxidase inhibitor phenelzine (Nardil) has been found to be effective for SAD; however, because of its interaction with other medications, foods, and beverages, it is reserved for patients who do not respond to other treatment interventions (Blanco et al., 2010). Tricyclic antidepressants have not been found to be effective for SAD (Davidson et al., 2009), and the antidepressant bupropion (Wellbutrin) has not been widely studied (Blanco et al.).

Among anticonvulsants, gabapentin has been found to reduce symptoms of SAD for some patients, but the response rate is low, 45% (Schneier, 2006). Older patients showed a greater response to gabapentin than younger patients (Blanco et al., 2010). Pregabalin at high doses—600 mg/day—has been found to reduce symptoms of SAD and to improve social avoidance (Blanco et al., 2010; Pande, Feltner, Jefferson, et al., 2004).

Clinical trials with small numbers of patients with SAD suggest that atypical antipsychotics olanzapine and quetiapine may relieve some symptoms (Barnett, Kramer, Casat, et al., 2002; Schutters, van Megen, & Westenberg, 2005). Risperidone, when used as augmentation, has been found to reduce symptoms of SAD (Simon, Hoge, Fischmann, et al., 2006).

Combined Pharmacotherapy and Psychotherapy

CBT and medications when used alone have similar response rates: approximately 50% in the acute treatment of SAD (Otto, Pollack, Gould, et al., 2000). There does not appear to be any benefit of combining psychotherapy and pharmacotherapy because a combination of CBT and medications had a response rate similar to that of each used alone (Davidson, Foa, Huppert, et al., 2004; Hollander & Simeon, 2008).

A new approach to combined treatment is to administer the glutamatergic *N*-methyl-D-aspartate (NMDA) receptor agonist, D-cycloserine, with psychotherapy. D-cycloserine is an antibiotic that is used in the treatment of tuberculosis; however, in addition to antibiotic activity, the drug also affects brain functioning by increasing the effectiveness of fear-reduction strategies. It has been found to be effective in helping people to overcome phobias. Hofmann, Meuret, Smits, et al. (2006) reported that those who received D-cycloserine, in comparison to those who received a placebo, had much less social anxiety during the exposure interventions.

Pharmacotherapy for Nongeneralized SAD

First choices for nongeneralized SAD—which is also known as performance anxiety—are beta blockers or benzodiazepines (Davidson et al., 2009). Beta blockers decrease distress by reducing autonomic arousal, such as tachycardia, palpitations, tremors, sweating, and dry mouth (Dubovsky, 2005). Beta blockers such as metoprolol (Lopressor), atenolol (Tenormin), and propranolol (Inderal) are effective when taken about 45 minutes before a performance. They control stage fright with few side effects. Although benzodiazepines may decrease performance anxiety, they may have an adverse effect on performance and mental focus (Hollander & Simeon, 2008). Dubovsky (p. 383) suggests trying a test dose and having the patient visualize the situation.

Psychosocial Interventions for SAD

Psychosocial interventions used for SAD include social skills training and relaxation training. Social skills training is based on the assumption that an individual's social anxiety is caused by a lack of social skills, and this lack produces negative reactions from others and leads to the individual's experiencing feelings of failure and rejection. Social skills training provides information about correct social behaviors. The correct social behaviors are modeled, and then patients practice the skills in real situations that have caused them distress in the past. The information available on the outcome of social skills training for SAD suggests that it is effective and that the benefit was maintained for 2 years after the treatment ended (Turner, Beidel, & Cooley-Quille, 1995).

Relaxation strategies teach individuals with SAD how to relax, encourage them to practice the relaxation techniques in non-anxiety-producing situations, and then prompt them to use relaxation techniques as they gradually expose themselves to anxiety-producing situations. The intervention is a combination of using relaxation techniques and exposure to feared stimuli. There is no empirical evidence of the effect of relaxation intervention when used alone for SAD (Hollander & Simeon, 2008).

Course

SAD onset is in midadolescence (van Ameringen et al., 2003). The onset may be sudden—e.g., occurring after a humiliating social experience—but more often, SAD develops over a long time and there may be no precipitating event (Hollander & Simeon, 2008). The course is often lifelong, and it is marked by severe anxiety, limitation of academic, vocational, and social functioning, dropping out of school, and dissatisfaction with life (Ollendick & Hirshfeld-Becker, 2002; Ramsawh, Raffa, Edelen, et al., 2009; Shields, 2004). Approximately half of patients with SAD recover (Hollander & Simeon, 2011). The outcomes are less favorable for patients with SAD who have comorbid depression, other anxiety disorders, and personality disorders (Hollander & Simeon, 2011; Keller, 2003).

Key Points

- SAD is a common disorder that is stressful, impairing, and treatable, but it is frequently unrecognized.
- Patients with SAD have often had the symptoms for 10 years or longer before being correctly diagnosed, and most do not receive treatment (Gross, Olfson, Gameroff, et al., 2005).
- Evidence-based treatments for SAD include cognitive behavioral therapies that include exposure and cognitive restructuring and pharmacotherapy.
- Drugs approved by the FDA for treatment of SAD include the SSRIs paroxetine (Paxil), sertraline (Zoloft), and fluvoxamine CR (Luvox CR) and the SNRI venlafaxine SR (Effexor SR) (Davidson et al., 2009).
- Trials of the use of anticonvulsant medications, such as pregabalin (Lyrica), suggest that they may be effective in reducing symptoms of SAD.
- Among those receiving treatment, the treatment is often suboptimal in terms of amount and length of treatment (Keller, 2003).
- The consequences of untreated SAD are a life of "missed opportunity": people with untreated SAD may not complete high school or succeed in a career, and they often have a life of disabilities, depression, and substance abuse (van Ameringen et al., 2003, p. 569).
- For society, the consequences of untreated SAD include loss of social and occupational functioning and decreased productivity (van Ameringen et al., 2003).

Case Study 10-1 describes a patient with SAD.

Panic Disorder

Panic disorder is characterized by panic attacks that occur repeatedly, great concern about the possibility of future panic attacks, and avoidance of situations that might trigger a panic attack (Pollack, Smoller, Otto, et al., 2010; Shrestha, Natarajan, & Coplan, 2010). *Panic* is the outward evidence of an underlying constitutional vulnerability for anxiety—probably a genetic vulnerability—that is evidenced in an abnormally sensitive fear network (Gorman, Shear, Cowley, et al., 2004). *Panic attacks* are biological events, and their origin lies in brain dysfunction (Andrews, Charney,

CASE STUDY 10-1

A Patient With Social Anxiety Disorder

Gail Stevens, a 34-year-old single Caucasian woman who lives with her parents, has been referred by her primary care physician to the Behavioral Health Clinic for depression that has responded only partially to treatment with the SSRI sertraline.

Assessment reveals that the patient is an only child whose parents had been in their early 40s when she was born. She had been a shy child, and school had been difficult for her. She had become very anxious when she had to take tests and had avoided participating in sports or other school activities. She had two close friends in school and continues to see them. After graduating from high school, she had worked as a receptionist in her parents' art restoration business, but she had difficulty talking with customers and became anxious when she tried to answer their questions. She took online courses so that she could work as a bookkeeper in her parents' business. Her parents sold the business 4 months ago and are planning to move to a smaller place as soon as they can sell their house. Gail is now unemployed and facing the need to find a job.

Gail denies any past history of psychiatric disorder, psychiatric treatment, or suicide ideation. In school, her teachers made accommodations for her shyness. She says that her mother and father are perfectionists who tend to keep to themselves.

Gail appears to be her stated age. She is well-groomed and appropriately dressed. She has a worried expression and twists her hands as she sits on the edge of her chair. Her speech is slow with an anxious tone. She denies any current medical problems. There has been no change in her appetite, weight, energy, or daily activities. She says that she has trouble falling asleep and that she needs a glass or two of sherry to help her fall asleep. She says that she has been depressed off and on since she turned 30, but it has gotten worse since she became unemployed. She worries about finding a job; how hard it will be to go for an interview; and, if hired, how she will she be able to work with strangers.

Questions

1. What differential diagnoses might the psychiatric advanced practice nurse be considering as she takes the history?
2. Based on a diagnosis of social anxiety disorder, what are the treatment options?

Answers to these questions can be found at the end of this chapter.

Sirovatka, et al., 2009). Panic attacks are fairly common, with a lifetime prevalence of 28% among the general population in the United States (Kelly, Jorm, & Kitchener, 2009). They also occur frequently in certain psychiatric disorders: panic disorder, specific phobias, SAD, PTSD, mood disorders, and substance-related disorders (Hollander & Simeon, 2008).

Panic attacks usually begin with patients suddenly unable to catch their breath. They may feel dizzy, light-headed, or faint. Panic attacks are associated with somatic sensations, such as palpitations, pounding heart, sweating, trembling, shortness of breath, feeling of smothering, choking, chest pain or discomfort, nausea, numbness, or chills. Individuals with panic attacks experience cognitive symptoms, such as a sudden onset of intense fear, a feeling of terror, or a sense of doom in the absence of real danger. They may experience derealization (feeling that things are not real) or depersonalization (feeling that one is detached from oneself). Many patients with panic attacks hyperventilate, leading to decreased cerebral blood flow and symptoms of dizziness, confusion, and derealization. Patients experiencing a panic attack often think that they are having a heart attack or fear that they are about to die or are going crazy (Hollander & Simeon, 2008).

Although the first panic attack seems to come out of nowhere, there are often prodromal signs, such as anxiety, hypochondriacal fears, dependence on others, and avoidance behaviors. The first panic attack is usually part of a stressful situation, such as exposure to life-threatening illnesses or accidents, loss of personal relationships, or separation from family (Hollander & Simeon, 2008). It may occur while using drugs such as marijuana, lysergic acid diethylamide (LSD), cocaine, or amphetamines. These events may act as triggers to provoke panic attacks in individuals who are already vulnerable to developing them. Even after these conditions end, the panic attacks may continue to occur (Hollander & Simeon).

Most panic attacks last 5 to 20 minutes with peak intensity of anxiety occurring about 10 minutes after the first symptoms, which are usually intense fear and apprehension (Pollack et al., 2010). Some patients who describe the panic attacks as "lasting all day" may be experiencing waves of panic attacks that they perceive as continuous, or they may feel agitated after the panic attack and interpret it as a continuation of the panic attack (Hollander & Simeon, 2008). Patients with panic attacks are often very worried about the consequences of repeated panic attacks. They fear that they may lose their job or their role in the family. They develop anticipatory anxiety, which is apprehension about the possible time and occasion of the next panic attack. They often relate the previous panic attack to certain situations and avoid similar situations (Hollander & Simeon). They may avoid all situations that they think might trigger another attack (Gorman et al., 2004).

Patients with panic attacks may also develop agoraphobia characterized by multiple fears and avoidance behaviors. The fears include fear of leaving home; fear of living alone; fear of being away from home; and fear of being unable to escape or get help. For example, they may fear using public transportation, traveling through tunnels, or being on bridges, in elevators, or in crowds of people. Some patients with panic attacks with agoraphobia are able to face feared situations when they are accompanied by a relative or friend, but for some patients the agoraphobia may be so severe that they are afraid to leave their homes even with a friend and may even be afraid to stay at home alone (Hollander & Simeon, 2008).

After having a panic attack, factors that increase the risk of the patient's developing panic disorder include experiencing the sensations during the attack as a catastrophe; having many severe physical symptoms during the attack; and the presence of other psychiatric disorders (Kelly et al., 2009). Panic disorder is characterized by

- Recurrent, unexpected panic attacks
- Worry about having additional attacks
- Concern about the consequences that the attacks will have (such as "going crazy")
- Changes in behavior that are related to the attacks

Panic disorder is associated with

- Impaired social and occupational functioning (Sherbourne, Wells, & Judd, 1996)
- Poor physical health
- Substance abuse
- Financial dependency
- Diminished quality of life (Katerndahl & Realini, 1997; Rapaport, Clary, Fayyad, et al., 2005; Stein, Roy-Byrne, Craske, et al., 2005)
- Increased risk for suicide attempts (Goodwin & Roy-Byrne, 2006; Johnson, Weissman, & Klerman, 1990)

Epidemiology

Prevalence

The 12-month prevalence of panic disorder is 2.1% of the U.S. general population (Grant, Hasin, Stinson, et al., 2006), with women having twice the rate of men (Pollack et al., 2010). Women are three times more likely to have panic disorder with agoraphobia than men (Pollack et al). Panic disorder is more common in never-married persons and is less common in persons who have completed college.

Onset

The age of onset is considered to be between the early 20s (Gorman et al., 2004) and early 30s (Hollander & Simeon, 2008); however, approximately 50% of patients with panic disorder reported having had childhood anxiety disorders such as overanxious disorder, social phobia, or separation anxiety disorder (Pollack, Otto, Majcher, et al., 1996).

Culture

In most cultures, it is acceptable for women to say that they are fearful or anxious and to avoid situations that cause them fear. Men are usually expected to hide their fears and to face situations rather than avoid them.

Risk Factors

Risk factors for the development of panic disorder include female gender; being Native American, middle-aged, widowed, separated, or divorced; having a low income; having experienced separation, loss, or illness of a significant other; being a victim of sexual assault or interpersonal violence (Hollander & Simeon, 2008); and having a childhood history of experiencing physical abuse, sexual abuse, or both (Goodwin, Fergusson, & Horwood, 2005). Exposure to stressors, such as financial or work problems, starting college, or moving to start a new job, has been found to be a risk factor for development of panic disorder (Taylor, 2000). Intoxication and the use of sedatives, marijuana, cocaine, LSD, and amphetamines have also been found to increase the risk of developing panic disorder (Hollander & Simeon).

Etiology

Explanations of the etiology for panic disorder include genetically influenced vulnerability, developmental theories, psychodynamic theories, and the role of experienced factors.

Genetically Influenced Vulnerability

A high rate of panic disorder exists among first-degree relatives of patients with panic disorder (Smoller, 2008). There is a strong genetic influence for both panic disorder and agoraphobia. For example, heritability accounts for 43% of the variance of panic disorder and 38% of the variance for agoraphobia (Smoller, Sheidley, & Tsuang, 2008). Similar to depression, panic disorder has demonstrated anticipation (a decrease in the age of onset and an increase in severity of symptoms for succeeding generations). Thus, in a family with a history of panic disorder, the younger generation may experience an earlier onset and more severe symptoms than the previous generation (Battaglia, Bertella, Bajo, et al., 1998).

Developmental Theories

Behavioral inhibition, an attribute of genetically influenced temperament, can be defined as an increased state of arousal and inhibition of behavior in the face of new challenges, unfamiliar situations, or uncertainty about what is expected. During childhood, children with inhibited temperament are likely to be shy and fearful and tend to constrict their behavior in new or unfamiliar situations (Rosenbaum, Biederman, Gersten, et al., 1988). Physical signs of inhibited temperament include a higher heart rate and large papillary response to stress that suggests increased activation of the locus ceruleus and a low limbic threshold to arousal. Children with inhibited temperament show more fear-like responses to separations. They have higher rates of anxiety disorders, and the rate increases as they grow older. Separation anxiety in childhood has been linked with adult panic disorder, and school phobia has been linked with agoraphobia (Pollack & Smoller, 1995). However, only 30% of children with inhibited temperament develop anxiety disorders.

Psychodynamic Theories

Psychoanalytical theories propose that anxiety signals the ego to mobilize defense mechanisms such as repression to counteract an internal danger and restore equilibrium. Panic attacks arise from previous unsuccessful attempts to manage anxiety (Hollander & Simeon, 2008). Klein (1981) based his theory of the development of panic attacks on Bowlby's (1973) theory of attachment and separation. (See Chapter 1 for more on attachment theory.) Klein proposed that attachment of an infant to his or her mother is a genetically programmed biological response as well as a learned response; he also proposed that panic disorder and agoraphobia resulted from nonsupportive patterns of family interactions, which he described as having

1. A controlling, domineering parent who keeps the child close to him or her
2. Quarrels and violent behavior between parents
3. Threats of physical harm to one of the parents by the other that results in a child who is afraid to leave home for fear that something dreadful will happen to one of the parents
4. Threats of abandonment of the child or threats of being ejected from the family for bad behavior
5. Overprotective parents who keep the child at home for fear of the child's being harmed

Taylor, Wald, and Asmundson (2007) noted that individuals who are born with neurophysiological vulnerabilities that predispose them to panic disorder are further sensitized by poor parenting, which leads to the child's perception of not being protected. Not being protected leads to feelings of anger at the parents. The child fears that if the anger is expressed it will lead to abandonment. This fear leads to other fears related to separation and independence; it also leads to an impaired ability to modulate angry emotional responses. In adulthood, conflicts such as life stressors reactivate the fear of loss of attachments and of being abandoned.

Experienced Factors

Patients with panic disorder have a greater rate of childhood abuse than patients with GAD or SAD (Safren, Gershuny, Marzol, et al., 2002). For example, among women with panic disorder, 60% had a history of childhood sexual abuse, compared to 31% for women with other forms of anxiety disorder. As adults, patients with panic attacks have a higher rate of adverse life events (losses, marital conflicts, miscarriages, or death of a significant other) in the months before a panic attack than control subjects (Craske, Miller, Rotunda, et al., 1990; Hollander & Simeon, 2008).

Biological Basis

The neuroanatomical hypothesis of panic disorder proposes that panic originates from an abnormally sensitive fear network that involves the prefrontal cortex, insula, hippocampus, amygdala, hypothalamus, thalamus, and brainstem (Bremner & Charney, 2010; Hollander & Simeon, 2008). (See Chapter 9 for information about the fear/anxiety circuit.) Figure 10-3 shows activation of the amygdala, hypothalamus, and brainstem in a patient with panic disorder.

Gorman, Kent, Sullivan, et al. (2000) noted that the cortical processing of information is defective in patients with panic disorder, resulting in misinterpretation of physiological triggers and a misreading of bodily sensations. This misinterpretation activates the fear network and leads to panic. Structural abnormalities, functional abnormalities, and chemical abnormalities all contribute to the biological basis for panic disorder.

Structural Abnormalities

Abnormalities of brain structures—such as in the hippocampus, amygdala, and brainstem—have been found in patients with panic disorder. Patients with panic disorder have decreased density of neurons in the parahippocampal area, which is an area that is part of the hippocampus and the limbic system (Massana, Serra-Grabulosa, Salgado-Pineda, et al., 2003a). This area of the brain receives information from the association areas of the cortex and from the thalamus, and it is involved in learning, emotions, and social behavior.

Patients with panic disorder also have a decreased volume of the amygdala (Massana, Serra-Grabulosa, Salgado, et al., 2003b). The amygdala, through its connections with the hypothalamus, influences regulation of autonomic, endocrine, and immune responses to stimuli; and through its projections to the brainstem, it influences breathing (Hollander & Simeon, 2008). The amygdala also integrates sensory information with previously stored information from similar experiences to determine the significance of the stimulus, e.g., is the stimulus good or bad, is it safe or dangerous. The amygdala then triggers responses based on the determined significance of the stimulus (Amiel et al., 2009).

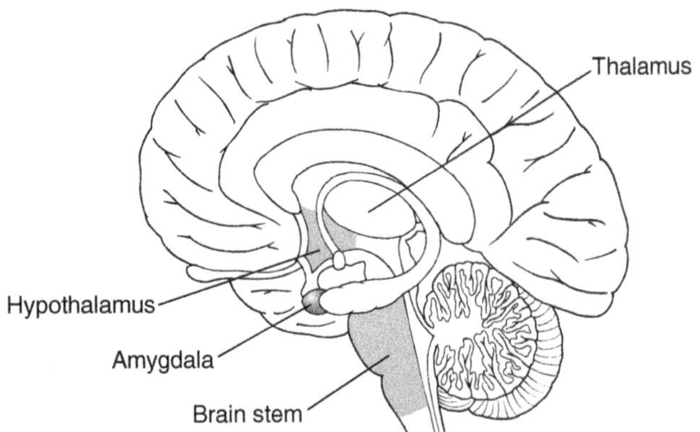

FIGURE 10-3: Neuroanatomical model of the brain in panic disorder that shows activation of the amygdala, hypothalamus, and brainstem (Gorman, Kent, Sullivan, et al., 2000).

Reprinted from Stein, D. J. (2000). False alarm! How to conquer the anxiety disorders. Cape Town, South Africa: University of Stellenbosch. Used with permission.

Increased density of the gray matter volume of the brainstem that controls breathing has been found in patients with panic disorder. That increased density of the neurons suggests greater activity of the brainstem in patients with panic disorder (Protopopescu, Pan, Tuescher, et al., 2006).

Functional Abnormalities

Klein (1993) proposed that panic disorder is caused by carbon dioxide hypersensitivity. When the brain's suffocation monitoring system detects a lack of useful air, it signals the brain's suffocation alarm system. Whereas fear of suffocation is an extremely intense and common fear, in panic disorder, a faulty suffocation alarm system may misinterpret situations as having no exit, causing carbon dioxide hypersensitivity. A biological marker for panic disorder is represented by the induction of panic-like attacks using carbon dioxide inhalation. Hypersensitivity to carbon dioxide occurs in 75% of patients with panic disorder, and its rate is increased in first-degree relatives in comparison to controls (Marazziti & Rotondo, 1999). These findings suggest a genetic influence in the development of hypersensitivity to carbon dioxide.

Abnormalities of the brainstem, which controls functions such as respiration, blood pressure, and digestion, are thought to play an important role in the pathophysiology of panic disorder (Abelson, Weg, Nesse, et al., 2001). Evidence of dysfunction of the brainstem in panic disorder is provided by the finding that patients with panic disorder have irregular breathing patterns: irregular volume, irregular frequency, and a sighing pattern of breathing. These irregular breathing patterns are stable, and they are neither influenced by induced hyperventilation nor reduced by cognitive interventions. In other words, hyperventilation does not cause panic attacks. Rather, panic attacks are precipitated when exposure to carbon dioxide causes transient cerebral hypercapnia (greater than normal amounts of carbon dioxide in the blood) that stimulates the brainstem carbon dioxide receptors, with resulting hyperventilation and panic (Hollander & Simeon, 2008). Thus, brainstem dysregulation may play a more important role in panic disorder than do higher-level brain regulatory circuits (Abelson et al., 2001).

Chemical Abnormalities

Chemical abnormalities of the serotonin, GABA, and benzodiazepine receptors may provide a biological basis for panic disorder:

- ***Serotonin.*** Serotonin is involved in regulation of mood, impulse control, sleep, vigilance, eating, libido, and cognitive functions and in modulation of anxiety and fear. The serotonin system is regulated through different serotonin receptors. In patients with panic disorder, three brain areas in the center of the brain are lacking a key component of a neurochemical messenger system that regulates emotion: the anterior and posterior cingulate areas and the midbrain. The density of the serotonin 1A receptor is reduced by 33% in the anterior cingulate and posterior cingulate areas, which are associated with regulation of anxiety, and by 41% in the midbrain, where serotonin 1A stimulation regulates the synthesis and release of serotonin (Neumeister, Bain, Nugent, et al., 2004). These findings suggest that the heritability of panic disorder may be due to genes that increase the risk by coding for decreased expression of the serotonin 1A receptor (Neumeister et al.). This theory of serotonergic dysregulation is supported by the fact that administration of medications—such as the SSRIs that increase availability of serotonin—is associated with improvement of panic disorder symptoms; however, at this time, there is not sufficient evidence to say that the SSRIs modify the serotonin 1A receptor (Akimova et al., 2009).

- ***GABA.*** GABA is the most important and most widely available *inhibitory* neurotransmitter. Glutamate is the most prominent *excitatory* neurotransmitter. The balance between the GABA system and the glutamate system is crucial for optimal functioning. If GABA overwhelms the glutamate system, then sedation and forgetfulness occur. If GABA is in short supply, then glutamate-influenced activities—such as arousal, restlessness, insomnia, and anxiety—may occur (Shrestha et al., 2010).
- ***Benzodiazepine receptor.*** The benzodiazepine receptor is linked to a receptor for the inhibitory neurotransmitter GABA. Binding of a benzodiazepine to the benzodiazepine receptor increases the action of GABA and results in a calming effect. Overactivity of the insula, which is involved in visceral-somatic functions, owing to decreased inhibition by GABA may result in some of the symptoms seen in panic disorder (Shrestha et al., 2010). It is believed that abnormal GABA functioning contributes to the development of panic disorder (Goddard, Mason, Appel, et al., 2004; Hollander & Simeon, 2008).

Clinical Presentation

The clinical evolvement of panic disorder is in stages:

1. Subpanic stage, in which the patient experiences tachycardia, light-headedness, and shortness of breath.
2. Panic attack stage, with fear of loss of control, freezing, or flight.
3. Hypochondriasis stage, in which patients fear that the panic symptoms are related to a physical illness and hence undergo numerous diagnostic tests and consult with many physicians.
4. Anticipatory anxiety stage, in which patients worry about future attacks.
5. Phobic avoidance stage (agoraphobia), in which the patient avoids places or situations where escape might be difficult, where a panic attack might be embarrassing, or where help might be unavailable. They may avoid bridges, tunnels, elevators, buses, trains, crowded rooms, waiting in line, and stores (Pollack et al., 2010). When the fear of triggers spreads to more things and to fear of not being able to escape or get help, patients begin to avoid all situations that might trigger a panic attack. These behaviors are called "agoraphobic avoidance" (Pollack et al., p. 369).

Individuals with panic disorder often go to an emergency room or primary care setting for the first panic attack, thinking that they are having a heart attack (Deacon, Lickel, & Abramowitz, 2008; Hollander & Simeon, 2011). Their symptoms may include extreme fear and a sense of impending doom and death; cardiovascular symptoms, such as palpitations, chest pain, and paresthesia (numbing, tingling, or a pins-and-needles feeling); and cognitive symptoms, such as apprehension, depersonalization, or fear of losing their mind (Black & Andreasen, 2011). They are examined and tested to rule out heart attack and other physical health problems. Usually the results of these tests are negative and the patient is reassured that nothing is wrong and sent home (Hollander & Simeon). However, the panic attacks often recur once or twice a week and may leave the patient feeling exhausted and drained for up to 2 days. Seventy percent of patients with panic disorder have contacted at least 10 physicians—neurologists, cardiologists and gastroenterologists—without a correct diagnosis being made (McBride & Austin, 1996), and many patients with panic disorder have been ill for 8 to 10 years before coming for psychiatric treatment.

Because of their panic symptoms, anticipatory anxiety, and avoidance behaviors, patients with panic disorder have greater impairment of social, vocational, and role functioning and lower quality of life than the general population (Cramer et al., 2005; Simon, Otto, Korbly, et al., 2002). They are often depressed and are at risk for alcohol or substance abuse; impaired marital, parenting, work, and social functioning; and suicide. In clinical settings, 75% of patients with panic disorder have been found to have at least mild symptoms of agoraphobia (Pollack et al., 2010). Some patients with panic disorders and agoraphobia may develop such a fear of having a panic attack outside the safety of their homes that they become housebound (Pollack et al.). In the United States, patients with symptoms of panic disorder make up 20% of emergency room visits (Swinson, Cox, & Woszczyna, 1992) and half of all visits to primary care providers (Katon, 1996). The majority of patients with panic disorder receive their care in primary care settings, where their panic disorder is often not recognized or is misdiagnosed and treatment is inadequate (Marcks, Weisberg, & Keller, 2009); for example, nearly half of patients with panic disorder receiving care in primary care settings do not receive treatment that would help them (Deacon et al., 2008; Roy-Byrne, Russo, Dugdale, et al., 2002).

Comorbidity

Patients with panic disorder have high rates of comorbid medical disorders (Sareen, Cox, Clara, et al., 2005). They also have high rates of Axis I psychiatric disorders, Axis II personality disorders, impairment of functioning, and social problems (Pollack et al., 2010).

Medical Disorders

Frequently co-occurring medical illnesses include cardiovascular illnesses (Sareen et al., 2005); respiratory illnesses (Simon & Fischmann, 2005); irritable bowel syndrome; asthma; chronic fatigue syndrome; hypothyroidism; migraine headaches; mitral valve prolapse; and the syndrome of joint hypermobility (Coplan & Gorman, 2002; Gulpek, Bayraktar, Akbay, et al., 2004). Joint hypermobility syndrome, which is an inherited connective tissue condition (lax connective tissue), occurs in approximately 70% of patients with panic disorder in contrast to 15% of healthy control subjects (Martin-Santos, Bulbena, Porta, et al., 1998). The incidence of mitral valve prolapse is increased in patients with panic disorder (Coplan & Gorman), especially among those with joint hypermobility. Some of the symptoms of panic disorder and mitral valve prolapse are the same—dyspnea (less frequent in mitral valve prolapse), palpitations, and chest pain (less frequent in panic disorder)—but in mitral valve prolapse there is rarely choking, dizziness, derealization, hot or cold flashes, sweating, trembling, or fear of dying or going crazy (Hollander & Simeon, 2008). There is some controversy about the actual rate of occurrence of mitral valve prolapse among patients with panic disorder (Andreasen & Black, 2006; Hollander & Simeon, 2011; Katerndahl, 1993).

Psychiatric Disorders

Among patients with panic disorder, the comorbidity of Axis I psychiatric disorders is 80.3%, and the comorbidity of Axis II personality disorders is 33.9% (Ozkan & Altindag, 2005). The lifetime prevalence of major depressive disorder among patients with panic disorder is 50% to 60%, with major depressive disorder preceding panic disorder in about one-third of patients. Comorbid depression increases the risk for suicide in patients with panic disorder (Vickers & McNally, 2004). Other comorbid psychiatric disorders include SAD, GAD, PTSD, OCD, bipolar disorder, and alcohol abuse (Pollack et al., 2010). The most frequently occurring personality disorders are the borderline, dependent, and avoidant personality disorders (Starcevic, Bogojevic, Marinkovic, et al., 1999). Psychiatric advanced practice nurses need to be aware that suicide ideation is a serious comorbid condition among patients with panic disorder, with the risk for suicide higher among patients with panic disorder who have comorbid depression, personality disorders, or alcohol or substance abuse (Gorman et al., 2004; Ozkan & Altindag, 2005; Pilowsky, Olfson, Gameroff, et al., 2006).

Impaired Functioning and Social Problems

In comparison to the general population, patients with panic disorder have higher rates of impaired role functioning, such as trouble carrying out normal daily activities (Pollack et al., 2010). They have more problems with marital relationships and more impairment of social and vocational functioning. For example, in one study, 43% of patients with panic disorder were unable to work full time, and 25% were unemployed (Ettigi, Meyerhoff, Chirban, et al., 1997). They are more likely to be dependent on others for financial support (Roy-Byrne, Stein, Russo, et al., 1999).

Differential Diagnosis

Panic disorder with and without agoraphobia (Table 10-5 and Table 10-6) must be differentiated from medical conditions, psychiatric disorders, and substance use. It must also be differentiated from medical conditions, medications, and substances that cause anxiety (see Table 10-1).

TABLE 10-5 DIFFERENTIAL DIAGNOSIS OF PANIC DISORDER WITH AGORAPHOBIA

Other Psychiatric Disorder	Differentiating Characteristics of Other Psychiatric Disorder
Substance-induced anxiety disorder	Panic attacks are due to the direct physiological effects of a substance or medication
Panic attacks occurring as part of another anxiety disorder (social phobia, specific phobia, obsessive-compulsive disorder, post-traumatic stress disorder)	Panic attacks are either situationally bound or situationally predisposed (in comparison to unexpected panic attacks of panic disorder)
Separation anxiety disorder	Onset is in childhood and is characterized by anxiety and avoidance that is focused on separation concerns (e.g., being away from home and family)
Avoidance in delusional disorder	Related to delusional concerns

Sources: First, Frances, & Pincus, 2002; Hollander & Simeon, 2011.

TABLE 10-6 **DIFFERENTIAL DIAGNOSIS OF PANIC DISORDER WITHOUT AGORAPHOBIA**

Other Psychiatric Disorder	Differentiating Characteristics of Other Psychiatric Disorder
Panic disorder with agoraphobia	Characterized by recurrent unexpected panic attacks preceding the onset of agoraphobia
Social phobia	Characterized by avoidance of performance in social situations in which the individual would be exposed to the scrutiny of others
Specific phobia	Characterized by avoidance of a specific fear object or situation that is not related to worries about being able to escape if panic symptoms develop
Being housebound related to major depressive disorder	Feelings of apathy, fatigue, loss of capacity to experience pleasure, or worry about crying in public
Avoidance in delusional disorder	Related to delusion (e.g., being followed)
Avoidance in obsessive-compulsive disorder	Behavior is intended to prevent triggering an obsession or compulsion (avoiding items seen as dirty or dangerous)
Separation anxiety disorder	Characterized by avoidance of situations that involve being away from home or close relatives
Avoidance related to realistic concerns about a general medical condition	Behavior is appropriated given the nature of the general medical condition (e.g., worry about fainting)
Somatization disorder	Somatic symptoms are episodic (e.g., they occur with panic attacks)

Sources: First, Frances, & Pincus, 2002; Hollander & Simeon, 2011.

Treatment

Both individual psychotherapy and pharmacotherapy have been found to be effective in treating panic disorder (Hollander & Simeon, 2008). However, some patients view psychotherapy as being more inconvenient, more likely to be a financial problem, and more stigmatizing than pharmacotherapy (Marcks et al., 2009). At the present time, a combination of psychotherapy and pharmacotherapy is the most frequently used approach to treating patients with panic disorder (Black & Andreasen, 2011).

In addition to a comprehensive psychiatric assessment, screening instruments can be used to measure the presence of anxiety symptoms, the severity of panic disorder symptoms, and the severity of agoraphobic avoidance behaviors. *The Anxiety Sensitivity Index (ASI)* (Reiss, Peterson, Gursky, et al., 1986) is a 16-item self-report questionnaire that evaluates whether patients interpret symptoms of anxiety as threatening, as a source of embarrassment, or as a loss of control. It is a valid screen for panic disorder. The *Panic Disorder Severity Scale (PDSS)* (Shear, Brown, Barlow, et al., 1997) is a brief, seven-item instrument intended to assess severity of symptoms. The severity of agoraphobic avoidance behaviors can be measured with the *Mobility Inventory for Agoraphobia (MI)* (Chambless, Caputo, Jasin, et al., 1985), which asks patients to rate the degree to which they avoid 26 situations such as trains or supermarkets that frequently cause anxiety. Screening instruments can be used to provide a baseline measure of severity of symptoms and to monitor response to treatment.

Treatment for panic disorder should address five core problem areas:

1. Symptoms of panic attacks
2. Anticipatory anxiety
3. Phobias related to the panic attacks
4. Impaired functioning
5. Overall well-being (Ballenger, Davidson, Lecrubier, et al., 1998; Davidson et al., 2009)

Treatment plans should be based on assessment of the patient's clinical status, functioning, stressors, social support, living situation, and basic needs (Gorman et al., 2004). Treatment of panic disorder includes the use of psychotherapy, pharmacotherapy, and psychosocial interventions that include education about the illness and support.

Psychotherapy

Psychotherapy for panic disorder usually combines in vivo exposure and cognitive interventions (Hofmann et al., 2010). The foundation of treatment is the theory that panic disorder is based on cognitive and behavioral factors that can be changed to prevent panic attacks. Cognitive treatment seeks to change how the patient interprets bodily sensations. The goal of in vivo exposure is the reduction of anxiety, and it requires patients to expose themselves to feared situations until anxiety is diminished. Models of psychotherapy that are used in the treatment of patients with panic disorder include CBT, cognitive behavioral group therapy (CBGT), psychodynamic therapy, exposure therapy, and supportive psychotherapy.

Cognitive Behavioral Therapy and Cognitive Behavioral Group Therapy

Among the different models of psychotherapy, CBT is considered to be the first line of psychotherapy for panic disorder and has been found to be comparable in effectiveness to first-line pharmacotherapy treatment (Hollander & Simeon, 2008). CBT usually includes

1. Psychoeducation that provides an explanation of the symptoms
2. Continuous monitoring, in which patients are taught to monitor their panic attacks and to record their thoughts, e.g., to use a daily diary

3. Breathing retraining to reduce hyperventilation
4. Cognitive restructuring that teaches the patient to consider evidence and alternative explanation for their symptoms and not to use catastrophic anticipation
5. Exposure to triggers that helps the patient to tolerate exposure to feared events

CBT is usually administered over 12 to 15 weeks and requires a strong commitment and active participation by the patient. The intensity of CBT—measured by the number of therapy sessions, the number of follow-up booster phone calls, and the number of coping and exposure strategies—appears to be related to the degree of improvement achieved (Craske, Roy-Byrne, Stein, et al., 2006). Among patients with panic disorder who complete treatment in which in vivo exposure is used, 60% to 75% improve (Mitte, 2005).

CBT appears to have long-term benefits for patients with panic disorder. Fava, Rafanelli, Grandi, et al. (2001) found that 10 years after treatment with CBT, 62% of the patients were in remission. However, panic disorder is less responsive to CBT than other anxiety disorders are (Hofmann & Smits, 2009), and one out of four patients drops out of treatment (Hofmann & Smits).

CBT is also effective in a group format (Telch, Lucas, Schmidt, et al., 1993) and as group therapy in combination with medication (Nagy, Krystal, Wood, et al., 1989). More recently, CBGT has been found to be effective for patients with panic disorder who had not benefited from pharmacotherapy. CBGT consisting of 12 sessions resulted in reduction of general and anticipatory anxiety and improvement of quality of life (Heldt, Blaya, Isolan, et al., 2006).

Psychodynamic Therapy

Psychodynamic therapy is based on the theory that conflicts are the basis of panic symptoms (Milrod, Busch, Cooper, et al., 1997). In panic disorder, it is thought that unconscious conflict related to separations experienced in childhood may be the basis for symptoms of anxiety in adulthood when separations are imagined or threatened (Hollander & Simeon, 2008). The goal of psychodynamic therapy is to identify and change the patient's core conflicts. Explanation of symptoms is placed in the context of the patient's life history and present situation. Reports of case studies suggest that psychodynamic therapy is effective for some patients with panic disorder (Gorman et al., 2004). In a randomized controlled clinical trial, psychodynamic therapy was found to be more effective than a control intervention of applied relaxation training: there was a greater reduction of panic attacks, anxiety, and avoidance and there was improvement of functioning and quality of life (Milrod, Leon, Busch, et al., 2007). Psychodynamic therapy has been found to be useful in combined therapy with the antidepressant medication clomipramine (Spiegel & Hofmann, 2002).

Exposure Therapy

Using in vivo exposure (i.e., being in the actual feared situation) is more effective for agoraphobia than the older approach of using imaginal exposure with muscle relaxation. Exposure therapy for agoraphobia begins with creating a hierarchy of feared situations. Patients are encouraged to enter the situations starting with the least feared, or the one that is least likely to provoke anxiety. Hoffmann et al. (2010) reported that meta-analysis of treatment studies has shown that 60% to 75% of patients completing in vivo exposure treatment experienced clinical improvement.

Supportive Psychotherapy

Supportive psychotherapy is helpful for patients with panic disorder who still use avoidance behaviors even though medication may have reduced the panic attacks. Some patients are able to benefit from being in a group with other patients who have overcome similar avoidance behaviors (Hollander & Simeon, 2008).

Pharmacotherapy

The goals of pharmacotherapy for panic disorder are (1) to reduce or eliminate panic attacks, avoidance behavior, and anticipatory anxiety and (2) to manage comorbid conditions (Pollack, 2005). Choice of medication depends on the patient's history of response to medication, potential for tolerating side effects of the medication, presence of comorbid psychiatric or medical illnesses, history of substance abuse, and presenting symptoms (Davidson & Connor, 2004). The patient should be told that in the beginning the medication will block the panic attacks, but it may not prevent anticipatory anxiety and the use of avoidance behaviors (Hollander & Simeon, 2008). Pharmacotherapy for panic disorder includes first-line, second-line, and third-line pharmacotherapy; augmentative medications; combined pharmacotherapy and psychotherapy; and long-term pharmacotherapy.

First-line Pharmacotherapy

The SSRIs and SNRIs are considered to be the first line of pharmacotherapy for the treatment of panic disorder (Bandelow & Baldwin, 2010; Davidson et al., 2009; Hollander & Simeon, 2008).

- ***SSRIs.*** Although the FDA has approved only some of the SSRIs—specifically, paroxetine, sertraline, and fluoxetine—it is generally accepted that all of the SSRIs are equally effective in the treatment of panic disorder (Stein & Campbell-Sills, 2007). The following SSRIs have been reported to be effective in managing panic disorder: citalopram, paroxetine, sertraline, fluvoxamine, fluoxetine, and escitalopram oxalate (Bandelow & Baldwin, 2010; Davidson et al., 2009). Cost and previous response to a medication may guide selection of a specific SSRI (Hollander & Simeon, 2008). Benefits usually are evidenced by 4 weeks, and patients may experience a full response by 8 to 12 weeks (Gorman et al., 2004).

Because discontinuation symptoms—e.g., dizziness, lack of coordination, headache, irritability, and nausea—resemble some of the symptoms of panic attacks, the SSRIs must be tapered off when discontinued (Black, Wesner, Bowers, et al., 1993), and patients should be warned against stopping their medications abruptly. CBT added to the treatment plan during withdrawal from benzodiazepines and antidepressant medications can reduce the risk of rebound panic attacks (Schmidt, Wollaway-Bickel, Trakowski, et al., 2002).

- *SNRIs.* Venlafaxine has FDA approval for the treatment of panic disorder. It has been found to reduce the number of panic attacks and improve symptoms of anticipatory anxiety, fear, and avoidance (Bradwejn, Ahokas, Stein, et al., 2005).

Some patients with panic disorder are sensitive to antidepressant medications. They may feel jittery and agitated and have trouble sleeping. These symptoms are transient, and patients should be told that these symptoms do not signify the onset of a panic attack. A benzodiazepine may be used with an SSRI in the beginning to manage the activating properties of the SSRI (Bandelow & Baldwin, 2010). The benzodiazepine is then tapered off after 4 weeks of antidepressant treatment using a 3-week taper (Hollander & Simeon, 2008). To avoid patients' terminating treatment, small doses of antidepressants—lower than the dose used for major depressive disorder—should be used in the beginning and should be combined with education about panic disorder and the effects of medications. The dose should be increased by small amounts every 1 to 2 weeks (Bandelow & Baldwin). Having patients call after each increase to report their progress prevents them from worrying if side effects are severe enough for them to call to report them (Dubovsky, 2005). Benefit usually begins in 2 to 4 weeks, although it may take 6 to 8 weeks for some patients (Bandelow & Baldwin).

Second-line Pharmacotherapy

TCAs such as clomipramine (Anafranil), imipramine, desipramine (Norpramin), and nortriptyline (Aventyl, Pamelor) are considered to be the second line of treatment for panic disorder, and continued treatment with TCAs for 18 months or longer has been found to be associated with reduced risk for relapse (Gorman et al., 2004). Although TCAs, which keep more of both serotonin and norepinephrine available, are as effective as the SSRIs in treating panic disorder, they are considered to be the second line of treatment because (1) they are more difficult for patients to tolerate than the SSRIs (Bandelow & Baldwin, 2010; Davidson et al., 2009; Dubovsky, 2005) and (2) TCAs have more troublesome side effects, such as cardiovascular problems, weight gain, and potential lethality in overdose (Stein & Campbell-Sills, 2007). TCAs must be tapered off when discontinued because discontinuation symptoms resemble some of the symptoms of panic attacks, including dizziness, impairment of coordination, headache, irritability, and nausea (Davidson et al.).

If there is a poor response to other antidepressants or if there is a comorbid atypical depression or social phobia, then the monoamine oxidase inhibitor (MAOI) antidepressants—phenelzine (Nardil) and tranylcypromine (Parnate)—have been found to be effective for panic disorder and for panic disorder with depression (Hollander & Simeon, 2008). Patients receiving MAOIs need education about dietary restrictions and about the interaction of MAOIs with other drugs and with over-the-counter cold medications (Dubovsky, 2005). MAOIs are reserved for patients who do not respond to other treatment modalities (Bandelow & Baldwin, 2010).

Reboxetine (Vestra), which is an SNRI, has been found to be effective for patients with panic disorder who have not responded to SSRIs or to benzodiazepines (Versiani, Cassano, Perugi, et al., 2002). Mirtazapine has also been found to be effective in the treatment of panic disorder (Carpenter, Leon, Yasmin, et al., 1999; Ribeiro, Busnello, Kauer-Sant'Anna, et al., 2001).

In summarizing the use of antidepressant medications for patients with panic disorder, it should be noted that full remission of panic attacks usually requires 8 to 12 weeks of treatment. Patients should be kept on full dose for at least 6 months to prevent early relapse. After 6 months, the dose can be tapered to half the usual dose and then, gradually, the dose can be reduced every few months until the minimum dose required to keep the patient symptom free is reached (Hollander & Simeon, 2008).

Third-line Pharmacotherapy: Benzodiazepines

Although antidepressants comprise the first two lines of treatment for panic disorder, benzodiazepines are also effective and may be used when the patient has a poor response to antidepressants or marked anticipatory anxiety or avoidance behaviors. Benzodiazepines such as alprazolam, lorazepam, clonazepam, and diazepam are known to be effective in blocking panic attacks and have the most rapid onset of action (Bandelow & Baldwin, 2010; Schatzberg, Cole, & DeBattista, 2007). Improvement of symptoms takes about 1 week with benzodiazepines in comparison to 4 to 6 weeks for antidepressant medications.

The effect of benzodiazepines differs from that of antidepressant medications. For example, benzodiazepines do not reduce the depression that is often present with panic disorder (Bandelow & Baldwin, 2010). Because side effects include drowsiness, weakness, slurred speech, cognitive impairment, and memory loss (Bandelow & Baldwin; Gorman et al., 2004), patients should be told not to drive when taking these medications. Another concern is the finding that alprazolam has been reported to induce mania (Dubovsky, 2005).

The major problem associated with the use of benzodiazepines is the development of dependence (Davidson et al., 2009). Many patients experience difficulty in discontinuing alprazolam (Rickels, Schweizer, Weiss, et al., 1993). Alprazolam XR, an extended-release formulation of alprazolam, does not cause the sudden increases of plasma levels of alprazolam and seems to cause less sedation and less impairment of cognitive and motor functioning. It may cause less clock-watching as patients anticipate the next dose. However, long-term use carries the same risk for dependence and the same withdrawal response as the original formulation of alprazolam (Rickels, 2004).

The benzodiazepine clonazepam blocks panic attacks and has been found to have other benefits, such as improved quality of life and increased work productivity (Jacobs, Davidson, Gupta, et al., 1997). It is a better choice than alprazolam because it is longer acting and less dangerous and there is less risk of the patient's experiencing withdrawal symptoms (Hollander & Simeon, 2008). Studies have shown that the addition of clonazepam for patients who are receiving SSRIs speeds up treatment response (Pollack, Simon, Worthington, et al., 2003). When clonazepam is used with SSRIs, it is used briefly—for 3 weeks—and then discontinued (Goddard, Brouette, Almai, et al., 2001).

In terminating benzodiazepines, a long, slow taper over weeks or months is used (Davidson et al., 2009). Some patients may experience a return of their original anxiety symptoms, which is known as rebound anxiety. However, rebound anxiety is transient, usually lasting only 48 to 72 hours. Clinicians monitoring termination of benzodiazepines need to be available to provide support and reassurance for patients as they go through the process. The addition of CBT has been found to be helpful in tapering off benzodiazepines (Davidson et al.; Hofmann, Rief, & Spiegel, 2010). Self-help groups are also helpful (Davidson et al.). Withdrawal signs include insomnia, agitation, anxiety, and rarely seizures. When seizures occur with the termination of benzodiazepines, it usually happens 5 to 7 days after the medication has been stopped.

Several researchers believe that the risk of benzodiazepine dependency is overstated (Hollander & Simeon, 2008; Schatzberg et al., 2007). They have said that most patients with panic disorder maintain benefits without needing an increased dose of the benzodiazepine over time, i.e., they do not develop tolerance. They have suggested that the risk for dependence is primarily among patients who are at risk for addiction. Therefore, benzodiazepines are contraindicated in patients with a history of substance abuse (Gorman et al., 2004).

Medications Used for Augmentation

Venlafaxine and buspirone have been suggested as augmentative medications for panic disorder (Gorman et al., 2004). For patients who have not responded to monotherapy with SSRIs, adding the atypical antipsychotic olanzapine has been found to result in a marked increase in response (Sepede, Mancini, Salerno, et al., 2006). Augmentation with olanzapine was associated with a 75% decrease in panic attacks and anticipatory anxiety in patients who had not responded to other forms of treatment (Hollifield, Thompson, Ruiz, et al., 2005).

Combined Pharmacotherapy and Psychotherapy

Early studies about the use of combined CBT and medications were inconclusive. More recent evidence suggests that there is a benefit from providing CBT with medications for panic disorder (Craske, Golinelli, Stein, et al., 2005). Improvement occurs earlier if the patient receives both medication and psychotherapy than if either is used alone (Furukawa, Watanae, & Churchill, 2006); improvement is seen in anxiety, social avoidance, and functioning (Craske et al.).

Psychodynamic therapy in combination with medication has also been found to be associated with improved long-term outcomes (Wiborg & Dahl, 1996). It is generally accepted that the combination of psychotherapy and pharmacotherapy produces better results than pharmacotherapy or psychotherapy alone (Furukawa et al., 2006). While waiting for the benefits of combined psychotherapy and pharmacotherapy, benzodiazepines may be used for severe panic attacks or high levels of anticipatory anxiety. In combined therapy, medications are continued for the acute phase, usually for 12 weeks.

Long-term Pharmacotherapy

Because there is a high rate of relapse (30% to 90%) when antidepressant medications are discontinued (Gorman et al., 2004), treatment is usually maintained for 12 to 24 months, then slowly tapered until discontinuation (Bandelow & Baldwin, 2010; Davidson et al., 2009). There is evidence of further improvement with longer treatment. For example, in a 4-year study of patients with panic disorder, greater improvement was found among those who continued on medication for 4 years in comparison to those who continued on medication for only 1 year (Katschnig, Amering, Stolk, et al., 1995).

Psychosocial Interventions

Patients with panic disorder tend to avoid activities and situations that may trigger a panic attack. Avoidance behaviors often result in withdrawal from social, vocational, and community activities. LeDoux and Gorman (2001) stated that psychosocial interventions have the potential to help patients to re-engage with their environment. They stated that patients with anxiety disorders should be encouraged to replace passive avoidance behaviors with active avoidance behaviors, e.g., they can replace withdrawal and inactivity with simple activities that bring pleasure and are not stressful, such as walking, reading for pleasure, or helping a friend. Psychosocial interventions that have been found to be beneficial as adjunctive interventions for patients with panic disorder include panic control treatment (PCT), marital and family therapy, bibliotherapy, education, and self-help interventions (Gorman et al., 2004).

Panic Control Treatment

PCT includes several elements: educating the patient about panic attacks, monitoring panic symptoms, teaching anxiety management skills, and providing cognitive restructuring and in vivo exposure (Gorman et al., 2004). Patients are taught how to reduce both arousal and hyperventilation. Cognitive restructuring is used to change thoughts about anxiety and panic with a focus on changing automatic thoughts about the danger of panic attacks. Patients are also exposed slowly to increasing amounts of bodily sensations that are similar to those experienced in a panic attack.

PCT has been found to be associated with a reduction of panic attacks, level of anxiety, and avoidance behaviors (Barlow, Esler, & Vitali, 1998). Studies of the outcome of PCT have shown that approximately 86% of patients with panic disorder were free of panic attacks after 3 to 4 months of treatment and, at the 2-year follow-up, 81% of patients were free of panic attacks (Craske, Brown, & Barlow, 1991).

PCT has been found to be more effective than the benzodiazepine alprazolam and the TCA imipramine (Barlow, Gorman, Shear, et al., 2000). A recent study has shown that PCT is effective in treating veterans with PTSD and comorbid panic disorder. Among a group receiving 10 individual sessions of PCT, 63% were panic free after treatment, whereas in the comparison group that received psychoeducational supportive treatment, 19% of the group was panic free after treatment (Teng, Bailey, Chaison, et al., 2008).

Marital and Family Therapy

Symptoms of panic disorder or panic disorder with agoraphobia can disrupt daily patterns of family living and may place the patient in the role of being the one who stays home and assumes all the family chores. These disorders may also put family members in the caretaker role. Family members may be angry and frustrated with the patient, or they may be accustomed to the patient's staying home and do not welcome treatment that changes the status quo (Gorman et al., 2004). There is little research on the efficacy of marital and family therapy for panic disorder, but the data that are available suggest that including the spouse or partner in treatment is effective (Gorman et al.).

Bibliotherapy

Bibliotherapy is a form of self-directed treatment that uses a manual for CBT to reduce panic attacks (Barlow et al., 1998). In comparison with a group of patients with panic disorder who were on a waiting list, patients receiving bibliotherapy had a reduced frequency of panic attacks, panic thoughts, anticipatory anxiety, avoidance, and depression (Wright, Clum, Roodman, et al., 2000). Later studies have found that bibliotherapy in combination with minimal telephone contact with a therapist reduces panic symptoms and avoidance behaviors (Febbraro, 2005).

Education

Education is provided for patients with panic disorder to help them understand and manage their illness. Education about panic disorder and treatment includes

- Providing the patient with an explanation of symptoms
- Teaching the patient to monitor the panic attacks and record events, emotions, and thoughts associated with the panic attacks in a daily diary
- Implementing cognitive restructuring that assists the patient to consider evidence related to the panic attacks and alternative explanations to prevent catastrophic anticipation (i.e., expecting the worse outcome)
- Providing support during exposure to triggers (Gorman et al., 2004)

Education about both panic attacks and the duration of a panic attack has the potential to reduce patients' anxiety and distress during panic attacks. It has an important augmentative role in the treatment of panic disorder. The effectiveness of education has been found to be greater among patients with less severe symptoms (Baillie & Rapee, 2004).

Self-Help Interventions

In an early study, it was found that exposure therapy that was self-administered using a manual or a computer was as effective for agoraphobia as therapy with a therapist (Ghosh & Marks, 1987). This approach has been expanded to include computer-assisted and self-directed CBT. Patients with panic disorder in a 10-week Internet self-help program with weekly telephone calls were compared to patients on a waiting list. Among patients in the self-help group, 77% no longer met criteria for panic disorder, whereas all of the patients on the waiting list did meet the criteria (Calbring, Bohman, Brunt, et al., 2006). A similar study found that 94% of the patients in an Internet CBT self-help group who received minimal therapist support by e-mail for 10 weeks no longer met criteria for panic disorder, and at 6 months, 82% no longer met criteria for panic disorder (Bergstrom, Andersson, Karlsson, et al., 2009). Internet- and computer-based CBT are interventions that may reduce barriers (lack of access to services and stigma) to receiving treatment for panic disorder (Reger & Gahm, 2009).

Course

Panic disorder is a chronic debilitating illness. It has an adverse effect on patients' physical and mental health and quality of life that is equal to the adverse effect of major depression and is greater than the adverse effect of certain medical conditions (Candilis, McLean, Otto, et al., 1999). Patients with panic disorder with agoraphobia and co-occurring personality disorders have even poorer outcomes (Black, Wesner, Gabel, et al., 1994). Despite the availability of effective psychotherapy and pharmacotherapy for panic disorder, over 40% of individuals with panic disorder do not receive treatment (Wang, Lane, Olfson, et al., 2005). Studies of long-term outcomes of patients who received treatment for panic disorder have found that 30% of patients are well; 40% to 50% are improved but have some symptoms; and 20% to 30% have the same symptoms or worse symptoms (Gorman et al., 2004; Hollander & Simeon, 2008). Among patients who achieved remission, approximately half relapsed at some time during the following 2 years despite continued pharmacotherapy (Simon, Safren, Otto, et al., 2002).

Key Points

- Panic disorder is characterized by panic attacks, by great concern about future panic attacks, and by avoidance of situations that might trigger a panic attack.
- Panic attacks may be triggered by stressful situations or by drugs such as marijuana, LSD, cocaine, or amphetamines.
- Risk factors for development of panic disorder include genetic influences, neurodevelopmental abnormalities of the brain, female gender, insecure attachment patterns, childhood history of separations, losses, and sexual abuse.
- Patients with panic disorder often present in emergency rooms with physical symptoms similar to the symptoms of a heart attack.
- Panic disorders are frequently misdiagnosed and inadequately treated in emergency and primary care settings.
- Consequences of failed diagnoses and inadequate treatment include repeated visits to doctors and emergency rooms; extensive medical examinations; disability; dropping out of school; unemployment; and increased rates of depression, substance use, and suicide.
- Consequences for society are costly owing to loss of time from work and increased use of health services.
- Psychiatric advanced practice nurses must be able to identify panic disorder and provide appropriate psychotherapy, pharmacotherapy, and psychosocial interventions that will relieve distress and promote recovery.
- First-line psychotherapy combines in vivo exposure to feared situations and cognitive interventions.
- First-line pharmacotherapy includes SSRIs and SNRIs.

Resources

Organizations

Anxiety Disorders Association of America (ADAA)
11900 Parklawn Drive, Suite 100
Rockville, MD 20852
301-231-9350
http://www.nimh.nih.gov
National Anxiety Foundation
3135 Custer Drive
Lexington, KY 40517-4001
606-272-7166
http://lexington-online.com/nafmasthead.html
Social Anxiety Research Clinic
http://www.columbia-socialanxiety.org
Social Anxiety/Social Phobia Association
http://www.social-phobia.org
Center for the Neuroscience of Fear and Anxiety
http://www.cns.nyu.edu/CNFA/
Phobias
www.nlm.nih.gov/medlineplus/phobias.html
Clinical anxiety scales can be found in Box 10-2.

BOX 10-2 Clinical Rating Scales for Anxiety Disorders

- *Fear Questionnaire (FQ):* A 24-item instrument developed to assess outcome of work with patients with phobic disorders—agoraphobia, blood-injection-injury phobia, social phobia (Marks & Mathews, 1978).
- *Social Avoidance and Distress Scale (SAD):* A 28-item scale developed to measure stress in social situations and avoidance of social situations that cause stress (Watson & Friend, 1969).
- *Social Anxiety Thoughts Questionnaire (SAT):* A 21-item scale designed to measure frequency of thoughts associated with social distress or anxiety (Hartman, 1984).
- *Liebowitz Social Anxiety Scale:* A 24-item scale that measures the severity of social anxiety (can be used to measure response to treatment) (Liebowitz, 1987).
- Self-report questionnaire: A 21-item questionnaire for identifying cognitive targets for treatment planning as well as assessing change in cognition associated with psychotherapeutic intervention (Hartman, 1984). (Available from Dr. L. M. Hartman. Addiction Research Foundation, 33 Russell Street, Toronto, Ontario, Canada.)
- *Hamilton Anxiety Rating Scale:* A 14-item scale administered by a clinician, used for assessment of severity of overall anxiety in patients with diagnosed anxiety or depressive disorders and monitoring outcome of treatment (Hamilton, 1959). (Available from Anxiety Disorders Prevention program, Western Psychiatric Institute and Clinic, 3811 O'Hara Street, Pittsburgh, PA 15213.)
- *Panic Disorder Severity Scale:* A 7-item clinician-administered or self-report rating scale designed to measure panic frequency, distress during panic, panic-focused anticipatory anxiety, phobic avoidance of situations, phobic avoidance of physical sensations, impairment in work functioning, and impairment in social functioning (Shear, Brown, Barlow, et al., 1997).
- *Panic Attack Symptoms Questionnaire (PASQ):* A 33-item instrument designed to measure duration (severity) of symptoms during panic attacks; able to differentiate between patients experiencing panic attacks and those with anxiety disorders not experiencing panic attacks (Clum, Broyles, Borden, et al., 1990).

Movies

Demme, J. (Producer), & Jonze, S. (Director). (2002). *Adaptation* [Motion picture]. United States: Columbia Pictures.

Movie depicting generalized anxiety disorder

Bruckheimer, J. (Producer), & McNally, D. (Director). (2000). *Coyote ugly* [Motion picture]. United States: Touchstone Pictures.

Movie depicting social anxiety disorder

Block, B. (Producer), & Meyers, N. (Director). (2003). *Something's gotta give* [Motion picture]. United States: Columbia Pictures Industries, Inc., and Warner Bros. Entertainment Inc.

Movie depicting panic attacks (Wedding, Boyd, & Niemiec, 2010)

Scorsese, M. (Director). (2006). *The departed* [Motion picture]. United States: Warner Bros.

Cassavetes, Z. R. (Director). (2007). *Broken English* [Motion picture]. United States: HDNET Films.

References

Abelson, J. L., Weg, J. G., Nesse, R. M., et al. (2001). Persistent respiratory irregularity in patients with panic disorder. *Biological Psychiatry, 49*(7), 588-595.

Akimova, E., Lanzenberger, R., & Kasper, S. (2009). The serotonin-1A receptor in anxiety disorders. *Biological Psychiatry, 66*(7), 627-635.

Alfano, C. A., Ginsburg, G. S., & Kingery, J. N. (2007). Sleep-related problems among children and adolescents with anxiety disorders. *Journal of American Academy of Child and Adolescent Psychiatry, 46,* 224-232.

Al-Kubaisy, T., Marks, I. M., Logsdail, S., et al. (1992). Role of exposure homework in phobia reduction: A controlled study. *Behavior Therapy, 23,* 599-621.

Allgulander, C. (2010). Novel approaches to treatment of generalized anxiety disorder. *Current Opinion in Psychiatry, 23,* 37-42.

Allgulander, C., Bandelow, B., Hollander, E., et al. (2003). WCA recommendations for the long-term treatment of generalized anxiety disorder. *CNS Spectrums, 8*(8 Suppl 1), 53-61.

Allgulander, C., Hackett, D., & Salinas, E. (2001). Venlafaxine extended release (ER) in the treatment of generalized anxiety disorder: Twenty-four week placebo-controlled dose-ranging study. *British Journal of Psychiatry, 179,* 15-22.

American Psychiatric Association. (2000). *Diagnostic and statistical manual of mental disorders* (4th ed., Text Revision). Washington, DC: American Psychiatric Association.

Amiel, J. M., Mathew, J. J., Garakani, A., et al. (2009). Neurobiology of anxiety disorders. In A. F. Schatzberg & C. B. Nemeroff (Eds.), *The American psychiatric publishing textbook of psychopharmacology* (4th ed.) (pp. 965-985). Washington, DC: American Psychiatric Publishing, Inc.

Anderson, I. M., & Palm, M. E. (2006). Pharmacological treatments for worry: Focus on generalized anxiety disorder. In G. C. L. Davey & A. Wells (Eds.), *Worry and its psychological disorders: Theory, assessment and treatment.* West Sussex, UK, John Wiley & Sons.

Andersson, G., Carlbring, P., Holmstrom, A., et al. (2006). Internet-based self-help with therapist feedback and in vivo group exposure for social phobia: A randomized controlled trial. *Journal of Consulting and Clinical Psychology, 74*(4), 677-686.

Andreasen, N. C., & Black, D. W. (2006). *Introductory textbook of psychiatry* (4th ed.). Washington, DC: American Psychiatric Publishing, Inc.

Andrews, G., Charney, D. S., Sirovatka, M. S., et al. (Eds.). (2009). *Stress-induced and fear circuitry disorders.* Washington, DC: American Psychiatric Publishing, Inc.

Antai-Otong, D. (2008). Social anxiety disorder: characteristics, course, and pharmacological management prevalence. *Perspectives in Psychiatric Care, 44*(1), 48-53.

Antonacci, D. J., Davis, E., Bloch, R. M., et al. (2010). CAM for your anxious patient: What the evidence says. *Current Psychiatry, 9*(10), 43-52.

Aquizerate, B., Martin-Guehl, C., & Tignol, J. (2004). Neurobiology and pharmacotherapy of social phobia. *Encephale, 30*(4), 301-313.

Asakura, S., Tajima, O., & Koyama, T. (2007). Fluvoxamine treatment of generalized social anxiety disorder in Japan: A randomized double-blind, placebo-controlled study. *International Journal of Neuropsychopharmacology, 10,* 263-274.

Baillie, A. J., & Rapee, R. M. (2004). Predicting who benefits from psychoeducation and self help for panic attacks. *Behaviour Research and Therapy, 42,* 513-527.

Ball, J. G., Kuhn, A., Wall, D., et al. (2005). Selective serotonin reuptake inhibitor treatment for generalized anxiety disorder: A double-blind, prospective comparison between paroxetine and sertraline. *Journal of Clinical Psychiatry, 66*(1), 94-99.

Ballenger, J. C., Davidson, J. R. T., Lecrubier, Y., et al. (1998). Consensus statement on panic disorder from the International Consensus Group on Depression and Anxiety. *Journal of Clinical Psychiatry, 59*(Suppl 8), 47-54.

Ballenger, J. C., Davidson, J. R. T., Lecrubier, Y., et al. (2001). Consensus statement on generalized anxiety disorder from the International Consensus Group on Depression and Anxiety. *Journal of Clinical Psychiatry, 62*(Suppl 11), 53-58.

Bandelow, B., & Baldwin, D. S. (2010). Pharmacotherapy for panic disorder. In D. J. Stein, E. Hollander, & B. O. Rothbaum (Eds.), *The American psychiatric publishing textbook of anxiety disorders* (2nd ed.) (pp. 399-416). Washington, DC: American Psychiatric Publishing, Inc.

Barbour, K. A., Edenfield, T. M., & Blumenthal, J. A. (2007). Exercise as a treatment for depression and other psychiatric disorders: A review. *Journal of Cardiopulmonary Rehabilitation and Prevention, 27*(6), 359-367.

Barlow, D. H., Esler, J. L., & Vitali, A. E. (1998). Psychosocial treatments for panic disorders, phobias, and generalized anxiety disorder. In P. E. Nathan & J. M. Gorman (Eds.), *A guide to treatments that work* (pp. 288-318). New York: Oxford University Press.

Barlow, D. H., Gorman, J. M., Shear, M. K., et al. (2000). Cognitive-behavioral therapy, imipramine, or their combination for panic disorder: A randomized controlled trial. *Journal of the American Medical Association, 283,* 2525-2536.

Barnett, S. D., Kramer, M. L., Casat, C. D., et al. (2002). Efficacy of olanzapine in social anxiety disorder: A pilot study. *Journal of Psychopharmacology, 16,* 365-368.

Battaglia, M., Bertella, S., Bajo, S., et al. (1998). Anticipation of age at onset in panic disorder. *American Journal of Psychiatry, 155*(5), 590-595.

Becker, E. S., Rinck, M., Turke, V., et al. (2007). Epidemiology of specific phobia subtypes: Findings from the Dresden Mental Health Study. *European Psychiatry, 22,* 69-74.

Behar, E., DiMarco, I. O., Hekler, E. B., et al. (2009). Current theoretical models of generalized anxiety disorder (GAD): Conceptual review and treatment implications. *Journal of Anxiety Disorders, 23*(8), 1011-1023.

Bergstrom, J., Andersson, G., Karlsson, A., et al. (2009). An open study of the effectiveness of Internet treatment for panic disorder delivered in a psychiatric setting. *Nordic Journal of Psychiatry, 63*(1), 44-50.

Bielski, R. J., Bose, A., & Chang, C. C. (2005). A double-blind comparison of escitalopram and paroxetine in the long-term treatment of generalized anxiety disorders. *Annuals of Clinical Psychiatry, 17,* 65-69.

Birmaher, B., Khetarpal, S., Brent, D., et al. (1997). The *Screen for Child Anxiety Related Emotional Disorders (SCARED):* Scale construction and psychometric characteristics. *Journal of American Academy of Child and Adolescent Psychiatry, 36,* 545-553.

Black, D. W., & Andreasen, N. C. (2011). *Introductory textbook of psychiatry* (5th ed.). Washington, DC: American Psychiatric Publishing, Inc.

Black, D. W., Wesner, R., Bowers, W., et al. (1993). A comparison of fluvoxamine, cognitive therapy and placebo in the treatment of panic disorder. *Archives of General Psychiatry, 50,* 44-50.

Black, D. W., Wesner, R. B., Gabel, J., et al. (1994). Predictors of short-term treatment response in 66 patients with panic disorder. *Journal of Affective Disorders, 30*(4), 233-242.

Blanco, C., Schneier, F. R., Vesga-Lopez, O., et al. (2010). Pharmacotherapy for social anxiety disorder. In D. J. Stein, E. Hollander, & B. O. Rothbaum (Eds.), *The American psychiatric publishing textbook of anxiety disorders* (2nd ed.) (pp. 471-499). Washington, DC: American Psychiatric Publishing, Inc.

Bogels, S., & Stein, M. B. (2009). Social phobia. In G. Andrews, D. S. Charney, P. J. Sirovatka, et al. (Eds.), *Stress-induced and fear circuitry disorders* (pp. 59-75). Washington, DC: American Psychiatric Publishing, Inc.

Bonne, O., Grillon, C., Vythilingam, M., et al. (2004). Adaptive and maladaptive psychobiological responses to severe psychological stress: Implications for the discovery of novel pharmacotherapy. *Neuroscience & Biobehavioral Reviews, 28*(1), 65-94.

Borge, F., Hoffart, A., Sexton, H., et al. (2008). Residential cognitive therapy versus residential interpersonal therapy for social phobia: A randomized clinical trial. *Journal of Anxiety Disorders, 32*(6), 991-1010.

Borkovec, T. D., Alcaine, O., Behar, E. (2004). Avoidance theory of worry and generalized anxiety disorder. In R. G. Heimberg, C. L. Turk, & D. S. Mennin (Eds.), *Generalized anxiety disorder: Advances in research and practice* (pp. 77-108). New York: Guilford Press.

Borkovec, T. D., Newman, M. G., Pincus, A. L., et al. (2002). A component analysis of cognitive-behavioral therapy for generalized anxiety disorder and the role of interpersonal problems. *Journal of Consulting and Clinical Psychology, 70*(2), 288-298.

Bowlby, J. (1973). *Attachment and loss* (Vol 2. Separation: Anxiety and anger). New York: Basic Books.

Bradwejn, J., Ahokas, A., Stein, D. J., et al. (2005). Venlafaxine extended-release capsules in panic disorder: Flexible-dose, double-blind, placebo-controlled study. *British Journal of Psychiatry, 187*, 352-359.

Brantley, P. J., Mehan, D. J. Jr., Ames, S. C., et al. (1999). Minor stressors and generalized anxiety disorders among low-income patients attending primary care clinics. *Journal of Nervous and Mental Disorders, 187*, 435-440.

Bremner, J. D., & Charney, D. S. (2010). Neural circuits in fear and anxiety. In E. Hollander, & B. O. Rothbaum (Eds.), *The American psychiatric publishing textbook of anxiety disorders* (2nd ed.) (pp. 55-67-56). Washington, DC: American Psychiatric Publishing, Inc.

Breslau, J., Aguilar-Gaxiola, S., Kendler, K. S., et al. (2006). Specifying race-ethnic differences in risk for psychiatric disorder in a USA national sample. *Psychological Medicine, 36*, 57-68.

Britton, J. C., Gold, A. L., Deckersbach, T., et al. (2009). Functional MRI study of specific animal phobia using an event-related emotional counting stroop paradigm. *Depression and Anxiety, 26*, 796-805.

Brown, E. S., Fulton, M. K., Wilkeson, A., et al. (2000). The psychiatric sequelae of civilian trauma. *Comprehensive Psychiatry, 41*, 19-23.

Calbring, P., Bohman, S., Brunt, S., et al. (2006). Remote treatment of panic disorder: A randomized trial of internet-based cognitive-behavior therapy supplemented with telephone calls. *American Journal of Psychiatry, 163*, 2119-2125.

Candilis, P. J., McLean, R. Y., Otto, M. W., et al. (1999). Quality of life in patients with panic disorder. *Journal of Nervous & Mental Disease, 187*(7), 429-434.

Carducci, B. J., & Zimbardo, P. G. (1995). Are you shy? *Psychology Today, 28*, 34-40.

Carpenter, L. L., Leon, Z., Yasmin, S., et al. (1999). Clinical experience with mirtazapine in the treatment of panic disorder. *Annuals of Clinical Psychiatry, 11*, 81-86.

Carter, N. J., & McCormack, P. L. (2009). Duloxetine: A review of its use in the treatment of generalized anxiety disorder. *CNS Drugs, 23*(6), 523-541.

Carter S. A., & Wu, K. D. (2010). Symptoms of specific and generalized social phobia: An examination of discriminant validity and structural relations with mood and anxiety symptoms. *Behavior Therapy, 41*(2), 254-265.

Cassidy, J. (1995). Attachment and generalized anxiety disorder. In D. Cicchetti & S. Toth (Eds.), *Rochester symposium on developmental psychopathology* (Vol. 6. Emotion, cognition and representation) (pp. 343-370). New York: University of Rochester Press.

Cassidy, J., Lichtenstein-Phelps, N. J., Sibrava, C. L., et al. (2009). Generalized anxiety disorder: Connections with self-reported attachment. *Behavior Therapy, 40*, 23-38.

Chambless, D. L., Caputo, G. C., Jasin, S. E., et al. (1985). The mobility inventory for agoraphobia. *Behavioral Research and Therapy, 23*, 35-44.

Clark, D. M. (2005). A cognitive perspective on social phobia. In W. R. Crozier & L. E. Alden (Eds.), *The essential handbook of social anxiety for clinicians* (pp. 193-218). West Sussex, UK: John Wiley & Sons, Ltd.

Clum, G. A., Broyles, S., Borden J., et al. (1990). Validity and reliability of the Panic Attack Symptoms and Cognition Questionnaire. *Journal of Psychopathology and Behavioral Assessment, 12*, 233-245.

Cohen, L. S., Nonacs, R., & Viguera, A. C. (2004). In T. Stern, G. L. Fricchione, N. H. Cassem, et al. (Eds.), *The Massachusetts General Hospital handbook of general hospital psychiatry* (5th ed.) (pp. 593-611). St. Louis: Mosby.

Connor, K. M., Davidson, J. R., Chung, H., et al. (2006). Multidimensional effects of sertraline in social anxiety disorder. *Depression & Anxiety, 23*(1), 6-10.

Connor, K. M., Davison, J. R., Churchill, L. E., et al. (2000). Psychometric properties of the Social Phobia Inventory (SPIN). New self-rating scale. *British Journal of Psychiatry, 176*, 379-386.

Connor, K. M., Kobak, K. A., Churchill, L. E., et al. (2001). MINI-SPIN: A brief screening assessment for generalized social anxiety disorder. *Depression and Anxiety, 14*, 137-140.

Coplan, J. D., & Gorman, J. M. (2002). Pathogenesis of panic disorder. In D. J. Stein & E. Hollander (Eds.), *The American psychiatric publishing textbook of anxiety disorders* (pp. 247-256). Washington, DC: American Psychiatric Publishing, Inc.

Covin, R., Quimet, A. J., Seeds, P. M., et al. (2008). A meta-analysis of CBT for pathological worry among clients with GAD. *Journal of Anxiety Disorders, 22*, 108-116.

Cox, B. J., MacPherson, P. S. R., & Enns, M. W. (2005). Psychiatric correlates of childhood shyness in a nationally representative sample. *Behavioral Research and Therapy, 43*, 1019-1027.

Cramer, V., Torgersen, S., & Kringlen, E. (2005). Quality of life and anxiety disorders: A population study. *Journal of Nervous and Mental Disease, 193*(3), 196-202.

Craske, M. G., Brown, T. A., & Barlow, D. H. (1991). Behavioral treatment of panic disorder: A two-year follow-up. *Behavior Therapy, 22*, 289-304.

Craske, M. G., Golinelli, D., Stein, M. B., et al. (2005). Does the addition of cognitive behavioral therapy improve panic disorder treatment outcome relative to medication alone in the primary-care setting? *Psychological Medicine, 35*(11), 1645-1654.

Craske, M. G., Miller, P. P., Rotunda, R., et al. (1990). A descriptive report of features of initial unexpected panic attacks in minimal and extensive avoiders. *Behaviour Research & Therapy, 28*(5), 395-400.

Craske, M. G., Roy-Byrne, P., Stein, M. B., et al. (2006). CBT intensity and outcome for panic disorder in a primary care setting. *Behavior Therapy, 37*(2), 113-119.

Crozier, W. R., & Alden, L. E. (2005a). Constructs of social anxiety. In W. R. Crozier & L. E. Alden (Eds.), *The essential handbook of social anxiety for clinicians* (pp. 1-23). West Sussex, UK: John Wiley & Sons, Ltd.

Crozier, W. R., & Alden, L. E. (2005b). The development of social anxiety. In W. R. Crozier & L. E. Alden (Eds.), *The essential handbook of social anxiety for clinicians* (pp. 28-32). West Sussex, UK: John Wiley & Sons, Ltd.

Culpepper, L. (2009). Generalized anxiety disorder and medical illness. *Journal of Clinical Psychiatry, 70*(Suppl 2), 20-24.

Davidson, J. R. T. (2009). First-line pharmacotherapy approaches for generalized anxiety disorder. *Journal of Clinical Psychiatry, 70*(Suppl 2), 25-31.

Davidson, J. R., Bose, A., Korotzer, A., et al. (2004). Escitalopram in the treatment of generalized anxiety disorder: Double-blind, placebo controlled flexible-dose study. *Depression and Anxiety, 19*(4), 234-240.

Davidson, J. R. T., & Connor, K. M. (2004). Treatment of anxiety disorders. In A. F. Schatzberg & C. B. Nemeroff (Eds.), *Textbook of psychopharmacology* (3rd ed.) (pp. 913-934). Washington, DC: American Psychiatric Publishing, Inc.

Davidson, J. R. T., Connor, K. M., & Zhang, W. (2009). Treatment of anxiety disorders. In A. F. Schatzberg & C. B. Nemeroff (Eds.), *The American psychiatric publishing textbook of psychopharmacology* (pp. 1171-1199). Washington, DC: American Psychiatric Publishing, Inc.

Davidson, J. R., Foa, E. B., Huppert, J. D., et al. (2004). Fluoxetine, comprehensive cognitive behavioral therapy, and placebo in generalized social phobia. *Archives of General Psychiatry, 61*, 1005-1013.

Deacon, B., Lickel, J., & Abramowitz, J. S. (2008). Medical utilization across the anxiety disorders. *Anxiety Disorders, 22*, 344-350.

Dobson, K. S., & Dozois, D. J. A. (2010). Historical and philosophical bases of the cognitive-behavioral therapies. In K. S. Dobson (Ed.), *Handbook of cognitive-behavioral therapies* (3rd ed.) (pp. 3-38). New York: Guilford Press.

Dubois, O., Salamon, R., Germain, C., et al. (2010). Balneotherapy versus paroxetine in the treatment of generalized anxiety disorder. *Complementary Therapies in Medicine, 18*, 1-7.

Dubovsky, S. (2005). *Clinical guide to psychotropic medications.* New York: W. W. Norton & Company.

Dugas, M. J., Savard, P., Gaudet, A., et al. (2007). Can the components of a cognitive model predict the severity of generalized anxiety disorder? *Behavioral Therapy, 38*, 169-178.

DuPont, R. L., DuPont, C. M., & Rice, D. P. (2002). Economic costs of anxiety disorders. In D. J. Stein & E. Hollander (Eds.), *The American psychiatric publishing textbook of anxiety disorders* (pp. 475-484). Washington, DC: American Psychiatric Publishing, Inc.

Durham, R. C., Chambers, J. A., MacDonald, R. R., et al. (2003). Does cognitive behavioral therapy influence the long-term outcome of generalized anxiety disorder? An 8-14 year follow-up of two clinical trials. *Psychological Medicine, 33*, 499-509.

Emmelkamp, P. M. G., & Wittchen, H. U. (2009). Specific phobias. In G. Andrews, D. S. Charney, P. J. Sirovatka, et al. (Eds.), *Stress-induced and fear circuitry disorders* (pp. 77-101). Washington, DC: American Psychiatric Publishing, Inc.

Eng, W., & Heimberg, R. G. (2006). Interpersonal correlates of generalized anxiety disorder: Self-versus other perception. *Journal of Anxiety Disorders, 29*(3), 380-387.

Ettigi, P., Meyerhoff, A. S., Chirban, J. T., et al. (1997). The quality of life and employment in panic disorder. *Journal of Nervous & Mental Disease, 185*(6), 368-372.

Fava, G. A., Rafanelli, C., Grandi, S., et al. (2001). Long-term outcome of panic disorder with agoraphobia treated by exposure. *Psychological Medicine, 31*, 891-898.

Fava G. A., Ruini, C., Rafanelli, C., et al. (2005). Well-being therapy of generalized anxiety disorder. *Psychotherapy and Psychosomatics, 74*(1), 26-30.

Febbraro, G. (2005). An investigation into the effectiveness of bibliotherapy and minimal contact interventions in the treatment of panic attacks. *Journal of Clinical Psychology, 61*(6), 763-779.

Feltner, D. E., Crockatt, J. G., Dubovsky, S. J., et al. (2003). A randomized double-blind, placebo-controlled, fixed-dose, multicenter study of pregabalin in patients with anxiety disorder. *Journal of Clinical Psychopharmacology, 23*, 240-249.

First, M. B., Frances, A., & Pincus, H. A. (Eds.). (2002). *DSM-IV-TR handbook of differential diagnosis.* Washington, DC: American Psychiatric Publishing, Inc.

First, M. B., & Tasman, A. (Eds.). (2004). *DSM-IV-TR mental disorders: Diagnosis, etiology and treatment.* West Sussex, UK: John Wiley & Sons, Ltd.

Fisher, P. L. (2006). The efficacy of psychological treatments for generalized anxiety disorder. In G. C. L. Davey & A. Wells (Eds.), *Worry and its psychological disorders: Theory, assessment and treatment.* West Sussex, UK: Wiley & Sons.

Fisher, P. L., & Durham, R. C. (1999). Recovery rates in generalized anxiety disorder following psychological therapy: An analysis of clinically significant change in the STAI-T across outcome studies since 1990. *Psychological Medicine, 29*, 1425-1434.

Foa, E. B., Huppert, J. D., & Cahill, S. P. (2006). Emotional processing theory: An update. In B. O. Rothbaum (Ed.), *Pathological anxiety: Emotional processing in etiology and treatment* (pp. 3-24). New York: Guilford Press.

Fricchione, G. (2004). Generalized anxiety disorder. *The New England Journal of Medicine, 35*(7), 675-682.

Friedman, S. (1997). *Cultural issues in the treatment of anxiety.* New York: Guilford Press.

Furmark, T. (2009). Neurobiological aspects of social anxiety disorder. *Israel Journal of Psychiatry and Related Sciences, 46*(1), 5-12.

Furukawa, T. A., Watanae, N., & Churchill, R. (2006). Psychotherapy plus antidepressant for panic disorder with and without agoraphobia: Systematic review. *British Journal of Psychiatry, 188*, 305-312.

Fyer, A. J., & Brown, T. A. (2009). Stress-induced and fear circuitry anxiety disorders: Are they a distinct group? In G. Andrews, D. S. Charney, P. J. Sirovatka, et al. (Eds.), *Stress-induced and fear circuitry disorders* (pp. 125-135). Washington, DC: American Psychiatric Publishing, Inc.

Gabbard, G. O. (2005). *Psychodynamic psychiatry in clinical practice* (4th ed.). Washington, DC: American Psychiatric Publishing, Inc.

Gambi, F., De-Berardis, D., Campanella, D., et al. (2005). Mirtazapine treatment of generalized anxiety disorder: A fixed dose, open label study. *Journal of Psychopharmacology, 19*, 483-487.

Gamble, A. L., Harvey, A. G., & Rapee, R. M. (2010). Specific phobia. In D. J. Stein, E. Hollander, & B. O. Rothbaum (Eds.), *The American psychiatric publishing textbook of anxiety disorders* (2nd ed.) (pp. 525-543). Washington, DC: American Psychiatric Publishing, Inc.

Ghosh, A., & Marks, I. M. (1987). Self-treatment of agoraphobia by exposure. *Behavior Therapy, 18*, 3-16.

Goddard, A. W., Brouette, T., Almai, A., et al. (2001). Early co-administration of clonazepam with sertraline for panic disorder. *Archives of General Psychiatry, 58*, 681-686.

Goddard, A. W., Mason, G. F., Appel, M., et al. (2004). Impaired GABA neuronal response to acute benzodiazepine administration in panic disorder. *American Journal of Psychiatry, 161*, 2186-2193.

Goodnick, P. J., Puig, A., DeVane, C. L., et al. (1999). Mirtazapine in major depression with comorbid generalized anxiety disorder. *Journal of Clinical Psychiatry, 60*, 446-448.

Goodwin, R. D., Fergusson, D. M., & Horwood, L. J. (2005). Childhood abuse and familial violence and the risk of panic attacks and panic disorder in young adulthood. *Psychological Medicine, 35*, 881-890.

Goodwin, R. D., & Roy-Byrne, P. P. (2006). Panic and suicidal ideation and suicide attempts: Results from the National Comorbidity Survey. *Depression and Anxiety, 23*, 124-132.

Gorman, J. M., Kent, J. M., Sullivan, G. M., et al. (2000). Neuroanatomical hypothesis of panic disorder, revised. *American Journal of Psychiatry, 157*, 493-505.

Gorman, J., Shear, K., Cowley, D., et al. (2004). Practice guideline for the treatment of patients with panic disorder. In *American psychiatric association practice guidelines for the treatment of psychiatric disorders: Compendium 2004* (pp. 613-1707). Washington, DC: American Psychiatric Publishing, Inc.

Grant, B. F., Hasin, D. S., Stinson, F. S., et al. (2006). The epidemiology of DSM-IV panic disorder and agoraphobia in the United States: Results from the national epidemiologic survey on alcohol and related conditions. *Journal of Clinical Psychiatry 67*, 363-364.

Gross, R., Olfson, M., Gameroff, M. J., et al. (2005). Social anxiety disorder in primary care. *General Hospital Psychiatry, 27*, 161-168.

Gulpek, D., Bayraktar, E., Akbay, S. P., et al. (2004). Joint hypermobility syndrome and mitral valve prolapse in panic disorder. *Progress in Neuro-Psychopharmacology & Biological Psychiatry, 28*, 969-973.

Hales, R. E., Yudofsky, S. C., & Gabbard, G. O. (Eds.) (2011). *Essential of psychiatry* (3rd ed.). Washington, DC: American Psychiatric Publishing, Inc.

Hamilton, M. (1959). The assessment of anxiety states by rating. *British Journal of Medical Psychology, 32*, 50-55.

Hansen, S. (2004). Managing anxiety disorders in women. *The Female Patient, 29*, 23-30.

Hartford, J., Kornstein, S., Liebowitz, M., et al. (2007). Duloxetine as an SNRI treatment for generalized anxiety disorder: Results from a placebo and active-controlled trial. *International Clinical Psychopharmacology, 22*, 167-174.

Hartman, L. M. (1984). Cognitive components of anxiety. *Journal of Clinical Psychology, 40*, 137-139.

Heimberg, R. G., Hope, D. A., Dodge, C. S., et al. (1990). DSM-III-R subtypes of social phobia: Comparison of generalized social phobics and public speaking phobics. *Journal of Nervous and Mental Disease, 178*, 172-179.

Heldt, E., Blaya, C., Isolan, L., et al. (2006). Quality of life and treatment outcome in panic disorder: Cognitive behavior group therapy effects in patients refractory to medication treatment. *Psychotherapy & Psychosomatics, 75*(3), 183-186.

Hermann, A., Schafer, A., Walter, B., et al. (2009). Emotion regulation in spider phobia: Role of the medial prefrontal cortex. *SCAN, 4*, 257-267.

Hettema, J. M., Neale, M. C., & Kendler, K. S. (2001). A review and meta-analysis of the genetic epidemiology of anxiety disorders. *American Journal of Psychiatry, 158*, 1568-1578.

Hettema, J. M., Prescott, C. A., & Kendler, K. S. (2004). Genetic and environmental sources of covariation between generalized anxiety disorder and neuroticism. *American Journal of Psychiatry, 161*, 1581-1587.

Hibbard, M. R., Uysal, S., Kepler, K., et al. (1998). Axis I psychopathology in individuals with traumatic brain injury. *The Journal of Head Trauma Rehabilitation, 13*(4), 24-39.

Hirshfeld-Becker, D. R., Biederman, J., Henin, A., et al. (2007). Behavioral inhibition in preschool children at risk is a specific predictor of middle childhood social anxiety: A five-year follow-up. *Journal of Deviant Behavior in Pediatrics, 28,* 225-233.

Hoffman, E. J., & Mathew, S. J. (2008). Anxiety disorders: A comprehensive review of pharmacotherapies. *Mount Sinai Journal of Medicine, 75,* 248-262.

Hofmann, S. G., Meuret, A. E., Smits, J. A., et al. (2006). Augmentation of exposure therapy with D-cycloserine for social anxiety disorder. *Archives of General Psychiatry, 63,* 298-304.

Hofmann, S. G., Rief, W., & Spiegel, D. A. (2010). Psychotherapy for panic disorder. In D. J. Stein, E. Hollander, & B. O. Rothbaum (Eds.), *The American psychiatric publishing textbook of anxiety disorders* (2nd ed.) (pp. 417-433). Washington, DC: American Psychiatric Publishing, Inc.

Hofmann, S. G., & Smits, J. A. (2008). Pitfalls of meta-analysis. *Journal of Nervous and Mental Disorders, 196*(9), 716-717.

Hofmann, S. G., & Smits, J. A. J. (2009). Cognitive-behavioral therapy for adult anxiety disorders: A meta-analysis of randomized placebo-controlled trials. *Journal of Clinical Psychiatry, 43,* 634-641.

Hollander, E., & Simeon, D. (2008). Anxiety disorders. In R. E. Hales, S. C. Yudofsky, & G. O. Gabbard (Eds.), *The American psychiatric publishing textbook of psychiatry* (5th ed.) (pp. 505-605). Washington, DC: American Psychiatric Publishing, Inc.

Hollander, E., & Simeon, D. (2011). Anxiety disorders. In R. E. Hales, S. C. Yudofsky, & G. O. Gabbard (Eds.), *Essentials of psychiatry* (3rd ed.) (pp. 185-228). Washington, DC: American Psychiatric Publishing, Inc.

Hollifield, M., Thompson, P. M., Ruiz, J. E., et al. (2005). Potential effectiveness and safety of olanzapine in refractory panic disorder. *Depression and Anxiety, 21,* 33-40.

Huppert, J. D., & Sanderson, W. C. (2002). Psychotherapy for generalized anxiety disorder. In D. J. Stein & E. Hollander (Eds.), *The American psychiatric publishing textbook of anxiety disorders* (pp. 163-178). Washington, DC: American Psychiatric Publishing, Inc.

Huppert, J. D., & Sanderson, W. C. (2010). Psychotherapy for generalized anxiety disorder. In D. J. Stein, E. Hollander, & B. O. Rothbaum (Eds.), *The American psychiatric publishing textbook of anxiety disorders* (2nd ed.) (pp. 219-238). Washington, DC: American Psychiatric Publishing, Inc.

Jacobs, R. J., Davidson, J. R., Gupta, S., et al. (1997). The effects of clonazepam on quality of life and work productivity in panic disorder. *American Journal of Managed Care, 2,* 1187-1196.

Jetty, R. V., Charney, D. S., & Goddard, A. W. (2001). Neurobiology of generalized anxiety disorder. *Psychiatric Clinics of North America, 24*(1), 75-97.

Johnson, J. G., Cohen, P., Pine, D. S., et al. (2000). The association between cigarette smoking and anxiety disorders during adolescence and early adulthood. *Journal of the American Medical Association, 284,* 2348-2351.

Johnson, J. G., Weissman, M. M., & Klerman, G. L. (1990). Panic disorder, comorbidity, and suicide attempts. *Archives of General Psychiatry, 47,* 805-808.

Josephs, L. (1994). Psychoanalytic and related interpretations. Related disorders. In B. B. Wolman & G. Stricker (Eds.), *Anxiety and related disorders: A handbook* (pp. 11-19). New York: Wiley Interscience.

Kagan, J., & Snidman, N. (1991). Temperament factors in human development. *The American Psychologist, 46*(8), 856-862.

Kandel, E. R., Schwartz, J. H., & Jessell, T. M. (2000). *Principles of neural science* (4th ed.). New York: McGraw Hill.

Kasper, S., Stein, D. J., Loft, H., et al. (2005). Escitalopram in the treatment of social anxiety disorder: Randomised, placebo-controlled, flexible-dosage study. *British Journal of Psychiatry, 186,* 222-226.

Katerndahl, D. A. (1993). Panic and prolapse. Meta-analysis. *Journal of Nervous & Mental Disease, 181*(9), 539-544.

Katerndahl, D. A., & Realini, J. P. (1997). Quality of life and panic-related work disability in subjects with infrequent panic and panic disorder. *Journal of Clinical Psychiatry, 58,* 153-158.

Katon, W. (1996). Panic disorder: Relationship to high medical utilization, unexplained physical symptoms, and medical costs. *Journal of Clinical Psychiatry, 57,* 11-18.

Katschnig, H., Amering, M., Stolk, J. M., et al. (1995). Long-term follow-up after a drug trial for panic disorder. *British Journal of Psychiatry, 167*(4), 487-494.

Katzman, M. A. (2009). Current considerations in the treatment of generalized anxiety disorder. *CNS Drugs, 23*(2), 103-120.

Keeton, C. P., Kolos, A. C., & Walkup, J. T. (2009). Paediatric generalized anxiety disorder: Epidemiology, diagnosis, and management. *Paediatric Drugs, 11*(3), 171-183.

Keller, M. B. (2003). The lifelong course of social anxiety disorder: A clinical perspective. *Acta Psychiatrica Scandinavica, Supplementum, 417,* 85-94.

Kelly, C. M., Jorm, A. F., & Kitchener, B. A. (2009). Development of mental health first aid guidelines for panic attacks: A Delphi study. *BMC Psychiatry, 9,* 49.

Kessler, R. C., Berglund, P., Demler, O., et al. (2005a). Lifetime prevalence and age-of-onset distributions of DSM-IV disorders in the National Comorbidity Survey Replication. *Archives of General Psychiatry, 62,* 593-602.

Kessler, R. C., Brandenburg, N., Lane, M., et al. (2005b). Rethinking the duration requirement for generalized anxiety disorder: Evidence from the National Comorbidity Survey Replication. *Psychological Medicine, 35*(7), 1073-1082.

Kessler, R. C., Stang, P., Wittchen, H. U., et al. (1999). Lifetime comorbidities between social phobia and mood disorders in the US National Comorbidity Survey. *Psychological Medicine, 29,* 555-567.

Khan, A. Y., & Macaluso, M. (2009). Duloxetine for the treatment of generalized anxiety disorder: A review. *Neuropsychiatric Disease and Treatment, 5,* 23-31.

Kirkwood, G., Rampes, H., Tuffrehy, V., et al. (2005). Yoga for anxiety: A systematic review of the research evidence. *British Journal of Sports Medicine, 39*(12), 884-891.

Klein, D. (1981). Anxiety reconceptualized. In D. F. Klein & J. G. Rabkin (Eds.), *Anxiety: New research and changing concepts* (pp. 235-263). New York: Raven Press.

Klein, D. (1993). False suffocation alarms, spontaneous panics and related conditions: An integrative hypothesis. *Archives of General Psychiatry, 50*(4), 306-318.

Klinger, E., Bouchard, S., Legeron, P., et al. (2005). Virtual reality therapy versus cognitive behavior therapy for social phobia: A preliminary controlled study. *Cyberpsychology and Behavior, 8,* 76-88.

Krijn, M., Emmelkamp, P. M. G., Biemond, R., et al. (2004a). Treatment of acrophobia in virtual reality: The role of immersion and presence. *Behaviour Research & Therapy, 42*(2), 229-239.

Krijn, M., Emmelkamp, P. M. G., Olafsson, R. P., et al. (2004b). Virtual reality exposure therapy of anxiety disorders: A review. *Clinical Psychology Review, 24,* 259-281.

Kroenke, K., Spitzer, R. L., Williams, J., et al. (2007). Anxiety disorders in primary care: Prevalence, impairment, comorbidity and detection. *Annals of Internal Medicine, 146,* 317-325.

Lader, M., Stender, K., Burger, V., et al. (2004). Efficacy and tolerability of escitalopram in 12 and 24 week treatment of social anxiety disorder: Randomised, double-blind, placebo-controlled fixed-dose study. *Depression & Anxiety, 19,* 241-248.

Lang, A. J. (2004). Treating generalized anxiety disorder with cognitive-behavioral therapy. *Journal of Clinical Psychiatry, 65*(Suppl 13), 14-19.

Lavie, C. J., & Milani, R. V. (2004). Generalized anxiety disorder. *The New England Journal of Medicine, 35*(21), 2239.

LeDoux, J. E. (2002). *Synaptic self: How our brains become who we are.* New York: Viking Press.

LeDoux, J. E., & Gorman, J. M. (2001). A call to action: Overcoming anxiety through active coping. *The American Journal of Psychiatry, 158*(12), 1953-1955.

Lenze, E. J., Rollman, B. L., Shear, M. K., et al. (2009). Escitalopram for older adults with generalized anxiety disorder. *Journal of the American Medical Association, 301*(3), 295-303.

Le Roux, H., Gatz, M., & Wetherell, J. L. (2005). Age at onset of generalized anxiety disorder in older adults. *American Journal of Geriatric Psychiatry, 13*(1), 23-30.

Liebowitz, M. R. (1987). Social phobia. *Modern Problems in Pharmacopsychiatry, 22,* 141-173.

Lightfoot, J. D., Seay, S., & Goddard, A. W. (2010). Pathogenesis of generalized anxiety disorder. In D. J. Stein, E. Hollander, & B. O. Rothbaum (Eds.),

The American psychiatric publishing textbook of anxiety disorders (2nd ed.) (pp. 173-192). Washington, DC: American Psychiatric Publishing, Inc.

Lipsitz, J. D., Gur, M., Vermes, D., et al. (2008). A randomized trial of interpersonal therapy versus supportive therapy for social anxiety disorder. *Depression and Anxiety, 25,* 542-553.

Lorberbaum, J. P., Kose, S., Johnson, M. R., et al. (2004). Neuronal correlates of speech anticipatory anxiety in generalized social phobia. *Neuroreport, 15*(18), 2701-2705.

Lydiard, R. B. (2002). When does shyness become a disorder? *Current Psychiatry, 1*(3), 41-44.

Marazziti, D., & Rotondo, A. (1999). Genetics of panic disorder. *CNS Spectrums, 4*(6), 62-70.

Marcks, B. A., Weisberg, R. B., & Keller, M. B. (2009). Psychiatric treatment received by primary care patients with panic disorder with and without agoraphobia. *Psychiatric Services, 60*(5), 823-830.

Marks, I. M., & Mathews, A. M. (1978). Brief standard self-rating for phobic patients. *Behaviour Research and Therapy, 17,* 263-267.

Martin, L. T., Kubzansky, L. K., & LeWinn, K. Z. (2007). Childhood cognitive performance and risk of generalized anxiety disorder. *International Journal of Epidemiology, 36,* 769-775.

Martin-Santos, R., Bulbena, A., Porta, M., et al. (1998). Association between joint hypermobility syndrome and panic disorder. *American Journal of Psychiatry, 155,* 1578-1583.

Massana, G., Serra-Grabulosa, J. M., Salgado-Pineda, P., et al. (2003a). Parahippocampal gray matter density in panic disorder: A voxel-based morphometric study. *American Journal of Psychiatry, 160*(3), 566-568.

Massana, G., Serra-Grabulosa, J. M., Salgado-Pineda, P., et al. (2003b). Amygdalar atrophy in panic disorder patients detected by volumetric magnetic resonance imaging. *NeuroImage, 19*(1), 80-90.

Mathew, R. J., Amiel, J. M., Coplan, J. D., et al. (2005). Open-label trial of riluzole in generalized anxiety disorder. *American Journal of Psychiatry, 162,* 2370-2381.

McBride, A. B., & Austin, J. K. (1996). Integrating the behavioral and biological sciences: Implications for practice, education and research. In A. B. McBride & J. K. Austin (Eds.), *Psychiatric-mental health nursing: Integrating the behavioral and biological sciences* (pp. 425-434). Philadelphia: W. B. Saunders Company.

Mendlewicz, J., Papadimitriou, G., & Wimotte, J. (1993). Family study of panic disorder: Comparison to generalized anxiety, panic/agoraphobia, and obsessive-compulsive disorders. *Psychiatric Genetics, 3,* 73-78.

Mennin, D. S., Heimberg, R. G., Turk, C. L., et al. (2005). Preliminary evidence for an emotion dysregulation model of generalized anxiety disorder. *Behavior Research and Therapy, 43,* 1281-1310.

Milrod, B. (2009). Psychodynamic psychotherapy outcome for generalized anxiety disorder. *American Journal of Psychiatry, 166*(8), 841-844.

Milrod, B., Busch, F., Cooper, A., et al. (1997). *Manual of panic-focused psychodynamic psychotherapy.* Washington, DC: American Psychiatric Publishing, Inc.

Milrod, B., Leon, A. C., Busch, F., et al. (2007). A randomized controlled clinical trial of psychoanalytic psychotherapy for panic disorder. *American Journal of Psychiatry, 164,* 265-272.

Mitte, K. (2005). A meta-analysis of the efficacy of psycho- and pharmacotherapy in panic disorder with and without agoraphobia. *Journal of Affective Disorders, 88,* 27-45.

Morreale, M., Tancer, M. E., & Uhde, T. W. (2010). Pathogenesis of social anxiety disorder. In D. J. Stein, E. Hollander, & B. O. Rothbaum (Eds.), *The American psychiatric publishing textbook of anxiety disorders* (2nd ed.) (pp. 453-469). Washington, DC: American Psychiatric Publishing, Inc.

Muehlbacher, M., Nickel, M. K., Nickel, C., et al. (2005). Mirtazapine treatment of social phobia in women: A randomized, double-blind, placebo-controlled study. *Journal of Clinical Psychopharmacology, 25,* 580-583.

Nagy, L. M., Krystal, J. H., Woods, W. W., et al. (1989). Clinical and medication outcome after short-term alprazolam and behavioral group treatment in panic disorder. 2.5 year naturalistic follow-up study. *Archives of General Psychiatry, 46*(11), 993-999.

Neal-Barnett, A. M., & Smith, J. (1997). African Americans. In S. Friedman (Ed.), *Cultural issues in the treatment of anxiety* (pp. 154-174). New York: Guilford Press.

Nelson, J. C. (2009). Tricyclic and tetracyclic drugs. In A. F. Schatzberg & C. B. Nemeroff (Eds.), *The American psychiatric publishing textbook of psychopharmacology* (4th ed.) (pp. 263-287). Washington, DC: American Psychiatric Publishing, Inc.

Neumeister, A., Bain, E., Nugent, A. C., et al. (2004). Reduced serotonin type 1A receptor binding in panic disorder. *The Journal of Neuroscience, 24*(3), 589-591.

Ogliari, A., Citterio, A., Zanoni, A., et al. (2006). Genetic and environmental influences on anxiety dimensions in Italian twins evaluated with the SCARED questionnaire. *Anxiety Disorders, 20,* 760-777.

Olfson, M., Fireman, B., Weissman, M. M., et al. (1997). Mental disorders and disability among patients in primary care group practice. *American Journal of Psychiatry, 154,* 1734-1740.

Ollendick, T. H., & Hirshfeld-Becker, D. R. (2002). The developmental psychopathology of social anxiety disorder. *Biological Psychiatry, 51,* 44-58.

Otto, M. W., Pollack, M. H., Gould, R. A., et al. (2000). A comparison of the efficacy of clonazepam and cognitive-behavioral group therapy for the treatment of social phobia. *Journal of Anxiety Disorders, 14,* 345-358.

Ozkan, M., & Altindag, A. (2005). Comorbid personality disorders in subjects with panic disorder: Do personality disorders increase clinical severity? *Comprehensive Psychiatry, 46,* 20-26.

Pande, A. C., Feltner, D. E., Jefferson, J. W., et al. (2004). Efficacy of the novel anxiolytic pregabalin in social anxiety disorder: A placebo-controlled, multicenter study. *Journal of Clinical Psychopharmacology, 24,* 141-149.

Panksepp, J. (2004). *Textbook of biological psychiatry.* Hoboken, NJ: Wiley-Liss.

Papp, L. A. (2010). Phenomenology of generalized anxiety disorder. In D. J. Stein, E. Hollander, & B. O. Rothbaum (Eds.), *The American psychiatric publishing textbook of anxiety disorders* (2nd ed.) (pp. 159-171). Washington, DC: American Psychiatric Publishing, Inc.

Parsons, T. D., & Rizzo, A. A. (2008). Affective outcomes of virtual reality exposure therapy for anxiety and specific phobias: A meta-analysis. *Journal of Behavior Therapy and Experimental Psychiatry, 39,* 250-261.

Paulesu, E., Sambugaro, E., Torti, T., et al. (2010). Neural correlates of worry in generalized anxiety disorder and in normal controls: A functional MRI study. *Psychological Medicine, 40,* 117-124.

Pietrini, F., Godini, L., Lazzeretti, L., et al. (2010). Neuroimaging and neurobiology of social anxiety. *Rivista di Psichiatria, 45*(6), 349-360.

Pilowsky, D. J., Olfson, M., Gameroff, M. J., et al. (2006). Panic disorder and suicidal ideation in primary care. *Depression and Anxiety, 23,* 11-16.

Pittler, M. H., & Ernst, E. (2003). Kava extract for treating anxiety. *The Cochrane Database Systematic Review,* (1). CD003383.

Pollack, M. H. (2005). The pharmacotherapy of panic disorder. *Journal of Clinical Psychiatry, 66*(Suppl 4), 23-27.

Pollack, M. H. (2009). Refractory generalized anxiety disorder. *Journal of Clinical Psychiatry, 70*(Suppl 2), 32-38.

Pollack, M. H., Kornstein, S. G., Spann, M. E., et al. (2008). Early improvement during duloxetine treatment of generalized anxiety disorder. *Journal of Psychiatric Research, 42*(4), 1176-1184.

Pollack, M. H., Otto, M. W., Majcher, D., et al. (1996). Relationship of childhood anxiety to adult panic disorder: Correlates and influence on course. *American Journal of Psychiatry, 153,* 376-381.

Pollack, M. H., Simon, N. M., Worthington, J. J., et al. (2003). Combined paroxetine and clonazepam treatment strategies compared to paroxetine monotherapy for panic disorder. *Journal of Psychopharmacology, 17,* 276-282.

Pollack, M. H., & Smoller, J. W. (1995). The longitudinal course and outcome of panic disorder. *Psychiatric Clinics of North America, 18*(4), 785-801.

Pollack, M. H., Smoller, J. W., Otto, M. W., et al. (2010). Phenomenology of panic disorder. In D. J. Stein, E. Hollander, & B. O. Rothbaum (Eds.), *The American psychiatric publishing textbook of anxiety disorders* (2nd ed.) (pp. 367-379). Washington, DC: American Psychiatric Publishing, Inc.

Pollack, M. H., Zaninelli, R., Goddary, A., et al. (2001). Paroxetine in the treatment of generalized anxiety disorder: Results of a placebo-controlled, flexible-dosage trial. *Journal of Clinical Psychiatry, 62,* 350-357.

Pontoski, K. E., Heimberg, R. G., Turk, C. L., et al. (2010). Psychotherapy for social anxiety disorder. In D. J. Stein, E. Hollander, & B. O. Rothbaum (Eds.), *The American psychiatric publishing textbook of anxiety disorders* (2nd ed.) (pp. 501-521). Washington, DC: American Psychiatric Publishing, Inc.

Poulton, R., Pine, D. S., & Harrington, H. L. (2009). Continuity and etiology of anxiety disorders. In G. Andrews, D. S. Charney, P. J. Sirovatka, et al. (Eds.), *Stress-induced and fear circuitry disorders* (pp. 105-123). Washington, DC: American Psychiatric Association.

Protopopescu, X., Pan, H., Tuescher, O., et al. (2006). Increased brainstem volume in panic disorder: A voxel-based morphometric study. *Neuroreport, 17*(4), 361-363.

Ramsawh, H. J., Chavira, D. A., & Stein, M. B. (2010). Phenomenology of social anxiety disorder. In D. J. Stein, E. Hollander, & B. O. Rothbaum (Eds.), *The American psychiatric publishing textbook of anxiety disorders* (2nd ed.) (pp. 437-452). Washington, DC: American Psychiatric Publishing, Inc.

Ramsawh, H. J., Raffa, S. D., Edelen, M. O., et al. (2009). Anxiety in middle adulthood: Effects of age and time on the 14-year course of panic disorder, social phobia, and generalized anxiety disorder. *Psychological Medicine, 39*, 615-624.

Rapaport, M. H., Clary, C., Fayyad, R., et al. (2005). Quality-of-life impairment in depressive and anxiety disorders. *American Journal of Psychiatry, 162*, 1171-1178.

Rapee, R. (1997). Potential role of childrearing practices in the development of anxiety and depression. *Clinical Psychology Review, 17*, 47-67.

Rauch, S. L., Savage, C. R., Alpert, N. M., et al. (1995). A positron emission tomographic study of simple phobic symptom provocation. *Archives of General Psychiatry, 52*, 20-28.

Reger, M., & Gahm, G. (2009). A meta-analysis of the effects of Internet-and computer-based cognitive-behavioral treatments for anxiety. *Journal of Clinical Psychology, 65*(1), 53-75.

Reiss, S., Peterson, R. A., Gursky, D. M., et al. (1986). Anxiety sensitivity, anxiety frequency, and the prediction of fearfulness. *Behavioral Research and Therapy, 24*, 1-8.

Ressler, K. J., Rothbaum, B. O., Tannenbaum, L., et al. (2004). Cognitive enhancers as adjuncts to psychotherapy: Use of D-cycloserine in phobic individuals to facilitate extinction of fear. *Archives of General Psychiatry, 61*, 1136-1144.

Reynolds, C. R., & Paget, K. D. (1981). Factor analysis of the *Revised Children's Manifest Anxiety Scale* for blacks, whites, males and females with a national normative sample. *Journal of Consulting and Clinical Psychology, 49*, 352-359.

Ribeiro, L., Busnello, J. V., Kauer-Sant'Anna, M., et al. (2001). Mirtazapine versus fluoxetine in the treatment of panic disorder. *Brazilian Journal of Medical Biological Research, 34*, 1303-1307.

Rickels, K. (2004). Alprazolam extended-release in panic disorder. *Expert Opinion on Pharmacotherapy, 5*(7), 1599-1661.

Rickels, K., DeMartinis, N., Garcia-Espana, F., et al. (2000). Imipramine and buspirone in treatment of patients with generalized anxiety disorder who are discontinuing long-term benzodiazepine therapy. *American Journal of Psychiatry, 157*, 1973-1979.

Rickels, K., Mangano, R., & Khan, A. (2004). A double-blind, placebo-controlled study of a flexible dose of venlafaxine ER in adult outpatients with generalized social anxiety disorder. *Journal of Clinical Psychopharmacology, 24*(5), 488-496.

Rickels, K., & Rynn, M. (2002). Pharmacotherapy of generalized anxiety disorder. *Journal of Clinical Psychiatry, 63*(Suppl 14), 9-16.

Rickels, K., Schweizer, E., Weiss, S., et al. (1993). Maintenance drug treatment for panic disorder, II: Short and long-term outcome after drug taper. *Archives of General Psychiatry, 50*, 61-68.

Rickels, K., Zaninelli, R., McCafferty, J., et al. (2003). Paroxetine treatment of generalized anxiety disorder: A double-blind, placebo-controlled study. *American Journal of Psychiatry, 160*(4), 749-756.

Rocca, P., Fonzo, V., Scotta, M., et al. (1997). Paroxetine efficacy in the treatment of generalized anxiety disorders. *Acta Psychiatrica Scandinavica 95*, 444-450.

Rodebaugh, T. L., Holaway, R. M., & Heimberg, R. G. (2004). The treatment of social anxiety disorder. *Clinical Psychology Review, 24*(7), 883-908.

Roemer, L., Molina, S., & Borkovec, T. D. (1997). An investigation of worry content among generally anxious individuals. *Journal of Nervous and Mental Disorders, 185*, 314-319.

Rosenbaum, J. F., Biederman, J., Gersten, M., et al. (1988). Behavioral inhibition in children of parents with panic disorder and agoraphobia. A controlled study. *Archives of General Psychiatry, 45*(5), 463-470.

Rothbaum, B. O., Hodges, L., Anderson, P. L., et al. (2002). Twelve-month follow-up of virtual reality and standard exposure therapies for the fear of flying. *Journal of Consulting and Clinical Psychology, 70*, 428-432.

Rowa, K., & Anthony, M. M. (2005). Psychological treatments for social phobia. *Canadian Journal of Psychiatry, 50*(6), 308-316.

Roy-Byrne, P., Russo, J., Dugdale, D. C., et al. (2002). Under-treatment of panic disorder in primary care: Role of patient and physician characteristics. *Journal of the American Board of Family Practice, 15*(6), 443-450.

Roy-Byrne, P. P., Stein, M. B., Russo, J., et al. (1999). Panic disorder in the primary care setting: Comorbidity, disability, service utilization, and treatment. *Journal of Clinical Psychiatry, 60*(7), 492-499.

Ruscio, A. M., & Borkovec, T. D. (2004). Experience and appraisal of worry among high worriers with and without GAD. *Behavior Research & Therapy, 42*(12), 1469-1482.

Ruscio, A. M., Brown, T. A., Chiu, W. T., et al. (2008). Social fears and social phobia in the SA: Results from the National Comorbidity Survey Replication. *Psychological Medicine, 38*, 15-28.

Ruscio, A. M., Lane, M., Roy-Byrne, P., et al. (2005). Should excessive worry be required for a diagnosis of generalized anxiety disorder? Results from the US National Comorbidity Survey Replication. *Psychological Medicine, 35*(12), 1761-1772.

Rynn, M. A., & Brawman-Mintzer, O. (2004). Generalized anxiety disorder: Acute and chronic treatment. *CNS Spectrums, 9*(10), 716-723.

Rynn, M., Russell, J., Erickson, J., et al. (2008). Efficacy and safety of duloxetine in the treatment of generalized anxiety disorder: A flexible-dose, progressive-titration, placebo-controlled trial. *Depression and Anxiety, 25*, 182-189.

Sadock, B., & Sadock, V. (2007). *Kaplan & Sadock's synopsis of psychiatry: Behavioral sciences clinical psychiatry* (10th ed.). Philadelphia: Wolters Kluwer/Lippincott Williams & Wilkins.

Safren, S. A., Gershuny, B. S., Marzol, P., et al. (2002). History of childhood abuse in panic disorder, social phobia and generalized anxiety disorder. *The Journal of Nervous and Mental Disease, 190*(7), 453-456.

Salzer, A. L., Pincus, J., Hoyer, R., et al. (2008). Interpersonal subtypes within generalized anxiety disorder. *Journal of Personality Assessment, 90*, 292-299.

Sareen, J., Cox, B. J., Afifi, T. O., et al. (2005). Anxiety disorders and risk for suicidal ideation and suicide attempts: A population-based longitudinal study of adults. *Archives of General Psychiatry, 62*, 1249-1257.

Sareen, J., Cox, B. J., Clara, I., et al. (2005). The relationship between anxiety disorders and physical disorders in the U.S. National Comorbidity Survey. *Depression and Anxiety, 21*, 193-202.

Schatzberg, A. F., Cole, J. O., & DeBattista, C. (Eds.). (2007). *Manual of clinical psychopharmacology* (6th ed.). Washington, DC: American Psychiatric Publishing, Inc.

Schmidt, L. A., Polak, C. P., & Spooner, A. L. (2005). Biological and environmental contributions to childhood shyness: A diathesis-stress model. In W. R. Crozier & L. E. Alden (Eds.), *The essential handbook of social anxiety for clinicians* (pp. 33-55). West Sussex, UK: John Wiley & Sons, Ltd.

Schmidt, N. B., Wollaway-Bickel, K., Trakowski, J. H., et al. (2002). Antidepressant discontinuation in the context of cognitive behavioral treatment for panic disorder. *Behavior Research and Therapy, 40*, 67-73.

Schneier, F. R. (2006). Social anxiety disorder. *The New England Journal of Medicine, 355*(10), 1029-1036.

Schutters, S. I., van Megen, H. J., & Westenberg, H. G. (2005). Efficacy of quetiapine in generalized social anxiety disorder: Results from an open label study. *Journal of Clinical Psychiatry, 66*, 540-542.

Sepede, G., Mancini, E., Salerno, R. M., et al. (2006). Olanzapine augmentation in treatment resistant panic disorder: A 12-week, fixed-dose, open-label trial. *Journal of Clinical Psychopharmacology, 26*, 45-49.

Shah, S. G., Klumpp, H., Angstadt, M., et al. (2009). Amygdala and insula response to emotional images in patients with generalized social anxiety disorder. *Journal of Psychiatry & Neuroscience, 34*(4), 296-302.

Sharma, I., Azmi, S. L. A., & Settiwar, R. M. (1991). Evaluation of the effect of pranayama in anxiety state. *Alternative Medicine, 3*, 227-235.

Shear, M. K., Brown, T. A., Barlow, D. H., et al. (1997). Multicentre collaborative Panic Disorder Severity Scale. *American Journal of Psychiatry, 154*, 1571-1575.

Sheikh, J. L. L. (1992). Anxiety disorders and their treatment. *Clinical Geriatric Medicine, 8*, 411-426.

Shelton, C. T. (2004). Diagnosis and management of anxiety disorders. *Journal of the American Osteopathic Association, 104*(3 Suppl 3), S2-S5.

Sherbourne, C. D., Wells, K. B., & Judd, L. L. (1996). Functioning and well-being of patients with panic disorder. *American Journal of Psychiatry, 153*, 213-218.

Shields, M. (2004). Social anxiety disorder—beyond shyness. *Health Reports, 15*(Supp l), 45-61.

Shrestha, R., Natarajan, N., & Coplan, J. D. (2010). Pathogenesis of panic disorder. In D. J. Stein, E. Hollander, & B. O. Rothbaum (Eds.), *The American psychiatric publishing textbook of anxiety disorders* (2nd ed.) (pp. 381-398). Washington, DC: American Psychiatric Publishing, Inc.

Silver, J. M., Kramer, R., Greenwald, S., et al. (2001). The association between head injuries and psychiatric disorders: Findings from the New Haven NIMH epidemiologic catchment area study. *Brain Injury, 15*(11), 935-945.

Simon, N. M., & Fischmann, D. (2005). The implications of medical and psychiatric comorbidity with panic disorder. *Journal of Clinical Psychiatry, 66*(Suppl 4), 8-15.

Simon, N. M., Hoge, E. A., Fischmann, D., et al. (2006). An open-label trial of risperidone augmentation for refractory anxiety disorders. *Journal of Clinical Psychiatry, 67*, 381-385.

Simon, N. M., Korbly, N. B., Worthington, J. J., et al. (2002). Citalopram for social anxiety disorder: An open-label pilot study in refractory and nonrefractory patients. *CNS Spectrums, 7*(9), 655-657.

Simon, N. M., Otto, M. W., Korbly, N. B., et al. (2002). Quality of life in social anxiety disorder compared with panic disorder and the general population. *Psychiatric Services, 53*(6), 714-718.

Simon, N. M., Safren, S. A., Otto, M. W., et al. (2002). Longitudinal outcome with pharmacotherapy in a naturalistic study of panic disorder. *Journal of Affective Disorders, 69*(1-3), 201-208.

Smith, K. L., Kirkby, K. C., Montgomery, I. M., et al. (1997). Computer-delivered modeling of exposure for spider phobia: Relevant versus irrelevant exposure. *Journal of Anxious Disorders, 11*, 489-497.

Smoller, J. W. (2008). Genetics of mood and anxiety disorders. In J. W. Smoller, B. R. Sheidley, & M. T. Tsuang (Eds.), *Psychiatric genetics: Applications in clinical practice* (pp. 131-177). Washington, DC: American Psychiatric Publishing, Inc.

Smoller, J. W., Sheidley, B. R., & Tsuang, M. T. (2008). *Psychiatric genetics: Applications in clinical practice.* Washington, DC: American Psychiatric Publishing, Inc.

Snyderman, S. H., Rynn, M. A., Bellew, K., et al. (2004). Paroxetine in the treatment of generalized anxiety disorder. *Expert Opinion on Pharmacotherapy, 5*(8), 1799-1806.

Spiegel, D. A., & Hofmann, S. G. (2002). Psychotherapy for panic disorder. In D. S. Stein and E. Hollander (Eds.), *American psychiatric publishing textbook of anxiety disorders* (pp. 273-285). Washington, DC: American Psychiatric Publishing, Inc.

Spitzer, R. L., Kroenke, K., Williams, J. B., et al. (2006). A brief measure for assessing generalized anxiety disorder: The GAD-7. *Archives of Internal Medicine*, 1092-1097.

Stahl, S. (2000). *Essential psychopharmacology: Neuroscientific basis and practical applications* (2nd ed.). Cambridge, UK: Cambridge University Press.

Starcevic, V., Bogojevic, G., Marinkovic, J., et al. (1999). Axis I and Axis II comorbidity in panic/agoraphobic patients with and without suicidal ideation. *Psychiatry Research, 88*(2), 153-161.

Stein, M. B. (2009). Neurobiology of generalized anxiety disorder. *Journal of Clinical Psychiatry, 70*(Suppl 2), 15-19.

Stein, M. B., & Campbell-Sills, L. (2007). Panic disorder. In G. O. Gabbard (Ed.), *Gabbard's treatments of psychiatric disorders* (4th ed.) (pp. 481-493). Washington, DC: American Psychiatric Publishing, Inc.

Stein, M. B., Fyer, A. J., Davidson, J. R. T., et al. (1999). Fluvoxamine treatment of social phobia (social anxiety disorder): A double-blind, placebo-controlled study. *American Journal of Psychiatry, 156*, 756-760.

Stein, M. B., & Kean, Y. M. (2000). Disability and quality of life in social phobia: Epidemiological findings. *American Journal of Psychiatry, 157*, 1606-1613.

Stein, M. B., Roy-Byrne, P. P., Craske, M. G., et al. (2005). Functional impact and health utility of anxiety disorders in primary care outpatients. *Medical Care, 43*, 1164-1170.

Stinson, F. S., Dawson, D. A., Chou, P. S., et al. (2007). The epidemiology of DSM-IV specific phobia in the USA: Results from the National Epidemiologic Survey on Alcohol and Related Conditions. *Psychological Medicine, 37*, 1047-1059.

Stuhlmiller, C., & Tolchard, B. (2009). Computer-assisted CBT for depression & anxiety. *Journal of Psychosocial Nursing, 47*(7), 32-39.

Swinson, R. P., Antony, M. M., Bleau, P., et al. (2006). Clinical practice guidelines. Management of anxiety disorders. *Canadian Journal of Psychiatry, 51*(Suppl 2), 1-92.

Swinson, R. P., Cox, B. J., & Woszczyna, C. B. (1992). Use of medical services and treatment for panic disorder with agoraphobia and for social phobia. *Canadian Medical Association Journal, 147*, 878-883.

Taylor, S. (2000). *Understanding and treating panic disorder: Cognitive-behavioral approaches.* New York: John Wiley & Sons.

Taylor, S., Wald, J., & Asmundson, J. (2007). Psychopathology of panic disorder. *Psychiatry, 5*, 188-192.

Telch, M. J., Lucas, R. A., Schmidt, N. B., et al. (1993). Group cognitive-behavioral treatment of panic disorder. *Behavioral Research Therapy, 31*, 279-287.

Teng, E., Bailey, S. D., Chaison, A. D., et al. (2008). Treating comorbid panic disorder in veterans with posttraumatic stress disorder. *Journal of Consulting & Clinical Psychology, 76*(4), 704-710.

Thase, M. E. (2006). Treatment of anxiety disorders with venlafaxine XR. *Expert Review of Neurotherapeutics, 6*(3), 269-282.

Tiihonen, J., Kuikka, J., Räsänen P., et al. (1997). Cerebral benzodiazepine receptor binding and distribution in generalized anxiety disorder: A fractal analysis. *Molecular Psychiatry, 2*, 463-471.

Turner, S. M., Beidel, D. C., & Cooley-Quille, M. R. (1995). Two-year follow-up of social phobics treated with social effectiveness therapy. *Behavior Research and Therapy, 33*, 553-555.

van Ameringen, M., Mancini, C., & Farvolden, P. (2003). The impact of anxiety disorders on education achievement. *Anxiety Disorders, 17*, 561-571.

van Ameringen, M., Mancini, C., Patterson, B., et al. (2010). Pharmacotherapy for generalized anxiety disorder. In D. J. Stein, E. Hollander, & B. O. Rothbaum (Eds.), *The American psychiatric publishing textbook of anxiety disorders* (2nd ed.) (pp. 193-218). Washington, DC: American Psychiatric Publishing, Inc.

van der Linden, G., van Heerden, B., Warwick, J., et al. (2000). Pharmacotherapy in social phobia: A single photon emission computed tomography before and after treatment with the selective serotonin reuptake inhibitor, citalopram. *Progress in Neuropsychopharmacological Biological Psychiatry, 24*, 419-438.

van Vliet, I. M., den Boer, J. A., & Westenberg, H. G. (1994). Psychopharmacological treatment of social phobia: A double-blind placebo-controlled study with fluvoxamine. *Psychopharmacology, 115*, 128-134.

Versiani, M., Cassano, G., Perugi, G., et al. (2002). Reboxetine, a selective norepinephrine reuptake inhibitor, is an effective and well tolerated treatment for panic disorder. *Journal of Clinical Psychiatry, 63*, 31-37.

Vickers, K., & McNally, R. J. (2004). Panic disorder and suicide attempt in the National Comorbidity Survey. *Journal of Abnormal Psychology, 113*, 582-591.

Voci, S. C., Beitchman, J. H., Brownlie, E. B., et al. (2006). Social anxiety in late adolescence: The importance of early childhood language impairment. *Journal of Anxiety Disorders, 20*(7), 915-930.

Wang, P. S., Lane, M., Olfson, M., et al. (2005). Twelve-month use of mental health services in the United States: Results from the National Comorbidity Survey Replication. *Archives of General Psychiatry, 62*, 629-640.

Warren, S. L., Huston, L., Egeland, B., et al. (1997). Child and adolescent anxiety disorders and early attachment. *Journal of American Academy of Child and Adolescent Psychiatry, 36*, 737-744.

Watson, D., & Friend, R. (1969). Measurement of social evaluation anxiety. *Journal of Consulting and Clinical Psychology, 33*, 448-457.

Wedding, D., Boyd, M. A., & Niemiec, R. M. (2010). *Movies and mental illness: Using films to understand psychopathology* (3rd ed.). Cambridge, MA: Hogrefe Publishing.

Weisberg, R. B. (2009). Overview of generalized anxiety disorder: Epidemiology, presentation, and course. *Journal of Clinical Psychiatry, 70*(Suppl 2), 4-9.

White, J. (1998b). Stresspac: Three year follow-up of a controlled trial of a self-help package for the anxiety disorders. *Behavioral and Cognitive Psychotherapy, 26,* 133-141.

Wiborg, I. M., & Dahl, A. A. (1996). Does brief dynamic psychotherapy reduce the relapse rate of panic disorder? *Archives of General Psychiatry, 53,* 689-694.

Windle, M., Windle, R. C., Scheidt, D. M., et al. (1995). Physical and sexual abuse and associated mental disorders among alcoholic inpatients. *American Journal of Psychiatry, 152,* 1322-1328.

Wittchen, H. U., Zhao, S., Kessler, R. C., et al. (1994). DSM-III-R generalized anxiety disorder in the National Comorbidity Survey. *Archives of General Psychiatry, 51,* 355-364.

Wright, J., Clum, G. A., Roodman, A., et al. (2000). A bibliotherapy approach to relapse prevention in individuals with panic attacks. *Journal of Anxiety Disorders, 14*(5), 483-499.

Wu, J. C., Buchsbaum, M. S., Hershey, T. G., et al. (1991). PET in generalized anxiety disorder. *Biological Psychiatry, 19,* 1181-1199.

Answers to Case Study 10-1 Questions

1. Differential diagnoses include avoidant personality disorder, dependent personality disorder, adjustment disorder with depression, and dysthymia.
2. Continue antidepressant medication because there is some response. Add cognitive behavioral therapy. Suggest psychosocial interventions such as community programs offering public speaking, job-hunting tips, and vocational counseling.

CHAPTER 11

Acute Stress Disorder and Post-traumatic Stress Disorder

Eris F. Perese, APRN-PMH

Exposure to traumatic events is a relatively common experience. In fact, 66% of the adults in the United States experience a traumatic event over their lifetime (Galea, Nandi, & Viahov, 2005). If the definition of a traumatic event is extended to include both direct exposure and indirect exposure, then 89% of the adults in the United States will have been exposed to at least one potentially traumatic event in their lifetime (Breslau, 2002; Breslau & Kessler, 2001; Breslau, Peterson, Poisson, et al., 2004). Potentially traumatic events include manmade or technological disasters, natural disasters, and personal events (Table 11-1). All of these types of events are unexpected, uncontrollable, or inescapable, but they differ in the scope of the population involved, in severity, in duration, in the degree of secondary traumatic events experienced, and in the rate of development of psychopathology (Modestin, Furrer, & Malti, 2005). Events intentionally caused by humans are associated with more severe responses than traumas arising from acts of nature because manmade traumatic events have the quality of deliberate, ruthless betrayal (Green, 1993; Neria, Nandi, & Galea, 2007). For example, individuals who experienced mass violence (terrorism and shooting sprees) had greater impairment—psychological problems, distress, health problems, and difficulty in adjusting to problems of living—than those who experienced natural disasters such as earthquakes (Norris, Friedman, Watson, et al., 2002a, 2002b).

Experiencing a traumatic event often changes individuals' basic assumptions about their vulnerability to injury or death, their status within a social group, their ability to meet their life goals, the reliability of an attachment, and their belief that there is an orderly relationship in the world between actions and outcomes (McFarlane, 2010). In addition to these changes in their perceptions of people, safety, and self-efficacy, the majority of individuals who have experienced a traumatic event demonstrate emotional responses of fear, anger, and sadness and cognitive responses such as denial, depersonalization (a feeling of unreality or detachment from one's self or one's body), or derealization (a feeling that other people or the world seems strange or unreal) (Horowitz, 2003). Children often experience physiological responses, such as gastrointestinal tract symptoms, respiratory tract symptoms, cardiovascular responses, and muscular responses such as numbness or tingling. They may have fears for their safety, fears of being separated from their family, and fears of abandonment. They may experience nightmares and have difficulty concentrating and remembering details. They are often depressed and lonely, and their view of themselves in relation to others is altered (Wiese & Burhorst, 2007).

The individual's developmental stage and coping skills and the availability of protective factors such as social support, stable networks, and material resources at the time of the trauma and following the trauma all affect an individual's early reactions to trauma (Brewin, Andrews, Rose, et al., 1999; Gaffney, 2008; Glass, Perrin, Campbell, et al., 2007). Most individuals who experience a potentially traumatic event demonstrate resilience (Reyes & Elhai, 2004), which means that they are able to respond adaptively by using coping strategies such as self-distraction, seeking emotional and instrumental support, venting their feelings, reframing the situation, planning, and using humor and religious beliefs. However, some individuals have difficulty responding adaptively (Schiller, Levy, Niv, et al., 2008), and they may develop psychopathology such as depression, anxiety disorders, adjustment disorder, substance misuse, acute stress disorder (ASD), and post-traumatic stress disorder (PTSD) (Forbes, Creamer, Phelps, et al., 2007; Kessler, Sonnega,

TABLE 11-1 POTENTIALLY TRAUMATIC EVENTS

Event Type	Examples	People Affected	Primary Effects	Secondary Effects
Technological/ Manmade disasters	Airplane crash, industrial explosion, bombings, terrorist attacks, combat, captivity	Circumscribed population	Physical injuries; threats to life; loss of loved ones	Financial losses; changes in roles and functioning
Natural disasters	Fire, earthquake, flood, tsunami, hurricane, tornado, ice storm	Large population	Loss of loved ones and property	Need to relocate; experiencing isolation, humiliation, and degradation (Neria et al., 2007; Shalev, 2002)
Personal traumatic events	Assault, rape, witnessing violent acts, being exposed to sudden death, being informed of a life-threatening illness, being a rescue worker	One individual, although the events may have an indirect effect on members of the individual's family and social network	Changes in sense of self-identity, safety, and predictability of life	Changes in activities to feel safe; alterations of life plans and sometimes, changes in religious commitment (Thielman, 2011)

Bromet, et al., 1995; Norris, et al., 2002a; Norris et al., 2002b; Yehuda & Sarapas, 2010). ASD and PTSD will be discussed in this chapter.

According to the *Diagnostic and Statistical Manual of Mental Disorders,* Fourth Edition, Text Revision *(DSM-IV-TR),* diagnosis of ASD or PTSD requires that the patient has undergone one of the following:

1. The patient has been exposed to an extremely traumatic event that involves actual or threatened death, serious injury, or threat to one's physical integrity.
2. The patient has witnessed an event that involves death, injury, or a threat to the physical integrity of another individual.
3. The patient has learned of unexpected or violent death, serious harm, or threat of death or injury that was experienced by a family member or other close associate (American Psychiatric Association, 2000, p. 463).

Among adults, traumatic events associated with the development of ASD or PTSD include incidents such as rape and assaults; ship, sea, and air disasters; earthquakes and floods; accidents; war; and terrorist attacks. Among adolescents, traumatic events associated with development of ASD include the above-listed events (Hollander & Simeon, 2011), and traumatic events associated with development of PTSD include death of a family member, serious illness, rape, childhood abuse, threat of violence, humiliation or bullying, abortion, near-drowning, and traffic accidents (Elklit & Petersen, 2008).

Normal response to stressors and traumatic events is described in Chapter 9. The fear/anxiety circuit is also described in Chapter 9. The concepts of allostasis and allostatic overload (also in Chapter 9) form the basis for psychiatric advanced practice nurses' understanding of the biological basis of ASD and PTSD.

Acute Stress Disorder (ASD)

ASD is characterized by symptoms of dissociation, intrusion, avoidance, and hyperarousal with impaired social and work functioning; it occurs within 4 weeks of exposure to a traumatic event (Marmar & Spiegel, 2007). The diagnosis of ASD was added to the *Diagnostic and Statistical Manual of Mental Disorders (DSM-IV)* in 1994 (American Psychiatric Association, 1994) to describe a response to a traumatic event in the first month after the event. At the time, the committee that was developing the *DSM-IV* hoped that adding the ASD diagnosis would enable clinicians to provide timely interventions that might prevent later development of PTSD (Black & Andreasen, 2011; Spiegel, 2005).

Criteria for Diagnosis of Acute Stress Disorder: Dissociation and Other Symptoms

Although the criteria for ASD and PTSD include many similar symptoms, the criteria for ASD require the presence of at least three dissociative symptoms (Black & Andreasen, 2011). It was thought that dissociation during a traumatic event hinders organization of memories associated with the traumatic event, and that this lack of organizing and processing of memories results in the development of PTSD (Koopman, Classen, Cardena, et al., 1995). Dissociative symptoms may occur in PTSD but need not be present for the diagnosis of PTSD.

Dissociation: The Key Characteristic of Acute Stress Disorder

Dissociation is a way of organizing information that serves as a defense mechanism to reduce anxiety (Gabbard, 2005). It refers to "a compartmentalization of experience" and can occur at the time of the trauma or after the trauma (van der

Kolk, van der Hart, & Marmar, 2006d, p. 306). Dissociation at the time of trauma may be an adaptive response to the acute stress experienced (Koopman, Classen, & Spiegel, 1996).

Disassociation occurs when individuals' cognitive capacities to modulate terror and horror are overwhelmed (Marmar & Spiegel, 2007). Gabbard (2005) said, "Dissociation allows individuals to retain an illusion of psychological control when they experience a sense of helplessness and loss of control over their bodies" (p. 284). Dissociation helps individuals to remove themselves from a traumatic event while it is occurring until they can place the event in perspective with the rest of their lives. Dissociation can be primary, secondary, or tertiary.

Primary Dissociation

In primary dissociation, sensory and emotional elements of the experience may not be integrated into an individual's memory and sense of self-identity. The traumatic experience does not become part of the individual's life story. Instead, the dissociated traumatic memories exist as upsetting intrusive recollections, nightmares, and flashbacks (van der Kolk et al., 2006d). Dissociative symptoms include

- Feelings of detachment, numbing, or lack of emotional responsiveness
- Decreased awareness of surroundings
- Derealization, which is an alteration in the perception or experience of the external world so that it seems strange or unreal, e.g., people may seem unfamiliar (American Psychiatric Association, 2000, p. 822)
- Depersonalization, which is an alteration in the perception or experience of the self so that one feels detached from oneself and as if one is an outside observer of one's mental processes or body, e.g., feeling like one is in a dream (American Psychiatric Association, 2000, p. 822)
- Dissociative amnesia, which is the inability to remember a significant aspect of the trauma (van der Kolk, 2006b)

Secondary Dissociation

Individuals may have further dissociative sensations, such as leaving their bodies at the moment of the trauma and observing what happens from a distance. This mechanism may serve to limit their pain or distress, but it puts them out of touch with the feelings and emotions related to the trauma. Trauma victims may report having had a sense of detachment from their body and an altered passage of time during the traumatic event (van der Kolk et al., 2006d).

Tertiary Dissociation

According to van der Kolk et al. (2006d), in tertiary dissociation, "people develop distinct ego states that contain the traumatic experience consisting of complex identities with distinct cognitive, affective and behavioral patterns" (p. 308). Thus, individuals develop distinct identities, which in the past were called multiple personalities. The development of fragments of identity is now called dissociative identity disorder (DID) (Maldonado & Spiegel, 2008). Some identities (sometimes called "alters") contain the pain, fear, and anger related to the traumatic experience, while other identities may contain other aspects of the traumatic event, such as shame, humiliation, and powerlessness. Some identities may remain unaware of the trauma and continue to carry out the routines of daily living. The goal of treatment is integration of painful memories and a more integrated state of memories, consciousness, and identity (Maldonado & Spiegel).

Other Symptoms of Acute Stress Disorder

In addition to dissociative symptoms, ASD is characterized by intrusive thoughts, recurrent images or dreams, flashbacks of the event, anxiety, sleep disturbances, restlessness, hyperarousal symptoms, and avoidance behaviors of at least 2 days' duration. For an individual to be diagnosed with ASD, his or her symptoms must occur within 1 month after exposure to an extreme traumatic stressor, and the symptoms must last for at least 2 days. The *DSM-IV-TR* (American Psychiatric Association, 2000) criteria for ASD state that the symptoms must markedly interfere with social or occupational functioning or prevent an individual from pursuing some necessary task. The symptoms may last from a minimum of 2 days to a maximum of 4 weeks and may include disorientation, confusion, intense agitation, and dazed detachment, sometimes followed by amnesia.

Acute stress response differs among different survivors. For example, in children, acute stress response to a severe traumatic event may include sleep disturbances, fear, anxiety, regressive symptoms, hallucinations, and delusions (Portnova, 2005). Among military combatants, early responses include severe anxiety, fear of death, crying, insomnia, numbing, fatigue, feelings of guilt about performing poorly in combat, a sense of loneliness and vulnerability, and disorientation (Solomon, Laror, & McFarlane, 2006).

Epidemiology

The prevalence of ASD is 14% to 33% among individuals who have experienced severe trauma (American Psychiatric Association, 2000, p. 470). The prevalence differs according to the type of traumatic event experienced, e.g., technological/manmade traumatic events, natural disasters, or personal traumatic events (Table 11-2).

Etiology

It is accepted that exposure to a traumatic event is the cause of ASD; however, Koenen, Harley, Lyons, et al. (2002) found that exposure to traumatic events is not random:

TABLE 11-2 DEVELOPMENT OF ACUTE STRESS DISORDER AFTER SPECIFIC TRAUMATIC EVENTS

Traumatic Event	Prevalence of Acute Stress Disorder in Victims	Source
Rape	70%–90%	First & Tasman, 2004
Ship or sea disaster	79%	Eriksson & Lundin, 1996
Earthquake	45%	Lima, Chavez, Samniego, et al., 1989
Burns (children)	30%	Stoddard, Saxe, Ronfeldt, et al., 2006
Learning the diagnosis of a life-threatening illness	28% (32% had subsyndromal symptoms)	Kangas, Henry, & Bryant, 2005
Parenting an infant in the neonatal intensive care unit	28%	Shaw, Deblois, Ikuta, et al., 2006
Violence/assault (adults seen in emergency room)	24% (21% had subsyndromal symptoms)	Elklit & Brink, 2003
Violence/assault (children seen in emergency room)	19.4% (24.7% met all criteria except dissociation [children may not have understood the term])	Meiser-Stedman, Yule, Smith, et al., 2005
Motor vehicle accident (adults)	16%	Bryant, Moulds, Guthrie, et al., 2003a
Motor vehicle accident (children)	11%–19%	Bryant, Mayou, Wigs, et al., 2004; Meiser-Stedman et al., 2005
Terrorist attack	12.4% those surveyed after the 9/11 attack on the World Trade Center	Norris et al., 2002b

some individuals are at higher risk. They found that increased risk for exposure to traumatic events was associated with family and individual risk factors, including parental depression and an individual's conduct disorder and/or substance-related disorder.

In a later study of exposure to traumatic events, Afifi, Asmundson, Taylor, et al. (2010) concluded that exposure to nonassaultive traumatic events (sudden death of a family member, earthquakes, fires, tornados, floods, or motor vehicle accidents) is random, but that exposure to assaultive traumatic events (robbery, captivity, being beaten up, sexual assault, and life-threatening events) is not random. Exposure to assaultive traumatic events is influenced by genetic heritability, which shapes the individual's choice of risky or nonrisky lifestyle practices and living situations; shared environmental factors (housing, family income, family size, and family smoking behavior); and nonshared environmental factors (illnesses, accidents, peer groups, and leisure activities). Specific influences include parental depression, parental antisocial behavior and less than high school education, and, in the individual, conduct disorder and substance-related disorder. Thus, some individuals are at higher risk of being exposed to traumatic events.

Similarly, the risk for developing ASD is not the same for all individuals who experience trauma. Those at increased risk include

- Females
- Individuals with psychiatric disorders
- Bereaved individuals
- Individuals with a high level of depressive symptoms
- Individuals with an avoidant coping style
- Children, especially if separated from their parents
- Individuals who are dependent on psychosocial support, such as older adults and handicapped people
- Workers who handle the bodies after the traumatic event
- Individuals with lower levels of social support (First & Tasman, 2004; Harvey & Bryant, 1998; Yasan, Guzel, Tamam, et al., 2009)

Clinical Presentation

Clinical presentation usually includes

- Physical symptoms (headaches or gastrointestinal problems)
- Emotional symptoms (fear, anxiety, and depression)
- Cognitive symptoms (reduced awareness; dissociative symptoms such as numbness, amnesia, reliving, depersonalization, and derealization; recurrent intrusive thoughts, dreams, and images; and poor concentration)
- Interpersonal symptoms (irritability with others and difficulty with trust and intimacy)
- Behavioral symptoms (avoidance of places or people that are reminders of the traumatic event, motor restlessness, and changes in sleep patterns) (Forbes et al., 2007; Spiegel, 2005)

Comorbidity

Comorbidities that frequently occur with ASD are injuries or burns that are associated with the traumatic event. ASD is often comorbid in patients with burns or life-threatening illnesses (see Table 11-2).

Differential Diagnosis

Other anxiety disorders, other psychiatric diagnoses, and other conditions must be considered as differential diagnoses (Black & Andreasen, 2011). Table 11-3 details the differential diagnoses for ASD and their individual characteristics.

Treatment

The first steps in treatment are assessment and meeting immediate needs. In evaluating patients who have been exposed to a traumatic event, the psychiatric advanced practice nurse uses the assessment process to build trust and to develop a therapeutic alliance (see Chapter 4). In assessing details of recent

TABLE 11-3 DIFFERENTIAL DIAGNOSIS OF ACUTE STRESS DISORDER

Other Disorder	Differentiating Characteristics of Other Disorder
Mental disorders due to a general medical condition or physical effects related to the stressful event such as injuries	Presence of a general medical condition that is causing the symptoms. ASD is not diagnosed if the symptoms are due to the physical effects of a stressful event.
Substance-induced disorder	Symptoms are due to the direct physiological effects of a substance (e.g., alcohol intoxication).
Brief psychotic disorder	Psychotic symptoms occur in response to a stressor.
Exacerbation of a mental disorder that was present before the exposure	Has no additional symptoms after the stressful event.
Post-traumatic stress disorder	Symptoms last more than 1 month after the stressful event.
Adjustment disorder with anxiety	The symptoms include nervousness, worry, or jitteriness but do not include dissociative symptoms. Symptoms do not meet the pattern of other mental disorders.
Malingering	Characterized by feigning of symptoms and should be ruled out when legal, financial, and other benefits play a role.

Sources: American Psychiatric Association, 2000, p. 471; First, Frances, & Pincus, 2002; First & Tasman, 2004.

traumatic events, the psychiatric advanced practice nurse must be aware of patients' capacity to participate. Patients should be given the opportunity to decide how deeply they are able to explore the details of the traumatic event. If patients experience increased distress in answering questions about a traumatic event immediately after exposure to the event, the assessment may be limited to evaluating the need for immediate medical care. After providing for patients' safety and stabilizing their medical condition, the psychiatric advanced practice nurse performs a complete psychiatric evaluation with specific assessment of symptoms associated with ASD: reexperiencing, avoidance or numbing, hyperarousal, and dissociation. The psychiatric advanced practice nurse assesses

- Recent or remote traumatic events, such as exposure to motor vehicle accidents, physical or sexual assault, natural disasters, technological disasters, and manmade disasters
- Pain
- Comorbid physical and psychiatric disorders
- Dangerousness to self or others
- Presence of stressors, such as impoverishment, bereavement, loss of loved ones and/or property, and fear of the perpetrator of the traumatic experience
- Basic needs, such as safe housing, food, clothing, transportation, and communication (e.g., telephone)
- Level of biopsychosocial functioning
- Availability of positive social support

The type of traumatic event experienced and the damage associated with the event affect the initial assessment. Common traumatic events include large-scale disasters; military service–related traumatic events; and assaultive, criminal system, or legal system traumatic events.

In a *large-scale disaster* that involves many people, the initial assessment may be a triage of physical injuries and psychological response. Psychiatric advanced practice nurses may screen for individuals at risk for developing ASD or PTSD and for individuals manifesting early symptoms of ASD or PTSD.

In evaluating exposure to traumatic events during *military service*, assessment includes

- Length of service and the presence or absence of disciplinary charges
- Awards received
- Previous referrals (if the individual had been referred for alcohol or substance use counseling, family violence counseling, or psychiatric evaluation)
- Frequency, duration, and effects of family separations
- Location and events related to combat

In evaluating victims of *assaultive events, criminal system events, and legal system events*, such as in motor vehicle accidents, assault, rape, or behaviors related to mental illness, one must keep in mind that ASD symptoms can be influenced by the legal process, payment of damages, or incarceration and/or release of a perpetrator. The evaluation process may also be influenced by victims' desire to profit from the experience.

During assessment, information can be collected by direct interview of the patient and his or her family, by review of medical records, and by the use of assessment instruments. Some instruments used during the initial assessment can also be used for ongoing monitoring of response to treatment (Box 11-1).

Data obtained during assessment form the basis for the case formulation that guides treatment. (See Chapter 5 for more information on case formulation.) The goals of treatment for ASD are to

- Reduce the severity of symptoms
- Prevent or treat trauma-related comorbid conditions
- Improve adaptive functioning by promoting resilience
- Prevent relapse
- Integrate the trauma into the patient's life experience
- Prevent the development of PTSD (Gaffney, 2008; Ursano, Bell, Friedman, et al., 2006a)

Interventions for achieving these goals that have been studied include psychological first aid (PFA), psychotherapy,

BOX 11-1 Instruments for Screening for Acute Stress Disorder

- *Acute Stress Disorder Interview (ASDI)* (Bryant, Harvey, Dang, et al., 1998). This is a structured clinical interview based on *DSM-IV* criteria for ASD that contains 19 items.
- *Brief COPE* (Carver, 1997). This is a measure of 14 coping strategies.
- *Brief Depression Rating Scale (BDRS)* (Kellner, 1986). This is an 8-item instrument that is designed to measure depression by clinical observation. It is not a self-report instrument.
- *Davidson Trauma Scale (DTS)* (Davidson, Book, Colket, et al., 1997a). This is a 17-item self-rating scale. Each item corresponds to a *DSM-IV-TR* symptom of PTSD.
- *Dissociative Experiences Scale (DES)* (Bernstein & Putman, 1986). This is a 28-item instrument that measures dissociation.
- *Harvard Trauma Questionnaire (HTQ)* (Mollica, Caspi-Yavin, Bollini, et al., 1992). This is a checklist that inquires about a variety of traumatic events and about emotional symptoms associated with the events.
- *Impact of Event Scale (IES)* (Horowitz et al., 1979). This is a 15-item scale that measures stress associated with traumatic events. It measures intrusive experiences such as ideas, feelings, or bad dreams and avoidance such as the avoidance of certain ideas, feelings and situations. It can be used to monitor change or response to treatment.
- *Perceived Stress Scale (PSS)* (Cohen, Kamarck, & Mermelstein, 1983). This is a 10-item instrument that measures the degree to which situations in one's life are appraised as stressful. It can be used as an outcome measure.
- *Positive and Negative Suicide Ideation Inventory (PANSI)* (Osman, Gutierrez, Kopper, et al., 1997). The PANSI is a 14-item instrument that has two subscales. One measures positive ideation and the other measures buffers against the possibility of suicide.
- *PTSD Checklist* (Weathers, Litz, Huska, et al., 1994). The PTSD Checklist is a 17-item self-report measure of the 17 *DSM-IV-TR* symptoms of PTSD.
- *Recent Life Changes Questionnaire (RLCQ)* (Rahe, 2000). This instrument measures changes in four domains: family, personal, work, and financial.

pharmacotherapy, psychosocial interventions, and interventions to prevent the development of PTSD.

Psychological First Aid (PFA)

The initial intervention for individuals experiencing trauma is usually a model of crisis intervention that focuses on the individual's biopsychosocial health (Bisson, Brayne, Ochberg, et al., 2007a; Cloak & Edwards, 2004; Frances, 2002). Psychological first aid is a well-known model of crisis intervention (Flannery & Everly, 2000). The key features of PFA are empathy, compassion, stabilizing the patient by reducing distress, and connecting the individual with resources (Reyes & Elhai, 2004). PFA includes the following strategies:

- Creating a sense of safety
- Comforting and consoling the individual
- Providing information
- Protecting the individual from further threat as much as possible
- Providing physical necessities, such as shelter
- Providing support for reality-based tasks
- Facilitating reunion with loved ones
- Allowing the individual to tell the story of the trauma
- Diffusing guilt
- Allowing the individual to express emotions after the danger or threat ends and panic subsides
- Linking the individual with systems of support
- Facilitating some beginning sense of mastery (Lundin, 1994; Marmar & Spiegel, 2007; Raphael, 1986)

Additional interventions are used to meet the individual's immediate needs for medical care, rest, nutrition, hydration, and control of pain that is related to the trauma (Ursano et al., 2006a). Providing information about the trauma helps the individual to recognize and accept the details of what happened; however, information needs to be given in a way that conveys hope and, at the same time, realistic expectations of what may happen. Support involves strengthening coping strategies and promoting use of adaptive defense mechanisms. Individuals do better when they recognize the need to take responsibility for a successful outcome, are actively involved in overcoming the problems associated with the traumatic event, and are involved in helping others (LeDoux & Gorman, 2001).

The frontline treatment for patients with ASD is multiple-session, trauma-focused cognitive behavioral therapy (CBT) (Bryant, Sackville, Dang, et al., 1999; Forbes et al., 2007). Pharmacotherapy may be used to relieve physical or psychological distress, insomnia, extremes of agitation, rage, or dissociation when the patient does not have the ability to use nonpharmacological interventions.

For military persons who have acute combat stress reactions, treatment is based on the PIE model, which has three principles: (1) **p**roximity, which means that the patient should be treated as close to the fighting as possible; (2) **i**mmediacy, which involves treating the patient as soon as possible after symptoms begin; and (3) **e**xpectancy, which emphasizes that the individual will return to combat. Treatment includes meeting patients' basic needs (e.g., providing food, drink, and the opportunity to sleep in a safe place) and offering a chance to talk about their experience. This model of intervention has been found to reduce the development of PTSD (Marmar & Spiegel, 2007).

Psychotherapy

The goal of psychotherapy is to help individuals acknowledge, tolerate, and put into perspective the traumatic experience (Maldonado & Spiegel, 2008). Brief CBT has been shown to lessen the severity of ASD symptoms and to reduce the development of PTSD (Ehlers & Clark, 2003). For children, although CBT has been found to be effective, better outcomes may be achieved if the treatment is delayed for several months after the acute traumatization (Cohen, 2003). A more complete discussion of CBT can be found in Chapter 7.

Pharmacotherapy

Immediately after the traumatic event, the goal of treatment is to reduce feelings of terror, horror, and panic associated with the event, because continuing distress increases consolidation of emotions and memories related to the event and thus may increase risk for PTSD (Marmar & Spiegel, 2007). Pharmacotherapy for acute responses to trauma has two goals: to reduce distress and to reduce the patient's risk of developing subsequent disorders such as PTSD, other anxiety disorders, and depression (Raskind, 2009). Benzodiazepines, antidepressants, antipsychotics, and beta-adrenergic blocking agents have all been used in reducing acute symptoms of distress and enabling patients to begin to cope with the trauma. Psychiatric advanced practice nurses may consider the use of these agents as an approach to reducing the symptoms of ASD or preventing ASD from developing following exposure to trauma.

Benzodiazepines

Antianxiety medications should be avoided if possible (Weigel, Purselle, D'Orio, et al., 2009). However, benzodiazepines may sometimes be used for short-term management of severe anxiety (Black & Andreasen, 2011). Although benzodiazepines may reduce anxiety and improve sleep, some researchers believe that they increase the likelihood of the patient's developing PTSD (Gelpin, Bonne, Peri, et al., 1996).

Antidepressants

Selective serotonin reuptake inhibitors (SSRIs) and other antidepressants may be used to reduce the symptoms of ASD (Shalev, 2002; Weigel et al., 2009). In early studies, the tricyclic antidepressant imipramine (Tofranil) was found to reduce intrusive and hyperarousal symptoms of PTSD in patients who had suffered severe burns (Robert, Blakeney, Villarreal, et al., 1999), and more recently, both imipramine and the SSRI fluoxetine (Prozac) have been found to be effective in reducing the symptoms of ASD in children with burns (Tcheung, Robert, Rosenberg, et al., 2005).

Antipsychotics

Risperidone (Risperdal) has been found to reduce flashbacks in survivors of physical trauma with ASD (Eidelman, Seedat, & Stein, 2000).

Beta-Adrenergic Blocking Agents

Researchers have studied the prevention or reduction of physiologic responses to triggers of the traumatic event with the use of modulators of adrenergic activity. According to Schoenfeld, Marmar, and Neylan (2004), "Sustained periods of increased adrenergic activity are thought to increase the risk of PTSD by initiating a process in which there is over-consolidation of memories of the traumatic event" (p. 523). Pitman and Delahanty (2005) have suggested that preventing noradrenergic hyperactivity by preventing presynaptic norepinephrine release with α_2-adrenergic agonists, such as opioids, or by blocking postsynaptic norepinephrine receptors with beta-adrenergic antagonists, such as propranolol (Inderal), may reduce aversive emotional memories and fear conditioning.

Propranolol, a nonselective beta-adrenergic blocker, appears to reduce the consolidation of emotional memories (Cahill, Prins, Weber, et al., 1994; Weigel et al., 2009). In studies of patients who were treated with propranolol and others who received a placebo within hours of a traumatic event, those receiving propranolol had fewer PTSD symptoms and less physiological reactions to triggers of the trauma (Pitman, Sanders, Zusman, et al., 2002; Vaiva, Ducrocq, Jezequel, et al., 2003). Use of propranolol within the first week of exposure to a traumatic event was associated with remission of symptoms of ASD in 63% of patients and partial response in 27.3% (Pastrana Jimenez, Catalina Romero, Garcia Dieguez, et al., 2007).

Psychosocial Interventions

Psychosocial interventions include psychoeducation and support, and self-activities to reduce distressful feelings.

Psychoeducation and Support

The benefit of providing education for acutely traumatized individuals to reduce the psychological sequelae of exposure to disaster or mass violence has not been established. For example, in one study, one group of patients with symptoms of ASD was offered a booklet of self-help information and another group was not offered the booklet. Symptoms of depression, anxiety, and PTSD in both groups decreased over time. There was no difference in outcome; however, patients receiving the booklet rated its usefulness very highly (Scholes, Turpin, & Mason, 2007). The study did not support the use of education as a strategy to prevent PTSD. Instead, promoting the use of the individual's own knowledge, judgment, support networks, coping strengths, and stress-reducing activities is believed to reduce the need for outside interventions (Wessely, 2005).

Self-Activities to Reduce Distressful Feelings

Following a traumatic experience, patients often feel anxious, agitated, restless, or uneasy. These feelings may be reduced by focusing the patient's attention on problem-solving activities and by encouraging engagement in activities that serve as distractions. LeDoux and Gorman (2001) suggested that engaging in active coping responses rather than using avoidance—i.e., doing something instead of nothing—reroutes the processing of thoughts and actions from passive fear responses to successful interactions with the environment. They recommended that clinicians encourage patients who have experienced traumatic events to engage in pleasurable activities.

Recent research findings support their recommendation. For example, among individuals who had experienced stressful life events, it was found that engaging in a greater number of daily pleasant activities was associated with lower rates of developing depression (Geschwind, Peeters, Jacobs, et al., 2010). Based on this research-based evidence, psychiatric advanced practice nurses should promote the use of daily pleasure-producing self-activities as protection against the development of depression after exposure to a traumatic event, in addition to promoting the use of stress-reducing activities. Pleasure-producing self-activities include

- Creative activities, such as crafts, painting, or drawing; reading fiction, mysteries, or inspirational writings; doing crossword puzzles, jigsaw puzzles, or playing games; gardening or fishing
- Exercise, such as walking, moving to music, or doing relaxation exercises
- Writing lists or plans, journals or records of the event, poems, or letters
- Listening to music or making music, such as playing the harmonica or guitar, or singing favorite songs
- Using spiritual resources, such as meditating, praying, reading affirmations, participating in rituals and ceremonies, or listening to spiritual programs on the radio
- Doing something routine, such as cleaning a drawer, calling a friend, walking the dog, or washing the car
- Wearing favorite clothes, jewelry, or fragrances
- Learning something new (Copeland, 2002)

Interventions to Prevent Development of Post-traumatic Stress Disorder

Factors that appear to increase the risk for developing PTSD among individuals with ASD include female gender, prior exposure to traumatic events, low levels of social support, stressful life events in year prior to trauma, a personal or family history of psychopathology, and experiencing new stressors after the original trauma (Nishith, Mechanic, & Resnick, 2000). The presence of trauma-related symptoms of excessive arousal, fear, dissociation, and depression are predictive of later development of PTSD (Bryant, Harvey, Guthrie, et al., 2000). Based on these known risk factors, interventions to prevent the development of PTSD focus on preventing or treating new stressors, reducing distress, modulating arousal, managing pain, and treating depression.

In the past, there was little evidence that treatment of ASD prevented the development of PTSD (First & Tasman, 2004). For example, the commonly used critical incident stress debriefing was not effective in preventing the development of PTSD (Carlier, 2000; Carlier, Voerman, & Gersons, 2000; Wessely, Rose, & Bisson, 2000) and may have delayed recovery (Carlier; Ehlers & Clark, 2003; Gray, Litz, & Papa, 2006; Mitchell & Everly, 2000; Rose, Bisson, & Wessely, 2002; Shalev, 2002). Recent evidence suggests that psychotherapy and pharmacotherapy have the potential to lower the risk that individuals with ASD will develop PTSD.

Psychotherapeutic Interventions That Prevent Post-traumatic Stress Disorder

Several studies provide evidence that psychotherapy for patients with ASD has the potential to prevent later development of PTSD. CBT that was provided for patients who developed ASD after automobile accidents and nonsexual assaults was associated with a lower rate of development of PTSD than that of the control group, who received supportive counseling that consisted of education about trauma and general problem-solving skills (Bryant, Moulds, Guthrie, et al., 2003a). Studies of combat treatment for acute stress symptoms, a model of psychological first aid, have shown that immediate care provided close to the front line with the expectation of a swift return to combat is associated with a rapid recovery and resumption of functioning, reduced rates of PTSD, and fewer social problems (Solomon, Shklar, & Mikulincer, 2005).

In a recent study of patients with ASD that compared prolonged exposure treatment (imaginal exposure in which patients talked about reliving the traumatic event and their emotional responses) and cognitive restructuring (identification and modification of patient's maladaptive appraisals of the traumatic event, response to the event, and view of the future), it was found that prolonged exposure therapy is more effective in preventing the development of symptoms of PTSD (Bryant, Mastrodomenico, Felmingham, et al., 2008).

Pharmacological Interventions That Prevent Post-traumatic Stress Disorder

Recently, pharmacotherapy has been studied as a way to prevent the development of PTSD in individuals at risk for developing it (Zhang & Davidson, 2010). Studies have shown the effectiveness of propranolol and opiates:

- ***Propranolol.*** Because noradrenergic activity is associated with persistent memories and symptoms of PTSD, the use of medications that reduce the release of norepinephrine or block the uptake of it at the norepinephrine receptors is being explored (Bennett, Zatzick, & Roy-Byrne, 2007; Weigel et al., 2009). Immediate treatment with propranolol, which is a nonselective beta-adrenergic blocker, has been reported to be effective in preventing later development of PTSD (Davidson & Connor, 2004; Marmar & Spiegel, 2007; Stein, 2005; Vaiva et al., 2003). However, propranolol was not found to reduce the risk of developing ASD among children who had experienced the trauma of severe burns (Sharp, Thomas, Rosenberg, et al., 2010), nor was it found to reduce the development of PTSD among soldiers with severe burns (McGhee, Maani, Garza, et al., 2009a).
- ***Opiates.*** The use of opiates to prevent PTSD is based on the assumptions that the opioid systems are

involved in modulating memories and that opiates modulate the release of norepinephrine following exposure to severe stressors (Bennett et al., 2007). Among young children (ages 1 to 4 years) with acute burns, treatment with morphine to manage pain was associated with a decreased rate of PTSD symptoms in the months that followed the burn trauma (Stoddard, Sorrentino, Ceranoglu, et al., 2009). Similarly, among military personnel injured in combat, the use of morphine during early treatment has been found to be associated with a reduced risk of their developing PTSD (Holbrook, Galarneau, Dye, et al., 2010). Currently, new pharmacological interventions for preventing PTSD from developing following ASD are targeting the norepinephrine and dopamine neurotransmitter systems that are involved in arousal and overconsolidation of traumatic memories (Stoddard et al., 2009).

Other agents are also used to prevent development of PTSD. Based on the evidence that early trauma-related symptoms of depression predict later development of PTSD (Bennett et al., 2007), antidepressant medications that are used to treat PTSD are also used to prevent the development of PTSD. Neuropeptide Y agonists are also being developed.

Course

Individuals may experience dissociative and cognitive symptoms of ASD during the traumatic event or immediately after. These symptoms tend to improve spontaneously over time, although approximately 80% of people with ASD develop PTSD (Bryant et al., 2000; Harvey & Bryant, 1998).

Key Points

- Exposure to trauma engages the brain's fear circuitry that promotes survival in the face of danger.
- Normal response to a traumatic event includes arousal, confusion, anxiety, panic, somatic complaints, and changes in eating, sleeping, thinking, and daily activities.
- Some individuals have a pathological response to trauma, including adjustment disorder, ASD, or PTSD.
- Symptoms of ASD include the normal responses to trauma and also symptoms of increased arousal, intrusive thoughts, avoidant behaviors, and dissociation, the latter of which is a cardinal symptom of ASD.
- ASD treatment includes psychological first aid and psychotherapy such as CBT. Pharmacotherapy is used for acute symptoms, and its use in preventing the development of PTSD is being studied.
- By definition, symptoms last for at least 2 days but no longer than 4 weeks. After 4 weeks, the diagnosis may become PTSD.

Resources

Organizations

Federal Emergency Management Agency (FEMA)
http://www.fema.gov

Substance Abuse and Mental Health Services Administration (SAMHSA), Center for Mental Health Services
www.samhsa.gov

National Mental Health Consumers' Self-Help Clearinghouse
1211 Chestnut Street, Suite 1100
Philadelphia, PA 19107
www.mhselfhelp.org/

Books

American Red Cross. (1997). *Disaster preparedness for people with disabilities.* www.redcross.org/disaster/safety/disability.html

Center for Mental Health Services. (1994). *Disaster response and recovery: A handbook for mental health professionals.* Copies are available at no charge from the Center for Mental Health Services, PO Box 42490, Washington, DC. http://www.mentalhealth.org

Movies

Strouse, J. C. (Director). (2007). *Grace is gone* [Motion picture]. United States: Weinstein Company.

Todd, F. (Director). (2001). *In the bedroom* [Motion picture]. United States: Miramax.

Source: Wedding, Boyd, & Niemiec, 2010.

Post-traumatic Stress Disorder

As previously noted, 89% of individuals in the United States have experienced a traumatic event in their lifetime (Breslau, et al., 2004), but only 10% of those who have experienced a traumatic event develop PTSD (Breslau, 2009). Posttraumatic stress disorder is the product of the interaction of the effects of a traumatic stressor with the attributes, biopsychosocial vulnerabilities, and protective resources of the individual exposed to the trauma (Miller, Wolf, Fabricant, et al., 2009, p. 278). The primary feature of PTSD is disturbance of memory, in which memories of the traumatic event are not processed and integrated with other information (McFarlane, 2010; van der Kolk & van der Hart, 1991); that is, traumatic memories continue to be reexperienced (Hollander & Simeon, 2008).

The effects of exposure to a traumatic stressor include changes in an individual's external reality through injuries, pain, and losses and changes in his or her internal reality through altered beliefs of safety, sense of self-efficacy, inability to trust, and view of life as fair (McFarlane, 2010). Symptoms of PTSD are part of the normal reaction to trauma, and for the majority of individuals who have experienced a traumatic event, their symptoms diminish in severity within 1 month and thus do not meet the criteria for PTSD; however, some individuals continue to have severe symptoms for more than 1 month after the trauma, which meets the criteria for the diagnosis of PTSD. Others may not develop PTSD for months or even years after the traumatic event (Adams & Boscarino, 2006; Yehuda & Sarapas, 2010).

In PTSD, failure of natural recovery is thought to be due to failure of fear extinction following a trauma. Individuals continue to experience emotional and physiological reactions to stimuli resembling the original traumatic event, and they try to avoid exposure to situations that trigger anxiety reactions (Rizzo, Reger, Gahm, et al., 2010). The avoidance behaviors of PTSD are associated with limitations of functioning in many areas (Brunello, Davidson, Deahl, et al., 2001; Kessler, 2000). For example, work impairment for individuals with PTSD resulting from time lost is similar to that for individuals with depression. PTSD is also associated with a diminished quality of life (Zatzick, Jurkovich, Gentilello, et al., 2002).

Epidemiology

The lifetime prevalence of PTSD in the general population is 6.8% (Kessler, Berglund, Demler, et al., 2005). The rate of development of PTSD varies according to type of traumatic stressor (McFarlane & de Girolamo, 2006); for example, the rate is higher for life-threatening events than for those that have less effect on survival (Kessler et al., 1995). The rate of development of PTSD is also influenced by the amount and closeness of exposure to the traumatic event; the degree of physical injury experienced; the severity of threat to life; the loss of loved ones and property; and the type of traumatic event (Neria et al., 2007; Pynoos, Steinberg, & Goenjian, 2006). The highest rates of PTSD are found among survivors of rape, military combat, captivity, and internment, and among those handling dead bodies (Breslau, 2001). In countries where war and disease are endemic, the rate of PTSD ranges from 9.4% to 37% of the population (Bleich, Gelkopf, & Solomon, 2003). The rate of PTSD is even higher among refugees. Two decades after resettlement in the United States, 62% of refugees from Cambodia and Laos still met the criteria for PTSD (Marshall, Schell, Elliott, et al., 2005). Table 11-4 presents rates of PTSD following exposure to specific traumatic events. The development of PTSD is also influenced by the presence of risk factors and protective and modulating factors.

TABLE 11-4 DEVELOPMENT OF POST-TRAUMATIC STRESS DISORDER AFTER SPECIFIC TRAUMATIC EVENTS

Traumatic Event	Prevalence of Post-traumatic Stress Disorder in Victims	Source
Rape	Within 2 weeks after attack, 94% At 35 days after attack, 65% At 3 months after attack, 47%	Rothbaum, Foa, Riggs, et al., 1992
Vietnam War	65% among those with high exposure; 28% among those with median exposure	Snow, Stellman, Stellman, et al., 1988
Iraq and Afghanistan military operations	14% of military personnel previously deployed had PTSD; rate may be low due to reluctance to disclose psychiatric symptoms that might harm military career	Marx, 2009
Prisoner of war	50%–70%	Basoglu, Paker, Paker, et al., 1994; Bauer, Priebe, Haring, et al., 1993
Refugee of war	50%–63%	Carlson & Rosser-Hogan, 1991; Hauff & Vaglum, 1993: Momartin, Silove, Manicavasagar, et al., 2004
Displacement by war	53.4%	Thapa & Hauff, 2005
Cruise ship crash (children)	51.5%	Yule, Bolton, Udwin, et al., 2000
Earthquake	32%–60%	Altindag, Ozwin, & Sir, 2005; Bodvarsdottir & Elklit, 2004; Lima et al., 1989
Terrorist attack	20%–40%	North, Pfefferbaum, Tiois, et al., 2004; Pfefferbaum, Seale, McDonald, et al., 2000; Pynoos, Frederick, Nader, et al., 1987; Schlenger & Jernigan, 2003; Shalev, 1992; Shalev & Freedman, 2005; Weisaeth, 1993
Road traffic accident (children)	25%	Schafer, Barkmann, Riedesser, et al., 2006
Road traffic accident (adults)	18.7%	Shalev & Freedman, 2005
Firefighting	21%	Galea et al., 2005; McFarlane, 1988
Intimate partner abuse (men)	20%	Faravelli, Giugni, Salvatori, et al., 2004
Intimate partner abuse (women)	24%	Faravelli, Giugni, Salvatori, et al., 2004
Assault	20.9%	Breslau, Kessler, Chilcoat, et al., 1998a
Disaster/rescue work	16.7%	Fullerton, Ursano, & Wang, 2004
Tsunami (children)	14%–39%	Neuner, Schauer, Catani, et al., 2006

Risk Factors

Risk factors associated with the development of PTSD that are related to the individual, to military service, and to the traumatic event have been identified (Brewin, Andrews, & Valentine, 2000; Keane, Marx, & Sloan, 2009; Yehuda & Sarapas, 2010).

Risk Factors Related to the Individual

Risk factors that are related to the individual are presented in Box 11-2.

Risk Factors Related to Military Service

Risk factors associated with military service are related to the individual and to psychological and social risk factors.

Risk Factors Related to the Individual

Among veterans of the Vietnam War, higher risk for developing PTSD was found to be associated with family instability, severe punishment in childhood, conduct disorder in childhood, greater war zone exposure, presence of dissociation around the time of the trauma, postwar traumas, and depression before, during, or after the war. Lower risk was associated with higher level of education, older age at entry into the war, higher socioeconomic status, positive relationship with the father, more social support at homecoming, and more social support later (Schnurr, Lunney, & Sengupta, 2004).

Psychological and Social Risk Factors

Among those who have been exposed to the trauma of war, the severity of response may be increased by the presence of daily stressors, such as poverty, inadequate housing, health problems, unemployment, social isolation, and lack of security (Miller & Rasmusssen, 2009). Among veterans returning home, emotional support and instrumental assistance at homecoming decreased the lifetime risk of PTSD (Schnurr et al., 2004). However, the presence of PTSD symptoms may erode social support resources. For example, a study by King, Taft, King, et al. (2007) suggested that the presence of PTSD symptoms among veterans has a negative influence on their social support resources.

Risk Factors Related to the Traumatic Event

Trauma that threatens the individual's life, humiliates the individual, causes physical injury, destroys the individual's social support system, is assaultive or violent, or involves rape is associated with increased risk of the individual's developing PTSD (Breslau, Kessler, Chilcoat, et al., 1998a; Keane et al., 2009). The presence of dissociation at the time of the trauma or shortly after the trauma also increases the risk of developing PTSD (Keane et al.). After the traumatic event, lack of emotional support or a negative response from the individual's social support network increases risk of the individual's developing PTSD (Keane et al.), as does the lack of tangible support to avoid reexperiencing the trauma, such as the support and resources needed by women assaulted by partners or family members (Brewin et al., 2000).

Protective Factors and Modulating Factors

Factors that protect an individual from developing PTSD are presented in Table 11-5.

Factors that modulate the influence or buffer the effects of traumatic events include culture, religion, and social support. Culture—through its values, traditions, and beliefs—influences how individuals evaluate the meaning of a traumatic event, e.g., whether it was a chance event, fate, or

BOX 11-2 Risk Factors for Development of Post-traumatic Stress Disorder Related to the Individual

Biological Risk Factors

- Female gender (Breslau, Chilcoat, Kessler, et al., 1999a; Keane et al., 2009; Seedat, Stein, & Carey, 2005)
- Genetic vulnerability to stress-related psychopathology, e.g., arousal, reexperiencing, and avoidance (True, Rice, Eisen, et al., 1993)
- Parental PTSD (3 times higher rate of PTSD in offspring [Yehuda, Halligan, & Bierer, 2001])
- Alterations in stress response systems related to exposure to stress during early development (Keane et al., 2009; Pine, 2003)
- Biological abnormalities: reduced hippocampal volume; increased startle response; abnormalities of serotonin transporter gene; decreased capacity to mobilize and sustain high levels of neuropeptide Y; and alterations (low levels) of cortisol (Friedman & Karam, 2009; Miller et al., 2009; Yehuda & Sarapas, 2010). It is thought that these biological risk factors may be due to abnormalities of prenatal brain development that impair the individual's response to traumatic stressors.

Psychological Risk Factors

- Early separation from parents (Breslau, Davis, Andreski, et al., 1991)
- Childhood abuse or neglect (Hetzel & McCanne, 2005; Koenen, Moffitt, Poulton, et al., 2007; Thompson, Crosby, Wonderlich, et al., 2003)
- Preexisting conduct disorder, anxiety or mood disorders, personality disorders, or alcohol- or drug-related problems (McFarlane, 2002)
- Negative self-appraisal (shame, guilt, or sense of incompetence)
- Presence of catastrophic thinking (thinking that events are much worse than the reality and that the outcome will be disastrous) (Bryant & Guthrie, 2005)

Social Risk Factors

- Multiple exposures to violence, traumas, and adversities in life (Keane et al., 2009; Kilpatrick, Ruggiero, Acierno, et al., 2003)
- Lower educational and economic status (Rhoads et al., 2007)
- Limited social support (Bennett et al., 2007)

TABLE 11-5 **FACTORS PROTECTIVE AGAINST THE DEVELOPMENT OF POST-TRAUMATIC STRESS DISORDER**

Protective Factor	How It Protects
Affiliation: sense of emotional attachment to family, friends, or others	Protects against being exposed to traumatic events (van der Kolk et al., 2006a). After exposure to traumatic event, affiliation helps in integrating effects of the experience.
Secure pattern of attachment	Individuals with a secure pattern of attachment exhibit fewer symptoms of PTSD following exposure to a traumatic event (Fraley, Fazzari, Bonanno, et al., 2006; Mikulincer, Florian, & Weller, 1993).
Basic needs met	In times of stress, individuals are sustained by having basic needs met (Hansell, 1976).
Financial support	Provides access to resources, services, and health care (Rhoads et al., 2007).
Social support (emotional)	Protects against the effects of exposure to traumatic events by validating the experience; e.g., support after a natural disaster (Rhoads et al., 2007; Ursano, Grieger, & McCarroll, 2006b).
Social support (tangible)	Tangible support (safe housing, child care, transportation, food, clothing, income) reduces PTSD among women who have experienced trauma (Glass et al., 2007).
Religion	Provides a purpose to life. Protects individuals from being overwhelmed by trauma by placing event in context of human suffering over time (McFarlane & van der Kolk, 2006).
Preparation for traumatic event	Protects by lessening fear of unknown, creating an expectation that the individual will cope, and fostering a sense of mastery that is transferable to other traumatic events (Ursano et al., 2007).
Mastery of prior traumatic events	Builds adaptive coping skills and resilience (Rhoads et al., 2007).

punishment (deVries, 2006; Mezzich, Caracci, Fabrega, et al., 2009). Culture provides a sanctioned approach for how stressful occasions, such as death and illnesses, will be managed and how help will be provided and accepted. The culture's rituals during losses and death regulate emotions and behaviors within time frames and promote the use of mature defense mechanisms and development of resilience. However, the buffering effect of culture may not be sufficient to blunt the shock of a severe traumatic event (deVries; Hobfoll & deVries, 1995).

Religion and spirituality often help people to deal with traumatic events (Ursano & Kilgore, 2011). For example, it has been found that individuals who had experienced trauma and who were strongly committed to their religious beliefs before the trauma were able to overcome the trauma and move on (Shaw, Joseph, & Linley, 2005). Other researchers have not found that religion prevents PTSD (Connor, Davidson, & Lee, 2003). However, to reflect the finding that religion does reduce symptoms of PTSD among individuals who are *committed* to their religion, Thielman (2011) suggested that revision of the *DSM-IV-TR* should include the following: "There is evidence that, for religiously committed patients, religious and spiritual coping strategies may promote reduction of posttraumatic stress symptoms and promote personal growth" (p. 110).

Social support has a preventive effect on the development of PTSD and a buffering effect in response to stressors. High levels of perceived social support are associated with decreased exposure to traumatic events and with reduced rates of anxiety and depression (Moak & Agrawal, 2009).

Etiology

Exposure to an extreme traumatic stressor is accepted as the cause of the development of PTSD (Keane et al., 2009; Ursano & Kilgore, 2011). Extreme traumatic stressors include but are not limited to the following: "military combat, violent personal assault (sexual assault, physical attack, robbery, mugging), being kidnapped, being taken hostage, terrorist attack, torture, incarceration as a prisoner of war or in a concentration camp, natural or manmade disasters, severe automobile accidents, or being diagnosed with a life-threatening illness" (American Psychiatric Association, 2000, pp. 463-464). An extreme traumatic stressor can also be witnessing such events. Children and adolescents experience the same traumatic events as adults (Pynoos, 1996; Pynoos et al., 2007). In addition, for children, exposure to photographs or media presentations of atrocities or of the mutilated bodies of family members or friends is a secondary risk for development of PTSD (Pynoos et al., 2006).

Biological Basis

Humans have the flexibility to integrate new information with old information, to organize that reprocessed information, to apply logic, to evaluate consequences, and to choose how to respond to a stimulus (LeDoux, 2002). After exposure to a traumatic event, most individuals demonstrate flexibility by engaging in *extinction learning;* that is, they link the conditioned stimuli—such as memories of the traumatic event—to safe consequences—such as the realization that the event occurred in the past and is not happening at the current moment—and in that way they inhibit the fear response (van der Kolk, 2006a). Extinction of fear or inhibition of fear does not mean erasing the fear; rather, a fear memory trace remains and can be reactivated (Fischer & Tsai, 2010).

Severe traumas may prevent individuals from processing and integrating the event, which does not allow them to cope with the trauma. Thus, memories of the trauma do not become part of their life story; instead, the trauma exists as isolated sensory, emotional, or motor imprints (van der

Kolk, 2004). The imprints of the trauma that remain may intrude on an individual's life as intense emotional reactions, aggressive behavior, or physical symptoms in response to reminders of the original trauma. The emotional reactions stay as fresh as they were during the traumatic event. The emotional reactions and the individual's responses to protect against those reactions are evidenced as PTSD symptoms.

In response to trauma, biological changes occur in brain structures, brain functioning, and neurotransmitter systems (Bremner, 2003; Bremmer & Charney, 2010). Although these biological changes usually return to the normal state after exposure to the stressor ends or the individual has achieved an adaptation to the stressor, in PTSD, biological changes last long after exposure to the stressor ends (see Chapter 9).

Abnormalities of Brain Structures and Functioning

Patients with PTSD may experience changes in structure and functioning of the thalamus, amygdala, hippocampus, anterior cingulate cortex, prefrontal cortex, and brain hemispheres (Rauch, Shin, Segal, et al., 2003; Weiss, 2007).

Thalamus

The thalamus, which transmits fearful stimuli—such as fearful memories, sights, and sounds—to the amygdala and to the frontal cortex, is enlarged and more active in those patients with PTSD who were born with a serotonin transporter gene deficiency. This serotonin transporter gene deficiency is thought to be a pre-existing vulnerability for the development of PTSD (Young, Bonkale, Holcomb, et al., 2008).

Amygdala

The amygdala is involved in evaluation of threatening stimuli, in fear conditioning, and in the memory of stressful events (Debiec & LeDoux, 2009; Shin, Rauch, & Pitman, 2006). There is some controversy about whether there are structural abnormalities in the amygdala in patients with PTSD, with some researchers reporting that patients with PTSD have a small amygdala (Woon & Hedges, 2009) and some reporting enlargement of the amygdala (Villarreal & King, 2001). It is known that the amygdala is overactive in response to fearful stimuli in patients with PTSD (Woon & Hedges) and that hyper-responsiveness of the amygdala results in an increase in signals sent to the brainstem, subcortical motor structures, and endocrine system and results in the symptoms that patients with PTSD experience: increased startle response, irritability, angry outbursts, and hypervigilance (Nutt & Malizia, 2004; Rauch & Drevets, 2009).

Hippocampus

The hippocampus—which is involved in forming conscious memories of facts and details, connecting those facts and details with other autobiographical information, and putting a time and place on an event (Nutt & Malizia, 2004)—is often smaller and less active in individuals who have experienced chronic traumatic events (Teicher, Tomoda, & Andersen, 2006; Villarreal & King, 2001; Woon & Hedges, 2009). Patients with PTSD and patients who experienced childhood abuse have been found to have deficits of hippocampal functioning that is believed to be linked to the smaller size of the hippocampus that is seen in both groups (DeBellis & Kuchibhatla, 2006; van der Kolk, 2006c). Nutt and Malizia suggested that a smaller or damaged hippocampus is less able to control an overactive amygdala.

However, not all research supports the finding of smaller hippocampi in individuals who have experienced severe trauma. For example, survivors of the Holocaust were not found to have smaller hippocampal volumes than nonexposed subjects (Golier, Yehuda, DeSanti, et al., 2005). Based on the finding that smaller hippocampal volume is present in combat veterans with PTSD and also in their noncombat-exposed identical twins, other researchers believe that smaller hippocampal volume is a pre-existing biological risk factor and thus not a result of exposure to a traumatic event (Pitman, Gilbertson, Gurvits, et al., 2006): that is, the pre-existing smaller size of the hippocampi of patients with PTSD increased their vulnerability to develop PTSD after exposure to a traumatic event.

Anterior Cingulate Cortex

The anterior cingulate cortex helps to integrate emotional and cognitive aspects of experiences, inhibits amygdala activity, and plays a role in extinguishing fear. It has been found to be smaller in patients with abuse-related PTSD (Kitayama, Quinn, & Bremner, 2006) and in combat veterans with PTSD (Woodward, Kaloupek, Streeter, et al., 2006).

Prefrontal Cortex

The prefrontal cortex—which processes information in order to compare previous experiences with the present experience, to plan actions, and to make decisions (van der Kolk, 2004)—is smaller in sexually abused children with PTSD (Bremner, 2002) and in children who have been deprived of normal socioemotional and cognitive stimulation (Perry, 2002). Imaging of the brains of patients with PTSD has shown that there is decreased activation of the medial prefrontal cortex that directly influences emotional arousal (Rauch & Drevets, 2009).

Neuroimaging of the brains of patients with PTSD showed that when patients were exposed to reminders of the traumatic event, there was increased cerebral blood flow in the right medial orbitofrontal cortex, insula, and amygdala and decreased blood flow in the left anterior prefrontal cortex, specifically in Broca's area, which is the area of the brain involved in communicating what one is thinking and feeling (i.e., Broca's area is involved in translating experiences into language—the ability to talk about the experience) (van der Kolk, 2006a). Van der Kolk wrote, "when people are reminded of a personal trauma, they activate brain regions that support intense emotions, while decreasing activity of brain structures involved in the inhibition of emotions and the translation of experience into communicable language"

(p. 278). They often experience a "speechless terror" (van der Kolk, 2006b, p. 234). Although the prefrontal cortex has the capacity to override automatic responses by inhibiting, organizing, and moderating them, when individuals who have been exposed to traumatic events are under stress, the higher brain areas involved in executive functioning—planning, anticipating consequences, inhibiting inappropriate responses—become less active.

Brain Hemispheres

Following exposure to a traumatic event, right hemispheric activity increases in areas that are associated with emotional appraisal, and left hemispheric activity decreases in areas that are involved in speech, cognitive analysis of traumatic events, and interpretation of the meaning of an experience. (See Chapter 2 for more information about lateralization of brain activities.) People who have been traumatized illustrate this altered brain functioning when they have difficulty putting the traumatic experience into words. They have difficulty verbalizing the event because the memory of the event exists as fragments of memories and as sensations and emotions related to the trauma rather than as a story with a distinguishable time frame.

In brief, the higher levels of brain functioning control the lower levels, but if the higher levels are not able to function, then the lower levels (the subcortical levels) control responses. For example, if the prefrontal cortex fails to dampen amygdala arousal, the lack of regulation may result in hypervigilance to trauma-related cues, increased startle response, flashbacks, intrusive memories, and misinterpretation of neutral stimuli (Frewen & Lanius, 2006). Knowledge of the pre-existing deficits of certain brain structures among individuals who develop PTSD and the effect that exposure to severe trauma has on the structures and functioning of the brain enables psychiatric advanced practice nurses to understand the symptoms of PTSD.

Abnormalities of Brain Neurochemistry

Traumatic events are processed by certain brain structures using neurotransmitter systems (Amiel, Mathew, Garakani, et al., 2009). It is believed that registering *factual* memories involves the neurotransmitters glutamate and gamma-aminobutyric acid (GABA), while registering *emotional* memories involves the neurotransmitters serotonin and norepinephrine in conjunction with activity of the amygdala (Nutt, 2000).

In response to exposure to a terrifying traumatic event, norepinephrine—which is involved in arousal, anxiety, and hypervigilance—is released into the brain cortex. Levels of norepinephrine are increased in patients with PTSD, and overaction of norepinephrine receptors in the prefrontal cortex is believed to be associated with the symptoms of hypervigilance, flashbacks, nightmares, and dissociation and to play a role in overconsolidation of trauma-related memories (Olszewski & Varrasse, 2005).

Norepinephrine is modulated by a neuropeptide, neuropeptide Y. Neuropeptide Y functions as an anxiolytic to reduce anxiety, as a neuroprotective agent in the hippocampus to nourish neurons and prevent cell death, and as a modulator of norepinephrine. In PTSD, levels of neuropeptide Y are reduced (Yehuda & Sarapas, 2010). Interestingly, among soldiers in very stressful survival training, those who were better able to mobilize neuropeptide Y coped better and performed better than those with low levels of neuropeptide Y (Morgan, Wang, Southwick, et al., 2000).

Levels of serotonin, which modulates stress and memory, are low in patients with PTSD. Low levels of serotonin are associated with some of the symptoms of PTSD, including anxiety, ruminations, irritability, impulsiveness, aggression, and suicidality (Olszewski & Varrasse, 2005).

Levels of cortisol are reduced in patients with PTSD, and there are alterations of the circadian rhythmicity of cortisol levels (Yehuda, 2009). Although the reasons are not well understood, it may be that cortisol-related alterations in PTSD reflect pre-existing biological vulnerability factors that increase an individual's likelihood of developing PTSD following trauma exposure (Yehuda & Sarapas, 2010).

Thus, alterations of brain structures and functioning–which may have been previously compromised by genetic influences, abnormalities of brain development, exposure to traumas, or abuse and alterations of neurotransmitter systems underlie the multiple physical, psychological, and social problems that are experienced by patients with PTSD (Nutt, 2000; Olszewski & Varrasse, 2005).

Clinical Presentation in Adults

According to the *DSM-IV-TR* criteria for PTSD, the individual must have been exposed to a traumatic event that involved serious injury, threat to life, or threat to the physical integrity of self or others, and the individual must have experienced intense fear, helplessness, or horror (American Psychiatric Association, 2000, p. 467). In addition, the individual must have persistent symptoms of reexperiencing, avoidance, and arousal; the symptoms must have been present for more than 1 month; and the symptoms must cause significant distress or impairment of functioning. The diagnosis of PTSD can be specified as *acute* if the symptoms have been present for less than 3 months; *chronic* if the symptoms have been present for 3 months or more; and *with delayed onset* if the onset of symptoms is 6 months or more after the traumatic event.

The key feature of PTSD in adults is an abnormality of memory, in which the traumatic experience is not integrated with other memories, experiences, perceptions, interpretations, and time frames. The *DSM-IV-TR* diagnostic criteria for PTSD propose that an overwhelming experience leaves a permanent effect on the individual's memory, and that the effect is responsible for the individual's impairment of autonomic activation and self-regulatory systems.

Abnormality of Memory

Abnormality of memory is manifested in the three distinguishing symptoms of PTSD (McFarlane, 2010):

- Reexperiencing of the trauma through intrusive symptoms, which include disturbing visual or sensory memories, dreams, nightmares, flashbacks, and recurrent, intense distress. These symptoms may occur spontaneously or in response to triggers (Black & Andreasen, 2011).
- Avoidance or numbing symptoms, which include avoiding thoughts, feelings, people, places, and activities that may trigger symptoms; feeling detached from others; loss of interest in usual activities; and inability to feel emotions such as intimacy, tenderness, or sexual interest (Hollander & Simeon, 2011; McFarlane, 2010).
- Arousal symptoms, which include irritability, angry outbursts, hypervigilance, increased startle response, and problems with memory, concentration, and sleeping (Hollander & Simeon, 2011; Olszewski & Varrasse, 2005).

Autonomic Activation System Impairment

Adult patients with PTSD often show signs of autonomic activation. Autonomic activation is a "hard-wired" response to stress that includes shortness of breath, tremulousness, racing heart, sweaty palms or cold sweats, dizziness, faintness, nausea, numbness or tingling, chills or hot flashes, dry mouth, and difficulty controlling bladder and bowel (Bracha, Williams, Haynes, et al., 2004, pp. 3-4).

Self-Regulatory System Impairment

The achievement of secure attachment patterns in childhood provides a basis for the development of a self-regulatory system that modulates arousal in response to stressors. This self-regulatory system functions later in life to manage responses to stressful situations and traumatic events. However, exposure to events that exceeded a child's capacity to adapt, such as maltreatment, may damage his or her self-regulatory system's ability to return to a normal state once the stressor has ended. As adults, individuals with damaged self-regulatory systems may have problems with the following:

- Regulation of anger, anxiety, and sexual impulses (Pitman, Orr, & Shalev, 1993; van der Kolk, Roth, Pelcovitz, et al., 1993)
- Focusing attention and impulse control when aroused (van der Kolk, 2006c)
- Uncontrollable feelings of rage, anger, and/or sadness (van der Kolk, 2006c)
- Relationships with others, such as distrust and social isolation (van der Kolk, 2006c)
- Self-destructive behaviors, such as self-cutting, suicide attempts, eating disorders, substance abuse, and other self-injurious behaviors (van der Kolk, 2006c)
- Dissociation, such as "spacing out" (van der Kolk, 2006c, p. 193)
- Identifying emotions or putting them into words, and using words to tell about the traumatic event (van der Kolk, 2006c)
- Self-identity, self efficacy, and worthiness (Herman, 1992; Verfaellie & Vasterling, 2009)
- Functioning following the trauma (van der Kolk, 2006c)

Subjective Feelings: Shame, Anger, Revenge, and Timelessness

Patients with PTSD may describe feelings of shame, anger, and revenge. The feelings of shame are related to being unable to protect themselves or to act in a way that fits with their expectations of themselves (Pynoos et al., 2006; van der Kolk, McFarlane, & van der Hart, 2002). Both anger and revenge include the perception that a traumatic event has harmed them, that the traumatic event was without justification, and that the event was due to the actions of another individual (Orth, Montada, & Maercker, 2006). However, revenge includes the quality of retaliation, e.g., punishing the perpetrator (Orth et al.). Revenge has been reported to occur in 41% to 46% of victims of crime (Cardozo, Kaiser, Gotway, et al., 2003). The presence of symptoms of anger and revenge and of problems forgiving self or others is associated with greater severity of PTSD symptoms (Connor et al., 2003; Witvliet, 2001; Witvliet, Phipps, Feldman, et al., 2004), and the symptoms of anger and revenge appear to increase over time, with the feelings of revenge becoming more maladaptive over time (Orth et al.).

Patients with PTSD tend to see similarities between present situations and previous trauma; in other words, their PTSD symptoms become timeless, with no beginning and no end. Patients cannot get over the past and thus they cannot take part in the present or plan for the future. They use maladaptive behaviors to avoid triggers, such as avoiding people, using drugs and alcohol, and emotionally withdrawing from friends. They may say that lack of energy, lack of interest, and impaired concentration limit their ability to readjust their lives.

Symptoms of Other Disorders

Patients may present with symptoms of other psychiatric disorders, such as depression, drug and alcohol abuse, and other anxiety disorders. They may also experience exacerbation of chronic physical illnesses (van der Kolk, 2004, p. 321). Case Study 11-1 describes a patient with PTSD, treatment interventions including virtual reality exposure, and outcomes.

Clinical Presentation in Children and Adolescents

The *DSM-IV-TR* criteria are the same for children and adolescents as for adults, with the exception that the response to the traumatic event may be expressed by disorganized or agitated behavior instead of intense fear, helplessness, or horror (American Psychiatric Association, 2000, p. 467).

CASE STUDY 11-1

A Patient With PTSD, Treatment Interventions Including Virtual Reality Exposure, and Outcomes

Mary is a 20-year-old college student who presented to the university counseling service with fear of driving on busy freeways, especially at night. The problem emerged 12 months ago after she was involved in a five-car accident while returning late from college. Another driver who swerved from the outside lane into her lane caused the accident. She was sideswiped by the car, and the resulting accident involved three other cars. No one was killed. However, one other driver had serious injuries. Mary had to be cut from her car, which took over 5 hours. Throughout the incident, Mary remembers thinking she was going to die. Before this, Mary had not experienced any significant anxiety and had been able to drive in any conditions. Since the accident, Mary has stopped driving; has become anxious, leading to avoidance of many situations; experiences poor sleep due to nightmares; is easily startled; and feels depressed. Mary's college work and social life are severely affected, and she is in danger of failing. She has been to her family practitioner, who has prescribed 50 mg of sertraline daily. Mary often forgets to take her medicine and believes it does not really help.

The counseling service referred Mary to the community psychiatric/mental health nurse, who helps Mary recognize that her fear of driving is a symptom of post-traumatic stress disorder. The nurse has suggested several approaches to Mary's problems. First, they work to improve sleep problems using a standard sleep hygiene approach. Second, she tackles her nondriving-related avoidances, such as agreeing to meet friends and go shopping. Finally, the nurse helped Mary to see the benefits and disadvantages of her medication. This discussion led to Mary's agreeing to take her medication regularly to see if it would help. After 2 months of weekly sessions, Mary began to show some general improvement. However, her fear of driving remained and she continued to struggle at college.

One week, Mary told the nurse about a TV program showing a virtual reality (VR) driving simulator treatment for people who have been in car accidents. The nurse stated she knew of this and would find out if it were available. The nurse was able to arrange a VR demonstration in the next session. After seeing how the simulator could help, Mary agreed to use it. Both the nurse and Mary were fitted with VR glasses, and different driving experiences were introduced. At first, Mary practiced quiet daytime driving and progressed to busy freeway night driving. Mary's anxiety about driving reduced quickly over 3 weeks. However, she still had not returned to driving. The nurse suggested that Mary repeat the VR exercises but in her own car. This involved graded live exposure. At first, Mary drove with friends and family in quiet times, moving to driving with others at night and then finally on her own at night. After 6 weeks, she had completely returned to driving, her college and social life was back to normal, and she experienced no anxiety.

Source: Barry Tolchard, PhD, MSC, RNM, RNLD

Children experience the same symptoms as adults, and the level of traumatic exposure is associated with the severity and course of their post-traumatic symptoms (Pynoos et al., 2006). Chronically abused children are at increased risk of developing PTSD, with about one-third of victims of childhood abuse (neglect, physical abuse, and sexual abuse) developing PTSD in their lifetime (Widom, 1999). Children who have been traumatized may have symptoms that reflect abnormal functioning of the brainstem, such as hypervigilance; increased muscle tone; low-grade temperature elevation; hypertension; increased startle response; and sleep disturbances (Perry & Pate, 1994).

Similar to adults with PTSD, children with PTSD may dissociate, which may be an adaptive or protective response for them in some situations but is maladaptive as a response for all new or challenging situations. Unlike adults, children with PTSD may experience "time skew" and "omen formation." Time skew refers to a child's putting the events associated with the trauma in incorrect time sequences. Omen formation refers to the child's belief that there were warning signs before the trauma but that the child was not alert enough to recognize the warning signs, and therefore the child should be more alert to warning signs to prevent another traumatic event from occurring (Hamblen & Barnett, 2009). Children with PTSD symptoms may avoid talking about the traumatic experience, have problems with schoolwork, be less interested in activities that they used to enjoy, and feel estranged from others (Dogan-Ates, 2010).

In adolescents with PTSD, symptoms resemble those of adults; however, adolescents are likely to engage in traumatic reenactment and to exhibit impulsive and aggressive behaviors (Hamblen & Barnett, 2009). Adolescents with PTSD frequently have comorbid major depressive disorder, panic disorder, generalized anxiety disorder, and substance use problems. Adolescents expect that they will have a short life span with negative outcomes. Their attitudes about career goals and marriage change and they do not make plans for their future (Dogan-Ates, 2010).

Subsyndromal Presentation of Post-traumatic Stress Disorder

Adults, adolescents, and children who have experienced serious illnesses, severe stressors such as abuse or devastating losses, or traumatic events often have subsyndromal symptoms of PTSD, which may not meet the criteria required for a diagnosis of PTSD. However, the PTSD symptoms often cause them great distress and they seek treatment for their distress.

The *DSM-IV-TR* (American Psychiatric Association, 2000) does not have a subcategory of *subsyndromal PTSD*, which is a term used by clinicians who often must diagnose and manage the care of patients seeking treatment who have some symptoms of PTSD but who do not meet the full criteria for the diagnosis of PTSD. Usually, these patients do not meet the criteria because of a lack of avoidance symptoms. For example, subsyndromal PTSD is believed to occur in 50% of patients with cancer, but they do not experience avoidance symptoms (Gurevich, Devins, & Rodin, 2002).

Subsyndromal PTSD is associated with disability that may be as severe as that of PTSD, including problems at home and at work, increased risk of binge drinking, a high rate of use of mental health services and increased risk of suicidal ideation (Shelby, Golden-Kreutz, & Andersen, 2008). McFarlane (2010) and others have stated that inclusion of subsyndromal PTSD as a subcategory of PTSD in the *DSM-V* would provide a diagnosis for patients with fluctuating symptoms of PTSD that meet the criteria at one time but not at another. Furthermore, because the majority of patients with *delayed-onset PTSD*, which has been found to occur in approximately one-fourth of patients with PTSD (Smid, Mooren, van der Mast, et al., 2009), has subsyndromal symptoms of PTSD within the first 6 months of the traumatic event (Carty, O'Donnell, & Creamer, 2006; Danielson, Macdonald, Amstadter, et al., 2010), adding subsyndromal PTSD to the next version of the *DSM* would help in defining interventions for these patients.

Comorbidity

Comorbidities of PTSD include medical, neurological, and psychiatric disorders.

Comorbid Medical Disorders

Patients with PTSD have higher rates of comorbid physical illnesses than patients with other anxiety disorders (Sareen, Cox, Clara, et al., 2005; Weisberg, Bruce, Machan, et al., 2002). In comparison to individuals who do not have PTSD, patients with PTSD have a two to three times greater risk for developing angina pectoris, heart failure, bronchitis, asthma, liver disease, peripheral arterial disease, and alcohol use disorder (Spitzer, Barnow, Volzke et al., 2009). Other frequent comorbid medical illnesses include metabolic/autoimmune conditions—such as diabetes, thyroid disease, and lupus—and joint conditions such as arthritis.

Comorbid Neurological Disorders

Frequently co-occurring neurological disorders include epilepsy, multiple sclerosis, and stroke (Boscarino, 2004; Sareen et al., 2005). Two neurological disorders, tension-type headaches and migraine headaches, have been found to be comorbid among 40% of veterans of Operation Iraqi Freedom and Operation Enduring Freedom who have PTSD (Afari, Harder, Madra, et al., 2009).

Comorbid Psychiatric Disorders

Eighty percent of individuals with PTSD have at least one comorbid psychiatric disorder (Kessler et al., 1995; Zhang & Davidson, 2010). Most frequently co-occurring psychiatric disorders are panic disorder, social phobia, simple phobia, generalized anxiety disorder, dysthymia, major depression, and substance-related disorders (McFarlane, 2010). In addition, approximately half of patients with PTSD have traits of personality disorders (Horowitz, 2003).

Medical Disorders and Comorbid Post-traumatic Stress Disorder

Patients with existing medical disorders may also have comorbid PTSD. Shemesh and Stuber (2006) identified the rate of PTSD in medically ill patients. To summarize their findings:

- Among patients with breast cancer, the rate of PTSD was 35%.
- Among patients with myocardial infarction, the rate of PTSD was 10% to 20%.
- Among patients with HIV infection, the rate of PTSD was 30% or more.
- Among patients with diabetes, there were self-reports of PTSD.
- Among children with cancer, the rate of PTSD was 35%.
- Among child recipients of solid organ transplants, such as heart and kidneys, the rate of PTSD was 16%.
- Among children with cardiac surgery, the rate of PTSD was 12%.

Patients with PTSD who have comorbid medical and psychiatric disorders tend to have more severe PTSD symptoms, are more likely to develop chronic PTSD, and require more support to manage daily living activities (Kluft, Bloom, & Kinzie, 2000).

Overall, patients with PTSD are high users of medical services but have poor health outcomes (Boscarino, 2004). They also have an increased risk for suicide (Kessler, 2000). For example, in comparison to individuals who have been exposed to traumatic events but do not develop PTSD, those who do develop PTSD are at a three times greater risk for attempted suicide (Wilcox, Storr, & Breslau, 2009).

Differential Diagnosis

The etiology and symptoms of PTSD overlap with symptoms of other psychiatric disorders. Severity of the stressor, duration of response, and type and level of symptoms differentiate other psychiatric disorders from PTSD. However, PTSD often co-occurs with other psychiatric disorders such as major depressive disorder, panic disorder, generalized anxiety disorder, and alcohol and substance use (Black & Andreasen, 2011; First & Tasman, 2004). The challenge for the psychiatric advanced practice nurse is to determine which psychiatric disorder is the primary disorder. Table 11-6 provides the differential diagnosis for PTSD.

TABLE 11-6 **DIFFERENTIAL DIAGNOSIS OF POST-TRAUMATIC STRESS DISORDER**

Other Disorder	Differentiating Characteristics of Other Disorder
Adjustment disorder	Characterized by a stressor of any level of severity and does not have a specific response pattern.
Other psychiatric disorders that may occur after exposure to an extreme stressor	Brief psychotic disorder. It has one or more symptoms of delusion, hallucinations, disorganized speech, disorganized or catatonic behavior. The symptom must last at least 1 day but less than 1 month.
Major depressive disorder	Similar symptoms of reduced interest, numbing, withdrawal from others, impaired concentration, insomnia, and irritability, but unlike PTSD does not have reexperiencing symptoms.
Acute stress disorder	Response is within 4 weeks of the stressor. If symptoms persist beyond 4 weeks and meet the criteria for PTSD, the diagnosis is changed to PTSD (Davidson & Connor, 2004). Dissociative symptoms are present in acute stress disorder.
Obsessive-compulsive disorder with intrusive thoughts	Symptoms are not related to an extreme stressor. Intrusive thoughts are recognized as inappropriate.
Malingering	Characterized by feigning of symptoms and should be ruled out when legal, financial, and other benefits are involved.
Generalized anxiety disorder	There is an overlap with symptoms of hyperarousal—being on edge, have poor concentration, irritability, and sleep disturbance—but PTSD requires the presence of additional symptoms of hypervigilance or exaggerated startle reflex, and the worry of PTSD is related to reexperiencing the trauma.
Panic disorder	Panic attacks are not related to the traumatic event, but occur unexpectedly.
Specific phobias	May follow a traumatic event but do not have intrusive or hyperarousal symptoms.
Complicated grief	Feelings of dejection, loss of interest, and reduction of normal activities. Trouble accepting the loss; anger or bitterness about the loss; emotional numbness; trouble feeling connected to others; and yearning for lost person and feeling as if there is no future without the lost person (Gray, Litz, & Papa, 2006). Symptoms of marked functional impairment, worthlessness, suicidal ideation, psychomotor retardation, or psychotic symptoms (Klein, Shankman, & McFarland, 2006).

Sources: Black & Andreasen, 2011, First et al., 2002; First & Tasman, 2004.

Treatment

One of the first steps in treatment is to help the patient to develop a sense of trust, safety, and separation from the traumatic event (Black & Andreasen, 2011, p. 201). The next step is a comprehensive evaluation

The overall goal of treatment for PTSD is to enable patients to regain control of their emotional responses and to place the trauma in the larger perspective of their lives as an event that happened at a certain time and that is unlikely to recur. The terrifying experience must become part of them. As stated in the Preface of *Traumatic Stress*, "the trauma must come to be personalized as an integrated aspect of one's personal history" (van der Kolk, McFarlane, & Weisaeth, 2006b, p. XVI). Specific goals of treatment for PTSD are to

- Reduce the core symptoms of reexperiencing, avoidance, numbing, and hyperarousal
- Reduce comorbidities and disability
- Reduce risk for suicide
- Improve coping with stressors of life
- Build resilience
- Improve functioning and quality of life
- Protect against relapse (Ursano et al., 2006a; Zhang & Davidson, 2010)

Because patients with PTSD frequently have co-occurring medical illnesses, depression, and substance-related disorders and impairment of interpersonal, social, and vocational functioning, a biopsychosocial approach to treatment that includes psychotherapy, pharmacotherapy, and psychosocial interventions is required (Cooper, Carty, & Creamer, 2005).

Assessment

The goal of assessment is to gain an understanding of the problems that the patient is experiencing, identify groups of symptoms that are responsive to treatment, and begin to consider treatment approaches for the patient's problems. Assessment includes a comprehensive psychiatric evaluation; laboratory testing, which is often used to rule out medical causes of psychiatric symptoms; and the use of assessment instruments or screening instruments. Data obtained with screening instruments provide a baseline measure of the presence and severity of psychiatric symptoms that can be used to monitor response to treatment.

According to Brewin (2005), brief screening instruments perform as well as longer and more complex measures in screening for PTSD. Some instruments measure specific symptoms of PTSD. For example, *The Impact of Event Scale* (Horowitz, Wilner, & Alvarez, 1979) can be used to monitor intrusive and avoidance symptoms; *The Positive States of Mind Scale* (Adler, Horowitz, Garcia, et al., 1998) can be used to assess functioning, such as being able to focus attention on a task; and *The Self-Regard Questionnaire* (Horowitz, Sonneborn, Sugahara, et al., 1995) can be used to assess sense of self-identity. Additional instruments that psychiatric advanced practice nurses may use in assessing patients for PTSD can be found in Box 11-3.

BOX 11-3 Instruments for Screening for Post-traumatic Stress Disorder

- *Beck Depression Inventory (BDI)* (Beck, Ward, Mendelson, et al., 1961)
- *Clinician Administered PTSD Scale (CAPS)* (Blake, Weathers, Nagy, et al., 1990). This scale is designed to assess the 17 symptoms of PTSD listed in the *DSM-IV-TR* (Blake, Weathers, Nagy, et al., 1995).
- *Coping Styles Questionnaire (CSQ)* (Roger, Jarvis, & Najarian, 1993). The CSQ is a trait-oriented measure in which preferences for particular coping styles are regarded as constitutive of the individual's personality. It measures four coping styles: emotional, avoidant, detached, and rational.
- *Core Bereavement Items (CBI)* (Burnett, Middleton, Raphael, et al., 1997). This 17-item scale assesses symptoms of complicated grief.
- *Harvard Trauma Questionnaire (HTQ)*. An instrument designed to measure psychiatric status of Cambodian refugees in the United States. Also used to measure trauma related to torture, escape, migration, and family separations (Mollica, Caspi-Yavin, Bollini, et al., 1992).
- *Impact of Event Scale (IES)* (Horowitz et al., 1979)
- *Medical Traumatic Stress Toolkit for Health Care Providers* (National Child Traumatic Stress Network: www.NCTSnet@org)
- *Perceived Stress Scale (PSS)* (Cohen et al., 1983)
- *PTSD Checklist* (Weathers, Litz, Huska, et al., 1994)
- *PTSD Inventory* (Solomon et al., 1994)
- *Recent Life Changes Questionnaire (RLCQ)* (Rahe, 2000)
- *Risk of Suicide Questionnaire (RSQ)* (Horowitz, Wang, Koocher, et al., 2001)
- *Short Screening Scale for DSM-IV Posttraumatic Stress Disorder* (Breslau et al., 1998b)
- *STRS (shortness of breath, tremulousness, racing heart, and sweating)* (Bracha et al., 2004)
- *Trauma Symptoms Checklist (TSC)* (Briere & Runtz, 1989)

Psychotherapy

People with PTSD become "stuck" on the trauma (van der Kolk, McFarlane, & van der Hart, 2006a, p. 419). They continue to reexperience the thoughts, feelings, actions, or images of the traumatic event. Stimuli resembling the event may cause anxiety, memories, or flashbacks. Individuals often avoid situations that may produce the same anxiety, but although they may avoid the anxiety, the link of fear to the stimulus of the original traumatic event remains (Amiel et al., 2009). The avoidance strategies that these individuals use to avoid anxiety often interfere with their social life, their ability to work, and their relationships with others (Basco, Glickman, Weatherford, et al., 2000). In brief, they use their time and energy to avoid the distress associated with thinking or talking about the trauma. In contrast to the normal process of reworking traumatic memories over time, placing them in context, and creating a tolerance for them, patients with PTSD organize their life around ways to avoid these memories, feelings, or sensations by using strategies such as

- Keeping away from situations, people, or emotions that remind them of the event
- Using alcohol or drugs that numb awareness of painful feelings
- Using dissociation to keep unpleasant experiences from conscious awareness
- Viewing the world as unmanageable
- Viewing themselves as unable to cope with present situations (van der Kolk et al., 2006a)

Psychotherapy has the potential to establish a sense of safety and control from which patients can examine the memories of the trauma. Verfaellie and Vasterling (2009) have said that memory does not work in isolation. "Recollection of personal past events is a construction of the past in light of current goals and attitudes rather than the retrieval of an actual record of past events" (p. 106). That is, memories and the maintenance of memories are influenced by the individual's goals, concerns, attitudes, and sense of self-identity. Psychotherapy can reduce the fear and anxiety related to the memories of the trauma and can help patients to make sense out of their lives. The model of psychotherapy that has been found to be most effective in the treatment of PTSD is exposure therapy (Cukor, Spitalnick, Difede, et al., 2009), although nonexposure psychotherapies are also used.

Exposure Therapies

Exposure therapy, considered to be the front line of treatment for PTSD (Cukor et al., 2009; Williams, Cahill, & Foa, 2010), is based on dual representation theory and learning theory. According to dual representation theory (Brewin, Dalgleish, & Joseph, 1996), during exposure to a traumatic event or immediately following it, information about the experience is processed and stored as different representations or images. This activity is due in part to hormonal responses to acute traumatic events that both *decrease* activity in brain structures involved in conscious memory processing and *increase* activity in brain structures involved in nonconscious memory processing.

One representation of the trauma, *verbally accessible knowledge*, will be of the individual's conscious experience of the trauma. It will contain some information about sensations associated with the traumatic event—such as emotions, bodily reactions, and meaning of the event—and it can be retrieved from the individual's memory (Brewin et al., 1996). Verbally accessible knowledge is made up of a series of autobiographical memories that can be changed as new information or new interpretations of old information are added.

Unconscious processing of the traumatic event will produce a second representation of the trauma called *situational accessible knowledge*, which cannot be deliberately retrieved. Individuals become aware of situational accessible knowledge when, in response to cues or triggers of the traumatic event, they experience symptoms of arousal, intrusive images, flashbacks, or dissociation (Brewin et al., 1996). Situational accessible knowledge remains unchanged and will continue to be reactivated by internal or external cues of the traumatic event causing symptoms of PTSD unless it is modified by treatment such as exposure therapy.

Learning theory proposes that fear, which is associated with specific stimuli, elicits the physiological response of anxiety. Anxiety is experienced as emotions and changes in functioning of the body—e.g., increased heart rate and respiration and changes in body temperature—and in cognition. For example, during times of acute distress, individuals often make errors in processing information. They may misperceive the event as more negative than it really is (Foa & Kozak, 1986), or they may overlook or ignore information that could be used to make an accurate assessment of the event, applying what is known as tunnel vision (Basco et al., 2000, p. A59). Individuals who experience anxiety may make guesses about what will happen in the future or what others will do in the future based on little evidence. Finally, they may oversimplify the situation by seeing it as all bad.

The therapeutic element of exposure therapy is thought to be the modification of the fear/anxiety response or the modification of the trauma memory through confrontation with the stimulus that elicits fear. In exposure therapy, confrontation activates the fear response, which is then modified by therapeutic interventions. Exposure therapy includes the use of imaginal exposure, simulated exposure, and in vivo or real-life exposure (Rizzo et al., 2010; Williams et al., 2010):

- Imaginal exposure involves revisiting the event mentally within a supportive therapeutic setting. The patient is able to begin to process trauma-relevant emotions and to extinguish traumatic memories by imagining a fear-arousing event and then using relaxation strategies and cognitive restructuring to overcome the anxiety (Basco et al., 2000).
- Simulated exposure is provided by virtual reality exposure (VRE) programs that immerse the patient in a simulation of the trauma environment with the intensity of the exposure controlled by the therapist.
- In vivo exposure involves confronting in real life trauma-related situations that the patient has been avoiding, usually starting with less anxiety-provoking situations (Basco et al., 2000).

Exposure therapy helps patients to develop less fear-based responses to internal and external cues. Exposure therapy helps patients to learn that

1. Being in a situation that reminds them of the original traumatic event is not dangerous
2. Remembering the traumatic event is not the same as experiencing it again
3. Anxiety will decrease in the presence of feared situations
4. Experiencing anxiety is not followed by loss of control

The goal of exposure therapy is to facilitate emotional processing of the traumatic event, which will lead to reduction of PTSD symptoms (Foa, Huppert, & Cahill, 2006).

Exposure therapies include CBT, eye movement desensitization and reprocessing (EMDR), trauma management therapy (TMT), structured writing therapy (SWT), and technology-based interventions such as Internet- and computer-based treatments and VRE therapy.

Cognitive Behavioral Therapy (CBT)

CBT is one of the most frequently used exposure therapies for PTSD. CTB proposes that trauma changes individuals' basic assumptions about the safety of the world they live in, their life experiences, their ability to evaluate situations, what their responses should be, and their sense of self-efficacy (Janoff-Bulman, 1992; McFarlane, 2010). CBT targets faulty beliefs and evaluation processes through repeated exposure or through techniques that focus on information processing without repeated exposure in an effort to desensitize the patient to trauma-related triggers. It includes education about the normal course of the response to a stressor, the symptoms of PTSD, reasons for recalling traumatic memories, and strategies for relaxation, such as deep breathing and progressive muscle relaxation (Bryant, Moulds, & Nixon, 2003b; Bryant et al., 1999; Ursano et al., 2006a). It also targets avoidance symptoms.

The principles of CBT are to extinguish fear through exposure and to learn new ways to counter that fear, such as new ways of thinking. The goal of CBT is to break the link between the stimulus and the anxiety response.

CBT uses cognitive strategies, such as thought stopping and cognitive restructuring. In thought stopping, the patient is taught to recognize repetitive thoughts and excessive worry, to stop the thought by self-talk (e.g., "Stop thinking about it"), and to replace the distressing thought with something pleasant. Cognitive restructuring helps the patient to gain a more realistic view of reality by replacing distorted thoughts with accurate interpretations. Cognitive restructuring requires the patient to recognize negative automatic thoughts that are caused by emotions associated with stressful situations and to use logic rather than emotions to evaluate the stressful situation and to problem solve. Behavioral strategies include relaxation training, controlled breathing techniques, progressive muscle relaxation, and exposure, either imaginal or in vivo (Basco et al., 2000).

The most important part of CBT for patients with PTSD is exposure, either through imagining the traumatic event or through actual exposure to similar stimuli so that the patient can confront memories of the event. The memories are activated in order to change the pathological aspect of the memories (Marmar & Spiegel, 2007, p. 520). There is evidence that CBT may speed recovery and prevent PTSD when therapy is given over a few sessions that begin 2 to 3 weeks after trauma exposure (Bryant et al., 1999; Bryant et al., 2003b; Ursano et al., 2006a).

OUTCOMES

For adults with PTSD, trauma-focused CBT (exposure and cognitive strategies that focus on the trauma) has been found to be more effective than no treatment (as seen represented by patients in a wait-list control group or in a usual treatment control group) for all symptoms of PTSD; it has also been found to improve symptoms of anxiety and depression (Bisson, Ehlers, Matthews, et al., 2007b). Among children and young adults with PTSD, trauma-focused CBT has been found to improve symptoms of PTSD and depression and to be associated with improvement of functioning (Smith, Yule, Perrin, et al., 2007). Other studies have shown that trauma-focused CBT is more effective than self-help booklets, relaxation exercises, or supportive counseling (Epp & Dobson, 2010). In a meta-analysis of pharmacological and physical interventions for adult PTSD, the results of one small study suggested that trauma-focused CBT is more effective than paroxetine (Paxil) for the treatment of chronic PTSD (National Collaborating Centre for Mental Health, 2005). This evidence of the effectiveness of trauma-focused CBT for patients with PTSD provides support for psychiatric advanced practice nurses to consider it as a first-line treatment for patients with PTSD.

Eye Movement Desensitization and Reprocessing (EMDR)

EMDR is an exposure-based therapy with multiple brief, interrupted exposures to traumatic material, use of eye movement strategies, and recall and verbalization of traumatic memories of an event or events (Ursano et al., 2006a). It is based on the model of Adaptive Information Processing (AIP) (Shapiro, 2001). AIP proposes that individuals have a physiological information processing system. As new information is processed, links between the new information and previously stored information are formed. AIP results in new learning and makes associated material available for use, thus relieving emotional distress. An assumption of AIP is that "information is understood to be stored in memory networks that contain related thoughts, images, emotions, and sensations with links between associated networks" (Shapiro & Maxfield, 2002, p. 935). According to the AIP model, if information related to a traumatic event is not processed, then the emotions, memories, and thinking related to the event are stored as they were initially experienced at the time of the event, and these stored emotions, memories, and thinking form the basis for the dysfunctional responses seen in individuals with PTSD. In other words, according to AIP, the intrusive symptoms of PTSD result from unprocessed sensory, emotional, and cognitive images of the traumatic event.

EMDR is based on the assumption that eye movements and other dual attention stimuli (tapping, touching, and finger clicking) enhance information processing. The patient is asked to focus on a disturbing image or memory and on the emotions and thinking connected with it while tracking the therapist's rapidly moving finger with his or her eyes (Seidler & Wagner, 2006). This is repeated until anxiety decreases. Then the patient generates a positive thought and links it to the scene while moving his or her eyes. Hogberg, Pagani, Sundin, et al. (2007) suggest that the sensory stimulus (the moving finger) is associated with "aspects of control, safety, relaxation, and attunement and thus functions as a positively valanced conditioned stimuli" (p. 59). The positive stimulus acts to counterbalance the conditioned fear response and other responses to reminders of the traumatic event.

Some researchers question the role of the eye movement component of EMDR (Pitman, Orr, Altman, et al., 1996). Davidson and Parker (2001) found that the saccadic eye movement component did not add to treatment efficacy. Their findings are supported by the research of Cahill, Carrigan, & Frueh (1999). Marmar & Spiegel (2007) also suggested that eye movement is not necessary for change to take place.

OUTCOMES

EMDR and CBT are equally effective in reducing symptoms of PTSD, and both are more effective than pharmacotherapy with SSRIs or anticonvulsant medications such as carbamazepine (Karatzias, Power, McGoldrick, et al., 2007; Seidler & Wagner, 2006). EMDR has been found to improve symptoms of depression and to improve functioning in addition to reducing symptoms of PTSD (Hogberg, Pagani, Sundin, et al., 2008). Van der Kolk, Spinazzola, Blaustein, et al. (2006c) pointed out that patients with adult-onset trauma such as combat or rape had a better response to EMDR than those with childhood-onset trauma such as physical abuse, sexual abuse, or both. The PTSD symptoms of patients with childhood-onset trauma responded better to pharmacotherapy with SSRIs than to EMDR.

Trauma Management Therapy (TMT)

TMT is a multicomponent treatment that was designed for use with combat-related PTSD. Although exposure therapy reduces PTSD symptoms of intrusion and physiological reactivity, it has not had an effect on the negative symptoms of PTSD (avoidance, social withdrawal, anger, emotional numbing, and difficulties with interpersonal relationships and employment) (Frueh, Turner, & Beidel, 1995). In order to treat more of the negative symptoms of PTSD, TMT (which incorporates exposure therapy and specific strategies to improve the negative symptoms of PTSD) has been used for veterans with PTSD (Frueh et al.). TMT includes education, exposure therapy, self-directed imaginal sessions, social skills training, anger management, emotional rehabilitation, and management of service-related issues such as an unwillingness to talk about some experiences or to trust those who had not served in the military.

OUTCOMES

The original TMT intervention was for 29 sessions over 17 weeks. In a study of veterans who completed the program, there was significant improvement of anxiety, flashbacks, nightmares, sleep difficulty, heart rate reactivity, and overall social functioning (Frueh, Turner, Beidel, et al., 1996). However, certain areas of functioning—such as expression of anger—did not show improvement (Frueh et al.).

Structured Writing Therapy (SWT)

SWT is another form of exposure therapy that has been used for patients with PTSD (Lange, Rietdijk, Hudcovicova, et al., 2003; Lange, van de Ven, Schrieken, et al., 2001). Similar to CBT, SWT uses imaginal exposure and cognitive restructuring. There are three phases of SWT: self-confrontation phase, cognitive reappraisal phase, and sharing phase. In the self-confrontation phase, patients write detailed accounts of the traumatic event, including sensory experiences, painful facts related to the trauma, and emotions experienced. In the cognitive reappraisal phase, patients write to an imagined close associate who experienced the same event with advice on how to deal with the event and its consequences. In the sharing phase, patients write about the traumatic event, its impact, and their coping efforts and share it with others.

OUTCOMES

In a study that compared SWT with CBT for the treatment of patients with ASD and PTSD, the two treatment modalities were equally effective. Both improved intrusive symptoms and symptoms of anxiety and depression. Both showed a trend to a decrease in avoidance behaviors. Neither modality was associated with a change in dissociation (van Emmerik, Kamphuis, & Emmelkam, 2008). A pre-test and post-test study examined the effectiveness of treating children with PTSD with writing therapy that was provided by trained therapists. The writing therapy included psychoeducation, exposure, cognitive restructuring, and promoting adequate coping skills. The child's written description of the experiences related to the traumatic event and written description of experiences related to cognitive restructuring, learning effective coping skills, and developing resilient behaviors became a part of their story line of the trauma with a beginning and an end. There was significant improvement of the children's PTSD symptoms and depressive symptoms (van der Oord, Lucassen, van Emmerik, et al., 2010).

Technology-Based Interventions

Technology-based treatments have been developed for patients with PTSD to overcome the obstacles of (1) lack of availability of treatment, (2) lack of financial resources to pay for the treatment, and (3) stigma attached to going to a psychiatrist or mental health clinic for treatment. Internet- and computer-based treatments have become a frequently used method of incorporating technology-based interventions into PTSD therapy. Some technological interventions—such as VRE—have been developed as a way to treat patients who have been unresponsive to other forms of treatment (Cukor et al., 2009).

Internet- and Computer-Based Treatments

In studies comparing patients with PTSD who underwent computer-based treatment with patients in a wait-list control group, a significant improvement of symptoms was found among the computer-based treatment groups (Reger & Gahm, 2009). In a study of a military population with PTSD, a cognitive behavioral Internet-delivered program called DE-STRESS was compared to the efficacy of an Internet-based supportive counseling intervention. The DE-STRESS program included exploration of triggers, the creation of a hierarchy of trauma triggers, stress management, in vivo exposure, trauma writing sessions, and relapse prevention. The patients receiving the DE-STRESS intervention had significantly greater decreases in symptoms of PTSD, depression, and anxiety than the group who participated in Internet-based supportive counseling (Litz, Engel, Bryant, et al., 2007).

Virtual Reality Exposure (VRE)

Virtual reality is being developed for the treatment of PTSD of military personnel who were deployed to Operation Iraqi Freedom and Operation Enduring Freedom (Cukor et al., 2009). Virtual reality combines real-time computer graphics and visual displays that enable patients to feel a sense of immersion in the virtual environments that simulate trauma environments and that can be controlled (Rizzo et al., 2010). Virtual reality does not depend on the patient's generating mental images, describing the images, and emotionally processing the traumatic event in an office or clinic setting; instead, virtual reality creates controllable, multisensory, interactive three-dimensional stimulus environments.

In the virtual reality environment, patients are able to expose themselves to and interact with the fear-producing environment while ultimately being in a safe environment. According to Cukor et al. (2009), "Repeated engagement with the fear structure in a safe therapeutic environment leads to a decrease in anxiety, through the processes of habituation and extinction, thereby allowing for the incorporation of new information" (p. 720).

Virtual reality has been used successfully for fear of flying and for fear of heights (Rizzo et al., 2010). The first virtual reality intervention for PTSD was known as Virtual Vietnam and included jungle scenery, Huey helicopters, rockets, explosions, and shouting. Twenty years after the Vietnam War, veterans of the Vietnam War with PTSD who had not responded to other treatments experienced significant reductions of PTSD symptoms after receiving Virtual Vietnam therapy (Rothbaum, Hodges, Ready, et al., 2001). Since then, other virtual environments have been created: the World Trade Center attack of 9/11, motor vehicle accidents, terrorist attacks, and a Virtual Iraq. Virtual Iraq includes a city that resembles a Middle Eastern city, desert roads, people, and a Humvee scenario. Sound such as gunfire and smells such as burning rubber, smoke, and diesel fuel can be added. Virtual Iraq has been found to reduce PTSD symptoms by 50% and also to reduce anxiety and depression (Yeh, Newman, Liewer, et al., 2009).

Nonexposure Psychotherapies

Nonexposure psychotherapies include interpersonal psychotherapy, brief trauma-focused or grief-focused therapy, psychodynamic psychotherapy, and psychological debriefing.

Interpersonal Psychotherapy

The symptoms of PTSD are often accompanied by problems with family relationships and problems with social and work relationships (Cukor et al., 2009). Interpersonal psychotherapy is a form of psychotherapy that focuses on the individual, his or her relationships, and his or her social functioning. Improvement in these areas is believed to lead to improvement of PTSD symptoms (Cukor et al.).

OUTCOMES

A pilot study found that patients with chronic PTSD who received 14 weeks of individual interpersonal therapy experienced improvement in their social relationships, and 69% experienced a 50% reduction of their symptoms of PTSD (Bleiberg & Markowitz, 2005). Although interpersonal therapy has been used in a group format for patients with PTSD, the results are not conclusive. One study found that patients experienced improvement in social functioning, depression, and well-being but only moderate improvement of PTSD symptoms (Robertson, Rushton, Batrim, et al., 2007). In a study of women with PTSD who received interpersonal therapy as a group intervention, it was found that the patients had more improvement in their PTSD symptoms and symptoms of depression than women in a wait-list control group (Krupnick, Green, Stockton, et al., 2008).

Brief Trauma-Focused or Grief-Focused Psychotherapy

Brief trauma-focused or grief-focused psychotherapy is a model that uses principles of interpersonal psychotherapy and CBT and includes psychoeducation to reconstruct the events before, during, and after the traumatic event to clarify misinterpretations; identify trauma reminders; elicit current stressors, losses, and changes resulting from traumatic events; assist with grieving; and promote normal activities and growth (Goenjian, Walling, Steinberg, et al., 2005).

OUTCOMES

Brief trauma-focused grief-focused psychotherapy has been found to be effective in reducing PTSD symptoms among adolescents following a disaster and also in preventing development of depression (Goenjian et al., 2005). The researchers suggest that implementing mental health interventions after disasters may reduce trauma-related psychopathology.

Psychodynamic Psychotherapy

In one psychodynamic psychotherapy approach, the individual's defenses and coping skills are viewed as products of his or her biopsychosocial development; therapy focuses on the meaning of the trauma for the individual in terms of prior psychological conflicts, developmental experiences, and relationships (Williams et al., 2010). The goal is to identify maladaptive coping and build new skills.

Another psychodynamic psychotherapy approach focuses on the effect of the traumatic experience on the individual's prior sense of self and altered perceptions of safety. With this approach, the goal is to help the individual maintain a sense of self-identity after the traumatic event and to reduce anxiety associated with triggers of the traumatic event.

OUTCOMES

Both approaches help in rebuilding trust, attachments, and the view of the world as a safe place (Marmar, 1991). A recent report says that psychodynamic therapy for patients with PTSD is associated with a reduction of PTSD symptoms, depression, and feelings of hostility and with improvement of social relationships (Tull, 2008).

Psychological Debriefing

There is considerable controversy about the effectiveness of debriefing (Robinson, 2008). Debriefing was developed by Jeffrey T. Mitchell in the 1970s as a way to help emergency service workers so that they did not become overwhelmed by their work. He introduced a group intervention that was designed to enable workers to talk about their stress and to receive support from others in the group. The group intervention was called Critical Incident Stress Debriefing (CISD). It was a supportive early intervention that was part of a Critical Incident Stress Management model, and it was to be linked with longer-term counseling or psychotherapy (Robinson, 2008).

Over time, debriefing was modified by many providers and used in situations and for individuals in ways that were not part of the original model. There is no evidence that psychological debriefing is effective in preventing PTSD or in improving social and occupational functioning (Bugg,

Turpin, Mason, et al., 2008; Rose et al., 2002; van Emmerik, Kamphuis, Hulsbosch, et al., 2002), and psychological debriefing may in fact increase symptoms of distress (Bisson, Jenkins, Alexander, et al., 1997; Foa & Meadows, 1997; Mayou, Ehlers, & Hobbs, 2000; National Collaborating Centre for Mental Health, 2005; Shalev, 2002). According to Spiegel (2005), two components of stress-debriefing approaches that have the potential to cause adverse responses are (1) the potential for arousing expectation of future emotional problems and (2) the potential for stirring up emotional reactions without providing strategies to restructure the meaning of the emotional experience and without providing support for managing the emotions. Another view is that stress debriefing provided by mental health professionals immediately after a traumatic event may get in the way in individuals who are seeking help and support from people they know, such as family members, friends, religious leaders, and family doctors (Wessely, 2005). Beekman, Cuijpers, van Marwijk, et al. (2006) stated that debriefing is ineffective in preventing PTSD. In short, empirical evidence doses do not support debriefing for survivors immediately following a traumatic event (Gray et al., 2006).

Other Interventions

Other treatment interventions for PTSD include behavioral activation, acupuncture, and imagery-based interventions.

Behavioral Activation

Behavioral activation is designed to help patients with PTSD symptoms of avoidance and social isolation. It uses a structured approach to increase patients' engagement in avoided activities and social activities.

OUTCOMES

From the outcome data available, Cukor et al. (2009) concluded that behavioral activation may be helpful when added to other treatment approaches; however, they also stated that the evidence does not indicate that behavioral activation addresses PTSD symptoms overall.

Acupuncture

In a pilot study of the use of acupuncture for patients with PTSD, patients displayed significant improvement in PTSD symptoms, depression, and anxiety. The improvement was comparable to those receiving group CBT, and the improvement was greater than the improvement displayed by patients in the wait-list control group (Hollifield, Sinclair-Lian, Warner, et al., 2007).

Imagery-Based Interventions

Guided imagery uses words, skills training, visualization, and meditation to help patients create either a new representation of what they want themselves to be or a new representation of their goals (Strauss, Calhoun, & Marx, 2009). Guided imagery has been used to help athletes improve their performance. It has also been used to help patients improve pain, headaches, hypertension, anxiety, and depression (Strauss et al., 2009). In a study of the use of guided imagery for female patients with PTSD, it was found that the patients experienced improvement of sleep and a decrease of severity of PTSD symptoms (Krakow, Hollifield, Johnston, et al., 2001). In a study of male combat veterans, guided imagery reduced anxiety and arousal and increased self-esteem, positive mood, and ability to concentrate (Root, Koch, Reyntjens, et al., 2002). Guided Imagery for Trauma (GIFT) and Imagery Rehearsal Therapy (IRT) are two forms of guided imagery that have been studied with relation to PTSD:

- GIFT is a clinician-facilitated self-management intervention that uses a manual. GIFT was designed to provide guided imagery to patients (1) with minimal clinical involvement, (2) at a low cost, and (3) to address frequent problems such as feelings of helplessness, vulnerability, and lack of power to bring about change. GIFT uses imagery audios to teach exercises that are designed to help patients learn better ways to manage their fears and hyperarousals. As they practice the exercises each day, the patients are able to replace trauma-related emotions with healthier emotions. In a study of 15 women with PTSD related to sexual trauma, there was a significant reduction of PTSD symptoms in the 10 women who completed the 12-week intervention (Strauss et al., 2009).
- IRT was developed to treat nightmares that followed exposure to traumatic events. Patients are taught how to create pleasant imagery to replace the imagery of the nightmares. They learn to generate new dreams with different characters and a nonthreatening or safe environment (Krakow, Hollifield, Schrader, et al., 2000). IRT has been found to be effective in improving nightmares in civilian populations who have experienced traumatic events such as sexual assault, but results have not been conclusive among veterans with PTSD (Cukor et al., 2009).

Summary of Psychotherapy Treatments for Post-traumatic Stress Disorder

Meta-analysis of 38 randomized controlled trials of psychological treatment for PTSD reported by Bisson et al. (2007b) showed that the two most effective interventions were trauma-focused CBT and EMDR. Both interventions are trauma-focused psychological treatments that address memories of the traumatic event, what that event means to the individual, and the consequences that the trauma has had on the individual's life (Marmar & Spiegel, 2007). Comparison of these two treatments has not shown superiority of one over the other (Seidler & Wagner, 2006). Seidler and Wagner recommended that a course of trauma-focused psychological treatment should be offered to everyone with chronic PTSD. For nonresponders, it may be beneficial to provide more than the usual 8 to 12 sessions, to try a different form of trauma-focused psychological treatment, or to add pharmacotherapy to the trauma-focused psychological treatment.

Pharmacotherapy

The goals of pharmacotherapy for patients with PTSD are to reduce core symptoms, restore functioning, improve quality of life, increase resilience to stress, treat comorbidities, and prevent relapse (Zhang & Davidson, 2010).

Pharmacotherapy is not considered to be the frontline treatment for PTSD (Marmar & Spiegel, 2007); however, in the period of time immediately after exposure to a traumatic event, severe hyperarousal symptoms may require pharmacotherapy. Pharmacotherapy is effective in treating some of the core symptoms of PTSD, such as intrusive reexperiencing of traumatic memories, avoidance of stimuli, numbing, anhedonia, and hyperarousal. Pharmacotherapy is also used in treating secondary symptoms such as impaired functioning, poor resistance to stress, and comorbid conditions (Zhang & Davidson, 2010) and may be used as an adjunctive intervention with psychotherapy (Stein, Ipser, & Seedat, 2006). The U.S. Food and Drug Administration (FDA) has approved only sertraline (Zoloft) and paroxetine for treatment of PTSD; all other drugs (Table 11-7) are used off-label (Antai-Otong, 2007, p. 57). For information on dosages, side effects, drug interactions, and augmentation, refer to a comprehensive psychopharmacology textbook.

Theoretical Basis for Pharmacotherapy

Increased levels of norepinephrine and epinephrine promote consolidation of the fear response caused by exposure to a severe traumatic event or by cues or memories of the event. Because patients with PTSD have overconsolidation of memories of the traumatic event, medications may be used to modulate these sensitized circuits and thereby decrease PTSD symptoms.

TABLE 11-7 MEDICATIONS USED TO TREAT POST-TRAUMATIC STRESS DISORDER

Medication	Outcomes	Treatment Considerations
Selective Serotonin Reuptake Inhibitors (SSRIs) SSRIs are effective for PTSD among civilian populations but less effective for combat trauma PTSD or chronic PTSD (Institute of Medicine, 2008; Mohamed & Rosenheck, 2008; Raskind, 2009). SSRIs are effective for daytime symptoms but not for sleep disturbances and nightmares (Stein, Pederson, Rothbaum, et al., 2008). "Only 40% to 50% of patients taking SSRIs for PTSD show major improvement" (Schatzberg, Cole, & DeBattista, 2007, p. 362)		
Fluoxetine (Prozac): Blocks serotonin reuptake pump; desensitizes serotonin receptors, especially 5-HT_{1A} receptor; increases norepinephrine and dopamine	Reduction of overall PTSD symptoms and improvement of intrusion and arousal symptoms (Connor, Sutherland, Tupler, et al., 1999; Martenyi, Brown, Zhang, et al., 2002). Reduction of avoidant and numbing symptoms (Davidson, Hughes, Blazer, et al., 1991; Nagy, Morgan, Southwick, et al., 1993). Decrease of vulnerability to stress and improved resilience (Connor et al., 1999). No difference between fluoxetine and placebo (van der Kolk et al., 2006c).	Not FDA approved for PTSD at this time (Ursano et al., 2006; Zhang & Davidson, 2010).
Sertraline (Zoloft)	Reduction of anger symptoms (Brady, Pearlstein, Asnis, et al., 2002; Davidson, Rothbaum, van der Kolk, et al., 2001b; Williams, Nieto, Sanford, et al., 2001). Improved functioning and quality of life (Rapaport, Endicott, & Clary, 2002; Raskind, Dobie, Danter, et al., 2000). Improvement of most symptoms and reduction of relapses (Davidson, Pearlstein, Londborg, et al., 2001a). May be associated with insomnia (Raskind, 2009).	FDA approved. Effective for short- and long-term treatment (Brady, Pearlstein, Asnis, et al., 2002; Davidson et al., 2001b) Female patients benefit more than male patients (Marmar & Spiegel, 2007). Use of sertraline for 9 months is associated with sustained improvement in 90% of patients (Londborg, Hegel, Goldstein, et al., 2001).
Paroxetine (Paxil): Blocks serotonin reuptake and desensitizes serotonin 1A receptors; mild anticholinergic action and mild blocking of norepinephrine reuptake	Overall improvement of PTSD symptoms, depression, and functioning (Cooper et al., 2005; Marshall, Beebe, Oldham, et al., 2001; Raskind, 2009; Tucker, Zaninelli, Yehuda, et al., 2001). Improvement of all symptom clusters of PTSD. No adverse effects on sleep (Raskind, 2009). Improvement of sleep disturbances and interpersonal difficulties (Marshall, Lewis-Fernandez, Blanco, et al., 2007). Increase in hippocampal volume; improvement in verbal declarative memory, cognition, and work performance (Bremner & Vermetten, 2004).	FDA approved. Abrupt discontinuation is associated with dizziness, nausea, stomach cramps, sweating, and tingling. Should be tapered when discontinued (Stahl, 2005; Ursano et al., 2006).
Fluvoxamine (Luvox)	Reduction of severity of PTSD symptoms (Cooper et al., 2005). Effective for intrusion, avoidance, arousal, and numbing (Zhang & Davidson, 2010).	Treatment effect achieved in 4 to 6 weeks.

Continued

TABLE 11-7 MEDICATIONS USED TO TREAT POST-TRAUMATIC STRESS DISORDER—continued

Medication	Outcomes	Treatment Considerations
Citalopram (Celexa): Blocks serotonin reuptake and desensitizes serotonin 1A autoreceptors; mild antagonist effect at H1 histamine receptors	Reduction of reexperiencing, and hyperarousal.	Not effective in improving avoidance and numbing (Schatzberg & Nemeroff, 2006). One study showed no superiority of citalopram over placebo (Tucker, Potter-Kimball, Wyatt, et al., 2003).
Tricyclic Antidepressants (TCAs)		
Imipramine (Tofranil)	Modest improvement (15% reduction of symptoms); effective for intrusive symptoms (Davidson, Kudler, Smith, et al., 1990; Kosten, Frank, Dan, et al., 1991).	Anticholinergic side effects. Effective for avoidance symptoms. Better response among veterans with less severe symptoms (Davidson, Kudler, Saunders, et al., 1993).
Amitriptyline (Elavil)	Moderate improvement (Davidson et al., 1990; Kosten et al., 1991).	Anticholinergic side effects.
Monoamine Oxidase Inhibitors (MAOIs)		
MAOIs Phenelzine (Nardil)	As effective as imipramine, a TCA, for intrusive symptoms (Kosten et al. 1991). Effective for intrusive symptoms (Hollander & Simeon, 2011).	Dietary and drug restrictions.
Other Antidepressants		
Venlafaxine (Effexor): Serotonin norepinephrine reuptake inhibitor	Improvement of PTSD symptoms and functioning (Schoenfeld et al., 2004) Improvement of reexperiencing and avoidance but not hyperarousal (Davidson, Baldwin, Stein, et al., 2006). Improvement of resilience (Davidson et al., 2006).	No FDA approval for PTSD. Onset of action: 2 to 4 weeks. Must be tapered when discontinued (Stahl, 2005).
Mirtazapine (Remeron): Dual norepinephrine and serotonin agent	Effective for PTSD and anxiety (Schoenfeld et al., 2004). Reduction of nightmares and insomnia (Lewis, 2002).	No FDA approval for PTSD. Onset of action is soon after starting medication for anxiety and sleep but is 2–4 weeks for depression (Bonne, Grillon, Vythilingam, et al., 2004).
Antianxiety Medications		
Benzodiazepines	Some reduction of anxiety and improvement of sleep, but rebound anxiety occurred (Braun, Greenberg, Dasberg, et al., 1990). No effect on core PTSD symptoms (Crockett & Davidson, 2002; Raskind, 2009; Ursano et al., 2006). Despite lack of evidence of efficacy for treatment of symptoms of PTSD, benzodiazepines are prescribed for 24% of veterans with PTSD (Raskind, 2009).	Risk of developing dependency; withdrawal symptoms (Risse, Whitters, Burke, et al., 1990). Use for augmentation, not monotherapy (Davidson & Connor, 2004). Evidence does not support use for PTSD (Zhang & Davidson, 2010).
Buspirone (Buspar)	Reduction of reexperiencing, avoidance, and intrusion (Schoenfeld et al., 2004).	Effective as augmentative agent for sleep disturbances in patients with PTSD (Maher, Rego, & Asnin, 2006).
Glutamatergic Agents		
Memantine (Namenda)	Reduction of arousal and conditioned responses (Bonne et al., 2004).	Improvement of delayed recall of memories (Battista, Hierholzer, & Khouzam, 2007).
Anticonvulsant Medications		
Carbamazepine (Tegretol)	Improvement of symptoms of reexperiencing, insomnia, hyperarousal, impulsivity, and violent behavior (Keck, McElroy, & Friedman, 1992).	Improvement of PTSD symptoms may be linked to reduction of stress-activated limbic kindling (Berlin, 2007).
Divalproex (Depakote)	Improvement of symptoms of reexperiencing, intrusive memories, flashbacks, and nightmares (Ursano et al., 2006).	Not effective for PTSD symptoms in combat veterans (Ravindran & Stein, 2009).
Topiramate (Topamax)	Reduction of nightmares (Berlant & van Kammen, 2002).	Reduced combat-related PTSD symptoms of nightmares and associated use of alcohol (Alderman, McCarthy, Condon, et al., 2009).
Lamotrigine (Lamictal)	Limited information.	As augmentative agent, improved reexperiencing symptoms and avoidance symptoms (Ravindran & Stein, 2009).

TABLE 11-7 MEDICATIONS USED TO TREAT POST-TRAUMATIC STRESS DISORDER—continued

Medication	Outcomes	Treatment Considerations
Gabapentin (Neurontin)	Improvement of nightmares and sleep disturbances (Marmar & Spiegel, 2007).	Used as augmentation for insomnia (Hamner, Brodrick, & Labbate, 2001).
Lithium	In open trials, improvement of irritability and intrusive symptoms were reported (Hollander & Simeon, 2011).	Used as augmentation for treatment-resistant anger and irritability (Forester, Schoenfeld, Marmar, et al., 1995).
Second-Generation Antipsychotic Medications For patients who have not responded to other treatment and for patients with PTSD with psychotic features (Raskind, 2009).		
Risperidone (Risperdal)	Improvement of intrusive thoughts, irritability, and other PTSD symptoms among combat veterans (Monnelly, Ciraulo, Knapp, et al., 2003). Improvement of PTSD symptoms among women with history of childhood abuse (Reich, Winternitz, Hennen, et al., 2004). Improvement of sleep disruptions among civilian trauma patients resistant to SSRIs (Rothbaum, Killeen, Davidson, et al., 2008).	When used as adjunctive medication for chronic combat-related PTSD, improved core symptoms and also anxiety and depressive symptoms (Bartzokis, Lu, & Turner, 2005).
Olanzapine (Zyprexa)	Improvement of irritability and psychotic symptoms (Hamner, Deitsch, Brodrick, et al., 2003; Monnelly et al., 2003).	Used as augmentation to other medications; e.g., patients resistant to treatment with SSRIs (Davidson & Connor, 2006; Ursano et al., 2006a). Adverse effect of weight gain (Raskind, 2009).
Quetiapine (Seroquel)	Improvement of sleep disruption symptoms in veterans with PTSD (Robert, Hamner, Chose, et al., 2005).	Adverse effects of weight gain and daytime sleepiness (Raskind, 2009).
Alpha-Adrenergic Antagonists, Alpha-Adrenergic Agonists, and Beta-Adrenergic Blockers May be helpful for chronic PTSD with anxious arousal.		
Prazosin (Minipress): An alpha-adrenergic antagonist	Improves sleep disturbances, nightmares, reexperiencing, avoidance, numbing, and hyperarousal (Raskind, Peskind, Kanter, et al., 2003; Taylor, Freeman, & Cates, 2008).	Improved nightmares associated with combat-related trauma and noncombat-related trauma. (Raskind et al., 2003; Taylor, Martin, Thompson, et al., 2008).
Propranolol (Inderal): a beta-adrenergic antagonist	Reduction of severity of responses to triggers, trauma-related nightmares, intrusive memories, hypervigilance, startle response, and expression of anger (Bonne et al., 2004; Brunet, Orr, Tremblay, et al., 2008; Kolb, Burris, Griffiths, 1984; Vaiva et al., 2003).	As early intervention to reduce risk of PTSD (Pitman et al., 2002; Vaiva et al., 2003).
Clonidine (Catapres): Alpha-agonist	Reduction of impulsive behaviors and intrusive thoughts. No reduction of avoidance and numbing.	Showed promise for PTSD sleep problems (Kinzie, Sack, & Riley, 1994).

Sources: Davidson & Connor, 2004; Marmar & Spiegel, 2007; Raskind, 2009; Schatzberg & Nemeroff, 2009; Ursano et al., 2006; Zhang & Davidson, 2010.

Medications Used To Treat Specific Symptoms of Post-traumatic Stress Disorder

Avoidance symptoms of PTSD and regulation of sleep are modulated by the serotonin pathways. Because medications that increase serotonergic transmission are clinically effective in treating PTSD (Marmar & Speigel, 2007), SSRIs are considered to be the first choice of pharmacotherapy for PTSD (Schatzberg & Nemeroff, 2009; Zhang & Davidson, 2010). SSRIs

- Ameliorate all three PTSD symptom clusters: reexperiencing, avoidance or numbing, and hyperarousal
- Are effective treatment for psychiatric disorders that are frequently comorbid with PTSD, including depression, panic disorder, social phobia, and obsessive-compulsive disorder
- May reduce anger and irritability
- May reduce clinical symptoms, such as suicidal impulsivity and aggressive behaviors
- Have relatively few side effects and are safer in overdose than tricyclic antidepressants or monoamine oxidase inhibitor antidepressants (Cooper et al., 2005)
- May increase resilience and reduce disability

All SSRIs increase serotonin functioning in the central nervous system and thereby regulate norepinephrine, thus modulating impulsive, aggressive, and suicidal behaviors. Use of the SSRIs—fluoxetine, sertraline, and paroxetine—is associated with (1) reduction of symptoms of anger and irritability in the first week (Davidson, Landerman, Farfel, et al., 2002) and (2) decrease in the core PTSD symptoms of reexperiencing, avoidance, and hyperarousal in 2 to 4 weeks. However, the response rate to SSRIs is about 60%, with only 30% of patients with PTSD achieving remission (Cukor, Olden, Lee, et al., 2010; Stein, Kline, & Matloff, 2002). It is significant that in four studies of veterans with chronic PTSD, SSRIs were associated with reduction of irritability, anger, anxiety, and depression but not with reduction of PTSD symptoms (Raskind, 2009). Discontinuation of medication is frequently associated with a return of symptoms (Zhang & Davidson, 2010).

While SSRIs are the medication of first choice for PTSD (Zhang & Davidson, 2010), mood stabilizers and atypical antipsychotics have also been investigated. Mood stabilizers are believed to reduce limbic system sensitization that may occur in the weeks following exposure to a severe traumatic event, and they are also effective for control of impulsive behavior and aggressive behavior and for problems with regulating emotions in patients who have not responded to SSRI treatment. According to Raskind (2009), mood stabilizers have not been found to be more effective than placebo for treatment of chronic PTSD. Atypical antipsychotics may be effective for treatment of patients with PTSD sleep difficulties, irritability, anger outbursts, intense flashbacks, and psychotic symptoms (Raskind).

New Pharmacotherapy Interventions

New approaches in the use of pharmacotherapy for PTSD include the use of D-cycloserine (Seromycin), propranolol, and prazosin (Minipress, Vasoflex).

- ***D-cycloserine***—a broad-spectrum antibiotic and cognitive enhancer—is being used with exposure therapy. It is a partial agonist at the *N*-methyl-D-aspartate (NMDA) glutamatergic receptor, which is involved in learning and memory. Antagonists at the NMDA glutamatergic receptor block fear extinction; because D-cycloserine facilitates NMDA receptor functioning in the amygdala, it thereby promotes fear extinction and new learning (Davis, Barad, Otto, et al., 2006). D-cycloserine has been found to reduce general social anxiety symptoms in patients who were exposed to feared social situations (Hofmann, Meuret, Smits, et al., 2006). Data support its use in augmenting exposure therapy and VRE (Cukor et al., 2010).
- ***Propranolol.*** As described in the section of this chapter on ASD, propranolol is a nonselective beta-adrenergic blocker that appears to have the ability to reduce the consolidation of emotional memories (Cahill et al., 1994; Weigel et al., 2009). In studies of patients who were treated with propranolol and others who received a placebo within hours of a traumatic event, those receiving propranolol had fewer PTSD symptoms and less physiological reactions to triggers of the trauma (Pitman et al., 2002; Vaiva et al., 2003).
- ***Prazosin,*** which is an antihypertensive medication, is an α_1-adrenergic receptor blocker. It inhibits adrenergic activity. Prazosin has been found to be effective in reducing nightmares among veterans with PTSD (Thompson, Taylor, McFall, et al., 2008). Prazosin was also found to improve overall clinical status and to improve reexperiencing, avoidance, and hyperarousal symptoms (Raskind, Peskind, Hoff, et al., 2007), and it has been found to be effective in reducing insomnia and sleep disturbances (Cukor et al., 2010; Taylor, Martin, Thompson, et al., 2008).

Ketamine's and morphine's effects on specific populations with PTSD have also been studied:

- ***Ketamine,*** a nonbarbituate anesthetic and an analgesic, acts as an antagonist at the NMDA receptor, and that action is thought to result in a disruption of the memory process. Ketamine is given intravenously to burn patients in some military hospitals. In one study that compared patients with burns who received ketamine to patients with burns who received opioids or nonopiod analgesics (Schonenberg, Reichwald, Domes, et al., 2008), it was found that patients with burns who received ketamine had a higher level of symptoms of dissociation, reexperiencing, avoidance, and hyperarousal. However, in another study, patients with burns who received ketamine during surgery had lower rates of PTSD than those who did not (McGhee, Maani, Garza, et al., 2009b).
- ***Morphine,*** an opiate, is known to relieve pain, but its role in preventing PTSD is not known. (Opiates were discussed in the section on ASD.) It has been suggested that morphine may inhibit norepinephrine in areas of the brain that are associated with consolidation of traumatic memories (Saxe, Stoddard, Courtney, et al., 2001). When given soon after exposure to a traumatic event, it has been found to prevent or reduce the development of PTSD. For example, in a study of children who had suffered burns, it was found that the administration of morphine was associated with prevention of the development of PTSD (Saxe et al.). In a recent study of injured servicemen, it was found that morphine administered soon after the injury, during resuscitation or trauma care, was associated with an approximately 50% reduction in development of PTSD later on (Holbrook et al., 2010).

Combining Pharmacotherapy and Psychotherapy

Pharmacotherapy may be used in combination with psychotherapy that focuses on exposure to the trauma-related stimulus and with psychosocial interventions that focus on self-regulation, social skills building, and cognitive restructuring (Marmar & Spiegel, 2007, p. 530).

Although there are not many studies of the efficacy of combining pharmacotherapy and psychotherapy, clinical experiences suggest that the two treatment interventions have a synergistic effect, such that the combined effect is greater than the effect of either intervention alone (Cooper et al., 2005). Combining pharmacotherapy and psychotherapy may improve the response to medication in patients who have not responded to medication (Otto, Hinton, Korbly, et al., 2003), and by reducing the symptoms of hyperarousal, they may be helpful for engaging patients in psychotherapy. Continuing psychotherapy when discontinuing medication may prevent relapse (Frommberger, Stieglitz, Nyberg, et al., 2004).

Psychosocial Interventions

Early supportive interventions are recommended as a first-line intervention at the time of the traumatic event (Ursano, Zhang, Li, et al., 2009). Psychosocial interventions that are used in the treatment of patients with PTSD include supportive interventions, interventions that promote self-regulation, cognitive restructuring, education, exercise, problem-solving therapy, using timelines and ladders, and social and family-based interventions.

Supportive Interventions

Support interventions—such as psychological first aid—are designed to restore self-efficacy, a sense of control, and mastery by encouraging individuals to rely on their own strengths, to use their internal resources, to ask for help from existing support networks, and to use their own judgment (Frances, 2002).

Self-Regulation

In PTSD, there is a dysregulation of arousal at the brainstem level. Because of this dysregulation, individuals must learn to control their physiological arousal in order to overcome the consequences of past exposure to a traumatic event. For example, some individuals with PTSD have impaired ability to perform self-soothing functions: they cannot relax or calm themselves. For these patients, psychosocial interventions that focus on promoting self-regulation may be helpful (Green & Shellenberger, 1991).

Self-regulation involves the control of physiological and psychological processes through the use of both internal and external resources and through choices that the individual makes. Individuals who do not assume the responsibility of self-regulation place themselves at risk of being controlled by others, by circumstances, by the environment, and by their habitual emotional responses and behaviors. Interventions and attributes used in developing self-regulation include the following:

- Problem-solving, which involves defining problems, planning, evaluating alternatives, and anticipating consequences (see Chapter 8 for more information on problem-solving)
- Self-efficacy, which means having confidence that one can do what needs to be done
- Relaxation, which could include breathing exercises and progressive muscle relaxation
- Cognitive coping skills, such as positive imagery, thoughts, expectations, and self-talk

Cognitive Restructuring

Cognitive restructuring helps individuals to learn that negative thinking can result in unhealthy physical and behavioral problems, disturbances of interpersonal relationships, and maladaptive coping, such as substance abuse. In cognitive restructuring, individuals are taught to recognize destructive thoughts, emotions, physical symptoms, and behaviors. They are then taught how to change their thinking. It is believed that changing negative thinking to more positive thinking will result in reduced stress and improved health and functioning (Rhoads, Pearman, & Rick, 2007). Although cognitive restructuring is effective for preventing PTSD among patients with ASD, it is less effective in treating PTSD than therapies that use prolonged exposure (Bryant et al., 2008).

Education

Education focuses on teaching normal physical and emotional responses to trauma so that patients can learn ways to reduce their response to the original event. Patients are taught how to manage emotional responses to triggers, anger, sleep disturbances, and dissociative symptoms. Patients are also taught stress-reduction strategies, active coping, and how to use their own self-strengths and networks to heal (Ursano et al., 2006a). Patient education includes changing lifestyle practices, such as reducing caffeine intake and smoking, and learning how to avoid exposure to new traumatic events by seeking safe living situations and avoiding abrasive or abusive social and romantic relationships (Kubany, Hill, Owens, et al., 2004). Education is presented in a clear, concrete manner to compensate for patients' anxiety, difficulties in concentrating, or impairment of memory (Olszewski & Varrasse, 2005). It is usually incorporated into other interventions. There is little information about the effectiveness of education alone.

Exercise

Among patients with PTSD who have not responded to other treatment interventions, exercise has been found to be associated with reduction of PTSD symptoms and also with reduction of symptoms of depression and anxiety. The benefits achieved with a 12-session aerobic exercise program were maintained at 1 month after participation in the program (Manger & Motta, 2005).

Using Timelines and Ladders

To help put traumatic events into perspective, a timeline can be developed. For children, the timeline can start with their birth and end with the current date. Then, significant events such as birthdays, first day of school, or a best friend moving away can be filled in. The timeline puts the traumatic event in concrete and historical perspective. Adults use the timeline by plotting positive and negative events and by identifying how they coped with each event. Then, using a ladder with several rungs, they place the lowest point of their life—often the traumatic event—at the bottom, and then they list their long-term goals—such as family, vocational goals, financial goals, and personal development goals—at the top; the adult then selects previously used coping strategies that he or she can use to meet his or her long-term goals (Busuttil, Turnbull, Neal, et al., 1995).

Social and Family-Based Treatments

Several family and couples treatment interventions have been developed to help the veterans of Operation Iraqi Freedom and Operation Enduring Freedom. Among veterans of

Operation Iraqi Freedom and Operation Enduring Freedom with PTSD, 75% have been found to have problems with marital relationships, aggression toward partners and children, sexual dysfunction, and emotional distancing (Sayers, Farrow, Ross, et al., 2009). In addition, these veterans often report feeling that they do not belong or that people do not understand them (Erbes, Polusny, MacDermid, et al., 2008).

One family-based intervention that has data about its efficacy is cognitive behavioral conjoint therapy, which is designed for couples when one or both have PTSD (Monson, Fredman, & Adair, 2008). The intervention uses a three-stage approach over 15 sessions: (1) psychoeducation and safety building; (2) confronting the avoidance behaviors, strengthening relationships, and improving communication; and (3) focusing on maladaptive thoughts around the trauma. The one available study found that whereas clinicians identified significant improvement in PTSD symptoms, the veterans did not. The veterans' significant others reported greater relationship satisfaction, and the veterans reported improvement in anxiety and depression (Monson, Schnurr, Stevens, et al., 2004).

Treatment Summary

Although approximately 60% to 80% of patients respond to treatment, only 30% or less experience remission (Masand, 2003). In a multidimensional meta-analysis of 26 studies of psychotherapy for PTSD, Bradley, Greene, Russ, et al. (2005) reported that among patients completing treatment, 67% no longer met the criteria for PTSD, although there continued to be residual symptoms. Treatment for combat-related PTSD showed the least change. Bradley et al. concluded that "a variety of treatments, primarily exposure, other cognitive behavior therapy approaches, and eye movement desensitization and reprocessing are highly efficacious in reducing PTSD symptoms" (p. 225).

Within pharmacotherapy, the strongest evidence is for the use of antidepressants. The SSRIs and selective norepinephrine reuptake inhibitors have been found to reduce core symptoms of PTSD, prevent relapse, reduce symptoms of some co-occurring psychiatric disorders, and promote resilience (Davidson, Connor, & Zhang, 2009). There is some evidence for the use of atypical antipsychotic medications as adjunctive medications. Evidence of benefit from use of mood stabilizers is inconclusive (Raskind, 2009; Zhang & Davidson, 2010).

Determining efficacy of treatment in clinical practice requires the use of instruments to establish a baseline of severity of symptoms and to monitor response to treatment. Instruments for outcome measurement can be found in Box 11-4. Other instruments that can be used to assess response to treatment can be found at American Psychological Association Web site (www.apa.org), American Psychiatric Association Web site (www.psych.org), and the International Society for Traumatic Stress Studies Web site (www.istss.org).

BOX 11-4 Instruments for PTSD Outcome Measurements

Instruments that can be used to evaluate PTSD treatment include

- *Treatment-outcome post-traumatic stress disorder scale (TOP-8)* (Davidson & Colket, 1997b). This 8-item scale measures response to treatment of symptoms from 3 clusters of PTSD symptoms.
- *Posttraumatic Symptoms Scale, a Self-report Version (PSS-SR)* (Foa, Riggs, Dancu, et al., 1993). This is a 17-item scale that can be used to measure changes in PTSD over time. Items correspond to *DSM-IV* symptom criteria for PTSD.

Course

In general, PTSD symptom distress is greatest within days and weeks of the trauma and then gradually declines over the following 12 months with a continued gradual decrease over the next 6 years (Rothbaum & Foa, 1994). However, some patients report that intrusive traumatic memories increase over time and are worse than the initial traumatic response because they cannot control them. Other symptoms that may increase over time include startle response, nightmares, irritability, and depression (First & Tasman, 2004). For some patients, there is a delayed onset, with symptoms appearing years later (Adams & Boscarino, 2006). Delayed onset of PTSD requires that symptoms of PTSD appear at least 6 months after exposure to the stressor; however, patients often have some symptoms or a subsyndromal level of symptoms soon after the traumatic event, although it may be months or years before the symptoms meet the criteria for PTSD (Andrews, Brewin, Philpott, et al., 2007).

The course of PTSD varies according to the type of traumatic event experienced. For survivors of technological disasters, the rate of PTSD was high (54%) 1 month after exposure to the disaster but decreased to 10% to 15% within 1 year (Neria et al., 2007). Some studies of survivors of natural disasters reported a decline in PTSD over time (van Griensven, Chakkraband, Thienkrua, et al., 2006), but other studies have reported an increase in PTSD symptoms over time (Neria et al., 2007).

For some patients, PTSD symptoms are unchanged. For example, among traumas such as rape, 16% of women continued to have PTSD 17 years after the rape (Kilpatrick, Saunders, Veronen, et al., 1987), and 15% of male Vietnam veterans still had PTSD 19 years after combat exposure (Kulka, Schlenger, Fairbank, et al., 1990). Poorer outcomes are associated with male gender; history of childhood trauma or multiple traumas in life or experiencing of interpersonal traumas; being injured during the trauma; suicide risk; comorbid psychiatric disorders; living alone; problems with anger; use of benzodiazepines as treatment for symptoms; and low levels of patient engagement in treatment (Williams et al., 2010). Higher levels of self-competence—which is made up of self-esteem; self-confidence in social, academic, or work abilities; a positive sense of self-efficacy ("can do"); and a sense of self-worth—are associated with more favorable outcomes (Perkonigg, Pfister, Stein, et al., 2005). About 50% of patients with PTSD have a full recovery, and about 50% develop a chronic form of the illness (First & Tasman, 2004; Perkonigg et al.) that is characterized by depression and/or alcohol abuse, limitation of functioning, decreased productivity, diminished quality of life, and suicide attempts (Black & Andreasen, 2011; Kessler, 2000; Ursano et al., 2006a; Warshaw, Fierman, Pratt, et al., 1993). Nearly one-half of patients with subsyndromal PTSD still have symptoms of PTSD 3 years after the trauma, and many go on to develop PTSD (Perkonigg et al.).

Key Points

- In their lifetime, 90% of Americans are exposed to traumatic events that are severe enough to cause PTSD.
- Only 10% of those exposed to severe traumatic events develop PTSD.
- Risk factors for developing PTSD depend on individual attributes, such as lower academic achievement and prior exposure to traumas; biological risk factors, such as smaller hippocampus; family factors, such as substance abuse, conflict, and poverty; circumstances surrounding the trauma, such as trauma that threatens life; and events following the trauma, such as lack of emotional and instrumental support.
- Protective factors include affiliation, having a secure pattern of attachment, having needs met, and having social support, culture, religion, and prior mastery of traumatic events.
- A core feature of PTSD is the continued presence of traumatic memories that cause reexperiencing such as flashbacks, hyperarousal, and avoidance or numbing.
- There is a high rate of comorbid medical and psychiatric disorders, including substance abuse and suicidality.
- Effective treatment for PTSD includes psychotherapy and pharmacotherapy. Psychosocial interventions are helpful with some symptoms.
- Exposure therapies such as cognitive behavioral therapy and eye movement desensitization and reprocessing have been found to be equally effective in treating PTSD.
- Selective serotonin reuptake inhibitors and selective norepinephrine reuptake inhibitors are considered to be the first choice in pharmacotherapy.
- Psychosocial interventions that restore self-efficacy and sense of mastery include self-regulation, cognitive restructuring, education, exercise, and problem-solving training.
- New treatment approaches include imagery-based interventions and technology-based interventions (e.g., virtual reality therapy).
- Although 50% of patients with PTSD achieve remission, for others, PTSD is a chronic disorder with distressful symptoms, impaired functioning, and diminished quality of life.

Resources

Organizations

National Center for Posttraumatic Stress Disorder
http://www.ncptsd.va.gov
Posttraumatic Stress Disorder Alliance
http://www.ptsdalliance.org

Movies

Haggis, P. (Director). (2007). *In the Valley of Elah* [Motion picture]. United States: Warner Independent Pictures.

Stone, O. (Director), and Stone, O., & Kitman, H. (Producers). (1989). *Born on the Fourth of July* [Motion picture]. United States: Universal Pictures.

Demme, J. (Director). (2004). *The Manchurian Candidate* [Motion picture]. United States: Paramount Pictures.

SOURCE: WEDDING, BOYD, & NIEMIEC, 2010.

References

Adams, R. E., & Boscarino, J. A. (2006). Predictors of PTSD and delayed PTSD after disaster: The impact of exposure and psychosocial resources. *Journal of Nervous and Mental Disorders, 194*, 485-493.

Adams, R. E., Boscarino, J. A., & Galea, S. (2006). Alcohol use, mental health status and psychological well-being 2 years after the World Trade Center attacks in New York City. *American Journal of Drug and Alcohol Abuse, 32*(12), 203-222.

Adler, N. E., Horowitz, M., Garcia, A., et al. (1998). Additional validation of a scale to assess positive states of mind. *Psychosomatic Medicine, 60*, 26-32.

Afari, N., Harder, L. H., Madra, N. J., et al. (2009). PTSD, combat injury, and headache in veterans returning from Iraq/Afghanistan. *Headache, 49*(9), 1267-1276.

Afifi, T. O., Asmundson, G., Taylor, S., et al. (2010). The role of genes and environment on trauma exposure and posttraumatic stress disorder symptoms: A review of twin studies. *Clinical Psychology Review, 30*(1), 101-112.

Alderman, C. P., McCarthy, L. G., Condon, J. T., et al. (2009). Topiramate in combat-related posttraumatic stress disorder. *Annals of Pharmacotherapy, 43*(4), 635-641.

Altindag, A., Ozwin, S., & Sir, A. (2005). One-year follow-up study of posttraumatic stress disorder among earthquake survivors in Turkey. *Comprehensive Psychiatry, 46*, 328-333.

American Psychiatric Association. (2000). *Diagnostic and statistical manual of mental disorders* (4th ed., text rev.). Washington, DC: American Psychiatric Publishing, Inc.

Amiel, J. M., Mathew, S. J., Garakani, A., et al. (2009). Neurobiology of anxiety disorders. In A. F. Schatzberg & C. B. Nemeroff (Eds.), *The American psychiatric publishing textbook of psychopharmacology* (4th ed.) (pp. 965-985). Washington, DC: American Psychiatric Publishing, Inc.

Andrews, B., Brewin, C. R., Philpott, R., et al. (2007). Delayed-onset posttraumatic stress disorder: A systematic review of the evidence. *American Journal of Psychiatry, 164*, 1319-1326.

Antai-Otong, D. (2007). Pharmacologic management of posttraumatic stress disorder. *Perspectives in Psychiatric Care, 43*(1), 55-57.

Bartzokis, G., Lu, P. H., & Turner, J. (2005). Adjunctive risperidone in the treatment of chronic combat related posttraumatic stress disorder. *Biological Psychiatry, 57*, 474-479.

Basco, M. R., Glickman, M., Weatherford, P., et al. (2000). Cognitive-behavioral therapy for anxiety disorders: Why and how it works. *Bulletin of the Menninger Clinic, 64*(3, Suppl A), A52-A70.

Basoglu, M., Paker, M., Paker, O., et al. (1994). Psychological effects of torture: A comparison of tortured with nontortured political activists in Turkey. *American Journal of Psychiatry, 151*, 76-81.

Battista, M. A., Hierholzer, R., & Khouzam, H. (2007). Pilot trial of memantine in the treatment of posttraumatic stress disorder. *Psychiatry: Interpersonal and Biological Processes, 70*(2), 167-174.

Bauer, M., Priebe, S., Haring, B., et al. (1993). Long-term sequelae of political imprisonment in East Germany. *Journal of Nervous and Mental Disease, 181*, 257-262.

Beck, A. T., Ward, C. H., Mendelson, M., et al. (1961). An inventory for measuring depression. *Archives of General Psychiatry, 4*, 561-571.

Beekman, A. T. F., Cuijpers, P., van Marwijk, W. W. J., et al. (2006). The prevention of psychiatric disorders. *Nederlands Tijdschrift voor Geneeskunde, 150*(8), 419-423.

Bennett, W. R. M., Zatzick, D., & Roy-Byrne, P. (2007). Can medications prevent PTSD in trauma victims? *Current Psychiatry, 6*(9), 47-53.

Berlant, J., & van Kammen, D. P. (2002). Open-label topiramate as primary or adjunctive therapy in chronic civilian posttraumatic stress disorder: A preliminary report. *Journal of Clinical Psychiatry, 63*, 15-20.

Berlin, H. A. (2007). Antiepileptic drugs for the treatment of posttraumatic stress disorder. *Current Psychiatry Reports, 9*(4), 291-300.

Bernstein, E. M., & Putman, F. W. (1986). Development, reliability and validity of a dissociation scale. *Journal of Nervous and Mental Disease, 174*, 727-735.

Bisson, J. I., Brayne, M. M. A., Ochberg, F. M., et al. (2007a). Early psychosocial intervention following traumatic events. *The American Journal of Psychiatry, 164*(7), 1016-1019.

Bisson, J. I., Ehlers, A., Matthews, R., et al. (2007b). Psychological treatments for chronic post-traumatic stress disorder: Systematic review and meta-analysis. *British Journal of Psychiatry, 190*, 97-104.

Bisson, J. I., Jenkins, P. L., Alexander, J., et al. (1997). Randomized controlled trial of psychological debriefing for victims of acute burn trauma. *British Journal of Psychiatry, 171*, 78-81.

Black, E. W., & Andreason, N. C. (2011). *Introductory textbook of psychiatry* (5th ed.). Washington, DC: American Psychiatric Publishing, Inc.

Blake, D. D., Weathers, F. W., Nagy, L. M., et al. (1990). A clinician rating scale for assessing current and lifetime PTSD: The CAPS-1. *Behavioral Therapy, 18*, 187-188.

Blake, D. D., Weathers, F. W., Nagy, L. M., et al. (1995). The development of a Clinician-Administered PTSD Scale. *Journal of Traumatic Stress, 8*, 75-90.

Bleiberg, K. L., & Markowitz, J. C. (2005). A pilot study of interpersonal psychotherapy for posttraumatic stress disorder. *American Journal of Psychiatry, 162*(1), 181-183.

Bleich, A., Glekopf, M., & Solomon, Z. (2003). Exposure to terrorism, stress-related mental health symptoms, and coping behaviors among a nationally representative sample in Israel. *Journal of the American Medical Association, 290*, 612-620.

Bodvarsdottir, I., & Elklit, A. (2004). Psychological reactions in Icelandic earthquake survivors. *Scandinavian Journal of Psychology, 45*, 3-13.

Bonne, O., Grillon, C., Vythilingam, M., et al. (2004). Adaptive and maladaptive psychobiological responses to severe psychological stress: Implications for the discovery of novel pharmacotherapy. *Neuroscience and Biobehavioral Reviews, 28*, 65-94.

Bosoglu, M., Paker, M., Paker, O., et al. (1994). Psychological effects of torture: A comparison of tortured with nontortured political activists in Turkey. *American Journal of Psychiatry, 151*, 76-81.

Boscarino, J. A. (2004). Posttraumatic stress disorder and physical illness: Results from clinical and epidemiologic studies. *Annals of the New York Academy of Sciences, 1032*, 141-153.

Bracha, H. S., Williams, A. E., Haynes, S. N., et al. (2004). The STRS (shortness of breath, tremulousness, racing heart and sweating): A brief checklist for acute distress with panic-like autonomic indicators; development and factor structure. *Annals of General Hospital Psychiatry, 3*, 8

Bradley, R., Greene, J., Russ, E., et al. (2005). A multidimensional meta-analysis of psychotherapy for PTSD. *American Journal of Psychiatry, 162*(2), 214-217.

Brady, K., Pearlstein, T., Asnis, G. M., et al. (2002). Efficacy and safety of sertraline treatment of posttraumatic stress disorder: A randomized controlled trial. *Journal of the American Medical Association, 183*, 1837-1844.

Braun, P., Greenberg, D., Dasberg, H., et al. (1990). Core symptoms of posttraumatic stress disorder unimproved by alprazolam treatment. *Journal of Clinical Psychiatry, 51*, 236-238.

Bremner, J. D. (2002). Neuroimaging of childhood trauma. *Seminars in Clinical Neuropsychiatry, 7*, 104-112.

Bremner, J. D. (2003). Functional neuroanatomical correlates of traumatic stress revisited 7 years later, this time with data. *Psychopharmacology Bulletin, 37*(2), 6-25.

Bremner, J. D., & Charney, D. S. (2010). Neural circuits in fear and anxiety. In D. J. Stein, E. Hollander, & B. O. Rothbaum (Eds.), *Textbook of anxiety disorders* (2nd ed.) (pp. 55-71). Washington, DC: American Psychiatric Publishing, Inc.

Bremner, J. D., & Vermetten, E. (2004). Neuroanatomical changes associated with pharmacotherapy in posttraumatic stress disorder. *Annals of the New York Academy of Sciences, 1032*, 154-157.

Breslau, N. (2001). The epidemiology of posttraumatic stress disorder: What is the extent of the problem? *Journal of Clinical Psychiatry, 62*(Suppl 17), 16-22.

Breslau, N. (2002). Epidemiologic studies of trauma, posttraumatic stress disorder and other psychiatric disorders. *Canadian Journal of Psychiatry, 47*, 923-929.

Breslau, N. (2009). The epidemiology of trauma, PTSD, and other posttrauma disorders. *Trauma Violence & Abuse, 10*(3), 198-210.

Breslau, N., Chilcoat, H. D., Kessler, R. C., et al. (1999). Vulnerability to assaultive violence: Further specification of the sex difference in posttraumatic stress disorder. *Psychological Medicine, 29*, 813-821.

Breslau, N., Davis, G. C., Andreski, P., et al. (1991). Traumatic events and posttraumatic stress disorder in an urban population of young adults. *Archives of General Psychiatry, 48*, 216-222.

Breslau, N., & Kessler, R. C. (2001). The stressor criterion in DSM-IV posttraumatic stress disorder: An empirical investigation. *Biological Psychiatry, 50*, 699-704.

Breslau, N., Kessler, R. C., Chilcoat, H. D., et al. (1998a). Trauma and posttraumatic stress disorder in the community: The 1996 Detroit Area survey of trauma. *Archives of General Psychiatry, 55*, 626-632.

Breslau, N., Kessler, R. C., & Peterson, E. L. (1998b). Posttraumatic stress disorder assessment with a structured interview: Reliability and concordance with a standardized clinical interview. *International Journal of Methods in Psychiatric Research, 7*, 121-127.

Breslau, N., Peterson, E. L., Kessler, R. C., et al. (1999). Short screening scale for DSM-IV posttraumatic stress disorder. *American Journal of Psychiatry, 156*, 908-911.

Breslau, N., Peterson, E. L., Poisson, L. M., et al. (2004). Estimating post-traumatic stress disorder in the community: Lifetime perspective and the impact of typical traumatic events. *Psychological Medicine, 34*, 889-898.

Brewin, C. R. (2005). Systematic review of screening instruments for adults at risk of PTSD. *Journal of Traumatic Stress, 18*(1), 53-62.

Brewin, C. R., Andrews, B., & Rose, S. (2003). Diagnostic overlap between acute stress disorder and PTSD in victims of violent crime. *American Journal of Psychiatry, 160*, 783-785.

Brewin, C. R., Andrews, B., Rose, S., et al. (1999). Acute stress disorder and posttraumatic stress disorder in victims of violent crimes. *American Journal of Psychiatry, 156*, 360-366.

Brewin, C. R., Andrews, B., & Valentine, J. D. (2000). Meta-analysis of risk factors for posttraumatic stress disorder in trauma-exposed adults. *Journal of Counseling and Clinical Psychology, 68*(5), 748-766.

Brewin, C. R., Dalgleish, T., & Joseph, S. (1996). A dual representation theory of posttraumatic stress disorder. *Psychological Review, 103*, 670-686.

Briere, J., & Runtz, M. G. (1989). The Trauma Symptoms Checklist (TSD-33): Early data on a new scale. *Journal of Interpersonal Violence, 4*, 151-163.

Brunello, N., Davidson, J. R., Deahl, M., et al. (2001). Posttraumatic stress disorder: Diagnosis and epidemiology, comorbidity and social consequences, biology and treatment. *Neuropsychobiology, 43*(3), 150-162.

Brunet, A., Orr, S. P., Tremblay, J., et al. (2008). Effect of post-retrieval propranolol on psychophysiologic responding during subsequent script-driven traumatic imagery in post-traumatic stress disorder. *Journal of Psychiatric Research, 42*(6), 503-506.

Bryant, R. A., & Guthrie, R. M. (2005). Maladaptive appraisals as a risk factor for posttraumatic stress: A study of trainee firefighters. *Psychological Science, 16*(10), 749-752.

Bryant, R. A., Harvey, A. G., Dang, S. T., et al. (1998). Assessing acute stress disorder: Psychometric properties of a structured clinical interview. *Psychological Assessment, 10*, 215-220.

Bryant, R. A., Harvey, A. G., Guthrie, R. M., et al. (2000). A prospective study of psychophysiological arousal, acute stress disorder and posttraumatic stress disorder. *Journal of Abnormal Psychology, 109*, 341-344.

Bryant, R. A., Mastrodomenico, J., Felmingham, K. L., et al. (2008). Treatment of acute stress disorder. *Archives of General Psychiatry, 65*(6), 659-667.

Bryant, B., Mayou, R., Wiggs, L., et al. (2004). Psychological consequences of road traffic accidents for children and their mothers. *Psychological Medicine, 34*, 335-346.

Bryant, R. A., Moulds, M. M., Guthrie, R. M., et al. (2003a). Treating acute stress disorder following mild traumatic brain injury. *The American Journal of Psychiatry, 160*(3), 585-587.

Bryant, R. A., Moulds, M. M., Nixon, R. V., et al. (2003b). Cognitive behaviour therapy of acute stress disorder: A four-year follow-up. *Behavioral Research and Therapy, 41*, 489-494.

Bryant, R. A., Sackville, T., Dang, S. T., et al. (1999). Treating acute stress disorder: An evaluation of cognitive behavior therapy and supportive counseling techniques. *American Journal of Psychiatry, 156*, 1780-1786.

Bugg, A., Turpin, G., Mason, S., et al. (2008). A randomized controlled trial of the effectiveness of writing as a self-help intervention for traumatic injury patients at risk of developing post-traumatic stress disorder. *Behaviour Research and Therapy, 47*(1), 6-12.

Burnett, P., Middleton, W., Raphael, B., et al. (1997). Measuring core bereavement phenomena. *Psychological Medicine, 27*(1), 49-57.

Busuttil, W., Turnbull, G. J., Neal, L. A., et al. (1995). Incorporating psychological debriefing techniques within a brief group psychotherapy programme for the treatment of post-traumatic stress disorder. *British Journal of Psychiatry, 167*, 495-502.

Cahill, S. P., Carrigan, M. H., Frueh, B. C. (1999). Does EMDR work? And if so, why? A critical review of controlled outcome and dismantling research. *Journal of Anxiety Disorders, 13*, 5-33.

Cahill, L., Prins, B., Weber, M., et al. (1994). Beta-adrenergic activation and memory for emotional events. *Nature, 371*, 702-704.

Cardozo, B. L., Kaiser, R., Gotway, C. A., et al. (2003). Mental health, social functioning, and feelings of hatred and revenge of Kosovar Albanians one year after the war in Kosovo. *Journal of Traumatic Stress, 16*, 351–360.

Carlier, I. V. (2000). Critical incident stress debriefing. In R. Yehuda (Ed.), *International handbook of human response to trauma. The Plenum series on stress and coping* (pp. 379-387). New York: Kluwer Academic/Plenum Publishers.

Carlier, I. V., Voerman, A. E., & Gersons, B. P. (2000). The influence of occupational debriefing on posttraumatic stress symptomatology in traumatized police officers. *British Journal of Medical Psychology, 73*, 87-98.

Carlson, E. B., & Rosser-Hogan, R. (1991). Trauma experiences, posttraumatic stress, dissociation, and depression in Cambodian refugees. *American Journal of Psychiatry, 148*, 1548-1551.

Carty, J., O'Donnell, M. L., & Creamer, M. (2006). Delayed-onset PTSD: A prospective study of injury survivors. *Journal of Affective Disorders, 90*(2-3), 257-261.

Carver, C. S. (1997). You want to measure coping but your protocol's too long: Consider the Brief COPE. *International Journal of Behavioral Medicine, 4*, 92-100.

Cloak, N. L., & Edwards, P. (2004). Psychological first aid: Emergency care for terrorism and disaster survivors. *Current Psychiatry, 3*(5), 13-23.

Cohen, J. A. (2003). Treating acute posttraumatic reactions in children and adolescents. *Biological Psychiatry, 53*, 827-833.

Cohen, S., Kamarck, T., & Mermelstein, R. (1983). A global measure of perceived stress. *Journal of Health and Social Behavior, 24*, 385-396.

Connor, K. M., Davidson, J. R. T., & Lee, L. (2003). Spirituality, resilience and anger in survivors of violent trauma: A community survey. *Journal of Traumatic Stress, 16*(5), 487-494.

Connor, K. M., Sutherland, S. M., Tupler, L. A., et al. (1999). Fluoxetine in post-traumatic stress disorder: Randomized, double-blind study. *British Journal of Psychiatry, 175*, 17-22.

Cooper, J., Carty, J., & Creamer, M. (2005). Pharmacotherapy for posttraumatic stress disorder: Empirical review and clinical recommendations. *Australian and New Zealand Journal of Psychiatry, 39*, 674-682.

Copeland, M. E. (2002). *Dealing with the effects of trauma: A self-help guide.* Rockville, MD: U.S. Department of Health and Human Services, Substance Abuse and Mental Health Services Administration, Center for Mental Health Services.

Crockett, B. A., & Davidson, J. R. T. (2002). Pharmacotherapy for posttraumatic stress disorder. In D. J. Stein & E. Hollander (Eds.), *The American psychiatric publishing textbook of anxiety disorders* (pp. 387-402). Washington, DC: American Psychiatric Publishing, Inc.

Cukor, J., Olden, M., Lee, F., et al. (2010). Evidence-based treatments for PTSD, new directions, and special challenges. *Annals of the New York Academy of Sciences, 1208*(2), 82.

Cukor, J., Spitalnick, J., Difede, J., et al. (2009). Emerging treatments for PTSD. *Clinical Psychology Review, 29*, 715-726.

Danielson, C. K., Macdonald, A., Amstadter, A. B., et al. (2010). Risky behaviors and depression in conjunction with—or in the absence of—lifetime history of PTSD among sexually abused adolescents. *Child Maltreatment, 15*(1), 101-107.

Davidson, J., Baldwin, D., Stein, D. J., et al. (2006). Treatment of posttraumatic stress disorder with venlafaxine extended release: A 6-month randomized controlled trial. *Archives of General Psychiatry, 63*(10), 1158-1165.

Davidson, J. R., Book, S. W., Colket, J. T., et al. (1997a). Assessment of a new self-rating scale for post-traumatic stress disorder. *Psychological Medicine, 27*, 153-160.

Davidson, J. R., & Colket, J. T. (1997b). The eight-item treatment-outcome post-traumatic stress disorder scale: A brief measure to assess treatment outcomes in post-traumatic stress disorder. *International Clinical Psychopharmacology, 12*(1), 41-45.

Davidson, J. R., & Connor, K. M. (2004). Treatment of anxiety disorders. In A. F. Schatzberg & C. B. Nemeroff (Eds.), *The American psychiatric publishing textbook of psychopharmacology* (3rd ed.) (pp. 913-934). Washington, DC: American Psychiatric Publishing, Inc.

Davidson, J. R., Connor, K. M., & Zhang, W. (2009). Treatment of anxiety disorders. In A. F. Schatzberg & C. B. Nemeroff (Eds.), *The American psychiatric publishing textbook of psychopharmacology* (4th ed.) (pp. 1171-1199). Washington, DC: American Psychiatric Publishing, Inc.

Davidson, J. R., Hughes, D., Blazer, D. G., et al. (1991). Post-traumatic stress disorder in the community: An epidemiological study. *Psychological Medicine, 21*, 713-721.

Davidson, J. R., Kudler, H., Saunders, W. B., et al. (1993). Predicting response to amitriptyline in posttraumatic stress disorder. *American Journal of Psychiatry, 150*, 1024-1029.

Davidson, J. R., Kudler, H., Smith, R., et al. (1990). Treatment of posttraumatic stress disorder with amitriptyline and placebo. *Archives of General Psychiatry, 47*, 259-266.

Davidson, J. R., Landerman, L. R., Farfel, G. M., et al. (2002). Characterizing the effects of sertraline in post-traumatic stress disorder. *Psychological Medicine, 32*, 661-670.

Davidson, J. R., Pearlstein, T., Londborg, P., et al. (2001a). Efficacy of sertraline in preventing relapse of post-traumatic stress disorder: Results of a 28-week double-blind, placebo-controlled study. *American Journal of Psychiatry, 158*, 1974-1981.

Davidson, J. R., Rothbaum, B. O., van der Kolk, B. A., et al. (2001b). Multicenter double-blind comparison of sertraline and placebo in the treatment of posttraumatic stress disorder. *Archives of General Psychiatry, 58*, 485-492.

Davidson, P. R., & Parker, K. C. H. (2001). Eye movement desensitization and reprocessing (EMDR): A meta-analysis. *Journal of Consulting and Clinical Psychology, 69*, 305-316.

Davis, M., Barad, M., Otto, M., et al. (2006). Combining pharmacotherapy with cognitive behavioral therapy: Traditional and new approaches. *Journal of Traumatic Stress, 19*(5), 571-620.

DeBellis, M. D., & Kuchibhatla, M. (2006). Cerebellar volumes in pediatric maltreatment-related posttraumatic stress disorder. *Biological Psychiatry, 60*(7), 697-703.

Debiec, J., & LeDoux, J. (2009). The amygdala and the neural pathways of fear. In P. J. Shiromani, T. M. Keane, & J. E. LeDoux (Eds.), *Post-traumatic stress disorder: Basic science and clinical practice* (pp. 23-38). New York: Humana Press.

deVries, M. W. (2006). Trauma in cultural perspective. In B. A. van der Kolk, A. C. McFarlane, & L. Weisaeth (Eds.), *Traumatic stress: The effects of overwhelming experience on mind, body, and society* (pp. 300-413). New York: Guilford Press.

Dogan-Ates, A. (2010). Developmental differences in children's and adolescents' post-disaster reactions. *Issues in Mental Health Nursing, 31,* 470-476.

Ehlers, A., & Clark, D. M. (2003). Early psychological interventions for adult survivors of trauma: A review. *Biological Psychiatry, 53,* 817-826.

Eidelman, I., Seedat, S., & Stein, D. J. (2000). Risperidone in the treatment of acute stress disorder in physically traumatized in-patients. *Depression and Anxiety, 11,* 187-188.

Elklit, A., & Brink, I. (2003). Acute stress disorder in physical assault victims visiting a Danish emergency ward. *Violence and Victims, 18*(4), 461-472.

Elklit, A., & Petersen, T. (2008). Exposure to traumatic events among adolescents in four nations. *Torture, 18*(1), 2-11.

Epp, A. M., & Dobson, K. S. (2010). The evidence base for cognitive-behavioral therapy. In K. S. Dobson (Ed.), *Handbook of cognitive-behavioral therapies* (3rd ed.) (pp. 39-73). New York: Guilford Press.

Erbes, C. R., Polusny, M. A., MacDermid, S. M., et al. (2008). Couple therapy with combat veterans and their partners. *Journal of Clinical Psychology, 64*(8), 972-983.

Eriksson, N., & Lundin, T. (1996). Early traumatic stress reactions among Swedish survivors of the M. S. Estonia disaster. *The British Journal of Psychiatry, 169*(6), 713-716.

Faravelli, C., Giugni, A., Salvatori, S., et al. (2004). Psychopathology after rape. *American Journal of Psychiatry, 16*(8), 1483-1485.

First, M. B., Frances, A., & Pincus, H. A. (2002). *DSM-IV-TR handbook of differential diagnosis.* Washington, DC: American Psychiatric Publishing, Inc.

First, M. B., & Tasman, A. (2004). *DSM-IV-TR mental disorders: Diagnosis, etiology, and treatment.* West Sussex, UK: John Wiley & Sons, Ltd.

Fischer, A., & Tsai, L-H (2010). Counteracting molecular pathways regulating the reduction of fear: Implications for the treatment of anxiety diseases. In P. J. Shiromani, T. M. Keane, & J. E. LeDoux (Eds.), *Post-traumatic stress disorder: Basic science and clinical practice* (pp. 79-103). New York: Humana Press.

Flannery, R. B., Jr., & Everly, G. S., Jr. (2000). Crisis intervention: A review. *International Journal of Emergency Mental Health, 2,* 119-125.

Foa, E. B., Huppert, J. D., & Cahill, S. (2006). Emotional processing theory: An update. In B. O. Rothbaum (Ed.), *Pathological anxiety: Emotional processing in etiology and treatment* (pp. 3-24). New York: Guilford Press.

Foa, E. B., & Kozak, M. J. (1986). Emotional processing of fear: Exposure to corrective information. *Psychological Bulletin, 99*(1), 20-35.

Foa, E. B., & Meadows, E. A. (1997). Psychosocial treatments for posttraumatic stress disorder: A critical review. *Annual Review of Psychology, 48,* 449-480.

Foa, E. B., Riggs, D. S., Dancu, C. V., et al. (1993). Reliability and validity of a brief instrument for assessing post-traumatic stress disorder. *Journal of Traumatic Stress, 6,* 459-473.

Forbes, D., Creamer, M. C., Phelps, A. J., et al. (2007). Treating adults with acute stress disorder and post-traumatic stress disorder in general practice: A clinical update. *The Medical Journal of Australia, 187*(2), 120-123.

Forester, P. L., Schoenfeld, F. B., Marmar, C. R., et al (1995). Lithium for irritability in posttraumatic stress disorder. *Journal of Traumatic Stress, 8,* 143-149.

Fraley, R. C., Fazzari, D. A., Bonanno, G. A., et al. (2006). Attachment and psychological adaptation in high exposure survivors of the September 11th attack on the World Trade Center. *Personality & Social Psychology Bulletin, 32*(4), 538-551.

Frances, K. (2002). *Crisis intervention: A handbook of immediate person-to-person help* (4th ed.). Springfield, IL: Charles C Thomas Publisher, Ltd.

Frans, O., Rimmo, P. A., Aberg, L., et al. (2005). Trauma exposure and post-traumatic stress disorder in the general population. *Acta Psychiatrica Scandinavica, 111*(4), 291-299.

Frewen, P., & Lanius, R. (2006). Toward a psychobiology of post-traumatic self-dysregulation: Reexperiencing, hyperarousal, dissociation, and emotional numbing. *Annals of the New York Academy of Sciences, 1071,* 110-124.

Friedman, M. J., & Karam, E. G. (2009). Posttraumatic stress disorder. In G. Andrews, D. S. Charney, P. J. Sirovatka, et al. (Eds.), *Stress-induced and fear circuitry disorders* (pp. 3-29). Washington, DC: American Psychiatric Publishing, Inc.

Frommberger, U., Stieglitz, R. D., Nyberg, E., et al. (2004). Comparison between paroxetine and behaviour therapy in patients with posttraumatic stress disorder (PTSD): A pilot study. *International Journal of Psychiatry in Clinical Practice, 8,* 19-23.

Frueh, B. C., Turner, S. M., & Beidel, D. C. (1995). Exposure therapy for combat-related PTSD: A critical review. *Clinical Psychology Review, 15,* 799-817.

Frueh, B. C., Turner, S. M., Beidel, D. C., et al. (1996). Trauma management therapy: A preliminary evaluation of a multicomponent behavioral treatment for chronic combat-related PTSD. *Behavior Research Therapy, 34*(7), 533-543.

Fullerton, C. S., Ursano, R. J., & Wang, L. M. S. (2004). Acute stress disorder, posttraumatic stress disorder and depression in disaster or rescue workers. *American Journal of Psychiatry, 161*(8), 1370-1376.

Gabbard, G. O. (2005). *Psychodynamic psychiatry in clinical practice* (4th ed.). Washington, DC: American Psychiatric Publishing, Inc.

Gaffney, D. (2008). Families, schools, and disaster: The mental health consequences of catastrophic events. *Family Community Health, 31*(1), 44-53.

Galea, S., Nandi, A., & Viahov, D. (2005). The epidemiology of post-traumatic stress disorder after disasters. *Epidemiological Review, 27,* 78-91.

Gelpin, E., Bonne, O., Peri, T., et al. (1996). Treatment of recent trauma survivors with benzodiazepines: A prospective study. *Journal of Clinical Psychiatry, 57,* 390-394.

Geschwind, N., Peeters, F., Jacobs, N., et al. (2010). Meeting risk with resilience: High daily life reward experience preserves mental health. *Acta Psychiatrica Scandinavica, 122*(2), 129-138.

Glass, N., Perrin, N., Campbell, J., et al. (2007). The protective role of tangible support on post-traumatic stress disorder symptoms in urban women survivors of violence. *Research in Nursing & Health, 30*(5), 558-568.

Goenjian, A. K., Walling, D., Steinberg, A. M., et al. (2005). A prospective study of posttraumatic stress and depressive reactions among treated and untreated adolescents 5 years after a catastrophic disaster. *American Journal of Psychiatry, 162*(12), 2302-2308.

Golier, J. A., Yehuda, R., DeSanti, S., et al. (2005). Absence of hippocampal volume differences in survivors of the Nazi Holocaust with and without PTSD. *Psychiatry Research, 139,* 53-64.

Gray, M. J., Litz, B. T., & Papa, A. (2006). Crisis debriefing: What helps, and what might not. *Current Psychiatry, 5*(10), 17-29.

Green, M. M., McFarlane, A. C., Hunter, C. E., et al. (1993). Undiagnosed posttraumatic stress disorder following motor vehicle accidents. *Medical Journal of Australia, 159*(8), 529-534.

Green, J., & Schellenberger, R. (1991). *The dynamics of health & wellness: A biopsychosocial approach.* Fort Worth, TX: Holt, Rinehart and Winston, Inc.

Gray, M. J., Litz, B. T., & Papa, A. (2006). Crisis debriefing: what helps, and what might not. *Current Psychiatry, 5*(10), 17-20, 25-29.

Gurevich, M., Devins, G. M., & Rodin, G. M. (2002). Stress response syndromes and cancer. *Psychosomatics, 43,* 259-281.

Hamblen, J., & Barnett, E. (2009). *PTSD in children and adolescents.* United States Department of Veterans Affairs, National Center for PTSD. Retrieved from http://www.ptsd.va.gov/professional/pages/ptsd_in_children_and__adolescents_overview_ for _professionals

Hamner, M. B., Brodrick, P. S., & Labbate, L. A. (2001). Gabapentin in PTSD: A retrospective clinical series of adjunctive therapy. *Annals of Clinical Psychiatry, 13*(3), 141-146.

Hamner, M. B., Deitsch, S. E., Brodrick, P. S., et al. (2003). Quetiapine treatment in patients with posttraumatic stress disorder: An open trial of adjunctive therapy. *Journal of Clinical Psychopharmacology, 23,* 15-20.

Hansell, N. (1976). *The person-in-distress.* New York: Human Sciences Press.

Harvey, A. G., & Bryant, R. A. (1999). The relationship between acute stress disorder and posttraumatic disorder: A two year prospective evaluation. *Journal of Consulting and Clinical Psychology, 67,* 985-988.

Harvey, A. G., & Bryant, R. A. (2002). Acute stress disorder: A synthesis and critique. *Psychological Bulletin, 128*(6), 886-902.

Hauff, E., & Vaglum, P. (1993). Vietnamese boat refugees: The influence of war and flight traumatization on mental health on arrival in the country of resettlement. *Acta Psychiatrica Scandinavica, 88,* 162-168.

Herman, J. L. (1992). *Trauma and recovery*. New York: Basic Books.

Hetzel, M. D., & McCanne, T. R. (2005). The rates of peritraumatic dissociation, child physical abuse and child sexual abuse in the development of posttraumatic stress disorder and adult victimization. *Child Abuse & Neglect, 29*(8), 915-930.

Hobfoll, S. E., & deVries, M. W. (Eds.). (1995). *Extreme stress and communities: When culture fails.* Norwell, MA: Kluwer.

Hofmann, S. G., Meuret, A. E., Smits, J. A., et al. (2006). Augmentation of exposure therapy with D-cycloserine for social anxiety disorder. *Archives of General Psychiatry, 63*(3), 298-304.

Hogberg, G., Pagani, M., Sundin, O., et al. (2007). On treatment with eye movement desensitization and reprocessing of chronic post-traumatic stress disorder in public transportation workers—A randomized controlled trial. *Nordic Journal of Psychiatry, 61*(1), 54-61.

Hogberg, G., Pagani, M., Sundin, O., et al. (2008). Treatment of post-traumatic stress disorder with eye movement desensitization and reprocessing: Outcome is stable in 35-month follow-up. *Psychiatry Research, 159*(1), 101-108.

Holbrook, T. L., Galarneau, M. R., Dye, J. L., et al. (2010). Morphine use after combat injury in Iraq and posttraumatic stress disorder. *The New England Journal of Medicine, 362*(2), 110-117.

Hollander, E., & Simeon, D. (2008). Anxiety disorders. In R. E. Hales, S. C. Yudofsky, & G. O. Gabbard (Eds.), *The American psychiatric publishing textbook of psychiatry* (5th ed.) (pp. 505-607). Washington, DC: American Psychiatric Publishing, Inc.

Hollander, E., & Simeon, D. (2011). Anxiety disorders. In R. E. Hales, S. C. Yudofsky, & G. O. Gabbard (Eds.), *Essentials of psychiatry* (3rd ed.) (pp. 185-228). Washington, DC: American Psychiatric Publishing, Inc.

Hollifield, M., Sinclair-Lian, N., Warner, T., et al. (2007). Acupuncture for posttraumatic stress disorder: A randomized controlled pilot trial. *Journal of Nervous & Mental Disease, 195*(6), 504-513.

Horowitz, M. J. (2003). *Treatment of stress response syndromes.* Washington, DC: American Psychiatric Publishing, Inc.

Horowitz, M., Sonneborn, D., Sugahara, C., et al. (1995). Self-regard: A new measure. *American Journal of Psychiatry, 153*, 382-385.

Horowitz, L. M., Wang, P. S., Koocher, G. P., et al. (2001). Detecting suicide risk in a pediatric emergency department: Development of a brief screening tool. *Pediatrics, 107*, 1133-1137.

Horowitz, M. J., Wilner, N., & Alvarez, W. (1979). Impact of event scale: A measure of subjective stress. *Psychosomatic Medicine, 41*, 209-218.

Institute of Medicine (2008). *Treatment of posttraumatic stress disorder: An assessment of the evidence.* Washington, DC: National Academies Press.

Janoff-Bulman, R. (1992). *Shattered assumptions: Towards a new psychology of trauma.* New York: Free Press.

Kangas, M., Henry, J. L., & Bryant, R. A. (2005). The relationship between acute stress disorder and posttraumatic stress disorder following cancer. *Journal of Consulting and Clinical Psychology, 73*(2), 360-364.

Karatzias, A., Power, K., McGoldrick, T., et al. (2007). Predicting treatment outcome on three measures for post-traumatic stress disorder. *European Archives of Psychiatry Clinical Neuroscience, 257*, 240-246.

Keane, T. M., Marx, B. P., & Sloan, D. M. (2009). Post-traumatic stress disorder: Definition, prevalence, and risk factors. In P. J. Shiromani, T. M. Keane, & J. E. LeDoux (Eds.), *Post-traumatic stress disorder: Basic science and clinical practice* (pp. 1-19). New York: Humana Press.

Keck, P. E., Jr., McElroy, S. L., & Friedman, L. M. (1992). Valproate and carbamazepine in the treatment of panic and posttraumatic stress disorders, withdrawal states and behavioral dyscontrol syndromes. *Journal of Clinical Psychopharmacology, 12*, 36S-41S.

Kellner, M. (1986). The brief depression rating scale. In N. Sartorius & T. A. Ban (Eds.), *Assessment of depression* (pp. 179-183). New York: Springer-Verlag.

Kessler, R. C. (2000). Posttraumatic stress disorder: The burden to the individual and to society. *Journal of Clinical Psychiatry, 61*(Suppl 5), 4-12.

Kessler, R. C., Berglund, P., Demler, O., et al. (2005). Lifetime prevalence and age of onset distributions of DSM-IV disorders in the National Comorbidity Survey Replication. *Archives of General Psychiatry, 62*, 592-602.

Kessler, R. C., Sonnega, R., Bromet, E. J., et al. (1995). Posttraumatic stress disorder in the National Comorbidity Survey. *Archives of General Psychiatry, 52*, 1048-1060.

Kilpatrick, D. G., Ruggiero, K. J., Acierno, R., et al. (2003). Violence and risk of PTSD, major depression, substance abuse/dependence and comorbidity: Results from the National Survey of Adolescents. *Journal of Counseling & Clinical Psychology, 71*(4), 692-700.

Kilpatrick, D. G., Saunders, B. E., Veronen, L. J., et al. (1987). Criminal victimization: Lifetime prevalence, reporting to police, and psychological impact. *Crime and Delinquency, 33*, 479-489.

King, D. W., Taft, C. T., King, L. A., et al. (2007). Directionality of the association between social support and posttraumatic stress disorder: A longitudinal investigation. *Journal of Allied Social Psychology, 36*, 2980-2992.

Kinzie, J. D., Sack, R. L., & Riley, C. M. (1994). The polysomnographic effects of clonidine on sleep disorders in posttraumatic stress disorder: A pilot study with Cambodian patients. *Journal of Nervous and Mental Disorders, 182*, 585-587.

Kitayama, N., Quinn, S., & Bremner, J. D. (2006). Smaller volume of anterior cingulate cortex in abuse-related posttraumatic stress disorder. *Journal of Affective Disorders, 90*, 171-174.

Klein, D. N., Shankman, S. A., & McFarland, B. R. (2006). Classification of mood disorders. In D. J. Stein, D. J. Kupfer, & A. F. Schatzberg (Eds.), *The American psychiatric publishing textbook of mood disorders* (pp. 17-32). Washington, DC: American Psychiatric Publishing, Inc.

Kluft, R. P., Bloom, S. L., & Kinzie, J. D. (2000). Treating traumatized patients and victims of violence. *New Direction in Mental Health Services, 86*, 79-102.

Koenen, K. C., Harley, R., Lyons, M., et al. (2002). A twin registry study of familial and individual risk factors for trauma exposure and posttraumatic stress disorder. *The Journal of Nervous and Mental Disease, 190*(4), 209-218.

Koenen, K. C., Moffitt, T. E., Poulton, R., et al. (2007). Early childhood factors associated with the development of post-traumatic stress disorder: Results from a longitudinal birth cohort. *Psychological Medicine, 37*, 181-192.

Kolb, L. C., Burris, B. C., & Griffiths, S. (1984). Propranolol and clonidine in the treatment of the chronic post traumatic stress disorders of war. In B. van der Kolk (Ed.), *Post-traumatic stress disorder: Psychological and biological sequelae.* Washington, DC: American Psychiatric Publishing, Inc.

Koopman, C., Classen, C., Cardena, E., et al. (1995). When disaster strikes, acute stress disorder may follow. *Journal of Traumatic Stress, 8*, 29-46.

Koopman, C., Classen, C., & Spiegel, D. (1996). Dissociative responses in the immediate aftermath of the Oakland/Berkeley firestorm. *Journal of Traumatic Stress, 9*, 521-540.

Kosten, R. T., Frank, J. B., Dan, E., et al. (1991). Pharmacotherapy for posttraumatic stress disorder using phenelzine or imipramine. *Journal of Nervous and Mental Diseases, 179*, 366-370.

Krakow, B., Hollifield, M., Johnston, L., et al. (2001). Imagery rehearsal therapy for chronic nightmares in sexual assault survivors with posttraumatic stress disorder: A randomized controlled trial. *Journal of the American Medical Association, 286*, 537-545.

Krakow, B., Hollifield, M., Schrader, R., et al. (2000). A controlled study of imagery rehearsal for chronic nightmares in sexual assault survivors with PTSD: A preliminary report. *Journal of Traumatic Stress, 13*(4), 589-609.

Krupnick, J. L., Green, B. L., Stockton, P., et al. (2008). Group interpersonal psychotherapy for low-income women with posttraumatic stress disorder. *Psychotherapy Research, 18*(5), 497-507.

Kubany, E. S., Hill, E. E., Owens, J. A., et al. (2004). Cognitive trauma therapy for battered women with PTSD (CTT-BW). *Journal of Consulting Clinical Psychology, 72*, 3-18.

Kulka, R. A., Schlenger, W. E., Fairbank, J. A., et al. (1990). *Trauma and the Vietnam War Generation: Report of findings from the National Vietnam Veterans Readjustment Study.* New York: Brunner/Mazel.

Lange, A., Rietdijk, D., Hudcovicova, M., et al. (2003). Interapy: A controlled randomized trial of the standardized treatment of posttraumatic stress through the internet. *Journal of Counseling and Clinical Psychology, 71*(5), 901-909.

Lange, A., van de Ven, J. P., Schrieken, B., et al. (2001). Interapy, treatment of posttraumatic stress through the internet: A controlled trial. *Journal of Behavioral Therapy and Experimental Psychiatry, 32*, 73-90.

LeDoux, J. E. (2002). *Synaptic self: How our brains become who we are.* New York: Viking Press.

LeDoux, J. E., & Gorman, J. M. (2001). A call to action: Overcoming anxiety through active coping. *American Journal of Psychiatry, 158*(12), 1953-1995.

Lewis, J. (2002). Mirtazepine for PTSD. *American Journal of Psychiatry, 159,* 1948-1949.

Lima, B. R., Chavez, H., Samniego, N., et al. (1989). Disaster severity and emotional disturbance: Implications for primary mental health care in developing countries. *Acta Psychiatrica Scandinavica, 79,* 74-82.

Litz, B. T., Engel, C. C., Bryant, R. A., et al. (2007). A randomized, controlled proof-of-concept trial of an internet-based, therapist-assisted self-management treatment for posttraumatic stress disorder. *American Journal of Psychiatry, 164*(11), 1676-1683.

Londborg, P. D., Hegel, M. T., Goldstein, S., et al. (2001). Sertraline treatment of posttraumatic stress disorder: Results of 24 weeks of open-label continuation treatment. *Journal of Clinical Psychiatry, 62,* 325-331.

Lundin, T. (1994). The treatment of acute trauma: Posttraumatic stress disorder prevention. *Psychiatric Clinics of North American, 17,* 385-391.

Maher, M. J., Rego, S. A., & Asnis, G. M. (2006). Sleep disturbances in patients with posttraumatic stress disorder: Epidemiology, impact and approaches to management. *CNS Drugs, 20*(7), 567-590.

Maldonado, J. R., & Spiegel, D. (2008). Dissociative disorders. In R. E. Hales, S. C. Yudofsky, & G. O. Gabbard (Eds.), *The American psychiatric publishing textbook of psychiatry* (5th ed.) (pp. 665-710). Washington, DC: American Psychiatric Publishing, Inc.

Manger, T. A., & Motta, R. W. (2005). The impact of an exercise program on posttraumatic stress disorder, anxiety and depression. *International Journal of Emergency Mental Health, 7*(1), 49-57.

Marmar, C. R. (1991). Brief dynamic psychotherapy of post-traumatic stress disorder. *Psychiatry Annuals, 21,* 405-414.

Marmar, C. R., & Spiegel, D. (2007). Posttraumatic stress disorder and acute stress disorder. In G. O. Gabbard (Ed.), *Gabbard's treatments of psychiatric disorders* (4th ed.) (pp. 517-536). Washington, DC: American Psychiatric Publishing, Inc.

Marshall, R. D., Beebe, K. L., Oldham, M., et al. (2001). Efficacy and safety of paroxetine treatment for chronic PTSD: A fixed-dose, placebo-controlled study. *American Journal of Psychiatry, 158,* 1982-1988.

Marshall, R. D., Lewis-Fernandez, R., Blanco, C., et al. (2007). A controlled trial of paroxetine for chronic PTSD, dissociation, and interpersonal problems in mostly minority adults. *Depression and Anxiety, 24,* 77-84.

Marshall, G. N., Schell, T. L., Elliott, M. N., et al. (2005). *Mental health of Cambodian refugees two decades after resettlement in the United States* (Vol. 294). Chicago: American Medical Association.

Martenyi, F., Brown, E. B., Zhang, H., et al. (2002). Fluoxetine versus placebo in posttraumatic stress disorder. *Journal of Clinical Psychiatry, 63,* 199-206.

Marx, B. P. (2009). Posttraumatic stress disorder and Operations Enduring Freedom and Iraqi Freedom: Progress in a time of controversy. *Clinical Psychology Review, 29*(8), 671-673.

Masand, P. S. (2003). Tolerability and adherence issues in antidepressant therapy. *Clinical Therapy, 25,* 2289-2304.

Mayou, R. A., Ehlers, A., & Hobbs, M. (2000). Psychological debriefing for road traffic accident victims. *British Journal of Psychiatry, 176,* 589-593.

McFarlane, A. C. (1988). The longitudinal course of posttraumatic morbidity: The range of outcomes and their predictors. *Journal of Nervous and Mental Disease, 176,* 4-14.

McFarlane, A. C. (2002). Phenomenology of posttraumatic stress. In D. J. Stein, E. Hollander, & B. O. Rothbaum (Eds.), *Textbook of anxiety disorders* (2nd ed.) (pp. 547-565). Washington, DC: American Psychiatric Publishing, Inc.

McFarlane, A. C. (2010). Phenomenology of posttraumatic stress disorder. In D. J. Stein, E. Hollander, & B. O. Rothbaum (Eds.), *Textbook of anxiety disorders* (2nd ed.) (pp. 547-565). Washington, DC: American Psychiatric Publishing, Inc.

McFarlane, A. C., & de Girolamo, G. (2006). The nature of traumatic stressors and the epidemiology of posttraumatic reactions. In B. A. van der Kolk, A. C. McFarlane, & L. Weisaeth (Eds.), *Traumatic stress: The effects of overwhelming experience on mind, body, and society* (pp. 129-154). New York: Guilford Press.

McFarlane, A. C., & van der Kolk, B. A. (2006). Trauma and its challenge to society. In B. A. van der Kolk, A. C. McFarlane, & L. Weisaeth (Eds.), *Traumatic stress: The effects of overwhelming experience on mind, body, and society* (pp. 24-46). New York: Guilford Press.

McGhee, L. L., Maani, C. V., Garza, T. H., et al. (2009a). The effect of propranolol on posttraumatic stress disorder in burned service members. *Journal of Burn Care Research, 30,* 92-97.

McGhee, L. L., Maani, C. V., Garza, T. H., et al. (2009b). The correlation between ketamine and posttraumatic stress disorder in burned service members. *The Journal of Trauma, Injury, Infection and Critical Care, 64,* S195-S199.

McNally, R. J. (2003). Psychological mechanisms in acute response to trauma. *Biological Psychiatry, 53,* 779-788.

Meiser-Stedman, R., Yule, W., Smith, P., et al. (2005). Acute stress disorder and posttraumatic stress disorder in children and adolescents involved in assaults or motor vehicle accidents. *American Journal of Psychiatry, 162,* 1381-1383.

Mezzich, J. E., Caracci, G., Fabrega, H., et al. (2009). Cultural formulation guidelines. *Transcultural Psychiatry, 46*(3), 383-405.

Mikulincer, M., Florian, V., & Weller, A. (1993). Attachment styles, coping strategies and posttraumatic psychological distress: The impact of the Gulf War in Israel. *Journal of Personality and Social Psychology, 64,* 817-826.

Miller, K. E., & Rasmussen, A. (2009). War exposure, daily stressors, and mental health in conflict and post-conflict settings. Bridging the divide between trauma-focused and psychosocial frameworks. *Social Science & Medicine, 70*(2010), 8-16.

Miller, M. W., Wolf, E. J., Fabricant, L., et al. (2009). Low basal cortisol and startle responding as possible biomarkers of PTSD: The influence of internalizing and externalizing comorbidity. In P. J. Shiromani, T. M. Keane, & J. E. LeDoux (Eds.), *Post-traumatic stress disorder: Basic science and clinical practice* (pp. 277-293). New York: Humana Press.

Mitchell, J. T., & Everly, G. S. (2000). Critical incident stress management and critical incident stress debriefings: Evolution, effects and outcomes. In J. P. Wilson (Ed.), *Psychological debriefing: Theory, practice and evidence* (pp. 71-90). New York: Cambridge University Press.

Moak, Z. B., & Agrawal, A. (2009). The association between perceived interpersonal social support and physical and mental health: Results from the national epidemiological survey on alcohol and related conditions. *Journal of Public Health, 32*(2), 191-201.

Modestin, J., Furrer, R., & Malti, T. (2005). Different traumatic experiences are associated with different pathologies. *Psychiatric Quarterly, 76*(1), 19-32.

Mohamed, S., & Rosenheck, R. (2008). Pharmacotherapy of PTSD in the U.S. Department of Veterans Affairs: Diagnostic-and symptom-guided drug selection. *Journal of Clinical Psychiatry, 69,* 959-965.

Mollica, R. F., Caspi-Yavin, Y., Bollini, P., et al. (1992). The *Harvard Trauma Questionnaire:* Validating a cross-cultural instrument for measuring torture, trauma and post-traumatic stress disorder in Indochinese refugees. *Journal of Nervous & Mental Disease, 180*(2), 111-116.

Momartin, S., Silove, D., Manicavasagar, V., et al. (2004). Complicated grief in Bosnian refugees: Associations with posttraumatic stress disorder and depression. *Comprehensive Psychiatry, 45*(6), 475-482.

Monnelly, E. P., Ciraulo, D. A., Knapp, C., et al. (2003). Low-dose risperidone as adjunctive therapy for irritable aggression in posttraumatic stress disorder. *Journal of Clinical Psychopharmacology, 23,* 193-196.

Monson, C. M., Fredman, S. J., & Adair, K. C. (2008). Cognitive-behavioral conjoint therapy for PTSD: Application to Operation Enduring and Iraqi Freedom service members and veterans. *Journal of Clinical Psychology, 64*(8), 958-971.

Monson, C. M., Schnurr, P. P., Stevens, S. P., et al. (2004). Cognitive-behavioral couple's treatment for posttraumatic stress disorder: Initial findings. *Journal of Traumatic Stress, 17*(4), 341-344.

Morgan, C. A., Wang, S., Southwick, S. M., et al. (2000). Plasma neuropeptide-Y concentrations in humans exposed to military survival training. *Biological Psychiatry, 47,* 902-909.

Nagy, L. M., Morgan, C. A., Southwick, S. M., et al. (1993). Open prospective trial of fluoxetine for posttraumatic stress disorder. *Journal of Clinical Psychopharmacology, 13,* 107-113.

National Collaborating Centre for Mental Health. (2005). *Clinical guideline 26, Post-traumatic stress disorder: The management of PTSD in adults and children in primary and secondary care.* London: National Institute for Clinical Excellence.

Neria, Y., Nandi, A., & Galea, S. (2007). Post-traumatic stress disorder following disasters: A systematic review. *Psychological Medicine, 38,* 467-480.

Neuner, F., Schauer, E., Catani, C., et al. (2006). Post-tsunami stress: A study of posttraumatic stress disorder in children living in three severely affected regions in Sri Lanka. *Journal of Traumatic Stress, 19*(3), 339-347.

Nishith, P., Mechanic, M. B., & Resick, P. A. (2000). Prior interpersonal trauma: The contribution to current PTSD symptoms in female rape victims. *Journal of Abnormal Psychology, 109*, 20-25.

Norris, F. H., Friedman, M. J., Watson, P. J., et al. (2002a). 60,000 disaster victims speak: Part I: An empirical review of the empirical literature, 1981-2001. *Psychiatry, 65*(3), 207-239.

Norris, F. H., Friedman, M. J., & Watson, P. (2002b). 60,000 disaster victims speak: Part II. Summary and implications of the disaster mental health research. *Psychiatry, 65*(3), 240-251.

North, C. S., Nixon, S. J., Shariat, S., et al. (1999). Psychiatric disorders among survivors of the Oklahoma City bombing. *Journal of the American Medical Association, 282*, 755-762.

North, C. S., Pfefferbaum, B., Tiois, L., et al. (2004). The course of posttraumatic stress disorder in a follow-up study of survivors of the Oklahoma City bombing. *Annals of Clinical Psychiatry, 16*(4), 209-215.

Nutt, D. J. (2000). The psychobiology of posttraumatic stress disorder. *Journal of Clinical Psychiatry, 61*(Suppl 50), 24-29.

Nutt, D. J., & Malizia, A. L. (2004). Structural and functional brain changes in posttraumatic stress disorder. *Journal of Clinical Psychiatry, 65*(Suppl 1), 11-17.

Olszewski, T., & Varrasse, J. (2005). The neurobiology of PTSD: Implications for nursing. *Journal of Psychosocial Nursing and Mental Health Services, 43*(6), 40-47.

Orth, U., Montada, L., & Maercker, A. (2006). Feelings of revenge, retaliation motive and posttraumatic stress reactions in crime victims. *Journal of Interpersonal Violence, 21*(2), 229-243.

Osman, A., Gutierrez, P. M., Kopper, B. A., et al. (1997). The positive and negative suicide ideation inventory: Development and validation. *Psychological Reports, 82*(3 part 1), 783-793.

Otto, M. W., Hinton, D., Korbly, N. B., et al. (2003). Treatment of pharmacotherapy-refractory posttraumatic stress disorder among Cambodian refugees: A pilot study of combination treatment with cognitive-behavior therapy vs sertraline alone. *Behaviour Research and Therapy, 41*, 1271-1276.

Pastrana Jimenez, J. I., Catalina Romero, C., Garcia Dieguez, N., et al. (2007). Pharmacological treatment of acute stress disorder with propranolol and hypnotics. *Actas Espanolas de Psiquiatria, 35*(6), 351-358.

Perkonigg, A., Pfister, H., Stein, M. B., et al. (2005). Longitudinal course of posttraumatic stress disorder and posttraumatic stress disorder symptoms in a community sample of adolescents and young adults. *American Journal of Psychiatry, 162*, 1320-1327.

Perry, B. D. (2002). Childhood experiences and the expression of genetic potential: What childhood neglect tells us about nature and nurture. *Brain and Mind, 3*, 79-100.

Perry, B. D., & Pate, J. E. (1994). Neurodevelopment and the psychobiological roots of post-traumatic stress disorder. In L. F. Koziol & C. E. Stout (Eds.), *The neuropsychology of mental disorders: A practical guide* (pp. 129-146). Springfield, IL: Charles C Thomas Publisher, Ltd.

Pfefferbaum, B., Seale, T. W., McDonald, N. B., et al. (2000). Posttraumatic stress two years after the Oklahoma City bombing in youths geographically distant from the explosion. *Psychiatry, 63*, 358-370.

Pine, D. S. (2003). Developmental psychobiology and response to threats: Relevance to trauma in children and adolescents. *Biological Psychiatry, 53*, 796-808.

Pitman, R. K., & Delahanty, D. L. (2005). Conceptually driven pharmacologic approaches to acute trauma. *CNS Spectrums, 10*(2), 99-106.

Pitman, R. K., Gilbertson, M. W., Gurvits, T. V., et al. (2006). Clarifying the origin of biological abnormalities in PTSD through the study of identical twins discordant for combat exposure. *Annals of the New York Academy of Sciences, 1071*, 242-254.

Pitman, R. K., Orr, S. P., Altman, B., et al. (1996). Emotional processing and outcome of imaginal flooding therapy in Vietnam veterans with chronic posttraumatic stress disorder. *Comprehensive Psychiatry, 37*, 409-418.

Pitman, R. K., Orr, S., & Shalev, A. (1993). Once bitten, twice shy: Beyond the conditioning model of PTSD. *Biological Psychiatry, 33*, 145-146.

Pitman, R. K., Sanders, K. M., Zusman, R. M., et al. (2002). Pilot study of secondary prevention of posttraumatic stress disorder with propranolol. *Biological Psychiatry, 51*, 189-192.

Portnova, A. A. (2005). Acute mental disorders in children and adolescents held as hostages by the terrorists in Beslan [Russian]. *Zhurnal Nevrologii I Psikhiatrii Imeni S. S. Korsakova, 105*(6), 10-15.

Pynoos, R. S. (1996). Exposure to catastrophic violence and disaster in childhood. In C. R. Pfeffer (Ed.), *Severe stress and mental disturbance in children* (pp. 181-208). Washington, DC: American Psychiatric Publishing, Inc.

Pynoos, R. S., Frederick, C., Nader, K., et al. (1987). Life threat and posttraumatic stress in school-age children. *Archives of General Psychiatry, 44*, 1057-1063.

Pynoos, R. S., Steinberg, A. M., & Goenjian, A. (2006). Traumatic stress in childhood and adolescence: Recent developments and current controversies. In B. A. van der Kolk, A. C. McFarlane, & L. Weisaeth (Eds.), *Traumatic stress: The effects of overwhelming experience on mind, body, and society* (pp. 351-358). New York: Guilford Press.

Rahe, R. H. (2000). Recent life changes questionnaire (RLCQ). In T. H. Holmes (Ed.), *American psychiatric association task force for the handbook of psychiatric measures* (pp. 235-237). Washington, DC: American Psychiatric Publishing, Inc.

Rapaport, M. H., Endicott, J., & Clary, C. M. (2002). Posttraumatic stress disorder and quality of life: Results across 64 weeks of sertraline treatment. *Journal of Clinical Psychiatry, 63*, 59-65.

Raphael, B. (1986). *When disaster strikes.* New York: Basic Books.

Raskind, M. A. (2009). Pharmacologic treatment of PTSD. In P. J. Shiromani, T. M. Keane, & J. E. LeDoux (Eds.), *Post-traumatic stress disorder: Basic science and clinical practice* (pp. 337-361). New York: Humana Press.

Raskind, M. A., Dobie, D. J., Danter, E. D., et al. (2000). Posttraumatic stress disorder and quality of life: Results across 64 weeks of sertraline treatment. *Journal of Clinical Psychiatry, 63*, 59-65.

Raskind, M. A., Peskind, E. R., Hoff, D. J., et al. (2007). A parallel group placebo controlled study of prazosin for trauma nightmares and sleep disturbance in combat veterans with posttraumatic stress disorder. *Biological Psychiatry, 61*, 928-934.

Raskind, M. A., Peskind, E. R., Kanter, E. D., et al. (2003). Reduction of nightmares and other PTSD symptoms in combat veterans by prazosin: A placebo-controlled study. *American Journal of Psychiatry, 160*, 371-373.

Rauch, S. L., & Drevets, W. C. (2009). Neuroimaging and neuroanatomy of stress-induced and fear circuitry disorders. In G. Andrews, D. S. Charney, P. J. Sirovatka, et al. (Eds.), *Stress-induced and fear circuitry disorders* (pp. 215-254). Washington, DC: American Psychiatric Publishing, Inc.

Rauch, S., Shin, L., Segal, E., et al. (2003). Selectively reduced regional cortical volumes in posttraumatic stress disorder. *Neuroreport, 14*(7), 913-916.

Ravindran, L. N., & Stein, M. B. (2009). Pharmacotherapy of PTSD: Premises, principles and priorities. *Brain Research, 1299*(1), 24-39.

Reger, M. A., & Gahm, G. A. (2009). A meta-analysis of the effects of internet- and computer-based cognitive-behavioral treatments for anxiety. *Journal of Clinical Psychology, 65*(1), 53-75.

Reich, D. B., Winternitz, S., Hennen, J., et al. (2004). A preliminary study of risperidone in the treatment of posttraumatic stress disorder related to childhood abuse in women. *Journal of Clinical Psychiatry, 65*, 1601-1606.

Reyes, G., & Elhai, J. D. (2004). Psychosocial interventions in the early phases of disasters. *Psychotherapy, Theory, Research, Practice, Training, 41*(4), 399-411.

Rhoads, J., Pearman, T., & Rick, S. (2007). Clinical presentation and therapeutic interventions for posttraumatic stress disorder post-Katrina. *Archives of Psychiatric Nursing, 21*(5), 249-256.

Risse, S. C., Whitters, A., Burke, J., et al. (1990). Severe withdrawal symptoms after discontinuation of alprazolam in eight patients with combat-induced posttraumatic stress disorder. *Journal of Clinical Psychiatry, 51*, 206-209.

Rizzo, A., Reger, G., Gahm, G., et al. (2010). Virtual reality exposure therapy for combat-related PTSD. In P. J. Shiromani, T. M. Keane, & J. E. LeDoux (Eds.), *Post-traumatic stress disorder: Basic science and clinical practice* (pp. 375-399). New York: Humana Press.

Robert, R., Blakeney, P. E., Villarreal, C., et al. (1999). Imipramine treatment in pediatric burn patients with symptoms of acute stress disorder: A pilot study. *Journal of the American Academy of Child and Adolescent Psychiatry, 38*, 873-882.

Robert, S., Hammer, M. B., Chose, S., et al. (2005). Quetiapine improves sleep disturbances in combat trauma veterans with PTSD: Sleep data from a prospective open-label study. *Journal of Clinical Psychopharmacology, 25,* 387-388.

Robertson, M., Rushton, P., Batrim, D., et al. (2007). Open trial of interpersonal psychotherapy for chronic posttraumatic stress disorder. *Australian Psychiatry, 15*(5), 375-379.

Robinson, R. (2008). Reflections on the debriefing debate. *International Journal of Emergency Mental Health, 10*(4), 253-260.

Roger, D., Jarvis, G., & Najarian, B. (1993). Detachment and coping: The construction and validation of a new scale for measuring coping strategies. *Personality and Individual Differences, 15*(3), 619-623.

Root, L. P., Koch, E. I., Reyntjens, J. O., et al. (2002, November). *Trauma-specific guided imagery: A systematic evaluation of an adjunct intervention to group psychotherapy.* Abstract presented at International Society for Traumatic Stress Studies Annual meeting, Baltimore, MD.

Rose, S., Bisson, J., & Wessely, S. (2002). Psychological debriefing for preventing posttraumatic stress disorder (PTSD). *The Cochrane Database of Systematic Reviews,* (2). CD000560.

Rothbaum, B. O., & Foa, E. B. (1994). Subtypes of posttraumatic stress disorder and duration of symptoms. In J. R. T. Davidson & E. B. Foa (Eds.), *Posttraumatic stress disorder: DSM-IV and beyond* (pp. 23-35). Washington, DC: American Psychiatric Publishing, Inc.

Rothbaum, B. O., Foa, E. B., Riggs, D. S., et al. (1992). A prospective examination of post-traumatic stress disorder in rape victims. *Journal of Traumatic Stress, 5*(3), 455-475.

Rothbaum, B. O., Hodges, L. F., Ready, D., et al. (2001). Virtual reality exposure therapy for Vietnam Veterans with posttraumatic stress disorder. *Journal of Clinical Psychiatry, 62*(8), 617-622.

Rothbaum, B. O., Killeen, T. K., Davidson, J. R. T., et al. (2008). Placebo-controlled trial of risperidone augmentation for selective serotonin reuptake inhibitor-resistant civilian posttraumatic stress disorder. *Journal of Clinical Psychiatry, 69,* 520-525.

Sareen, J., Cox, B. J., Clara, I., et al. (2005). The relationship between anxiety disorders and physical disorders in the U.S. National Comorbidity Survey. *Depression and Anxiety, 21,* 193-202.

Saxe, G., Stoddard, F., Courtney, D., et al. (2001). Relationship between acute morphine and the course of PTSD in children with burns. *Academy of Child and Adolescent Psychiatry, 40*(8), 915-921.

Sayers, S. L., Farrow, V. A., Ross, J., et al. (2009). Family problems among recently returned military Veterans referred for a mental health evaluation. *The Journal of Clinical Psychiatry, 70*(2), 163-170.

Schafer, I., Barkmann, C., Riedesser, P., et al. (2006). Posttraumatic syndromes in children and adolescents after road traffic accidents-a prospective cohort study. *Psychopathology, 39*(4), 259-264.

Schatzberg, A. F., Cole, J. O., & DeBattista, C. (Eds.). (2007). *Manual of clinical psychopharmacology* (6th ed.). Washington, DC: American Psychiatric Publishing, Inc.

Schatzberg, A. F., & Nemeroff, C. B. (Eds.). (2006). *Essentials of clinical psychopharmacology.* Washington, DC: American Psychiatric Publishing, Inc.

Schatzberg, A. F., & Nemeroff, C. B. (Eds.). (2009). *The American psychiatric publishing textbook of psychopharmacology* (4th ed.). Washington, DC: American Psychiatric Publishing, Inc.

Schiller, D., Levy, I., Niv, Y., et al. (2008). From fear to safety and back: Reversal of fear in the human brain. *The Journal of Neuroscience, 28*(45), 11517-11525.

Schlenger, W. E., & Jernigan, N. E. (2003). Mental health issues in disasters and terrorist attacks. *Ethnicity & Disease, 13*(3 Suppl 3), S3-89-93.

Schnurr, P. P., Lunney, C. A., & Sengupta, A. (2004). Risk factors for the development versus maintenance of posttraumatic stress disorder. *Journal of Trauma Stress, 17,* 85-95.

Schoenfeld, F. B., Marmar, C. R., & Neylan, T. C. (2004). Current concepts in pharmacotherapy for posttraumatic stress disorder. *Psychiatric Services, 55*(5), 519-531.

Scholes, C., Turpin, G., & Mason, S. (2007). A randomized controlled trial to assess the effectiveness of providing self-help information to people with symptoms of acute stress disorder following a traumatic injury. *Behaviour Research & Therapy, 45*(11), 2527-2536.

Schonenberg, M., Reichwald, U., Domes, C., et al. (2008). Ketamine aggravates symptoms of acute stress disorder in a naturalistic sample of accident victims. *Journal of Psychopharmacology, 2295,* 493-497.

Seedat, S., Stein, D. J., & Carey, P. D. (2005). Posttraumatic stress disorder in women: Epidemiological and treatment issues. *CNS Drugs, 19*(5), 411-427.

Seidler, G. H., & Wagner, F. E. (2006). Comparing the efficacy of EMDR and trauma-focused cognitive-behavioral therapy in the treatment of PTSD: A meta-analytic study. *Psychological Medicine, 36,* 1515-1522.

Shalev, A. Y. (1992). Posttraumatic stress disorder among injured survivors of a terrorist attack: Predictive value of early intrusion and avoidance symptoms. *Journal of Nervous Diseases, 180,* 505-509.

Shalev, A.Y. (2002). Acute stress reactions in adults. *Biological Psychiatry, 51*(7), 532-543.

Shalev, A. Y., & Freedman, S. (2005). PTSD following terrorist attacks: A prospective evaluation. *American Journal of Psychiatry, 162*(6), 1188-1191.

Shapiro, E. (2001). *Eye movement desensitization and reprocessing: Basic principles, protocols and procedures* (2nd ed.). New York: Guilford Press.

Shapiro, E., & Maxfield, L. (2002). Eye movement desensitization and reprocessing (EMDR): Information processing in the treatment of trauma. *Psychotherapy in Practice, 58*(8), 933-946.

Sharp, S., Thomas, C., Rosenberg, L., et al. (2010). Propranolol does not reduce risk for acute stress disorder in pediatric burn trauma. *The Journal of Trauma, Injury, Infection, and Critical Care, 68*(1), 193-197.

Shaw, R. J., Deblois, T., Ikuta, L., et al. (2006). Acute stress disorder among parents of infants in the neonatal intensive care nursery. *Psychosomatics, 47*(3), 206-212.

Shaw, A., Joseph, S., & Linley, P. A. (2005). Religion, spirituality, and posttraumatic growth: A systematic review. *Mental Health, Religion, and Culture, 8,* 1-11.

Shaw, R. J., Deblois, T., Ikuta, L., et al. (2006). Acute stress disorder among parents of infants in the neonatal intensive care nursery. *Psychosomatics, 47*(3), 206-212.

Shelby, R. A., Golden-Kreutz, D. M., & Andersen, B. L. (2008). PTSD diagnoses, subsyndromal symptoms, and comorbidities contribute to impairments for breast cancer survivors. *Journal of Traumatic Stress, 21*(2), 165-172.

Shemesh, E., & Stuber, M. L. (2006). Posttraumatic stress disorder in medically ill patients: What is known, what needs to be determined, and why is it important. *CNS Spectrums, 11*(2), 106-117.

Shin, L. M., Rauch, S. L., & Pitman, R. K. (2006). Amygdala, medial prefrontal cortex and hippocampal function in PTSD. *Annals of the New York Academy of Sciences, 1079,* 67-79.

Smid, G. E., Mooren, T., van der Mast, R., et al. (2009). Delayed posttraumatic stress disorder: Systematic review, meta-analysis, and meta-regression analysis of prospective studies. *Journal of Clinical Psychiatry, 70*(11), 1572-1582.

Smith, P., Yule, W., Perrin, S., et al. (2007). Cognitive-behavioral therapy for PTSD in children and adolescents: A preliminary randomized controlled trial. *Journal of American Academy of Child and Adolescent Psychiatry, 48*(8), 1051-1061.

Snow, B. R., Stellman, J. M., Stellman, S. D., et al. (1988). Posttraumatic stress disorder among American Legionnaires in relation to combat experience in Vietnam: Associated and contributing factors. *Environmental Research, 47,* 175-192.

Solomon, Z., Laror, N., & McFarlane, A. C. (2006). Acute posttraumatic reactions in soldiers and civilians. In B. A. van der Kolk, A. C. McFarlane, & L. Weisaeth (Eds.), *Traumatic stress: The effects of overwhelming experience on mind, body, and society* (pp. 102-114). New York: Guilford Press.

Solomon, Z., Neria, Y., Ohry, A., et al. (1994). PTSD among Israeli former prisoners of war and soldiers with combat stress reaction: A longitudinal study. *American Journal of Psychiatry, 151,* 554-559.

Solomon, Z., Shklar, R., & Mikulincer, M. (2005). Frontline treatment of combat stress reactions: A 20-year longitudinal evaluation study. *American Journal of Psychiatry, 162,* 2309-2314.

Spiegel, D. (2005). Treatment of acute traumatic stress reactions. *Journal of Trauma & Dissociation: The Official Journal of the International Society for the Study of Dissociation, 6*(2), 101-108.

Spitzer, C., Barnow, S., Volzke, H., et al. (2009). Trauma, posttraumatic stress disorder, and physical illness: Findings from the general population. *Psychosomatic Medicine, 71,* 1012-1017.

Stahl, S. (2005). *Essential psychopharmacology: The prescriber's guide.* New York: Cambridge University Press.

Stein, M. (2005, November 2-5). *Pharmacoprevention of adverse psychiatric sequelae of physical injury.* Paper presented at 21st Annual Meeting of the International Society for Traumatic Stress Studies. Toronto, Ontario, Canada.

Stein, D. J., Ipser, J. C., & Seedat, S. (2006). Pharmacotherapy for post-traumatic stress disorder (PTSD). *The Cochrane Database of Systematic Reviews,* (1). CD002795.

Stein, M. B., Kline, N. A., & Matloff, J. L. (2002). Adjunctive olanzapine for SSRI-resistant combat-related PTSD: A double-blind, placebo-controlled study. *American Journal of Psychiatry, 159,* 1777-1779.

Stein, D. J., Pederson, R., Rothbaum, B. O., et al. (2008). Onset of activity and time to response on individual CAPS-SX 17 items in patients treated for posttraumatic stress disorder with venlafaxine ER: A pooled analysis. *International Journal of Neuropsychopharmacology, 11,* 1-9.

Stoddard, F. J., Saxe, G., Ronfeldt, H., et al. (2006). Acute stress symptoms in young children with burns. *Journal of American Academy of Child & Adolescent Psychiatry, 45*(1), 87-93.

Stoddard, F. J., Sorrentino, E. A., Ceranoglu, T. A., et al. (2009). Preliminary evidence for the effects of morphine on posttraumatic stress disorder symptoms in one-to-four year olds with burns. *Journal of Burn Care Research, 30,* 836-843.

Strauss, J. L., Calhoun, P. S., & Marx, C. E. (2009). Guided imagery as a therapeutic tool in posttraumatic stress disorder. In P. J. Shiromani, T. M. Keane, & J. E. LeDoux (Eds.), *Post-traumatic stress disorder: Basic science and clinical practice* (pp. 363-373). New York: Humana Press.

Taylor, H. R., Freeman, M. K., & Cates, M. E. (2008). Prazosin for treatment of nightmares related to posttraumatic stress disorder. *American Journal of Health-System Pharmacy, 65*(8), 716-722.

Taylor, F. B., Martin, P., Thompson, C., et al. (2008). Prazosin effects on sleep measures and clinical symptoms in civilian trauma posttraumatic stress disorder: A placebo-controlled study. *Biological Psychiatry, 63,* 629-632.

Tcheung, W. J., Robert, R., Rosenberg, L., et al. (2005). Early treatment of acute stress disorder in children with major burn injury. *Pediatric Critical Care Medicine, 6*(6), 676-681.

Teicher, M. H., Tomoda, A., & Andersen, S. L. (2006). Neurobiological consequences of early stress and childhood maltreatment: Are results from human and animal studies comparable? *Annals of the New York Academy of Sciences, 1071,* 313-323.

Thapa, S. B., & Hauffa, E. (2005). Psychological distress among displaced persons during an armed conflict in Nepal. *Social Psychiatry and Psychiatric Epidemiology, 40*(8), 672-679.

Thielman, S. B. (2011). Religion and spirituality in the description of posttraumatic stress disorder. In J. R. Peteet, F. G. Lu, & W. E. Narrow (Eds.), *Religious and spiritual issues in psychiatric diagnosis: A research agenda for DSM-V* (pp. 105-117). Washington, DC: American Psychiatric Publishing, Inc.

Thompson, K. M., Crosby, R. D., & Wonderlich, S. A., et al. (2003). Psychopathology and sexual trauma in childhood and adulthood. *Journal of Traumatic Stress, 16,* 35-38.

Thompson, C. E., Taylor, F. B., McFall, M. E., et al. (2008). Non-nightmare distressed awakenings in Veterans with posttraumatic stress disorder: Response to prazosin. *Journal of Traumatic Stress, 21*(4), 417-420.

True, W. R., Rice, J., Eisen, S. A., et al. (1993). A twin study of genetic and environmental contributions to liability for posttraumatic stress symptoms. *Archives of General Psychiatry, 50,* 257-264.

Tucker, P., Potter-Kimball, R., Wyatt, D. B., et al. (2003). Can physiologic assessment and side effects tease out differences in PTSD trials? A double-blind comparison of citalopram, sertraline, and placebo. *Psychopharmacology Bulletin, 37,* 135-149.

Tucker, P., Zaninelli, R., Yehuda, R., et al. (2001). Paroxetine in the treatment of chronic posttraumatic stress disorder: Results of a placebo-controlled flexible dosage trial. *Journal of Clinical Psychiatry, 62,* 860-888.

Tull, M. (2008). Psychodynamic treatment of PTSD. Retrieved from http://ptsd.about.com/od/treatment/a/psychodynamic.htm

Ursano, E. J., Bell, E. S., Friedman, M., et al. (2006a). Practice guideline for the treatment of patients with acute stress disorder and posttraumatic stress disorder. In *American Psychiatric Association practice guidelines for the treatment of psychiatric disorders: Compendium 2006* (pp. 1003-1095). Washington, DC: American Psychiatric Publishing, Inc.

Ursano, R. J., Grieger, T. A., & McCarroll, J. E. (2006b). Prevention of posttraumatic stress: Consultation training and early treatment. In B. A. van der Kolk, A. C. McFarlane, & L. Weisaeth (Eds.), *Traumatic stress: The effects of overwhelming experience on mind, body, and society* (pp. 441-462). New York: Guilford Press.

Ursano, R. J., & Kilgore, J. A. (2011). Commentary on "Religion and spirituality in the description of posttraumatic stress disorder": Posttraumatic stress disorder, life threat, religion and spirituality. In J. R. Peteet, F. G. Lu, & W. E. Narrow (Eds.), *Religious and spiritual issues in psychiatric diagnosis: A research agenda for DSM-V* (pp. 119-122). Washington, DC: American Psychiatric Publishing, Inc.

Ursano, R. J., Zhang, L., Li, H., et al. (2009). PTSD and traumatic stress from gene to community and bench to bedside. *Brain Research, 1293,* 2-12.

Vaiva, G., Ducrocq, F., Jezequel, K., et al. (2003). Immediate treatment with propranolol decreases posttraumatic stress disorder two months after trauma. *Biological Psychiatry, 54,* 947-949.

van der Kolk, B. A. (2004). Psychobiology of posttraumatic stress disorder. In J. Panksepp (Ed.), *Textbook of biological psychiatry* (pp. 319-344). Hoboken, NJ: John Wiley & Sons, Inc.

van der Kolk, B. A. (2006a). Clinical implications of neuroscience research in PTSD. *Annals of the New York Academy of Sciences, 1071,* 277-293.

van der Kolk, B. A. (2006b). The body keeps the score: Approaches to the psychobiology of posttraumatic stress disorder. In B. A. van der Kolk, A. C. McFarlane, & L. Weisaeth (Eds.), *Traumatic stress: The effects of overwhelming experience on mind, body, and society* (pp. 214-241). New York: Guildford Press.

van der Kolk, B. A. (2006c). The complexity of adaptation to trauma: Self-regulation, stimulus discrimination and characterological development. In B. A. van der Kolk, A. C. McFarlane, & L. Weisaeth (Eds.), *Traumatic stress: The effects of overwhelming experience on mind, body, and society* (pp. 182-213). New York: Guilford Press.

van der Kolk, B. A. (2006d). Trauma and memory. In B. A. van der Kolk, A. C. McFarlane, & L. Weisaeth (Eds.), *Traumatic stress: The effects of overwhelming experience on mind, body, and society* (pp. 279-302). New York: Guilford Press.

van der Kolk, B., McFarlane, A. C., & van der Hart, O. (2002). Psychotherapy for posttraumatic stress disorder and other trauma-related disorders. In D. J. Stein & E. Hollander (Eds.), *The American psychiatric publishing textbook of anxiety disorders* (pp. 403-411). Washington, DC: American Psychiatric Publishing, Inc.

van der Kolk, M. A., McFarlane, A. C., & van der Hart, O. (2006a). A general approach to treatment of posttraumatic stress disorder. In B. A. van der Kolk, A. C. McFarlane, & L. Weisaeth (Eds.), *Traumatic stress: The effects of overwhelming experience on mind, body, and society* (pp. 417-440). New York: Guilford Press.

van der Kolk, B. A., McFarlane, A. C., & Weisaeth, L. (Eds.). (2006b). *Traumatic stress: The effects of overwhelming experience on mind, body, and society* (pp. IX-XVIII). New York: Guilford Press.

van der Kolk, B., Roth, S., Pelcovitz, D., et al. (1993). *Complex PTSD: Results of the PTSD field trials for DSM-IV.* Washington, DC: American Psychiatric Publishing, Inc.

van der Kolk, B. A., Spinazzola, J., Blaustein, M. E., et al. (2006c). A randomized clinical trial of Eye Movement Desensitization and Reprocessing (EMDR), fluoxetine, and pill placebo in the treatment of posttraumatic stress disorder: Treatment effects and long-term maintenance. *Journal of Clinical Psychiatry, 68*(1), 37-46.

van der Kolk, B., & van der Hart, O. (1991). The intrusive past: The flexibility of memory and the engraving of trauma. *American Image, 48*(4), 425-454.

van der Kolk, B., van der Hart, O., & Marmar, C. R. (2006d). Dissociation and information processing in posttraumatic stress disorder. In B. A. van der Kolk, A. C. McFarlane, & L. Weisaeth (Eds.), *Traumatic stress: The effects of overwhelming experience on mind, body, and society* (pp. 303-327). New York: Guilford Press.

van der Oord, S., Lucassen, S., van Emmerik, A. A. P., et al. (2009). Treatment of posttraumatic stress disorder in children using cognitive behavioural writing therapy. *Clinical Psychology and Psychotherapy, 17,* 240-249.

van Emmerik, A. A., Kamphuis, J. H., Hulsbosch, A. M., et al. (2002). Single session debriefing after psychological trauma: A meta-analysis. *Lancet, 360,* 766-771.

van Emmerik, A. A., Kamphuis, J. H., Hulsbosch, A. M., et al. (2008). Treating acute stress disorder and posttraumatic stress disorder with cognitive behavioral therapy or structured writing therapy: A randomized controlled trial. *Psychotherapy and Psychosomatics, 77*(2), 93-100.

van Griensven, F., Chakkraband, M. L., Thienkrua, W., et al. (2006). Mental health problems among adults in tsunami-affected areas in Southern Thailand. *Journal of the American Medical Association, 296,* 537-548.

Verfaellie, M., & Vasterling, J. J. (2009). Memory in PTSD: A neurocognitive approach. In P. J. Shiromani, T. M. Keane, & J. E. LeDoux (Eds.), *Post-traumatic stress disorder: Basic science and clinical practice* (pp. 105-130). New York: Humana Press.

Villarreal, G., & King, C. Y. (2001). Brain imaging in posttraumatic stress disorder. *Seminars in Clinical Neuropsychiatry, 6*(2), 131-145.

Warshaw, M. G., Fierman, E., Pratt, L., et al. (1993). Quality of life and dissociation in anxiety disorder patients with histories of trauma or PTSD. *American Journal of Psychiatry, 150,* 1512-1516.

Weathers, F. W., Litz, B. T., Huska, J., et al. (1994). *PTSD Checklist (PCL) for DSM-IV.* Boston: Boston National Center for PTSD, Behavioral Science Division.

Wedding, D., Boyd, M. A., & Niemiec, R. M. (2010). *Movies and mental illness 3: Using films to understand psychopathology* (3rd ed.). Cambridge, MA: Hogrefe Publishers.

Weigel, M. B., Purselle, D. C., D'Orio, B., et al. (2009). Treatment of psychiatric emergencies. In A. F. Schatzberg & C. B. Nemeroff (Eds.), *The American psychiatric publishing textbook of psychopharmacology* (4th ed.) (pp. 1287-1308). Washington, DC: American Psychiatric Publishing, Inc.

Weisaeth, L. (1993). Torture of a Norwegian ship's crew: Stress reactions, coping and psychiatric after effects. In J. P. Wilson & B. Raphael (Eds.), *International handbook of traumatic stress syndromes* (pp. 743-750). New York: Plenum Press.

Weisberg, R. B., Bruce, S. E., Machan, J. T., et al. (2002). Nonpsychiatric illness among primary care patients with trauma histories and posttraumatic stress disorder. *Psychiatric Services, 53*(7), 848-854.

Weiss, S. J. (2007). Neurobiological alterations associated with traumatic stress. *Perspectives in Psychiatric Care, 43*(3), 114-121.

Wessely, S. (2005). Victimhood and resilience. *The New England Journal of Medicine, 353,* 548-550.

Wessely, S., Rose, S., & Bisson, J. (2000). Brief psychological interventions ("debriefing") for trauma-related symptoms and the prevention of post traumatic stress disorder. *The Cochrane Database Systematic Review,* (2). CD000560.

Widom, C. S. (1999). Posttraumatic stress disorder in abused and neglected children grown up. *The American Journal of Psychiatry, 156*(8), 1223-1229.

Wiese, E., & Burhorst, I. (2007). The mental health of asylum-seeking and refugee children and adolescents attending a clinic in the Netherlands. *Transcultural Psychiatry, 44*(4), 596-613.

Wilcox, H. C., Storr, C. L., & Breslau, N. (2009). Posttraumatic stress disorder and suicide attempts in a community sample of urban American young adults. *Archives of General Psychiatry, 66*(3), 305-311.

Williams, M. T., Cahill, S. P., & Foa, E. B. (2010). Psychotherapy for posttraumatic stress disorder. In D. J. Stein, E. Hollander, & B. O. Rothbaum (Eds.), *Textbook of anxiety disorders* (2nd ed.) (pp. 603-626). Washington, DC: American Psychiatric Publishing, Inc.

Williams, J. E., Nieto, F. J., Sanford, C. P., et al. (2001). Effects of an angry temperament on coronary heart disease risk: The Atherosclerosis Risk in Communities Studies. *American Journal of Epidemiology, 154,* 230-235.

Witvliet, C. V. (2001). Forgiveness and health: Review and reflections on a matter of faith, feelings and physiology. *Journal of Psychology and Theology, 29,* 212-224.

Witvliet, C. V. O., Phipps, K. A., Feldman, M. E., et al. (2004). Posttraumatic mental and physical health correlates of forgiveness and religious coping in military veterans. *Journal of Traumatic Stress, 17*(3), 269-273.

Woodward, S. H., Kaloupek, D. G., Streeter, C. C., et al. (2006). Decreased anterior cingulate volume in combat-related PTSD. *Biological Psychiatry, 59,* 582-587.

Woon, F., & Hedges, D. W. (2009). Amygdala volume in adults with posttraumatic stress disorder: A meta-analysis. *Journal of Neuropsychiatry and Clinical Neuroscience, 21*(1), 215-212.

Yasan, A., Guzel, A., Tamam, Y., et al. (2009). Predictive factors for acute stress disorder and posttraumatic stress disorder after motor vehicle accidents. *Psychopathology, 42*(4), 236-241.

Yeh, S. C., Newman, B., Liewer, M. C., et al. (2009). Application development and clinical results from a Virtual Iraq System for the treatment of Iraq War PTSD. Proceedings of the IEEE VR 2009 Conference, Lafayette, IL.

Yehuda, R. (2009). Stress hormones and PTSD. In P. J. Shiromani, T. M. Keane, & J. E. LeDoux (Eds.), *Post-traumatic stress disorder: Basic science and clinical practice* (pp. 257-275). New York: Humana Press.

Yehuda, R., Halligan, S. L., & Bierer, L. M. (2001). Relationship of parental trauma exposure and PTSD to PTSD, depressive and anxiety disorders in offspring. *Journal of Psychiatric Research, 35,* 261-270.

Yehuda, R., & Sarapas, C. (2010). Pathogenesis of posttraumatic stress disorder and acute stress disorder. In D. J. Stein, E. Hollander, & B. O. Rothbaum (Eds.), *Textbook of anxiety disorders* (2nd ed.) (pp. 567-581). Washington, DC: American Psychiatric Publishing, Inc.

Young, K. A., Bonkale, W. L., Holcomb, L. A., et al. (2008). Major depression, 5HTTLPR genotype, suicide, and antidepressant influences on thalamic volume. *British Journal of Psychiatry, 192*(4), 285-289.

Yule, W., Bolton, D., Udwin, O., et al. (2000). The long-term psychological effects of a disaster experienced in adolescence: I. The incidence and course of PTSD. *Journal of Child Psychology and Psychiatry, 41,* 503-511.

Zatzick, D. F., Jurkovich, G. J., Gentilello, L., et al. (2002). Posttraumatic stress, problem drinking and functional outcomes after injury. *Archives of Surgery, 137*(2), 200-205.

Zhang, W., & Davidson, J. R. T. (2010). Pharmacotherapy for posttraumatic stress disorder. In D. J. Stein, E. Hollander, & B. O. Rothbaum (Eds.), *Textbook of anxiety disorders* (2nd ed.) (pp. 583-602). Washington, DC: American Psychiatric Publishing, Inc.

CHAPTER 12

Obsessive-Compulsive Disorder and Obsessive-Compulsive Spectrum Disorders

Eris F. Perese, APRN-PMH

Obsessive-compulsive disorder (OCD) has traditionally been included with anxiety disorders; however, some researchers believe that OCD is not an anxiety disorder, pointing out that OCD does not share the same fear/anxiety circuitry of other anxiety disorders (Bartz & Hollander, 2006; Higgins & George, 2007; Stein, 2008). (Fear/anxiety circuitry is discussed in Chapters 9 and 10.) Previously it was proposed that OCD was part of a compulsive-impulsive spectrum of disorders, with impulsive disorders, such as pathological gambling, at one end of the spectrum and obsessive-compulsive spectrum disorders (OCSDs), such as OCD and other repetitive behavioral disorders, at the other end (Eisen, Yip, Mancebo, et al., 2010; Hollander & Wong, 1995). Now it is being suggested that disorders that are related to OCD by their repetitive thoughts and behaviors should be classified as obsessive-compulsive related disorders (OCRDs) rather than OCSDs (Hollander, Kim, Braun, et al., 2009); it is also being recommended that OCD and OCSD or OCRD should be separate categories in the proposed revision of the *Diagnostic and Statistical Manual of Mental Disorders (DSM-V)* (Hollander, Rosen, and the IOCDC Spectrum Work Group, 1999; Phillips, Stein, Rauch, et al., 2010). Additionally, it is being recommended that hoarding—which is included in the current version of the *Diagnostic and Statistical Manual of Mental Disorders* (4th ed., Text Revision) *(DSM-IV-TR)* (American Psychiatric Association, 2000) as a diagnostic criterion for obsessive-compulsive personality disorder and, if extreme, as a symptom of OCD—should have a separate category or should be included as a separate disorder within the OCSD or OCRD category (Mataix-Cols, Frost, Pertusa, et al., 2010). Based on these considerations, OCD, OCSD (currently the more-used term), and hoarding are presented in this textbook separately from anxiety disorders.

Obsessive-Compulsive Disorder

The characteristic symptoms of OCD, obsessions and compulsions, have been described throughout history and across many cultures (Snider & Swedo, 2004a; Stanley & Wand, 1995). They have been integrated into art, with descriptions of individuals with OCD symptoms included in Shakespearian tragedies (Murphy, Timpano, Wheaton, et al., 2010).

Obsessions are intrusive, unwanted mental occurrences (thoughts, ideas, ruminations, images, fears, impulses, or urges) that cause anxiety and distress (Hollander & Simeon, 2008). Eighty percent to ninety percent of the general population experience intrusive thoughts, or thoughts that are similar to the obsessional content of patients with OCD (Abramowitz, Schwartz, & Moore, 2003). Individuals who do not have OCD recognize that these thoughts are senseless and push them away, but patients with OCD equate thoughts with actions. Abramowitz and Deacon (2005) described this phenomenon as "thought-action fusion" (p. 126). Patients with OCD believe that negative thoughts and doubts are the same as the corresponding behavior and that the thoughts make the event more likely to happen (Abramowitz, Whiteside, Lynam, et al., 2003). Because they believe that certain thoughts may be harmful, they feel that they must stop the thoughts in order to prevent the harmful event from occurring (Abramowitz & Deacon).

Compulsions are acts or behaviors—such as repeated cleaning, checking, arranging, or counting—that temporarily reduce anxiety or distress associated with obsessions. According to Hollander and Simeon (2008), "A compulsive ritual is a behavior that usually reduces discomfort but is carried out in a pressured or rigid fashion" (p. 552). Similar to patients with other anxiety disorders, such as panic disorder, patients with OCD use safety-seeking behaviors: behavioral rituals, neutralizing acts, avoidance, and suppression of negative thoughts. Safety-seeking behaviors reduce the patient's distress for a short time, but in the long run, they maintain or strengthen the obsessions and the urge to perform rituals or neutralizing behaviors (Abramowitz & Deacon, 2005).

Patients with OCD tend to have low self-esteem, few friends, and problems with family relationships (Micallef & Blin, 2001). They need to be certain of things and in control in order to cope with their environment, to keep it safe. They resist change because change, both positive and negative, brings stress. They have a need for perfection because of their fears of the consequences of not achieving perfection. Often they have curtailed their education and efforts to advance in their work. They are ashamed of their thoughts and behaviors and try to hide them. They keep their symptoms secret for fear that others will think that they are crazy (Collie, 2005, p. 37).

Overall, patients with OCD have impairment of functioning in their roles as spouse/partner, parent, worker, and neighbor (Pinto, Manceabo, Eisen, et al., 2006), and they often experience financial difficulties due to problems with employment (Huppert, Simpson, Nissenson, et al., 2009). For example, Ruscio, Stein, Chiu, et al. (2010) found that 80% of patients with OCD experienced impairment of functioning in home management, relationships, and social activities. Patients with OCD have diminished quality of life, and 13% of those with OCD symptoms have made suicide attempts (Hollander, Kwon, Stein, et al., 1996). OCD, with its unwanted intrusive obsessions and compulsive behaviors, has a severe negative impact not only on the lives of patients but also on their families (Collie, 2005; Flament, Whitaker, Rapoport, et al., 1988). For example, in a study of families with a member with OCD, 88% of the family members reported that they give up things, forego activities, and make adjustments or accommodations to the family member's illness. Sometimes, they feel "bullied" by the family member into doing things to accommodate his or her obsessions and compulsions (Gabbard, 2005, p. 268).

The dimensional model and the subtype model (Box 12-1) offer a way for psychiatric advanced practice nurses to understand the genetic, neurobiological, natural history, and treatment response of OCD. Specifiers supply information about the degree of insight that patients have about their illness (Leckman, Mataix-Cols, & Rosario-Campos, 2005). In the current version of the *DSM-IV-TR*

BOX 12-1 Dimensional Model and Subtype Model of Obsessive-Compulsive Disorder

Dimensional Model

The *DSM-IV-TR* presents OCD as a unitary syndrome (American Psychiatric Association, 2000). However, many researchers consider OCD to be heterogeneous (Pato, Pato, & Pauls, 2002), and a heterogeneous nature is supported by the recent finding that although symptoms in each dimension share some genetic influences, each symptom dimension has unique genetic influences (Katerberg, Delucchi, Stewart, et al., 2010). The dimensional model proposes that OCD is composed of sets of dimensions, with each dimension caused by a combination of factors—genetic, structural, functional, neurochemical, experienced, and others. Each combination makes a specific contribution to the development of OCD. The dimensional model conceptualizes OCD as composed of sets of symptoms related to threat detection and harm avoidance (Leckman et al., 2005). The dimensional model is supported by the stability of symptoms in adults across time; e.g., although the obsessions may change, they tend to stay in the same dimension. The dimensions are as follows:

- Obsessions that include aggressive, sexual, religious, or somatic obsessions and checking compulsions. Comorbidities frequently associated with this dimension of OCD include anxiety disorders and depression (Hasler, LaSalle-Ricci, Ronquillo, et al., 2005).
- Symmetry obsessions; ordering, counting, and repeating compulsions; and the need to have things "just right" (Murphy et al., 2010, p. 133). Comorbidities frequently associated with this dimension of OCD include tic disorders, bipolar disorder, obsessive-compulsive personality disorder, panic disorder, and agoraphobia.
- Contamination obsessions and cleaning compulsions. Comorbidities frequently associated with this disorder include eating disorders.
- Hoarding obsessions and collecting compulsions. Comorbidities frequently associated with this dimension of OCD include personality disorders. Comorbidities among men include generalized anxiety disorders and tic disorders, and comorbidities among women include social phobia, post-traumatic stress disorder, BDD, nail biting, and skin picking (Leckman, Grice, Boardman, et al., 1997; Leckman et al., 2010).

Subtype Model

Subtypes are based on the agents that affect the brain circuitry involved in OCD. Based on the subtype model, treatments are expected to have a similar effect on disorders within the same subtype.

The subtypes include clusters defined by the following:

- Personality traits.
- Age of onset: Symptoms present before puberty. Patients with early-onset OCD tend to respond well to CBT in combination with SSRIs (Pediatric OCD Treatment Study [POTS] Team, 2004).
- Presence of tics and/or family history of tics: Presence of tics tends to reduce response to SSRIs in children but may not in adults (March, Franklin, Leonard, et al., 2007). Patients with tics may respond to antipsychotic augmentation (Bloch et al., 2006).
- Infection-based (PANDAS).

(American Psychiatric Association, 2000), OCD can be described with the specifier "with poor insight" (p. 463) (patient believes that obsessions are true). Researchers have recommended that specifiers in the next revision of the *DSM* include "with good insight or fair insight" (to indicate that the patient recognizes that the OCD symptoms may not be true), "with poor insight," and "with delusional beliefs" (Leckman, Denys, Simpson, et al., 2010).

Epidemiology

Prevalence

At one time, OCD was thought to be extremely rare (Rosenberg, Russell, & Fougere, 2005), but the 1984 National Epidemiologic Catchment Area Survey surprised the mental health profession when it revealed that OCD is the fourth most common psychiatric disorder (Robins, Helzer, Weissman, et al., 1984), and Murray and Lopez (1996) reported that it is the tenth leading cause of disability worldwide. The worldwide prevalence is 1% to 3% of children and adults (Snider & Swedo, 2004a). Leckman et al. (2010) reported a 1.2% rate of OCD in the general population, but they found that 28.2% of the general population had experienced symptoms of obsessions and compulsions that did not meet the criteria for OCD. They found that the most frequently occurring symptoms were checking, hoarding, and ordering. This finding suggests that subclinical OCD may occur in more than one-quarter of the U.S. population and hence may be present in many of the patients that psychiatric advanced practice nurses see in their practice.

Age of Onset

Symptoms of OCD usually begin in adolescence or early adulthood but can begin earlier, as young as 2 to 4 years of age (Snider & Swedo, 2004a). A subtype of OCD that begins before puberty and is characterized by an episodic course with severe exacerbations has been linked to infections caused by the group A beta-hemolytic streptococcal infection. That subtype is one of the pediatric autoimmune neuropsychiatric disorders associated with streptococcal infections (PANDAS). One-third to one-half of adults with OCD developed the disorder during childhood or adolescence (DeVeaugh-Geiss, Moroz, Biedeman, et al., 1992), with 21% of cases starting by age 10 (Kessler, Berglund, Demler, et al., 2005) and 70% before age 30 (Hollander & Simeon, 2008).

Gender

Women develop OCD more frequently than men, but in clinical populations the prevalence is often equal (Attiullah, Eisen, & Rasmussen, 2000). Males tend to have an earlier onset (ages 5 to 15 years) (Lensi, Cassano, Correddu, et al., 1996; Noshirvani, Kasvikis, Marks, et al., 1991), whereas females have a later onset (ages 26 to 35 years) (Noshirvani et al.). Among patients with OCD with comorbid psychiatric disorders such as schizophrenia, delusional disorder, or schizotypal personality disorder, the rate is higher for men (Eisen & Rasmussen, 1993). In children and adolescents with OCD, the rate is equal for males and females.

Marital Status

Some studies have found that about half of patients with OCD never married (Eisen et al., 2010; Rasmussen & Eisen, 1991). Among patients with OCD who married, there was a higher rate for separation or divorce (Zetin & Kramer, 1992). Patients with OCD who are married have a higher rate of remission than patients with OCD who are not married (Steketee, Eisen, Dyck, et al., 1999). This suggests that social support, especially support from a spouse or partner, may be important in achieving optimal outcomes.

Risk Factors

Risk factors for the development of OCD include prenatal, perinatal, and postnatal factors (Vasconcelos, Sampaio, Hounie, et al., 2007); environmental factors (infections, childhood abuse, traumatic events, and stressful life events); psychiatric disorders; and treatment of schizophrenia with atypical antipsychotics (Grisham, Anderson, & Sachdev, 2008).

Prenatal, Perinatal, and Postnatal Risk Factors

Prenatal factors found to be associated with OCD include (1) maternal use of medications or procedures to conceive and (2) the presence of maternal medical problems during the pregnancy such as excess weight gain; edema of the hands, feet, or face; hyperemesis; and use of medications. Perinatal risk factors include premature rupture of the membranes, prolonged labor, and Cesarean delivery. Immediate postnatal factors include factors related to preterm birth and jaundice (Vasconcelos et al., 2007).

Infections

There appears to be a relationship between exposure to streptococcal infections and development of OCD and symptoms of Tourette's syndrome (TS) among some children (Swedo, 2002). The development of OCD and symptoms of TS is known as pediatric autoimmune neuropsychiatric disorder associated with streptococcal infections (PANDAS) (Grisham et al., 2008, p. 109). There is some question as to whether PANDAS are due to the environmental risk factor of infection, because there is an increased rate of OCD and TS in the relatives of children with PANDAS (Lougee, Perlmutter, Nicolson, et al., 2000), suggesting a genetic influence. OCD has also been found to occur in patients with rheumatic fever with and without Sydenham's chorea, and OCSD has been found in adults with a history of rheumatic fever (de Alvarenga, Flores, Torres, et al., 2009). It is thought that abnormal immune response to streptococcal infections with abnormal antibody production may lead to autoimmune destruction of the striatum (a part of the basal ganglia that filters out extraneous stimuli and controls motor behaviors) in the presence of infection (Rauch, Cora-Locatelli, & Greenberg, 2002a; Snider & Swedo, 2004b; Swedo & Grant, 2005).

Childhood Abuse

Studies suggest that physical and sexual abuse during childhood is a risk factor for the development of OCD (Lochner, du Toit, Zungu-Dirwayi, et al., 2002).

Traumatic Events

Injury to the brain following accidents that involve the head have been found to be followed by the rapid onset (days to a few months) of new cases of OCD. Patients who experience head trauma are at a twofold risk of developing OCD in comparison to individuals without head injuries (Silver, Kramer, Greerwald, et al., 2001). For example, it has been found that children with OCD have experienced more traumatic events than children without OCD (Gothelf, Aharonovsky, Horesh, et al., 2004).

Stressful Life Events

Adults with OCD have identified stressful life events associated with the onset of OCD. Stressful events include pregnancy, childbirth, significant losses, promotion to a new job, sexual problems, and physical illnesses (Yorulmaz, Gencoz, & Woody, 2009).

Psychiatric Disorders

The presence of a psychiatric disorder appears to be a risk factor for the development of OCD. For example, posttraumatic stress disorder (PTSD) has been found to be followed by OCD (Brown, Campbell, Lehman, et al., 2001), and OCD following PTSD is associated with later onset, symmetry obsessions (either believing that arranging things in a set way prevents harm or feeling driven to arrange things to keep one's environment perfect), tic disorders, and anxiety and depression. The presence of anxiety, depression, and substance use has been found to be higher among adolescents who develop OCD in comparison to those who do not develop OCD (Douglass, Moffitt, Dar, et al., 1995).

Atypical Antipsychotics

Following treatment with atypical antipsychotics, some patients with schizophrenia have been found to develop OCD (McDougle, Epperson, & Price, 1996). For example, Sa, Hounie, Sampaio, et al. (2009) found that patients treated with haloperidol (Haldol) and clozapine (Clozaril) developed symptoms of OCD, with the patients receiving clozapine having more severe symptoms.

Etiology

It is known that genetic vulnerability and infections are associated with the development of OCD. Theories of the etiology of OCD include evolutionary theory, false alarm theory, cognitive theory, and unified theory.

Genetics

The genetic influence (heritability) of OCD is 68% less than the 70% to 80% for bipolar disorder or schizophrenia and more than the 43% for panic disorder (Smoller, Sheidley, & Tsuang, 2008). Within the symptoms of OCD, obsessions have 33% heritability and compulsions 26% heritability (Jonnal, Gardner, Prescott, et al., 2000). Family studies suggest that there is a genetic predisposition for OCD, OCSD, and movement disorders such as tics. For example, among the family members of patients with OCD, 16% to 18% also have OCD (Dougherty, Rauch, & Greenberg, 2010). It is likely that several genes are involved in OCD (Pato, Pato, Kennedy, et al., 1999). Three genes thought to be involved are genes for the serotonin transporter; genes involved in the dopamine D_4 receptor (in OCD with tics); and genes involved with the enzyme catechol-*O*-methyltransferase (levels of this enzyme have been found to be lower in males with OCD) (Hollander & Simeon, 2008).

Infections

Following the early reports of Grimshaw (1964) that patients with obsessional behaviors often had a history of Sydenham's chorea, which is a neurological manifestation of rheumatic fever, researchers began to study the link between OCD and autoimmune phenomena. They found evidence of an association between obsessive-compulsive behaviors and a history of Sydenham's chorea and speculated that the immune system plays a role in OCD (Swedo, 1994; Wilcox & Nasrallah, 1986). In one study, it was found that over 70% of children with Sydenham's chorea had an abrupt onset of OCD symptoms, such as repetitive, unwanted thoughts and behaviors, 2 to 4 weeks before the onset of the chorea (Swedo, Leonard, Schapiro, et al., 1993). Children who had group A beta-hemolytic streptococcal infections experienced exacerbation of their OCD symptoms, especially symptoms of emotional lability, separation anxiety, and attention difficulties (Swedo, Leonard, Garvey, et al., 1998).

Evolutionary Theory

Polimeni, Reiss, and Sareen (2005) proposed that OCD is linked to ancient behavioral specialization (division of labor) that was designed to promote effectiveness in meeting the needs of the group and thus ensuring survival of the species. They suggested that symptoms of OCD are vestigial behaviors once needed by hunting and gathering people who faced three main threats: attacks by other tribes, disease, and starvation. The compulsions of OCD—checking, cleaning, counting, hoarding, and requiring precision or perfection—could, at one time in evolution, have been protective against the threats faced. For example:

- Washing protects against dirt and illness
- Checking maintains safety
- Hoarding secures food for future need (Mataix-Cols, Rosario-Campos, & Leckman, 2005)

False Alarm Theory

Based on the theory that learned habits and responses are maintained in the basal ganglia (Saint-Cyr, Taylor, & Nicholson, 1995) and that the basal ganglia are involved in the pathology of OCD, others have described the symptoms of OCD as the result of "false alarms" related to evolutionary precautionary responses (Stein & Bouwer, 1997). Polimeni et al. (2005) suggested that pathology caused by gene mutations, neurodevelopmental abnormalities, or infections such as streptococcal infections can lead to errors in these vestigial behaviors and to the development of the symptoms of OCD.

Cognitive Theory

Cognitive theory proposes that obsessions are caused by misinterpretations of the importance or significance of intrusive thoughts or impulses; obsessions will last as long as the misinterpretations last; and obsessions will weaken or fade as the interpretations are changed (Lambrecq, Rotge, Guebl, et al., 2009; Rachman, 1997). Patients with OCD have characteristic patterns of dysfunctional beliefs:

- They have a sense of excessive responsibility.
- They tend to overestimate the importance of a change or threat.
- They seek perfectionism and are intolerant of uncertainty.
- They place great importance on controlling their thoughts.
- They tend to remember negative things and ignore positive things.
- They have a faulty evaluation of the consequences.
- They lack the ability to ignore intrusive thoughts (Lambrecq et al., 2009).

Rachman (1997) stated that intrusive thoughts are the raw material from which obsessions are made. He also said that patients with OCD may have had early life experiences in which they were taught that they were responsible for harmful things' happening. Patients with OCD interpret their obsessions as being very important, revealing, threatening, dangerous, or catastrophic. They fear the consequences to themselves that the obsessions may bring—rejection by others, being declared insane, or being condemned to hell.

Unified Theory

In the unified theory, the brain is viewed as the sum of its subsystems (Yaryura-Tobias, 1998). The theory proposes that OCD and OCSDs are on a continuum. The etiology and maintenance of the symptoms of the disorders are located within the brain and its circuitry.

Biological Basis

Although OCD was previously considered to have primarily a psychological etiology, it is now thought to have a biological etiology. The biological basis of OCD is believed to involve a brain circuit, the cortico-striato-thalamo-cortical (CSTC) circuit, which is different from the fear/anxiety circuit that is involved in anxiety (Stein & Rauch, 2010).

In CSTC circuitry, the loop begins in the cortical area of the brain, the frontal lobe, and extends to the cingulate cortex (an area in the frontal lobe that has many functions, including error detection), then to the caudate nucleus (part of the striatum of the basal ganglia), then to the thalamus, and back to the cortical area. CSTC circuitry is involved in sensorimotor functioning, emotional and motivational functioning, inhibition of responses, working memory, and executive functioning (Rauch et al., 2002a). Abnormalities of structures within the CSTC circuitry such as abnormalities of the orbitofrontal cortex and the basal ganglia have been found to underlie the symptoms of OCD (Rotge, 2010). Support for the biological basis of OCD comes from research related to (1) the basal ganglia, (2) neuropsychological abnormalities, (3) abnormalities of brain structures and functioning and abnormalities of neurotransmitter systems, and (4) response to treatment (Trivedi, 1996).

Basal Ganglia

The basal ganglia are involved in planning and executing motor strategies (e.g., the basal ganglia facilitate some movements and suppress others) (Kandel, Schwartz, & Jessell, 1995). The basal ganglia are thought to be the primary site of pathology of OCD (Rosenberg et al., 2005). Symptoms of OCD are thought to result from disturbances of the basal ganglia's functioning in filtering and suppressing cortical input. The basal ganglia are five interconnected nuclei (a group of cells in the central nervous system with a common function): caudate nucleus, putamen, globus pallidus, subthalamic nucleus, and substantia nigra. The caudate nucleus and the putamen together are known as the striatum. The striatum receives input from afferent connections (pathways that send signals to the central nervous system) (Kandel et al., 1995). The striatum also receives input from the cerebral cortex. The striatum processes the information, filtering out extraneous input before the information is transmitted to the thalamus, which is the relay center for all sensory pathways to the cerebral cortex (Gold, Berman, Randolph, et al., 1996). By controlling the information going from the thalamus to the cortex, the striatum regulates the content and quality of information processed in the cortex of the brain (Rauch et al., 2002a).

It has long been known that the striatum is involved in fixed-action patterns or inherited motor sequences, such as grooming and nest building (MacLean, 1973), but more recently it has been found that the striatum is involved in motor and cognitive procedural functions (Stein & Rauch, 2010); additionally, because the striatum includes the nucleus accumbens, it is thought that the striatum is involved in reward responses (Higgins & George, 2007). Studies have shown that the head of the caudate nucleus and the pathway that connects the caudate with areas of the prefrontal cortex (the area of the brain involved in integrating positive and negative emotions with information) and with the anterior cingulate cortex (the area of the brain involved in monitoring decisions and behavioral responses during conflict and uncertainty) are hyperactive in OCD (D'Alessandro, 2009; Sachdev & Malhi, 2005). This hyperactivity may result in inadequate inhibition of the thalamus, which leads to deficits in gaiting of information going to the cerebral cortex.

Abnormalities of the basal ganglia's ability to filter and suppress information going to the brain's cortex are believed to be one of the causes of OCD (Insel, 1992). When the functioning of the basal ganglia is impaired, the cortex is flooded with information that otherwise would have been processed before reaching the cortex. This hypothesis is supported by evidence that higher rates of OCD have been found in patients with disorders that affect the basal ganglia, including Huntington's disease, TS, PANDAS, and postencephalitis parkinsonism (Rosenberg et al., 2005). Several researchers have described increased basal ganglia volume in patients with PANDAS that they propose is related to inflammation of the basal ganglia (Giedd, Rapoport, Garvery, et al., 2000).

Neuropsychological Abnormalities

Neuropsychological abnormalities found in patients with OCD include history of birth injury, growth delays or delays in achieving developmental milestones, history of head trauma, abnormal electroencephalograms, abnormal auditory evoked potentials, and high rates of soft neurological signs. For example, patients with OCD have more soft neurological signs, especially in the areas of coordination, visuospatial functioning, involuntary movements, and mirror movements than patients without OCD (Hollander, Schiffman, Cohen, et al., 1990; Khanna, 1991; Stein & Rauch, 2010). These soft neurological signs reflect impairment of frontal brain functioning and brain functioning required for complex motor tasks, such as fine motor coordination and visuospatial functioning (Andreasen & Black, 2006; Hollander et al., 1990). These findings suggest that neurodevelopmental abnormalities may underlie deficits in functioning of the CSTC circuitry (Hollander & Simeon, 2008; Stein & Rauch, 2010).

Abnormalities of Brain Structures, Functioning, and Neurochemistry

Studies of brain structures and functioning of patients with OCD are not consistent, but they do suggest that there are abnormalities of brain structures with resulting impairment of functioning (Jenike, Breiter, Baer, et al., 1996). Structural abnormalities include

- Loss of neurons in the orbitofrontal cortex, cingulate cortex, amygdala, and thalamus
- Enlargement of the ventricles
- Reduction of white matter volume (myelin)
- Abnormalities of the corpus callosum (Stein & Rauch, 2010)

Functional abnormalities include increased activity of the CSTC circuitry in response to obsessions (Lambrecq et al., 2009), with different parts of the circuitry showing increased activity during different rituals (washing, checking, or hoarding) (Higgins & George, 2007). Abnormalities of functioning are evidenced as problems with nonverbal memory, ability to use coping strategies, visuospatial skills, and executive functioning (Dougherty et al., 2010; Howieson & Lezak, 2010). Functional impairment can also be elicited on neurological examination. For example, patients with OCD, in comparison to controls without psychiatric illnesses, evidence more impairment of fine motor coordination and sensory and visuospatial functioning and more involuntary movements (Hollander et al., 1990).

The symptoms of OCD are linked with activation of specific brain structures—the orbitofrontal cortex, anterior cingulate cortex, striatum, thalamus, lateral frontal and temporal cortexes, amygdala, and insula—and their functioning (Saxena, Bota, & Brody, 2001), with different symptom clusters linked to specific areas (Rauch, Whalen, Dougherty, et al., 1998) (Table 12-1).

TABLE 12-1 ABNORMALITIES OF BRAIN STRUCTURES AND FUNCTIONING IN OBSESSIVE-COMPULSIVE DISORDER

Brain Structure	Normal Function	Structural and Functional Abnormalities in Obsessive-Compulsive Disorder
Basal ganglia	Facilitate some movements and suppress others (Kandel et al., 1995). Cerebral cortex sends messages to the basal ganglia, which pass the signal to the thalamus. Thalamus filters the information and sends it back to the cerebral cortex (Higgins & George, 2007).	Decreased volume of basal ganglia in OCD (Rosenberg, Kevashan, O'Hearn, et al., 1997). Increased volume of basal ganglia in patients with PANDAS (Giedd et al., 2000). Abnormalities of ability to filter and suppress information (Insel, 1992). Impaired gaiting of stimuli with resulting hyperexcitability and lack of inhibitory control; e.g., cortex is flooded with information (Rossi, Bartalini, Ulivelli, et al., 2005).
Caudate nucleus	Involved in inhibition, executive functioning, language, memory, and emotions (Hurley, Fisher, & Taber, 2010).	Head of caudate nucleus is hyperactive in OCD.
Striatum (caudate nucleus and putamen and nucleus accumbens)	Receives input; processes information before it is transmitted to the thalamus. Filters out extraneous information from going to the cerebral cortex; controls behavior (Aouizerate, Guehl, Cuny, et al., 2004).	Inhibition of the thalamus by the striatum is not adequate in OCD.

TABLE 12-1 ABNORMALITIES OF BRAIN STRUCTURES AND FUNCTIONING IN OBSESSIVE-COMPULSIVE DISORDER—continued

Brain Structure	Normal Function	Structural and Functional Abnormalities in Obsessive-Compulsive Disorder
Globus pallidus	Output from the basal ganglia. Conveys information to the thalamus.	Reduction of inhibition by the global pallidus in OCD is associated with increased stimulation of the frontal cortex by the thalamus; e.g., the presence of intrusive obsessions (Rauch et al., 2002a).
Paralimbic system (orbitofrontal cortex, cingulate cortex, anterior temporal area, parahippocampal areas, and insular cortex) (Rauch et al., 2002).	Connects cortical areas with the limbic system. Gives emotional meaning to information being processed. Modulates arousal and emotions. Involved in anxiety and autonomic responses (Rauch et al., 2002a). Determines the significance of consequences of actions (Aouizerate et al., 2004).	Repetitive thoughts and behaviors associated with OCD (Aouizerate et al., 2004).
Thalamus	Integrates information and perceptions (Baxter, Saxena, Brody, et al., 1996). It is inhibited by striatum.	Without inhibition by the striatum, the thalamus overstimulates the cortex. In children with OCD, the volume of thalamus is increased. It is reduced following treatment with SSRIs (Gilbert, Moore, Keshavan, et al., 2000). In adults with OCD, the gray matter of thalamus is increased. It is decreased with SSRIs and with psychotherapy (Baxter et al., 1996; Kim, Lee, Kim, et al., 2001; Rosenberg, MacMaster, Keshavan, et al., 2000). Research studies show that thalamic stimulation is associated with compulsive behaviors.
Hippocampus	Compares predicted events with actual events.	When there is a conflict or mismatch between predicted and actual events, there may be a lack of purposeful behaviors and occurrence of behaviors that are related to monitoring the environment, such as checking.
Amygdala	Emotional appraisal; fear modulation of anxiety.	Volume of amygdala is reduced in OCD (Szeszko, Robinson, Alvir, et al., 1999). May be involved in maintaining compulsive behaviors (Rausch et al., 1998).
Anterior cingulate cortex (within frontal cortex)	Focuses attention. Assigns emotional importance to stimuli. Involved in problem-solving, error detection, and choosing among multiple response options (D'Alessandro, 2009; Laraia, 2006; Saxena & Maidment, 2004) Involved in reward expectancy and with expectancy of moral violations (Shidara & Richmond, 2002).	In OCD, there is increased volume of gray matter; increased glucose metabolism; increased activation (Baxter et al., 1996). Hyperactivity leads to overactive monitoring of actions and to feeling the need to correct performance repeatedly (Ursu, Stenger, Shear, et al., 2003). Anterior cingulate cortex hyperactivity may be part of the pathogenesis of OCD due to the false errors generated by the action-monitoring system that causes patients to feel the need to correct their actions repeatedly.
Posterior cingulate cortex	Involved in processing visual events, spatial orientation, memory, and emotional stimuli (Laraia, 2006, p. 11).	Decreased volume of gray matter (Valente, Miguel, Castro, et al., 2005). Treatment with SSRIs was associated with increased activity of posterior cingulate cortex (Rauch, Jenike, Alpert, et al., 2002b).
Prefrontal cortex	Cognitive functions such as planning, organizing and controlling. Inhibition of responses. Verifying actions (Rauch et al., 2002a).	Reduction of orbitofrontal volume (Baxter et al., 1992; Szesko et al., 1999). Disinhibition, disorganization, inflexibility, perseveration, and stereotypy (Rauch et al., 2002a).

SSRI, selective serotonin reuptake inhibitors; PANDAS, pediatric autoimmune neuropsychiatric disorders associated with streptococcal infections.

Neurotransmitter Systems Associated With Obsessive-Compulsive Disorder

Several neurotransmitter systems are involved in the communication among the brain structures involved in OCD. At one time, based on observations that the symptoms of OCD responded to treatment with selective serotonin reuptake inhibitors (SSRIs), it was thought that the serotonergic system was the primary neurotransmitter system involved in OCD and that SSRIs corrected a deficit of the serotonergic system (Stein & Rauch, 2010). It is now accepted that other neurotransmitters—such as dopamine, glutamate, and gamma-aminobutyric acid (GABA)—are involved (Table 12-2) (Rauch et al., 2002a; Stein & Rauch, 2010).

TABLE 12-2 ABNORMALITIES OF NEUROTRANSMITTERS IN OBSESSIVE-COMPULSIVE DISEASE

Neurotransmitter	Location/Normal Function	Abnormalities in Obsessive-Compulsive Disease
Serotonin	Striato-thalamo-cortical communication (Micallef & Blin, 2001). Serotonin is believed to play a role in regulating impulsivity, suicidality, aggression, anxiety, learning, and social dominance.	Dysregulation of serotonin may be involved in repetitive obsessions and compulsions of OCD (Hollander & Simeon, 2008).
Dopamine	Striatum.	Overactivity of dopaminergic system possibly due to lack of serotonin inhibition (Snider & Swedo, 2004a). Dopaminergic system may be involved in tics and Tourette's syndrome (Stein & Rauch, 2010).
Glutamate	Glutamatergic tract projects from orbitofrontal and cingulate cortex to caudate nucleus and ventral striatum (nucleus accumbens; e.g., pleasure and reward).	Possible hyperglutamatergic condition in prefrontal cortex (Micallef & Blin, 2001). Recent studies using magnetic resonance spectroscopy have shown increased levels of glutamate in several regions involved in hyperactive cortico-striato-limbic-thalamic circuitry (Pittenger, Krystal, & Coric, 2006).
GABA	Caudate nucleus sends GABA-ergic inhibitory projections to the globus pallidus, which sends inhibitory projections to the thalamus, which sends projections to the cortex.	Inhibition of the caudate nucleus may cause the globus pallidus to have a less inhibitory effect on the thalamus, which may result in greater activity of the CSTC circuit (Baxter et al., 1992). Inhibition of the caudate nucleus may decrease inhibition of the globus pallidus and thalamus, thus increasing activity of the orbitofrontal-cingulate-caudate pallido-thalamic neural circuitry (Trivedi, 1996).
N-Acetyl-aspartate	Localized in mature neuronal cells.	Reduced amounts suggest neuronal dysfunction or loss of neurons (Tsai & Coyle, 1995). Reduced levels in OCD are found in the caudate nucleus (Bartha, Stein, Williamson, et al., 1998), in the anterior cingulate cortex (Ebert, Speck, Konig, et al., 1997), and in the medial thalamus (Fitzgerald, Moore, Paulson, et al., 2000), suggesting neuronal loss in the CSTC circuitry of patients with OCD.
Neuropeptides	Involved in memory, grooming, and maternal, sexual, and aggressive behaviors and possibly in stereotyped behaviors (McDougle, Barr, Goodman, et al., 1999).	Arginine vasopressin and somatostatin may be involved in OCD.

CSTC, cortico-striato-thalamo-cortical; GABA, gamma-aminobutyric acid.

Treatments That Support the Biological Basis of Obsessive-Compulsive Disorder

Outcomes following pharmacotherapy, psychotherapy, and psychosurgery support the neurobiological basis of OCD. Both pharmacotherapy with SSRIs and behavioral therapy have reduced hyperactivity of the caudate, orbitofrontal lobes, and cingulate cortex in patients with symptoms of OCD (Baxter, Schwartz, Bergman, et al., 1992). Cognitive behavioral therapy (CBT) has been shown to result in similar changes in cerebral metabolism (Schwartz, 1998). Recently, Saxena, Gorbis, O'Neill, et al. (2009) found that brief intensive daily CBT resulted in functional changes, changes in brain activity in 4 weeks, and changes in brain glucose metabolism in specific regions. The changes correlated with improvement in OCD symptoms. Neurosurgical interventions directly interrupt the CSTC loop. The outcomes of these neurosurgical procedures support the involvement of CSTC circuitry in the production of symptoms of OCD (Stein & Rauch, 2010).

Clinical Presentation

It was formerly believed that patients with OCD were always aware of the unreasonableness of their obsessions (had insight) and that they struggled against them and often tried to hide them rather than seek treatment. Based on the observation that not all patients with OCD had good insight into the unreasonableness of their obsessions, the specifier "OCD with poor insight" was added to the criteria for OCD in the *DSM-IV-TR* (American Psychiatric Association, 2000). More recently, it has been accepted that insight in patients with OCD may be good, poor, or absent (delusional thinking) (Eisen & Rasmussen, 2002). Although the average age of onset of OCD symptom is 14.5 years, patients often wait 10 years before seeking treatment from their primary care physician. When they do seek treatment, they are often diagnosed as having generalized anxiety disorder or depression, and another 6 years may pass before they are referred for a psychiatric evaluation and correctly diagnosed with OCD (Hollander et al., 1996).

During the psychiatric evaluation, patients with OCD often describe obsessions as a sudden intrusion of unwanted thoughts or distressing images that are associated with a sense of dread and an urge to carry out an activity that will reduce the distress (Leckman et al., 2005). There is usually no precipitating stressful event. They may describe an episode characterized by intrusive thoughts that are anxiety provoking, such as fear of contamination and germs or fear of harm to themselves or others (McKay & Robbins, 2009). They may describe compulsions and repetitive behaviors, such as constant checking, washing, touching, or counting (Hollander et al., 1996; Rosqvist & Norling, 2008; Summerfeldt, 2008). Patients may have chapped hands from repeated washing or dental problems from excessive teeth cleaning. They may describe problems at work related to their need for constant checking and perfectionism that interferes with completing assignments on time.

Clinical Symptoms

Obsessions

Obsessions can involve preoccupation with contamination; preoccupation with symmetry (exactness, precision); pathologic doubting or uncertainty (concern that as a result of their carelessness they will be responsible for a dire event); somatic obsessions (fear of developing a serious life-threatening illness, such as cancer); saving or hoarding; preoccupation with harm to self and others; preoccupation with sexual or violent thoughts; or a sense that something unpleasant may happen if a particular ritual is not performed (Jenike, 2001).

The four most common obsessions among adults are contamination (57.5%), pathological doubt (56.0%), need for symmetry (47.8%), and sexual or aggressive obsessions (45.5%). The next most common obsessions are hoarding (29.4%) and somatic obsessions (26.3%) (Eisen et al., 2010, p. 267).

- *Contamination.* Contamination obsessions are the most frequent of the obsessions encountered in treatment settings. They are usually fear of dirt or germs, but they can include fear of things in the environment, such as toxins, or can include fear of bodily wastes (Attiullah et al., 2000). Patients fear the consequence of touching a contaminated object. They often fear that they will harm others or make them ill. Patients use avoidance to prevent contact and excessive washing after contact with something they consider to be contaminated (Attiullah et al.; Eisen & Rasmussen, 2002).
- *Pathological doubt.* Patients with pathological doubt dread causing a dire event by their carelessness. They worry about leaving the stove on and consequently causing a fire that may destroy the house. They may doubt their own perceptions. They often use checking rituals and may use avoidance behaviors, such as not leaving the house so that there is no possibility of leaving it unlocked (Attiullah et al., 2000).
- *Need for symmetry.* The need for symmetry is an urge to arrange things perfectly or to perform actions in an exact sequence. Patients with a need for symmetry have an urge to repeat actions until they feel "just right" (Eisen & Rasmussen, 2002, p. 181). Patients with this obsession often have magical thinking. They believe that if they do ordering and arranging rituals, then they can prevent harm to their loved ones. Some patients have obsessive slowness. They take a very long time to perform a task. Each small step of a task must be done perfectly, and they lose track of the bigger goal to be achieved. Patients with symmetry obsessions and compulsions describe feeling uneasy rather than fearful or anxious when things are not arranged or ordered just so. They have increased uneasiness or a sense of tension until they perform the acts of ordering or arranging things so that they are perfect. Or, they may feel the need to "even up" (Eisen & Rasmussen, 2002, p. 181) by performing the same act on both sides of an object. Eisen et al. (2010) said that this sensation of uneasiness is more similar to that of patients with tics than to the anxiety experienced by patients with other subcategories of OCD. Patients with extreme perfectionism or obsessional slowness may not respond to behavioral therapy.
- *Sexual and aggressive obsessions.* Patients fear that they may commit a sexually inappropriate act or harm others, or they fear that they have already committed such acts. Watching reports of unsolved murders on television may make them very anxious. They use checking, seeking reassurance, and confession to police and priests to reduce anxiety. They may use avoidance behaviors, such as removing sharp knives and scissors to reduce their fears that they may hurt someone. They may think that they deserve to be punished (Attiullah et al., 2000).
- *Hoarding.* There are few studies of hoarding among humans, in contrast to the many studies of hoarding among animals. Human hoarding does not usually involve hoarding food. The most commonly hoarded items are newspapers, magazines, junk mail, old clothes, notes or lists, and old receipts (Laraia, 2006). The fear that underlies the behavior seems to be a fear of making the wrong decision (e.g., discarding something useful or something that could be needed in the future) (Feusner & Saxena, 2005).

Hoarding obsession occurs among 11% of children with OCD (Rapoport, 1989) and among 18% to 42% of adults with OCD (Laraia, 2006; Rasmussen & Eisen, 1989). Patients with OCD and hoarding tend to have higher levels of anxiety and depression; tics; social anxiety; and dependent, schizotypal, and obsessive-compulsive personality disorders than patients with OCD who do not have hoarding (Baer, 1994; Laraia,

2006). Patients with hoarding obsessions have more severe OCD symptoms and greater impairment of social and vocational functioning than patients with other obsessions (Frost, Steketee, Williams, et al., 2000). Patients with OCD and hoarding obsessions often do not have insight into their symptoms and think that hoarding is reasonable behavior.

Patients with OCD and hoarding have lower levels of metabolism in the anterior cingulate cortex and thalamus (Laraia, 2006). Lower activity in the anterior and posterior cingulate cortexes may underlie the problems patients with OCD have in making decisions and focusing attention. These findings support the reasoning that OCD with hoarding may have a neurobiological basis that is different from that of other categories of OCD.

- *Somatic obsessions.* Somatic obsessions are irrational fears of developing a serious life-threatening illness (e.g., cancer, venereal disease, AIDS) (Attiullah et al., 2000). Patients with somatic obsessions often use checking rituals—checking the body for signs and symptoms of illness.

Compulsions

Compulsions include repetitive physical behaviors, mental rituals, or both, such as checking; ordering; arranging; counting; repeating rituals; cleaning; hoarding; collecting; repeating specific prayers or protective thoughts; needing to ask repeatedly; needing to confess; and mental compulsions (silent counting, reviewing, or praying) (de Silva, Menzies, & Shafran, 2003). Most adults and children with OCD have multiple obsessions and compulsions (First & Tasman, 2005). In children, the most common compulsions are washing and repeating rituals (Rapoport, 1989). Noshirvani et al. (1991) found that early onset (ages 5 to 15 years) was associated with more checking compulsions and late onset (ages 26 to 35 years) with more washing compulsions. Table 12-3 lists obsessions and their characteristics, associated compulsions, and potential biological bases.

TABLE 12-3 OBSESSIONS IN OBSESSIVE-COMPULSIVE DISORDER: THEIR CHARACTERISTICS, ASSOCIATED COMPULSIONS, AND BIOLOGICAL BASIS

Obsession	Characteristics	Associated Compulsions	Biological Basis
Contamination (most frequent obsession encountered in treatment settings)	Fear of dirt or germs; fear of things in the environment such as toxins; fear of bodily wastes (Attiullah et al., 2000). Fear that touching a contaminated object will bring harm to others or make them ill.	Patients use avoidance to prevent contact and wash excessively (Attiullah et al., 2000; Eisen & Rasmussen, 2002).	Increased cerebral blood flow in bilateral anterior cingulate cortex and left orbitofrontal cortex. Activation of brain regions involved in emotions and disgust (visual regions and insular cortex) (Phillips, Marks, Senior, et al., 2000).
Pathological doubt	Worry that one will cause a dire event by carelessness; e.g., worry about leaving the stove on and causing a fire that may destroy the house.	They may doubt their own perceptions and use checking rituals. They may use avoidance behaviors such as not leaving the house so that there is no possibility of leaving it unlocked (Attiullah et al., 2000).	Reduced gray matter volume in the right amygdala (Pujol, Soriano, Alonso, et al., 2004). Checking symptoms correlate with increased blood flow in the striatum (Rauch et al., 1998). Checking: activation in frontal-striatal regions and thalamus (Phillips et al., 2000).
Need for symmetry	A feeling of *uneasiness* when things are not arranged or ordered just so. An urge to arrange things perfectly or to perform actions in an exact sequence or an urge to repeat actions until they feel "just right" (Eisen & Rasmussen, 2002, p. 181). Some individuals with this obsession have magical thinking. Some have obsessive slowness. They take a long time to perform a task.	They perform the acts of ordering or arranging things so that they are perfect. Or, they may feel the need to "even up" by performing the same act on both sides of an object (Eisen & Rasmussen, 2002, p. 181). They fear consequences to their loved ones and do ordering and arranging rituals to prevent harm to their loved ones. Each small step of a task must be done perfectly. They lose track of the bigger goal to be achieved.	Reduced cerebral blood flow in the striatum (Rauch et al., 1998).
Somatic obsessions	Irrational fears of developing a serious life threatening illness. Fears frequently are of cancer, venereal disease, and AIDS (Attiullah et al., 2000).	Patients with somatic obsessions often use checking rituals—checking the body for signs and symptoms of illness.	Abnormalities of BDNF, which modulates the glutamate system that is involved in symptoms of OCD (Katerberg, Lochner, Cath, et al., 2007). Abnormalities of serotonin transporter gene (Katerberg et al., 2007).

TABLE 12-3 OBSESSIONS IN OBSESSIVE-COMPULSIVE DISORDER: THEIR CHARACTERISTICS, ASSOCIATED COMPULSIONS, AND BIOLOGICAL BASIS—continued

Obsession	Characteristics	Associated Compulsions	Biological Basis
Hoarding (occurs among 20% to 30% of patients with OCD) (Frost, Krause, & Steketee, 1996)	Fear of making the wrong decisions and discarding something useful or needed in the future (Feusner & Saxena, 2005), Four key features: 1. Difficulty discarding 2. Excessive acquiring 3. Clutter 4. Impaired ability to function and loss of use of home for family activities. Excessive collection of things (paper, magazines, junk mail, old clothes, notes, and receipts) (Laraia, 2006) or animals to the point that they interfere with tasks of daily living, interpersonal relationships, vocational functioning, and even safety and health (Best-Lavigniac, 2006; Gilliam & Tolin, 2010).	Saving things but without an organizational system or proper storage. Acquiring more items. Failing to discard useless items. Cluttering living spaces of home with acquisitions. Restriction of family, social, and work activities (Gilliam & Tolin, 2010).	Reduced glucose metabolism (less activity) in the posterior cingulate gyrus and the dorsal anterior cingulate cortex (Saxena, Brody, Maidment, et al., 2004). Increased cerebral blood flow in the striatum; e.g., activation in frontal-striatal regions and thalamus.
Sexual or aggressive obsessions.	Fear that they might harm others or commit a sexually unacceptable act. Think that they deserve to be punished (Attiullah et al., 2000).	Use checking, confession to priests or police, or reassurance rituals (First & Tasman, 2005). Use avoidance such as removing potential harmful objects such as knives or scissors.	Abnormalities of BDNF, which modulates the glutamate system that is involved in symptoms of OCD (Katerberg et al., 2007).

BDNF, brain-derived neurotropic factor.

The occurrence of obsessions or compulsions alone is rare, but compulsions may occur without obsessional thoughts. In such instances, the compulsions are more tic-like. The individual has to do them until the feeling of anxiety is quieted. Compulsions may change over time, but they tend to remain in the same dimension (Mataix-Cols, Rauch, Baer, et al., 2002; Rufer, Fricke, Moritz, et al., 2006) (see Box 12-1 for dimensional categories). Compulsions include both repetitive physical behaviors and mental rituals, and some patients with OCD use neutralizing strategies to reduce distress (Box 12-2).

Family Accommodation to OCD

Family accommodation refers to the family's participation or assistance in the patient's rituals. It is present among 60% of families who have a family member with OCD (Albert, Bogetto, Maina, et al., 2010). Family members with accommodation behaviors often experience anxiety, depression, distress, and a sense of burden. Accommodation behaviors include

- Providing reassurance
- Participating in rituals, most frequently those associated with contamination, washing or checking, or both
- Providing supplies used in the patient's rituals
- Assisting in avoidance behaviors
- Assuming the patient's responsibilities or tasks

BOX 12-2 Compulsions: Physical Behaviors, Mental Rituals and Neutralizing Strategies

Physical Behaviors
- Checking
- Ordering
- Arranging
- Counting
- Repeating rituals
- Cleaning
- Hand washing
- Hoarding
- Collecting

Mental Rituals
- Repeating specific prayers, words, or protective thoughts
- Need to ask
- Need to confess
- Mental compulsions (silent counting, reviewing, or praying)

Neutralizing Strategies
- Seeking reassurance from others
- Overanalyzing
- Using rational self-talk
- Replacing a bad thought with a good thought
- Performing brief mental or behavioral acts to remove the thought
- Using a distracting activity
- Thought stopping

Sources: deSilva, Menzies, & Shafran, 2003; and Ladouceur et al., 2000.

- Modifying work schedules, leisure activities, and family relations to fit with the patient's rituals
- Agreeing with the patient with regard to rituals because of fear of abuse if they do not (Albert et al., 2010)

The presence of accommodation by the family or by a family member is associated with greater severity of the patient's symptoms and the patient's poorer response to treatment. Family accommodation is one component of the clinical presentation and needs to be part of the treatment plan (Albert et al., 2010).

Comorbidity

Two-thirds of patients with OCD have comorbid Axis I psychiatric disorders (Murphy et al., 2010). The most common comorbid psychiatric disorders are major depression, dysthymia, panic disorder, separation anxiety disorder, generalized anxiety disorder, social anxiety disorder, schizophrenia, schizoaffective disorder, adjustment disorder, and eating disorders (Attiullah et al., 2000). Approximately half of patients with OCD have comorbid Axis II psychiatric disorders (personality disorders), with dependent, avoidant, and obsessive-compulsive personality disorders being the most common (Dougherty et al., 2010; Eisen & Rasmussen, 2002; Wiegartz & Rasminsky, 2005). Among patients with OCD and symptoms of schizotypal personality disorder, there is a tendency for an earlier age of onset of OCD, a greater number of comorbidities, and a higher rate of learning disabilities. They tend to have aggressive and somatic obsessions and to have compulsions of counting and arranging (Sobin, Blundell, Weiller, et al., 2000).

Among neurological comorbid conditions, approximately 20% of patients with OCD have a lifetime history of tics, and 5% to 10% have a history of TS (Leckman, Walker, Goodman, et al., 1994). Patients with OCD and coexisting tic disorders are more likely to have touching, tapping, counting, hoarding, blinking, and staring compulsions and obsessions with symmetry, ordering, and somatic or religious content (Leckman et al., 1994); patients with tic disorders are most likely to have OCD symptoms of symmetry and ordering (Eisen & Rasmussen, 2002; Petter, Richter, & Sandor, 1998).

Differential Diagnosis

Other psychiatric disorders that are characterized by repetitive behaviors and thoughts include TS, trichotillomania, kleptomania, hypochondriasis, panic disorder, generalized anxiety disorder, and obsessive-compulsive personality disorder (Micallef & Blin, 2001) (Table 12-4). Case Study 12-1 presents a patient with OCD and comorbid psychiatric, medical, and social health problems.

Treatment

The first step in treatment is a comprehensive psychiatric assessment. The psychiatric assessment provides the base of information that will be used in developing a plan of treatment that addresses the pattern and severity of the patient's symptoms and the patient's unmet needs, strengths and weaknesses, stressors, social support, and family situation. During the psychiatric assessment, if the diagnosis of OCD is considered, the psychiatric advanced practice nurse should follow the National Institute for Health and Clinical

TABLE 12-4 DIFFERENTIAL DIAGNOSIS OF OBSESSIVE-COMPULSIVE DISORDER

Other Disorder	Differentiating Characteristics
Obsessive-compulsive personality disorder	Does not have obsessions or compulsions. Involves pervasive pattern of orderliness, perfectionism, and control. It is more likely to have restricted affect, excessive devotion to work, and rigidity; in OCD, the obsessions are preoccupying and distressing and impair functioning (Eisen et al., 2010).
Anxiety disorder due to general medical condition	Presence of a general medical condition that involves the basal ganglia, such as Sydenham's chorea and Huntington's disease. OCD tends to occur earlier than medical conditions (Sadock & Sadock, 2007).
Substance-induced anxiety disorder	Due to direct physiological effects of a substance, including medications (American Psychiatric Association, 2000).
Body dysmorphic disorder or eating disorder	Recurrent thoughts are related to a preoccupation with appearance or body weight (First & Tasman, 2004).
Phobia	Thoughts are related to a feared specific object (Eisen et al., 2010).
Social anxiety disorder (SAD)	Fears are circumscribed and related to specific triggers such as social situations. Patients are able to avoid the situations causing anxiety (Eisen et al., 2010).
Hypochondriasis	Recurrent thoughts are related to fear that one has a serious illness (First & Tasman, 2004).
Kleptomania, pathological gambling ,and trichotillomania (like OCD, characterized by impulsive behaviors)	The behaviors are associated with gratification, whereas in OCD the behaviors just relieve anxiety (First & Tasman, 2004).
Major depressive disorder	The thoughts are brooding and ego-syntonic. In depression, there are more likely to be ruminations that focus on past losses. Black and Andreasen (2011) wrote, "Whereas the depressed patient tends to focus on past events, the obsessional patient focuses on the prevention of future events" (p. 195). The ruminations tend to focus on past losses.

TABLE 12-4 DIFFERENTIAL DIAGNOSIS OF OBSESSIVE-COMPULSIVE DISORDER—continued

Other Disorder	Differentiating Characteristics
Generalized anxiety disorder (GAD)	In patients with GAD, the worries are everyday worries and are ego-syntonic. The worry is excessive but thinking is realistic. Patients with GAD usually do not develop rituals (Eisen et al., 2010).
Post-traumatic stress disorder (PTSD)	In PTSD, intrusive thoughts and images are replays of actual events (First & Tasman, 2004).
Delusional disorder or psychotic disorder not otherwise specified	In schizophrenia, the patient has a fixed conviction or delusional disorder that cannot be shaken and also usually has other psychotic symptoms such as paranoia or hallucinations (Jenike, 2001). In contrast, patients with OCD may be able to recognize that their ideas are unfounded and unwanted (Black & Andreasen, 2011).
Tic or stereotypical movement disorder	Movements are not done to neutralize an obsession (American Psychiatric Association, 2000).
Driven behaviors associated with other disorders; e.g., paraphilias	Individual gets pleasure from activity; may want to stop because of consequences (First & Tasman, 2004).
Nonpathological superstitions and repetitive behaviors	Does not result in distress or impairment of functioning (First & Tasman, 2004).

CASE STUDY 12-1

A Patient With OCD and Comorbid Psychiatric, Medical, and Social Health Problems

Lona Peters is a 38-year-old single Caucasian woman. She never married, lives alone, and works as a secretary in the research center of the University. Her primary care physician referred her for a psychiatric consultation because of her recent panic attack.

Lona appears well groomed, conservatively dressed, of normal weight for her height, and older than her stated age. On entering the office, before sitting down, she arranges the chair to align it with the edge of the desk and folds her raincoat precisely before placing it on her lap with her gloves and purse centered on the coat. She says that she has come to get help to prevent further panic attacks. The panic attack that she experienced happened at work, and she was mortified at losing control and not being able to stop the attack. She was sure that she was having a heart attack.

History reveals that she is an only child. Her father had been in the Navy, and they had moved every 2 years. She says that she dreaded relocating because she feared that she would lose her things. When her father retired, her parents moved to Pensacola, Florida, and she visits them there. She says that, from what her mother has told her, she had been a forceps delivery and a good baby. She had walked and talked at the normal time. She says that she was a quiet child and adds with pride that, unlike most children, she kept her toys in perfect condition in the boxes in which they came. As a child, she had several bad throat infections and then had her tonsils removed. After that, her health had been good until 2 months ago, when she began feeling down and having problems falling asleep. Her primary physician prescribed sertraline. She said that the sertraline may have helped a little, but she still has difficulty falling asleep.

She denies any health problems, has not been treated for any psychiatric problems, and denies any thoughts of suicide. She does not know of any psychiatric disorders in the family or of anyone having panic attacks. She describes her father as a stern man and a heavy drinker and her mother as a worrier.

On questioning about events or situations that have changed in her life, she describes changes at work that have been very upsetting for her. She said that it had always been her custom to go to work an hour and a half early so that she could arrange her desk and the material that she knew she would be working on just right. About 3 months ago, the director of the department whom she had known for 14 years retired, and the new director instituted a change of work assignments. The secretaries were expected to work together on sections of grants that had highest priority. Lona found the uncertainty of not knowing what she would be expected to do each day very disturbing. She was accustomed to working alone. She believed that there was a right way to do an assignment and that whatever she was doing had to be perfect before she could hand it in. She often stayed late to check her work or do it over because she felt responsible for the success of the project.

When asked about other changes in her life and what she did for enjoyment, Lona hesitated and said that the clutter, which had accumulated as a result of her habit of saving newspapers, receipts, and telephone books in case she needed them, made her ashamed to invite people to visit her. She no longer participated in the book club that she had once enjoyed because she did not want the group to come to her home. Now, she is worried about what would happen if she had a panic attack and had to call for help.

Questions

1. What type of obsessions is the patient experiencing?
2. What comorbid biopsychosocial health problems are present?
3. What treatment would you recommend?

Answers to these questions can be found at the end of this chapter.

Excellence (NICE) (2005) guidelines for the treatment of OCD, which recommend using six screening questions:

1. Do you wash or clean a lot?
2. Do you check things a lot?
3. Is there any thought that keeps bothering you that you would like to get rid of but can't?
4. Do your daily activities take a long time to finish?
5. Are you concerned about orderliness or symmetry?
6. Do these problems trouble you?

HEYMAN, MATAIX-COLS, FINEBERG, 2006, P. 426 (DERIVED FROM THE ZOHAR-FINEBERG OBSESSIVE COMPULSIVE SCREEN).

If a diagnosis of OCD is generated, the psychiatric advanced practice nurse may use the Yale-Brown Obsessive Compulsive Scale (Y-BOCS) (Goodman, Price, Rasmussen, et al., 1989a, 1989b), which is a 10-item scale, to evaluate the severity of the illness. It may also be used to monitor change of the OCD symptoms over time. If a scale is not used, the psychiatric advanced practice nurse should document the number of hours in the day that the patient spends on obsessions and on performing compulsive behaviors. The items and situations that the patient avoids should also be documented. This information provides a baseline for measuring the effectiveness of treatment (American Psychiatric Association, 2007).

OCD is a chronic disorder, but 50% of patients will improve with treatment ("Treating obsessive-compulsive disorder," 2009). The overall goals of treatment are to (1) reduce frequency and intensity of symptoms, (2) minimize the symptoms' interference with the patient's life, (3) improve functioning, and (4) improve quality of life (family, social, work/school, parenting, and leisure activities domains) (American Psychiatric Association, 2007; First & Tasman, 2005).

First-line treatment for OCD includes serotonin reuptake inhibitors (SRIs) and CBT (Davidson, Connor, & Zhang, 2009; Fineberg & Craig, 2010; Greist & Baer, 2002). About 25% of patients with OCD refuse behavioral therapy because they fear that it will be too anxiety provoking (Lucey, Butcher, Clare, et al., 1994; McDonald & Blizard, 1988), and about 25% of patients with OCD refuse medications (Greist & Baer, 2002). Whereas either CBT or pharmacotherapy can be offered first as monotherapy for adults, CBT is recommended as the first-line treatment for children and adolescents because of the possible adverse effects of SSRIs (Heyman et al., 2006). In deciding which treatment modality to use, the psychiatric advanced practice nurse takes into consideration the severity of the patient's symptoms, the presence and treatment of co-occurring psychiatric and medical disorders, the history of past response to treatment, the patient's preferences, and the availability of treatment modalities such as CBT.

Pharmacotherapy

Both SSRIs and SRIs are effective in treating OCD. The first line of treatment for patients with OCD is a 12-week trial of an SSRI. Fluvoxamine (Luvox), fluoxetine (Prozac), sertraline (Zoloft), and paroxetine (Paxil) have U.S. Food and Drug Administration (FDA) approval for treatment of OCD (Davidson et al., 2009). However, all of the SSRIs have proved to be effective in the treatment of OCD. Their side effects—including nausea, sleepiness, insomnia, tremor, and sexual dysfunction—tend to be less troublesome for the patient than the side effects of the SRI clomipramine (Anafranil), which include dry mouth, constipation, sedation, weight gain, nausea, tremor, orthostatic hypotension, sexual dysfunction, prolonged QT interval, risk for seizures at high doses, and risk of death by overdose (American Psychiatric Association, 2007; Hollander & Simeon, 2008).

- ***SSRIs.*** The dose of SSRIs that is used for OCD may need to be higher than the dose used for depression, and the time to response may be longer (Black & Andreasen, 2011; Davidson & Connor, 2004; Fineberg & Craig, 2010): response time may be 3 months (Dubovsky, 2005). Goodman (2002) suggested that improvement of symptoms with SSRIs may be due to increased serotonin activity in the orbitofrontal cortex. Approximately 70% of patients receiving SSRIs will have a response (defined by Fineberg, Tonnoir, & Lemming [2006] as a 25% or greater improvement on the Y-BOCS from the baseline score), and 40% will achieve remission (Fineberg & Craig, 2010). Poor response to SSRIs is associated with some subtypes of OCD, such as OCD with obsessional slowness, pathological doubting, and checking (Goodman).
- ***SRI: Clomipramine.*** Clomipramine was one of the first medications studied for treatment of OCD. It has FDA approval. A tricyclic antidepressant, clomipramine differs from other tricyclic antidepressants in that it has a potent serotonin reuptake-inhibiting effect (it is not selective for serotonin). Although clomipramine and the SSRIs are considered to be equally effective in the treatment of OCD (Flament & Bisserbe, 1997; Greist & Jefferson, 2007; Koran, McElroy, Davidson, et al., 1996; Zohar & Judge, 1996), the relatively low level of side effects of the SSRIs in comparison to the more numerous side effects of clomipramine make clomipramine a second-line choice for treatment (Goodman, 2002). However, it is often used when patients do not respond to SSRIs (Davidson & Connor, 2004).

Nonresponse to Pharmacotherapy

Response to treatment is usually determined by scores on the 10-item Y-BOCS (Goodman et al., 1989a, 1989b): the presence of no OCD symptoms is scored as 0, and the presence of extreme symptoms is scored as 40. Nonresponse to treatment is also called *treatment resistance*, and the term is used to describe lack of response to at least two trials of SSRIs. *Treatment refractory* or *treatment intractable* refers to a greater degree of nonresponsiveness, such as failure to respond to a variety of OCD treatment strategies

(Goodman, 2002). Reasons for treatment resistance include incorrect dosage, incorrect length of treatment time, lack of patient adherence to treatment, and differences of underlying OCD neuropathology. The presence of psychosocial factors, such as stressors or lack of support, is associated with lower rates of response to treatment. The presence of certain comorbid conditions—such as Axis II disorders (schizotypal or avoidant personality disorder), medical disorders, and chronic tic disorder—is associated with a poorer outcome (Baer, Jenike, Black, et al., 1992; Black & Noyes, 1997; Jenike, Baer, & Minichiello, 1986).

Switching, Augmentation, and Combination

Before considering switching or augmentation, patients should have a 12-week trial of a medication (Fineberg & Craig, 2010). If there is some response to an SSRI without too many troublesome side effects, the first step may be to *increase* the dose to the highest recommended dose (Goodman, 2002). If there is no improvement following a trial with one SSRI, switching to another SSRI may be tried. Clomipramine should be tried if the patient does not respond to the SSRIs.

Augmentation includes the use of fluvoxamine with clomipramine in patients who have shown a partial response to clomipramine, because fluvoxamine increases the availability of clomipramine (Szegedi, Wetzel, Leal, et al., 1996). While benzodiazepines are not effective as monotherapy (Hollander, Kaplan, & Stahl, 2003), the benzodiazepine clonazepam (Klonopin), which has anxiolytic properties and serotonergic effects, has been added to clomipramine, with mixed benefits (Pigott, L'Heureux, Rubinstein, et al., 1992).

In combination therapy, patients who are refractory to SSRI and SRI treatment have been found to benefit from the addition of an agent from another class of medication such as antipsychotics (Fineberg & Craig, 2010). For example, haloperidol and risperidone (Risperdal) have been found to be effective, but olanzapine (Zyprexa) and quetiapine (Seroquel) have been found to be less effective (Davidson et al., 2009). For patients with OCD and comorbid tic disorders, adding haloperidol to fluvoxamine has been found to be beneficial (McDougle, Goodman, Leckman, et al., 1994). In a review of effectiveness of adding antipsychotics for treatment of refractory OCD, Bloch, Landeros-Weisenberger, Kelmendi, et al. (2006) concluded that patients should be treated for at least 3 months of maximally tolerated therapy with an SSRI or SRI before an antipsychotic is added. They noted that only one-third of treatment-refractory OCD patients showed response to added antipsychotics and that patients with OCD and comorbid tics were the ones who were most likely to benefit.

Novel Drug Treatment

Clomipramine administered intravenously as initial loading has been used and may have a greater effect than oral loading (Koran, Sallee, & Pallanti, 1997). Inositol, a second-messenger precursor that is believed to be involved in the maintenance of cell membranes and the regulation of the action of serotonin within the brain cells, has been found to be associated with a reduction of OCD symptoms in some studies (Fux, Levine, Aviv, et al., 1996), but this is not supported by others (Fux, Benjamin, & Belmaker, 1999). Venlafaxine (Effexor) has been found to be effective by some clinicians (Goodman, 2002) but not by others (Fineberg & Craig, 2010).

Long-term Treatment

Long-term treatment for patients who have responded during an acute phase to a medication usually includes maintenance of the patient on that medication for 1 to 2 years with a gradual discontinuation after that time (American Psychiatric Association, 2007; Greist, Bandelow, Hollander, et al., 2003). The relapse rate with sudden discontinuation of medication is as high as 90% (Pato et al., 1990). Therefore, discontinuation should include a gradual taper to reduce discontinuation symptoms of vertigo, dizziness, headache, vivid dreams, and irritability and to reduce the risk of relapse (Goodman, 2002).

Other Somatic Interventions

Other somatic interventions include electroconvulsive therapy (ECT), repetitive transcranial magnetic stimulation (rTMS), neurosurgical interventions, and deep brain stimulation (Fineberg & Craig, 2010). ECT may be useful for patients with OCD and depression who are at risk for suicide (Goodman, 2002). However, there is no consensus that ECT and rTMS are effective treatments for OCD (Fineberg & Craig, 2010; "Treating obsessive-compulsive disorder," 2009). (See Chapter 13 for more information on ECT and rTMS.)

Neurosurgical approaches, such as anterior cingulotomy, subcaudate tractotomy, and anterior capsulotomy, have been reported to be helpful for refractory OCD (Greist & Jefferson, 2007). For example, among patients with refractory OCD who received neurosurgical treatment, 25% to 30% showed marked improvement (Baer, Rauch, Ballantine, et al., 1995; Jernicke, Baer, Ballantine, et al., 1991). Neurosurgical approaches are considered to be the option of last resort. Criteria for surgery include extensive trials of medication and behavioral therapy and a combination of therapies. Risks include seizures and personality changes ("Treating obsessive-compulsive disorder," 2009).

Deep brain stimulation, a nondestructive and reversible neuromodulary technique, has recently been approved by the FDA for the treatment of severe OCD. In this procedure, a surgeon places electrodes in the brain and connects them to a small electrical generator in the chest. The device distributes electrical pulses deep within the brain to suppress the symptoms associated with severe OCD. It is used for patients with severe OCD who have not responded well to medications or psychotherapy (Dyess, 2009). Deep brain stimulation benefits about 50% of patients with refractory

OCD (Bear, Fitzgerald, Rosenfeld, et al., 2010). At the present time, deep brain stimulation is an expensive treatment option that is not readily available.

Psychotherapy

Psychotherapists seek to change thoughts and feelings and expect that these changes will be followed by changes in behavior and functioning (Greist & Baer, 2002). Behavioral therapists seek to change behaviors, and they expect that changes in behavior will be followed by a reduction of distressful thoughts and feelings and improved functioning.

Cognitive Behavioral Therapy (CBT)

CBT that uses exposure and response prevention (ERP), which is described below, is considered to be the front-line treatment for OCD, based on the evidence generated in research studies (American Psychiatric Association, 2007). Standard CBT uses *weekly* sessions and requires 8 to 12 weeks for improvement of OCD symptoms. Intensive CBT uses *daily* sessions and requires 4 weeks for improvement of OCD symptoms (Saxena et al., 2009). OCD symptoms improved in 60% to 80% of patients who received intensive CBT (Saxena et al.).

Exposure and Response Prevention Therapy

ERP therapy, a variant of CBT, includes (1) daily exposure to cues that are usually avoided because they induce discomfort and compulsive rituals, (2) maintaining exposure and not ritualizing for at least an hour, and (3) 10 to 20 hours of treatment. The response rate is 70% to 80% after 20 sessions. For example, Foa and Kozak (1996) found that 76% of patients with OCD had a good response to ERP and that the benefits were maintained 2 years after the treatment. There is evidence that ERP is more effective if it includes discussion of feared consequences and dysfunctional beliefs (Vogel, Stiles, & Gotestam, 2004).

Behavioral Therapy

Behavioral therapy alone is effective for patients with mild symptoms of OCD and for those who do not want to take medications ("Treating obsessive-compulsive disorder," 2009). The goal of behavioral therapy is to gradually extinguish a conditioned behavioral response. Effective behavioral therapy for OCD consists of in vivo ERP (prevention of ritual behaviors in response to the exposure) (Abramowitz, 1996). Performance of ritual behaviors shows early improvement, whereas reduction of obsessions and anxiety may take 3 months (Greist & Jefferson, 2007). However, behavioral therapy is not effective for 25% of patients with OCD, including those with depression, those who lack insight, or those with poor compliance with homework assignments (Greist, 1994).

Supportive Psychotherapy

Supportive psychotherapy is characterized by empathy, support for the individual's strengths, education about the illness, and optimism for improvement. It is useful as part of the treatment of OCD (Greist & Jefferson, 2007).

Combination of Psychotherapy and Pharmacotherapy

The evidence supports the premise that combination of SSRIs and SRI and ERP therapy is better for some patients with OCD (Fineberg & Craig, 2010). Combination approach is indicated for

- Treatment of patients with OCD who have a comorbidity that may interfere with ERP therapy (e.g., depression or anxiety disorders that respond to medication)
- Enhancing adherence to ERP
- Treatment of partial responders to monotherapy (SSRIs, SRIs, or ERP)
- Reducing relapse associated with SSRIs and SRIs
- Treatment of severe OCD (Simpson & Liebowitz, 2005)

Psychosocial Interventions

Psychosocial interventions are used to reduce patients' distress, enhance response to pharmacotherapy and psychotherapy, and improve quality of life. They are often directed at meeting patients' needs, improving patients' ability to cope, increasing their knowledge of their illness and treatment, and facilitating their social and vocational role functioning. Psychosocial interventions that psychiatric advanced practice nurses may implement include

- Providing information about OCD, medications, and adherence to treatment
- Identifying triggers that increase the symptoms, such as nonprescription medications, nicotine, caffeine, and alcohol
- Encouraging the use of bibliotherapy
- Teaching coping strategies, such as habit reversal or thought stopping
- Coordinating the patient's care with other care providers (American Psychiatric Association, 2007; Berghuis, Jongsma, & Bruce, 2008)
- Enhancing social support (Abramowitz, 2010).

Psychiatric advanced practice nurses may make referrals for financial resources, housing assistance, family therapy, self-help groups, or community resources. For example, guided self-help may be effective in mild OCD. It can be accomplished with computer programs or self-help manuals (Table 12-5).

Course

In one 11-year follow-up study of patients with childhood-onset OCD, 36% still had OCD. Among those who still had OCD, 70% had at least one other psychiatric disorder, such as an anxiety disorder or a mood disorder (Wewetzer, Jans, Muller, et al., 2001). In a meta-analysis of 16 long-term follow-up studies of children with OCD, Stewart, Geller, Jenike, et al. (2004) found that the persistence rate of OCD was 41% and that five studies reported high levels of problems with peers, employment, and social relationships. In a recent study of children with OCD who received CBT alone, an SSRI alone,

TABLE 12-5 SELF-HELP INTERVENTIONS AND OUTCOMES

Intervention	Outcomes
Bibliotherapy	Fritzler, Hecker, & Losee (1997) reported improvement of OCD using the self-help book *When Once Is Not Enough* (Steketee & White, 1990) and five face-to-face sessions with a clinician.
Brief exposure and response prevention (ERP) instructions given by therapist on the telephone	Patients with OCD receiving telephone-administered ERP supplemented with the workbook *Brain Lock* (Schwartz & Beyette, 1997) improved significantly and maintained improvement (Taylor, Thordarson, Maxfield, et al., 2003).
Computer-aided cognitive behavioral therapy	Effective in reducing checking compulsion (Baer, Minichiello, & Jenike, 1987).
Computer-aided vicarious exposure	Effective in improving two compulsions, washing and checking (more improvement of washing) (Clark, Kirby, Daniels, et al., 1998; Kirby, Berrios, Daniels, et al., 2000).
Behavior therapy (BT Steps)	Interactive computer program that helps patients work on ERP. Patients receiving computer-guided ERP improved more than the group receiving relaxation therapy but not as much as the patients receiving therapist-guided ERP (Greist & Baer, 2002).

or combined treatment with an SSRI and CBT, 53.6% achieved clinical remission after 12 weeks of combined treatment (Pediatric Obsessive Compulsive Disorder Treatment Study (POTS) Team, 2004). The authors of the study noted that in one setting, CBT was as effective as the combined treatment.

Long-term follow-up studies of patients with OCD are rare. In a 3-year follow-up study of patients who received treatment for 3 years with SSRIs or SRIs, only 38% achieved remission, and 33% were found to be treatment resistant (Catapano, Perris, Masella, et al., 2006). Predictors of poorer outcome were longer duration of OCD, greater severity of OCD symptoms initially, and presence of schizotypal personality disorder (Catapano et al., 2006). In the longest follow-up study of patients with OCD, a 47-year follow-up study in Sweden, Skoog and Skoog (1999) found that 83% of the patients had improved, with 20% achieving full remission, 28% achieving partial recovery, and 35% continuing to meet the criteria for OCD but with some improvement of symptoms. Many showed improvement in social functioning. Higher functioning (a higher Global Assessment of Functioning score at baseline) correlated with better prognosis; however, some symptoms, such as rituals and magical obsessions, were associated with less favorable outcomes. The content of the obsessions and compulsions changed over time for two-thirds of the patients. However, the obsessions and compulsions tended to change within the same cluster rather than moving to another cluster (Mataix-Cols et al., 2002).

In summary, the course of OCD is usually chronic, with 50% to 55.6% of patients having a constant or progressive illness, 25% to 33% having a fluctuating course, and less than 15% having a fluctuating course with periods of remission (Hollander & Simeon, 2008, p. 558). Poorer outcomes are associated with onset before age 20, longer duration of illness, presence of both obsessions and compulsions, lower level of social functioning, and magical thinking (Hollander & Simeon).

Key Points

- OCD is characterized by obsessions and compulsions.
- Obsessions are intrusive, unwanted thoughts, ideas, images, fears, impulses, or urges.
- Compulsions are acts or behaviors that reduce anxiety or distress associated with the obsessions.
- OCD usually begins in adolescence or early adulthood, but symptoms may be present in early childhood.
- Risk factors include genetic vulnerability; prenatal, perinatal, and postnatal factors; environmental factors; traumatic events; and stressful life events.
- Symptoms of OCD are thought to be due to abnormalities of the CSTC circuit with involvement of the basal ganglia.
- Common obsessions are contamination, pathological doubt, need for symmetry, somatic obsessions, and hoarding.
- Common compulsions are washing, checking, ordering/arranging precisely, counting, hoarding, praying, and repeating rituals.
- The family may feel burdened by the extensive accommodations that they make for the affected member's obsessions and compulsions.
- Frontline treatment includes SSRIs and CBT.
- OCD is a chronic illness.

Obsessive-Compulsive Spectrum Disorders

In the past 10 years, there has been increasing focus on OCSDs (Snider & Swedo, 2004a; Stein, 2008). OCSDs are a group of disorders that are related to OCD by their repetitive thoughts and behaviors but are distinct from OCD (Phillips et al., 2010) in that the obsessions and compulsions differ from those of OCD and differ within subcategories of OCSD. Although OCSDs share certain features with OCD—such as age of onset, clinical course, family history, and comorbidities (Hollander, Friedberg, Wasserman, et al., 2005; Rasmussen, 1994; Ravindran, da Silva,

Ranvindran, et al., 2009)—the biological processes of OCD and OCSD represent different disruptions of development and functioning and thus may require different treatment approaches (Stein & Lochner, 2006).

There is lack of consensus as to which disorders should be included in the category of OCSDs (Phillips et al., 2010; Wetterneck, Teng, & Stanley, 2010). In an early approach, OCSDs were divided into four subgroups of diagnostic clusters; inclusion of disorders within the clusters was broad and included some impulse-control disorders (Hollander et al., 1999; Hollander et al., 2005):

1. *Preoccupation with bodily sensations or appearance,* which included body dysmorphic disorder (BDD), depersonalization, anorexia nervosa, and hypochondriasis (HYP)
2. *Impulsive disorders,* which included sexual compulsions, pathological gambling, trichotillomania (TTM), skin picking, self-injurious behavior, kleptomania, and compulsive shopping
3. *Neurological disorders* that affect the basal ganglia, which included autism, Sydenham's chorea, torticollis, and TS
4. *Schizo-obsessive disorders,* which included patients with schizophrenia, among whom 10% to 25% have comorbid OCD (Rasmussen & Tsuang, 1986)

Some researchers included eating disorders and dissociative disorders as OCSDs (Hollander & Wong, 1995; Hollander & Wong, 1999); however, other researchers have stated that although there is evidence to support inclusion of tic disorders, HYP, BDD, and TTM (Bienvenu, Samuels, Riddle, et al., 2000; Ketay, Stein, & Hollander, 2010), there is *not* sufficient evidence to include sexual compulsions, pathological gambling, eating disorders, and depersonalization disorder (Jaisoorya, Reddy, & Srinath, 2003).

In a recent survey of world experts on OCD, it was agreed that based on available evidence, if a new category of OCSD was included in the *DSM-V*, it should be kept narrow. In sum:

- There was strong support for inclusion of BDD, TTM, and tic disorders
- There was moderate support for inclusion of HYP and obsessive-compulsive personality disorder
- There was little support for inclusion of autism or addictions (Mataix-Cols, Pertusa, & Leckman, 2007)
- It was also recommended that impulse-control disorders, such as pathological gambling and shopping, not be considered as part of the OCSDs (Phillips et al., 2010).
- There is support for including hoarding in the *DSM-V* as either a separate disorder ("hoarding disorder") or an OCSD (Mataix-Cols et al., 2010)

Examples of OCSDs from the four subgroups listed above will be discussed in this section. Because of the strong support for including hoarding as a separate disorder, probably within the OCSDs, and because psychiatric advanced practice nurses often manage the care of patients with hoarding, it will be discussed separately.

Epidemiology

While there is no prevalence rate for OCSDs, according to Hollander (1993), when OCD is included as part of the OCSDs, the prevalence is 10% of the general population. Research on the risk factors for the development of OCSDs has been limited (Sampaio, Miguel, Borcato, et al., 2009).

Etiology

The OCSDs are thought to have a genetic basis, and recent studies suggest that genetic mutations underlie the excessive grooming and self-injurious behaviors of some of the OCSDs (Graybiel & Saka, 2002). Family studies suggest a genetic association between OCD and some but not all of the OCSDs (Hollander et al., 2005). For example, Bienvenu et al. (2000) found an elevated prevalence of BDD, HYP, and TTM among family members of patients with OCD.

Biological Basis

The neurocircuitry in OCD and that in OCSD show similar abnormalities. It is thought that the orbitofrontal-subcortical circuits mediate certain symptoms common to both OCD and OCSD, including preoccupation with danger, violence, hygiene, order, and sex.

Clinical Presentation, Comorbidity, Treatment, and Course

Clinical presentation varies among the four clusters of OCSDs:

1. Preoccupation with bodily sensations or appearance
2. Impulsive disorders
3. Neurological disorders
4. Schizo-obsessive disorders (Hollander et al., 2005)

Preoccupation With Bodily Sensations or Appearance Cluster

This cluster includes disorders with symptoms related to body image, bodily sensitization, and body weight. It has included HYP, BDD, eating disorders such as anorexia nervosa and binge eating, and depersonalization disorder. Because at this time only HYP and BDD are widely accepted as belonging to this cluster, discussion in the following section is limited to these two disorders.

Hypochondriasis

In HYP, the patient is obsessed with the fear of having a physical illness despite lack of medical evidence (Fallon & Feinstein, 2001; Fallon, Qureshi, Laje, et al., 2000). The fears are based on misinterpretation of bodily signs or symptoms and are repetitive, intrusive, and distressing. The compulsions associated with HYP include checking the body, checking with others, and seeking medical evaluations and screening tests (Fallon et al.), searching for information about the feared illness, trying herbal remedies, and avoiding situations because of fear of contacting the illness (Taylor & Asmundson, 2008).

Epidemiology

Ten percent to twenty percent of the general population have been found to have unfounded fears about illness that persist despite reassurances (Kellner, 1987). While the prevalence of HYP in the general population is low, 0.05% to 0.4% (Lieb, Zimmermann, Friis, et al., 2002), the rate is 8.2% to 15% among patients with OCD (Phillips et al., 2010). Risk factors include early childhood maltreatment (physical and sexual abuse) (Barsky, Wool, Barnett, et al., 1994) and stressful life events, such as having a serious illness or the loss of a family member (Barsky & Klerman, 1983).

Etiology and Biological Basis

Preliminary studies suggest that HYP does not have a strong degree of heritability (Fallon et al., 2000). Development of HYP is thought to be due to learning experiences that promote misinterpretation of bodily sensations. Likely learning experiences include parental modeling of behaviors in which illness relieves them of responsibilities; parental overprotection that implies that the child is frail and at risk for becoming ill; and parental reinforcement of the child's illness behaviors (Taylor & Asmundson, 2008). Studies of brain functioning of patients with HYP suggest widespread (frontal, striatal, and temporal) response to words associated with threat, indicating abnormality in attention functioning (van den Heuvel, Veltman, Groenewegen, et al., 2005).

Clinical Presentation

Patients with HYP may have an obsessional anxiety about their health, about becoming ill, and about the long-term consequences to their health and well-being. They tend to misinterpret normal changes in their body's functioning, such as in response to a difference in the daily schedule. They may describe somatic fears and avoidance behaviors (Leibbrand, Hiller, & Fichter, 2000). They have poor insight into their illness and are unable to tolerate uncertainty. As a consequence, they often engage in "doctor shopping" by going to many physicians in the hope of finding help for the illness that they think they have (Taylor & Asmundson, 2008, p. 306).

Comorbidity

Comorbidities include OCD, social anxiety disorder, generalized anxiety disorder, panic disorder, pain disorders, and somatoform disorder (Phillips et al., 2010).

Treatment

Treatment for HYP includes SSRIs (paroxetine, fluoxetine, fluvoxamine), CBT (Fallon, Liebowitz, Salman, et al., 1993; Fallon, Qureshi, Schneier, et al., 2003), and psychosocial interventions (Taylor & Asmundson, 2008). Trials of fluoxetine and fluvoxamine have found them to be effective, but the length of time to response is long, 6 weeks or longer. CBT, which challenges patients' misinterpretation of symptoms and attempts to modify behaviors that maintain their symptoms such as checking their body or seeking reassurance from a friend or a physician, has been found to be effective relative to a wait-list control group (Warwick, Clark, & Salkovskis, 1996). SSRIs and CBT have been found to be equally effective (Greeven, van Balkom, Visser, et al., 2007). Psychosocial interventions include helping patients to meet their basic needs such as sleep and exercise, psychoeducation, and stress management (Taylor & Asmundson).

Course

Age of onset is 19 to 23 years (Kessler et al., 2005). Over time, one-fourth of patients do poorly, two-thirds have a chronic fluctuating course, and one-tenth experience recovery (Yutzy & Parish, 2008).

Clinical Implications

First-line treatments are individual CBT and behavioral therapy. There is preliminary evidence to support the use of SSRIs for HYP and for HYP with depression (Ravindran et al., 2009). Pharmacotherapy and CBT may be presented as supplements to the patient's continued medical care. Gradually, the emphasis is shifted from physical symptoms to social or interpersonal problems. Hospitalization, medical tests, and medications are avoided as much as possible (Yutzy & Parish, 2008).

Body Dysmorphic Disorder

In BDD, patients have a preoccupation with an imagined defect in appearance or a minor physical abnormality, often of the face, or with the thought that they are ugly overall (Allen & Hollander, 2000; Yutzy & Parish, 2008). They have high ideals of attractiveness and compare themselves to those idealized standards rather than to the general population (Gleaves & Ambwani, 2008). They also overestimate others' response to their imagined deficit (Ravindran et al., 2009). Patients' core beliefs include the thought that they are inadequate, worthless, or unlovable (Veale, Boocock, Gournay, et al., 1996a). There are obsessive thoughts about their appearance and compulsions that include seeking reassurance; checking their appearance in mirrors, store windows, and other reflective surfaces; attempting to conceal the defect with makeup or clothing; and seeking cosmetic surgery (Phillips, 2007). Some patients with BDD avoid all reflective surfaces. Patients with BDD may diet to correct imagined defects and read about ways to correct their imagined defect (Gleaves & Ambwani, 2008). Patients may spend 3 hours a day or more thinking about their imagined defect, and they may spend hours camouflaging the imagined defect before they will leave their home (Phillips, 2005). The preoccupation causes significant clinical distress and impairment of social, occupational, or other important areas of functioning (American Psychiatric Association, 2000).

A recent manifestation of BDD is "muscle dysmorphia," in which patients' preoccupation is that they are not lean enough or muscular enough (Gleaves & Ambwani,

2008, p. 289). They may avoid situations in which their body is on display, and they may engage in workout sessions to correct their imagined defects or use anabolic steroids, despite knowing the dangers (Cafri, Thompson, Ricciardelli, et al., 2005).

Epidemiology

BDD occurs in approximately 2% of nonclinical populations (Rich, Rosen, & Orosan, 1992) and 12% of psychiatric outpatients (Zimmerman & Matia, 1998). It is present on the average in 15% to 20% of patients with OCD (Phillips et al., 2010) and in 12% of patients seeking dermatological or cosmetic treatment (Phillips, Dufresne, Wilkel, et al., 2000). BDD is associated with impairment of work, social, and intimate relationships. For example, 75% of patients with BDD never marry, and there is a high divorce rate among those who do marry; additionally, one-third become housebound (Phillips, 1995). They are often unemployed, socially isolated, and in poor financial circumstances and lack social support (Gleaves & Ambwani, 2008). Risk factors include perfectionist personality traits (Buhlmann, Etcoff, & Wilhelm, 2008) and history of childhood abuse and neglect (Didie, Tortolani, Pope, et al., 2006).

Etiology and Biological Basis

There is some evidence of genetic influence and of abnormalities of the serotonergic system (Phillips & Kaye, 2007). There is some evidence of abnormalities of the frontal-striatal and temporo-parieto-occipital systems (Perugi & Frare, 2005). There is evidence of impairment of cognitive functioning, in that patients with BDD misinterpret neutral facial expressions as angry and have deficits in memory and executive functioning (Phillips & Kaye). Neziroglu, Roberts, and Yaryura-Tobias (2004) proposed that individuals with a genetic vulnerability for anxiety disorders who are teased or mocked during puberty about physical changes of a facial or body feature may feel shame and disgust associated with that feature. These feelings of shame and disgust are strengthened by avoidance behaviors that the individual uses to reduce distress.

Clinical Presentation

Patients are often referred for psychiatric evaluation by plastic surgery, dermatology, and otorhinolaryngology clinics (De Leon, Bott, & Simpson, 1989). Patients are frequently too embarrassed to describe their preoccupation and will present with symptoms of depression, anxiety, or social withdrawal. They tend to have poor insight, and 27% to 60% have delusional beliefs (Mancuso, Knoesen, & Castle, 2010). They may report difficulties in social and occupational functioning. As many as 48% to 76% of patients with BDD may seek facial cosmetic surgery (Crerand, Sarwer, Magee, et al., 2004), but in 81% of the cases, surgery does not improve the overall symptoms of BDD (Veale, Gournay, Dryden, et al., 1996b). Patients may also describe depressive symptoms and suicidal ideation.

Comorbidity

Comorbidities include depression, social phobia, OCD, and substance-related disorders (Gunstad & Phillips, 2003). The rate of comorbid substance use is approximately 50% (Phillips, Menard, Fay, et al., 2005). In addition, patients with BDD are at increased risk for suicide (Phillips, 2007). For example, the lifetime suicide attempt rate has been estimated at 22% to 24% (Veale et al., 1996a).

Treatment

Patient response to clomipramine is seen in a reduction in preoccupation with appearance, checking behaviors, and depression (Hollander et al., 1999). Patients also respond to SSRIs, such as fluvoxamine (Phillips, McElroy, Dwight, et al., 2001), fluoxetine (Phillips, Albertini, & Rasmussen, 2002), and citalopram (Celexa) (Phillips & Najjar, 2003), with a reduction in intensity of appearance concerns and time spent on preoccupation with an imagined defect (Gleaves & Ambwani, 2008). However, response to SSRIs is often partial, with 40% to 50% of patients not responding to SSRIs as monotherapy (Phillips, Gunderson, Mallya, et al., 1998). Reports of results of CBT that includes ERP have been mixed. When CBT is used alone, 20% to 30% of patients with BDD do not respond. The combination of SSRIs and CBT is associated with a greater response than either treatment alone (Saxena, Winograd, Dunkin, et al., 2001).

Course

Adolescence is the typical time of onset of BDD, with a mean age of onset of 16 to 17 years (Phillips et al., 2005). However, patients often are not correctly diagnosed for many years, until their early or mid 30s (Phillips & Diaz, 1997). BDD is a chronic illness with waxing and waning of symptoms (Phillips, McElroy, Keck, et al., 1993).

Clinical Implications

BDD is characterized by fear, preoccupation with the body, obsessive thoughts, and strong convictions of physical abnormalities (Fallon et al., 2000). Each of these features is taken into consideration in planning treatment (Phillips et al., 2010).

Impulsive Disorder Cluster

In disorders of impulsivity, the patient's actions are impulsive and linked to negative consequences, but the patient lacks control over them (Hollander et al., 2005). The impulses cause a sense of tension or arousal, and the actions cause pleasure, gratification, or a sense of release (McElroy, Pope, Keck, et al., 1995). TTM and skin-picking are widely accepted as impulse disorders within OCSD and will be discussed in the following section.

Trichotillomania

Trichotillomania is the term used to describe recurrent pulling out of one's hair. It is a distressing, chronic condition. There is increased tension before the act and relief of tension afterward (O'Sullivan, Mansueto, Lerner, et al., 2000). Patients tend to have good insight into their illness (Lochner, Seedat, du Toit, et al., 2005). Triggers can be negative affect, such as hyperarousal or boredom. TTM has also been found to be linked with sedentary or contemplative activities, such as watching TV (Christenson, Ristvedt, & Mackenzie, 1993).

Epidemiology

TTM occurs in 0.6% to 3.4% of the general population (Woods, Adcock, & Conelea, 2008) and in 10% to 13% of the college-age population (Rothbaum, Shaw, Morris, et al., 1993). Onset is in middle childhood or early adolescence (Woods et al.). Risk factors include having family members with OCD and possibly early exposure to trauma (Lochner, Simeon, Niehaus, et al., 2002).

Etiology and Biological Basis

Studies of genetic influence and abnormalities of the cortico-striato-thalamic circuitry in TTM are inconclusive (Phillips et al., 2010). Decreased activity in the frontal and parietal lobes, which has been found in patients with TTM, responds to treatment with SSRIs, suggesting involvement of the serotonergic system (Woods et al., 2008).

Clinical Presentation

The key feature is hair pulling that results in hair loss from the scalp, eyebrows, eyelashes, and pubic area (Cohen, Stein, Simeon, et al., 1995). The hair pulling may be accompanied by ritual behaviors, such as eating the hair (Phillips et al., 2010). There are two kinds of hair pulling: nonfocused and focused. Nonfocused hair pulling is present in approximately 75% of adult TTM patients. It has an automatic quality and the patient may not be aware of the behavior. Focused hair pulling involves a conscious effort to reduce a sense of tension by pulling out hair (Woods et al., 2008). Patients with TTM often keep the behavior secret. They experience embarrassment over the loss of hair and tend to limit social activities. They frequently have a negative body image and experience distress over their inability to control the hair pulling (Woods et al).

Comorbidity

Approximately 82% of patients with TTM have a comorbid psychiatric disorder or had one in the past (Hollander, Berlin, & Stein, 2008). The most common Axis I comorbid psychiatric disorders are mood disorders, anxiety disorders, and substance abuse disorders. The most common Axis II disorders are histrionic, borderline, and obsessive-compulsive personality disorders (Christenson, Chernoff-Clementz, & Clementz, 1992).

Treatment

In a systematic review of behavioral treatment and pharmacotherapy for TTM, habit reversal therapy (HRT), a CBT technique, was found to be the most effective intervention (Bloch, Landeros-Weisenberger, Dombrowski, et al., 2007). HRT has four main components:

1. *Self-monitoring:* The patient keeps a record of hair-pulling behavior: when, where, and in what situations.
2. *Awareness training:* The patient is taught to be aware of hair-pulling behavior and high-risk situations that trigger hair pulling.
3. *Stimulus control:* The patient learns techniques to decrease the opportunities for hair pulling and techniques to make it harder to do (e.g., wearing gloves).
4. *Stimulus-response intervention or competing-response intervention:* Patients learn activities to substitute when they feel the desire to pull hair—activities that make it physically impossible to engage in hair pulling at the same time (Bloch et al., 2007).

Reports of effectiveness of SSRIs are inconclusive (Hollander et al., 2008). For example, in one study, escitalopram (Lexapro) was found to benefit 50% of patients (Gadde, Ryan Wagner, Connor, et al., 2007), but in another study, fluoxetine was found to be less effective than CBT or the control (patients on the wait list) (van Minnen, Hoogduin, Keijsers, et al., 2003). Some studies have found clomipramine to be more effective than SSRIs (Bloch et al., 2007). The combination of sertraline and individual HRT has been found to be more effective than either treatment alone (Dougherty, Loh, Jenike, et al., 2006). Patients who have not responded to treatment with SSRIs have responded to augmentation of the SSRI with an atypical antipsychotic such as risperidone (Epperson, Fasula, Wasylink, et al., 1999). Some response to mood stabilizers has been reported (Lochner, Seedat, Niehaus, et al., 2006). Results of naltrexone (ReVia, Depade) are inconsistent (Ravindran et al., 2009).

Course

Onset is in childhood or early adolescence and it has a chronic course (Rasmussen, & Eisen, 1997). In a recent study in which patients received a combination of HRT and cognitive therapy, 66% of those who completed 10 sessions over 12 weeks had a significant reduction of hair pulling and improvement of symptoms of depression and anxiety (Twohig & Woods, 2004).

Clinical Implications

Some of the symptoms of TTM and OCD overlap. There are some features shared with skin-picking disorder, but there is less similarity to impulse-control disorders (Phillips et al., 2010). Overall, the SRIs have limited efficacy in TTM, although clomipramine has been found to be effective. Cognitive therapy, especially individual HRT, has been found to be effective, although the results may wear off over time (Ravindran et al., 2009).

Skin Picking

Skin picking, also called psychogenic excoriation or dermatotillomania (Wetterneck et al., 2010), is repetitive picking, scratching, or gouging the skin that results in tissue damage or infected lesions. It is habitual, ritualistic, tension-reducing, and ego-syntonic (behavior, thoughts, and attitudes are viewed by the self as acceptable and consistent with personality) (Black & Andreasen, 2011, p. 600), rather than ego-dystonic (behavior, thoughts, and attitudes are viewed by self as repugnant and not consistent with personality) (Black & Andreasen, 2011, p. 600) (Simeon, Stein, & Hollander, 1995).

Epidemiology

There is little epidemiological information about skin picking, but one study found that it is present in 2.7% to 4.6% of college students (Teng, Woods, Twohig, et al., 2002) and 1.4 to 5.4% of the general population (Odlaug & Grant, 2010). It occurs more often in women than men, and the age of onset is about 15 years (Keuthen, Koran, Aboujaoude, et al., 2010).

Etiology

Etiology is unknown. It is proposed that skin picking is related to emotion dysregulation. Patients used repetitive behaviors to regulate negative affect; that is, they avoid certain thoughts or feelings by using repetitive behaviors, even though the behaviors are detrimental to their health (Wetterneck et al., 2010).

Clinical Presentation

Individuals with pathological skin picking are often unaware that it is a treatable disorder (Odlaug & Grant, 2008). They are ashamed and embarrassed by their skin picking and may describe a sense of tension and nervousness before skin picking or when they try to resist the urge to skin pick. They may have severe skin excoriations, infections, and scarring. Nail biting is often present (Odlaug & Grant).

Comorbidity

Skin picking is often comorbid with OCD, mood disorders, and other anxiety disorders. Other comorbid conditions include BDD, substance abuse, eating disorders, and personality disorders (Wetterneck et al., 2010).

Treatment

One study found that fluoxetine reduced skin-picking behavior (Simeon, Stein, Gross, et al., 1997); however, in a more recent study, 42.1% of patients with skin-picking behavior receiving escitalopram responded only partially or not at all. Clomipramine has been found to be more effective (Leonard, Lenane, Swedo, et al., 1991). One trial study has found lamotrigine (Lamictal) to be effective (Grant, Odlaug, & Kim, 2007). There have been no reports on CBT for skin-picking behavior, but individual HRT has been found to be effective (Teng, Woods, Twohig, 2006; Twohig, Woods, Marcks, et al., 2003).

Clinical Implications

There is preliminary support for the use of clomipramine and strong support for the use of behavioral therapy (Ravindran et al., 2009).

New Treatment Approach for Impulse-Control Disorders

A different treatment approach for impulse-control disorders is a treatment package called Acceptance and Commitment Therapy (Hayes, Strosahl, & Wilson, 1999), which addresses the underlying dynamic of avoidance. It uses acceptance and mindfulness to help patients to verbally process their experienced emotions rather than avoid them. It has been found to reduce TTM symptoms, but no studies are available for skin picking (Wetterneck et al., 2010).

Neurological Disorder Cluster

Disorders within the neurological cluster include tic disorders, such as TS and PANDAS. In these neurological disorders, changes in functioning of the basal ganglia are evidenced in repetitive and stereotyped behaviors. There may also be obsessions and compulsions that differ from those of OCD.

Tourette's Syndrome

Gorman, Thompson, Plessen, et al. (2010) have defined TS as a childhood-onset neuropsychiatric disorder defined by motor and vocal tics that persist for longer than 1 year (p. 36). To meet the criteria for TS, there must be multiple motor tics and at least one vocal tic, and the tics must occur many times a day for a period of more than 1 year. Onset must be before 18 years of age.

Tics may be simple or complex. Simple motor tics may involve single head movements or a movement in a limb that involves only a few muscles. Examples of simple tics are neck jerking, eye blinking, or facial grimacing (Wetterneck et al., 2010). Simple vocal tics include grunting, sniffing, snorting, barking, coughing, or throat clearing. Complex tics include jumping, touching, repeatedly smelling an object, or copropraxia (involuntary vulgar or obscene gesturing). Complex vocal tics include expression of single words or phrases, changes in pitch or volume, and coprolalia (involuntary use of obscene words) (Wetterneck et al., p. 143). In comparison to patients with OCD, who usually experience a mental stimulus or thought before engaging in a compulsion, patients with TS often experience a sensory stimulus, such as a tickle, itch, tingle, or pressure, prior to engaging in the tic (Leckman et al., 1994). Some patients experience an urge or a feeling of something not being "just right" (Wetterneck et al., p. 143).

Epidemiology

The prevalence of TS is 0.5% to 1% of the general population (Pauls, 2003). The onset of TS is before 18 years of age; median age is 5.5 years (Pauls, Raymond, Stevenson, et al., 1991). It is considered to be a family disorder, with heritability of 90% (Smoller et al., 2008). In addition to genetic influence, risk factors include adverse circumstances of birth, such as maternal abuse of caffeine, nicotine, and alcohol during pregnancy; neonatal anoxia; maternal stress during pregnancy; and delivery by forceps (Sampaio et al., 2009). Other risk factors include psychosocial stressors that may interact with genetic vulnerability (Lin, Katsovich, Ghebremichael, et al., 2007).

Etiology and Biological Basis

In addition to a genetic influence, TS is associated with a maternal history of pregnancy complications and childhood streptococcal infections. Biological changes include structural abnormalities of the caudate nucleus and the basal ganglia and abnormalities of dopamine activity (Wetterneck et al., 2010). There are also changes in the amygdala, hippocampus, and cerebellum that are not present in OCD (Chamberlain, Menzies, Fineberg, et al., 2008).

Clinical Presentation

In addition to motor and vocal tics, children with TS may present with repetitive behaviors such as mental play, echophenomena, and touching and self-injurious behaviors (Cath, Spinhoven, Hoogduin, et al., 2001) and with anxiety disorders. For example, 29% of children with TS have a comorbid anxiety disorder (panic disorder, agoraphobia, separation anxiety, and overanxious disorder) (Kurlan, Como, Miller, et al., 2002). They may also have sleep disturbances, nightmares, and oppositional behavior (Hickey & Wilson, 2000). Aggressive behaviors and explosive tantrums occur in 42% to 66% of children with TS (Alsobrook & Pauls, 1997). Learning difficulties, such as attention deficit, problems with memorization, and visuospatial impairment, occur in one-third of children with TS (Wodrich, Benjamin, & Lachar, 1997). Children may experience rejection by their classmates and loneliness (Wodrich et al.).

Comorbidity

There is a high rate of comorbid psychiatric disorders in patients with TS. For example, the cormorbidity rate of OCD is 23% to 50% (Miguel, Ferrao, Rosario, et al., 2008). Other comorbidities include attention deficit-hyperactivity disorder and anxiety disorders (Wetterneck et al., 2010).

Treatment

Pharmacotherapy and behavioral interventions, such as HRT, are frequently used to treat tic disorders.

Pharmacotherapy includes the use of beta-blockers, antipsychotics, and other agents. Patients with TS have been found to respond to an atypical antipsychotic such as risperidone, with a reduction of number and severity of tic symptoms (Scahill, Leckman, Schultz, et al., 2003). However, the reduction rate is only 20% to 50% (Robertson, 2000).

HRT is effective in reducing tics (Bloch et al., 2007; Piacentini & Chang, 2006). In HRT, patients are taught to be aware of the situations in which their tics occur; then they are taught a competing response that is incompatible with the tic and uses muscles antagonistic to those used in the tic. Family members provide support for use of the competing responses. HRT has been found to reduce tics by up to 90% (Himle, Woods, Piacentini, et al., 2006).

Not all patients with tic disorders respond to medications or perform the competing responses consistently. Patients with tic disorders and comorbid attention deficit-hyperactivity disorder or OCD may have more difficulty using HRT.

Course

The age of onset of tics is around 7 years (Freeman, Fast, Burd, et al., 2000). Simple tics develop before complex tics, and motor tics develop before vocal tics (O'Connor & Leclerc, 2008). The tics associated with TS usually improve during adolescence, and by age 18 years, nearly 90% of patients have only mild tics or none at all (Pappert, Goetz, Louis, et al., 2003). However, although the tics may improve, older adolescents with TS have been found to have impairment of psychosocial functioning and increased rates of attention deficit disorder, conduct disorder, major depressive disorder, learning disorders, OCD, and other anxiety disorders (Gorman et al., 2010).

Pediatric Autoimmune Neuropsychiatric Disorders Associated With Streptococcal Infections

Streptococcal diseases are acute infections that range from pharyngitis and upper respiratory infections to delayed sequelae, such as Sydenham's chorea. Sydenham's chorea and other pediatric autoimmune neuropsychiatric disorders (PANDAS) are believed to be "an autoimmune, delayed neuropsychiatric manifestation of streptococcal infection" (Williams, Grant, & Kim, 2008, p. 96). Symptoms of PANDAS include the obsessions and compulsions of OCD and the involuntary movements of TS and Sydenham's chorea. There is also a history of a group A streptococcus (GAS) infection (Williams et al.).

Epidemiology

Age of onset of OCD symptoms has been reported to be 6.3 years, and age of onset of tic symptoms is later, 7.4 years of age (Swedo et al., 1998). Prevalence is higher in males. Multiple GAS infections are associated with increased incidence of PANDAS (Mell, Davis, & Owens, 2005).

Etiology and Biological Basis

It is thought that development of PANDAS is linked to genetic vulnerability, exposure to a GAS infection, and an autoimmune reaction with damage to the basal ganglia (Snider & Swedo, 2004b). Biological changes include increased volume of the basal ganglia (Williams et al., 2008). One theory of the development of PANDAS focuses on a process called "molecular mimicry" (Williams et al., p. 100). According to this theory, in response to a GAS infection, the body creates antibodies. Because proteins of the cell wall of the GAS bacteria are similar to the proteins of the basal ganglia (Dale & Heyman, 2002), the antibodies set off an immune reaction that damages the basal ganglia, thus causing the symptoms of OCD (National Institute of Mental Health Pediatrics and Developmental Neuroscience Branch, 2010; Williams et al., 2008).

Clinical Presentation

Symptoms begin abruptly in patients with PANDAS and may appear overnight (Williams et al., 2008). Symptoms include moodiness, irritability, sadness, anxiety about being separated from parents, sleep disturbances, and joint pain (National

Institute of Mental Health, 2010). There may be complaints of bladder problems, such as the need for frequent voiding, although the pain or fever that is normally associated with a bladder infection may be absent. There may also be deterioration of handwriting skills that may resemble the choreiform hand movements associated with Sydenham's chorea (Williams et al., 2008). Other features of Sydenham's chorea, a disorder that occurs in association with rheumatic fever, are involuntary and uncoordinated movements, muscular weakness, problems with concentration, mood swings, and obsessions such as violent or aggressive obsessions and contamination obsessions. Compulsions include checking, washing, and ordering (Snider & Swedo, 2003).

Treatment

Treatment includes antibiotics for GAS infection, antiobsessional medications such as SSRIs, and CBT.

Course

PANDAS have an episodic course with a slow gradual improvement. If patients have another GAS infection, their symptoms may reappear or worsen (National Institute of Mental Health, 2010).

Schizo-obsessive Cluster

Researchers have noted an overlap between the symptoms of OCD and schizophrenia and the schizophrenia spectrum disorders. For example, the symptom of magical thinking is common in both OCD and schizophrenia, and the types of obsessions and compulsions are similar. Among patients with schizophrenia, the presence of OCD symptoms is associated with greater severity of symptoms of schizophrenia—higher levels of positive symptoms and emotional discomfort and greater impairment of executive functioning (Lysaker, Marks, Picone, et al., 2000). Among patients with OCD, the presence of symptoms of schizophrenia is associated with poorer response to multimodal CBT, poorer response to pharmacotherapy (McKay & Gruner, 2008), and a poorer outcome (Skoog & Skoog, 1999). It is often difficult to differentiate between the symptoms of obsession with poor insight and the delusions of schizophrenia because patients with OCD of the schizo-obsessive cluster may have thought-action fusion and delusional or psychotic symptoms (Hollander et al., 1999).

Epidemiology

Among patients with schizophrenia, as many as 30% to 59% have significant obsessive or compulsive symptoms (Berman, Kalinowski, Berman, et al., 1995); however, the number of patients who meet the criteria for a diagnosis of OCD is much less, approximately 14% (Bottas, Cooke, & Richter, 2005). Eisen, Beer, Pato, et al. (1997) found that 7.8% of patients with schizophrenia or schizoaffective disorder who were directly interviewed met the criteria for OCD. Among patients with a diagnosis of OCD, approximately half have some symptoms of schizophrenia, such as magical thinking or ideas of reference (Sobin et al., 2000).

Etiology and Biological Basis

There is considerable overlap of abnormalities of brain structure and functioning among patients with OCD and among those with schizophrenia. The degree of impairment of functioning among patients with comorbid OCD and schizophrenia appears to be greater than that of patients with OCD alone but less than that of patients with schizophrenia alone (Bottas et al., 2005).

Clinical Presentation

Patients with schizophrenia and OCD have information-processing deficits, such as difficulty maintaining attention, problems with memory, and deficits of executive functioning (McKay & Gruner, 2008). They may have peculiarities of speech, paranoid ideation, constricted affect, and deficits of social skills (McKay & Gruner). In addition, patients with schizophrenia and comorbid OCD tend to have poorer social and vocational functioning (Fenton & McGlashan, 1986; Poyurovsky, Hramenkov, Isakov, et al., 2001) than patients with schizophrenia who do not have OCD, and they are higher users of health-care services (Berman et al., 1995).

Treatment

Treatment of the schizo-obsessive subgroup of OCSD may require the use of a combination of a typical antipsychotic and SSRIs or SRIs (Bottas et al., 2005; Woo, Canuso, Wojcik, et al., 2009) and CBT that uses an ERP approach (McKay & Gruner, 2008). Some researchers believe that the newer atypical antipsychotics, especially olanzapine and clozapine, make the symptoms of OCD worse (Ongur & Goff, 2005).

Course

Obsessive-compulsive symptoms are more difficult to treat when the patient also has schizophrenia or symptoms of schizophrenia (McKay & Gruner, 2008).

Hoarding: Compulsive Hoarding

As stated previously, in the *DSM-IV-TR* (American Psychiatric Association, 2000), hoarding, which occurs when a patient is unable to discard worn-out or worthless objects, even when they have no sentimental value (p. 729), is one of the criteria for obsessive-compulsive personality disorder; if the hoarding is excessive, the diagnosis of OCD rather than obsessive-compulsive personality disorder should be considered (p. 728). The *DSM-IV-TR* wording creates confusion in that compulsive hoarding often occurs independent of OCD symptoms or other obsessive-compulsive personality disorder symptoms (Mataix-Cols et al., 2010). Compulsive hoarding was originally used "to differentiate normal saving and collecting from excessive, impulsive or pathological hoarding" (Mataix-Cols et al., p. 557). It now is used to describe hoarding behaviors that are due to fears of losing items that could be valuable or impossible to replace or because of excessive emotional attachment to the items.

Although hoarding is not identified as a mental disorder, patients continue to present with the disorder, and researchers continue to study compulsive hoarding. As part of their research on compulsive hoarding, Frost and Hartl (1996) developed a set of diagnostic criteria that is summarized as follows:

- The individual has difficulty discarding or parting with personal belongings, strong urges to save things, and distress when urged to discard things (p. 343).
- Accumulated items fill up and clutter all areas of the home, prevent use of space, and create unsafe living situations for the patient and family (p. 341).
- Symptoms create distress or impairment of functioning in family, social, and work environments (p. 341).

Later, the original three criteria of Frost and Hartl (1996) were supplemented with two additional criteria:

- Symptoms are not due to a general medical condition, such as a brain injury.
- Hoarding is not limited to hoarding due to an obsession, lack of motivation, depression, delusions related to schizophrenia or other psychotic disorder, cognitive impairment due to dementia, restricted interests in autistic disorder, and food storing in Prader-Willi syndrome (Mataix-Cols et al., 2010, p. 558). Specifiers that describe the hoarding behavior include the following:
  - "With excess acquisition" for patients whose symptoms include excess acquiring by buying, collecting, or stealing items that are not needed or when there is no space for them. Not all compulsive hoarders engage in excessive acquisition (Mataix-Cols et al., 2010, p. 558).
  - "With good or fair insight" if the patient recognizes that hoarding is problematic.
  - "With poor insight" if the patient is mostly convinced that the hoarding is not problematic.
  - "Delusional" when the patient is completely convinced that the hoarding, acquiring, and inability to discard items is not problematic, even when presented with evidence to the contrary (Mataix-Cols et al., 1010, p. 558).

Epidemiology

The estimated prevalence of compulsive hoarding is 5% of the general population (Samuels, Bienvenu, Grados, et al., 2008). It is associated with impairment of family, social, and vocational functioning and frequently endangers the health and welfare of patients and their families (Gilliam & Tolin, 2010; Mataix-Cols et al., 2010). In retrospective studies, onset of hoarding symptoms has been reported to occur in childhood or adolescence with an average age of 12 to 13 years. Compulsive hoarding occurs at about the same rate in men and women (Pertusa, Fullana, Singh, et al., 2008). The symptoms of compulsive hoarding that are found among the population in the United States are similar to those found in other countries, such as Japan, India, South Africa, and Brazil (Mataix-Cols et al., 2010).

Etiology and Biological Basis

There is a genetic influence on compulsive hoarding, and there are abnormalities of brain structures that are involved in executive functioning, decision making, attention, organization, and regulation of emotions. Compulsive hoarding is linked to impaired functioning of emotional and cognitive processes:

- Deficits of information processing related to problems with memory, organizing, and making decisions
- Emotional attachment to possessions
- Avoidance of decision making and other stressful situations
- Erroneous beliefs about the value of possessions, their responsibility for keeping and protecting possessions, the consequences of discarding items, and the need to collect items (Grisham, Brown, Savage, et al., 2007; Hartl, Frost, Allen, et al., 2004; Wincze, Steketee, & Frost, 2007).

Clinical Presentation

Among patients with compulsive hoarding, the fear of losing something important and the urge or compulsion to save or collect things are considered to be ego-syntonic and part of normal life. They are not considered by the patient to be distressful or unpleasant, and acquiring items may be experienced as exciting and pleasurable. Patients may describe themselves as perfectionists and may report problems with their memory. Patients' distress may be related to

- Fear of not being able to remember something if they cannot see it, and fear of losing important items
- Anxiety about being criticized for not protecting and saving things
- Sadness or anger at being forced to discard what they have collected

On clinical presentation, patients may be experiencing family conflict that is associated with their hoarding behaviors, social isolation, impairment of work functioning, and financial problems (Gilliam & Tolin, 2010). They may be facing legal problems if their living environment has been found to be unsanitary, unhealthy, or unsafe (Frost & Tolin, 2008).

Comorbidity

Between 25% and 36% of patients with compulsive hoarding have comorbid anxiety disorders (social phobia and generalized anxiety disorder) and depression (Frost, Steketee, Tolin, et al., 2010). The comorbidity rate of OCD with compulsive hoarding is approximately 12% (Frost, Steketee, & Grisham, 2004). Patients with hoarding and comorbid OCD obsessions that are related to hoarding often collect items of similar shapes, buy certain numbers of things, save rotting food, and refuse to discard anything (Pertusa et al., 2008).

Treatment

The goals of treatment of compulsive hoarding are twofold: (1) to reduce the clutter in the patient's environment to ensure safety and allow living areas to be used for daily living activities and (2) to help the patient develop skills to maintain a constant number of possessions, e.g., to reduce acquiring behaviors (Frost & Tolin, 2008). Treatment includes pharmacotherapy, CBT, and multicomponent CBT.

Hoarding has been found to have a poorer response to treatment than some of the other subcategories of OCD (Winsberg, Cassic, & Koran, 1999). Treatment for OCD with hoarding includes the use of SSRIs or SRIs at high doses for 12 weeks. If there is no response, an atypical antipsychotic such as risperidone or olanzapine may be used in a low dose as an adjunctive medication. If SSRIs are not effective, a serotonin-norepinephrine reuptake inhibitor may be used.

Treatment of OCD with hoarding also includes (1) CBT that uses an EPR approach and (2) psychosocial interventions that include the following strategies:

- Education of patients about hoarding to increase their insight and motivation
- Facilitation of the patients' awareness that they must make decisions, organize, store, and discard the hoarded items and education about how to do it
- Assistance for patients to reduce incoming clutter
- Education of patients about how to organize their belongings, tasks, and time
- Assistance for patients to identify activities to replace hoarding and collecting activities (Feusner & Saxena, 2005)

The multicomponent CBT model is based on the belief that hoarding is due to information-processing deficits, problematic beliefs and behaviors, emotional distress, and avoidance behaviors (Steketee, Frost, Tolin, et al., 2010). The model proposes (1) that strong negative emotional reactions to possessions (anxiety, grief, and guilt) lead to avoidance of discarding and organizing and (2) that strong positive emotions (joy, pleasure, excitement, and euphoria) reinforce saving and acquiring of possessions (Steketee & Frost, 2003). The multicomponent CBT model includes the following interventions:

- Motivational interviewing is used during assessment and, when needed, for homework noncompliance and attendance problems.
- Cognitive skills training are provided in organizing, decision making, and problem-solving.
- Patients are gradually exposed to nonacquring and discarding situations.
- Cognitive therapy is provided for problematic hoarding-relevant beliefs.
- Strategies for managing stressors without using hoarding behaviors are developed for each patient.

Patients with severe clutter or physical disabilities that make it difficult for them to clear the clutter receive one or two sessions of 3 to 6 hours each in which the therapists and others help the patient in sorting, organizing, and discarding. These sessions occur late in the therapy program, after the patient has learned how to organize, make decisions, and discard. The sessions are directed by the patient (Steketee et al., 2010). In comparison to a wait-list control group, 70% of patients who received 26 weeks of the multicomponent CBT intervention had significant improvement in symptoms of hoarding. However, only 24% were rated as very much improved. The researchers note that 37% of those with hoarding problems declined to participate in the intervention.

Course

Compulsive hoarding is a chronic illness that begins early in life. The onset of symptoms and exacerbation of symptoms have been found to be linked with stressful or traumatic life events, and the symptoms tend to get worse over time without treatment (Tolin, Meuneir, Frost, et al., 2010). Compulsive hoarding is associated with high rates of comorbid psychiatric and medical problems and impairment of family, social, and vocational functioning (Gilliam & Tolin, 2010). The symptoms of hoarding become worse as patients age, and hoarding may become part of their identity and the primary purpose in their lives (Mataix-Cols et al., 2010).

Clinical Implications

Obstacles to adherence to treatment include patients' belief that things must be perfect, anxiety created by others touching of their things, inability to organize items into categories, and their feeling that the task of decluttering their environment is overwhelming.

Key Points

Hypochondriasis

- The patient is obsessed with the fear of having a physical illness despite lack of medical evidence of an illness.
- Patients seek repeated medical evaluations of the feared illness.
- There is a high rate of comorbid disorders: somatization disorder, panic disorder, depressive disorder, generalized anxiety disorder, and panic disorder.
- Treatment is with SSRIs and CBT.

Body Dysmorphic Disorder

- The patient is preoccupied with an imagined defect in appearance or a minor physical abnormality.
- There is a high rate of comorbid OCD, depression, substance abuse, and suicidal ideation.

- As many as 48% to 76% of patients seek cosmetic surgery for the imagined defect.
- Cosmetic surgery does not change the patient's preoccupation with the defect.
- Treatment is with SSRIs, but response may be partial; a combination of SSRIs and CBT is more effective.

Trichotillomania

- The key feature is pulling out hair.
- There is a high rate of comorbid psychiatric disorders: mood, anxiety, and substance-related disorders.
- Treatment includes habit reversal therapy; SSRIs have limited efficacy.

Skin Picking

- Skin picking is also called psychogenic excoriation or dermatotillomania.
- It is a form of self-injurious behavior that is habitual, ritualistic, and tension reducing.
- There is a high rate of comorbid OCD, mood disorders, BDD, and other anxiety disorders.
- Treatment includes habit reversal therapy.

Tourette's Syndrome

- This is a childhood-onset disorder with motor and vocal tics.
- Patients often have sensation of something not being just right.
- There is a high rate of comorbid OCD, sleep disturbances, learning difficulties, and explosive tantrums.
- Treatment is with pharmacotherapy including beta-blockers, antipsychotics, and other agents. Habit reversal therapy is effective in reducing tics.
- Tics may diminish by the late teen years, but patients often have problems with psychosocial functioning.

Pediatric Autoimmune Neuropsychiatric Disorders Associated With Streptococcal Infections (PANDAS)

- Patients may have a genetic vulnerability.
- There may be separation anxiety, obsessions of contamination, and compulsions of washing, checking, and ordering.
- Treatment includes antibiotics for GAS infection, antiobsessional medications such as SSRIs, and CBT.
- The disorder follows an episodic course with recurrences related to other infections.

Schizo-obsessive Subtype of OCD

- Among patients with schizophrenia, approximately half have OCD symptoms.
- Patients have information-processing deficits and often manifest peculiar speech and paranoid thoughts.
- Treatment includes antipsychotics, SRIs, and CBT.

Hoarding

- Compulsive hoarding is associated with strong urge to save things and difficulty discarding things; cluttering of living spaces that creates an unsafe and unhealthy living situation; and impairment of family, social, and work functioning.
- Compulsive hoarding is thought to involve deficits of information processing.
- Goals of treatment are to reduce clutter and teach skills to reduce acquiring behaviors.
- Treatment follows a multicomponent CBT model that includes the following interventions: motivational interviewing; cognitive skills training in organizing, decision making, and problem-solving; gradual exposure to nonacquiring and discarding situations; cognitive therapy for problematic hoarding-relevant beliefs; and strategies for managing stressors without using hoarding behaviors.
- It is a chronic illness.

Resources

Organizations

The Obsessive-Compulsive Foundation
P.O. Box 70
Milford, CT 06460-0070
203-878-5669
www.ocfoundation.org

National Institute for Health and Clinical Excellence (NICE)

Tourette Syndrome Association, Inc.
42-40 Bell Blvd.
Bayside, NY 11361
www.tsa-usa.org

Trichotillomania Learning Center
207 McPherson St., Suite H
Santa Cruz, CA 95060-5863
www.trich.org

Books

Rapoport, J. (1991). *The boy who couldn't stop washing*. New York: Penguin Books.

Schwartz, J. M., & Beyette, B. (1997). *Brain lock: Free yourself from obsessive-compulsive behavior.* New York: Harper Perennial.

Steketee, G., & White, K. (1990). *When once is not enough: Help for obsessive-compulsives.* Oakland, CA: New Harbinger Publications.

Veale, D., & Willson, R. (2005). *Overcoming obsessive compulsive disorder.* London: Constable & Robinson.

A self-help book suitable for adults and older teenagers.

Hyman, B., & Pedrick, C. (2005). *The OCD workbook: Your guide to breaking free from obsessive-compulsive disorder.* Oakland, CA: New Harbinger Publications.

Movies

Winick, G. (Director). (1999). *The tic code.* [Motion picture]. United States: Universal Pictures.

Depicts Tourette's syndrome.

Shergold, A. (Director). (2004). *Dirty, filthy love.* [Motion picture]. England.

Depicts OCD and Tourette's syndrome.

Brooks, J. L. (Director). (1997). *As good as it gets.* [Motion picture]. United States: Tristar Pictures.

Depicts OCD.

I have Tourette's but Tourette's doesn't have me (2005). [Documentary]. United States: HBO Pictures.

Depicts Tourette's syndrome.

Scorsese, M. (Director). (2004). *The aviator.* [Motion picture]. United States: Miramax.

Depicts OCD.

Allen, W. (Director). (1986). *Hannah and her sisters* [Motion picture]. United States: Orion.

Depicts hypochondriasis

SOURCE: WEDDING, BOYD, & NIEMIEC, 2010.

References

Abramowitz, J. S. (1996). Variants of exposure and response prevention in the treatment of obsessive-compulsive disorder: A meta-analysis. *Behavior Therapy, 27,* 583-560.

Abramowitz, J. S. (2010). Psychological treatment for obsessive-compulsive disorder. In D. J. Stein, E. Hollander, & B. O. Rothbaum (Eds.), *Textbook of anxiety disorders* (2nd ed.) (pp. 339-354). Washington, DC: American Psychiatric Publishing, Inc.

Abramowitz, J. S., & Deacon, B. J. (2005). Obsessive-compulsive disorder: Essential phenomenology and overlap with other anxiety disorders. In J. S. Abramowitz & A. C. Houts (Eds.), *Concepts and controversies in obsessive-compulsive disorder* (pp. 119-135). New York: Springer.

Abramowitz, J. S., Schwartz, S. A., & Moore, K. M. (2003). Obsessional thoughts in postpartum females and their partners: Content, severity and relationship with depression. *Journal of Clinical Psychology in Medical Settings, 10,* 157-164.

Abramowitz, J. S., Whiteside, S., Kalsy, S. A., et al. (2003). Thought control strategies in obsessive-compulsive disorder: A replication and extension. *Behaviour Research and Therapy, 41*(5), 529-540.

Abramowitz, J. S., Whiteside, S., Lynam, D., et al. (2003). Is thought-action fusion specific to obsessive-compulsive disorder: A mediating role of negative affect. *Behaviour Research and Therapy, 41*(9), 1069-1079.

Albert, U., Bogetto, F., Maina, G., et al. (2010). Family accommodation in obsessive-compulsive disorder: Relation to symptom dimensions, clinical and family characteristics. *Psychiatry Research, 179,* 204-211.

Allen, A., & Hollander, E. (2000). Body dysmorphic disorder. *Psychiatric Clinics of North America, 23,* 617-628.

Alsobrook, J. P., & Pauls, D. L. (1997). The genetics of Tourette's syndrome. *Neurology Clinics, 15,* 381-393.

American Psychiatric Association (2000). *Diagnostic and statistical manual of mental disorders* (4th ed., text rev.). Washington, DC: American Psychiatric Publishing, Inc.

American Psychiatric Association (2007). *Practice guideline for the treatment of patients with obsessive-compulsive disorder.* Washington, DC: American Psychiatric Association. Available online at http://www.psych.org/psych-practi/treatg/pg/prac-guide.cfm

Andreasen, N. C., & Black, D. W. (2006). *Introductory textbook of psychiatry* (4th ed.). Washington, DC: American Psychiatric Publishing, Inc.

Aouizerate, B., Guehl, D., Cuny, E., et al. (2004). Pathophysiology of obsessive-compulsive disorder: A necessary link between phenomenology, neuropsychology, imagery and physiology. *Progress in Neurobiology, 72,* 195-221.

Attiullah, N., Eisen, J. L., & Rasmussen, S. A. (2000). Clinical features of obsessive-compulsive disorder. *Psychiatric Clinics of North America, 23*(3), 469-491.

Baer, L. (1994). Factor analysis of symptom subtypes of obsessive-compulsive disorder and their relationship to personality and tic disorders. *Journal of Clinical Psychiatry, 55,* 18-23.

Baer, L., Jenike, M. A., Black, D. W., et al. (1992). Effect of axis II diagnosis on treatment outcome with clomipramine (Anafranil) in 55 patients with obsessive-compulsive disorder. *Archives of General Psychiatry, 49,* 862-866.

Baer, L., Minichiello, W. E., & Jenike, M. A. (1987). Use of a portable-computer program in behavioral treatment of obsessive-compulsive disorder. *American Journal of Psychiatry, 144,* 1101.

Baer, L., Rauch, S. L., Ballentine, T., et al. (1995). Cingulotomy for untreatable obsessive-compulsive disorder. *Archives of General Psychiatry, 52,* 384-392.

Barsky, A. J., & Klerman, G. L. (1983). Overview: Hypochondriasis, bodily complaints, and somatic styles. *American Journal of Psychiatry, 140*(3), 273-283.

Barsky, A. J., Wool, C., Barnett, M. C., et al. (1994). Histories of childhood trauma in adult hypochondriacal patients. *American Journal of Psychiatry, 151,* 397-401.

Bartha, R., Stein, M. B., Williamson, P. C., et al. (1998). A short echo 1 H spectroscopy and volumetric MRI study of the corpus striatum in patients with obsessive-compulsive disorder and comparison subjects. *American Journal of Psychiatry, 155,* 1584-1591.

Bartz, J. A., & Hollander, E. (2006). Is obsessive-compulsive disorder an anxiety disorder? *Progress in Neuropsychopharmacological and Biological Psychiatry, 30,* 338-352.

Baxter, L. R., Jr., Saxena, S., Brody, A. L., et al. (1996). Brain mediation of obsessive-compulsive disorder symptoms: Evidence from functional brain imaging studies in the human and nonhuman primate. *Seminars in Clinical Neuropsychiatry, 1,* 32-47.

Baxter, L. R., Jr., Schwartz, J. M., Bergman, K. S., et al. (1992). Caudate glucose metabolic rate changes with both drug and behavior therapy for obsessive compulsive disorder. *Archives of General Psychiatry, 49,* 681-689.

Bear, R. E., Fitzgerald, R., Rosenfeld, J. V., et al. (2010). Neurosurgery for obsessive compulsive disorder: Contingency approaches. *Journal of Clinical Neuroscience, 17*(1), 1-5.

Berghuis, D. J., Jongsma, A. E., & Bruce, T. J. (2008). *The severe and persistent mental illness treatment planner* (2nd ed.). Hoboken, NJ: John Wiley & Sons, Inc.

Berman, L., Kalinowski, A., Berman, S. M., et al. (1995). Obsessive and compulsive symptoms in schizophrenia. *Comprehensive Psychiatry, 36,* 6-10.

Best-Lavigniac, J. (2006). Hoarding as an adult: Overview and implications for practice. *Journal of Psychosocial Nursing & Mental Health Services, 44*(1), 48-51.

Bienvenu, O. J., Samuels, J. F., Riddle, M. A., et al. (2000). The relationship of obsessive-compulsive disorder to possible spectrum disorders: Results from a family study. *Biological Psychiatry, 48,* 287-293.

Black, E. W., & Andreasen, N. C. (2011). *Introductory textbook of psychiatry* (5th ed.). Washington, DC: American Psychiatric Publishing, Inc.

Black, D., & Noyes, R. (1997). Obsessive-compulsive disorder and Axis II. *International Review of Psychiatry, 18,* 111-118.

Bloch, M. H., Landeros-Weisenberger, A., Dombrowski, P., et al. (2007). Systematic review: Pharmacological and behavioural treatment for trichotillomania. *Biological Psychiatry, 62,* 839-846.

Bloch, M. H., Landeros-Weisenberger, A., Kelmendi, B., et al. (2006). A systematic review: Antipsychotic augmentation with treatment refractory obsessive-compulsive disorder. *Molecular Psychiatry, 11*(7), 622-632.

Bottas, A., Cooke, R. G., & Richter, M. A. (2005). Comorbidity and pathophysiology of obsessive-compulsive disorder in schizophrenia: Is there evidence for a schizo-obsessive subtype of schizophrenia? *Journal of Psychiatry and Neuroscience, 30*(3), 187-193.

Brown, T. A., Campbell, L. A., Lehman, C. L., et al. (2001). Current and lifetime comorbidity of the DSM-IV anxiety and mood disorders in a large clinical sample. *Journal of Abnormal Psychology, 110,* 585-599.

Buhlmann, U., Etcoff, N. L., & Wilhelm, S. (2008). Facial attractiveness ratings and perfectionism in body dysmorphic disorder and obsessive-compulsive disorder. *Journal of Anxiety Disorders, 22,* 540-547.

Cafri, G., Thompson, J. K., Ricciardelli, L., et al. (2005). Pursuit of the muscular ideal: Physical and psychological consequences and putative risk factors. *Clinical Psychology Review, 25,* 215-239.

Catapano, F., Perris, F., Masella, M., et al. (2006). Obsessive-compulsive disorder: A 3-year prospective follow-up study of patients treated with serotonin reuptake inhibitors OCD follow-up study. *Journal of Psychiatric Research, 40,* 502-510.

Cath, D. C., Spinhoven, P., Hoogduin, C. A., et al. (2001). Repetitive behaviors in Tourette's syndrome and OCD with and without tics: What are the differences? *Psychiatry Research, 101,* 171-185.

Chamberlain, S. R., Menzies, L. A., Fineberg, N. A., et al. (2008). Grey matter abnormalities in trichotillomania; morphometric magnetic resonance imaging study. *British Journal of Psychiatry, 193,* 216-221.

Christenson, G. A., Chernoff-Clementz, E., & Clementz, B. A. (1992). Personality and clinical characteristics in patients with trichotillomania. *Journal of Clinical Psychiatry, 53*, 407-413.

Christenson, G. A., Ristvedt, S. L., & Mackenzie, T. B. (1993). Identification of trichotillomania cue profiles. *Behaviour Research and Therapy, 31*, 315-320.

Clark, D. M., Kirby, K. C., Daniels, B. A., et al. (1998). A pilot study of computer-aided vicarious exposure for obsessive-compulsive disorder. *Australian and New Zealand Journal of Psychiatry, 32*(2), 268-275.

Cohen, J. A. (2003). Treating acute posttraumatic reactions in children and adolescents. *Biological Psychiatry, 53*, 827-833.

Cohen, L. J., Stein, D. J., Simeon, D., et al. (1995). Clinical profile, comorbidity, and treatment history in 123 hair pullers: A survey study. *Journal of Clinical Psychiatry, 56*, 319-326.

Collie, R. (2005). *Obsessive-compulsive disorder: A guide for family, friends and pastors.* New York: The Haworth Pastoral Press.

Crerand, C. E., Sarwer, D. B., Magee, L., et al. (2004). Rate of body dysmorphic disorder among patients seeking facial plastic surgery. *Psychiatric Annals, 34*, 958-965.

Dale, R. C., & Heyman, I. (2002). Post-streptococcal autoimmune psychiatric and movement disorders in children. *British Journal of Psychiatry, 181*, 188-190.

D'Alessandro, T. M. (2009). Factors influencing the onset of childhood obsessive compulsive disorders. *Pediatric Nursing, 35*(1), 43-46.

Davidson, J. R. T., & Connor, K. M. (2004). Treatment of anxiety disorders. In A. F. Schatzberg & C. B. Nemeroff (Eds.), *The American psychiatric publishing textbook of psychopharmacology* (3rd ed.) (pp. 913-934). Washington, DC: American Psychiatric Publishing, Inc.

Davidson, J. R., Connor, K. M., & Zhang, W. (2009). Treatment of anxiety disorders. In A. F. Schatzberg & C. B. Nemeroff (Eds.), *The American psychiatric publishing textbook of psychopharmacology* (4th ed.) (pp. 1171-1199). Washington, DC: American Psychiatric Publishing, Inc.

de Alvarenga, P. G., Flores, A. C., Torres, A. R., et al. (2009). Higher prevalence of obsessive-compulsive spectrum disorders in rheumatic fever. *General Hospital Psychiatry, 31*, 178-180.

De Leon, J., Bott, A., & Simpson, G. M. (1989). Dysmorphophobia: Body dysmorphic disorder or delusional disorder, somatic subtype? *Comprehensive Psychiatry, 30*, 457-472.

de Silva, P., Menzies, R. G., & Shafran, R. (2003). The spontaneous decay of compulsive urges: The case of covert compulsions. *Behaviour Research and Therapy, 41*, 129-137.

DeVeaugh-Geiss, J., Moroz, G., Biedeman, J., et al. (1992). Clomipramine (Anafranil) hydrochloride in childhood and adolescent obsessive-compulsive disorder—a multicenter trial. *Journal of American Academy of Child and Adolescent Psychiatry, 31*, 45-49.

Didie, E. R., Tortolani, C. C., Pope, G. G., et al. (2006). Childhood abuse and neglect in body dysmorphic disorder. *Child Abuse and Neglect, 30*, 1015-1105.

Dougherty, D. D., Loh, R., Jenike, M. A., et al. (2006). Single modality versus dual modality treatment for trichotillomania: Sertraline, behavioral therapy, or both. *Journal of Clinical Psychiatry, 67*, 1086-1092.

Dougherty, D. D., Rauch, S. L., & Greenberg, B. D. (2010). Pathophysiology of obsessive-compulsive disorders. In D. J. Stein, E. Hollander, & B. O. Rothbaum (Eds.), *Textbook of anxiety disorders* (2nd ed.) (pp. 287-309). Washington, DC: American Psychiatric Publishing, Inc.

Douglass, H. M., Moffitt, T. E., Dar, R., et al. (1995). Obsessive-compulsive disorder in a birth cohort of 18-year olds: Prevalence and predictors. *Journal of American Academy of Child and Adolescent Psychiatry, 34*, 1424-1431.

Dubovsky, S. (2005). *Clinical guide to psychotropic medications.* New York: W. W. Norton & Company.

Dyess, D. (2009, February). FDA approves implant device for OCD treatment. *Health News.*

Ebert, D., Speck, O., Konig, A., et al. (1997). 1H-magnetic resonance spectroscopy in obsessive-compulsive disorder: Evidence for neuronal loss in the cingulate gyrus and the right striatum. *Psychiatric Research, 74*, 173-176.

Eisen, J. L., Beer, D. A., Pato, M. T., et al. (1997). Obsessive-compulsive disorder in patients with schizophrenia or schizoaffective disorder. *American Journal of Psychiatry, 154*, 271-273.

Eisen, J. L., & Rasmussen, S. A. (1993). Obsessive-compulsive disorder with psychotic features. *Journal of Clinical Psychiatry, 54*, 373-379.

Eisen, J. L., & Rasmussen, S. A. (2002). Phenomenology of obsessive-compulsive disorder. In D. J. Stein & E. Hollander (Eds.), *The American psychiatric publishing textbook of anxiety disorders* (pp. 173-189). Washington, DC: American Psychiatric Publishing, Inc.

Eisen, J. L., Yip, A. G., Mancebo, M. C., et al. (2010). Phenomenology of obsessive-compulsive disorder. In D. J. Stein, E. Hollander, & B. O. Rothbaum (Eds.), *Textbook of anxiety disorders* (2nd ed.) (pp. 261-286). Washington, DC: American Psychiatric Publishing, Inc.

Epperson, C. N., Fasula, D., Wasylink, S., et al. (1999). Risperidone addition in serotonin reuptake inhibitor-resistant trichotillomania: Three cases. *Journal of Child and Adolescent Psychopharmacology, 9*, 43-49.

Fallon, B. A., & Feinstein, S. (2001). Hypochondriasis. In K. A. Phillips (Ed.), *Somatoform and factitious disorders* (pp. 27-65). Washington, DC: American Psychiatric Publishing, Inc.

Fallon, B. A., Liebowitz, M. R., Salman, E., et al. (1993). Fluoxetine for hypochondriacal patients without major depression. *Journal of Clinical Psychopharmacology, 13*, 438-441.

Fallon, B. A., Qureshi, A., Laje, G., et al. (2000). Hypochondriasis and its relationship to obsessive-compulsive disorder. *Psychiatric Clinics of North America, 23*, 605.

Fallon, B. A., Qureshi, A., Schneier, F. R., et al. (2003). An open trial of fluvoxamine for hypochondriasis. *Psychosomatics, 44*, 298-303.

Fenton, W. W., & McGlashan, T. H. (1986). The prognostic significance of obsessive-compulsive symptoms in schizophrenia. *American Journal of Psychiatry, 143*, 437-441.

Feusner, J., & Saxena, S. (2005). Compulsive hoarding: Unclutter lives and homes by breaking anxiety. *Current Psychiatry, 4*(3), 12-26.

Fineberg, N. A., & Craig, K. J. (2010). Pharmacotherapy for obsessive-compulsive disorder. In D. J. Stein, E. Hollander, & B. O. Rothbaum (Eds.), *Textbook of anxiety disorders* (2nd ed.) (pp. 311-337). Washington, DC: American Psychiatric Publishing, Inc.

Fineberg, N. A., Tonnoir, B., & Lemming, O. (2006). Escitalopram predicts relapse of obsessive-compulsive disorder. *European Neuropsychopharmacology*, dol.10,1016, Jeuroneuro, 2006, 11.005.

First, M. B., & Tasman, A. (2004). *DSM-IV-TR mental disorders: Diagnosis, etiology and treatment.* West Sussex, UK: John Wiley & Sons, Ltd.

Fitzgerald, K. D., Moore, G. J., Paulson, L. D., et al. (2000). Proton spectroscopic imaging of the thalamus in treatment-naive pediatric obsessive-compulsive disorder. *Biological Psychiatry, 47*, 174-182.

Flament, M. F., & Bisserbe, J. D. (1997). Pharmacologic treatment of obsessive-compulsive disorder: Comparative studies. *Journal of Clinical Psychiatry, 58*(Suppl 12), 18-22.

Flament, M. F., Whitaker, A., Rapoport, J. L., et al. (1988). Obsessive-compulsive disorder in adolescence: An epidemiological study. *Journal of American Academy of Child and Adolescent Psychiatry, 27*, 764-771.

Foa, E. B., & Kozak, M. J. (1996). Psychological treatment for obsessive-compulsive disorder. In M. R. Mavissakalian & R. F. Prien (Eds.), *Long-term treatments of anxiety disorders* (pp. 285-309). Washington, DC: American Psychiatric Press, Inc.

Freeman, R. D., Fast, D. K., Burd, L., et al. (2000). An international perspective on Tourette syndrome: Selected findings from 3,500 individuals in 22 countries. *Developmental Medicine and Child Neurology, 42*(7), 436-447.

Fritzler, B. K., Hecker, J. E., & Losee, M. D. (1997). Self-directed treatment with minimal therapist contact: Preliminary findings for obsessive-compulsive disorder. *Behaviour Research and Therapy, 35*, 627-631.

Frost, R. O., & Hartl, T. L. (1996). A cognitive-behavioral model of compulsive hoarding. *Behavioral Research and Therapy, 34*, 341-350.

Frost, R. O., Krause, M. S., & Steketee, G. (1996). Hoarding and obsessive-compulsive symptoms. *Behavior Modification, 20*(1), 116-132.

Frost, R. O., Steketee, G., & Grisham, J. (2004). Measurement of compulsive hoarding: Saving inventory-revised. *Behavioral Research and Therapy, 42*, 1163-1182.

Frost, R. O., Steketee, G., Tolin, D., et al. (2010, June 2-5). *Diagnostic comorbidity in hoarding and OCD.* World Congress of Behavioral and Cognitive Therapies, Boston.

Frost, R. O., Steketee, G., Williams, L. F., et al. (2000). Mood, personality disorders symptoms and disability in obsessive-compulsive hoarders, a comparison with clinical and non-clinical controls. *Behavioral Research and Therapeutics, 38,* 1071-1081.

Frost, R. O., & Tolin, D. F. (2008). Compulsive hoarding. In J. S. Abramowitz, D. McKay, & S. Taylor (Eds.), *Clinical handbook of obsessive-compulsive disorder and related problems* (pp. 76-94). Baltimore: The Johns Hopkins University Press.

Frost, R. O., Tolin, D. F., Steketee, G., et al. (2009). Excessive acquisition in hoarding. *Journal of Anxiety Disorders, 23*(5), 632-639.

Fux, M., Benjamin, J., & Belmaker, R. H. (1999). Inositol versus placebo augmentation of serotonin reuptake inhibitors in the treatment of obsessive-compulsive disorder: A double blind crossover study. *International Journal of Neuropsychopharmacology,* 193-195.

Fux, M., Levine, J., Aviv, A., et al. (1996). Inositol treatment of obsessive-compulsive disorder. *American Journal of Psychiatry, 153,* 1219-1221.

Gabbard, G. (2005). *Psychodynamic psychiatry in clinical practice* (4th ed.). Washington, DC: American Psychiatric Publishing, Inc.

Gadde, K. M., Ryan Wagner, H., Connor, K. M., et al. (2007). Escitalopram treatment of trichotillomania. *International Clinical Psychopharmacology, 22,* 39-42.

Giedd, J. N., Rapoport, J. L., Garvery, M. A., et al. (2000). MRI assessment of children with obsessive-compulsive disorder or tics associated with streptococcal infection. *American Journal of Psychiatry, 157,* 281-283.

Gilbert, A. R., Moore, G. J., Keshavan, M. S., et al. (2000). Decrease in thalamic volumes of pediatric obsessive-compulsive disorder patients taking paroxetine. *Archives of General Psychiatry, 57,* 449-456.

Gilliam, C. M., & Tolin, D. F. (2010). Compulsive hoarding. *Bulletin of the Menninger Clinic, 74*(2), 93-121.

Gleaves, D. H., & Ambwani, S. (2008). Body dysmorphic disorder. In J. S. Abramowitz, D. McKay, & S. Taylor (Eds.), *Clinical handbook of obsessive-compulsive disorder and related problems* (pp. 288-303). Baltimore: The Johns Hopkins University Press.

Gold, J. M., Berman, K. F., Randolph, C., et al. (1996). PET validation of a novel prefrontal task: Delayed response alternation. *Neuropsychology, 10,* 3-10.

Goodman, W. K. (2002). Pharmacotherapy for obsessive-compulsive disorder. In D. J. Stein & E. Hollander (Eds.), *The American psychiatric publishing textbook of anxiety disorder* (pp. 207-219). Washington, DC: American Psychiatric Publishing, Inc.

Goodman, W. K., Price, L. H., Rasmussen, S. A., et al. (1989a). The Yale-Brown obsessive compulsive scale (Y-BOCS), I: Development, use and reliability. *Archives of General Psychiatry, 46,* 1006-1011.

Goodman, W. K., Price, L. H., Rasmussen, S. A., et al. (1989b). The Yale-Brown obsessive compulsive scale (Y-BOCS), II: Validity. *Archives of General Psychiatry, 46,* 1012-1016.

Gorman, D. A., Thompson, N., Plessen, K. J., et al. (2010). Psychosocial outcome and psychiatric comorbidity in older adolescents with Tourette syndrome: Controlled study. *The British Journal of Psychiatry, 197,* 36-44.

Gothelf, D., Aharonovsky, O., Horesh, N., et al. (2004). Life events and personality factors in children and adolescents with obsessive-compulsive disorder and other anxiety disorders. *Comprehensive Psychiatry, 45,* 192-198.

Grant, J. E., Odlaug, B. L., & Kim, S. W. (2007). Lamotrigine treatment of pathologic skin picking: An open-label study. *Journal of Clinical Psychiatry, 68,* 1384-1391.

Graybiel, A. M., & Saka, E. (2002). A genetic basis for obsessive grooming. *Neuron, 33,* 1-2.

Greeven, A., van Balkom, A. J., Visser, S., et al. (2007). Cognitive behavior therapy and paroxetine in the treatment of hypochondriasis: A randomized controlled trial. *American Journal of Psychiatry, 164,* 91-99.

Greist, J. H. (1994). Behavior therapy for obsessive compulsive disorder. *Journal of Clinical Psychiatry, 55*(Suppl), 60-68.

Greist, J. H., & Baer, L. (2002). Psychotherapy for obsessive-compulsive disorder. In D. J. Stein & E. Hollander (Eds.), *The American psychiatric publishing textbook of anxiety disorders* (pp. 221-233). Washington, DC: American Psychiatric Publishing, Inc.

Greist, J. H., Bandelow, B., Hollander, E., et al; World Council of Anxiety. (2003). WCA recommendations for the long-term treatment of obsessive-compulsive disorder in adults. *CNS Spectrums, 8*(8 Suppl 1), 7-16.

Greist, J. H., & Jefferson, J. W. (2007). Obsessive-compulsive disorder. *Focus, 5,* 283-298.

Grimshaw, L. (1964). Obsessional disorder and neurological illness. *Journal of Neurology, Neurosurgery and Psychiatry, 27,* 229-231.

Grisham, J. R., Anderson, T. M., & Sachdev, P. S. (2008). Genetic and environmental influences on obsessive-compulsive disorder. *European Archives of Psychiatry and Clinical Neuroscience, 258,* 107-116.

Grisham, J. R., Brown, T. A., Savage, C. R., et al. (2007). Neuropsychological impairment associated with compulsive hoarding. *Behavioral Research and Therapy, 45,* 1471-1483.

Gunstad, J., & Phillips, K. A. (2003). Axis I comorbidity in body dysmorphic disorder. *Comprehensive Psychiatry, 44,* 270-276.

Hartl, T. L., Frost, R. O., Allen, G. J., et al. (2004). Actual and perceived memory deficits in individuals with compulsive hoarding. *Depression and Anxiety, 20,* 59-69.

Hasler, G., LaSalle-Ricci, V. H., Ronquillo, J. G., et al. (2005). Obsessive-compulsive disorder symptom dimensions show specific relationships to psychiatric comorbidity. *Psychiatry Research, 135,* 121-132.

Hayes, S. C., Strosahl, K., & Wilson, K. G. (1999). *Acceptance and commitment therapy: An experiential approach to behavior change.* New York: Guilford Press.

Heyman, I., Mataix-Cols, D., & Fineberg, N. A. (2006). Obsessive-compulsive disorder. *British Medical Journal, 333,* 424-429.

Hickey, T., & Wilson, L. (2000). Tourette syndrome: Symptom severity, anxiety, depression, stress, social support, and ways of coping. *Irish Journal of Psychology, 21,* 78-87.

Higgins, E. S., & George, M. S. (2007). The neuroscience of clinical psychiatry: The pathophysiology of behavior and mental illness. Philadelphia: Wolters Kluwer/Lippincott, Williams & Wilkins.

Himle, M. B., Woods, D. W., Piacentini, J. C., et al. (2006). Brief review of habit reversal training system for Tourette syndrome. *Journal of Child Neurology, 21,* 719-725.

Hollander, E. (1993). Obsessive-compulsive spectrum disorders: An overview. *Psychiatric Annals, 23,* 355-358.

Hollander, E., Berlin, H. A., & Stein, D. J. (2008). Impulse-control disorders not elsewhere classified. In R. E. Hales, S. C. Yudofsky, & G. O. Gabbard (Eds.), *The American psychiatric publishing textbook of psychiatry* (5th ed.) (pp. 777-820). Washington, DC: American Psychiatric Publishing, Inc.

Hollander, E., Friedberg, J., Wasserman, D., et al. (2005). Venlafaxine in treatment resistant obsessive-compulsive disorder. *Journal of Clinical Psychiatry, 64,* 546-550.

Hollander, E., Kaplan, A., & Stahl, S. M. (2003). A double-blind, placebo controlled trial of clonazepam in obsessive-compulsive disorder. *World Journal of Biological Psychiatry, 4,* 30-34.

Hollander, E., Kim, S., Braun, A., et al. (2009). Cross-cutting issues and future directions for the OCD spectrum. *Psychiatry Research, 170,* 3-6.

Hollander, E., Kwon, J. H., Stein, D. J., et al. (1996). Obsessive-compulsive and spectrum disorders: Overview and quality of life issues. *Journal of Clinical Psychiatry, 57*(Suppl 8), 3-6.

Hollander, E., Rosen, J., & the IOCDC Spectrum Work Group. (1999). OC spectrum disorders: The impulsive and schizo-obsessive clusters. *CNS Spectrums,* 4(Suppl 3), 16-21.

Hollander, E., Schiffman, E., Cohen, B., et al. (1990). Signs of central nervous system dysfunction in obsessive-compulsive disorder. *Archives of General Psychiatry, 47,* 27-32.

Hollander, E., & Simeon, D. (2008). Anxiety disorders. In R. E. Hales, S. C. Yudofsky, & G. O. Gabbard (Eds.), *The American psychiatric publishing textbook of psychiatry* (5th ed.) (pp. 505-607). Washington, DC: American Psychiatric Publishing, Inc.

Hollander, E., & Wong, C. M. (1995). Introduction: Obsessive-compulsive spectrum disorder. *Journal of Clinical Psychiatry, 56,* 3-6.

Hollander, E., & Wong, C. M. (1999). Spectrum boundary and subtyping issues: Implications for treatment refractory obsessive-compulsive disorder. In W. K. Goodman, M. V. Rudorger, & J. Masser (Eds.), *Obsessive-compulsive disorder: Contemporary issues in treatment.* Mahwah, NJ: Lawrence Erlbaum Associates, Inc.

Howieson, D. B., & Lezak, M. D. (2010). The neuropsychological evaluation. In S. C. Yudofsky & R. E. Gales (Eds.), *Essentials of neuropsychiatry and behavioral neurosciences* (2nd ed.) (pp. 29-54). Washington, DC: American Psychiatric Publishing, Inc.

Huppert, J. D., Simpson, H. B., Nisssenson, K. J., et al. (2009). Quality of life and functional impairment in obsessive-compulsive disorder: A comparison of patients with and without comorbidity, patients in remission, and healthy controls. *Depression and Anxiety, 26,* 39-45.

Hurley, R. A., Fisher, R. E., & Taber, K. H. (2010). Clinical and functional imaging in neuropsychiatry. In S. C. Yudofsksy & R. E. Hales (Eds.), *Essentials of neuropsychiatry and behavioral neurosciences* (2nd ed.) (pp. 55-93). Washington, DC: American Psychiatric Publishing, Inc.

Insel, T. R. (1992). Toward a neuroanatomy of obsessive-compulsive disorder. *Archives of General Psychiatry, 49,* 739-744.

Jaisoorya, T. S., Reddy, Y. C., & Srinath, S. (2003). The relationship of obsessive-compulsive disorder to putative spectrum disorders: Results from an Indian study. *Comprehensive Psychiatry, 44,* 317-323.

Jenike, M. (2001). An update in obsessive-compulsive disorder. *Bulletin of the Menninger Clinic, 65*(1), 4-25.

Jenike, M., Baer, L., Ballantine, H. L., et al. (1991). Cingulotomy for refractory obsessive-compulsive disorder: A long-term follow-up of 33 patients. *Archives of General Psychiatry, 48,* 548-555.

Jenike, M. A., Baer, L., & Minichiello, W. E. (Eds.). (1986). *Obsessive-compulsive disorders: Theory and management.* Littleton, MA: PSG Publishing.

Jenike, M. A., Breiter, H. C., Baer, L., et al. (1996). Cerebral structural abnormalities in obsessive-compulsive disorder: A quantitative morphometric magnetic resonance imaging study. *Archives of General Psychiatry, 53,* 625-632.

Jones, E. F. (1997). Cortical development and thalamic pathology. *Schizophrenia Bulletin, 23,* 483-501.

Jonnal, A. H., Gardner, C. O., Prescott, C. A., et al. (2000). Obsessive and compulsive symptoms in a general population sample of female twins. *American Journal of Medical Genetics, 96,* 701-796.

Kandel, E. R., Schwartz, J. H., & Jessell, T. M. (1995). *Essentials of neural science and behavior.* Norwalk, CT: Appleton & Lange.

Katerberg, H., Delucchi, K. L., Stewart, E., et al. (2010). Symptom dimensions in OCD: Item-level factor analysis and heritability estimates. *Behavioral Genetics, 40,* 505-517.

Katerberg, H., Lochner, C., Cath, D., et al. (2007). The role of brain-derived neurotropic factor (BDNF) Val66met variant in the phenotypic expression of obsessive compulsive disorder (OCD). *American Journal of Medical Genetics. Part B, Neuropsychiatric Genetics, 150B*(8), 1050-1062.

Kellner, R. (1987). Hypochondriasis and somatization. *Journal of the American Medical Association, 258*(19), 2718-2722.

Kessler, R. C., Berglund, P., Demler, O., et al. (2005). Lifetime prevalence and age-of-onset distributions of DSM-IV disorders in the national Comorbidity Survey Replication. *Archives of General Psychiatry, 62,* 593-602.

Ketay, S., Stein, D. J., & Hollander, E. (2010). The obsessive-compulsive spectrum of disorders. In D. J. Stein, E. Hollander, & B. O. Rothbaum (Eds.), *Textbook of anxiety disorders* (2nd ed.) (pp. 355-364). Washington, DC: American Psychiatric Publishing, Inc.

Keuthen, N. J., Koran, L. M., Aboujaoude, E., et al. (2010). The prevalence of pathologic skin picking. *Comprehensive Psychiatry, 51*(2), 183-186.

Khanna, S. (1991). Soft neurological signs in obsessive-compulsive disorder. *Biological Psychiatry, 29*(Suppl), 442.

Kim, J. J., Lee, M. C., Kim, J., et al. (2001). Gray matter abnormalities in obsessive-compulsive disorder: Statistical parametric mapping of segmented magnetic resonance images. *British Journal of Psychiatry, 179,* 330-334.

Kirby, K. C., Berrios, G. E., Daniels, B. A., et al. (2000). Process-outcome analysis in computer-aided treatment of obsessive-compulsive disorder. *Comprehensive Psychiatry, 41*(4), 259-265.

Koran, L. M., McElroy, S. L., Davidson, J. R. T., et al. (1996). Fluvoxamine (Luvox) versus clomipramine (Anafranil) for obsessive-compulsive disorder: A double-blind comparison. *Journal of Clinical Psychopharmacology, 16,* 121-129.

Koran, L. M., Sallee, R. R., & Pallanti, S. (1997). Rapid benefit of intravenous pulse loading of clomipramine (Anafranil) in obsessive-compulsive disorder. *American Journal of Psychiatry, 154,* 396-401.

Kurlan, R., Como, P. G., Miller, B., et al. (2002). The behavioral spectrum of tic disorders: A community-based study. *Neurology, 59*(3), 414-420.

Ladouceur, R., Freeston, M. H., Rheaume, J., et al. (2000). Strategies used with intrusive thoughts: A comparison of OCD patients with anxious and community controls. *Journal of Abnormal Psychology, 109*(2), 179-187.

Lambrecq, V., Rotge, J-Y, Guebl, D., et al. (2009). Lesions in the associative striatum improve obsessive-compulsive disorder. *Biological Psychiatry, 65,* e11-e12.

Laraia, M. T. (2006). Keep it, repeat it, berate it: Differential diagnosis and treatment of OCD and compulsive hoarding. *APNA News, 18*(1), 10-13.

Leckman, J. F., Denys, D., Simpson, H. B., et al. (2010). Obsessive-compulsive disorder: A review of the diagnostic criteria and possible subtypes and dimensional specifiers for DSM-V. *Depression and Anxiety, 27,* 507-527.

Leckman, J., Grice, D., Boardman, J., et al. (1997). Symptoms of obsessive-compulsive disorder. *American Journal of Psychiatry, 154,* 911-917.

Leckman, J., Mataix-Cols, D., & Rosario-Campos, M. C. (2005). Symptom dimensions in OCD: Developmental and evolutionary perspectives. In J. S. Abramowitz & A. C. Houts (Eds.), *Concepts and controversies in obsessive-compulsive disorder* (pp. 3-25). New York: Springer.

Leckman, J. F., Walker, D. E., Goodman, W. K., et al. (1994). "Just right" perceptions associated with compulsive behavior in Tourette's syndrome. *American Journal of Psychiatry, 151,* 675-680.

Leibbrand, R., Hiller, W., & Fichter, M. M. (2000). Hypochondriasis and somatization: Two distinct aspects of somatoform disorders? *Journal of Clinical Psychology, 56,* 63-72.

Lensi, P., Cassano, G. B., Correddu, G., et al. (1996). Obsessive-compulsive disorder: Familial-developmental history, symptomatology, comorbidity and course with special reference to gender-related differences. *British Journal of Psychiatry, 169,* 101-107.

Leonard, H. L., Lenane, M. C., Swedo, S. E., et al. (1991). A double-blind comparison of clomipramine and desipramine treatment of severe onychophagia (nail biting). *Archives of General Psychiatry, 199,* 821-827.

Lieb, R., Zimmermann, P., Friis, R. H., et al. (2002). The natural course of DSM-IV somatoform disorders and syndromes among adolescents and young adults: A prospective-longitudinal community study. *European Psychiatry, 17,* 321-331.

Lin, H., Katsovich, L., Ghebremichael, M., et al. (2007). Psychosocial stress predicts future symptom severities in children and adolescents with Tourette syndrome and/or obsessive-compulsive disorder. *Journal of Child Psychology and Psychiatry, 48,* 157-166.

Lochner, C., du Toit, P. L., Zungu-Dirwayi, N., et al. (2002). Childhood trauma in obsessive-compulsive disorder, trichotillomania, and controls. *Depression and Anxiety, 15,* 66-68.

Lochner, C., Seedat, S., du Toit, P. L., et al. (2005). Obsessive-compulsive disorder and trichotillomania: A phenomenological comparison. *BMC Psychiatry, 13*(5), 2.

Lochner, C., Seedat, S., Niehaus, D. J., et al. (2006). Topiramate in the treatment of trichotillomania: an open-label pilot study. *International Clinical Psychopharmacology, 21*(5), 255-259.

Lochner, C., Simeon, D., Niehaus, D. J., et al. (2002). Trichotillomania and skin-picking: A phenomenological comparison. *Depression and Anxiety, 15*(2), 83-86.

Lougee, L., Perlmutter, S. J., Nicolson, R., et al. (2000). Psychiatric disorders in first-degree relatives of children with pediatric autoimmune neuropsychiatric disorders associated with streptococcal infections (PANDAS). *Journal of American Academy of Child and Adolescent Psychiatry, 39,* 1120-1126.

Lucey, J. V., Butcher, F., Clare, A. W., et al. (1994). The clinical characteristics of patients with obsessive-compulsive disorder: A descriptive study of an Irish sample. *Irish Journal of Psychological Medicine, 11,* 11-14.

Lysaker, P. H., Marks, K. A., Picone, J. B., et al. (2000). Obsessive and compulsive symptoms in schizophrenia. *Journal of Nervous and Mental Disease, 188,* 78-83.

MacLean, P. D. (1973). *A tribune concept of the brain and behavior.* Toronto, Ontario, Canada: University of Toronto Press.

Mancuso, S., Knoesen, N., & Castle, D. J. (2010). Delusional vs nondelusional body dysmorphic disorder. *Comprehensive Psychiatry, 51,* 177-182.

March, J. S., Franklin, M. E., Leonard, H., et al. (2007). Tics moderate treatment outcome with sertraline but not cognitive-behavior therapy in pediatric obsessive-compulsive disorder. *Biological Psychiatry, 61*(3), 344-347.

Mataix-Cols, D., Frost, R. O., Pertusa, A., et al. (2010). Hoarding disorder: A new diagnosis for DSM-V? *Depression and Anxiety, 27,* 556-572.

Mataix-Cols, D., Pertusa, A., & Leckman, J. F. (2007). Issues for DSM-V: How should obsessive-compulsive and related disorders be classified? *American Journal of Psychiatry, 164,* 1313-1314.

Mataix-Cols, D., Rauch, S. L., Baer, L., et al. (2002). Symptom stability in adult obsessive-compulsive disorder: Data from a naturalistic two-year follow-up study. *American Journal of Psychiatry, 159*, 263-268.

Mataix-Cols, D., Rosario-Campos, M. C., & Leckman, J. F. (2005). A multidimensional model of obsessive-compulsive disorder. *The American Journal of Psychiatry, 162*(2), 228-238.

McDonald, R., & Blizard, R. (1988). Quality assurance of outcome in mental health care: A model for routine use in clinical settings. *Health Trends, 20*(4), 111-114.

McDougle, C. J., Barr, L. C., Goodman, W. K., et al. (1999). Possible role of neuropeptides in obsessive compulsive disorder. *Psychoneuroendocrinology, 24*(1), 1024.

McDougle, C. J., Epperson, C. N., & Price, L. H. (1996). Obsessive-compulsive symptoms with neuroleptics. *Journal of the American Academy of Child & Adolescent Psychiatry, 35*(7), 837-888.

McDougle, C. J., Goodman, W. K., Leckman, J. F., et al. (1994). Haloperidol addition in fluvoxamine (Luvox)-refractory obsessive-compulsive disorder: A double blind, placebo-controlled study in patients with and without tics. *Archives of General Psychiatry, 51*, 302-308.

McElroy, S. L., Pope, H. G., Keck, P. E., et al. (1995). Disorders of impulse control. In E. Hollander, & D. Stein (Eds.), *Impulsivity and aggression* (pp. 109-136). New York: Wiley.

McKay, D., & Gruner, P. (2008). Obsessive-compulsive disorder and schizotypy. In J. S. Abramowitz, D. McKay, & S. Taylor (Eds.), *Clinical handbook of obsessive-compulsive disorder and related problems* (pp. 126-138). Baltimore: The Johns Hopkins University Press.

McKay, D., & Robbins, R. (2009). Fears of contamination. In J. S. Abramowitz, D. McKay, & S. Taylor (Eds.), *Clinical handbook of obsessive-compulsive disorder and related problems* (pp. 18-29). Baltimore: The Johns Hopkins University Press.

Mell, L. K., Davis, R. L., & Owens, D. (2005). Association between streptococcal infection and obsessive-compulsive disorder, Tourette's syndrome, and tic disorder. *Pediatrics, 116*, 56-60.

Micallef, J., & Blin, O. (2001). Neurobiology and clinical pharmacology of obsessive-compulsive disorder. *Clinical Neuropharmacology, 24*(4), 191-207.

Miguel, E. C., Ferrao, Y. A., Rosario, M. C., et al. (2008). The Brazilian Research Consortium on Obsessive-Compulsive Spectrum Disorders: Recruitment, assessment instruments, methods for the development of multicenter collaborative studies and preliminary results. *Brazil Journal of Psychiatry, 30*, 185-196.

Murphy, D. L., Timpano, K. R., Wheaton, M. G., et al. (2010). Obsessive-compulsive disorder and its related disorders: A reappraisal of obsessive-compulsive spectrum concepts. *Dialogues in Clinical Neuroscience, 12*(2), 131-148.

Murray, C. J. L., & Lopez, A. D. (1996). *The global burden of disease.* Cambridge, MA: Harvard School of Public Health.

National Institute for Health and Clinical Excellence (NICE) Guidelines for OCD. (2005). OCD-UK www.ocdjuk.org/nice. Retrieved 6/18/2010.

National Institute of Mental Health Pediatrics and Developmental Neuroscience Branch (2010). *PANDAS.* Retrieved from Intramural. nimh.nih.gov/pdn/web.htm

Neziroglu, F., Roberts, M., & Yaryura-Tobias, J. A. (2004). A behavioral model for body dysmorphic disorder. *Psychiatric Annals, 34*, 915–920.

Noshirvani, H. F., Kasvikis, Y., Marks, I. M., et al. (1991). Gender-divergent etiological factors in obsessive-compulsive disorder. *British Journal of Psychiatry, 158*, 260-263.

O'Connor, K. P., & Leclerc, J. (2008). Tourette syndrome and chronic tic disorders. In J. S. Abramowitz, D. McKay, & S. Taylor (Eds.), *Clinical handbook of obsessive-compulsive disorder and related problems* (pp. 270-287). Baltimore: The Johns Hopkins University Press.

Odlaug, B. L., & Grant, J. E. (2008). Trichotillomania and pathologic skin picking: Clinical comparison with an examination of co-morbidity. *Annals of Comprehensive Psychiatry, 20*(2), 57-63.

Odlaug, B. L., & Grant, J. E. (2010). Pathologic skin picking. *American Journal of Drug and Alcohol Abuse, 35*(5), 296-303.

Ongur, D., & Goff, D. C. (2005). Obsessive-compulsive symptoms in schizophrenia: Associated clinical features, cognitive function and medication status. *Schizophrenia Research, 75*, 349-362.

O'Sullivan, R. L., Mansueto, C. S., Lerner, E. A., et al. (2000). Characterization of trichotillomania. A phenomenological model with clinical relevance to obsessive-compulsive spectrum disorders. *Psychiatric Clinics of North America, 23*(3), 587-604.

Pappert, E. J., Goetz, C. G., Louis, E. D., et al. (2003). Objective assessments of longitudinal outcome in Gilles de la Tourette's syndrome. *Neurology, 61*(7), 936-940.

Pato, M. T., Pato, C. N., Kennedy, J. L., et al. (1999). Summary of the genetics of obsessive-compulsive disorder. Proceedings of the third IODCC. *CNS Spectrums, 4*(5, Suppl 3), 22-24.

Pato, M. T., Pato, C. N., & Pauls, D. L. (2002). Recent findings in the genetics of OCD. *Journal of Clinical Psychiatry, 63*(Suppl 6), 30-33.

Pauls, D. L. (2003). An update on the genetics of Gilles de la Tourette syndrome. *Journal of Psychosomatic Research, 55*(1), 7-12.

Pauls, D. L., Raymond, C. L., Stevenson, J. M., et al. (1991). A family study of Gilles de la Tourette syndrome. *American Journal of Human Genetics, 48*, 154-163.

Pediatric Obsessive Compulsive Disorder Treatment Study (POTS) Team. (2004), Cognitive-behavior therapy, sertraline, and their combination for children and adolescents with obsessive-compulsive disorder: The Pediatric OCD Treatment Study (POTS) randomized controlled trial. *Journal of the American Medical Association, 292*(16), 1969-1976.

Pertusa, A., Fullana, M. A., Singh, S., et al. (2008). Compulsive hoarding: OCD symptom, distinct clinical syndrome, or both? *American Journal of Psychiatry, 165*, 1289-1298.

Perugi, G., & Frare, F. (2005). Body dysmorphic disorder. In M. Maj, H. S. Akiskal, J. E. Mezzich, et al. (Eds.), *Evidence and experience in psychiatry* (Vol. 9) (pp. 191-221). Chichester, UK: John Wiley & Sons.

Petter, T., Richter, M. A., & Sandor, P. (1998). Clinical features distinguish patients with Tourette's syndrome and obsessive-compulsive disorder from patients with obsessive-compulsive disorder without tics. *Journal of Clinical Psychiatry, 59*, 456-459.

Phillips, K. A. (1995). Body dysmorphic disorder: Clinical features and drug treatment. *CNS Drugs, 3*, 30-40.

Phillips, K. A. (2005). *The broken mirror: Understanding and treating body dysmorphic disorder.* New York: Oxford University Press.

Phillips, K. A. (2007). Body dysmorphic disorder. In G. O. Gabbard (Ed.), *Gabbard's treatments of psychiatric disorders* (4th ed.) (pp. 613-620). Washington, DC: American Psychiatric Publishing, Inc.

Phillips, K. A., Albertini, R. S., & Rasmussen, S. A. (2002). A randomized placebo-controlled trial of fluoxetine in body dysmorphic disorder. *Archives of General Psychiatry, 59*, 381-388.

Phillips, K. A., & Diaz, S. F. (1997). Gender differences in body dysmorphic disorder. *Journal of Nervous and Mental Diseases, 185*, 570-577.

Phillips, K. A., Dufresne, R. G., Jr., Wilkel, C. S., et al. (2000). Rate of body dysmorphic disorder in dermatology patients. *Journal of the American Academy of Dermatology, 42*, 436-441.

Phillips, K. A., Gunderson, C. G., Mallya, G., et al. (1998). A comparison study of body dysmorphic disorder and obsessive-compulsive disorder. *Journal of Clinical Psychiatry, 59*, 568-575.

Phillips, K. A., & Kaye, W. H. (2007). The relationship of body dysmorphic disorder and eating disorders in obsessive-compulsive disorder. *CNS Spectrums, 12*, 347-358.

Phillips, M. L., Marks, I. M., Senior, C., et al. (2000). A differential neural response in obsessive-compulsive patients with washing compared with checking symptoms to disgust. *Psychological Medicine, 30*, 1037-1050.

Phillips, K. A., McElroy, S. L., Dwight, M. M., et al. (2001). Delusionality and response to open-label fluvoxamine in body dysmorphic disorder. *Journal of Clinical Psychiatry, 62*, 87-91.

Phillips, K. A., McElroy, S., Keck, P. E., Jr., et al. (1993). Body dysmorphic disorder: 30 Cases of imagined ugliness. *American Journal of Psychiatry, 150*, 302-308.

Phillips, K. A., Menard, W., Fay, C., et al. (2005). Demographic characteristics, phenomenology, comorbidity, and family history in 200 individuals with body dysmorphic disorder. *Psychosomatics, 46*, 317-325.

Phillips, K. A., & Najjar, F. (2003). An open-label study of citalopram in body dysmorphic disorder. *Journal of Clinical Psychiatry, 64*, 715-720.

Phillips, K. A., Stein, D. J., Rauch, S. L., et al. (2010). Should an obsessive-compulsive spectrum grouping of disorders be included in DSM-V? *Depression and Anxiety, 27*, 528-555.

Piacentini, J. C., & Chang, S. W. (2006). Behavioral treatments for tic suppression: Habit reversal training. *Advances in Neurology, 99*, 227-233.

Pigott, T., L'Heureux, F., Rubinstein, C. S., et al. (1992, May 2-7). *A controlled trial of clonazepam augmentation in OCD patients with clomipramine (Anafranil) or fluoxetine (NR 82) in 1992 New Research Program and Abstracts.* Presented at the American Psychiatric Association 145th Annual Meeting, Washington, DC.

Pinto, A., Manceabo, M. C., Eisen, J. L., et al. (2006). The Brown longitudinal obsessive compulsive study: Clinical features and symptoms of the sample at intake. *Journal of Clinical Psychiatry, 67,* 703-711.

Pittenger, C., Krystal, J. H., & Coric, V. (2006). Glutamate-modulating drugs as novel pharmacotherapeutic agents in the treatment of obsessive-compulsive disorder. *NeuroRx, 3*(1), 69-81.

Polimeni, J., Reiss, J. P., & Sareen, J. (2005). Could obsessive-compulsive disorder have originated as a group-selected adaptive trait in traditional societies? *Medical Hypotheses, 65,* 655-664.

Poyurovsky, M., Hramenkov, S., Isakov, V., et al. (2001). Obsessive-compulsive disorder in hospitalized patients with chronic schizophrenia. *Psychiatry Research, 102,* 49-57.

Pujol, J., Soriano, M. C., Alonso, P., et al. (2004). Mapping structural brain alterations in obsessive-compulsive disorder. *Archives of General Psychiatry, 61,* 720-730.

Rachman, S. (1997). A cognitive theory of obsessions. *Behavior Research and Therapeutics, 35*(9), 793-802.

Rapoport, J. L. (Ed). (1989). *Obsessive-compulsive disorder in children and adolescents.* Washington, DC: American Psychiatric Association.

Rasmussen, S. A. (1994). Obsessive-compulsive spectrum disorders. *Journal of Clinical Psychiatry, 55,* 89-91.

Rasmussen, S. A., & Eisen, J. L. (1989). Clinical features and phenomenology of obsessive compulsive disorder. *Psychiatric Annals, 19,* 67-73.

Rasmussen, S. A., & Eisen, J. L. (1991). Phenomenology of obsessive-compulsive disorder. In J. Insel & S. Rasmussen (Eds.), *Psychobiology of obsessive compulsive disorder* (pp. 743-758). New York: Springer-Verlag.

Rasmussen, S. A., & Eisen, J. L. (1997). Treatment strategies for chronic and refractory obsessive-compulsive disorder. *Journal of Clinical Psychiatry, 58,* 9-13.

Rasmussen, S. A., & Tsuang, M. T. (1986). Epidemiology and clinical features of obsessive-compulsive disorder. In M. A. Jenike, L. Baer, & W. E. Minichiello (Eds.), *Obsessive-compulsive disorder: A theory of management* (pp. 23-44). Littleton, MA: PSG Publishing.

Rauch, S. L., Cora-Locatelli, G., & Greenberg, B. D. (2002a). Pathogenesis of obsessive-compulsive disorder. In D. J. Stein & E. Hollander (Eds.), *The American psychiatric publishing textbook of anxiety disorders* (pp. 191-205). Washington, DC: American Psychiatric Publishing, Inc.

Rauch, S. L., Jenike, M. A., Alpert, N. M., et al. (2002b). Predictors of fluvoxamine response in contamination-related obsessive compulsive disorder: A PET symptom provocation study. *Neuropsychopharmacology, 27,* 782-791.

Rauch, S. L., Whalen, P. J., Dougherty, D. D., et al. (1998). Neurobiological models of obsessive-compulsive disorders. In M. Jenike (Ed.), *Obsessive-compulsive disorders: Practical management* (pp. 222-253). Boston: Mosby.

Ravindran, A. V., da Silva, T. L., Ravindran, L. N., et al. (2009). Obsessive-compulsive spectrum disorders: A review of the evidence-based treatments. *The Canadian Journal of Psychiatry, 54,* 331-343.

Rich, N., Rosen, J. C., & Orosan, P. G. (1992, November 2). *Prevalence of body dysmorphic disorder in non-clinical populations.* Presented at the 26th annual convention of the Association for the Advancement of Behavior Therapy, Boston.

Robertson, M. M. (2000). Tourette syndrome, associated conditions and the complexities of treatment. *Brain, 123*(Pt 3), 425-462.

Robins, L. N., Helzer, J. E., Weissman, M. M., et al. (1984). Lifetime prevalence of specific psychiatric disorders in three sites. *Archives of General Psychiatry, 41,* 949-958.

Rosenberg, D. R., Keshavan, M. S., O'Hearn, K. M., et al. (1997). Frontostriatal measurement in treatment-naïve children with obsessive-compulsive disorder. *Archives of General Psychiatry, 54,* 824-830.

Rosenberg, D. R., MacMaster, F. P., Keshavan, M. S., et al. (2000). Decreases in caudate glutamatergic concentrations in pediatric obsessive-compulsive disorder patients taking paroxetine. *Journal of the American Academy of Child and Adolescent Psychiatry, 39,* 1096-1103.

Rosenberg, D. R., Russell, A., & Fougere, A. (2005). Neuropsychiatric models of OCD. In J. S. Abramowitz & A. C. Houts (Eds.), *Concepts and controversies in obsessive-compulsive disorder* (pp. 209-228). New York: Springer.

Rosqvist, J., & Norling, D. C. (2008). Compulsive checking. In J. S. Abramowitz, D. McKay, & S. Taylor (Eds.), *Clinical handbook of obsessive-compulsive disorder and related problems* (pp. 30-43). Baltimore: The Johns Hopkins University Press.

Rossi, S., Bartalini, S., Ulivelli, M., et al. (2005). Hypofunctioning of sensory gating mechanisms in patients with obsessive-compulsive disorder. *Biological Psychiatry, 57*(1), 16-20.

Rotge, J-Y. (2010). Anatomical alterations and symptom-related functional activity in obsessive-compulsive disorder are correlated in the lateral orbitofrontal cortex. *Biological Psychiatry, 67,* e37-e38.

Rothbaum, B. O., Shaw, L., Morris, R., et al. (1993). Prevalence of trichotillomania in a college freshman population. *Journal of Clinical Psychiatry, 54*(2), 72-73.

Rufer, M., Fricke, S., Moritz, S., et al. (2006). Symptom dimensions in obsessive-compulsive disorder: Prediction of cognitive behavior therapy outcome. *Acta Psychiatrica Scandinavica, 113,* 440-446.

Ruscio, A. M., Stein, D. J., Chiu, W. T., et al. (2010). The epidemiology of obsessive-compulsive disorder in the National Comorbidity Survey Replication. *Molecular Psychiatry, 15,* 53-63.

Sa, A. R., Hounie, A. G., Sampaio, A. S., et al. (2009). Obsessive-compulsive symptoms and disorder in patients with schizophrenia treated with clozapine or haloperidol. *Comprehensive Psychiatry, 50,* 437-442.

Sachdev, P., & Malhi, G. S. (2005). Obsessive-compulsive behaviour: A disorder of decision making. *Australian and New Zealand Journal of Psychiatry, 39*(9), 757-763.

Sadock, B. J., & Sadock, V. A. (2007). *Kaplan & Sadock's synopsis of psychiatry: Behavioral sciences/clinical psychiatry* (10th ed.). Philadelphia: Lippincott, Williams & Wilkins.

Saint-Cyr, J. A., Taylor, A. E., & Nicholson, K. (1995). Behavior and the basal ganglia. In W. J. Weiner & A. E. Lang (Eds.), *Behavioral neurology of movement disorders.* New York: Raven Press.

Sampaio, A. S., Miguel, E. C., Borcato, S., et al. (2009). Perinatal risk factors and obsessive-compulsive spectrum disorders in patients with rheumatic fever. *General Hospital Psychiatry, 31,* 288-291.

Samuels, J., Bienvenu, O. J., Grados, M. A., et al. (2008). Prevalence and correlates of hoarding behavior in a community-based sample. *Behaviour Research and Therapy, 46,* 836-844.

Saxena, S., Bota, R. G., & Brody, A. L. (2001). Brain-behavior relationships in obsessive-compulsive disorder. *Seminars in Clinical Neuropsychiatry, 6,* 82-101.

Saxena, S., Brody, A., Maidment, K., et al. (2004). Cerebral glucose metabolism in obsessive-compulsive hoarding. *The American Journal of Psychiatry, 161,* 1038-1048.

Saxena, S., Gorbis, E., O'Neill, J., et al. (2009). Rapid effects of brief intensive cognitive-behavioral therapy on brain glucose metabolism in obsessive-compulsive disorder. *Molecular Psychiatry, 14,* 197-205.

Saxena, S., & Maidment, K. (2004). Treatment of compulsive hoarding. *Journal of Clinical Psychology/In Session, 60*(11), 1143-1154.

Saxena, S., Winograd, A., Dunkin, J. J., et al. (2001). A retrospective review of clinical characteristics and treatment response in body dysmorphic disorder versus obsessive-compulsive disorder. *Journal of Clinical Psychiatry, 62,* 67-72.

Scahill, L., Leckman, J. F., & Schultz, R. T. (2003). A placebo-controlled trial of risperidone in Tourette syndrome. *Neurology, 60,* 1130-1135.

Schwartz, J. M., & Beyette, B. (1997). *Brain lock: Free yourself from obsessive-compulsive behavior.* New York: Harper Perennial.

Schwartz, J. M. (1998). Neuroanatomical aspects of cognitive-behavioural therapy response in obsessive-compulsive disorder. An evolving perspective in brain and behaviour. *The British Journal of Psychiatry. Supplement.* (35), 38-44.

Shidara, M., & Richmond, B. J. (2002). Anterior cingulate: Single neuronal signals related to degree of reward expectancy. *Science, 296,* 1709-1711.

Silver, J. M., Kramer, R., Greerwald, S., et al. (2001). The association between head injuries and psychiatric disorders: Findings from the New Haven NIMH Epidemiologic Catchment Area Study. *Brain Injury, 15,* 935-945.

Simeon, D., Stein, D. J., Gross, S., et al. (1997). A double-blind trial of fluoxetine in pathologic skin picking. *Journal of Clinical Psychiatry, 58,* 341-347.

Simeon, D., Stein, D. J., & Hollander, E. (1995). Depersonalization disorder and self-injurious behavior. *Journal of Clinical Psychiatry, 56*(Suppl 4), 36-39.

Simpson, H. B., & Liebowitz, M. R. (2005). Combining pharmacotherapy and cognitive-behavioral therapy in the treatment of OCD. In J. S. Abramowitz & A. C. Houts (Eds.), *Concepts and controversies in obsessive-compulsive disorder* (pp. 359-376). New York: Springer.

Skoog, G., & Skoog, I. (1999). A 40-year follow-up of patients with obsessive-compulsive disorder. *Archives of General Psychiatry, 56,* 121-127.

Smoller, J. W., Sheidley, B. R., & Tsuang, M. T. (2008). *Psychiatric genetics: Applications in clinical practice.* Washington, DC: American Psychiatric Publishing, Inc.

Snider, L. A., & Swedo, S. E. (2003). Childhood-onset obsessive-compulsive disorder and tic disorders: Case report and literature review. *Journal of Child and Adolescent Psychopharmacology, 13,* S81-S88.

Snider, L. A., & Swedo, S. E. (2004a). Nature and treatment of obsessive-compulsive disorder. In J. Panksepp (Ed.), *Textbook of biological psychiatry* (pp. 367-392). New York: Wiley-Liss.

Snider, L. A., & Swedo, S. E. (2004b). PANDAS: Current status and directions for research. *Molecular Psychiatry, 9,* 900-907.

Sobin, C., Blundell, M. C., Weiller, F., et al. (2000). Evidence of a schizotypy subtype in OCD. *Journal of Psychiatric Research, 34,* 15-24.

Stanley, D., & Wand, R. (1995). Obsessive-compulsive disorder: A review of the cross-cultural epidemiological literature. *Transcultural Psychiatric Research Review, 32,* 103-136.

Stein, D. J. (2008). Psychobiology of anxiety disorders and obsessive-compulsive spectrum disorders. *CNS Spectrums, 13*(9), 23-28.

Stein, D. J., & Bouwer, C. (1997). A neuro-evolutionary approach to the anxiety disorders. *Journal of Anxiety Disorders, 11*(4), 409-429.

Stein, D. J., & Lochner, C. (2006). Obsessive-compulsive spectrum disorders: A multidimensional approach. *Psychiatric Clinics of North America, 29,* 343-351.

Stein, D. J., & Rauch, S. L. (2010). Neuropsychiatric aspects of anxiety disorders. In S. C. Yudofsky & R. E. Hales (Eds.), *Essentials of neuropsychiatry and behavioral neurosciences* (2nd ed.) (pp. 479-493). Washington, DC: American Psychiatric Publishing, Inc.

Steketee, G., Eisen, J., Dyck, I., et al. (1999). Predictors of course in obsessive-compulsive disorder. *Psychiatry Research, 89,* 229-238.

Steketee, G., & Frost, R. O. (2003). Compulsive hoarding: Current status of the research. *Clinical Psychology Review, 23,* 905-927.

Steketee, G., Frost, R. O., Tolin, D. F., et al. (2010). Waitlist-controlled trial of cognitive behavior therapy for hoarding disorder. *Depression and Anxiety, 27,* 476-484.

Steketee, G., & White, K. (1990). *When once is not enough.* Oakland, CA: New Harbinger Publications.

Stewart, S. E., Geller, D. A., Jenike, M., et al. (2004). Long-term outcome of pediatric obsessive-compulsive disorder: A meta-analysis and qualitative review of the literature. *Acta Psychiatrica Scandinavica, 110,* 4-13.

Summerfeldt, L. J. (2008). Ordering, incompleteness, and arranging. In J. S. Abramowitz, D. McKay, & S. Taylor (Eds.), *Clinical handbook of obsessive-compulsive disorder and related problems* (pp. 44-60). Baltimore: The Johns Hopkins University Press.

Swedo, S. E. (1994). Sydenham's chorea: A model for childhood autoimmune neuropsychiatric disorders. *Journal of the American Medical Association, 272,* 1788-1791.

Swedo, S. E. (2002). Pediatric autoimmune neuropsychiatric disorders associated with streptococcal infections (PANDAS). *Molecular Psychiatry, 7,* S24-S25.

Swedo, S. E., & Grant, P. J. (2005). Annotation: PANDAS: A model for human autoimmune disease. *Journal of Child Psychology and Psychiatry, 46,* 227-234.

Swedo, S. E., Leonard, H., Garvey, M., et al. (1998). Pediatric autoimmune neuropsychiatric disorders associated with streptococcal infections: Clinical description of the first 50 cases. *American Journal of Psychiatry, 155,* 264-271.

Swedo, S. E., Leonard, H. L., & Schapiro, M. B., et al. (1993). Sydenham's chorea: Physical and psychological symptoms of St. Vitus' dance. *Pediatrics, 91,* 706-713.

Szegedi, A., Wetzel, H., Leal, M., et al. (1996). Combination treatment with clomipramine (Anafranil) and fluvoxamine (Luvox): Drug monitoring, safety and tolerability data. *Journal of Clinical Psychiatry, 57,* 257-264.

Szeszko, P. R., Robinson, D., Alvir, J. M., et al. (1999). Orbital frontal and amygdala volume reductions in obsessive-compulsive disorder. *Archives of General Psychiatry, 56,* 913-919.

Taylor, S., & Asmundson, G. J. G. (2008). Hypochondriasis. In J. S. Abramowitz, D. McKay, & S. Taylor (Eds.), *Clinical handbook of obsessive-compulsive disorder and related problems* (pp. 304-315). Baltimore: The Johns Hopkins University Press.

Taylor, S. Thordarson, D. S., Maxfield, L., et al. (2003). Comparative efficacy, speed and adverse effects of three PTSD treatments: Exposure therapy, EMDR and relaxation training. *Journal of Consulting and Clinical Psychology, 71*(2), 330-338.

Teng, E. J., Woods, D. W., Twohig, M. P., et al. (2002). Body focused repetitive behavior problems: Prevalence in a non-referred population and differences in somatic awareness. *Behavior Modification, 26,* 340-360.

Teng, E. J., Woods, D. W., & Twohig, M. P. (2006). Habit reversal as a treatment for chronic skin picking: A pilot investigation. *Behavior Modification, 30,* 411-422.

Tolin, D., Meunier, S. A., Frost, R. O., et al. (2010). Course of compulsive hoarding and its relationship to life events. *Depression and Anxiety, 27*(9), 829-838.

Treating obsessive-compulsive disorder (March, 2009). Harvard Mental Health Letter. Cambridge, MA: Harvard Health Publications.

Trivedi, M. H. (1996). Functional neuroanatomy of obsessive-compulsive disorder. *Journal of Clinical Psychiatry, 57*(Suppl 8), 23-63.

Tsai, G., & Coyle, J. T. (1995). N-Acetylaspartate in neuropsychiatric disorders. *Progress in Neurobiology, 46,* 531-540.

Twohig, M. P., & Woods, D. W. (2004). A preliminary investigation of acceptance and commitment therapy and habit reversal as a treatment for trichotillomania. *Behavior Therapy, 35,* 803-820.

Twohig, M. P., Woods, D. W., Marcks, B. A., et al. (2003). Evaluating the efficacy of habit reversal: Comparison with a placebo control. *Journal of Clinical Psychiatry, 64,* 40-48.

Ursu, S., Stenger, V. A., Shear, M. K., et al. (2003). Overactive action monitoring in obsessive-compulsive disorder: Evidence from functional magnetic resonance imaging. *Psychological Science: A Journal of the American Psychological Society, 14,* 347-353.

Valente, A. A., Miguel, E. C., Castro, C. C., et al. (2005). Regional gray matter abnormalities in obsessive-compulsive disorder: A voxel-based morphometry study. *Biological Psychiatry, 58,* 479-487.

van den Heuvel, O. A., Veltman, D. J., Groenewegen, H. J., et al. (2005). Disorder-specific neuroanatomical correlates of attentional bias in obsessive-compulsive disorder, panic disorder, and hypochondriasis. *Archives of General Psychiatry, 62*(8), 922-933.

van Minnen, A., Hoogduin, K. A., Keijsers, C. P., et al. (2003). Treatment of trichotillomania with behavioural therapy or fluoxetine: A randomized, waiting-list controlled study. *Archives of General Psychiatry, 60,* 517-522.

Vasconcelos, M. S., Sampaio, A. S., Hounie, A. G., et al. (2007). Prenatal, perinatal, and postnatal risk factors in obsessive-compulsive disorder. *Biological Psychiatry, 61,* 301-307.

Veale, D., Boocock, A., Gournay, K., et al. (1996a). Body dysmorphic disorder: A survey of fifty cases. *British Journal of Psychiatry, 169,* 196-201.

Veale, D., Gournay, K., Dryden, W., et al. (1996b). Body dysmorphic disorder: A cognitive behavioural model and pilot randomized controlled trial. *Behavioral Research and Therapy, 34,* 717-729.

Vogel, P. A., Stiles, T. C., & Gotestam, K. G. (2004). Adding cognitive therapy elements to exposure therapy for obsessive compulsive disorder: A controlled study. *Behavioural and Cognitive Psychotherapy, 32,* 275-290.

Warwick, H., Clark, D., & Salkovskis, P. (1996). A controlled trial of cognitive-behavioral treatment of hypochondriasis. *British Journal of Psychiatry, 169,* 189-195.

Wedding, D., Boyd, M. A., & Niemiec, R. M. (2010). *Movies and mental illness 3: Using films to understand psychopathology* (3rd ed.). Cambridge, MA: Hogrefe Publishing.

Wetterneck, C. T., Teng, E. J., & Stanley, M. A. (2010). Current issues in the treatment of OC spectrum conditions. *Bulletin of the Menninger Clinic, 74*(2), 141-166.

Wewetzer, C., Jans, T., Muller, B., et al. (2001). Long-term outcome and prognosis of obsessive-compulsive disorder with onset in childhood or adolescent. *European Child & Adolescent Psychiatry, 10*(1), 37-46.

Wiegartz, P. S., & Rasminsky, S. (2005). Treating OCD in patients with psychiatric comorbidity. *Current Psychiatry Online, 4*(4), 57.

Wilcox, J. A., & Nasrallah, H. A. (1986). Sydenham's chorea and psychosis. *Neuropsychobiology, 15,* 13-14.

Williams, K. A., Grant, J. E., & Kim, S. W. (2008). The PANDAS subgroup of obsessive-compulsive disorder. In J. S. Abramowitz, D. McKay, & S. Taylor (Eds.), *Clinical handbook of obsessive-compulsive disorder and related problems* (pp. 95-108). Baltimore: The Johns Hopkins University Press.

Wincze, J. P., Steketee, G., & Frost, R. O. (2007). Categorization in compulsive hoarding. *Behavioral Research and Therapy, 45,* 63-72.

Winsberg, M. D., Cassic, K. S., & Koran, L. M. (1999). Hoarding in obsessive-compulsive disorder: A report of 20 cases. *Journal of Clinical Psychiatry, 60*(9), 391-397.

Wodrich, D. L., Benjamin, E., & Lachar, D. (1997). Tourette's syndrome and psychopathology in a child psychiatry setting. *Journal of the American Academy of Child and Adolescent Psychiatry, 36*(11), 1618-1624.

Woo, T-U., Canuso, C. M., Wojcik, J. D., et al. (2009). Treatment of schizophrenia. In A. F. Schatzberg & C. B. Nemeroff (Eds.), *The American psychiatric publishing textbook of psychopharmacology* (4th ed.) (pp. 1135-1169). Washington, DC: American Psychiatric Publishing, Inc.

Woods, D. W., Adcock, A. C., & Conelea, C. A. (2008). Trichotillomania. In J. S. Abramowitz, D. McKay, & S. Taylor (Eds.), *Clinical handbook of obsessive-compulsive disorder and related problems* (pp. 205-221). Baltimore: The Johns Hopkins University Press.

Yaryura-Tobias, J. A. (1998). The unified theory of obsessive-compulsive disorder. *CNS Spectrums, 3*(7), 54-60.

Yorulmaz, O., Gencoz, T., & Woody, S. (2009). Vulnerability factors in OCD symptoms: Cross-cultural comparisons between Turkish and Canadian samples. *Clinical Psychology and Psychotherapy, 17,* 110-121.

Yutzy, S. H., & Parish, B. S. (2008). Somatoform disorders. In R. E. Hales, S. C. Yudofsky, & G. O. Gabbard (Eds.), *The American psychiatric publishing textbook of psychiatry* (5th ed.) (pp. 609-642). Washington, DC: American Psychiatric Publishing, Inc.

Zimmerman, M., & Matia, J. (1998). Body dysmorphic disorder in psychiatric outpatients: Recognition, prevalence, comorbidity, demographic, and clinical correlates. *Comprehensive Psychiatry, 39,* 265-270.

Zohar, J., & Judge, R. (1996). Paroxetine versus clomipramine in the treatment of obsessive-compulsive disorder. *British Journal of Psychiatry, 169,* 468-474.

Answers to Case Study 12-1 Questions

1. Obsessions of symmetry and saving/hoarding.
2. Comorbid biopsychosocial health problems include but are not limited to obsessive-compulsive personality disorder, panic attacks, symptoms of depression, sleep disturbance, impairment of vocational functioning, social isolation, and acquisition behaviors.
3. Treatment recommendations might include the following:
    - Gradually increasing the dose of the SSRI that she is currently taking or changing to another SSRI.
    - Adding cognitive behavioral therapy (CBT).
    - Using a multicomponent CBT model to address hoarding and acquisition behaviors.
    - Using psychosocial interventions for panic attacks, such as restricting caffeine, bibliotherapy, education, and self-help interventions.
    - Using sleep hygiene strategies.
    - Using psychosocial interventions for social isolation such as support groups.

UNIT V

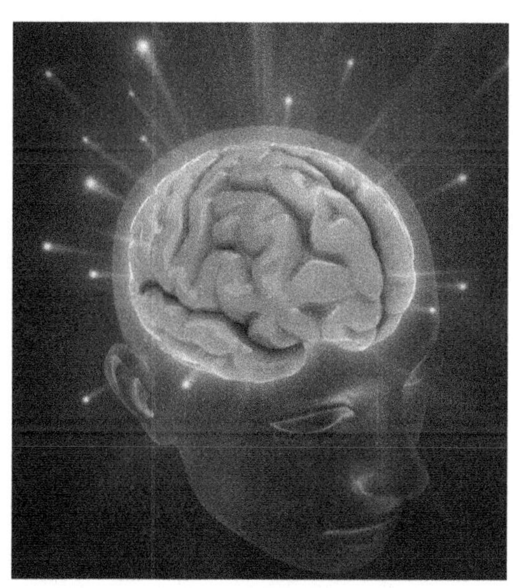

Psychiatric Disorders: Mood Disorders

CHAPTER 13

Depressive Disorders

Eris F. Perese, APRN-PMH

Depressive disorders include major depressive disorder, dysthymic disorder, and major depressive disorder not otherwise specified (*Diagnostic and Statistical Manual of Mental Disorders, Fourth Edition, Text Revision [DSM-IV-TR]*, American Psychiatric Association, 2000). Depressive disorders are not just illnesses that involve feelings of sadness or unhappiness; rather, depressive disorders reflect disturbances of brain subsystems that regulate mood, pleasure/reward, sleep, appetite, and cognitive, motor, social, and sexual functioning (Krishnan & Nestler, 2008).

Depressive disorders take a toll on the whole individual, on the family, and on society (Charney, Manji, & Husseini, 2004). The cost to patients is evidenced in impaired functioning, loss of income, and diminished quality of life (Simon, 2003; Whooley, Kiefe, Chesney, et al., 2002). The effects of depression on families include marital problems, care-providing burden on partners and other family members (Simon, 2003), and adverse effects on the emotional, behavioral, and cognitive development of children in the family (Lumley & Austin, 2001). The cost of depression to society is related to both increased use of medical services (Katon, 2003) and decreased productivity due to time lost from work (Brennan, Hammen, Andersen, et al., 2000). However, identifying depressive disorders and providing appropriate treatment can move patients toward recovery and reduce the burden associated with these disorders (Black & Andreasen, 2011).

Major Depressive Disorder (MDD)

Major depressive disorder (MDD) has a clinical course marked by one or more major depressive episodes. Major depressive episodes are characterized by the presence of depressed mood, lack of interest in usual activities, marked weight loss or gain, sleep disturbances, agitation, fatigue or loss of energy, feelings of worthlessness or inappropriate guilt, difficulty concentrating or making decisions, thoughts of death or suicide, and impairment of social and vocational functioning (Belmaker & Agam, 2008). (See the *DSM-IV-TR* [American Psychiatric Association, 2000] for specific criteria for major depressive disorder, single episode; for major depressive disorder, recurrent; for specifiers of severity and duration; and for subcategories.)

In the past, MDD was thought of as an episodic, one-time event. The current view is that MDD is a chronic illness and that the first episode is often followed by other episodes or by symptoms of depression that do not reach the severity of the criteria for a diagnosis of MDD (Bresee, Gotto, & Rapaport, 2009). Some researchers have proposed that MDD is part of a continuum that includes minor depression, subsyndromal depressive symptoms, dysthymia, and double depression (dysthymia and coexisting major depression) (Maddux & Rapaport, 2004).

Epidemiology

Prevalence

The prevalence of MDD is 6.6% for 1 year and 16.2% for lifetime among the U.S. adult population (Kessler, Berglund, Demler, et al., 2003). Until age 13, depression is equally common among boys and girls; after age 13, the rate doubles for females (Costello, Pine, Hammen, et al., 2002). The prevalence of MDD is approximately twice as high in women as in men (Kessler & Walters, 1998), and that rate is similar across most countries and cultures (Kornstein & Sloan, 2006). The difference cannot be attributed to women's seeking more medical attention for depression, because the prevalence difference has been found to be the same in community samples of men and women (Kornstein, 1997). The time of increased risk for depression for women coincides approximately with the childbearing years. The reasons for the increased risk are not known, but it may be due to the interaction between psychosocial factors and neuroendocrine changes (Cyranowski, Frank, Young, et al., 2000).

The age of onset of MDD is early adulthood—in the late 20s (Goodwin, Jacobi, Bittner, et al., 2006)—with a mean age of 27 years (First & Tasman, 2004). Onset of MDD after the age of 50 is frequently due to medical conditions such as Parkinson's disease, dementia, brain lesions, or strokes, or it may be due to the use of medications such as antihypertensives or corticosteroids (Joska & Stein, 2008). The presence of anticipation, ethnic and cultural factors, risk factors, and protective factors influence the development of MDD.

Anticipation

Earlier age of onset and increased lifetime prevalence of MDD suggest that anticipation is occurring in depressive disorders (Costello et al., 2002; Kessler et al., 2003; Klerman & Weissman, 1989; Williams & Neighbors, 2006). Anticipation refers to the earlier onset and increased severity of a genetic disorder that shows change from one generation to the next (Battaglia, Bertella, Bajo, et al., 1998).

Anticipation is associated with a mutation that induces variation in gene expression or sometimes gene shutdown. The mechanism of anticipation has been well described in several neurological disorders such as Huntington's ataxia, fragile X syndrome, and certain types of muscular dystrophy. Anticipation in depressive disorders may be influenced by changes in population demographics, changes in the structure of the family, and changes in occupational and employment patterns. Lambert (2006) has proposed that technology, by reducing the amount of physical effort and manual labor required to meet basic needs, may contribute to anticipation in depression by reducing the activation of brain areas involved in motivation, problem-solving, coping, and pleasure and by causing changes in neurochemistry, such as lower levels of serotonin. Lambert suggested that, in addition to its contribution to anticipation, lack of daily physical effort and manual labor may lead to symptoms of depression and decreased resilience in response to stressful events.

Ethnic and Cultural Factors

MDD has been identified in all the countries where it has been studied (Weissman, Bland, Canino, et al., 1996). Depression rates appear higher in cultures that emphasize individuals' responsibility for self-development, while depression rates appear lower in cultures where self-development is viewed as a socially shaped process with high priority placed on goals of social harmony and solidarity (Kirmayer & Jarvis, 2006). Some MDD symptoms are common across cultures, such as the symptoms of insomnia, lack of energy, problems with concentration, thoughts of death, muscular and skeletal pain, and fatigue (Sayer, Kirmayer, & Taillefer, 2003; Weissman et al.); however, because emotions evolve from social situations and are influenced by the individual's cultural world (White, 2000), patients describing their symptoms of depression may use "cultural idioms of distress; e.g., nerves, a darkness in life" (Kirmayer & Jarvis, p. 705; Kirmayer, Young, & Robbins, 1994).

Risk Factors

Risk factors for the development of MDD include the following:

- Female gender
- Personality traits of hypersensitivity to negative stimuli
- Prior episodes of anxiety or depression
- Family history of major depressive disorder
- Childhood maltreatment (neglect or abuse)
- History of suicide attempts
- Postpartum period
- Comorbid medical illnesses
- Lack of social support
- Active alcohol or substance abuse
- Widowed, separated, or divorced marital status
- Lower socioeconomic status
- Lower educational achievement
- Unemployment (more so for men than women)
- Stressful life events that cause loss, humiliation, loss of self-esteem, or feelings of entrapment (Blazer, Kessler, & McGonagle, 1994; First & Tasman, 2004; Goodwin et al., 2006; Joska & Stein, 2008; Mayberg, 2004; Weich, Churchill, Lewis, et al., 1997; Williams & Neighbors, 2006)

Protective Factors

Factors protective against the development of MDD include the following:

- *Resilience* is a characteristic of individuals that enables them to overcome the effects of a stressful event and gain mastery over it. (See Chapter 1 for more information on resilience.) Resilience is shaped by individuals' neurobiological responses to stress, adaptive social behaviors, sense of self-efficacy, faith, and ability to reframe obstacles that must be overcome. The attribute of resilience has been reported to offer protection against the development of depression (Edward, 2005).
- *Social support*—in the form of emotional support from family, close friends, or a supportive marital relationship—is believed to protect against the development of depression (Brown, 2002; Williams & Neighbors, 2006). A social network may reduce the risk for depression by decreasing the number and severity of life events and by preventing maladaptive interpretations of stressful events and negative thinking, thus promoting resilience (Johnson, Alloy, Panzarella, et al., 2001). (See Chapter 8 for more information on social support.)
- *Religion* offers protection by providing a network of potential friends, furnishing a meaning for events, providing ways to interpret stressful life events that reduce their impact, and promoting altruism.

Following religious practices by one's self (alone) does not serve as a buffer to depression, but religious practices that include interaction or involvement with others are associated with decreased rates of depression (Williams & Neighbors, 2006).

Etiology

The etiology of MDD has been studied with regard to evolutionary theory, genetic influence, the kindling model, the dysregulation of neurotransmitters model, and psychosocial theories of depression.

Evolutionary Theory

The evolutionary theory of depression proposes that experiencing depression after a loss is a positive way of adaptation. A state of depression allows individuals to consider what they have lost—e.g., property, status, role, or resources—and to think about how the loss can be regained or prevented in the future. During the period of depression, individuals may consider how much energy to expend in consideration of the diminished likelihood of regaining the lost object or how to go forward without the lost object. According to evolutionary theory, temporary depression following a loss may be protective (Nesse, 2006).

Genetic Influence

Genetic influence accounts for approximately 37% of the variance of MDD (Belmaker & Agam, 2008; Berrettini, 2006), a rate that is lower than the 84% heritability of bipolar disorder and schizophrenia (McGuffin, Rijsdisk, Andrew, et al., 2003; Smoller, Sheidley, & Tsuang, 2008). It is thought that the development of MDD is due to the interaction of multiple genes with environmental factors, such as stressful events (aan het Rot, Mathew, & Charney, 2009; Goodwin et al., 2006). How individuals react to stressful events depends on their ability to regulate the responses of the corticolimbic neurocircuits, which are molded early in life by temperament, caregiver nurturing, and life experiences and that are unique to each individual (Kaufman, Plotsky, Nemeroff, et al., 2000; Kendler, Neale, Kessler, et al., 1992).

Genetic influence may act through its effect on temperament by creating sensation-seeking traits or fearful, cautious traits (Nesse, 2006). These genetically determined traits influence individuals' choice of life experiences, which may lead to exposure to stressful situations or events—such as risky lifestyle practices, problems with interpersonal relationships, and financial difficulties—that are believed to be associated with the development of MDD (aan het Rot et al., 2009; Kessler, 1997).

Recent studies have identified the serotonin transporter gene as being involved in depression. This gene is associated with (1) reduced availability of the serotonin transporter, (2) reduced production of serotonin, and (3) impairment of emotional circuitry development with resulting hyperactivity of the amygdala, which is associated with anxiety and depression ("The 2006 Progress Report on Brain Research," 2006). These studies suggest that genetics may influence the development of depression through alterations in the availability of serotonin, which is the neurotransmitter system targeted by antidepressant medications such as the selective serotonin reuptake inhibitors (SSRIs).

Kindling Model

The kindling model provides a way for understanding the tendency of unipolar and bipolar affective disorders to recur (Post, 1992). According to the kindling model, events or experiences have long-lasting effects on brain structure, functioning, and chemistry. Each episode of depression produces neurobiological changes, such as alteration of the receptors for dopamine, acetylcholine, norepinephrine, serotonin, and neuropeptides; decreased thyroid activity; disruptions of sleep; abnormal hypothalamic-pituitary-adrenal axis responses; and decreased production of growth hormone (Post, 1992). Whereas the first episode of depression is likely to be associated with a major psychosocial stressor, such as loss of a loved one, there may be no stressors associated with recurrent episodes. This finding suggests that if enough stressor-related episodes occur, cycles of depression begin to occur without psychosocial stressors. The kindling model provides a way to understand the transition from episodes of depression that are caused by the impact of stressors to episodes that are not triggered by stressors.

Dysregulation of Neurotransmitters Model

Another model for understanding depression is the dysregulation of neurotransmitters theory, which proposes that there is impaired ability of neurons involved in emotional and cognitive circuitries to tolerate abnormal levels of certain neurotransmitters (Delgado & Moreno, 2006). For example, decreased levels of serotonin are associated with symptoms of depression, such as disruptions of appetite, sleep, and sexual functioning, and with the behavioral symptoms of impulsivity, aggression, and suicide. Decreased levels of norepinephrine are associated with fatigue, apathy, cognitive disturbances, slowness in information processing, and poor memory (Delgado & Moreno, 2006). Alterations of dopamine may be involved in psychomotor retardation and lack of pleasure.

Neuropeptides are also believed to be involved in depression. Neuropeptides may act directly as neurotransmitters or by inhibiting or modifying the release of serotonin, dopamine, norepinephrine, and acetylcholine. Alterations of neuropeptides such as corticotropin-releasing factor (CRF), arginine vasopressin, oxytocin, galanin, somatostatin, substance P, and orexin (hypocretin) are believed to play a role in depression, although their actions are not well understood (Belzung, Yalcin, Griebel, et al., 2006).

Psychosocial Theories of Depression

There are five main psychosocial theories of depression: cognitive theory, interpersonal theory, learned helplessness theory, attachment theory, and developmental theory.

- *Cognitive theory.* Beck (1976) described individuals with depression as having a negative view of themselves, their life situations, and their future. Beck's cognitive theory proposed that one's automatic assumptions determine feelings, such as those associated with depression; it also proposed that a negative self-view elicits negative responses from others.
- *Interpersonal theory.* In interpersonal theory, depression is viewed as the result of a disturbance in interpersonal relationships that impairs the individual's ability to cope with difficult situations, leading to depression.
- *Learned helplessness theory.* Learned helplessness theory proposes that individuals learn in inescapable, painful, or uncontrollable situations that they cannot escape the stressor with any action of their own, and they generalize this learning to all situations; that is, all of life will be the same and they cannot change negative events (Abramson, Metalsky, & Alloy, 1989; Seligman, 1975).
- *Attachment theory.* In attachment theory, it is postulated that the mother's failure to soothe and provide security for the infant results in a lack of modulation of the effect of cortisol on the infant's brain development, with subsequent hypersensitivity of the circuitry that is involved in emotions and cognition (Statham, 1998).
- *Developmental theory.* Developmental theory is based on the belief that early adverse experiences lay the foundation for later mental disorders, such as depression. For example, adverse experiences—including childhood losses, neglect, and abuse—are associated with increased rates of major depression in adulthood (Bifulco & Brown, 1998; Brown, 1993; Jaffee, Moffitt, Caspi, et al., 2002). (Early adverse experiences are discussed in Chapter 3 and Chapter 19.) Developmental theory also proposes that buffering provided by responsive caregivers may decrease the risk of depression among children who have been exposed to adverse experiences (Nachmias, Gunnar, Mangelsdorf, et al., 1996).

In summary, evidence suggests that an individual's vulnerability to developing depression may be due to the excessive reaction of neural circuits involved in the response to stress (Gillespie, Garlow, & Binder, 2009). It is believed that depression results from the interaction of a combination of factors: (1) genetically influenced responses to stress, (2) exposure to early life stress, such as trauma, abuse, or loss of a parent, and (3) the presence of ongoing stressors, such as death of a loved one, divorce, or loss of a job (Bresee et al., 2009; Charney et al., 2004).

Biological Basis

Response to stress consists of a series of events that have long-lasting consequences. (See Chapter 9 for more information about the stress response.) Exposure to stress triggers neurochemical activity—such as increased amounts of cortisol—and sets into motion intracellular changes at the level of gene transcription that cause enduring changes of neurotransmitters, receptors, and neuropeptides (McEwen, 1998). These changes may result in long-term synaptic adaptations, alterations of brain structures, and impairment of functioning (Post, 1992). The current focus of neurobiological research on depression has shifted from the interaction between neurotransmitters and cell receptors to changes of gene expression and changes of brain structures and their functioning.

Abnormalities of Brain Structures

Structural abnormalities of the brains of patients with MDD that are thought to be due to prenatal brain development include enlargement of the ventricles, prominence of the sulci, and decreased volume of the prefrontal cortex (Charney, 2002; Davidson, Lewis, Allory, et al., 2002), the amygdala (Sheline, Gado, & Price, 1998), and the hippocampus (Bremmer, Narayan, Anderson, et al., 2000; Rajkowska, 2006).

At the cell level, abnormalities of the brain include fewer neurons in the subgenual prefrontal cortex, which is an area of the prefrontal cortex ventral to the genu of the corpus callosum that is located 2½ inches behind the bridge of the nose. The subgenual prefrontal cortex modulates acute sadness and has a role in regulating negative mood. In individuals with depression, there is decreased blood flow and decreased glucose metabolism in that region, indicating reduced activity (Drevets, Price, Simpson, et al., 1997; Rajkowska, Halaris, & Selemon, 2001). Individuals with MDD also have decreased density of glial cells in the prefrontal cortex, in the cingulate cortex, and in the amygdala (Mayberg, 2006).

It is not known whether abnormalities of brain structures (atrophy of brain structures, diminished dendritic branching of the neural cells, and decreased density of glial cells) are due to abnormalities of neurodevelopment, are the effect of the illness, or are due to biochemical changes related to increased levels of cortisol that are associated with exposure to stressors (Rajkowska, 2006).

Abnormalities of Brain Functioning

When a sad mood is induced in individuals without depression, blood flow and metabolic activity *increase* in the frontal cortex, blood flow *increases* in the left amygdala, and blood flow *decreases* in the right amygdala (Pardo, Pardo, & Raichle, 1993). In contrast, individuals who are depressed have

- *Reduced* blood flow and metabolic activity in the frontal cortex and in the basal ganglia, indicating less brain activity in these areas (Joska & Stein, 2008; Soares & Mann, 1997)

- *Increased* blood flow and metabolism in the amygdala, orbital cortex, and thalamus, indicating more brain activity in these areas (Sackeim, 2001)

Thus, in patients with depression, the structures that are thought to be involved in emotional expression are activated, and those that are thought to modulate attention and sensory processing—the prefrontal cortex, cingulate cortex, and corpus callosum—are less active (Davidson et al., 2002).

Abnormalities of Brain Chemistry

Previously, depression was thought to be due to dysregulation of the norepinephrine system, the serotonin system, or both (Joska & Stein, 2011), but now it is thought that cascades of neurotransmitters (serotonin, norepinephrine, dopamine, glutamate, gamma-amminobutyric acid [GABA], and cortisol) play a role in regulation of stress and depression (aan het Rot et al., 2009):

- Serotonin regulates the neurovegetative signs of depression, which are sleep, pain, appetite, and sexual functioning (Joska & Stein, 2011; Maes, Scharpe, & Meltzer, 1995).
- Norepinephrine modulates behavior and attention and gives the emotional component to memories (Cahill, McGaugh, Weinberger, et al., 2001).
- Dopamine is thought to be linked to anhedonia (lack of pleasure in usual activities), which is often experienced by patients with depression. Dopamine in the limbic areas is regulated by serotonin (Duman, 2004), and in individuals with depression, there may be dysregulation of dopamine systems that may result in certain symptoms of depression such as psychomotor retardation, flat affect, and lack of pleasure (Gillespie et al., 2009; Hasler, Drevets, Manji, et al., 2004). Abnormalities of dopamine receptors are believed to influence the effect of past stressful life events on current mood (Dunlop & Nemeroff, 2007).
- Glutamate, an excitatory neurotransmitter, is involved in learning, memory, and synaptic plasticity. Glutamate is essential for brain activity, but too much glutamate is toxic to neurons (Higgins & George, 2007). Levels of glutamate are elevated in individuals with depression (Gillespie et al., 2009). Experimental studies have found that ketamine, a glutamate receptor antagonist, has a rapid but transient antidepressant effect (Zarate, Singh, Carlson, et al., 2006).
- GABA acts as an inhibitor and regulates other neurotransmitter systems; that is, it quiets overactive neurons (Higgins & George, 2007). GABA is decreased in individuals with depression and in their relatives who do not have depression, suggesting a genetic influence on the GABA system (Bjork, Moeller, Kramer, et al., 2001; Gillespie et al., 2009).
- Cortisol mobilizes energy and the fight-or-flight response. Prolonged elevated rates of cortisol are associated with impairment of memory and atrophy of the hippocampus (Higgins & George, 2007). Levels of cortisol are elevated in individuals with depression who were exposed to stressors as children; also, cortisol levels are elevated in these individuals during episodes of depression (Carroll, Cassidy, Naftolowitz, et al., 2007; Gillespie et al., 2009). The dexamethasone suppression test (DST) was used in the past to diagnose depression by detecting the body's resistance to cortisol suppression (Copolov, Rubin, Stuart, et al., 1989). It is not used as frequently now because of its limited sensitivity (positive in only 40% to 50% of depressed patients) (Wallach, 2000). More information about DST can be found in Box 13-1.

Neuropeptides are also involved in depression. Patients with MDD have been found to have lower levels of

BOX 13-1 Cortisol and the Dexamethasone Suppression Test (DST)

Acute stress and chronic stress deplete norepinephrine, serotonin, and acetylcholine and they increase cortisol secretion. Even anticipated stress or imagined losses may precipitate increased cortisol activity and may produce other abnormalities of biochemical functioning (Post, 1992).

In individuals who are depressed, there are increased brain levels of corticotropin-releasing factor (CRF), which is released from the hypothalamus and is the major regulator of the hypothalamic-pituitary-adrenal axis. CRF causes increased activity of the adrenal glands that secrete cortisol. Depression associated with increased levels of cortisol reflects an underlying dysfunction or dysregulation of the body's ability to suppress cortisol or turn off cortisol secretion.

The dexamethasone suppression test (DST) was used in the past to diagnose depression. Dexamethasone is a synthetic glucocorticoid. When normal individuals receive dexamethasone, their body's production of cortisol is suppressed. The DST detects resistance to cortisol feedback and nonsuppression of cortisol that was considered to be a marker for MDD; however, nonsuppression also occurs in medical illnesses, with use of medications such as barbiturates and carbamazepine, with alcohol use, with malnutrition, and with infections (Wallach, 2000).

Because the DST is positive in only 40% to 50% of patients with depression (Wallach, 2000) and can be influenced by many factors—including comorbid psychiatric disorders, such as anxiety disorders and somatoform disorder (Veen, Derijk, Giltay, et al., 2009)—it has limited clinical application (Kim et al., 2008).

(1) somatostatin, which has antianxiety and antidepressant actions (Bissette & Myers, 1992), (2) neuropeptide Y, which modulates emotional behaviors (Carvajal, Dumont, Quirion, 2006), and (3) brain-derived neurotropic factor, which plays a role in neuron survival, synaptic plasticity, and fear-related memories (Gillespie et al., 2009).

Thyroid Abnormalities

The thyroid gland regulates the basal metabolic rate and thus affects the functioning of every organ. Hyperthyroidism is manifested as irritability, insomnia, weight loss, and agitation (Demet, Ozmen, Deveci, et al., 2002). In contrast, hypothyroidism, which is the most common endocrine disorder associated with depression, is manifested in symptoms such as fatigue, memory impairment, irritability, depression, and loss of interest in sex (Chueire, Silva, Perotta, et al., 2003).

In overt hypothyroidism, the thyroid gland is seriously damaged and produces extremely low levels of the hormone thyroxine. However, most cases of hypothyroidism are caused by a slowly developing condition known as symptomless autoimmune thyroiditis, which affects women more frequently than men and runs in families. About 0.5% of the general population has overt hypothyroidism, but subclinical hypothyroidism affects 3 to 8.5% of the general population (Zagaria, 2010). Among patients with MDD, the prevalence of subclinical hypothyroidism is 9% (Joffee & Levitt, 1992). However, among patients with chronic depression and treatment-resistant depression, the rate of hypothyroidism and subclinical hypothyroidism is 22% (Hickie, Bennett, Mitchell, et al., 1996). Subclinical hypothyroidism increases vulnerability to depression and reduces effectiveness of antidepressant medications. Some clinicians advise treating the hypothyroidism for a week and then adding an antidepressant if the depression has not improved.

Insulin Resistance

In patients with depressive disorders there is a high prevalence of insulin resistance, which is a metabolic abnormality in which the body becomes insensitive to normal amounts of insulin and secretes increasingly greater amounts (Pearson, Schmidt, Patton, et al., 2010; Rasgon & Kenna, 2005). There is also an increased rate of depression among patients with polycystic ovary syndrome, which consists of androgen hypersecretion, insulin resistance, and chronic anovulation (Rasgon, Rao, Hwang, et al., 2003; Teede, Deeks, & Moran, 2010).

Clinical Presentation

Clinical presentation of MDD includes the signs and symptoms included in the *DSM-IV-TR* criteria for major depressive episode, with sleep disturbances being one of the most frequent symptoms (occurring in 80% of patients with depression) (Buysse, Germain, Nofzinger, et al., 2006). Organizing the signs and symptoms of MDD into behavioral domains—mood, circadian/vegetative, cognitive, and motor—provides a basis for targeting treatment and evaluating outcomes (Box 13-2).

In addition to symptoms identified in Box 13-2, patients with MDD also present with a variety of biopsychosocial health problems. For example, patients with MDD have increased rates of medical illnesses and risk for suicide; they also have impaired functioning that may be manifested in time lost from work, reduced productivity in

BOX 13-2 Behavioral Domains of Major Depressive Disorder and Associated Major Depressive Disorder Symptoms

Mood

- Recurrent episodes of depressed mood
- Sadness
- Discouragement
- Anhedonia
- Hopelessness
- Suicidality
- Anxiety
- Irritability
- Dysphoria

Circadian/Vegetative

- Low energy
- Decreased drive
- Decreased libido
- Insomnia or hypersomnia
- Early morning wakening
- Changes in weight (more than 5% in 1 month)
- Loss of appetite, or may have a craving for carbohydrates

Cognitive

- Poor attention
- Inability to concentrate
- Easily distracted
- Decreased motivation
- Apathy
- Excessive guilt
- Memory loss that may resemble dementia
- Recurrent thoughts of death (not just fear of dying)
- Thoughts that others would be better off if they were dead
- Perception of themselves as worthless and responsible for adverse events
- Ruminations over past failures
- Inappropriate guilt

Motor

- Restlessness
- Agitation
- Hand-wringing
- Pulling at skin or clothes
- Inability to sit still
- Pacing
- Slowed speech, thinking, and movements

Sources: American Psychiatric Association, 2000; First & Tasman, 2004; Joska & Stein, 2011; Mayberg, 2004.

other areas of their lives, and problems with interpersonal relationships (Bresee et al., 2009). Patients with MDD have smaller social support networks than individuals without depression, and within their social networks they report deficits of emotional support, e.g., a lack of caring, empathy, love, and trust. They also have a higher rate of illnesses, stressful life events, and arguments or conflicts with family or partners (Skarsater, Agren, & Dencker, 2001).

Severity Specifiers

On clinical presentation, if the patient meets the criteria for having a major depressive episode, specifiers are used to describe the status and the features of the current episode. Specifiers include severity, clinical status, longitudinal course, and type of major depressive episodes.

In the *DSM-IV-TR*, an episode of MDD is classified as mild, moderate, severe without psychotic features, severe with psychotic features, or chronic (American Psychiatric Association, 2000):

- **Mild:** Symptoms meet the minimum level required to make the diagnosis; there is only minor impairment of functioning.
- **Moderate:** Symptoms are in excess of the minimum required to make the diagnosis; there is greater impairment of functioning.
- **Severe without psychotic features:** Several symptoms are in excess of the minimal requirements; the symptoms markedly interfere with social or occupational functioning or with relationships with others. In severe episodes, the individual may be unable to function socially or occupationally or to maintain self-care.
- **Severe with psychotic features:** Delusions or hallucinations are present and should be identified as mood-congruent (personal inadequacy, guilt, disease, death, nihilism, or deserving of punishment) or mood-incongruent (persecutory delusions, thought insertion, thought broadcasting, and delusions of control). Mood-congruent delusions and hallucinations occur more frequently than mood-incongruent ones (Flores & Schatzberg, 2006). Patients with MDD, severe depression, and psychotic features, have severely impaired functioning and are often a danger to themselves (suicide) or are a danger to others and require immediate hospitalization.
- **Chronic:** This specifier can be applied to the current or most recent major depressive episode if full criteria for a major depressive episode have been met continuously for at least the past 2 years (American Psychiatric Association, 2000, p. 417).

The level of suicidal ideation and suicidal behaviors should be considered in determining severity (Karasu, Gelenberg, Merriam, et al., 2006, p. 800).

When comparing the MDD specifiers "severe with psychotic features" and "without psychotic features," it is helpful to note that a patient with MDD *with* psychotic features is likely to have

- A younger age of onset
- More severe depression
- More symptoms of paranoia
- More rumination
- More feelings of guilt and thoughts of sin
- More psychomotor agitation
- More feelings of worthlessness
- More suicidal ideation
- More impairment of functioning (physical, psychological, and social)
- Higher rates of relapse, of suicide, and of mortality from other causes (Flores & Schatzberg, 2006)

MDD with psychotic features occurs in 20% of patients with severe MDD (Black & Andreasen, 2011). The impairment of attention, verbal-memory functioning, executive functioning, and psychomotor speed functioning among patients with MDD with psychotic features resembles that of patients with schizophrenia, although the impairment is less severe (Flores & Schatzberg, 2006).

Clinical Status Specifiers

Clinical status specifiers include "in partial remission" and "in full remission." The specifier "in partial remission" is used if the symptoms of MDD are present but do not meet criteria fully or if there is a period of time without any significant symptoms of a major depressive episode lasting less than 2 months following the end of an episode. The specifier "in full remission" is used if no significant signs or symptoms of the disturbance have been present for a period of 2 months (American Psychiatric Association, 2000, pp. 412-413).

Longitudinal Course Specifiers

The longitudinal course specifiers "with inter-episode recovery" and "without inter-episode recovery" describe the course of illness of individuals with recurrent MDD. "With inter-episode recovery" is used if full remission is attained between the two most recent mood episodes. "Without inter-episode recovery" is used if full remission is *not* attained between the two most recent mood episodes (American Psychiatric Association, 2000, p. 425).

MDD with seasonal pattern, known as *seasonal affective disorder* (SAD), can also be a longitudinal specifier. More on SAD can be found in Box 13-3.

Major Depressive Episode Specifiers

Major depressive episode specifiers include MDD with catatonic features, MDD with melancholic features, MDD with atypical features, and MDD with postpartum onset (American Psychiatric Association, 2000, p. 376).

Major Depressive Disorder With Catatonic Features

MDD with catatonic features is characterized by immobility, mutism, echolalia (repeating words or phrases that

BOX 13-3 Seasonal Affective Disorder

Seasonal affective disorder (SAD) is characterized by symptoms that appear in the fall or winter and improve in the spring. This pattern of onset and remission of episodes must have occurred during the last 2 years without any nonseasonal episodes occurring during this period (American Psychiatric Association, 2000, p. 426).

The prevalence of SAD in the United States is associated with geographical location or latitude. For example, the prevalence of SAD for people in Sarasota, Florida, is 1.4% whereas the prevalence for people in Nashua, New Hampshire, is 9.7% (Mersch, Middendorp, Bouhuys, et al., 1999).

The onset of SAD is in the early 20s, although patients may have experienced depressive symptoms that did not meet the criteria for major depression in previous winter months. The rate is higher among women of childbearing age (Kasper, Wehr, Bartko, et al., 1989).

Symptoms of SAD include overeating, carbohydrate craving, weight gain, lethargy, oversleeping, and feelings of sadness, anxiety, and irritability. There is often impairment of occupational and social functioning (Lam et al., 2006). The physical symptoms often appear first (Rosenthal & Rosenthal, 2006).

SAD has a genetic influence and is believed to be related to three areas of alteration: dysregulation in the serotonin system, dysregulation of the circadian rhythms, and abnormal processing of environmental light by the eyes (Rosenthal & Rosenthal, 2006). Light serves as a zeitgeber, or time cue, and helps to establish and reset underlying biological rhythms, including the circadian rhythm of various hormones and the sleep-wake and rest-activity rhythms.

Comorbidities of SAD include anxiety disorders and personality disorders.

someone else has said), posturing, negativism (resistance to passive movement or repeatedly turning away from the examiner), mannerisms (repeated movements that have no purpose), and stereotypies (repeated movements or behaviors that are not goal directed) (Klein, Shankman, & McFarland, 2006a).

Major Depressive Disorder With Melancholic Features

MDD with melancholic features is characterized by (1) loss of pleasure in all or almost all activities, (2) lack of response to a pleasurable event, and (3) three of the following: diurnal variation, where depression is worse in the morning; early morning awakening; slowed motor activity or agitation; loss of appetite; weight loss; and expressions of inappropriate guilt (Klein et al., 2006a). Melancholic depression is more likely to occur with severe major depressive episodes and in MDD with psychotic features (American Psychiatric Association, 2000).

Major Depressive Disorder With Atypical Features

MDD with atypical features is characterized by mood reactivity; for instance, the individual's mood improves when something good or pleasant happens. It is also characterized by the following features:

- An unusually excessive need for sleep
- A feeling that the arms or legs are heavy and leaden
- Overeating, with cravings for carbohydrate, sweets, and chocolate
- Weight gain
- Inability to anticipate pleasure, but no loss of actual ability to experience pleasure once involved in an activity
- Anxiety
- Rejection sensitivity
- A fluctuating course in response to events
- Impairment of functioning, such as loss of time at work and missed school and social activities
- Changes of relationships due to perceived rejection (Potter, Padich, Rudorfer, et al., 2006; Stewart, Quitkin, & Davies, 2006)

Atypical depression is often comorbid with bipolar disorder (Angst, Gamma, Sellaro, et al., 2002), substance abuse (Markowitz, Moran, Kocsis, et al., 1992), and Axis II personality disorders such as avoidant, histrionic, and borderline personality disorders (Perugi, Akiskal, Lattanzi, et al., 1998). Patients with early onset of atypical depression—before age 20—tend to have lower levels of cortisol, a more severe chronic course, and poor response to tricyclic antidepressants. Those with late onset—after age 20—tend to be more similar to those with depressive disorders with melancholic features and have elevated levels of cortisol and a less chronic depression (Stewart et al., 2006).

Major Depressive Disorder With Postpartum Onset

The *DSM-IV-TR* (American Psychiatric Association, 2000) states that the specifier "with postpartum onset" can be applied to the most recent major depressive episode, manic episode, or mixed episode in a major depressive disorder, in bipolar I disorder, or in bipolar II disorder in a postpartum patient; it may also be applied to a brief psychotic disorder if the onset of symptoms is within 4 weeks after childbirth. *DSM-IV-TR* (American Psychiatric Association, 2000) criteria require that the onset of depression be within 4 weeks of delivery and that the postpartum patient present with depression for 2 weeks or with loss of interest or pleasure in daily activities that is a change from previous behavior and that causes impairment in everyday functioning. In addition, at least four of the following symptoms must be present: weight change in the absence of dieting; insomnia or hypersomnia; psychomotor agitation or retardation, fatigue, or loss of energy; feelings of worthlessness or guilt; decreased ability to think or concentrate; and recurrent thoughts of death or suicide (American Psychiatric Association, 2000). The onset of MDD with postpartum features can present with or without psychotic features.

Postpartum depression may also be the depressive phase of a bipolar disorder. In addition to the symptoms that are often present in patients with MDD with postpartum onset, patients with postpartum depression that is part of the depressive phase of bipolar disorder may have symptoms of distractibility, racing thoughts, highly irritable mood, hostility, increased talkativeness, risky behavior, elevated mood, and impulsive behaviors (Akiskal, Benazzi, Perugi, et al., 2005; Bifulco, Figueiredo, Guedeney, et al., 2004).

In practice, clinicians often think of symptoms of altered mood that occur during the postpartum period as including "baby blues," MDD with postpartum onset, and postpartum psychosis (Doucet, Dennis, Letourneau, 2009).

Baby Blues

Approximately 85% of mothers experience postpartum blues ("baby blues"), in which symptoms are mild, are transient, and usually occur within the first 2 days of delivery (Doucet et al., 2009). Symptoms of the baby blues that usually resolve without treatment include tearfulness, mood lability, irritability, and anxiety. However, because the symptoms may peak on the fifth, sixth, or seventh day after delivery, mothers and their families should be taught about postpartum blues so that they will understand what is happening and realize that it is a transient condition that responds to support, reassurance, and assistance caring for the baby so that the mother is not sleep deprived (Burt & Stein, 2008).

Major Depressive Disorder With Postpartum Onset

In MDD with postpartum onset, experienced by about 13% of new mothers, depression occurs within the first 4 weeks postpartum (Burt & Stein, 2008; Sit et al., 2006). Risk factors for MDD with postpartum onset are a prior postpartum mood episode, prior history of a mood disorder, family history of mood disorder, and history of drug or alcohol abuse. For example, women who have had previous postpartum depression are at 50% to 60% risk of another major depressive episode with postpartum onset (Burt & Stein, 2008). MDD with postpartum onset is more likely to occur among women with low levels of social support, among women in conflicted marriages, among women who were ambivalent about the pregnancy, and among women who are single parents, have a low self-esteem, and are experiencing financial difficulties and child care stress (Beck, 2001; Kornstein & Sloan, 2006). Other risk factors that are related to the mother include having an insecure attachment pattern, a history of childhood separation from parents, or childhood sexual abuse; being a single parent; experiencing a significant loss or recent move that decreased social support; and having the "baby blues" (Bifulco et al., 2004; Cullen-Drill, Smith, & Morris, 2008).

In MDD with postpartum onset, mild hypomanic symptoms in the early postpartum period are common (Heron, Craddock, & Jones, 2005). Other symptoms include depressed mood, anhedonia, lack of interest in the baby, appetite changes, fear or thoughts of hurting the baby, anxiety, agitation, inability to sleep, irritability, and thoughts of death or suicide (Driscoll, 2006). Treatment options include psychotherapy, psychosocial interventions, and electroconvulsive therapy (ECT) for women who wish to breastfeed and are concerned about the effects of pharmacotherapy.

Postpartum Psychosis

MDD with postpartum onset *with psychotic features* is one of several disorders that can cause postpartum psychosis. Other disorders that can cause postpartum psychosis include bipolar I disorder, bipolar II disorder, schizoaffective disorder, unspecified functional psychosis, and brief psychotic disorder (Doucet et al., 2009). Evidence suggests that postpartum psychosis is most frequently due to bipolar disorder (Sit et al., 2006). Because of the risk that antidepressants will exacerbate manic symptoms in these patients, Bergink and Koorengevel (2010) recommended that all cases of psychotic depression with an onset within 4 weeks of delivery be considered to be bipolar depression.

In MDD with postpartum onset and with psychotic features, symptoms include delusions, hallucinations, mania, or mixed features. There may be severe ruminations; delusional thoughts about the infant that may include thinking that the baby is persecuting the mother or is a changeling (an infant believed to have been substituted for another) (Brockington, 1996). Delusional thoughts may be paranoid, grandiose, or bizarre. There may be disorganized behaviors. These symptoms are associated with increased risk of infanticide, danger of injury to other children, and risk of suicide for the mother (Burt & Stein, 2008; Sit et al., 2006). For example, Andrea Yates, who was experiencing MDD with postpartum onset with psychotic features, had made serious suicide attempts and eventually killed all five of her children by drowning them in the bathtub (Yardley, 2002). Factors that increase the risk of infanticide include situations that put the mother under severe stress, such as financial problems, housing problems, conflict with spouse, abuse, and lack of social support (Mugavin, 2005). Postpartum psychosis is a psychiatric emergency that requires hospitalization (Burt & Stein, 2008). Treatment options include pharmacotherapy, such as the use of mood stabilizers or antipsychotics (Sharma, 2002, 2008), and ECT (Forray & Ostroff, 2007).

Comorbidity

Medical, Neurological, and Psychiatric Comorbidities

Among patients with MDD, there is a high rate of co-occurring medical illnesses such as cancer, diabetes, pain, AIDS, respiratory diseases, and cardiovascular diseases; neurological disorders such as Parkinson's disease and stroke; and psychiatric disorders such as anxiety disorders, dementia, schizophrenia, substance abuse, and suicide (aan het Rot et al., 2009; Boland, 2006; Bresee et al., 2009). In addition, unhealthy lifestyle practices such as smoking, obesity, and inactivity appear to be linked with depression (Rosal, Ockene, Ma, et al., 2001), and depression appears to be linked with nonadherence to medical treatment and lack of self-care (DiMatteo, Lepper, & Croghan, 2000). More information on the medical, neurological, and psychiatric comorbidities of MDD can be found in Box 13-4. Suicide, a comorbidity of MDD, is discussed below.

Suicide

Suicide is the result of many factors: genetic influence, gender, biopsychosocial health problems, availability of means to commit suicide, and lack of protective factors (Box 13-5). Results of family and twin studies indicate that the amount of genetic variance for suicide is 43%, in the moderate range (Glatt, Faraone, & Tsuang, 2008; Smoller et al., 2008). Women make more suicide attempts (3 times more often than men), but men commit suicide more often (3.7 times more often than women). Depression or other psychiatric disorders—including substance-related disorders—are present in more than 90% of individuals who commit suicide (Cavanagh, Carson, Sharpe, et al., 2003). The most frequent method of suicide is the use of firearms (51.6%), followed by hanging (22.6%) and ingestion of poisons (17.9%) (Simon, 2008). The purpose of evaluating risk for suicide is to determine what appropriate actions should be taken to prevent it—e.g., medication, psychiatric referral, consultation, or immediate hospitalization (Folse, Eich, Hall, et al., 2006; Muzina, 2007; Simon, 2011)—and to identify risk factors that can be modified or removed and protective factors that can be mobilized to support the patient (Simon, 2008).

Risk Factors

General risk factors for suicide include

- Being widowed, divorced, separated, or incarcerated (Muzina, 2007).
- Lack or loss of social supports (Muzina, 2007)

BOX 13-4 Comorbidity of Medical, Neurological, and Psychiatric Disorders With Major Depressive Disorder

Medical Disorders

- ***Trauma:*** 17% to 25% of patients with head injury have MDD (Holsinger, Steffens, Phillips, et al., 2002).
- ***Stroke***: Among post-stroke patients, 50% have symptoms of depression and 10% to 27% have MDD (First & Tasman, 2004; Whyte & Mulsant, 2002).
- ***Cerebrovascular disease:*** Even without a clinical stroke, cerebrovascular disease is related to the development of depression, the so-called vascular depression that is characterized by loss of interest, apathy, cognitive impairment, and motor retardation.
- ***Cardiac disease:*** Among patients with congestive heart failure, 17% to 37% have MDD (Freedland, Carney, & Skala, 1995).
- ***Coronary artery disease:*** 40% to 65% of patients with post-myocardial infarction have MDD (Freedland et al., 1995).
- ***Cancer:*** MDD occurs in 25% to 50% of patients with cancer (First & Tasman, 2004).
- ***Chronic fatigue syndrome:*** 46% to 75% of patients with chronic fatigue syndrome experience MDD (Hawk, Jason, & Torres-Harding, 2006).
- ***Diabetes:*** The rate of depression is three times greater among persons with diabetes than among the general population (First & Tasman, 2004).
- ***Dialysis:*** 10% to 40% of patients on dialysis have depressive symptoms.
- ***HIV:*** Among persons with HIV, the lifetime rate of depression is 22% to 45% (Dew, Reynolds, Houck, et al., 1997).

Neurological Disorders

- ***Alzheimer's disorder:*** 15% to 20% have MDD, and 50% have depressive symptoms (Krishan, Delong, Kraemer, et al., 2002).
- ***Epilepsy:*** About 33% of people with epilepsy have MDD (Kanner, 2003).
- ***Multiple sclerosis:*** Of people with multiple sclerosis, 41% have depressive symptoms, and 29% have moderate to severe depression (Chwastiak, Ehde, Gibbons, et al., 2002).
- ***Parkinson's disease:*** 50% of patients with Parkinson's disease have MDD (First & Tasman, 2004).

Psychiatric Disorders

- ***Dysthymia***: 20% to 40% of patients with MDD meet criteria for dysthymia (Goodwin et al., 2006).
- ***Anxiety disorders:*** Anxiety disorders precede the onset of MDD about 50% of the time. Among patients with MDD, 30% to 40% have generalized anxiety disorder and 10% to 20% have panic attacks.
- ***Alcohol- and drug-related disorders:*** Among patients with MDD, 27% have a comorbid substance-related disorder—16.5% alcohol and 18% substance abuse—with the two often overlapping (Richards et al., 1999).
- ***Eating disorders:*** 50% to 75% of persons with eating disorders have MDD (First & Tasman, 2004).
- ***Personality disorders:*** 30% to 40% of persons with MDD have a comorbid personality disorder (First & Tasman, 2004).
- ***Suicide:*** 70% to 90% of people who commit suicide have a depressive illness (Thomas, Insel, & Charney, 2003).

BOX 13-5 Biopsychosocial Suicide Risk Factors, Preventive Factors, and Protective Factors

Biopsychosocial Risk Factors

Risk Factors Significant Within 1 Year Prior to Suicide

Alcohol abuse
Anxiety
Depressive turmoil
Global insomnia
Inability to concentrate
Loss of pleasure and interest
Panic attacks

Risk Factors Significant Within 2 Years or More

Hopelessness
Prior suicide attempts
Suicidal ideation

Other Risk Factors

Agitation
Drug abuse
Family history of mental illness
Impulsivity
Physical illness

Social Problems That Are Risk Factors

Availability of guns
Family problems: spouse, partner, children
Financial problems
Living situation
Work or academic problems

Demographic Factors That Contribute to Suicide Risk

White race
Imprisoned
Living alone
Male gender
Rural residence

Preventive Factors

Belonging to a desired group
Fear of social disapproval
Having reasons for living such as a sense of responsibility to family
Life satisfaction
Married status
Material resources
Moral objections to suicide
Parenthood
Plans for the future
Problem-solving skills
Resilience
Social support

Protective Factors

Adherence to treatment for medical, psychiatric, and substance abuse disorders
Availability of care for medical, psychiatric, and substance abuse disorders
Being pregnant or having children at home
Family and community support
Having moral/religious/spiritual values

Adapted from Joiner et al., 2005; Simon, 2008; Westefeld et al., 2006.

- Presence of medical illness such as multiple sclerosis, Huntington's disease, systemic lupus erythematosus, and AIDS (Muzina, 2007)
- Feelings of depression and hopelessness, having fewer reasons for living, and having more aggressive and impulsive behaviors in general but especially with regard to interpersonal relationships (Mann & Currier, 2006)
- Impulsivity or agitation (Simon, 2011)
- A history of comorbid borderline personality disorder, smoking, substance use, or alcohol abuse
- Childhood head injuries and childhood abuse
- Family history of suicide (Mann, Watermaux, Haas, et al., 1999)
- Depressive episodes, panic attacks, substance abuse, or command hallucinations (Simon, 2011)
- Prior suicide attempts and suicidal ideation (Murphy, Wetzel, Robins, et al., 1992)
- Loss of social support or employment, decrease of socioeconomic status, and sense of hopelessness (Muzina, 2007)
- Availability of lethal means (e.g., guns or drugs) (Simon, 2008)

Short-term risk factors for suicide are acute risk factors that occur close to the time of a suicide, although they may have been present for 1 year before suicide. They include

- Panic attacks
- Severe anxiety
- Loss of pleasure
- Moderate alcohol abuse
- Depressive turmoil
- Inability to concentrate
- Global insomnia (which is difficulty falling asleep, difficulty staying asleep, and feeling that sleep is not refreshing at least two or three times a week)
- Making arrangements for children or pets, updating wills, and making financial arrangements for bills (Fawcett, Scheftner, Fogg, et al., 1990; Hall, Platt, Hall, et al., 1999; Okun, Kravitz, Sowers, et al., 2009; Simon, 2011)

Joiner, Pfaff, and Acres (2002) have said that everyone needs to belong to a valued group and that the loss of a sense of belonging increases the risk for suicide. For example, young adults—young, intoxicated, single males who are in jail or a holding center for their first-time violation—are often placed in isolation, where some commit suicide by hanging themselves. The rate of suicide of jail inmates is approximately four times higher than that of prison inmates and nine times greater than that of the general population (Metzner & Hayes, 2006). Psychiatric advanced practice nurses can measure suicidal ideation among adolescents and young adults (especially those in forensic settings) with the brief self-report screening tool (4 questions) shown in Figure 13-1 (Joiner et al., 2002).

(A) 0 I do not have thoughts of killing myself.
1 Sometimes I have thoughts of killing myself.
2 Most of the time I have thoughts of killing myself.
3 I always have thoughts of killing myself.

(B) 0 I am not having thoughts of suicide.
1 I am having thoughts about suicide but have not formulated any plans.
2 I am having thoughts about suicide and am considering possible ways of doing it.
3 I am having thoughts about suicide and formulated a definite plan.

(C) 0 I am not having thoughts about suicide.
1 I am having thoughts about suicide but have these thoughts completely under my control.
2 I am having thoughts about suicide but have these thoughts somewhat under my control.
3 I am having thoughts about suicide but have little or no control over these thoughts.

(D) 0 I am not having impulses to kill myself.
1 In some situations I have impulses to kill myself.
2 In most situations I have impulses to kill myself.
3 In all situations I have impulses to kill myself.

FIGURE 13-1: **Depressive Symptom Index—Suicidality Subscale (DSI-SS).** In the DSI-SS, patients are asked to circle the sentence or number in each A, B, C, and D category that best fits their state of mind. Scores range from 0 to 3 for each category. A score of 3 out of 12 was considered to suggest a risk for suicide.
Source: Joiner, T. E., Plaff, J. J., & Acres, J. G. (2002). A brief screening tool for suicidal symptoms in adolescents and young adults in general health settings: Reliability and validity data from the Australian National General Practice Youth Suicide Prevention Project. *Behaviour Research and Therapy, 40* (4), 471-481. doi: 10.1016/S0005-7967(01)00017-1. | DSI-SS reprinted with permission of Elsevier Limited.

Some of the risk factors for suicide are modifiable with treatment. For example, treating anxiety, depression, panic attacks, substance abuse, and severe insomnia could reduce risk for suicide (Simon, 2011). Although sleep hygiene has traditionally played a primary role in the treatment of insomnia, a recent study by Edinger, Olsen, Stechuchak, et al. (2009) found that cognitive behavioral therapy (CBT) was more effective in treating global insomnia than sleep hygiene.

Protective Factors

Factors protective against suicide include having problem-solving skills, being satisfied with life, being resilient, having social support, belonging to a desired group, being married, having material resources, and having reasons for living such as a sense of responsibility to family, plans for the future, fear of social disapproval, and moral objections to suicide (Joiner et al., 2002; Simon, 2008; Westefeld, Button, Haley, et al., 2006). Other factors that have been found to be protective are being pregnant or having young children at home and having moral/religious/spiritual values (Simon, 2008). Spirituality offers protection through the belief that there is a meaning to life, and religion offers protection through traditions and practices that shape an individual's behaviors and views of life events (Dervic, Gruenbaum, Burke, et al., 2006). For example, in a group of 100 patients who had made serious suicide attempts, 51% had no religious belief or affiliation, 33% were Protestant, 15% were Catholic, and 1% were Muslim (Hall et al., 1999). Because firearms are frequently used in suicide and because suicide is often an impulsive act, safe storage of firearms is a crucial protective measure against suicide (Shenassa, Rogers, Spalding, et al., 2004; Simon, 2008). Psychiatric advanced practice nurses can measure protective factors against suicidal behavior with the *Reasons for Living Inventory (RFLI)* (Linehan, Goldstein, Nielsen, et al., 1983). Psychiatric advanced practice psychiatric nurses should also be knowledgeable about interventions for threatened suicide or suicidal behaviors (Box 13-6) and the myths regarding suicide (Box 13-7).

Differential Diagnosis

Depression is (1) a clinical feature of several disorders, (2) secondary to some medications and substances, and (3) part of a response to some life events. Hence, in making the diagnosis of MDD, other psychiatric disorders, substance abuse disorders, normal grieving, physical sources, medical conditions, and medications must be considered. Information regarding the psychiatric differential diagnosis for MDD can be found in Table 13-1. Information regarding the physical causes, medical conditions, and medications or drugs associated with MDD can be found in Box 13-8.

Treatment

Assessment, Phases, and Goals

Assessment

Treatment for MDD is based on a comprehensive psychiatric assessment. A comprehensive psychiatric assessment provides information for diagnosis, case formulation, and planning of appropriate interventions.

Psychiatric Interview and Mental Status Examination

A key component of the comprehensive psychiatric assessment is the psychiatric interview, which includes

BOX 13-6 Interventions for Threatened Suicide or Suicidal Behaviors

Talk openly about the patient's well-being and concerns for his or her safety.
Be willing to listen.
Be nonjudgmental.
Don't ask why.
Don't be sworn to secrecy.
Offer hope that there are alternatives to the situation.
Remove lethal items (guns, pills, ropes, alcohol, and other drugs).
Get help to prevent the suicide from the primary clinician, crisis services, hospital psychiatric emergency room, or police.

BOX 13-7 Myths About Suicide

Psychiatric advanced practice nurses should know the myths about suicide and include them in health teaching for family members. The following are common incorrect beliefs:

Myth: Asking about suicide will put the idea in the patient's head.

Reality: Not true. Asking people if they are thinking about suicide does not put the idea into their head.

Myth: With suicide, there are talkers and there are doers.

Reality: Not true. Most people who die by suicide have talked about their intent.

Myth: If someone really wants to commit suicide, then you cannot do anything about it.

Reality: Not true. Suicide is often an impulsive act in response to a crisis. Help the patient find a way of coping with the underlying problem.

Myth: The patient has signed a No Harm Contract, so s/he will not commit suicide.

Reality: No guarantee. The strength of contract is based on strength of alliance between patient and care provider.

Myth: Multiple self-injurious behaviors mean that the patient is trying to get attention and is not suicidal.

Reality: Not true. Multiple prior suicide attempts increase the likelihood of dying by suicide.

Sources: Barrero, 2008; Caruso, K. (n.d.).

TABLE 13-1 DIFFERENTIAL DIAGNOSIS OF MAJOR DEPRESSIVE DISORDER

Psychiatric Disorder	Differentiating Characteristics
Bipolar I or bipolar II disorder	Includes one or more manic, mixed, or hypomanic episodes. MDD is not diagnosed if a manic, mixed, or hypomanic episode has ever been present.
Mood disorder due to a general medical condition	Requires the presence of an etiological general medical condition.
Substance-induced mood disorder	Is due to the direct physiological effects of a substance. MDD is not diagnosed if the major depressive-like episodes are due to the direct physiological effects of a substance (including medication).
Dysthymic disorder	Includes patients who are usually ill for years with symptoms that are less severe than those of major depressive disorder. There is no psychosis and usually no suicidal ideation.
Schizophrenia	Occurs when mood is empty or there is more apathy. Greater impairment of functioning.
Dementia	Is characterized by a premorbid history of declining cognitive functioning.
Adjustment disorder with depressed mood	Is characterized by depressive symptoms that occur in response to a life stressor that occurred within the last 3 months.
Bereavement	Occurs in response to the loss of a loved one; is not characterized by functional impairment, suicidal ideation, psychotic symptoms, or psychomotor retardation.
Complicated grief	Occurs in response to the loss of a loved one. Characterized by 1 year or more of intense intrusive thoughts, distressing yearnings, excessive feelings of being alone or empty, avoiding tasks reminiscent of the deceased, sleep disturbances, and loss of interest in personal activities (Horowitz, Siegel, Holen, et al., 1997).
Nonpathological periods of sadness	Is characterized by short duration, few associated symptoms, and lack of significant functional impairment or distress.

Sources: Black & Andreasen, 2011; First, Frances, & Pincus, 2002; Joska & Stein, 2011; Morrison, 2007.

demographic information about the patient; chief complaint; history of the present illness; past history; family history; social history; and general medical history.

Mental status examination is also part of the comprehensive assessment. It includes an evaluation of the appearance and attitude of patient; level of motor activity; thought and speech; mood and affect; perception; orientation; memory; fund of general information; ability to do mathematical calculations and to read and write; visuospatial ability, such as ability to draw the face of a clock; attention; ability to do abstract thinking; and judgment and insight (Andreasen & Black, 2006). Based on the patient's chief complaint, the psychiatric advanced practice nurse begins to develop a provisional diagnosis and differential diagnoses. More detailed questioning about the chief complaint and other symptoms will be used to rule out the differential diagnoses. Depressive symptoms that would be queried in detail include the following:

- **Dysphoric mood:** Ask patients if they feel sad, discouraged, or anxious or are experiencing a feeling of tense irritability. Ask if they have times when they do not care about anything or cannot seem to enjoy anything.
- **Changes in appetite or weight:** Ask patients if they have gained or lost more weight than is usual for them.

BOX 13-8 Physical Sources, Medical Conditions, and Medications or Drugs Associated With Major Depressive Disorder

Physical Sources

- Food allergies
- Hypoglycemia
- Lack of exercise
- Nutritional deficiencies
- Poisoning with heavy metals (mercury, lead, aluminum, cadmium, and thallium)
- Premenstrual syndrome
- Selenium toxicity
- Sleep disturbances

Medical Conditions

- Brain tumors
- Cancer: pancreatic cancer and lung cancer
- Cardiac conditions, e.g., congestive heart failure, ischemic heart disease, myocardial infarction
- Chronic inflammation
- Chronic pain
- Diabetes
- Epilepsy
- Fibromyalgia
- Head injury
- Infections: AIDS, influenza, infectious mononucleosis, Lyme disease, syphilis (late stage), tuberculosis, viral hepatitis, viral pneumonia
- Liver disease
- Lung disease
- Multiple sclerosis
- Parkinson's disease
- Rheumatoid arthritis
- Stroke
- Thyroid diseases
- Systemic lupus erythematosus

Medications or Drugs

- Amphetamines (withdrawal from)
- Anabolic steroids
- Antihistamines
- Anti-inflammatory agents
- Antipsychotic drugs
- Benzodiazepines
- Beta-blockers
- Cimetidine (Tagamet)
- Corticosteroids (adrenal hormone agents)
- Cycloserine (an antibiotic)
- High blood pressure medications
- Indomethacin (Indocin)
- Marijuana
- Opioids
- Oral contraceptives
- Phencyclidine
- Ranitidine (Zantac)
- Reserpine (Serpasil)
- Thiazide diuretics
- Tranquilizers and sedative-hypnotics
- Vinblastine (anticancer drug)

Sources: Boland & Keller (2004 [adapted from Charney, Berman, & Miller, 1998]); Medical illness and depression. HealthyPlace.com. http://www.healthyplace.com/depression/main/medical_illness_and_depression/menu_id_68/ November 29, 2007; Joska & Stein, 2008.

- **Changes in sleep habits**: Ask if they have trouble getting to sleep, awaken in the middle of the night, or awaken in the early morning. Also ask if they have been sleeping more than usual and how much they sleep in a 24-hour period.
- **Psychomotor activity:** Patients may have the need to keep moving and may show hand-wringing, fidgeting, or pacing. Ask if they feel restless or agitated.
- **Psychomotor retardation**: Patients may experience difficulty moving or feel slowed down. Determine if their speech is slowed.
- **Loss of interest or pleasure**: Patients may have lost interest in usual activities or a decrease in sexual drive. Ask if they have noticed a change in desire to do things that they used to enjoy.
- **Loss of energy**: Patients may complain of having less energy or of becoming tired easily. Ask if they feel more tired than usual or have less energy than usual.
- **Feelings of worthlessness:** Patients may complain of feeling worthless and may have feelings of self-reproach or excessive guilt. Ask patients if they feel down on themselves. Ask if they feel guilty about something and, if so, ask what it is that they feel guilty about.
- **Diminished ability to think or concentrate:** Patients may complain of difficulty thinking or concentrating. Ask if they have had trouble making decisions.
- **Recurrent thoughts of death or suicide:** Patients may have thoughts about death or suicide or may have a wish to be dead. Ask if they have been thinking about death or taking their own life. If yes, ask specifically (1) how they plan to do it, (2) when they plan to do it, (3) where do they plan to do it, and (4) if they have the means to do it.
- **Quality of the mood:** Ask patients if their depressed mood is different from a depressed mood that they may have experienced before, such as after the death of a loved one. How is it different or similar?
- **Nonreactivity of mood:** Patients' depressed mood stays the same even after something good or pleasurable happens. Ask if the depressed mood gets better after they talk with a friend or do something enjoyable.
- **Diurnal variation:** Patients' moods shift during the day. Ask patients if they feel worse in the morning and then the mood gradually improves or if they feel the same all the time (Andreasen & Black, 2006).

As part of a comprehensive psychiatric assessment, rating scales and laboratory tests can help psychiatric advanced practice nurses in making the diagnosis of MDD.

Rating Scales

Psychological tests and rating scales are used to add information to the assessment and to provide a basis for treatment planning. Psychological tests are standardized methods of looking at behaviors in a reliable way (Clarkin, Howieson, & McClough, 2008). Psychological tests include the *Wechsler Adult Intelligence Scale* (Wechsler, 1955) and the *Minnesota Multiphasic Personality Inventory-2* (Hathaway & McKinley, 1989). Behavior rating scales are standardized instruments that allow observers to rate the behavior of patients in specific areas (Clarkin et al.). The following rating scales are frequently used in the assessment of patients who present with symptoms of MDD:

- *Brief Psychiatric Rating Scale* (Overall & Gorham, 1962). An 18-item scale administered by a clinician that measures the severity of general psychopathology, including mood symptoms, in patients with moderate to severe psychiatric disorders.
- *Hamilton Rating Scale for Depression (Ham-D)* (Hamilton, 1960, 1967). A 17-item scale administered by an interviewer that measures the severity of depressive symptoms in patients with MDD and can be used to monitor response to treatment.
- *Beck Depression Inventory (BDI)* (Beck, Ward, Mendelsohn, et al., 1961). A 21-item self-report scale that measures the severity of depression.
- *Hospital Anxiety and Depression Scale (HADS)* (Zigmond & Snaith, 1983). A 14-item self-report scale that has two subscales—one that measures anxiety and one that measures depression—and was designed to measure mood disorders in medically ill patients.
- *Edinburgh Postnatal Depression Scale (EPDS)* (Cox, Holden, & Sagaovsky, 1987). A 10-item self-report scale that measures severity of depression.
- *Geriatric Depression Scale (GDS-15)* (Yesavage & Brink, 1983). A 30-item self-report screening test used to measure depression in older adults.
- *Suicide Intent Scale* (Beck, Schuyler, & Herman, 1974). A 20-item scale administered by a clinician and designed for use with patients who survive a suicide attempt. It measures the intensity of a suicide attempter's desire to die at the time of the suicide attempt and can be used to assess the severity of the suicide attempt.
- *Suicide Probability Scale* (Cull & Gill, 1986). A 36-item scale with four subscales: hopelessness, suicidal ideation, negative self-esteem, and hostility.

Laboratory Tests

It is recommended that laboratory screening be part of the assessment of adult patients with new-onset mood symptoms such as depression or mania. Laboratory screening frequently includes the following:

- Complete blood count with differential and platelets
- Serum chemistries/vitamins including liver and renal function tests
- Thyroid-stimulating hormone test
- Rapid plasma reagin (a screening blood test for syphilis)
- Urinalysis
- Urine toxicology screen for drugs of abuse
- Serum alcohol level
- Urine pregnancy test
- HIV serology (Kim, Schulz, Wilde, et al., 2008)

These tests are used to determine if the patient is pregnant and if there are any medical disorders, nutritional deficits, infections, or substances causing the symptoms of depression.

Use of imaging procedures—such as computed tomography and magnetic resonance imaging—is usually limited to identifying medical causes of psychiatric disorders such as trauma, stroke, or brain tumors. There is little justification for their use in the routine screening of psychiatric patients (Agzarian, Chryssidis, Davies, et al., 2006).

Phases of Treatment

Treatment is considered to have three phases:

- Acute treatment, which usually lasts for 6 to 8 weeks
- Continuation treatment, which usually lasts for another 4 to 9 months
- Maintenance treatment, which may last 5 years for patients with recurrent depression (Chen, Hansen, Gaynes, 2010; Kupfer, 1993)

In the acute phase, the focus of treatment is remission, and treatment includes psychotherapy, pharmacotherapy, and psychosocial interventions. Approximately 33% of patients achieve remission within 6 to 10 weeks of treatment (Bresee et al., 2009).

In the continuation phase, the treatment is the same as in the acute phase. The focus is to protect the patient from relapse, hold the gains made in symptom reduction, and improve functioning and quality of life (Bresee et al., 2009). When pharmacotherapy is discontinued after the acute phase, the risk of relapse is at least 50% (Thase, 1999). Maintenance therapy is indicated when there is a lifetime history of three or more episodes of MDD, presence of double depression, history of two or more severe episodes of MDD within the past 5 years, comorbid substance or anxiety disorders, and age greater than 60 years at onset of MDD (Bresee et al., p. 1104).

In the maintenance phase, the focus of treatment is on preventing a recurrence or a new episode of MDD, and the treatment that helped the patient to achieve remission is continued (Martinez, Marangell, & Martinez, 2008), although some researchers have found that the benefit of the medication may decrease and the patient may need to have the pharmacotherapy altered (Zimmerman & Thongy, 2007).

Goals of Treatment

The immediate goal of treatment of an episode of major depression is to achieve full remission (Bresee et al., 2009). *Remission* is defined as a state of minimal to no symptoms and return to normal functioning with the patient no longer meeting the criteria for the disorder for 2 months (Keller, 2003, p. 3154; Stahl, 2000). Remission is associated with better long-term outcomes—for example, diminished use of health-care services and improvement of physical health, functioning at work, social relationships, and quality of life (Simon, Revicki, Heiligenstein, et al., 2000). A return to a fully symptomatic state during remission is defined as *relapse* (Keller, 2003).

After remission, the goal of treatment is to achieve recovery. *Recovery* is an extended period of remission that indicates the end of a current episode. Recovery is defined as the absence of symptoms or the presence of only one or minimal symptoms of major depression for more than 2 months (Keller, 2003, p. 3154). Stahl says that if remission lasts 6 to 12 months, it is considered to be recovery. Appearance of a new episode of major depression during recovery is defined as *recurrence* (Keller, 2003).

The goals of treatment for MDD can be summarized as follows:

- Reducing symptoms
- Reducing risk of suicide
- Improving functioning, physical health, and quality of life
- Preventing recurrence
- Promoting recovery
- Decreasing adverse effects on the family

Interventions used to achieve treatment goals include *somatic* interventions and *nonsomatic* interventions. Treatment for MDD with specified features (catatonic, melancholic, atypical, and postpartum onset), for MDD with seasonal pattern, and for specific populations (children and adolescents, older adults, and veterans) will be discussed later in the chapter.

Somatic Interventions

Somatic therapies include pharmacotherapy, ECT, vagus nerve stimulation (VNS), repetitive transcranial magnetic stimulation (rTMS), deep brain stimulation (DBS), psychosurgery, epidural cortical stimulation (EpCS), light therapy, exercise, acupuncture, and sleep deprivation.

Pharmacotherapy

The goal of pharmacotherapy for all patients with MDD is remission—not just a response to treatment—which usually means a 50% reduction of symptoms as measured on a standard rating scale (Bresee et al., 2009). Stahl (2000) has said that clinicians should use the optimal dose and duration of treatment in the pursuit of recovery. Stahl has asked, "Why settle for silver, when you can go for gold?" (Stahl, 1999, p. 213). When antidepressant medications are continued for several years, the recurrence rate of MDD is about 10%; however, without continuation of medication, the recurrence rate is about 80% over 5 years. Significantly, 5% to 20% of patients with recurrent major depressive episodes who discontinue their medications develop a bipolar disorder.

Antidepressant medications used for MDD include SSRIs, serotonin-norepinephrine reuptake inhibitors (SNRIs), tricyclic antidepressants (TCAs), tetracyclic antidepressants, monoamine oxidase inhibitors (MAOIs), and atypical antidepressants. Most antidepressants increase synaptic levels of norepinephrine, serotonin, or both and sometimes increase levels of dopamine by inhibiting the reuptake or the action of monoamine oxidase (Nierenberg, Ostacher, Delgado, et al., 2007). Other actions of antidepressant medications have been proposed. It is hypothesized that antidepressant and antimanic medications influence neurogenesis (especially in the hippocampal area), increase the branching of neurons, promote cell growth, and protect neurons from stress-induced death (Warner-Schmidt & Duman, 2006) (see Chapter 2 for more information on neurogenesis).

In contrast to the "top-down" effect of psychotherapy, the mechanism of action of psychotropic medications is a "bottom-up cascade" effect (Mayberg, 2006, p. 225). In other words, the medications' effect is on the brainstem, limbic structures, and subcortical areas with secondary changes in cortical areas, whereas psychotherapy brings about changes in cortical areas that result in secondary changes to the subcortical, limbic, and brainstem areas. Pharmacotherapy is indicated for MDD for conditions that are unlikely to improve without medication; in situations in which there is risk of dangerous consequences, such as loss of employment or suicide; or if there is risk of relapse or recurrence. Some researchers believe that for maximum therapeutic benefit, pharmacotherapy should be accompanied by supportive interventions, education, and cognitive therapy (Delgado & Zarkowski, 2004).

Predictors of a *good response* to antidepressant medications include depression with melancholic features, short duration of depression, family history of depression, and patient's past history of a positive response to an antidepressant medication (Dubovsky, 2005, p. 119). Predictors of a *poor response* to antidepressant medications include depression with psychotic features, bipolar depression, active substance abuse, comorbid medical illnesses, comorbid personality disorders, and MDD with atypical depression (Dubovsky, p. 119). The choice of antidepressant should take into consideration the patient's gender and age, medical status, prior treatment history, and symptom profile. The severity and subcategory of MDD should also be taken into account (Boland & Keller, 2006).

Pharmacotherapy and Major Depressive Disorder Severity: Mild, Severe, and Psychotic

In patients with *mild depression*, antidepressants may not be needed (First & Tasman, 2004). Psychotherapy—CBT, interpersonal therapy, and dynamic psychotherapy—has been found to be equivalent to the use of antidepressant medications; however, medications may be used for mild depression if preferred by the patient (Karasu et al., 2006). Because response to both psychotherapy and pharmacotherapy is good, combining medications and therapy is not recommended for mild depression because it does not increase response (Dubovsky, 2005).

Among patients with *severe depression*, approximately 80% will have suicidal ideation (Hawton, 1992; Thase, 2000), and at the more extreme end of severe depression, patients may have impaired ability for self-care (Karasu et al., 2006). The SSRIs are thought to be as effective as the TCAs in treating severe depression and may be better tolerated (Dubovsky, 2005). They are also considered to be safer. For example, Thase (2000) warns of the potential lethality of TCAs in patients with suicidal ideation. For treatment of severe depression, Dubovsky suggests the use of mirtazapine (Remeron) and venlafaxine (Effexor); venlafaxine may be effective because of its effect on the reuptake of both serotonin and norepinephrine (Thase, 2000) and its effectiveness in reducing symptoms, improving functioning, and reducing relapse (Thase, Entsuah, & Rudolph, 2001). Reboxetine (Vestra) may be considered for its effect as an SNRI (Nemeroff, 2007). ECT has been found to be effective for severe depression (Dubovsky; McDonald, Meeks, McCall, et al., 2009).

Psychotic depression is one of the most difficult forms of depression to treat (Rothschild, 2003). There tends to be a low response rate (25%) when antidepressants are used alone and a low response rate (40%) when antipsychotics are used alone. A good response rate (70%) is achieved when a combination of antidepressants and antipsychotics is used, such as an antipsychotic and venlafaxine or mirtazapine. In studies of the use of atypical antipsychotics for the treatment of MDD with psychotic features, olanzapine (Zyprexa) as monotherapy was not found to be more effective than placebo; however, olanzapine combined with the antidepressant fluoxetine (Prozac) was more effective than placebo (Rothschild). Patients with MDD with psychotic features also respond well to ECT, with a response rate of 86% (Potter et al., 2006), and to amoxapine (Asendin), which is an antidepressant derivative of the antipsychotic loxapine (Loxitane) that has dopamine antagonist activity (Rothschild). The American Psychiatric Association Practice Guidelines for the treatment for MDD with psychotic features recommends the use of either ECT or a combination of an antidepressant with an antipsychotic medication (Karasu et al., 2006). ECT may be the first choice in some situations, such as in a patient with life-threatening symptoms, a patient with a history of good response to ECT, or an older patient (Flint & Rifat, 1998).

When considering pharmacotherapy for a patient, psychiatric advanced practice nurses should consider not only the severity of the MDD (discussed above), but also the features of the subcategory of depression that is present. In addition, they should be knowledgeable of the effects of switching, augmentation, and combining medications.

Pharmacotherapy and Subcategories of Depression

Subcategories of depression include bereavement, MDD with atypical features, MDD with melancholic features, MDD with catatonic features, MDD with postpartum onset, and MDD with seasonal pattern.

Antidepressants are not usually used for *bereavement* or uncomplicated grief. Antidepressants may be used if symptoms do not improve with support; if there is a past history of depression in response to loss; if there have been multiple depressive recurrences; or if persistent vegetative signs of depression have developed (Dubovsky, 2005). Pharmacotherapy may be delayed if assessment suggests that the depression associated with bereavement is due to an adjustment disorder, a medical condition, or a side effect of a medication or is associated with substance abuse.

MDD with atypical features responds to MAOIs such as tranylcypromine (Parnate) and phenelzine (Nardil) (Nelson, 2009) and to bupropion (Wellbutrin) (Schatzberg, Cole, & DeBattista, 2003). SSRIs such as fluoxetine are also effective (Dubovsky, 2005; Fava, Uebelacker, Alpert, et al., 1997; McGrath, Stewart, Janal, et al., 2000). Sertraline (Zoloft) has not been found to be more effective than placebo (Henkel, Mergl, Allgaier, et al., 2010). Atypical depression is less responsive to TCAs (Schatzberg et al.). The efficacy of cognitive therapy (CT) is equal to that of MAOIs in treating depressive disorders with atypical features (Jarrett, Schaffer, McIntire, et al., 1999), and CBT has also been found to be effective (Henkel et al.).

The first line of pharmacotherapy for *MDD with melancholic features* includes venlafaxine or mirtazapine because of their dual action in preventing the reuptake of both serotonin and norepinephrine, or reboxetine for its action in preventing reuptake of norepinephrine (Schatzberg et al., 2003). SSRIs, TCAs, MAOIs, and ECT have been found to be effective for depression with melancholic features (Nelson 2009). The TCAs and SSRIs have equal efficacy, although the TCA clomipramine (Anafranil) is more effective than paroxetine (Paxil) or citalopram (Celexa) in severely depressed patients (Nelson).

For *MDD with catatonic features*, acute treatment may include the use of a benzodiazepine such as lorazepam (Ativan). Clonazepam (Klonopin) may be substituted for lorazepam for longer treatment (Dubovsky, 2005). ECT is considered to be very effective (Dubovsky; Karasu et al., 2006; McDonald et al., 2009; Nobler & Sackeim,

2006). Lithium or lithium in combination with antidepressants may be used, and if psychotic symptoms are present, atypical antipsychotics may be used (First & Tasman, 2004).

Pharmacotherapy for *MDD with postpartum onset* includes the use of lithium (Dubovsky, 2005) and the use of SSRIs—fluoxetine, sertraline, venlafaxine, fluvoxamine (Luvox), and paroxetine—that have been found to be effective in decreasing the symptoms of depression with postpartum onset (Kornstein & Sloan, 2006; Yonkers, Lin, Howell, et al., 2008). However, one treatment issue for MDD with postpartum onset is that mothers who are breastfeeding may be reluctant to take medications that they fear may harm their infants. ECT is effective in treating postpartum depression and is one of the most effective treatments for severe and treatment-resistant postpartum depression (Forray & Ostroff, 2007). ECT is discussed later in the chapter.

For *MDD with postpartum onset and psychotic features*, treatment includes hospitalization of the patient to reduce risk of suicide, infant neglect, or infanticide; pharmacotherapy that includes the use of mood stabilizers, antipsychotics, and benzodiazepines; and ECT that is also effective (Burt & Stein, 2008).

Treatment for *MDD with seasonal pattern (SAD)* includes light therapy, pharmacotherapy, and psychotherapy (Rosenthal & Rosenthal, 2006). Light therapy affects both serotonin and norepinephrine neurotransmission. SAD has been found to respond to medications that increase availability of serotonin—sertraline and fluoxetine—and availability of norepinephrine—such as reboxetine (Rosenthal & Rosenthal, 2006). Because the symptoms of SAD are similar to those of MDD with atypical features and because atypical features are common in the depressive phase of bipolar disorder, the potential for developing mania or hypomania with treatment (medication, light, or psychotherapy) must be considered (First & Tasman, 2004).

Management of Pharmacotherapy

Approximately two-thirds of patients with depressive disorders experience some improvement following treatment with the first antidepressant that is used—that is, they experience at least a 50% reduction of their symptoms; however, less than 50% of patients achieve remission (Blier, 2006). To achieve remission and thus reduce the risk of relapse, it may be necessary to (1) substitute or switch medications, (2) augment medications, or (3) combine medications. Switching or substituting involves trying a different medication from the same class or from a different class of antidepressants. Augmentation involves adding a second agent that is not a monotherapy antidepressant drug. In general usage, augmentation implies the use of two medications. Combination involves keeping the first drug and adding a second recognized antidepressant monotherapy drug.

Switching Medications

When patients do not benefit adequately from an antidepressant, clinicians often switch to another antidepressant (Nierenberg et al., 2007). When deciding whether to switch or augment a first trial of an antidepressant drug, the advantages and disadvantages must be considered. Switching maintains monotherapy, but it will take time for the second drug to reach therapeutic effectiveness; in addition, the patient does not have the benefit of the response of the first drug even though it may not have been as effective as anticipated. Switching to another SSRI may be useful, but for other classes of antidepressants, switching within the same class may be less beneficial. In switching in older adults, the first medication should be tapered off over 1 to 2 weeks (Flint, 1997). Switching from a TCA to an SSRI does not require a washout period, but the first medications should be tapered at the time of the initiation of the second one. Switching to an MAOI requires a washout time, and switching from an MAOI to an SSRI, a TCA, or an atypical antidepressant requires a washout time (Nierenberg et al.). (Readers should refer to a comprehensive psychopharmacology textbook for specific washout times for each class of antidepressant.)

Augmenting Medications

Augmentation preserves the gain made by the first antidepressant, which means that no time is lost tapering the patient off one medication before starting another. Also, augmentation may produce a faster improvement than switching and thus reduce the adverse effect of depression on the brain and reduce the risk for suicide (Sheline, Sanghavi, Mintum, et al., 1999). Another consideration in choosing an augmenting agent is its ability to target a symptom of the depression such as insomnia. The disadvantages of augmentation include the risk for more drug interactions, the risk for more or different side effects, and the risk of patient nonadherence, because adding more medications may make patients less likely to take the medications (Nelson, 2001).

Because SSRIs are the first line for the treatment of MDD, augmentation often involves adding a medication or medications to the first trial of SSRI monotherapy. Medications used for augmentation include bupropion, which facilitates dopaminergic and noradrenergic neurotransmission (Brody & Serby, 2006); buspirone (Buspar); desipramine (Norpramin); atomoxetine (Strattera); and mirtazapine. Atypical antipsychotic medications that increase synaptic availability of serotonin, norepinephrine, and dopamine may be used (Shelton, 2006). The atypical antipsychotics—olanzapine, risperidone (Risperdal), quetiapine (Seroquel), and aripiprazole (Abilify)—have been found to be effective in augmenting SSRIs. Venlafaxine, a dual reuptake inhibitor of serotonin and norepinephrine, may be used in augmentation. If venlafaxine is not effective, an SNRI such as reboxetine can be used.

The augmenting drug may be selected to target a specific symptom. For example, for patients who lack energy, bupropion may be used. For patients with severe melancholic symptoms, bupropion or venlafaxine may be used. For agitation that is close to psychotic behavior, olanzapine or risperidone may be used. For symptoms of anxiety, mirtazapine or buspirone may be used. For patients who may have bipolar disorder, lithium can be used (Nelson, 2001).

Combining Medications

Combination strategies involve adding another medication with established efficacy for treatment of depression to an antidepressant that the patient is already taking (Nierenberg et al., 2007). Nierenberg et al. cautioned, "Neither SSRI's, venlafaxine, duloxetine, nor clomipramine should ever be combined with MAOI's" (p. 399). For patients who do not wish to take another antidepressant, thyroid hormone may be considered because of its supposed effect on adrenergic neurotransmission. It should not be used for patients with hypertension, coronary artery disease, or arrhythmia (Brody & Serby, 2006). Blier (2006) recommended that combined treatment be continued for 6 months before tapering off one of the drugs.

Medication Strategy

Because 50% to 85% of persons experience a second episode of depression 4 to 6 months after the first episode, the trend in managing pharmacotherapy is to maintain treatment. To prevent relapse, medications may be continued for 2 years after remission of MDD symptoms. Lifelong medication may be used for patients who have had three or more episodes of MDD; who have double depression; who have had at least two severe episodes in 5 years; who have comorbid substance use or anxiety disorders; and whose onset of MDD occurs after 60 years of age (Bresee et al., 2009). A decision to discontinue maintenance therapy should be based on consideration of the risk of recurrence, that is, the number of prior episodes, the severity of episodes, the presence of dysthymic symptoms, and comorbid psychiatric and medical disorders (Karasu et al., 2006).

Based on a review of the evidence, certain antidepressant medications—clomipramine, duloxetine (Cymbalta), escitalopram (Lepraxo), milnacipran (Savella), mirtazapine, and venlafaxine—have been found to have superior efficacy over other antidepressants (Montgomery, Baldwin, Blier, et al., 2007). In the treatment of *severe depression*, escitalopram and venlafaxine were found to have superior efficacy, and milnacipran and clomipramine were found to have possible superiority over other antidepressants (Montgomery et al.).

Electroconvulsive Therapy (ECT)

ECT is considered to be an effective treatment for depression that has not responded to pharmacotherapy, for psychotic depression, for mania, and for severe suicidality (Karasu et al., 2004). It is indicated for older adults, patients who are pregnant, and patients with multiple health problems (Baghai & Moller, 2008). The benefits of ECT include rapid response, less loss of time from work, no medication side effects, and no drug interactions. Adverse effects may include headache, nausea, muscle pain, and confusion after the treatment; memory loss; and impaired ability to learn new information that may last for several months (Black & Andreasen, 2011; Nahas, Lorberbaum, Kozel, et al., 2004).

The mechanism of action of ECT in achieving benefits is not known; it is known that ECT does not damage the brain. There is no damage to glial cells or to neurons (McClintock & Husain, 2011). One hypothesis suggests that the beneficial effect is due to an increase of levels of brain-derived neurotropic factor and neuronal sprouting (creation of new dendrites; see Chapter 2) (Duman, 1999; Duman, Heninger, & Nestler, 1997). ECT is thought to increase the potential of neurons to make new connections, especially in the hippocampus (Nobler & Sackeim, 2006, p. 321). Other hypotheses suggest that ECT results in decreased excitatory input to the prefrontal cortex or that the therapeutic effect is due to release of endogenous neuropeptides and neurotransmitters that decrease the excitability of the brain (Nobler & Sackeim).

ECT can be administered with either right (nondominant) unilateral or bilateral placement of electrodes. It has been proposed that right unilateral placement would result in less memory loss (note that memory function is localized on the left side for right-handed individuals). However, for the right unilateral placement to approach the greater efficacy of bilateral placement, higher amounts of energy must be applied—rates at which the loss of memory increases (McCall, Reboussin, Weiner, et al., 2000). To target the mood-regulating circuit, frontal placements are used, and electrodes are placed on the forehead above each eye. Bifrontal ECT has the same advantage as bilateral placement, but it may have fewer adverse effects on cognitive memory because it spares the temporal lobes and hippocampus (Nahas et al., 2004).

ECT has the highest rate of response of any form of antidepressant treatment (Karasu et al., 2006). Remission rates are 50% to 60%, and remission occurs within 2 to 3 weeks of treatment (Nahas & Anderson, 2011). Nahas and Anderson wrote, "ECT remains the gold standard for acute treatment of TRD [treatment resistant depression]" (p. 215); however, patients do need maintenance treatment with antidepressants after a successful course of ECT. For example, among patients who had achieved remission following ECT but who did not receive antidepressant therapy, all had relapsed 6 months after completion of ECT. In comparison, among those who received nortriptyline (Pamelor, Aventyl), the relapse rate was 60%, and among those who received nortriptyline and lithium, the relapse rate was 39%. Patients with recurrent, relapsing, or medication-resistant depression may require maintenance ECT (Nobler and Sackeim, 2006). In a small study, maintenance ECT was found to be effective in sustaining clinical improvement and caused limited memory impairment, with 5.7% of patients having severe memory problems and 17% having slight memory impairment (Abraham, Milev, Delva, et al., 2006).

Vagus Nerve Stimulation (VNS)

The vagus nerve is one of the 12 cranial nerves, which are direct extensions of the brain (George, Sackeim, Rush, et al., 2000). The vagus nerve has *efferent* fibers that control and regulate autonomic functions, such as heart rate and gastric activity, and it has *afferent* fibers that carry information from the head, neck, thorax, and abdomen to the brain. The right branch of the vagus nerve is involved in cardiac function and gastric activity. The left branch of the vagus nerve is composed of 80% afferent fibers that send information (1) to the forebrain, hypothalamus, and thalamic regions that control the insula and the orbitofrontal and prefrontal cortexes, and (2) to the amygdala, which consists of structures that are implicated in emotion recognition and mood regulation (George et al.). Beekwider and Beems (2010) said that "electrical stimulation of this structure in the cervical region allows direct modulative access to subcortical brain areas, requiring only minimally invasive surgery with low risks involved" (p. 130).

VNS uses a permanently implanted device to treat patients with medication-resistant depression—that is, patients who have not responded to at least four trials of antidepressant therapy (Marangell, Martinez, Martinez, et al., 2005). Mathews and Eljamel (2003) said that the intervention is similar to an implanted cardiac pacemaker. In VNS, the stimulation is directed to the afferent connections of the left cervical vagus nerve. VNS is achieved by coiling an electrode around the left vagus nerve in the neck at the level of the fifth to sixth cervical vertebrae (Beekwilder & Beems, 2010). A subcutaneous line connects the stimulating electrode to a bipolar pulse generator implanted in the left chest wall. The neurostimulation appears to disrupt or modulate abnormal activity of limbic brain structures and to change levels of neurotransmitters (serotonin, norepinephrine, glutamate, and GABA) (Burns & Stuart, 2000) without producing any cardiac effects (Tamminga, Nemeroff, Blakely, et al., 2002). VNS has been found to have antidepressant effects (George, Nahas, Bohning, et al., 2006) and is effective for treatment-resistant depression (Howland, Shutt, Berman, 2011) and for treatment-refractory depression (Mathews & Eljamel, 2003). For example, a VNS study conducted by Rush, George, Sackeim, et al. (2000) found a 40% to 50% reduction in depressive symptoms. Others have found that VNS is not effective for treatment-refractory depression (Marangell et al., 2005). For example, patients who had failed seven trials of antidepressants during treatment for MDD did not respond to VNS (Rush, Gullion, Basco, et al., 1996). VNS is not effective for psychotic depression (Dumitriu, Collins, Alterman, et al., 2008), and unlike ECT, it is not an emergency intervention. Benefits may not be seen for a year (Sackeim, Brannan, Rush, et al., 2007). A 1-year follow-up found that the response rate was 55% and the remission rate was 27% (Corcoran, Thomas, Phillips, et al., 2006). Adverse effects of VNS include coughing, alterations of the voice, or hoarseness (Beekwilder & Beems, 2010; Dubovsky, 2005).

Repetitive Transcranial Magnetic Stimulation (rTMS)

rTMS, which the U.S. Food and Drug Administration approved in 2008 for the treatment of depression (Fitzsimons, Disner, & Bress, 2009), acts on the principle that the brain is an electrical organ that transmits electrical signals from one nerve cell to another (George, 2003). In rTMS, changing magnetic fields induce electrical current to flow within the superficial cortex of the brain (George & Belmaker, 2006). Burns & Stuart (2000) described rTMS as "a non-invasive procedure in which a changing magnetic field is introduced into the brain to influence the brain's activity" (p. 203). Burns & Stuart explained the mechanism of action as follows: "...when an electric current is passed through a coil, a magnetic field is generated. If another conductive material, such as a neuron in the brain, is exposed to a changing magnetic field, a secondary electric field is activated within that material. This activation may result in neurochemical changes based on alterations in gene expression. TMS directly stimulates the brain to produce neurochemical changes" (p. 204).

Changes in brain activity are achieved by conducting a large current through a figure 8–shaped coil that is placed on the patient's scalp (Fitzsimons et al., 2009). Earplugs are used to prevent tinnitus or hearing loss (Burns & Stuart, 2000). A magnetic field that passes through the skull induces an electrical field in the cerebral cortex. It is thought that the magnetic field causes a current in the neurons (Kramer, 2000). rTMS activates the cortical interneurons rather than motor neurons (Delgado & Zarkowski, 2004). rTMS may not be appropriate for patients with metal objects in their bodies, with cardiac conditions, with history of seizures, with increased intracranial pressure, or with pacemakers or other implants (Burns & Stuart, 2000).

rTMS has been found to be beneficial for treatment-resistant depression (Howland et al., 2011). The therapeutic effect takes about 2 weeks to occur (George, Lisanby, & Sackeim, 1999). Six months after treatment with rTMS and ECT, the relapse rates were equivalent, indicating similar effectiveness (Dannon, Dolberg, & Schreiber, 2002). rTMS is indicated for patients who cannot tolerate psychopharmacotherapy and as an alternative to a second or third medication trial (O'Reardon, Solvason, Janicak, et al., 2007). Unlike ECT, rTMS is not associated with memory loss. Side effects include pain at the treatment site and risk for seizures.

Deep Brain Stimulation (DBS)

DBS is approved by the FDA for treatment of Parkinson's disease and severe obsessive-compulsive disorder but it has not been approved for the treatment of depression. However, some researchers have found it to be effective for treatment-resistant depression, causing improvement of symptoms and functioning (Malone, 2010), and to have fewer adverse cognitive effects than ECT or ablative neurosurgical procedures (Moreines, McClintock, & Holtzheimer, 2011). The theory behind the use of DBS for depression is that high-frequency DBS causes inhibition of neuronal activity (George et al.). A small electrode is passed into the brain through a hole in the skull and is connected to a pacemaker implanted in the chest. The pacemaker sends high-frequency electrical pulses directly into subcortical areas of the brain (Nahas & Anderson, 2011). The mechanism of change is not known, but Mayberg, Lozano, Voon, et al. (2005) suggested that depression involves integrated pathways that link cortical, subcortical, and limbic systems and that DBS may restore functioning of the circuitry (brainstem, hypothalamus, nucleus accumbens, and orbital medial and prefrontal cortexes) that is involved in depression. The immediate response to DBS described by patients is a sense of calm and relief and the disappearance of negative feelings, rather than the appearance of a positive mood (Mayberg et al.). Reports of small noncontrolled studies suggest that DBS is effective, with 35% of patients achieving remission at 6-month follow-up (Lozano, Mayberg, Giacobbe, et al., 2008).

Psychosurgery

Surgery is used only for patients with severe resistance to conventional multimodal therapies. The four stereotactic approaches that are used are anterior capsulotomy, cingulotomy, subcaudate tractotomy, and limbic leukotomy (lobotomy) (Cosgrove & Rauch, 1995; Nahas et al., 2004). Improvement varies by approach, from 55% for anterior capsulotomy to 78% for limbic leukotomy (Cosgrove & Rauch).

Epidural Cortical Stimulation (EpCS)

EpCS is an experimental procedure that involves surgical placement of electrodes beneath the skull but above the meninges over the anterior and midlateral prefrontal area of the brain, which is involved in integrating emotional and cognitive experiences and modulating subcortical brain activity. The goal is to modulate the activity of prefrontal-limbic networks and thus reduce treatment-resistant depression (Nahas & Anderson, 2011). The procedure is less invasive than DBS, and according to Nahas, Anderson, Borckardt, et al. (2010), the results are promising.

Light Therapy

Artificial bright light therapy is as effective as antidepressants for SAD (Lam, Levitt, Levitan, et al., 2006) and for chronic depression that has a seasonal exacerbation pattern (Dubovsky, 2005). Patients with postpartum depression have also been found to benefit from light therapy (Epperson, Terman, Terman, et al., 2004).

The beneficial effect of light therapy is by way of the eyes, not the skin. Patients need to be taught that for the treatment to be effective their eyes must be open during the treatment, and that tanning salons—where the skin is exposed to light but the eyes are protected—are not effective in treating depression. Light therapy is based on the finding that exposure to a minimum intensity of 2,500 lux, which is the luminance required to suppress nocturnal melatonin secretion, was effective in treating SAD (Levy, Wehr, Goodwin, et al., 1980). Later, Terman, Terman, Schlager, et al. (1990) demonstrated that higher-intensity light at 10,000 lux was more effective than 2,500 lux.

Light therapy is more effective when given in the morning (Rosenthal & Oren, 2007). Light may be administered in divided doses (Rosenthal & Oren), and it may be administered by light visors, light boxes, and dawn simulators (devices that gradually increase the light in the bedroom in the morning) (Phelps, 2009). Response to light therapy usually starts 2 to 3 days after light exposure (Dubovsky, 2005). Side effects include headache, eyestrain, nausea, irritation, and agitation (Rosenthal & Rosenthal, 2006). Predictors of a favorable response to light therapy are a history of hypersomnia, a high rate of vegetative symptoms, increased intake of sweet foods in the afternoon, and a history of mood improvement when going south in the winter (Terman, Amira, Terman, et al., 1996). There are case studies of the development of hypomania (Phelps, 2009) and mania and suicidality (Rosenthal & Oren) during treatment with light therapy.

Exercise

There is evidence that higher levels of physical activity are associated with lower levels of depressive symptoms (Stephens, 1988) and that exercise, as a therapeutic intervention, has a positive effect on depression (Barbour, Edenfield, & Blumenthal, 2007; Stathopoulou, Powers, Berry, et al., 2006). There are several hypotheses of how exercise affects depressive symptoms. The effect may be through the positive feedback that people receive from others for engaging in exercise with resulting increases of self-esteem and self-worth, or its action may be due to distraction, mastery of new skills, or increased social contact (Lawlor & Hopker, 2001). The effect may be related to changes in cortical activity of the brain or to changes in serotonin synthesis. However the effect is brought about, it is thought that exercise acts on the same pathways that are the target of antidepressant medications (Ransford, 1982).

Although the evidence supporting exercise as a treatment for depression is considered to be insufficient by some researchers (Smith & Hay, 2005), others believe that there is sufficient evidence to support the role of exercise in the treatment of depression (Wang, Qi, Wang, et al., 2008).

For example, participation in a 30-minute exercise program three times a week for 16 weeks has been found to be as effective as CBT and as effective as antidepressant treatment or a combination of exercise and antidepressant treatment and provides longer-lasting benefits (Babyak, Blumenthal, Herman, et al., 2000; Blumenthal, Babyak, Moore, et al., 1999; Trivedi, Greer, Grannemann, et al., 2006). Also, the reduction in depressive symptoms produced by aerobic exercise done at home has been found to be comparable to that produced by supervised exercise programs and antidepressant medication (Blumenthal, Babyak, Doraiswamy, et al., 2007).

Acupuncture

Some researchers suggest that acupuncture is effective for the treatment of depression (Meng, Luo, & Halbreicht, 2002; Wang et al., 2008), but there have been few studies reported. It has been found to be effective for older patients with depression who were receiving antidepressant medication but who were treatment resistant or had comorbid medical conditions, anxiety disorders, or negative thinking (Williams & Graham, 2006). It was not found to be effective as a monotherapy for MDD (Allen, Schnyer, Chambers, et al., 2006). Smith and Hay (2005), in their review, concluded that there is not enough evidence to determine the efficacy of acupuncture for the treatment of depression.

Sleep Deprivation

Sleep deprivation, which consists of keeping the patient awake for 24 hours without any naps, improves depression the next day in approximately 60% of patients (Wirz-Justice & Van den Hoofdakker, 1999), but the depression returns with return to the normal sleep pattern (Dubovsky, 2005). Sleep deprivation therapy may involve either deprivation of sleep during half of the night or deprivation of rapid eye movement sleep (Buysse, Germain, Nofzinger, et al., 2006). It reduces rapid eye movement latency of sleep, which is a symptom of depression (Wu, Buchsbaum, Gillin, et al., 1999). Positron emission tomography scans of patients' brains show increased activity in the anterior cingulate area of the brain (the limbic area of the brain that is involved in modulation of emotion) of patients who respond to sleep deprivation. Sleep deprivation has been found to be more effective when administered in conjunction with antidepressant medications. However, sleep deprivation can induce mania or hypomania in patients with bipolar disorder and should be used in combination with a mood stabilizer medication for these patients (Buysse et al.).

Nonsomatic Interventions

Nonsomatic interventions include various types of psychotherapy and psychosocial interventions.

Psychotherapy

Psychotherapy is frequently used for patients with MDD who have a history of childhood adversities or who have experienced recent stressful events (aan het Rot et al., 2009). Psychotherapies most commonly used are what Friedman & Thase (2007) called "depression-focused psychotherapies" (p. 409). Depression-focused psychotherapies are effective interventions for mild to moderately severe depression. They are nontraditional in that they do not focus on unconscious or neurotic conflicts and do not operate on the premise that the therapeutic relationship is the means of resolving conflict. The most common of the depression-focused psychotherapies are CT, CBT, and interpersonal therapy (IPT). CT, CBT, and IPT share the following six characteristics:

1. They assess patients' current state and problems.
2. They provide education about depression.
3. They instill hope.
4. They help patients to work themselves out of the depression.
5. Their goal is to relieve the symptoms of depression.
6. They are of short term, usually lasting 2 to 4 months.

While CT, CBT, and IPT share these six characteristics, they differ in terms of approach.

- CT was developed in response to clinicians' observations that patients with depression often presented with a pattern of hopelessness, pessimism, self-criticism, and irrational thinking such as overgeneralization, catastrophic thinking, maximizing and minimizing, black-or-white thinking, jumping to conclusions without evidence, personalization of events, and a negative focus that ignores evidence (Friedman & Thase, 2006). CT rests on the foundational belief that cognition determines emotions and behavior (Beck, 1976), and it assumes that patients are able to learn new ways of perceiving themselves, the world, and their future (Evans, Foa, Gur, et al., 2005).
- CBT focuses on education, behavioral assignments, and cognitive retraining. Symptom reduction is achieved through identification and correction of cognitive distortions—such as negative views of self and one's world and pessimistic views of the future—and often through behavioral interventions meant to increase socialization, build confidence, reduce avoidance of necessary tasks, and increase activities that move patients toward their goals (Maerov, 2006).
- IPT is based on the premise that depression is a consequence of individuals' difficulty in adapting to their environment. Interpersonal problems associated with depression occur most often in relation to role transitions (marriage or divorce, beginning or ending jobs, and relocation); grief (death of a loved one); interpersonal deficits (social isolation); and interpersonal disputes (conflicts with significant others) (Evans et al., 2005; Markowitz, 2006). IPT helps patients to solve life problems, reduce stressors, and strengthen their interpersonal functioning (Markowitz). The efficacy of IPT for the treatment of MDD appears to be similar to that of CBT and pharmacotherapy.

Another model of psychotherapy used for MDD is brief psychodynamic therapy. Brief psychodynamic therapy, which usually consists of 12 weekly sessions, focuses on a specific problem, such as moving away or changing jobs. The therapist links the problem to patterns in past relationships and to present relationships with the goal of helping the patient to overcome the fear of how others will respond (Gabbard, 2005). Brief psychodynamic therapy has been found to be as effective as CBT (Evans et al., 2005).

Psychotherapies that have been found to be effective in managing postpartum depression include (1) CBT directed toward infant management problems soon after delivery, (2) supportive therapy for 8 weeks, and (3) dynamic psychotherapy (Chabrol, Teissedre, Saint-Jean, et al., 2002). Other researchers have found IPT to be effective for postpartum depression, with 43.8% of the mothers achieving remission after 12 weeks of IPT ("Post-partum Depression: Use Interpersonal Therapy," 2003). O'Hara, Stuart, Gorman, et al. (2000) found that 1-hour sessions of IPT for 12 weeks reduced postpartum depression symptoms and improved social adjustment. Programs based on the principles of IPT appear to be effective in reducing the development of postpartum depression in women who are at risk (Zlotnick, Miller, Pearlstein, et al., 2006). For example, the ROSE Program (Reach Out, Stand strong, Essentials for new mothers) is an intervention of four hour-long group sessions that help women at risk for developing postpartum depression to improve their interpersonal relationships, change their expectations about the relationships, build and use social support networks, and master their transition to motherhood (Zlotnick et al., 2006). The low-income women who received the ROSE Program in addition to routine antenatal care were less likely to develop depression within 3 months after delivery than the women who received only routine antenatal care.

In summary, CT, CBT, and IPT have been found to be as effective as medications in treating depression with the exception of severe depression (Bresee et al., 2009; Karasu et al., 2006). Chronic depression may respond better to a combination of medication and psychotherapy (Bresee, et al.; Evans et al., 2005). Markowitz (2006) suggested reserving combined psychotherapy and pharmacotherapy for patients with chronic, severe, or treatment-resistant MDD. He also noted that combined therapy produces further gains over time in functioning and in resolving interpersonal problems.

Psychosocial Interventions

Psychosocial interventions are interventions designed to decrease symptom severity or distress, avoid hospitalizations, and improve psychosocial functioning and quality of life (Addington, Piskulic, & Marshall, 2010; Beebe, 2007; Mueser, Bond, & Drake, 2001). They often help patients to change dysfunctional thinking and lifestyle practices, to increase social support and socializing activities, and to learn new coping skills. For example, a group exercise intervention for postpartum patients—pram walking twice a week with other mothers—was more effective in reducing postpartum symptoms of depression than social support groups (Daley, MacArthur, & Winter, 2007). Another psychosocial intervention that has been found to reduce postpartum depression is to reduce sleep deprivation by providing child care so that the mothers can sleep.

Psychosocial interventions that psychiatric advanced practice nurses can use for patients with MDD include modifying cognitive responses; changing lifestyle practices; promoting social support; developing adaptive coping skills, such as problem-solving; teaching assertive communication skills; providing education for patients and for families; and bibliotherapy (Berghuis, Jongsma, & Bruce, 2008; Lau, 2008; Saeed, Bloch, Antonacci, et al., 2009). These psychosocial interventions are described in Chapter 8. In addition, some psychiatric advanced practice nurses have used aromatherapy to reduce symptoms of grief, anxiety, and depression (Butje, Repede, & Shattel, 2008).

Case Study 13-1 describes a woman with depressed mood.

CASE STUDY 13-1

A Woman With Depressed Mood

Alula Tarif's daughter, Leila, had called the community mental health clinic to request an evaluation for her mother. She said that she and her older brother live with her mother and that—though her brother does not think that there is anything wrong with their mother—she has become very worried about her mother's increasing complaints of fatigue, lack of energy, and loss of interest in life. She had bought her mother some multipurpose vitamins, but when she did not seem to improve, she had taken her mother to the primary care physician, who recommended that she be evaluated at the community mental health clinic. When Leila called for an appointment, she said that it was very important that her mother be seen by a woman doctor. An appointment was arranged with a female psychiatric nurse practitioner.

Alula Tarif enters the examining room hesitantly, holding the arm of her daughter, Leila. She is dressed in a black long skirt and long-sleeved loosely fitting tunic top and is wearing a headscarf that covers her hair and forehead. She appears much older than her stated age of 43 years. Her face is lined and there are dark circles under her eyes. She does not make eye contact and appears very anxious. She responds to the nurse's greeting with a nod. Leila explains that her mother speaks Kurdish, and although she understands a little English, she

Continued

CASE STUDY 13-1—continued

does not speak much English. The nurse asks Mrs. Tarif if she would like to have her arrange for an outside interpreter. When Leila translates the question, Mrs. Tarif becomes very agitated and prepares to leave unless Leila can stay and interpret for her.

History reveals the patient was born in Samsun, Turkey. She is the oldest of five children. Her mother died when she was 10 years old. She was told that her mother had "weak blood." Her father remarried, but Alula was expected to care for her brothers and sisters and to do the household chores. She was married at 16 years of age to Rashid, a merchant, who was 15 years older than she. The first of her two children, her son Nasim, was born a year later, and Leila was born the following year. At the time they moved to the United States, Mrs. Tarif was 20 years old. They moved into a neighborhood where there were other Kurdish families. Mrs. Tarif stayed at home with the children. Her social activities were limited to grocery shopping, at which time she was accompanied by her husband and later by her son. Her husband died 4 years ago and she has continued to keep house for her son and daughter.

During the interview, when asked if she had any illnesses or surgeries or suffered any accidents, traumas, or abuse as a child, she looks down at her hands in her lap and shakes her head no to each question. Her children were born at home and she does not remember any problems. When the nurses asks about present illnesses, surgeries, accidents, traumas, substance use, and any verbal, physical, or sexual abuse, her daughter becomes uneasy in the translating process and says quickly, "No, none of that." The patient says that she had been in good health, although she tires easily and has to rest between tasks, until about 4 months ago, when she began to have periods of crying and trouble sleeping, She has no desire to eat and thinks that she may have lost weight. She has no energy to cook or clean the house and has no interest in shopping for groceries that she used to enjoy. She sits in the house with the shades drawn and rocks in her favorite chair. Questioning about recent changes or events reveals that about 6 months ago her son had informed her that he was making arrangements to marry and that he and his wife would live with her and Leila.

Questions

1. What differential diagnoses would you consider?
2. What would be your diagnosis?
3. What treatment would you recommend?

Answers to these questions can be found at the end of this chapter.

Issues in Management of Major Depressive Disorder

Potential issues in the management of MDD can occur with patients who have MDD and medical problems, who are pregnant or breastfeeding, or who have treatment-resistant depression.

Patients With Major Depressive Disorder and Medical Problems

In considering which antidepressant to prescribe for patients with medical problems, Dubovsky (2005, p. 129) provided recommendations for which medications are preferred and which should be avoided:

- Patients with cardiac conduction problems should be treated with bupropion, citalopram, fluoxetine, fluvoxamine, paroxetine, and sertraline. TCAs should be avoided.
- Patients with congestive heart failure should be treated with bupropion and the SSRIs. TCAs, trazodone (Desyrel), and nefazodone (Sersone) should be avoided.
- Patients with dementia, delirium, or cognitive disorder should be treated with bupropion, fluoxetine, fluvoxamine, nefazodone, paroxetine, sertraline, trazodone, and venlafaxine. Amitriptyline (Elavil), clomipramine, imipramine (Tofranil), protriptyline (Vivactil), and trimipramine (Surmontil) should be avoided.
- Patients with diabetes type II should be treated with fluoxetine. Amitriptyline and doxepin should be avoided.
- Patients with chronic constipation should be treated with fluoxetine, fluvoxamine, sertraline, trazodone, and venlafaxine. Amitriptyline, doxepin, protriptyline, and trimipramine should be avoided.
- Patients with irritable bowel syndrome should be treated with amitriptyline, desipramine, doxepin, nortriptyline, phenelzine, and trazodone. There is no available information on medications to be avoided (Adapted from Dubovsky, 2005, p. 129).

Patients With Major Depressive Disorder Who Are Pregnant or Breastfeeding

Approximately 14% to 20% of pregnant women meet the criteria for MDD or for dysthymic disorder (Marcus, Flynn, Blow, et al., 2003). The goal of treatment is the welfare of two patients: mother and fetus. Depressed pregnant women have been found to have higher rates of drug, alcohol, and tobacco use; suicidal behaviors; neglect of prenatal care; and inadequate nutrition (Zuckerman, Amaro, Bauchner, et al., 1989). These factors may have adverse effects on the fetus. Some researchers have reported that women whose depression is not treated during pregnancy have higher rates of poor obstetrical outcomes, such as preterm delivery and low birth weight or small-for-gestational-age babies (Chung, Lau, Yip, et al., 2001; Federenko & Wadwha, 2004; Steer, Scholl, Hediger, et al., 1992). However, others have not found evidence that supports those findings (Yonkers, Wisner, Stewart, et al., 2009).

For the fetus, the goal is to minimize exposure to the effects of the mother's illness and to the effects of treatment of the mother's illness (Newport, Fernandez, Juric, et al.,

2009). Untreated maternal depression has been found to be associated with adverse cognitive, behavioral, and emotional outcomes for the infant (Luoma, Tamminen, Kaukonen, et al., 2001). During pregnancy, mild depression can be treated with psychotherapy, such as CBT or IPT (Kornstein & Sloan, 2006). For severe depression, hospitalization or ECT may be used (Kornstein & Sloan). In deciding whether to use pharmacotherapy, the risks to the fetus caused by treatment must be weighed against the risks of untreated illness to the mother and fetus. According to Kornstein & Sloan, "...antidepressants have not been found to be associated with an increased rate of major congenital malformations, spontaneous pregnancy loss, or behavioral teratogenicity relative to the baseline rate in the general population" (p. 692). However, adverse effects of prenatal exposure to antidepressants have been reported, and Simon, Cunningham, and Davis (2002) have described a transient neonatal SSRI syndrome consisting of jitteriness, lower Apgar scores, or respiratory problems. Based on a review of multiple studies, Dubovsky (2005) concluded that infants exposed to TCAs do not differ from nonexposed infants in gestational age, weight, or head circumference and that infants exposed to SSRIs have lower gestational age, lower birth weight, lower Apgar scores (only with third-trimester exposure), and slower psychomotor development than children of depressed mothers who did not take any antidepressant medications. No psychotropic drugs have been approved by the FDA for use during pregnancy or lactation (Newport et al.).

For patients who wish to breastfeed, the risks of exposure of the infant to medications and the risk of untreated illness to mother and infant must be evaluated. All psychotropic medications are excreted in breast milk (Kornstein & Sloan, 2006). There are some case studies that report respiratory depression and urinary retention in infants whose mothers were taking TCAs while breastfeeding; among the infants of mothers who were taking SSRIs while breastfeeding, there were symptoms of colic, sleep myoclonus, sedation, and activation (Dubovsky, 2005). However, there is no evidence of serious adverse effects related to exposure to antidepressant medications through breastfeeding (Kornstein & Sloan), although, Newport et al. (2009) reported, "The long-term neurobehavioral effects of infant exposure to psychotropic medications through breast-feeding are unknown" (p. 1399).

Patients With Treatment-Resistant Depression

About 30% to 40% of individuals with MDD do not benefit from pharmacotherapy or psychotherapy (Greden, 2001). Among those nonresponsive to treatment, the depression may have a strong genetic influence, be atypical, or be MDD with psychotic features. Treatment resistance may also be due to patients' nonadherence to the treatment plan (Brown, 2003-2004), or the treatment may be inadequate. Young, Klap, Sherbourne, et al. (2001) found that only 25% of patients with depression receive appropriate psychopharmacological or psychosocial treatment.

The Sequenced Treatment Alternatives to Relieve Depression (STAR*D) study of the NIMH examined four levels of treatment for patients with treatment-resistant depression (Howland, 2008; Insel, 2006). In Level 1, all patients received citalopram. If they did not improve, Level 2 was recommended. In Level 2, patients could choose to switch from citalopram to a new medication—sertraline, bupropion sustained release, or venlafaxine extended release—or they could add on to the citalopram. The options for adding on to the citalopram included cognitive psychotherapy, bupropion sustained release, or buspirone. If they did not improve, they moved to Level 3, where they could switch to another medication—mirtazapine or nortriptyline—or they could add on to their existing medication either lithium or triiodothyronine (T3), the latter of which is a medication used to treat thyroid conditions. If there was no improvement at Level 3, patients were moved to Level 4, where they were taken off medications and switched to one of two treatments—an MAOI, tranylcypromine, or a combination of venlafaxine extended release and mirtazapine.

The results showed that in Level 1, 33% of the patients reached remission and 10% to 15% responded. It took 6 weeks to reach remission. Response was best among highly educated, currently employed white women with low rates of comorbid disorders. In Level 2, 25% of patients in the switch group became symptom free, and 33% in the add-on group became symptom free. In Level 3, 12% to 20% of patients in the switch group became symptom free, and about 20% in the add-on group became symptom free. In Level 4, 7% to 10% of participants became symptom free.

To summarize, about half of the participants became symptom free after two treatment levels. Over the course of all four treatment levels, almost 70% of those who did not drop out became symptom free. Key points for psychiatric advanced practice nurses are that one in four patients who have not improved with a trial of one SSRI will improve when switched to another medication. One in three will improve if a new medication is added to the existing SSRI. The odds of being symptom free diminish with every additional treatment strategy (Howland, 2008).

Course

MDD is considered to be a chronic illness with persistence of subsyndromal symptoms and recurrent episodes (Bresee et al., 2009). MDD usually begins by age 30, but it may begin in adolescence (Joska & Stein, 2008). Symptoms of MDD may develop over days or weeks, although prodromal symptoms—such as generalized anxiety, panic attacks, phobias, or depressive symptoms that do not meet the criteria for diagnosis of MDD—may develop suddenly after a severe stressful event, such as death of a loved one, marital separation, or childbirth (Karasu et al., 2006; Mayberg, 2004). While about 80% of patients recover from a single depressive episode, those who have only a partial remission are at increased risk of experiencing recurrent depressive episodes. After the first episode of MDD, 50% to 60% of patients are likely to have a second episode (Angst, 1992). Among these, 70% will have a third episode, and among these, 90% will have a fourth episode (Angst), with episodes increasing in severity as they recur (Maj, Veltro, Pirozzi, et al., 1992). Approximately 20% will go on to develop a chronic form of depression (Black & Andreasen, 2011). Recurrent MDD is associated with increased risk for developing bipolar disorder (Goodwin & Jamison, 1990; Smith, Harrison, Muir, et al., 2005).

Serious complications of MDD include impairment of marital, parental, social, and vocational functioning that affects children, family members, coworkers, and employers; adverse effects on recovery from medical disorders such as myocardial infarction (Karasu et al., 2006); and risk for suicide (Black & Andreasen, 2011). Poor outcomes are associated with the presence of comorbid personality disorders, substance abuse, medical illnesses, sustained unemployment, or marital discord (First & Tasman, 2004; Williams & Neighbors, 2006).

Depressive Disorders in Special Populations

Depressive disorders occur across the life span. The prevalence, clinical manifestation, and treatment of depressive disorders vary among different populations: children and adolescents, older adults, and veterans.

Children and Adolescents

Depression in children and adolescents occurs as MDD, dysthymic disorder, depressive disorder not otherwise specified, adjustment disorder with depressed mood, and bipolar disorder with most recent episode depressed (Emslie, Mayes, Kennard, et al., 2006). Emslie et al. said that many of the symptoms of depression in children are similar to those of adults: "depressed or irritable mood, anhedonia, sleep and appetite disturbance, feelings of worthlessness or guilt, psychomotor disturbance, decreased concentration, decreased energy, and suicidal ideation" (p. 574).

According to the *DSM-IV-TR*, to be diagnosed with MDD, a child or adolescent must have a persistent depressed or irritable mood that lasts for at least 2 weeks and other symptoms such as wishing to be dead; suicidal thoughts or attempts; increases or decreases of appetite, weight, or sleep; and diminished energy, concentration, or sense of self-worth (American Psychiatric Association, 2000). Depression in children is a recurring illness with repeated relapses: for instance, one-third of children relapse within 2 years of the first episode. Childhood recurrent depression is associated with an increased risk of developing bipolar disorder, with 20% to 30% of depressed children developing bipolar disorder in their late teens or early twenties (Birmaher, Brent, & The AACAP Workgroup, 2007).

Epidemiology/Prevalence

Depression occurs in about 2% of children ages 7 to 12 years and in 6% to 9% of adolescents (Voelker, 2003). The rate of depression is similar for boys and girls until adolescence, and then it occurs twice as frequently in girls (Angold, Costello, & Worthman, 1998). The lifetime prevalence of MDD in adolescents is thought to be 20% (Williams, O'Connor, Eder, et al., 2009). It has been found that the onset of depressive disorders is occurring at a younger age (Birmaher, Ryan, Williamson, et al., 1996); as stated previously, this phenomenon is called anticipation.

Etiology

Etiology includes genetic influence, childhood maltreatment, and bereavement.

- ***Genetic influence.*** Children who have a parent with MDD have a 50% chance of developing depression before the age of 20, suggesting a moderate genetic influence ("Depression in Children," 2002).
- ***Childhood maltreatment.*** Depression in very young children is often linked with abuse, neglect, and unsupportive living situations (Nemeroff, 2003). McGuinness (2010) believes that early traumatic experiences make the child more vulnerable to stress and to the development of depression and anxiety by sensitizing the neural circuits of the central nervous system that are involved in stress and emotions.
- ***Bereavement.*** Children whose parents have died from suicide, accidental death, or sudden natural death have been found to have higher rates of new-onset depression and post-traumatic stress disorder (PTSD) during the first 9 months after the death (Melhem, Walker, Moritz, et al., 2008). Factors that appeared to protect against the development of depression included good self-esteem, positive coping, family cohesion, and social support (Brent, Melhem, Donohoe, et al., 2009).

Clinical Presentation

Depression presents differently in children and adolescents.

Children

Until age 3 years, signs of depression include feeding problems, tantrums, and lack of playfulness. From ages 3 to 5 years, children may be accident prone, have many fears, blame themselves for things, and be apologetic for small mistakes. From ages 6 to 8 years, they may show vague physical symptoms, exhibit aggressive behavior, or cling to their parents. At ages 9 to 12 years, they may worry about schoolwork and blame themselves for disappointing their parents.

Symptoms of childhood depression include sadness, anhedonia, and lack of energy; irritability, anger, and hostility; poor school performance; low self-esteem; fear of death; feelings of worthlessness; and somatic complaints (Birmaher et al., 2007; Voelker, 2003). In comparison to children who are not depressed, children with depression have more school-related problems with behavior, attitude, and academic achievement; lower levels of social skills; and more problems with family and peers (Emslie et al., 2006). Children tend to have fewer melancholic symptoms, delusions, and suicide attempts than adults (Birmaher et al.). Because children may not be able to describe their symptoms or may be unaware of them, depression rating scales such as *The Children's Depression Inventory* (Kovacs, 1981) and *The Children's Depression Rating Scale* (Poznanski, Cook, & Carroll, 1979) can be used to measure symptoms in children.

Adolescents

Among adolescents, symptoms of depression include depressed mood, self-deprecation, anger, restlessness, grouchiness, aggression, sulkiness, reluctance to participate in family activities, and hypersensitivity to criticism (Sadock & Sadock, 2007). They may be uncommunicative and annoying to others ("Depression in Children," 2002). They may show poor academic achievement, drop out of school, have problems with relationships with others, and exhibit delinquent behavior such as running away from home, reckless driving, promiscuity, stealing, and substance abuse (Lynch, Glod, & Fitzgerald, 2001). For adolescents, the *Reynolds Adolescent Depression Scale* (Reynolds, 1987), a self-reporting instrument, can be used to measure symptoms and feelings.

Depression is expressed differently among ethnic groups. For example, white adolescents most often cite problems with feeling lonely; black adolescents describe not being liked by their friends anymore; and Hispanic adolescents describe inability to have fun anymore (Emslie, Weinberg, Rush, et al., 1990). Clinical depression during adolescence increases the risk for (1) developing other psychiatric disorders, (2) impairment of functioning, and (3) suicide in adulthood (Lewinsohn, Rohde, & Seeley, 1998).

Comorbidity

Psychiatric Disorders

MDD and dysthmia in children are frequently accompanied by other psychiatric disorders. The most frequently occurring are anxiety disorders, followed in frequency by disruptive behavior disorders and attention deficit-hyperactivity disorder. Anxiety disorders are nine times more frequent in depressed children than in those without depression; conduct disorder and oppositional defiant disorder are six times more frequent; and attention deficit-hyperactivity disorder is five times more frequent (Angold, Costello, & Erkanli, 1999; Angold, Costello, & Worthman, 1998). Children and adolescents with depression also have high rates of comorbid medical conditions, including diabetes mellitus, asthma, and epilepsy (Emslie et al., 2006). Substance abuse is comorbid in 25% to 48% of adolescents with MDD and tends to follow the onset of depression (Emslie et al.; Birmaher et al., 2007). Suicidal ideation and suicide attempts are comorbid conditions among depressed children and adolescents.

Suicide

Suicide is the third most common cause of death in adolescents (National Center for Health Statistics, 2001). The most common cause of death in the 15- to 24-year-old age group is an accident due to high-risk behaviors, and the second most common is homicide (Arias, Anderson, Kung, et al., 2003). During the time from 1979 to 2001, suicide rates doubled for 5- to 14-year-olds but decreased in the 15- to 24-year-old age group (Pfeffer, 2006). However, within the 15- to 24-year-old age group, the suicide rate has since declined for white adolescents and increased for black adolescents (Pfeffer).

Firearms are the most frequently used means of committing suicide by both children and adolescents and among both genders. More males in both age groups commit suicide, but the rate of nonfatal suicide behaviors is higher in females. Four percent of boys and 15% of girls between the ages of 13 and 17 have attempted suicide. Among gay and lesbian adolescents in the same age range, the rates are 28% for boys and 21% for girls.

Risk Factors

Exposure to multiple negative life events before adolescence increases the risk for adolescent suicide. For example, childhood abuse is associated with a four to seven times greater risk of adolescent suicide (Johnson, Cohen, Gould, et al., 2002). Separation of family members, communication problems between the child and the parent, parental problems with the law, and school suspension of the child increase the risk for suicide (Pfeffer, 2006).

Specific risk factors for suicide include the presence of a psychiatric disorder, prior history of suicide attempts, impulsivity, family psychopathology, and family history of suicide (Pfeffer, 2006). For example, suicide by a parent or sibling increases the risk for adolescent suicide five times (Brent, Bridge, Johnson, et al., 1996; Gould, Fisher, Parides, et al., 1996).

Among adolescents, substance abuse, living alone, male gender, and being over 16 years of age are also risk factors (Simon, 2008). Other risk factors include current stressors such as school problems, loss of a romantic relationship, unwanted pregnancy, or an event that causes humiliation (Bhatia & Bhatia, 2007).

Emslie et al. (2006, p. 575) have said that 40% to 80% of adolescent suicide attempters were clinically depressed at the time of the attempt. Among children and adolescents who committed suicide, 90% had psychiatric disturbances, such as MDD, bipolar disorder, substance abuse, or personality disorders (Shaffer, Gould, Fisher, et al., 1996). Among teens, 33% of those who committed suicide had made previous attempts (Pfeffer, 2006).

Predictors of suicide in adolescents include lack of future planning, putting affairs in order, making suicidal statements such as "I won't be a problem for you much longer," and suddenly becoming cheerful after a period of depression (Pfeffer, 2006). Other predictors of suicide include high levels of suicidal ideation, depression, parent-child conflict, and the use of alcohol or drugs (Brent, Emslie, Clarke, et al., 2009). For example, adolescents with a mood disorder were 12 times more likely to commit suicide than those without. The highest risk was among those with MDD or bipolar disorder and comorbid substance abuse disorder. Among those with personality disorders, those with borderline personality disorder, histrionic personality disorder, and narcissistic personality disorder were at four times greater risk for suicidal ideation and suicidal behaviors than those without these three personality disorders (Johnson, Cohen, Skodol, et al., 1999; Pfeffer, 2006).

Protective Factors

Factors protecting against youth suicide include good problem-solving skills; a close, warm, supportive family; religious beliefs; a positive outlook for the future; and ability to identify reasons to live. Protection is also provided by the absence of certain factors, including depression, substance use, history of physical or sexual abuse, family history of suicide, exposure to media coverage of suicide, and access to firearms or toxic substances (Bhatia & Bhatia, 2007).

Suicide Prevention

Prevention of youth suicide includes both individual and group approaches. Children and adolescents coming for treatment of psychiatric symptoms should be screened for suicide risk. Families can be taught to

- Love and support each child
- Establish predictability, availability, and security within the family
- Foster open and honest communication
- Discipline constructively (Pfeffer, 2006)

Screening approaches—such as a self-report written survey to identify suicide risk by inquiring about psychiatric illness, psychiatric symptoms, and adverse life events—have been used for groups of youths or for school populations. If risk is identified, follow-up is done with a computer psychiatric diagnostic interview, face-to-face interview, and referral for evaluation. Self-report screening, when used alone, tends to over-identify youths at risk. The ability of these screening approaches to predict which adolescents are likely to commit suicide has not been determined (Pfeffer, Jiang, Kakuma, et al., 2000), and classroom interventions to prevent suicide have had mixed results (Shaffer, Garland, Vieland, et al., 1991).

Interventions to reduce risk of suicide include

1. Identifying a social support system for the child or adolescent that can monitor suicidal risk and access crisis treatment
2. Providing treatment such as CBT, IPT, dialectical behavioral therapy, or pharmacotherapy for underlying mood disorders (Pfeffer, 2006)

In addition, access to ways to commit suicide should be eliminated. For example, parents should be urged to remove firearms. However, parents' willingness to follow the recommendation to relinquish firearms has been found to be limited (Brent, Baugher, Mirmaher, et al., 2000). If firearms are not removed entirely, the parents must agree to secure firearms in a safe place or to make them inaccessible.

Treatment of Major Depressive Disorder in Children and Adolescents

For children and adolescents with mild to moderate depression, treatment with CBT and IPT appears to be as effective as treatment with medications (Asarnow, Jaycox, & Tompson, 2001; Weller, Sheikh, Laracy, et al., 2007). However, psychotherapy alone may not be helpful for adolescents with severe depression (Weller et al.). About 40% of adolescents with depression do not respond to medication or to psychotherapy (Weller et al.).

Monotherapy With Antidepressant Medications

In considering which antidepressants to use with children and adolescents:

- TCAs have been found to be no more effective than placebo (Wagner, 2006).
- At this time, only fluoxetine has been approved for use for depression in pediatric populations (Emslie et al., 2006).
- European studies of the use of SSRIs for depression in children and adolescents showed that citalopram, paroxetine, and escitalopram were no more effective than placebo.
- Sertraline was more effective than placebo (Wagner, 2006).
- Bupropion has been found to be associated with a 50% reduction of depression score from baseline (Glod & Manchester, 2000).
- In a study of the use of venlafaxine for children with MDD, there was no change from baseline to 8-week endpoint (Emslie, Wagner, Kutcher, et al., 2004).
- Response to mirtazapine was no different than response to placebo (Wagner, 2006).

In summary, more than half (60%) of adolescents with depression respond to SSRIs or psychotherapy. For those who do not respond, interventions include switching to another SSRI or switching to an SNRI such as mirtazapine or venlafaxine (Emslie et al., 2006).

Combined Pharmacotherapy and Psychotherapy

From their study of 439 adolescents with MDD, March, Silva, Petrycki, et al. (2004) found that after 12 weeks of treatment, 71% responded to the combination of fluoxetine and CBT; 60.6% responded to fluoxetine-only treatment; 43.2% responded to CBT only; and 34.8% respond to a placebo intervention. March et al. concluded that the combination of medication and CBT was superior to medication alone or therapy alone. The combination of medication and psychotherapy has been found to be the most effective intervention for treatment of adolescents with MDD and suicidal ideation (Strickland, 2007). Combined treatment usually includes psychosocial interventions such as case management, working closely with school personnel, and support and education for the family (Wagner, 2006).

In prescribing for children and adolescents, as for other patients, it must be determined if the patient is taking other botanical or nutritional agents. In a 1998 survey, 56% of pediatric patients were using botanical and nutritional therapies in addition to prescribed psychotropic medication, but only 43% of the parents had informed the prescribing physician of this fact (Horrigan, Sikich, Courvoisie, et al., 1998).

Based on a combined analysis of short-term trials of antidepressant medications (SSRIs, bupropion, venlafaxine, nefazodone, and mirtazapine) in children and adolescents with MDD, obsessive-compulsive disorder, and other psychiatric disorders that showed that the suicidal thinking and behavior (not suicides) was 4% among the children taking the antidepressant medications in comparison to 2% for children receiving placebo, the Food and Drug Administration directed manufacturers to add a "black box" warning. The warning describes the increased risk of suicidal thoughts and behaviors and the need for close monitoring. Hammad, Laughren, and Racoosin (2006), in their report on suicidality in children and adolescents treated with antidepressant drugs, point out that the overall risk for increased suicidality with the use of SSRIs for depression was 1.66 and that the overall risk for all drugs across all indications was 1.95. They concluded that "use of antidepressant drugs in pediatric patients is associated with a modestly increased risk of suicidality" (p. 332). In their review, Williams et al. (2009) said that the increased absolute risk for developing suicidality (thoughts or behaviors, but not completed suicide) was 2% for patients receiving antidepressant therapy.

Course

Ninety percent of children and adolescents recover from the first episode of MDD with minimal treatment, but recurrence rates are between 40% and 72% (Birmaher, Arbelaez, & Brent, 2002; Emslie, Rush, Weinberg, et al., 1998). Recurrence is associated with more severe depression, feelings of hopelessness and low self-esteem, family dysfunction, stressful life events, and suicidality at baseline (Emslie et al., 2006). Among those with childhood depression, 60% to 70% have a high risk of developing depression as adults (Fergusson & Woodward, 2002), and 20% to 40% have a high risk for developing bipolar disorder (Birmaher et al., 2007; Geller, Zimerman, Williams, et al., 2001). The presence of subsyndromal depression during adolescence also increases the risk for MDD in adulthood (Georgiades, Lewinsohn, Monroe, et al., 2006).

To summarize, depression in children severely impairs functioning with resulting adverse effects on their academic achievement, peer relationships, family relationships, and health (children with depression use health-care services more often than nondepressed children and adolescents) (Emslie et al., 2006, p. 575). They experience lower levels of self-esteem and satisfaction with life and increased rates of suicide. The risk for suicide is higher in those with a history of suicide attempts, comorbid psychiatric disorders, substance abuse, impulsivity, aggression, maltreatment, and abuse and in those to whom firearms are available (Birmaher et al., 2007). Depression during adolescence is associated with increased risk of recurrent episodes, other forms of psychopathology, long-term psychosocial impairment, and high rates of unemployment and suicide in adulthood (Georgiades et al., 2006).

Older Adults

Depression among older adults is associated with emotional and physical suffering, disability, and diminished quality of life (Antai-Otong, 2006; Bresee et al., 2009). Older adults (those over 65 years) with depression may be at high risk for suicide if they experience a sense of hopelessness that reflects their fear of being a burden because they are no longer able to carry out their roles of partner, parent, and breadwinner (Joiner, Brown, Wingate, et al., 2005). Among older adults, developing depression is associated with having chronic health problems, having a family history of mood disorders, having impairment of functioning, and having experienced financial losses or loss of a loved one.

There are also factors that protect older adults from depression or modulate its course (Antai-Otong, 2006). Buffering factors include having basic needs met—needs for appropriate housing, food, personal safety, transportation, financial resources, health care, sense of identity, connectedness to others, and a role in life (Perese, 1997)—and the presence of social support and religious or spiritual beliefs.

Epidemiology/Prevalence

About 3% of older adults living in the community have MDD, but 15% have subsyndromal depressive symptoms, with the rate being higher among women. The presence of symptoms of depression is much higher among older adults in nursing homes or in institutions, with 10% to 15% having MDD and 20% to 30% having depressive symptoms, in comparison to a rate of depressive symptoms of 11% in those living at home ("Elderly in Nursing Homes More Likely to be Depressed Than Those Living at Home," 2008; Parmelee, Katz, & Lawton, 1989).

Etiology

Late-life depression is associated with a lower rate of family history of depression (less genetic influence) and a greater frequency of brain abnormalities, such as those seen with ischemic cerebrovascular disease (Roose & Devanand, 2006). It is also associated with significant losses, social isolation, chronic illnesses, and reductions of functioning (Antai-Otong, 2006). Medications found to be associated with depression in older adults include benzodiazepines, steroids, beta-blockers, cimetidine, clonidine, and antiparkinsonian agents (Antai-Otong, 2006, p. 150).

Clinical Presentation

Depression among older adults is characterized by

- Feelings of helplessness
- Pessimism about the future
- Ruminating about problems
- Being critical and envious of others
- Loss of self-esteem
- Guilt feelings
- Somatic complaints
- Constipation
- Social withdrawal
- Loss of motivation (Weeks, McGann, Michaels, et al., 2003)

Comorbidity

Among older adults, frequently occurring comorbidities include medical disorders such as coronary heart disease, stroke, and cancer; neurological disorders such as Parkinson's disease; and psychiatric disorders such as Alzheimer's disease (Krishnan, Delong, Kraemer, et al., 2002).

Suicidal ideation and suicide attempts are also comorbid conditions among older adults with depression. According to the statistics on suicide, in 2005, Americans 65 years old or older had the highest suicide rates of any age group (Caruso, n.d.), and research studies have shown that 75% of older adults who commit suicide have seen their primary care physician within the last month of their life (Strickland, 2006). Strickland wrote, "One of the leading causes of suicide among the elderly is depression" (p. 14). Other risk factors for suicide include physical illnesses, especially those that affect sleeping; losses, such as death of a spouse or other important source of support; social isolation; and physical or psychological abuse (Barrero, 2008; Juurlink, Herrmann, Szalai, et al., 2004). Psychiatric advanced practice nurses have the knowledge and clinical expertise to identify older adults with depression and to provide interventions that will reduce symptoms of depression and reduce risk for suicide.

Treatment

Assessment

Treating depression in older adults requires a biopsychosocial assessment that includes a comprehensive psychiatric and physical history; information about medications, including over-the-counter drugs and complementary therapies; and identification of social problems such as unmet needs, social isolation, lack of social support, neglect, and abuse. Laboratory tests include complete blood count with differential, chemistries, electrolytes, urinalysis, blood urea nitrogen, creatinine clearance, renal and liver panels, thyroid function test (T3, T4), vitamin B_{12}, thiamine and folate, syphilis screening, drug levels when indicated, electrocardiogram, and toxicology screen.

Butcher and McGonigal-Kenney (2005) suggested that the following clinical rating scales be used to assess depression in older adults:

- *Hamilton Rating Scale for Depression (Ham-D)* (Hamilton, 1967)
- *Beck Depression Inventory (BDI)* (Beck et al., 1961)
- *Geriatric Depression Scale (GDS-15)* (Sheikh & Yesavage, 1986)
- The nine-item depression subscale *(PHQ-9)* from the PRIME-MD *Patient Health Questionnaire* (Kroenke, Spitzer, & Williams, 2001).

Treatment Interventions

Untreated depression among older adults is linked to increased morbidity and mortality, use of medical services, placement in nursing homes, and caregiver burden (Bresee et al., 2009; Flint, 1997; Weeks et al., 2003). Treatment of depression in older adults has been influenced by three commonly held but *erroneous* clinical beliefs:

- Older adults do not respond to antidepressant medications at the same rate or as robustly as younger patients.
- Older adults take longer to respond to antidepressant medications, and therefore a 12-week trial of a medication is required instead of the 4-week or 6-week trial used for other adults.
- Older adults experience a higher rate of side effects and adverse events (Roose, Pollock, & Devanand, 2004).

A review of recent studies of older adults with depression who were treated with antidepressant medications has found that older adults do not take longer to respond to antidepressant medications. There is no evidence to support the practice of a 12-week trial of an antidepressant medication for all patients over the age of 60 years. It is now accepted that if the antidepressant has not been effective at 4 or 6 weeks, clinicians can change medications without waiting 12 weeks (Roose et al., 2004).

Treatment for MDD in older adults includes psychotherapy and pharmacotherapy. The goals of treatment are to relieve symptoms, improve functioning and quality of life, and reduce recurrences (Reynolds, Dew, Pollock, et al., 2006). Treatment for MDD in older adults includes psychotherapy and pharmacotherapy.

Psychotherapy

Psychotherapy—such as CBT, IPT, and psychodynamic therapy—has the advantage of no medication-related side effects or drug interactions; it also has the advantage of providing social support, reducing the effect of stressors, and increasing coping skills. Pinquart, Duberstein, and Lyness (2006) concluded that there is no difference in effectiveness between pharmacotherapy and psychotherapy for older adults, and in a comparision of different types of psychotherapy, CBT was associated with greater improvement than other types of psychotherapy.

Pharmacotherapy

Older adults have decreased muscle-to-fat ratio and decreased efficiency of the hepatic system, which may lead to increased plasma levels of antidepressants and longer half-lives (Boland & Keller, 2006). Therefore, a lower dose may be used initially.

The SSRIs are the most frequently used antidepressants among older adults because they cause less orthostatic hypotension, have fewer anticholinergic effects (such as confusion and urinary retention), and have less risk of arrhythmias than TCAs. However, the SSRIs are associated with increased risk for impairment of balance and falls (Dubovsky, 2005).

In general, the TCAs and MAOIs are not used for older adults because of their side effects. One TCA antidepressant, nortriptyline, has been found to be effective in the treatment of older adults. It has fewer orthostatic hypotension and anticholinergic effects than other TCAs (Roose & Devanand, 2006). Bupropion and venlafaxine are effective for older depressed patients with cognitive impairment.

Among older adults, who often are receiving medications for multiple health problems, the SSRIs—citalopram and sertraline—are well tolerated and seem to produce fewer drug interactions. The remission rates associated with specific SSRIs are as follows: paroxetine, 38%; citalopram, 36%; fluoxetine, 35%; and sertraline, 29%. Other antidepressants that are known to have fewer drug interactions are venlafaxine, with a remission rate of 42%; mirtazapine, with a remission rate of 38%; and reboxetine (no remission rate available) (Roose et al., 2004).

Reynolds et al. (2006) emphasized that patients over the age of 70 years tend to have co-occurring medical illnesses such as hypertension, coronary artery disease, diabetes, hyperlipidemia, osteoarthritis, and chronic lung disease that may affect recurrence of major depressive episodes; they also emphasized that maintenance treatment of depression must be linked with management of coexisting illnesses.

Among older adults, 30% *do not respond* to an initial adequate trial of antidepressant medication and may require alternative treatment or augmentation that includes adding different antidepressants, lithium, methylphenidate, buspirone, or valproate (Depakote, Depakene). Augmentation may increase response, but it has the potential for increased interaction of medications. Switching from one class of antidepressants to another may benefit the patient. In switching, the first drug should be tapered off over 2 weeks before introduction of the new drug (Flint, 1997). Augmentation with exercise has also been found to be effective in improving efficacy of medications (Mather, Rodgriguez, Guthrie, et al., 2002). An alternative treatment that is effective for older adults who do not respond to antidepressant medications is ECT.

Veterans

Hoge, Lesikar, Guevara, et al. (2002) reported on the presence of mental disorders among United States military personnel and associated utilization of health care. Surprisingly, although PTSD is widely studied among military personnel, Hoge et al. found that the rate of hospitalizations for MDD was twice as high as that for PTSD; they also found that the rate of ambulatory visits for depression was the same as that for PTSD.

More recently, it has been reported that an estimated 25% to 30% of veterans of the wars in Iraq and Afghanistan have reported symptoms of a mental disorder, with 9.3% of the veterans ages 21 to 39 having experienced at least one major depressive episode in the previous year. This percentage was higher among those aged 21 to 25 years (12.1%) and among those aged 26 to 29 years (13.4%), and it was lower among those aged 30 to 34 years (7.5%) and among those aged 35 to 39 years (8.3%) (National Survey on Drug Use and Health, 2008). Female veterans were twice as likely as males to have experienced a major depressive episode. Among the veterans who experienced major depressive episodes, more than half (51.7%) reported impairment of functioning in four life domains: home management, work, close relationships with others, and socializing (National Survey on Drug Use and Health).

Kaplan, Huguet, McFarland, et al. (2007) concluded that veterans in the general U.S. population are at an increased risk of suicide: they are twice as likely to die from suicide as nonveterans. They stressed the need for all care providers to be aware of this risk.

Key Points

- MDD is a chronic and recurring illness.
- Theories of etiology include evolutionary theory, genetic influences, kindling model, dysregulation of neurotransmitters model, and psychosocial theories.

- Patients with MDD have changes in brain structures, functioning, and neurochemistry.
- Subclinical hypothyroidism increases vulnerability to developing MDD.
- MDD is specified as MDD with catatonic features, with melancholic features, with atypical features, and with postpartum onset.
- Suicide risk should be determined initially and reassessed frequently.
- Severely depressed, suicidal, or psychotic patients may require hospitalization.
- Patients with severe MDD—with and without psychosis—have high rates of suicidal ideation; at the more extreme end of severe depression, patients may have impaired ability for self-care.
- Pharmacotherapy and psychotherapy are comparable in efficacy for mild to moderate MDD.
- ECT is a safe, effective treatment option for treatment-resistant depression, MDD with postpartum onset, and MDD with psychotic features.

Dysthymic Disorder

Dysthymic disorder is a chronic unipolar depressive disorder with depressive symptoms present most of the day, more days than not, for 2 years (Bresee et al., 2009; McFarland & Klein, 2005). It is characterized by (1) a relatively mild level of symptoms such as anorexia, insomnia, decreased energy, low self-esteem, problems with concentrating, and feelings of hopelessness (Black & Andreasen, 2011), (2) a chronic course, and (3) disability (Stewart et al., 2006). Specific criteria for the diagnosis of dysthymic disorder can be found in the *DSM-IV-TR* (American Psychiatric Association, 2000).

Epidemiology/Prevalence

The prevalence of dysthymic disorder in adults is 6% (Joska & Stein, 2011; Kessler, 1994). It is more common in women, with a lifetime prevalence of 4.1% for women and 2.2% for men (Stewart et al., 2006). Individuals with dysthymic disorder are likely to be unmarried, to be younger than 45 years of age, and to have lower incomes (Weissman, Leaf, Bruce, et al., 1988).

Etiology

Family studies suggest that genetic influence is similar for dysthymic disorder and MDD. Other researchers believe that dysthymic disorder is a form of MDD or that it lies on a continuum with MDD (Bresee et al., 2009; Klein, Shankman, Lewinsohn, et al., 2004).

Clinical Presentation

Clinical presentation of dysthymic disorder can vary among different populations.

Children and Adolescents

Symptoms of dysthymic disorder among children and adolescents include irritability, pessimism, depression, low self-esteem, poor social skills, impairment of school performance and social interactions, changes in appetite, sleep problems, fatigue, problems with making decisions, and feelings of hopelessness (American Psychiatric Association, 2000, p. 378). Whereas the criteria for dysthymia for adults require depressed mood for most of the day, for more days than not, for at least 2 years, the criteria for children and adolescents include irritable mood lasting for at least 1 year (American Psychiatric Association, 2000). It has been reported that more than two-thirds of children with dysthymic disorder develop MDD (Kovacs, Akiskal, Gatsonis, et al., 1994), and more recently it has been reported by Sarafolean (2009) that the majority of children with dysthymia develop MDD within 5 years.

Adults

Among adults with dysthymic disorder, symptoms do not reach the severity of MDD; although their functional impairment is similar to that of patients with MDD (Stewart et al., 2006). Symptoms include sadness, irritability, negative thinking, low self-esteem, lack of energy, and decreased capacity to experience pleasure (Stewart et al., 2006). The essential features of dysthymic disorder are gloom, brooding, lack of joy in life, and preoccupation with perceived inadequacy. Patients with dysthymia may be chronically complaining, demanding, morose, self-deprecating, and sarcastic (Andreasen & Black, 2006). They have fewer objective symptoms, such as loss of appetite, loss of sexual desire, or psychomotor retardation or agitation. They do have symptoms of inertia, lethargy, and anhedonia that are worse in the morning (Sadock & Sadock, 2007). A major depressive episode may occur after the onset of dysthymia, and that occurrence is called double depression (Black & Andreasen, 2011; Moore & Bona, 2001).

Older Adults

Dysthymic disorder occurs in 2% to 7% of the elderly population (Roose & Devanand, 2006). The onset is after age 50. Unlike in dysthymic disorder in young adults, there are fewer comorbid Axis I and Axis II disorders.

Dysthymic disorder in the elderly does not appear to be a continuation of early adult dysthymic disorder. Instead, it is more often associated with health problems and losses, such as the loss of a role in retirement, the death of family members, or lost contact with old friends (Roose & Devanand, 2006). Signs and symptoms of dysthymia in the elderly include loss of interest, lack of energy, a sense of hopelessness or worthlessness, more physical illnesses (especially cardiovascular illnesses), and loneliness (Roose & Devanand). The course is often chronic, with increased risk for cardiovascular and cerebrovascular morbidity and mortality and increased risk for suicide (Roose & Devanand).

Clinicians often take a "pseudoempathic approach," in which they consider the depression to be a normal reaction to aging or illnesses associated with aging. As a result of this approach, older adults with dysthymic disorder often do not receive treatment (Roose & Devanand, 2006, p. 609).

Comorbidity

Comorbid Axis I diagnoses occur among approximately 61% of patients, with dysthymia with MDD, anxiety disorders, and substance-related disorders being the most common (Stewart et al., 2006). Substance-related disorders occur in approximately one-third of patients with dysthymic disorder (Richards, Musser, & Gershon, 1999).

An Axis II diagnosis of one or more personality disorders co-occurs among 60% of patients with dysthymic disorder, with borderline personality disorder, histrionic personality disorder, and avoidant personality disorder the most common (Stewart et al., 2006). An Axis III diagnosis of medical illness is present among 58% of patients with dysthymia (Pepper, Klein, Anderson, et al., 1995).

Differential Diagnosis

Differential diagnoses for dysthymic disorder include MDD, depressive symptoms associated with chronic psychotic disorders, mood disorder due to a general medical condition, substance-induced mood disorder, cyclothymic disorder, and nonpathological periods of sadness. More information about these differential diagnoses can be found in Table 13-2.

Treatment

Pharmacotherapy and psychotherapy—such as IPT and CBT—have been found to be effective in the treatment of dysthymic disorder (Blazer, 2011; First & Tasman, 2004).

Pharmacotherapeutic findings are as follows:

- Sertraline has been found to be more effective than IPT for adults with dysthymic disorder (Markowitz, Kocsis, Bleiberg, et al., 2005).
- Sertraline has been found to be effective in treating dysthymic disorder among adolescents (Nixon, Milin, Simeon, et al., 2001).
- Sertraline has been found to be effective for double depression (dysthymia and coexisting major depression) (Ros, 2004).
- The TCA imipramine has been found to be as effective as sertraline in treating dysthymia (Keller, Gelenberg, Hirschfeld, et al., 1998).
- Mirtazapine has been found to have a good response in patients with dysthymia (Dunner, Hendrickson, Bea, et al., 1999).
- Bupropion sustained release has been found to have a good response in patients with dysthymia (Hellerstein, Batchelder, Kreditor, et al., 2001).

There is little information about treatment for older adults with dysthymic disorder, and treatments that are effective for young adults with dysthymia may not be effective for elderly patients (Devanand, Nobler, Cheng, et al., 2005). One study found that paroxetine was more effective than problem-solving therapy among older adults; however, Roose and Devanand (2006) suggested that medication may be only slightly more effective than placebo in older adults. At this time, no pharmacotherapeutic treatment for dysthymic disorder in older adults has been found to have proven efficacy. Psychotherapy has shown limited efficacy. Group therapy in conjunction with antidepressant medications may be helpful (Roose & Devanand).

Course

The onset of dysthymic disorder is most often in late childhood or early adolescence. The rate of spontaneous remission of dysthymic disorder is low, with many patients continuing to have depressive symptoms, hospitalizations, and suicide attempts (Stewart et al., 2006). Dysthymic disorder tends to be chronic; approximately 50% of patients recover (Klein, Schwartz, Rose, et al., 2000); however, 75%

TABLE 13-2 DIFFERENTIAL DIAGNOSIS OF DYSTHYMIC DISORDER

Other Disorder	Differentiating Characteristics
Major depressive disorder (MDD)	Must have one or more major depressive episodes. Both dysthymic disorder and MDD can be diagnosed if onset of the major depressive episode occurs after the first 2 years of the dysthymic disorder.
Depressive symptoms associated with chronic psychotic disorders	Depressive symptoms occur exclusively during the psychotic disturbance.
Mood disorder due to a general medical condition	General medical condition is the cause of the depression.
Substance-induced mood disorder	Symptoms are due to direct physiological effects of a substance, which may include medications.
Cyclothymic disorder	There are periods of *hypomania* and depressive periods. Hypomania does not interfere with work or social activities; no impairment of functioning.
Nonpathological periods of sadness	Characterized by short duration, few symptoms, and lack of functional impairment or distress

Sources: Black & Andreasen, 2011; First, Frances, & Pincus, 2002.

of patients with dysthymic disorder will experience double depression (Klein et al., 2006b, p. 872). Over time, 20% of cases of dysthymic disorder progress to MDD; 15% to bipolar II disorder; and less than 5% to bipolar I disorder (Sadock & Sadock, 2007). Despite the fact that dysthymic disorder is considered to be less severe than MDD, patients with dysthymic disorder have been found to have more suicide attempts and more hospitalization than patients with MDD (Stewart et al., 2006). There is often impaired functioning that is manifested in marital problems or divorce, alcohol or substance abuse, and vocational underachievement (First & Tasman, 2004).

Key Points

- Dysthymia is similar to MDD, but symptoms are less severe, duration is longer (2 years), and there is no psychosis.
- Impairment of functioning is the same as that found in patients with MDD.
- The essential features of dysthymic disorder are gloom, brooding, lack of joy in life, and preoccupation with perceived inadequacy.
- Patients with dysthymia are at increased risk of developing MDD.
- Pharmacotherapy and psychotherapy are effective treatment interventions for dysthymia.

Depressive Disorder Not Otherwise Specified (Depressive Disorder NOS)

The category "depressive disorder NOS" includes disorders with depressive features that do not meet the criteria for MDD, dysthymia, adjustment disorder with depressed mood, or adjustment disorder with mixed anxiety and depressed mood. Examples of depressive disorder NOS include premenstrual dysphoric disorder; minor depressive disorder; recurrent brief depressive disorder; postpsychotic depressive disorder of schizophrenia; a major depressive episode superimposed on a delusional disorder; and instances when it is clear that a depressive disorder is present but it cannot be determined if it is primary or secondary to either a medical condition or substance use (*Recommended Changes in "Depressive Disorder Not Otherwise Specified" [code 311]*, 2010). Although depressive disorder NOS is a residual category for depressive disorders, it has been reported that the number of patients with depressive symptoms that do not meet the *DSM-IV-TR* criteria for depressive disorders is about the same as those that do meet the criteria (Zinbarg, Barlow, Liebowitz, et al., 1994). Patients with depressive disorder NOS have high levels of distress and impairment of functioning (Phillips, Zhang, Shi, et al., 2009; Preisig, Merikangas, & Angst, 2001) and increased risk for suicide (Phillips et al.). To meet the needs of these patients and the clinicians providing care for them, it is being recommended that revision of the *DSM-IV-TR* include the following categories:

- Depressive conditions not elsewhere classified (Depressive CNEC) (symptoms do not meet criteria for any mood disorder)
- Depressive CNEC with insufficient information to make a specific diagnosis (uncertainty about primary or secondary cause or patient unwilling to provide information)
- Subsyndromal Depressive CNEC (atypical presentation or prodromal symptoms)

It is anticipated that more specific categories would lead to more accurate identification of patients with depressive disorders and would provide a basis for making treatment decisions.

Summary

In conclusion, development of depressive disorders is thought to be due to the interaction of genetic influences, compromised neurodevelopment, and experienced factors that influence how individuals respond to stressful life events (aan het Rot et al., 2009). There appears to be a link between childhood adverse experiences—e.g., loss of a mother before 10 years of age, separation from parents, family conflict, living with parents with psychiatric disorders, and childhood maltreatment and abuse—and later development of depression; this link can be understood as a "conveyor belt" of adversities (Williams and Neighbors, 2006, p. 149). For example, loss of the mother before the age of 10 years increases the risk for neglect and abuse, decreased self-esteem, and decreased ability to interact with others, to form social support networks, and to choose supportive life partners. These factors appear to interact with genetic vulnerability to increase the risk of an individual's developing depression (Charney, 2002).

Psychiatric advanced practice nurses must be aware that depression is "intertwined" with social stressors, symptoms of other psychiatric disorders, and chronic medical illnesses, and that treatment requires a biopsychosocial approach (Bentley & Katon, 2006, p. 603). Designing patient-centered care that will move patients toward recovery depends on knowledge of patients' risk for developing a depressive disorder, their resilience (Wagnild & Collins, 2009), the availability of protective factors, the pathophysiology of their depressive disorders, and an awareness of which treatments benefit which patients. In their study of strategies used by psychiatric advanced practice nurses to treat adults with depression, Parrish, Peden, and Staten (2008) found that nurses used

- Partnering with the client using active listening
- CBT
- Medications
- Psychosocial interventions such as self-help strategies, bibliotherapy, positive feedback, and referral to other providers

At the beginning of treatment, psychiatric advanced practice nurses scheduled appointments every 2 weeks to strengthen a therapeutic relationship and then, after the patient was stabilized, scheduled monthly visits. They used the patients' self-assessment of progress and patients' self-report of reduction of symptoms from the symptoms listed in the criteria for depression in the *DSM-IV-TR* (American Psychiatric Association, 2000) to measure response to treatment. They also used the *Zung Self-Rating Depression Scale* (Zung, 1965) and the *Hamilton Rating Scale for Depression* (Hamilton, 1960). Some used a numerical rating scale—the *Depression Symptom Severity Scale* (Parrish et al., 2008, p. 238)—that ranges from 1 to 10, with 1 equaling severe and 9 to 10 equaling no symptoms. The psychiatric advanced practice nurses found that using a symptoms-reduction checklist and the numerical rating scale provided a quick and easy way to evaluate patients' progress.

Based on their knowledge of the etiology and pathophysiology of depressive disorders, psychiatric advanced practice nurses can provide psychotherapy, pharmacotherapy, and psychosocial interventions and can make appropriate referrals for other treatment interventions, such as ECT and other forms of brain stimulation. In addition, psychiatric advanced practice nurses have competencies that enable them to plan and institute preventive interventions against the development of depressive disorders and suicide across the life span.

Resources

Organizations

American Psychological Association (APA)
www.apa.org
PsychINFO
http://www.apa.org/psychinfor
National Suicide Hotline
1-800-273-TALK (8255)
Suicide Prevention Resource Center
www.sprc.org

Toolkits

Toolkits for use with individuals and families after suicide attempts: http://www.nami.org/suicidebrochures

Instruments

Health and Psychosocial Instruments (HAPI) at *http://www.ovid.com*
Hamilton Rating Scale for Depression (9HRSD, HAM-D)
Zung Self-Rating Depression Scale (20 items)
Beck Scale for Suicide Ideation (BSS) and Beck Hopelessness Scale (BHS)

Movies

Bereavement

Turteltaub, J. (Director). (1995). *While you were sleeping* [Motion picture]. United States: Hollywood Pictures.

Armstrong, G. (Director). (1994). *Little women* [Motion picture]. United States: Columbia Pictures.

Major Depressive Disorder and Suicide Attempt

Brest, M. (Director). (1992). *Scent of a woman* [Motion picture]. United States: Universal Pictures.

Source: Wedding, Boyd, & Niemiec, 2010.

References

aan het Rot, M., Mathew, S. J., & Charney, D. S. (2009). Neurobiological mechanisms in major depressive disorder. *Canadian Medical Association Journal, 180*(3), 305-313.

Abraham, G., Milev, R., Delva, N., et al. (2006). Clinical outcome and memory function with maintenance electroconvulsive therapy: A retrospective study. *The Journal of ECT, 22*(1), 43-45.

Abramson, L. Y., Metalsky, G. L., & Alloy, L. B. (1989). Hopelessness depression: A theory-based subtype of depression. *Psychological Review, 96,* 358-372.

Addington, J., Piskulic, D., & Marshall, C. (2010). Psychosocial treatments for schizophrenia. *Current Directions in Psychological Science, 19,* 260-263.

Agzarian, M. J., Chryssidis, S., Davies, R. P., et al. (2006). Use of routine computed tomography brain scanning of psychiatry patients. *Australasian Radiology, 50*(1), 27-28.

Akiskal, H. S., Benazzi, F., Perugi, G., et al. (2005). Agitated "unipolar" depression re-conceptualized as a depressive mixed state: Implications for the antidepressant-suicide controversy. *Journal of Affective Disorders, 85*(3), 245-258.

Allen, J. J., Schnyer, R. N., Chambers, A. S., et al. (2006). Acupuncture for depression: A randomized controlled trial. *Journal of Clinical Psychiatry, 67*(11), 1665-1673.

American Psychiatric Association. (2000). *Diagnostic and statistical manual of mental disorders* (4th ed., text rev.). Washington, DC: American Psychiatric Publishing, Inc.

Andreasen, N. C., & Black, D. W. (2006). *Introductory textbook of psychiatry* (4th ed.). Washington, DC: American Psychiatric Publishing, Inc.

Angold, A., Costello, E. J., & Erkanli, A. (1999). Comorbidity. *Journal of Child Psychology and Psychiatry, 40,* 57-87.

Angold, A., Costello, E. J., & Worthman, C. M. (1998). Puberty and depression: The roles of age, pubertal status and pubertal timing. *Psychological Medicine, 28,* 51-61.

Angst, J. (1992). How recurrent and predictable is depressive illness. In S. Montgomery & F. Rovillan (Eds.), *Long-term treatment of depression* (pp. 1-13). New York: John Wiley & Sons, Ltd.

Angst, J., Gamma, A., Sellaro, R., et al. (2002). Toward validation of atypical depression in the community: Results of the Zurich Cohort Study. *Journal of Affective Disorders, 72,* 125-138.

Antai-Otong, D. (2006). Antidepressants in late-life depression: Prescribing principles. *Perspectives in Psychiatric Care, 42*(2), 149-153.

Arias, E., Anderson, R. N., Kung, H. C., et al. (2003). Deaths: Final data from 2001. *National Vital Statistics Report, 52*(3), 1-115.

Asarnow, J. R., Jaycox, L. H., & Tompson, M. C. (2001). Depression in youth: Psychosocial interventions. *Journal of Clinical Child Psychology, 30,* 33-47.

Babyak, M., Blumenthal, J. A., Herman, S., et al. (2000). Exercise treatment for major depression: Maintenance of therapeutic benefit at 10 months. *Psychosomatic Medicine, 62,* 633-638.

Baghai, T. C., & Moller, H. J. (2008). Electroconvulsive therapy and its different indications. *Dialogues in Clinical Neuroscience, 10*(1), 105-117.

Barbour, K. A., Edenfield, T. M., & Blumenthal, J. A. (2007). Exercise as a treatment for depression and other psychiatric disorders: A review. *Journal of Cardiopulmonary Rehabilitation and Prevention, 27,* 359-367.

Barrero, S. A. P. (2008). Preventing suicide: A resource for the family. *Annals of General Psychiatry, 7,* 1.

Battaglia, M., Bertella, S., Bajo, S., et al. (1998). Anticipation of age at onset in panic disorder. *American Journal of Psychiatry, 155*(5), 590-595.

Beck, A. T. (1976). *Cognitive therapy and the emotional disorders.* New York: International Universities Press.

Beck, A. T., Schuyler, D., & Herman I. (1974). Development of suicidal intent scales. In A. T. Beck, H. P. Resnik, D. J. Lettien, et al. (Eds.), *Prevention of suicide.* Philadelphia: Charles Press.

Beck, A. T., Ward, C. H., Mendelsohn, M., et al. (1961). An inventory for measuring depression. *Archives of General Psychiatry, 4,* 561-571.

Beck, C. T. (2001). Predictors of postpartum depression: An update. *Nursing Research, 50*(5), 275-285.

Beebe, L. H. (2007). Beyond the prescription pad. *Journal of Psychosocial Nursing, 45*(3), 35-43.

Beekwilder, J. P., & Beems, T. (2010). Overview of the clinical applications of vagus nerve stimulation. *Journal of Clinical Neurophysiology, 27*(2), 130-138.

Belmaker, R. H., & Agam, G. (2008). Major depressive disorder. *The New England Journal of Medicine, 358,* 55-68.

Belzung, C., Yalcin, I., Griebel, G., et al. (2006). Neuropeptides in psychiatric diseases: An overview with a particular focus on depression and anxiety disorders. *CNS & Neurological Disorders-Drug Targets, 5,* 135-145.

Bentley, S., & Katon, W. J. (2006). Depression in primary care. In D. J. Stein, D. J. Kupfer, & A. F. Schatzberg (Eds.), *The American psychiatric publishing textbook of mood disorders* (pp. 623-637). Washington, DC: American Psychiatric Publishing, Inc.

Berghuis, D. J., Jongsma, A. E., & Bruce, T. J. (2008). *The severe and persistent mental illness treatment planner.* Hoboken, NJ: John Wiley & Sons, Inc.

Bergink, V., & Koorengevel, K. M. (2010). Postpartum depression with psychotic features. *American Journal of Psychiatry, 167*(4), 476-477.

Berrettini, W. (2006). Genetics of bipolar and unipolar disorders. In D. J. Stein, D. J. Kupfer, & A. F. Schatzberg (Eds.), *The American psychiatric publishing textbook of mood disorders* (pp. 235-247). Washington, DC: American Psychiatric Publishing, Inc.

Bhatia, S. K., & Bhatia, S. C. (2007). Childhood and adolescent depression. *American Family Physician, 75,* 73-80, 83-84.

Bifulco, A., & Brown, G. W. (1998). Cognitive coping response to crises and onset of depression. *Social Psychiatry and Psychiatric Epidemiology, 31,* 163-172.

Bifulco, A., Figueiredo, B., Guedeney, N., et al.; TCS-PND Group. (2004). Maternal attachment style and depression associated with childbirth: Preliminary results from a European and US cross-cultural study. *British Journal of Psychiatry. Supplement. 46,* s31-s37.

Birmaher, B., Arbelaez, C., & Brent, D. (2002). Course and outcome of child and adolescent major depressive disorder. *Child and Adolescent Psychiatric Clinics of North America, 11*(3), 619-637, x.

Birmaher, B., Brent, D., & The AACAP Work Group. (2007). Practice parameters for the assessment and treatment of children and adolescents with depressive disorders. *Journal of the American Academy of Child & Adolescent Psychiatry, 46*(11), 1503-1526.

Birmaher, B., Ryan, N. D., & Williamson, D. E., et al. (1996). Childhood and adolescent depression: A review of the past 10 years, part 1. *Journal of the American Academy of Child and Adolescent Psychiatry, 35,* 1427-1439.

Bissette, G., & Myers, B. (1992). Somatostatin in Alzheimer's disease and depression. *Life Sciences, 51,* 1389-1410.

Bjork, J. M., Moeller, F. G., Kramer, G. L., et al. (2001). Plasma GABA levels correlate with aggressiveness in relatives of patients with unipolar depressive disorder. *Psychiatry Research, 101*(2), 131-136.

Black, D. W., & Andreasen, N. C. (2011). *Introductory textbook of psychiatry* (5th ed.). Washington, DC: American Psychiatric Publishing, Inc.

Blazer, D. G., Kessler, R. C., & McGonagle, K. A. (1994). The prevalence and distribution of major depression in a national community sample. *American Journal of Psychiatry, 151,* 979-986.

Blazer, D. G. (2011). Treatment of seniors. In R. E. Hales, S. C. Yudofsky, & G. O. Gabbard (Eds.). *Essentials of psychiatry* (3rd ed.) (pp. 643-660). Washington, DC: American Psychiatric Publishing, Inc.

Blier, P. (2006). Medication combination and augmentation strategies in the treatment of major depression. In D. J. Stein, D. J. Kupfer, & A. F. Schatzberg (Eds.), *The American psychiatric publishing textbook of mood disorders* (pp. 509-525). Washington, DC: American Psychiatric Publishing, Inc.

Blumenthal, J. A., Babyak, M.A., Doraiswamy, M., et al. (2007). Exercise and pharmacotherapy in the treatment of major depressive disorder. *Psychosomatic Medicine, 69,* 587-596.

Blumenthal, J. A., Babyak, M. A., Moore, K. A., et al. (1999). Effects of exercise training on older patients with major depression. *Archives of Internal Medicine, 159,* 2349-2356.

Boland, R. (2006). Depression in medical illness (secondary depression). In D. J. Stein, D. J. Kupfer, & A. F. Schatzberg (Eds.), *The American psychiatric publishing textbook of mood disorders* (pp. 639-652). Washington, DC: American Psychiatric Publishing, Inc.

Boland, R. J., & Keller, M. B. (2004). Treatment of depression. In A. F. Schatzberg & C. B. Nemeroff (Eds.), *The American psychiatric publishing textbook of psychopharmacology* (pp. 847-864). Washington, DC: American Psychiatric Publishing, Inc.

Boland, R. J., & Keller, M. B. (2006). Treatment of depression. In A. F. Schatzberg & C. B. Nemeroff (Eds.), *Essentials of clinical psychopharmacology* (pp. 465-478). Washington, DC: American Psychiatric Publishing, Inc.

Bremmer, J. D., Narayan, M., Anderson, E. R., et al. (2000). Hippocampal volume reduction in major depression. *American Journal of Psychiatry, 157,* 115-118.

Brennan, P. A., Hammen, C., Andersen, M. J., et al. (2000). Chronicity, severity and timing of maternal depressive symptoms: Relationships with child outcomes at age 5. *Developmental Psychology, 36*(6), 759-766.

Brent, D. A., Baugher, M., Mirmaher, B., et al. (2000). Compliance with recommendations to remove firearms in families participating in a clinical trial for adolescent depression. *Journal of the Academy of Child and Adolescent Psychiatry, 39,* 1220-1226.

Brent, D. A., Bridge, J., Johnson, B. A., et al. (1996). Suicidal behavior runs in families: A controlled family study of adolescent suicide victims. *Archives of General Psychiatry, 53*(1), 1145-1152.

Brent, D. A., Emslie, G. J., Clarke, G. N., et al. (2009). Predictors of spontaneous and systematically assessed suicidal adverse events in the treatment of SSRI resistant depression in adolescents (TORDIA) study. *American Journal of Psychiatry, 166,* 418-426.

Brent, D. A., Melhem, N., Donohoe, M. B., et al. (2009). The incidence and course of depression in bereaved youth 21 months after the loss of a parent to suicide, accident, or sudden natural death. *American Journal of Psychiatry, 166,* 786-794.

Bresee, C., Gotto, J., & Rapaport, M. H. (2009). Treatment of depression. In A. F. Schatzberg & C. B. Nemeroff (Eds.), *The American psychiatric publishing textbook of psychopharmacology* (4th ed.) (pp. 1081-1111). Washington, DC: American Psychiatric Publishing, Inc.

Brockington, I. F. (1996). *Puerperal psychosis: Motherhood and mental health* (p. 200). New York: Oxford University Press.

Brody, D., & Serby, M. (2006). When antidepressants fail the patients. *The Clinical Advisor,* September, pp. 53-64.

Brown, A. B. (1993). Life events and affective disorder: Replications and limitations. *Journal of Psychosomatic Medicine, 55, 248-259.*

Brown, A. B. (Winter 2003-2004). New strategies for treatment-resistant depression. *NARSAD Research Newsletter, 15*(4), 37-40.

Brown, G. W. (2002). Social roles, context and evolution in the origins of depression. *Journal of Health and Social Behavior, 43,* 255-276.

Burns, C. M., & Stuart, G. W. (2000). New somatic treatment in psychiatric care: Transcranial magnetic stimulation and vagal nerve stimulation. *Journal of the American Psychiatric Nurses Association, 6*(6), 203-206.

Burt, V. K., & Stein, K. (2008). Treatment of women. In R. E. Hales, S. C. Yudofsky, & G. O. Gabbard (Eds.), *The American psychiatric publishing textbook of psychiatry* (5th ed.) (pp. 1489-1525). Washington, DC: American Psychiatric Publishing, Inc.

Butcher, H. K., & McGonigal-Kenney, M. (2005). Depression and dispiritedness in later life: A 'gray drizzle of horror' isn't inevitable. *American Journal of Nursing, 105*(12), 5261.

Butje, A., Repede, E., & Shattel, M. M. (2008). Healing scents: An overview of clinical aromatherapy for emotional distress. *Journal of Psychosocial Nursing, 46*(10), 47-52.

Buysse, D. J., Germain, A., Nofzinger, E. A., et al. (2006). Mood disorders and sleep. In D. J. Stein, D. J. Kupfer, & A. F. Schatzberg (Eds.), *The American psychiatric publishing textbook of mood disorders* (pp. 717-737). Washington, DC: American Psychiatric Publishing, Inc.

Cahill, L., McGaugh, J. L., & Weinberger, N. M., et al. (2001). The neurobiology of learning and memory: Some reminders to remember. *Trends in Neurosciences, 24*(10), 578-581.

Carroll, B. J., Cassidy, F., Naftolowitz, D., et al. (2007). Pathophysiology of hypercortisolism in depression. *Acta Psychiatrica Scandinavica* (Suppl 433), 90-103.

Caruso, K. (n.d.). *Elderly suicide*. Retrieved from http://www.suicide.org

Caruso, K. (n.d.). *Suicide myths*. Retrieved from http://www.suicide.org

Carvajal, C., Dumont, Y., & Quirion, R. (2006). Neuropeptide y: Role in emotion and alcohol dependence. *CNS and Neurological Disorders Drug Targets, 5*(2), 181-195.

Cavanagh, J. T., Carson, A. J., Sharpe, M., et al. (2003). Psychological autopsy studies of suicide: A systematic review. *Psychological Medicine, 33*, 395-405.

Chabrol, H., Teissedre, F., Saint-Jean, M., et al. (2002). Prevention and treatment of post-partum depression: A controlled randomized study on women at risk. *Psychological Medicine, 32*(6), 1039-1047.

Charney, D. (2002). Depression and anxiety disorders. *NARSAD Research Newsletter, 14*(1), 42-44.

Charney, D., Berman, R. M., & Miller, H. L. (1998). Treatment of depression. In A. G. Schatzberg & C. B. Nemeroff (Eds.), *The American psychiatric publishing textbook of psychopharmacology* (2nd ed.). Washington, DC: American Psychiatric Publishing, Inc.

Charney, D. S., Manji, H. K., & Husseini, K. (2004). Life stress, genes, and depression: Multiple pathways lead to increased risk and new opportunities for intervention. *Science's STKE: Signal Transduction Knowledge Environment, 2004*(225), re 5.

Chen, S-Y., Hansen, R. A., Gaynes, B. N., et al. (2010). Guideline-concordant antidepressant use among patients with major depressive disorder. *General Hospital Psychiatry, 32*, 36-37.

Chueire, V. B., Silva, E. T., Perotta, E., et al. (2003). High serum TSH levels are associated with depression in the elderly. *Archives of Gerontology and Geriatrics, 36*(3), 281-288.

Chung, T. K., Lau, T. K., Yip, A. S., et al. (2001). Antepartum depressive symptomatology is associated with adverse obstetric and neonatal outcomes. *Psychosomatic Medicine, 63*(5), 830-834.

Chwastiak, L., Ehde, D. M., Gibbons, L. E., et al. (2002). Depressive symptoms and severity of illness in multiple sclerosis: Epidemiologic study of a large community sample. *American Journal of Psychiatry, 159*, 1862-1868.

Clarkin, J. F., Howieson, D. B., & McClough, H. J. (2008). The role of psychiatric measures in assessment and treatment. In R. E. Hales, S. C. Yudofsky, & G. O. Gabbard (Eds.), *The American psychiatric publishing textbook of psychiatry* (5th ed.) (pp. 73-110). Washington, DC: American Psychiatric Publishing, Inc.

Copolov, D. L., Rubin, R. T., Stuart, G. W., et al. (1989). Specificity of the salivary cortisol dexamethasone suppression test across psychiatric diagnoses. *Biological Psychiatry, 25*, 879-874.

Corcoran, D. D., Thomas, P. O., Phillips, J., et al. (2006). Vagus nerve stimulation in chronic treatment-resistant depression: Preliminary findings of an open-label study. *British Journal of Psychiatry, 189*, 282-283.

Cosgrove, G. R., & Rauch, S. L. (1995). Psychosurgery. *Neurosurgery Clinics of North America, 6*, 167-176.

Costello, E. J., Pine, D. S., Hammen, C., et al. (2002). Development and natural history of mood disorders. *Biological Psychiatry, 52*(6), 529-542.

Cox, J. L., Holden, J. M., & Sagovsky, R. (1987). Detection of postnatal depression: Development of the 10 item Edinburgh Postnatal Depression Scale. *British Journal of Psychiatry, 150*, 782-786.

Cull, J. L. G., & Gill, W. S. (1986). *Suicide probability scale (SPS) manual*. Los Angeles: Western Psychological Services.

Cullen-Drill, M., Smith, M., & Morris, M. (2008). Postpartum bipolar depression: A case study. *Perspectives in Psychiatric Care, 44*(4), 267-274.

Cyranowski, J. M., Frank, E., Young, E., et al. (2000). Adolescent onset of the gender difference in lifetime rates of major depression: A theoretical model. *Archives of General Psychiatry, 57*, 21-27.

Daley, A. J., MacArthur, C., & Winter, H. (2007). The role of exercise in treating postpartum depression: A review of the literature. Retrieved from http://www.medscape.com/viewarticle/551030_print

Dannon, P., Dolberg, O., & Schreiber, S. (2002). Three and six month outcome following courses of either ECT or rTMS in a population of severely depressed individuals. *Biological Psychiatry, 51*, 687-690.

Davidson, R. J., Lewis, D. A., Allory, L. B., et al. (2002). Neural and behavioral substrates of mood and mood regulation. *Biological Psychiatry, 15*, 478-502.

Delgado, P. L., & Moreno, F. A. (2006). Neurochemistry of mood disorders. In D. J. Stein, D. J. Kupfer, & A. F. Schatzberg (Eds.), *The American psychiatric publishing textbook of mood disorders* (pp. 101-116). Washington, DC: American Psychiatric Publishing, Inc.

Delgado, P. L., & Zarkowski, P. (2004). Treatment of mood disorders. In J. Panksepp (Ed.), *Textbook of biological psychiatry* (pp. 231-266). Hoboken, NJ: Wiley-Liss, Inc.

Demet, M. M., Ozmen, B., Deveci, A., et al. (2002). Depression and anxiety in hyperthyroidism. *Archives of Medical Research, 33*(6), 552-556.

Depression in Children-Part I. (2002). *The Harvard Mental Health Letter, 18*(8), 1-3.

Dervic, K., Gruenbaum, M. F., Burke, A. K., et al. (2006). Protective factors against suicidal behavior in depressed adults reporting childhood abuse. *The Journal of Nervous and Mental Disease, 194*(12), 971-974.

Devanand, D. P., Nobler, M., Cheng, J., et al. (2005). Randomized double-blind, placebo-controlled trial of fluoxetine treatment for elderly patients with dysthymic disorder. *American Journal of Geriatric Psychiatry, 13*(1), 59-68.

Dew, M. A., Reynolds, C. F., Houck, P. R., et al. (1997). Temporal profiles of the course of depression during treatment: Predictors of pathways toward recovery in the elderly. *Archives of General Psychiatry, 54*, 1016-1023.

DiMatteo, M. R., Lepper, H. S., & Croghan, T. W. (2000). Depression is a risk factor for noncompliance with medical treatment: Meta-analysis of the effects of anxiety and depression on patient adherence. *Archives of Internal Medicine, 160*(14), 2101-2107.

Doucet, S., Dennis, D-L, Letourneau, N., et al. (2009). Differentiation and clinical implications of postpartum depression and postpartum psychosis. *Journal of Obstetric, Gynecologic, and Neonatal Nursing, 38*, 269-279.

Drevets, W. C., Price, J. L., Simpson, J. R., et al. (1997). Subgenual prefrontal cortex abnormalities in mood disorders. *Nature, 386*, 824-827.

Driscoll, J. (2006). Postpartum depression: The state of the science. *The Journal of Perinatal and Neonatal Nursing, 20*(1), 40-42.

Dubovsky, S. (2005). *Clinical guide to psychotropic medications*. New York: W. W. Norton & Company.

Duman, R. S. (1999). The neurochemistry of mood disorders: Preclinical studies. In D. S. Charney, E. J. Nestler, & B. S. Bunney (Eds.), *The neurobiology of mental illness* (pp. 333-347). New York: Oxford University Press.

Duman, R. S. (2004). Depression: A case of neuronal life and death? *Biological Psychiatry, 56*, 141-145.

Duman, R. S., Heninger, G. R., & Nestler, E. J. (1997). A molecular and cellular theory of depression. *Archives of General Psychiatry 54*, 597-606.

Dumitriu, D., Collins, K., Alterman, R., et al. (2008). Neurostimulatory therapeutics in management of treatment-resistant depression with focus on deep brain stimulation. *Mt. Sinai Journal of Medicine, 75*(3), 263-275.

Dunlop, B. W., & Nemeroff, C. B. (2007). The role of dopamine in the pathophysiology of depression. *Archives of General Psychiatry, 64*(3), 327-337.

Dunner, D. L., Hendrickson, H. E., Bea, C., et al. (1999). Dysthymic disorder; treatment with mirtazapine. *Depression and Anxiety, 10*, 8-72.

Edinger, J. D., Olsen, M. K., Stechuchak, K. M., et al. (2009). Cognitive behavioral therapy for patients with primary insomnia or insomnia associated predominantly with mixed psychiatric disorders: A randomized clinical trial. *Sleep, 32*(4), 499-510.

Edward, K-L. (2005). Resilience: A protector from depression. *American Psychiatric Nurses Association Journal, 11*(4), 241-243.

Elderly in nursing homes more likely to be depressed than those living at home. (2008). NewsInferno. Retrieved from newsinferno.com

Emslie, G. J., Mayes, T. L., Kennard, B. D., et al. (2006). Pediatric mood disorders. In D. J. Stein, D. J. Kupfer, & A. F. Schatzberg (Eds.), *The American psychiatric publishing textbook of mood disorders* (pp. 573-602). Washington, DC: American Psychiatric Publishing, Inc.

Emslie, G. J., Rush, A. J., Weinberg, W. A., et al. (1998). Fluoxetine in child and adolescent depression: Acute and maintenance treatment. *Depression and Anxiety, 7*, 32-39.

Emslie, G., Wagner, K. D., Kutcher, S., et al. (2004, October). *Paroxetine treatment in children and adolescents with major depressive disorder*. Poster presented at the 51st annual meeting of the American Academy of Child and Adolescent Psychiatry, Washington, DC.

Emslie, G. J., Weinberg, W. A., Rush, A. J., et al. (1990). Depressive symptoms by self-report in adolescence: Phase I of the development of a questionnaire for depression by self-report. *Journal of Child Neurology, 5,* 114-121.

Epperson, C. N., Terman, M., Terman, J. S., et al. (2004). Randomized clinical trial of bright light therapy for antepartum depression: Preliminary findings. *Journal of Clinical Psychiatry, 65,* 421-425.

Evans, D. L., Foa, E. B., Gur, R. E., et al. (2005). *Treating and preventing adolescent mental health disorders: What we know and what we don't know.* Oxford, UK: Oxford University Press.

Fava, M., Uebelacker, L., Alpert, J., et al. (1997). Major depressive subtypes and treatment response. *Biological Psychiatry, 42,* 568-576.

Fawcett, J., Scheftner, W. A., Fogg, L., et al. (1990). Time-related predictors of suicide in major affective disorder. *American Journal of Psychiatry, 147*(9), 1189-1194.

Federenko, I. S., & Wadhwa, P. S. (2004). Women's mental health during pregnancy influences fetal and infant developmental and health outcomes. *CNS Spectrums, 9*(3), 198-206.

Fergusson, D. M., & Woodward, L. J. (2002). Mental health, educational and social role outcomes of adolescents with depression. *Archives of General Psychiatry, 59,* 225-231.

First, M. B., Frances, A., & Pincus, H. A. (2002). *DSM-IV-TR handbook of differential diagnosis.* Washington, DC: American Psychiatric Publishing, Inc.

First, M. B., & Tasman, A. (2004). Comorbidity with medical illnesses. In M. B. First & A. Tasman (Eds.), *DSM-IV-TR mental disorders: Diagnosis, etiology & treatment.* West Sussex, UK: John Wiley & Sons, Ltd.

Fitzsimons, L., Disner, S. G., & Bress, J. N. (2009). Effective utilization and future directions for repetitive transcranial magnetic stimulation: A guide for psychiatric nurses. *Journal of American Psychiatric Nurses Association, 15*(5), 314-324.

Flint, A. (1997). Pharmacologic treatment of depression in late life. *Canadian Medical Association Journal, 157*(8), 1061-1067.

Flint, A. J., & Rifat, S. L. (1998). The treatment of psychotic depression in later life: A comparison of pharmacotherapy and ECT. *Journal of Geriatric Psychiatry, 13,* 23-28.

Flores, B. H., & Schatzberg, A. F. (2006). Psychotic depression. In D. J. Stein, D. J. Kupfer, & A. F. Schatzberg (Eds.), *The American psychiatric publishing textbook of mood disorders* (pp. 561-571). Washington, DC: American Psychiatric Publishing, Inc.

Folse, V., Eich, K. N., Hall, A. M., et al. (2006). Detecting suicide risk in adolescents and adults in an emergency department. *Journal of Psychosocial Nursing and Mental Health Services, 44*(3), 23-29.

Forray, A., & Ostroff, R. B. (2007). The use of electroconvulsive therapy in postpartum affective disorders. *Journal of ECT, 23,* 188-193.

Freedland, K. E., Carney, R. M., & Skala, J. A. (1995). The prevalence of depression and dysthymia in patients with congestive heart failure. *Psychosomatic Medicine, 57,* 62.

Friedman, E. S., & Thase, M. E. (2006). Cognitive-behavioral therapy for depression and dysthymia. In D. J. Stein, D. J. Kupfer, & A. F. Schatzberg (Eds.), *The American psychiatric publishing textbook of mood disorders* (pp. 353-371). Washington, DC: American Psychiatric Publishing, Inc.

Friedman, E. S., & Thase, M. E. (2007). Depression-focused psychotherapies. In G. O. Gabbard (Ed.), *Gabbard's treatments of psychiatric disorders* (4th ed.) (pp. 409-431). Washington, DC: American Psychiatric Publishing, Inc.

Gabbard, G. O. (2005). *Psychodynamic psychiatry in clinical practice* (4th ed.). Washington, DC: American Psychiatric Publishing, Inc.

Geller, B., Zimerman, B., Williams, M., et al. (2001). Adult psychosocial outcome of prepubertal major depressive disorder. *Journal of the American Academy of Child and Adolescent Psychiatry, 40,* 673-677.

George, M. S. (2003). Stimulating the brain. *Scientific American,* 67-73. Retrieved from www.sciam.com

George, M. S., & Belmaker, R. H. (2006). *Transcranial magnetic stimulation in clinical psychiatry.* Washington, DC: American Psychiatric Publishing, Inc.

George, M. S., Lisanby, S. H., & Sackeim, H. A. (1999). Transcranial magnetic stimulation: Applications in psychiatry. *Archives of General Psychiatry, 56,* 300-311.

George, M. S., Nahas, Z, Bohning, D. E., et al. (2006). Vagus nerve stimulation and deep brain stimulation. In D. J. Stein, D. J. Kupfer, & A. F. Schatzberg (Eds.), *The American psychiatric publishing textbook of mood disorders* (pp. 337-352). Washington, DC: American Psychiatric Publishing, Inc.

George, M. S., Sackeim, H. A., Rush, A. J., et al. (2000). Vagus nerve stimulation: A new tool for brain research and therapy. *Biological Psychiatry, 47,* 287-295.

Georgiades, K., Lewinsohn, P. M., Monroe, S. M. (2006). Major depressive disorder in adolescence: The role of subthreshold symptoms. *Journal of the American Academy of Child and Adolescent Psychiatry, 45*(8), 936-944.

Gillespie, C. F., Garlow, S. J., & Binder, E. B. (2009). Neurobiology of mood disorders. In A. F. Schatzberg & C. B. Nemeroff (Eds.), *The American psychiatric publishing textbook of psychopharmacology* (4th ed.) (pp. 903-944). Washington, DC: American Psychiatric Publishing, Inc.

Glatt, S. J., Faraone, S. V., & Tsuang, M. T. (2008). Psychiatric genetics: A primer. In J. W. Smoller, B. R. Sheidley, & M. T. Tsuang (Eds.), *Psychiatric genetics: Applications in clinical practice* (pp. 3-26). Washington, DC: American Psychiatric Publishing, Inc.

Glod, C. A., & Manchester, A. (2000). Prescribing patterns of advanced practice nurses: Contrasting psychiatric mental health CNS and NP practice. *Clinical Excellence for Nurse Practitioners, 4*(1), 22-29.

Goodwin, F. K., & Jamison, K. R. (Eds.). (1990). *Manic-depressive illness.* New York: Oxford University Press.

Goodwin, R. D., Jacobi, F., Bittner, A., et al. (2006). Epidemiology of mood disorders. In D. J. Stein, D. J. Kupfer, & A. F. Schatzberg (Eds.), *The American psychiatric publishing textbook of mood disorders* (pp. 33-54). Washington, DC: American Psychiatric Publishing, Inc.

Gould, M. S., Fisher, P., Parides, M., et al. (1996). Psychosocial risk factors of child and adolescent completed suicide. *Archives of General Psychiatry, 53,* 1155-1162.

Greden, J. F. (2001). The burden of recurrent depression: Causes, consequences, and future prospects. *Journal of Clinical Psychiatry, 62*(Suppl 22), 5-9.

Hall, R. C., Platt, D. E., & Hall, R. C. (1999). Suicide risk assessment: A review of risk factors for suicide in 100 patients who made severe suicide attempts. *Psychosomatics, 40*(1), 18-27.

Hamilton, M. (1960). A rating scale for depression. *Journal of Neurology, Neurosurgery, and Psychiatry, 23,* 56-62.

Hamilton, M. (1967). Development of a rating scale for primary depressive illness. *British Journal of Social and Clinical Psychology, 6,* 278-296.

Hammad, T. A., Laughren, T., & Racoosin, J. (2006). Suicidality in pediatric patients treated with antidepressant drugs. *Archives of General Psychiatry, 63*(3), 332-339.

Hasler, G., Drevets, W., Manji, H., et al. (2004). Discovering endophenotypes for major depression. *Neuropsychopharmacology, 29,* 1765-1781.

Hathaway, S. R., & McKinley, J. C. (1989). *Minnesota Multiphasic Personality Inventory-2.* Minneapolis MN: University of Minnesota Press.

Hawk, C., Jason, L. A., & Torres-Harding, S. (2006). Differential diagnosis of chronic fatigue syndrome and major depressive disorder. *International Journal of Behavioral Medicine, 13*(3), 244-251.

Hawton, K. (1992). Suicide and attempted suicide. In E. E. Paykel (Ed.), *Handbook of affective disorders* (pp. 635-650). New York: Guilford Press.

Hellerstein, D. J., Batchelder, S., Kreditor, D., et al. (2001). Bupropion sustained-release for the treatment of dysthymic disorder: An open-label study. *Journal of Clinical Psychopharmacology, 21,* 325-329.

Henkel, V., Mergl, R., Allgaier, A. K., et al. (2010). Treatment of atypical depression: Post-hoc analysis of a randomized controlled study testing the efficacy of sertraline and cognitive behavioral therapy in mildly depressed outpatients. *European Psychiatry: The Journal of the Association of European Psychiatrists, 25*(8), 491-498.

Heron, J., Craddock, N., & Jones, I. (2005). Postnatal euphoria. Are the highs an indicator of bipolarity? *Bipolar Disorders, 7,* 103-110.

Hickie, I., Bennett, B., Mitchell, P., et al. (1996). Clinical and subclinical hypothyroidism in patients with chronic and treatment resistant depression. *Australian and New Zealand Journal of Psychiatry, 30*(2), 246-252.

Higgins, E. S., & George, M. S. (2007). *The neuroscience of clinical psychiatry: The pathophysiology of behavior and mental illness.* Philadelphia: Wolters Kluwer-Lippincott Williams & Wilkins.

Hoge, C. W., Lesikar, S. E., Guevara, R., et al. (2002). Mental disorders among U.S. military personnel in the 1990's: Association with high levels of health care utilization and early military attrition. *American Journal of Psychiatry, 159,* 1576-1583.

Holsinger, T., Steffens, D., Phillips, C., et al. (2002). Head injury in early adulthood and the lifetime risk of depression. *Archives of General Psychiatry, 59,* 17-22.

Horowitz, M. J., Siegel, B., Holen, A., et al. (1997). Diagnostic criteria for complicated grief disorder. *The American Journal of Psychiatry, 154*(7), 904-910.

Horrigan, J. P., Sikich, L., Courvoisie, H. E., et al. (1998). Alternative therapies in the child psychiatric clinic. *Journal of Child and Adolescent Psychopharmacology, 8,* 249-250.

Howland, R. H. (2008). Sequenced treatment alternatives to relieve depression (STAR*D) Part 2: Study outcomes. *Journal of Psychosocial Nursing, 46*(10), 21-24.

Howland, R. H., Shutt, L. S., Berman, S. R., et al. (2011). The emerging use of technology for the treatment of depression and other neuropsychiatric disorders. *Annals of Clinical Psychiatry, 23*(1), 48-62.

Insel, T. (2006). Beyond efficacy: The STAR*D trial. *The American Journal of Psychiatry, 163*(1), 5-7.

Jaffee, S. R., Moffitt, T. E., Caspi, A., et al. (2002). Differences in early childhood risk factors for juvenile-onset and adult-onset depression. *Archives of General Psychiatry, 59,* 215-222.

Jarrett, R. B., Schaffer, M., McIntire, D., et al. (1999). Treatment of atypical depression with cognitive therapy or phenelzine: A double-blind, placebo-controlled trial. *Archives of General Psychiatry, 56*(5), 431-437.

Joffee, R. T., & Levitt, A. J. (1992). Major depression and subclinical (Grade 2) hypothyroidism. *Psychoneuroendocrinology, 17*(2-3), 215-221.

Johnson, J. G., Alloy, L. B., Panzarella, C., et al. (2001). Hopelessness as a mediator of the association between social support and depressive symptoms: Findings of a study of men with HIV. *Journal of Consulting & Clinical Psychology, 69,* 1056-1060.

Johnson, J. G., Cohen, P., Gould, M. S., et al. (2002). Childhood adversities, interpersonal difficulties and risk for suicide attempts during late adolescence and early adulthood. *Archives of General Psychiatry, 59,* 741-749.

Johnson, J. G., Cohen, P., Skodol, A. E., et al. (1999). Personality disorders in adolescence and risk of major mental disorders and suicidality during adulthood. *Archives of General Psychiatry, 56,* 805-811.

Joiner, T. E., Jr., Brown, J., & Wingate, J. S., et al. (2005). The psychology and neurobiology of suicidal behavior. *Annual Review of Psychology, 56,* 287-314.

Joiner, T. E., Jr., Pfaff, J. J., & Acres, J. G. (2002). A brief screening tool for the suicidal symptoms in adolescents and young adults in general health settings: Reliability and validity data from the Australian National General Practice Youth Suicide Prevention Program. *Behaviour Research and Therapy, 40*(4), 471-481.

Joska, J. A., & Stein, D. J. (2008). Mood disorders. In R. E. Hales, S. C. Yudofsky, & G. O. Gabbard (Eds.), *The American psychiatric publishing textbook of psychiatry* (5th ed.) (pp. 457-503). Washington, DC: American Psychiatric Publishing, Inc.

Joska, J. A., & Stein, D. J. (2011). Mood disorders. In R. E. Hales, S. C. Yudofsky, & G. O. Gabbard (Eds.), *Essentials of psychiatry* (3rd ed.) (pp. 151-183). Washington, DC: American Psychiatric Publishing, Inc.

Juurlink, D. N., Herrmann, N., Szalai, J. P., et al. (2004). Medical illness and the risk of suicide in the elderly. *Archives of Internal Medicine, 164,* 1179-1184.

Kanner, A. M. (2003). Depression in epilepsy: Prevalence, clinical semiology, pathogenic mechanisms and treatment. *Biological Psychiatry, 54,* 388-398.

Kaplan, M. S., Huguet, N., McFarland, B. H., et al. (2007). Suicide among male veterans: A prospective population-based study. *Journal of Epidemiology and Community Health, 61,* 619-624.

Karasu, T. B., Gelenberg, A., Merriam, A., et al. (2006). Practice guideline for the treatment of patients with major depressive disorder, Second Edition. In *American psychiatric association practice guidelines for the treatment of psychiatric disorders: Compendium 2006* (pp. 763-840). Washington, DC: American Psychiatric Publishing, Inc.

Kasper, S., Wehr, T. A., Bartko, J. J., et al. (1989). Epidemiological findings of seasonal changes in mood and behavior: A telephone survey of Montgomery County, Maryland. *Archives of General Psychiatry, 46,* 823-833.

Katon, W. J. (2003). Clinical and health services relationships between major depression, depressive symptoms, and general medical illness. *Biological Psychiatry, 54*(3), 216-226.

Kaufman, J., Plotsky, P. M., Nemeroff, C., et al. (2000). Effects of early adverse experiences on brain structure and function: Clinical implications. *Biological Psychiatry, 48*(8), 778-790.

Keller, M. (2003). Past, present, and future directions for defining optimal treatment outcome in depression: Remission and beyond. *Journal of the American Medical Association, 289*(23), 3152-3160.

Keller, M. B., Gelenberg, A. J., Hirschfeld, R. M. A., et al. (1998). The treatment of chronic depression, part 2: A double-blind, randomized trial of sertraline and imipramine. *Journal of Clinical Psychiatry, 59,* 598-607.

Kendler, K., Neale, M., Kessler, R., et al. (1992). Major depression and generalized anxiety disorder: Same genes, (partly) different environments? *Archives of General Psychiatry, 49,* 716-722.

Kessler, R. C. (1994). The National Comorbidity Survey of the United States. *International Review of Psychiatry, 6,* 365-376.

Kessler, R. C. (1997). The effects of stressful life events on depression. *Annual Review of Psychology, 48,* 191-214.

Kessler, R. C. (2003). Epidemiology of women and depression. *Journal of Affective Disorders, 74,* 5-13.

Kessler, R. C., Berglund, P., Demler, O., et al. (2003). The epidemiology of major depressive disorder: Results from the National Comorbidity Survey Replication (NCS-R). *Journal of the American Medical Association, 289,* 3095-3105.

Kessler, R. C., & Walters, E. E. (1998). Epidemiology of DSM-III-R major depression and minor depression among adolescents and young adults in the National Comorbidity survey. *Depression and Anxiety, 7,* 3-14.

Kim, H. F., Schulz, P. E., Wilde, E. A., et al. (2008). Laboratory testing and imaging studies in psychiatry. In R. E. Hales, S. C. Yudofsky, & G. O. Gabbard (Eds.), *The American psychiatric publishing textbook of psychiatry* (5th ed.) (pp. 19-72). Washington, DC: American Psychiatric Publishing, Inc.

Kirmayer, L. J., & Jarvis, G. E. (2006). Depression across cultures. In D. J. Stein, D. J. Kupfer, & A. F. Schatzberg (Eds.), *The American psychiatric publishing textbook of mood disorders* (pp. 699-715). Washington, DC: American Psychiatric Publishing, Inc.

Kirmayer, L. J., Young, A., & Robbins, J. M. (1994). Symptom attribution in cultural perspective. *Canadian Journal of Psychiatry, 39,* 584-595.

Klein, D. N., Schwartz, J. E., Rose, S., et al. (2000). Five-year course and outcome of dysthymic disorder: A prospective, naturalistic follow-up study. *American Journal of Psychiatry, 157,* 931-939.

Klein, D. N., Shankman, S. A., Lewinsohn, P. M., et al. (2004). Family study of chronic depression in a community sample of young adults. *American Journal of Psychiatry, 161,* 646-653.

Klein, D. N., Shankman, S. A., & McFarland, B. R. (2006a). Classification of mood disorders. In D. J. Stein, D. J. Kupfer, & A. F. Schatzberg (Eds.), *The American psychiatric publishing textbook of mood disorders* (pp. 17-32). Washington, DC: American Psychiatric Publishing, Inc.

Klein, D. N., Shankman, S. A., & Rose, S. (2006b). Ten-year prospective follow-up study of the naturalistic course of dysthymic disorder and double depression. *The American Journal of Psychiatry, 163*(5), 872-880.

Klerman, G., & Weissman, M. (1989). Increasing rates of depression. *Journal of the American Medical Association, 261,* 2229-2235.

Kornstein, S. G. (1997). Gender differences in depression: Implications for treatment. *Journal of Clinical Psychiatry, 58*(Suppl 15), 12-18.

Kornstein, S. G., & Sloan, D. M. (2006). Depression and gender. In D. J. Stein, D. J. Kupfer, & A. F. Schatzberg (Eds.), *The American psychiatric publishing textbook of mood disorders* (pp. 687-698). Washington, DC: American Psychiatric Publishing, Inc.

Kovacs, M. (1981). Rating scales to assess depression in school-aged children. *Acta Paedopsychiatrica, 46,* 305-315.

Kovacs, M., Akiskal, H. S., Gatsonis, C., et al. (1994). Childhood onset of dysthymic disorder: Clinical features and prospective naturalistic outcome. *Archives of General Psychiatry, 51,* 365-374.

Kramer, T. (2000). Transcranial magnetic stimulation and its effectiveness in affective disorders. Medscape Education. htttp://www.medscape.org/viewarticle/420840

Krishnan, K. R., Delong, M., Kraemer, H., et al. (2002). Comorbidity of depression with other medical diseases in the elderly. *Biological Psychiatry, 52*, 559-588.

Krishnan, V., & Nestler, E. J. (2008). The molecular neurobiology of depression. *Nature, 455*(16), 894-902.

Kroenke, K., Spitzer, R. L., & Williams, J. B. (2001). The PHQ-9: Validity of a brief depression severity measure. *Journal of General and Internal Medicine, 16*(9), 606-613.

Kupfer, D. J. (1993). Management of recurrent depression. *Journal of Clinical Psychiatry, 54*(Suppl), 29-33.

Lam, R. W., Levitt, A. J., Levitan, R. D., et al. (2006). The Can-SAD study: A randomized controlled trial of the effectiveness of light therapy and fluoxetine in patients with winter seasonal affective disorder. *American Journal of Psychiatry, 163*, 805-812.

Lambert, K. (2006). Rising rates of depression in today's society: Consideration of the roles of effort-based rewards and enhanced resilience in day-to-day functioning. *Neuroscience and Biobehavioral Reviews, 30*, 497-510.

Lau, M. A. (2008). New developments in psychosocial interventions for adults with unipolar depression. *Current Opinion in Psychiatry, 21*(1), 30-36.

Lawlor, D., & Hopker, S. W. (2001). The effectiveness of exercise as an intervention in the management of depression: Systematic review and metaregression analysis of randomized controlled trials. *British Medical Journal, 322*(7289), 763-767.

Levy, A. J., Wehr, T. A., Goodwin, F. K., et al. (1980). Light suppresses melatonin secretion in humans. *Science, 210*, 1267-1269.

Lewinsohn, P. M., Rohde, P., & Seeley, J. R. (1998). Major depressive disorder in older adolescents: Prevalence, risk factors and clinical implications. *Clinical Psychology Review, 18*, 765-794.

Linehan, M. M., Goldstein, J. L., Nielsen, S. L., et al. (1983). Reasons for staying alive when you are thinking of killing yourself: The reasons for living inventory. *Journal of Consulting and Clinical Psychology, 51*, 276-286.

Lozano, A. M., Mayberg, H. S., Giacobbe, P., et al. (2008). Subcallosal cingulate gyrus deep brain stimulation for treatment-resistant depression. *Biological Psychiatry, 64*, 461-467.

Lumley, J., & Austin, M. (2001). What interventions may reduce postpartum depression. *Current Opinion in Obstetrics and Gynecology, 13*(6), 605-611.

Luoma, I., Tamminen, T., Kaukonen, P., et al. (2001). Longitudinal study of maternal depressive symptoms and child well-being. *Journal of the American Academy of Child and Adolescent Psychiatry, 40*(12), 1367-1374.

Lynch, A., Glod, C. A., & Fitzgerald, F. (2001). Psychopharmacologic treatment of adolescent depression. *Archives of Psychiatric Nursing, 15*(1), 41-47.

Maddux, R. E., & Rapaport, M. H. (2004). Psychopharmacology and psychotherapy of subsyndromal depressions. In M. Fava & J. E. Alpert (Eds.), *Handbook of chronic depression* (pp. 183–206). New York: Marcel Dekker.

Maerov, P. J. (2006). Demystifying CBT: Effective, easy-to-use treatment for depression and anxiety. *Current Psychiatry, 5*(8), 27-39.

Maes, M., Scharpe, S., & Meltzer, H. Y. (1995). The serotonin hypothesis of major depression in psychopharmacology. In F. E. Bloom, D. J. Kupfer, B. S. Buney, et al. (Eds.), *The fourth generation of progress* (pp. 933-944). New York: Raven Press.

Maj, M., Veltro, F., Pirozzi, R., et al. (1992). Pattern of recurrence of illness after recovery from an episode of major depression: A prospective study. *American Journal of Psychiatry, 149*, 795-800.

Malone, D. A. (2010). Use of deep brain stimulation in treatment-resistant depression. *Cleveland Clinic Journal of Medicine, 77*(Suppl 3), S77-S80.

Mann, J. J., & Currier, D. (2006). Understanding and preventing suicide. In D. J. Stein, D. J. Kupfer, & A. F. Schatzberg (Eds.), *The American psychiatric publishing textbook of mood disorders* (pp. 485-496). Washington, DC: American Psychiatric Publishing, Inc.

Mann, J., Watermaux, C., Haas, G. L., et al. (1999). Toward a clinical model of suicidal behavior in psychiatric patients. *American Journal of Psychiatry, 156*(2), 181-189.

Marangell, L. B., Martinez, M., Martinez, J. M., et al. (2005). Vagus nerve stimulation: A new tool for treating depression. *Primary Psychiatry, 12*(10), 40-43.

March, J., Silva, S., Petrycki, S., et al.; Treatment for Adolescents with Depression Study Team. (2004). Fluoxetine, cognitive-behavioral therapy and their combination for adolescents with depression: Treatment for adolescents with depression study (TADS) randomized controlled trial. *Journal of the American Medical Association, 292*, 807-820.

Marcus, S. M., Flynn, H. A., Blow, F. C., et al. (2003). Depressive symptoms among pregnant women screened in obstetrics settings. *Journal of Women's Health, 12*, 373-380.

Markowitz, J. C. (2006). Interpersonal psychotherapy for depression and dysthymic disorder. In D. J. Stein, D. J. Kupfer, & A. F. Schatzberg (Eds.), *The American psychiatric publishing textbook of mood disorders* (pp. 373-388). Washington, DC: American Psychiatric Publishing, Inc.

Markowitz, J. C., Kocsis, J. H., Bleiberg, K. L., et al. (2005). A comparative trial of psychotherapy and pharmacotherapy for "pure" dysthymic patients. *Journal of Affective Disorders, 89*(1-3), 167-175.

Markowitz, J. C., Moran, M. E., Kocsis, J. H., et al. (1992). Prevalence and comorbidity of dysthymic disorder among psychiatric outpatients. *Journal of Affective Disorders, 24*, 63-71.

Martinez, M., Marangell, L. B., & Martinez, J. M. (2008). Psychopharmacology. In R. E. Hales, S. C. Yudofsky, & G. O. Gabbard (Eds.), *The American psychiatric publishing textbook of psychiatry* (5th ed.) (pp. 1053-1131). Washington, DC: American Psychiatric Publishing, Inc.

Mather, A. S., Rodriguez, C., Guthrie, M. F., et al. (2002). Effects of exercise on depressive symptoms in older adults with poorly responsive depressive disorder: Randomized controlled trial. *British Journal of Psychiatry, 180*, 411-415.

Matthews, K., & Eljamel, M. (2003). Vagus nerve stimulation and refractory depression: Please can you switch me on doctor? *The British Journal of Psychiatry, 183*, 181-183.

Mayberg, H. S. (2004). Depression: A neuropsychiatric perspective. In J. Panksepp (Ed.), *Textbook of biological psychiatry* (pp. 11-143). Hoboken, NJ: Wiley-Liss, Inc.

Mayberg, H. S. (2006). Brain imaging. In D. J. Stein, D. J. Kupfer, & A. F. Schatzberg (Eds.), *The American psychiatric publishing textbook of mood disorder* (pp. 219-234). Washington, DC: American Psychiatric Publishing, Inc.

Mayberg, H. S., Lozano, A. M., Voon, V., et al. (2005). Deep brain stimulation for treatment-resistant depression. *Neuron, 45*(5), 651-660.

McCall, W. V., Reboussin, D. M., Weiner, R. D., et al. (2000). Titrated moderately supra-threshold vs fixed high-dose right unilateral electroconvulsive therapy: Acute antidepressant and cognitive effects. *Archives of General Psychiatry, 57*, 438-444.

McClintock, S. M., & Husain, M. M. (2011). Electroconvulsive therapy does not damage the brain. *Journal of the American Psychiatric Nurses Association, 17*(3), 212-213.

McDonald, W. M., Meeks, T. W., McCall, W. V., et al. (2009). Electroconvulsive therapy. In A. F. Schatzberg & C. B. Nemeroff (Eds.). *The American psychiatric publishing textbook of psychopharmacology* (4th ed.) (pp. 861-899). Washington, DC: American Psychiatric Publishing, Inc.

McEwen, B. S. (1998). Protective and damaging effects of stress mediators. *The New England Journal of Medicine, 338*, 171-179.

McFarland, B. R., & Klein, D. N. (2005). Mental health service use by patients with dysthymic disorder: Treatment use and dropout in a 7 ½-year naturalistic follow-up study. *Comprehensive Psychiatry, 46*, 246-253.

McGrath, P. J., Stewart, J. W., Janal, M. N., et al. (2000). A placebo-controlled study of fluoxetine versus imipramine in the acute treatment of atypical depression. *American Journal of Psychiatry, 157*, 344-350.

McGuffin, P., Rijsdijk, F., Andrew, M., et al. (2003). The heritability of bipolar affective disorder and the genetic relationship to unipolar depression. *Archives of General Psychiatry, 60*(5), 497-502.

McGuinness, T. M. (2010). Childhood adversities and adult health. *Journal of Psychosocial Nursing, 48*(8), 15-18.

Melhem, N. M., Walker, M., Moritz, G., et al. (2008). Antecedents and sequelae of sudden parental death in offspring and surviving caregivers. *Archives of Pediatric and Adolescent Medicine, 162*(5), 403-410.

Meng, F., Luo, H., & Halbreicht, U. (2002). Concepts, techniques and clinical application of acupuncture. *Psychiatric Annals, 32*(1), 45-49.

Mersch, P. P., Middendorp, H. M., Bouhuys, A. L., et al. (1999). The prevalence of seasonal affective disorder in The Netherlands: A prospective and retrospective study of seasonal mood variation in the general population. *Biological Psychiatry, 45*, 1013-1022.

Metzner, J., & Hayes, L. (2006). Suicide prevention in jails and prisons. In R. Simon & R. Hales (Eds.), *Textbook of suicide assessment and management* (pp. 139–155). Washington, DC: American Psychiatric Publishing, Inc.

Montgomery, S. A., Baldwin, D. S., Blier, P., et al. (2007). Which antidepressants have demonstrated superior efficacy? A review of the evidence. *International Clinical Psychopharmacology, 22*, 323-329.

Moore, J. D., & Bona, J. R. (2001). Depression and dysthymia. *Medical Clinics of North America, 85*, 631-644.

Moreines, J. L., McClintock, S. M., & Holtzheimer, P. E. (2011). Neuropsychologic effects of neuromodulation techniques for treatment-resistant depression: A review. *Brain Stimulation, 4*(1), 17-27.

Morrison, J. (2007). *Diagnosis made easier: Principles and techniques for mental health clinicians.* New York: Guilford Press.

Mueser, K. T., Bond, G. R., & Drake, R. E. (2001). Community-based treatment of schizophrenia and other severe mental disorders: Treatment outcomes. *Medscape General Medicine, 3*(1). Retrieved from http://www.medscape.com/viewarticle/430529_print

Mugavin, M. E. (2005). A meta-synthesis of filicide classification systems: Psychosocial and psychodynamic issues in women who kill their children. *Journal of Forensic Nursing, 1*(2), 65-72.

Murphy, G. E., Wetzel, R. D., Robins, E., et al. (1992). Multiple risk factors predict suicide in alcoholism. *Archives of General Psychiatry, 49*, 459-462.

Muzina, D. J. (2007). Suicide intervention: How to recognize risk, focus on patient safety. *Current Psychiatry, 6*(9), 31-46.

Nachmias, M., Gunnar, M., Mangelsdorf, S., et al. (1996). Behavioral inhibition and stress reactivity: The moderating role of attachment security. *Child Development, 67*, 508-522.

Nahas, Z., & Anderson, B. S. (2011). Brain stimulation therapies for mood disorders: The continued necessity of electroconvulsive therapy. *Journal of the American Psychiatric Nurses Association, 17*(3), 214-216.

Nahas, Z., Anderson, B., Borckardt, J., et al. (2010). Bilateral epidural prefrontal cortical stimulation for treatment-resistant depression. *Biological Psychiatry, 67*(2), 101-109.

Nahas, Z., Lorberbaum, J. P., Kozel, F., et al. (2004). Somatic treatments in psychiatry. In J. Panksepp (Ed.), *Textbook of biological psychiatry* (pp. 521-548). Hoboken, NJ: John Wiley & Sons, Inc.

National Center for Health Statistics. (1999). *Death rates for 72 selected causes by 5-year groups, race, and sex: United States, 1979-1999.* Atlanta: Centers for Disease Control and Prevention.

National Survey on Drug Use and Health. (2008). Major depressive episodes and treatment for depression among veterans aged 21-39. Substance Abuse and Mental Health Services Administration, Office of Applied Sciences, Rockville, MD. Retrieved from www.oas.samhsa.gov/nhsda.htm.

Nelson, J. C. (2001). Augmentation strategies in SSRI-resistant depression patients. *CNS News Special Edition, Dec. 2001*, 55-58.

Nelson, J. C. (2009). Augmentation and combination strategies in resistant depression. *Journal of Clinical Psychiatry, 70*(6), e20.

Nemeroff, C. (2003, May). *The neurobiological consequences of child abuse.* Presentation at the 156th annual meeting of the APA, San Francisco.

Nemeroff, C. (2007). The burden of severe depression: A review of diagnostic challenges and treatment alternatives. *Journal of Psychiatric Research, 41*, 189-206.

Nesse, R. M. (2006). Evolutionary explanations for mood and mood disorders. In D. J. Stein, D. J. Kupfer, & A. F. Schatzberg (Eds.), *The American psychiatric publishing textbook of mood disorders* (pp. 159-178). Washington, DC: American Psychiatric Publishing, Inc.

Newport, D. J., Fernandez, S. V., Juric, S., et al. (2009). Psychopharmacology during pregnancy and lactation. In A. F. Schatzberg & C. B. Nemeroff (Eds.), *The American psychiatric publishing textbook of psychopharmacology* (4th ed.) (pp. 1373-1412). Washington, DC: American Psychiatric Publishing, Inc.

Nierenberg, A. A., Ostacher, M. J., Delgado, P. L., et al. (2007). Antidepressant and antimanic medications. In G. O. Gabbard (Ed.), *Gabbard's treatments of psychiatric disorders* (4th ed.) (pp. 385-407). Washington, DC: American Psychiatric Publishing, Inc.

Nixon, M., Milin, R., Simeon, J., et al. (2001). Sertraline effects in adolescent major depression and dysthymia: A six month open trial. *Journal of Child and Adolescent Psychopharmacology, 11*, 131-142.

Nobler, M. S., & Sackeim, H. A. (2006). Electroconvulsive therapy and transcranial magnetic stimulation. In D. J. Stein, D. J. Kupfer, & A. F. Schatzberg (Eds.), *The American psychiatric publishing textbook of mood disorders* (pp. 317-335). Washington, DC: American Psychiatric Publishing, Inc.

O'Hara, M. W., Stuart, S., Gorman, L., et al. (2000). Efficacy of interpersonal psychotherapy for postpartum depression. *Archives of General Psychiatry, 57*(11), 1039-1045.

Okun, M. L., Kravitz, H. M., Sowers, M. F., et al. (2009). Psychometric evaluation of the insomnia symptoms questionnaire: A self-report measure to identify chronic insomnia. *Journal of Clinical Sleep Medicine, 5*(1), 41-51.

O'Reardon, J. P., Solvason, H. B., Janicak, P. G., et al. (2007). Efficacy and safety of transcranial magnetic stimulation in the acute treatment of major depression: A multisite randomized controlled trial. *Biological Psychiatry, 62*, 1208-1216.

Overall, J. E., & Gorham, D. R. (1962). The brief psychiatric rating scale. *Psychological Report, 10*, 799-812.

Pardo, J. V., Pardo, P. J., & Raichle, M. D. (1993). Neural correlates of self-induced dysphoria. *American Journal of Psychiatry, 150*, 713-719.

Parker, G., Roy, K., Wilhelm, K., et al. (2001). Assessing the comparative effectiveness of antidepressant therapies: A prospective clinical practice study. *Journal of Clinical Psychiatry, 62*, 117-125.

Parmelee, P. A., Katz, I. R., & Lawton, M. P. (1989). Depression among institutionalized aged: Assessment and prevalence estimation. *Journal of Gerontology, 44*(1), M22-M29.

Parrish, E., Peden, A., & Staten, R. T. (2008). Strategies used by advanced practice psychiatric nurses in treating adults with depression. *Perspectives in Psychiatric Care, 44*(4), 232-240.

Pearson, S., Schmidt, M., Patton, G., et al. (2010). Depression and insulin resistance: Cross sectional associations in young adults. *Diabetes Care, 33*(5), 1128-1133.

Pepper, C. M., Klein, D. N., Anderson, R. L., et al. (1995). DSM-III-R Axis II comborbidity in dysthymia and major depression. *American Journal of Psychiatry, 152*, 239-247.

Perese, E. F. (1997). Unmet needs of persons with chronic mental illnesses: Relationship to their adaptation to community living. *Issues in Mental Health Nursing, 18*(1), 19-34.

Perry, P. J. (1996). Pharmacotherapy for major depression with melancholic features: Relative efficacy of tricyclic versus selective serotonin reuptake inhibitor antidepressants. *Journal of Affective Disorders, 39*, 1-6.

Perugi, G., Akiskal, H. S., Lattanzi, L., et al. (1998). The high prevalence of "soft" bipolar (II) features in atypical depression. *Comprehensive Psychiatry, 39*, 63-71.

Pfeffer, C. R. (2006). Suicide in children and adolescents. In D. J. Stein, D. J. Kupfer, & A. F. Schatzberg (Eds.), *The American psychiatric publishing textbook of mood disorders* (pp. 497-507). Washington, DC: American Psychiatric Publishing, Inc.

Pfeffer, C. R., Jiang, H., & Kakuma, R. (2000). Child-adolescent suicidal potential index (CASPI): A screen for risk for early onset suicidal behavior. *Psychological Assessment, 12*, 304-318.

Phelps, J. (2009). Light therapies for depression. Retrieved from http://www.psycheducation.org/depression/LightTherapy.htm

Phillips, M. R., Zhang, J. X., Shi, Q. C., et al. (2009). Prevalence associated disability and treatment of mental disorders in four provinces in China, 2001-2005: An epidemiological survey. *Lancet, 373*, 73-82.

Pinquart, M., Duberstein, P. R., & Lyness, J. (2006). Treatments for later-life depressive conditions: A meta-analytic comparison of pharmacotherapy and psychotherapy. *The American Journal of Psychiatry, 163*(9), 1493-1501.

Post, R. (1992). Transduction of psychosocial stress into the neurobiology of recurrent affective disorder. *American Journal of Psychiatry, 149*(8), 999-1010.

Potter, W. Z., Padich, R. A., Rudorfer, M. V., et al. (2006). Tricyclics, tetracyclics, and monoamine oxidase inhibitors. In D. J. Stein, D. J. Kupfer, & A. F. Schatzberg (Eds.), *The American psychiatric publishing textbook of mood disorders* (pp. 251-261). Washington, DC: American Psychiatric Publishing, Inc.

Poznanski, L. E., Cook, S. C., & Carroll, B. J. (1979). A depression rating scale for children. *Pediatrics, 64*(4), 442-450.

Preisig, M., Merikangas, K. R., & Angst, J. (2001). Clinical significance and comorbidity of subthreshold depression and anxiety in the community. *Acta Psychiatrica Scandinavica, 104,* 96-103.

Rajkowska, G. (2006). Anatomical pathology. In D. J. Stein, D. J. Kupfer, & A. F. Schatzberg (Eds.), *The American psychiatric publishing textbook of mood disorders* (pp. 179-195). Washington, DC: American Psychiatric Publishing, Inc.

Rajkowska, G., Halaris, A., & Selemon, L. D. (2001). Reductions in neuronal and glial density characterize the dorsolateral prefrontal cortex in bipolar disorder. *Biological Psychiatry, 49*(9), 741-752.

Ransford, C. P. (1982). A role for amines in the antidepressant effect of exercise: A review. *Medical Science and Sports Exercise, 14,* 1-10.

Rasgon, N. L., & Kenna, H. A. (2005). Insulin resistance in depressive disorders and Alzheimer's disease: Revisiting the missing link hypothesis. *Neurobiology of Aging, 26*(1 Suppl 1), 103-107.

Rasgon, N. L., Rao, R. C., Hwang, S., et al. (2003). Depression in women with polycystic ovary syndrome: Clinical and biochemical correlates. *Journal of Affective Disorders, 74,* 299-304.

Recommended Changes in "Depressive Disorder Not Otherwise Specified" (code 311). (2010). American Psychiatric Association. Retrieved from http://www.dsm5.org/Documents/Mood%20Disorders%20Work%20Group/Subdividing%20the%20NOS%20Depressive%20Dx.2JAN2010.pdf

Reynolds, C. F., Dew, M. A., Pollock, B. G., et al. (2006). Maintenance treatment of major depression in old age. *The New England Journal of Medicine, 354*(11), 1130-1138.

Reynolds, W. M. (1987). *Reynolds adolescent depression scale: Professional manual.* Odessa, FL: Psychological Assessment Resources.

Richards, S. S., Musser, W. S., & Gershon, S. (1999). *Maintenance pharmacotherapies for neuropsychiatric disorders.* Levittown, PA: Brunner/Mazel Publishers, Inc.

Roose, S. P., & Devanand, D. P. (2006). Geriatric mood disorders. In D. J. Stein, D. J. Kupfer, & A. F. Schatzberg (Eds.), *The American psychiatric publishing textbook of mood disorders* (pp. 603-619). Washington, DC: American Psychiatric Publishing, Inc.

Roose, S. P., Pollock, B. G., & Devanand, D. P. (2004). Treatment during late life. In A. F. Schatzberg & C. B. Nemeroff (Eds.), *Essentials of clinical psychopharmacology* (3rd ed.) (pp. 1083-1108). Washington, DC: American Psychiatric Publishing, Inc.

Ros, L. T. (2004). A case of "double" depression under outpatient treatment conditions. *World Journal of Biological Psychiatry, 5*(3), 161-163.

Rosal, M. C., Ockene, J. K., Ma, Y., et al. (2001). Behavioral risk factors among members of a health maintenance organization. *Preventive Medicine, 33,* 58-59.

Rosenthal, J. E., & Oren, D. A. (2007). Light therapy. In G. O. Gabbard (Ed.), *Gabbard's treatments of psychiatric disorders* (4th ed.) (pp. 467-476). Washington, DC: American Psychiatric Publishing, Inc.

Rosenthal, J. Z., & Rosenthal, N. E. (2006). Seasonal affective disorder. In D. J. Stein, D. J. Kupfer, & A. F. Schatzberg (Eds.), *The American psychiatric publishing textbook of mood disorders* (pp. 527-545). Washington, DC: American Psychiatric Publishing, Inc.

Rothschild, A. (2003). Challenges in the treatment of depression with psychotic features. *Biological Psychiatry, 53*(8), 680-690.

Rush, A. J., George, M. S., Sackeim, H. A., et al. (2000). Vagus nerve stimulation (VNS) for treatment-resistant depressions: A multicenter study. *Biological Psychiatry, 47,* 276-286.

Rush, A. J., Gullion, C. M., Basco, M. R., et al. (1996). The inventory of depressive symptomatology (IDS): Psychometric properties. *Psychological Medicine, 26*(3), 477-486.

Sackeim, H. (2001). Functional brain circuits in major depression and remission. *Archives of General Psychiatry, 58,* 649-650.

Sackeim, H. A., Brannan, S. K., Rush, A. J., et al. (2007). Durability of antidepressant response to vagus nerve stimulation (VNS). *International Journal of Neuropsychopharmacology, 10*(6), 817-826.

Sadock, B. J., & Sadock, V. A. (2007). *Kaplan & Sadock's synopsis of psychiatry: Behavioral sciences clinical psychiatry* (10th ed.). Philadelphia: Wolters Kluwer/Lippincott Williams & Wilkins.

Saeed, S. A., Bloch, R. M., Antonacci, D. J., et al. (2009). CAM for your depressed patients: 6 recommended options. *Current Psychiatry, 8*(10), 39-47.

Sarafolean, M. M. (2009). Depression in school-age children and adolescents: Characteristics, assessment and prevention. Retrieved from HealthyPlace, www.healthyplace.com

Sayer, K., Kirmayer, L. J., & Taillefer, S. (2003). Predictors of somatic symptoms in depressive disorder. *General Hospital Psychiatry, 25,* 108-114.

Schatzberg, A. F., Cole, J. O., & DeBattista, C. (2003). *Manual of clinical psychopharmacology* (4th ed.). Washington, DC: American Psychiatric Publishing, Inc.

Seligman, M. (1975). *Helplessness: On depression, development and death.* San Francisco: Freeman, 1975.

Shaffer, D., Garland, A., Vieland, V., et al. (1991). The impact of curriculum based suicide prevention programs for teenagers. *Journal of the American Academy of Child and Adolescent Psychiatry, 30,* 588-596.

Shaffer, D., Gould, M. S., Fisher, P., et al. (1996). Psychiatric diagnosis in child and adolescent suicide. *Archives of General Psychiatry, 53,* 339-348.

Sharma, V. (2002). Pharmacotherapy of postpartum depression. *Expert Opinion on Pharmacotherapy, 3*(10), 1421-1431.

Sharma, V. (2008). Treatment of post-partum psychosis: Challenges and opportunities. *Current Drug Safety, 3*(1), 76-81.

Sheikh, J. I., & Yesavage, J. A. (1986). Geriatric depression scale (GDS): Recent evidence and development of a shorter version. *Clinical Gerontology, 5,* 165-172.

Sheline, Y. I., Gado, M. H., & Price, J. L. (1998). Amygdala core nuclei volumes are decreased in recurrent major depression. *Neuroreport, 9,* 2023-2028.

Sheline, Y. I., Sanghavi, M., Mintum, M. A., et al. (1999). Depression duration but not age predicts hippocampal volume loss in medically healthy women with recurrent major depression. *Journal of Neuroscience, 19,* 5034-5043.

Shelton, R. C. (2006). Treatment–resistant depression: Are atypical antipsychotics effective and safe enough? *Current Psychiatry, 5*(10), 31-43.

Shenassa, E. D., Rogers, M. L., Spalding, K. L., et al. (2004). Safer storage of firearms at home and risk of suicide: A study of protective factors in a nationally representative sample. *Journal of Epidemiology and Community Health, 58,* 841-848.

Simon, G. E. (2003). Social and economic burden of mood disorders. *Biological Psychiatry, 54*(3), 208-215.

Simon, G. E., Cunningham, M. L., & Davis, R. L. (2002). Outcomes of prenatal antidepressant exposure. *American Journal of Psychiatry, 159,* 2005-2061.

Simon, G. E., Revicki, D., Heiligenstein, J., et al. (2000). Recovery from depression, work productivity, and health care costs among primary care patients. *General Hospital Psychiatry, 22*(3), 153-162.

Simon, R. I. (2008). Suicide. In R. E. Hales, S. C. Yudofsky, & G. O. Gabbard (Eds.), *The American psychiatric publishing textbook of psychiatry* (5th ed.) (pp. 1637-1654). Washington, DC: American Psychiatric Publishing, Inc.

Simon, R. I. (2011). Suicide. In R. E. Hales, S. C. Yudofsky, & G. O. Gabbard (Eds.), Essentials of psychiatry (pp. 699-717). Washington, DC: American Psychiatric Publishing, Inc.

Sit, D., Rothschild, A. J., & Wisner, K. L. (2006). A review of postpartum psychosis. *Journal of Women's Health, 15*(4), 352-369.

Skarsater, I., Agren, H., & Dencker, E. (2001). Subjective lack of social support and presence of dependent stressful life events characterize patients suffering from major depression compared with healthy volunteers. *Journal of Psychiatric and Mental Health Nursing, 8,* 107-114.

Smith, C. A., & Hay, P. P. J. (2005). Acupuncture for depression. *The Cochrane Database of Systematic Reviews,* (2). CD004046.

Smith, D. J., Harrison, N., Muir, W., et al. (2005). The high prevalence of bipolar spectrum disorders in young adults with recurrent depression: Toward an innovative diagnostic framework. *Journal of Affective Disorders, 94*(2-3), 167-178.

Smoller, J. W., Sheidley, B. R., & Tsuang, M. T. (2008). *Psychiatric genetics: Applications in clinical practice.* Washington, DC: American Psychiatric Publishing, Inc.

Soares, J. C., & Mann, J. J. (1997). The functional neuroanatomy of mood disorders. *Journal of Psychiatric Review, 31*(4), 393-432.

Stahl, S. (1999). Why settle for silver, when you can go for gold? Response vs recovery as the goal of antidepressant therapy. *Journal of Clinical Psychiatry, 60*(4), 213-214.

Stahl, S. (2000). *Essential psychopharmacology: Neuroscientific basis and practical applications* (2nd ed.). Cambridge, UK: Cambridge University Press.

Statham, A. (1998). Current evidence from animal investigations of a role for early mother-infant relationships in the aetiology of major depressive illness. *Neurosciences in Psychiatry, 1*(2), 40-44.

Stathopoulou, G., Powers, M. B., Berry, A. C., et al. (2006). Exercise interventions for mental health: A quantitative and qualitative review. *Clinical Psychology: Science and Practice, 13,* 179-193.

Steer, R. A., Scholl, T. O., Hediger, M. L., et al. (1992). Self-reported depression and negative pregnancy outcomes. *Journal of Clinical Epidemiology, 5,* 1093-1099.

Stephens, T. (1988). Physical activity and mental health in the United States and Canada: Evidence from four population surveys. *Preventive Medicine, 17,* 35-47.

Stewart, J. W., Quitkin, F. M., & Davies, C. (2006). Atypical depression, dysthymia and cyclothymia. In D. J. Stein, D. J. Kupfer, & A. F. Schatzberg (Eds.), *The American psychiatric publishing textbook of mood disorders* (pp. 547-559). Washington, DC: American Psychiatric Publishing, Inc.

Strickland, C. C. (2006). Suicide in America. *American Psychiatric Nurses Association News, 18*(4), 14.

Strickland, C. C. (2007). Selected new research tidbits. *American Psychiatric Nurses Association News, 19*(1), 12-13.

Tamminga, C. A., Nemeroff, C. B., Blakely, R. D., et al. (2002). Developing novel treatments for mood disorders: Accelerating discovery. *Biological Psychiatry, 52,* 589-609.

Teede, H., Deeks, A., & Moran, L. (2010). Polycystic ovary syndrome: A complex condition with psychological, reproductive, and metabolic manifestations that impact on health across the life span. *BMC Medicine, 8,* 41.

Terman, M., Amira, L., Terman, J. S., et al. (1996). Predictors of response and nonresponse to light treatment for winter depression. *American Journal of Psychiatry, 153*(11), 1423-1429.

Terman, J. S., Terman, M., Schlager, D., et al. (1990). Efficacy of brief, intense light exposure for treatment of winter depression. *Psychopharmacology Bulletin, 26*(1), 3-11.

Thrase, M. (1999). Redefining antidepressant efficacy toward long-term recovery. *Journal of Clinical Psychiatry, 60*(Suppl 6), 15-19.

Thase, M. (2000). Treatment of severe depression. *Journal of Clinical Psychiatry, 61*(Suppl 1), 17-25.

Thase, M. E., Entsuah, A. R., & Rudolph, R. L. (2001). Remission rates during treatment with venlafaxine or selective serotonin reuptake inhibitors. *British Journal of Psychiatry, 178,* 238-241.

The 2006 Progress Report on Brain Research (2006). Advances in Neuorimaging. The DANA Foundation. Retrieved from http://www.dana.org/news/publications/publication.aspx?id=4386

Thomas, R., Insel, M. D., & Charney, M. D. (2003). Research on major depression: Strategies and prevention. *Journal of the American Medical Association, 289*(23), 3167-3168.

Trivedi, M. H., Greer, T., Grannemann, B. D., et al. (2006). Exercise as an augmentation strategy for treatment of major depression. *Journal of Psychiatric Practice, 12*(4), 205-213.

Veen, G., Derijk, R. H., Giltay, E. J., et al. (2009). The influence of psychiatric comorbidity on the dexamethasone/CRH test in major depression. *European Neuropsychopharmacology, 19*(6), 409-415.

Voelker, R. (2003). Researchers probe depression in children. *Journal of the American Medical Association, 289*(23), 3078-3079.

Wagner, K. D. (2006). Treatment of childhood and adolescent disorders. In A. F. Schatzberg & C. B. Nemeroff (Eds.), *Essentials of clinical psychopharmacology* (pp. 949-1007). Washington, DC: American Psychiatric Publishing, Inc.

Wagnild, G., & Collins, J. A. (2009). Assessing resilience. *Journal of Psychosocial Nursing, 47*(12), 28-33.

Wallach, J. (2000). *Interpretation of diagnostic tests* (7th ed.) (p. 200). Philadelphia: Lippincott Williams & Wilkins.

Wang, H., Qi, H., Wang, B. S., et al. (2008). Is acupuncture beneficial in depression: A meta-analysis of 8 randomized controlled trials. *Journal of Affective Disorders, 111*(2), 125-134.

Warner-Schmidt, J. L., & Duman, R. S. (2006). Hippocampal neurogenesis: Opposing effects of stress and antidepressant treatment. *Hippocampus, 16,* 239-249.

Wechsler, D. (1955). *Manual for the Wechsler adult intelligence scale.* New York: The Psychological Corporation.

Wedding, D., Boyd, M. A., & Niemiec, R. M. (2010). *Movies and mental illness 3: Using films to understand psychopathology* (3rd ed.). Cambridge, MA: Hogrefe Publishers.

Weeks, S., McGann, P., Michaels, T., et al. (2003). Comparing various short-form geriatric depression scales leads to the GDS-5/15. *Journal of Nursing Scholarship, 35*(2), 133-137.

Weich, S., Churchill, R., Lewis, G., et al. (1997). Do socio-economic risk factors predict the incidence and maintenance of psychiatry disorder in primary care? *Psychological Medicine, 27,* 73-80.

Weissman, M. M., Bland, R. C., Canino, G. J., et al. (1996). Cross-national epidemiology of major depression and bipolar disorder. *Journal of the American Medical Association, 276*(4), 293-299.

Weissman, M. M., Leaf, P. J., Bruce, M. L., et al. (1988). The epidemiology of dysthymia in five communities: Rates, risks, comorbidity and treatment. *American Journal of Psychiatry, 145,* 815-819.

Weissman, M. M., & Olfson, M. (1995). Depression in women: Implications for health care research. *Science, 269,* 799-801.

Weller, E. B., Sheikh, R. M., Laracy, B. A., et al. (2007). Mood disorders and suicidal behavior. In G. O. Gabbard (Ed.), *Gabbard's treatments of psychiatric disorders* (4th ed.) (pp. 5-27). Washington, DC: American Psychiatric Publishing, Inc.

Westefeld, J. S., Button, C., Haley, J. T., et al. (2006). College student suicide: A call to action. *Death Studies, 30,* 931-956.

White, G. M. (2000). Representing emotional meaning: Category, metaphor, schema, discourse. In M. Lewis & J. M. Haviland-Jones (Eds.), *Handbook of emotions* (pp. 30-44). New York: Guilford Press.

Whooley, M. A., Kiefe, C., Chesney, M. A., et al. (2002). Depressive symptoms, unemployment, and loss of income: The CARDIA Study. *Archives of Internal Medicine, 162,* 2614-2620.

Whyte, E., & Mulsant, B. (2002). Post stroke depression: Epidemiology, pathophysiology and biological treatment. *Biological Psychiatry, 52*(3), 253-264.

Williams, D. R., & Neighbors, H. W. (2006). Social perspectives in mood disorders. In D. J. Stein, D. J. Kupfer, & A. F. Schatzberg (Eds.), *The American psychiatric publishing textbook of mood disorders* (pp. 235-247). Washington, DC: American Psychiatric Publishing, Inc.

Williams, J., & Graham, C. (2006). Acupuncture for older adults with depression—A pilot study to assess acceptability and feasibility. *International Journal of Geriatric Psychiatry, 21,* 599-600.

Williams, S. B., O'Connor, E. A., Eder, M., et al. (2009). Screening for child and adolescent depression in primary care settings: A systematic evidence review for the US Preventive Services Task Force. *Pediatrics, 123,* e716-e735.

Wirz-Justice, A., & Van den Hoofdakker, R. H. (1999). Sleep deprivation in depression: What do we know, where do we go? *Biological Psychiatry, 46,* 445-453.

Wu, J., Buchsbaum, F. S., Gillin, J. C., et al. (1999). Prediction of antidepressant effects of sleep deprivation on metabolic rates in ventral anterior cingulate and medial prefrontal cortex. *American Journal of Psychiatry, 156,* 1149-1158.

Yardley, J. (2002, March 13). Texas jury convicts mother who drowned her children. *New York Times.*

Yesavage, J. A., & Brink, T. L. (1983). Development and validation of a geriatric depression screening scale: A preliminary report. *Journal of Psychiatric Research, 17,* 37-49.

Yonkers, K. A., Lin, H., Howell, H. B., et al. (2008). Pharmacologic treatment of post-partum women with new-onset major depressive disorder: A randomized controlled trial with paroxetine. *Journal of Clinical Psychiatry, 69*(4), 659-665.

Yonkers, K. A., Wisner, K. L., Stewart, D. E., et al. (2009). The management of depression during pregnancy: A report from the American Psychiatric Association and the American College of Obstetricians and Gynecologists. *General Hospital Psychiatry, 31,* 403-413.

Young, A. S., Klap, R., Sherbourne, C. D., et al. (2001). The quality of care for depressive and anxiety disorders in the United States. *Archives of General Psychiatry, 58,* 55-61.

Zagaria, M. A. (2010). Subclinical hypothyroidism. *U. S. Pharmacy, 35*(6), 20-22.

Zarate, C. A., Jr., Singh, J. B., Carlson, P. J., et al. (2006). A randomized trial of an N-methyl-D-aspartate antagonist in treatment-resistant major depression. *Archives of General Psychiatry, 63*(8), 856-864.

Zigmond, A. S., & Snaith, R. P. (1983). The hospital anxiety and depression scale. *Acta Psychiatrica Scandinavica, 67,* 361-370.

Zimmerman, M., & Thongy, T. (2007). How often do SSRIs and other new generation antidepressants lose their effect during continuation treatment? Evidence suggesting the rate of true tachyphylaxis during continuation treatment is low. *Journal of Clinical Psychiatry, 68,* 1271-1276.

Zinbarg, R. E., Barlow, D. H., Liebowitz, M., et al. (1994). The DSM-IV field trial for mixed anxiety-depression. *American Journal of Psychiatry, 151,* 1153-1162.

Zlotnick, C., Miller, I. W., Pearlstein, T., et al. (2006). A preventive intervention for pregnant women on public assistance at risk for postpartum depression. *American Journal of Psychiatry, 163*(8), 1443-1445.

Zuckerman, B., Amaro, H., Bauchner, H., et al. (1989). Depressive symptoms during pregnancy: Relationship to poor health behaviors. *American Journal of Obstetrics and Gynecology, 160,* 1107-1111.

Zung, W. W. K. (1965). A self-rating depression scale. *Archives of General Psychiatry, 12,* 63-70.

Answers to Case Study 13-1 Questions

1. Differential diagnoses include anemia; bereavement; adjustment disorder with depressive features (chronic); dependent personality disorder; post-traumatic stress disorder related to possible abuse; major depressive disorder.
2. Major depressive disorder with melancholic features.
3. Treatment:
   - Psychotherapy: Cognitive behavioral therapy or interpersonal psychotherapy.
   - Pharmacotherapy: Wait to see if psychotherapy is effective. If not, use venlafaxine (Effecor) or mirtazapine (Remeron).
   - Psychosocial interventions:
     - Education: health, finances, and social interactions
     - Problem-solving therapy
     - Assertiveness training
     - Build a social support network
     - Anticipatory guidance
     - Exposure to outdoor light for 30 minutes each day
     - Mild exercise, such as walking

CHAPTER 14

Bipolar Disorders

Eris F. Perese, APRN-PMH

The bipolar disorders are complex, recurring, long-term psychiatric disorders characterized by instability of mood and disturbances of cognition, perception, and behavior (Beynon, Soares-Weiser, Woolacott, et al., 2008). Bipolar disorders affect individuals' functioning in many areas: parenthood, marital and social relationships, work, financial management, and maintaining personal safety. For example, during manic episodes, individuals may put their health, safety, and well-being at risk through excessive spending, risk-taking activities, self-neglect, inappropriate behaviors, and sexual indiscretions (Bauer & Pfennig, 2005; McColm, Brown, & Anderson, 2006). They may be abusive to their children and spouses, and their behaviors often result in marital conflict, financial disasters, and criminal activities that impact the entire family (Stimmel, 2004). Even in remission or periods of euthymia (normal mood state), 60% of patients with bipolar disorder continue to experience impairments in social and vocational functioning (Hirschfeld, Bowden, Gitlin, et al., 2006; Keck, McElroy, Strakowski, et al., 1998; Tohen, Hennen, Zarate, et al., 2000) that result in increased use of mental health services, inability to work, and need for financial assistance (Judd & Akiskal, 2002). The total economic burden (direct and indirect costs) of bipolar I and II disorders in the United States in 2009 was $151 billion (Dilsaver, 2011), which is close to the $174 billion in direct and indirect costs for diabetes in the United States in 2009 (*National Diabetes Fact Sheet*, 2011).

Bipolar disorders include bipolar I disorder, bipolar II disorder, cyclothymic disorder, and bipolar disorder not otherwise specified (Black & Andreasen, 2011).

Bipolar I disorder is characterized by the occurrence of one or more manic episodes or mixed episodes that are usually accompanied by major depressive episodes (American Psychiatric Association, 2000, p. 345). Bipolar I has six separate criteria sets:

1. Single manic episode
2. Most recent episode hypomanic
3. Most recent episode manic
4. Most recent episode mixed
5. Most recent episode depressed
6. Most recent episode unspecified

If the full criteria for bipolar I disorder are met, the disorder can be further defined as

- With specifiers that describe the severity (e.g., mild, moderate, severe without psychotic features, or severe with psychotic features)
- With catatonic features
- With postpartum onset (American Psychiatric Association, 2000, pp. 388-392)

The course of bipolar I disorder can be specified as with and without interepisode recovery, with seasonal pattern, or with rapid cycling. See the *DSM-IV-TR* (American Psychiatric Association, 2000) for specifiers for each criteria set.

Bipolar II disorder is characterized by one or more major depressive episodes that are accompanied by at least one hypomanic episode and the absence of a manic episode or a mixed episode. The symptoms cause distress or impairment of social or vocational functioning or functioning in another area (American Psychiatric Association, 2000, pp. 392-393). For bipolar II, the current or most recent episode may be specified as hypomanic or depressed. If the full criteria for a major depressive episode are met, the current clinical status or features can be specified as

- Mild, moderate, severe without psychotic features, or severe with psychotic features
- Chronic
- With catatonic features
- With melancholic features
- With atypical features
- With postpartum onset

If the full criteria for hypomanic or major depressive episode are not currently met, then the clinical status of the bipolar disorder—the current clinical status of the bipolar II disorder or features of the most recent major depressive episode (only if it is the most recent type of mood episode)—should be specified as

- In partial remission
- In full remission
- Chronic
- With catatonic features
- With melancholic features
- With atypical features
- With postpartum onset (American Psychiatric Association, 2000, p. 397)

The course of bipolar II disorder can be specified as with and without interepisode recovery, with seasonal pattern, or with rapid cycling (see Box 14-1 for more information on rapid cycling) (American Psychiatric Association, 2000, p. 397).

Cyclothymic disorder is a fluctuating mood disturbance characterized by numerous periods of hypomanic symptoms that do not meet the criteria for a manic episode and numerous periods of depressive symptoms that do not meet the criteria for a major depressive episode (American Psychiatric Association, 2000, pp. 398-400). There must be numerous periods of hypomanic symptoms and of depressive symptoms for at least 2 years for adults and 1 year for children and adolescents, and the symptoms must cause clinically significant distress or impairment of social, vocational, or other functioning, and there must have been numerous periods with depressive symptoms that did not meet the criteria for a major depressive episode (American Psychiatric Association, 2000, pp. 398-400).

The diagnosis of *bipolar disorder not otherwise specified* is given to disorders with bipolar features that do not meet the criteria for any specific bipolar disorder. For example, it is used to describe rapid alterations of mood that do not meet the duration criteria for manic, hypomanic, or major depressive episodes; hypomanic episodes without intercurrent depressive episodes; a manic or mixed episode superimposed on delusional disorder, residual schizophrenia, or psychotic disorder not otherwise specified; hypomanic episodes with chronic depressive symptoms that are too infrequent to qualify for a diagnosis of cyclothymic disorder;

BOX 14-1 Bipolar Disorder With Rapid Cycling

Rapid cycling in bipolar disorder can include depressive, manic, hypomanic, and mixed episodes that are separated by one of the following:

- Full or partial remission for at least 2 months
- A switch to an episode at the opposite end of polarity (mania to depressive or depressive to mania) (Ketter & Wang, 2010f). There must be four separate episodes per year (Schneck, Miklowitz, Calabrese, et al., 2004). Note that
- Depressive episodes must last 2 weeks or longer.
- Hypomanic episodes must last 4 days or longer.
- Manic episodes must last 1 week or longer or require hospitalization (American Psychiatric Association, 2000, 427-428).

The cycling may follow a random pattern. The rate of rapid cycling is the same for patients with bipolar I disorder and with bipolar II disorder: about 24% of patients with bipolar disorder develop rapid cycling at some time (Tondo, Baldessarini, Hennen, et al., 1998). Rapid cycling in bipolar II tends to have more depressive episodes (Hirschfeld et al., 2006). Among patients with rapid cycling, 70% to 90% are women (Lewis, 2004). *Ultra-rapid cycling* refers to at least one mood occurrence a day, whereas *ultradian cycling* is used to describe brief episodes of dysphoric hypomania and depression that occur several times during a day (Dubovsky, 2005; Kramlinger & Post, 1996).

Patients with bipolar disorder with rapid cycling tend to have an earlier age of onset of the disorder, more episodes over their lifetime, more depressive symptoms, more severe symptoms, and greater resistance to treatment; in fact, treatment-resistant depression is considered by some to be a hallmark of rapid-cycling bipolar disorder (Calabrese, Shelton, Bowden, et al., 2001). Risk factors for developing rapid cycling include female gender, diagnosis of bipolar II disorder, comorbid alcohol abuse, a family history of substance abuse, and patient's history of hypothyroidism (Frye & Salloum, 2006; Ketter & Wang, 2010f; Vieta, Calabrese, Hennen, et al., 2004).

Treatment

Bipolar disorder with rapid cycling is very challenging to treat. The first steps of treatment are (1) to identify and treat any underlying medical conditions or (2) to identify medications or substances that may be contributing to the rapid cycling, such as alcohol, caffeine, steroids, drugs, or antidepressants, or the presence of hypothyroidism. Because thyroid functioning is commonly associated with depression, thyroid hormones—thyroxin (T4) and triiodothyronine (T3)—are sometimes added to the medications given to patients who are not responding to antidepressants, patients with bipolar disorder who are not responding to mood stabilizers, and patients who have rapid cycling (Seidman, 2006b; Stahl, 2000).

Bipolar disorder with rapid cycling often does not respond well to lithium or carbamazepine. Although divalproex was originally thought to be effective for rapid-cycling bipolar disorder (Swann et al., 1999) its efficacy is now considered to be similar to that of lithium (Calabrese, Keck, MacFadden, et al., 2005). Atypical antipsychotics—olanzapine, quetiapine, risperidone, and aripiprazole—are effective in treating rapid cycling (Ketter & Wang, 2010f) and appear to have greater efficacy than lithium (Keck & McElroy, 2009). Pharmacotherapy for rapid cycling also includes combinations of lithium and divalproex, divalproex and atypical antipsychotics, or lithium and lamotrigine (Hirschfeld et al., 2006). Lamotrigine is often used when there are depressive features, and valproate is used when there are manic or hypomanic features (Hirschfeld et al., 2006). According to Dubovsky (2005), a combination of two or three mood stabilizers or a combination of anticonvulsants and lithium may be necessary.

and situations in which a bipolar disorder is present but it cannot be determined whether it is primary or secondary to a general medical condition or is substance induced (American Psychiatric Association, 2000, pp. 401-402).

This chapter will focus on bipolar I disorder and bipolar II disorder. Historically, researchers have assumed that bipolar II was milder than bipolar I; more recently, however, it has been found that the morbidity of bipolar II is equal to or exceeds that of bipolar I (Rabasseda, 2010). For example, there is no significant difference in the rate of attempted suicide by patients with bipolar I versus bipolar II disorders, and patients with bipolar II use more violent and lethal methods to commit suicide (Novick, Swartz, & Frank, 2010; Rabasseda). Based on this evidence of similar severities of bipolar I and bipolar II, the term "bipolar disorder" will include both bipolar I and bipolar II disorders, and characteristics and treatments of bipolar II that differ from bipolar I will be noted.

Epidemiology

Bipolar disorder is thought of as a chronic recurrent disorder, with half of patients experiencing recurring symptoms. Depressive symptoms or mixed symptoms are the most common, occurring 80% of the time, whereas manic or hypomanic symptoms occur 20% of the time (Baldassano, 2009). Bipolar disorder is associated with high rates of morbidity and disability (Keck & McElroy, 2009). For example, in 1990, the disability associated with bipolar disorder ranked sixth in the Global Burden of Disease Survey (Keck & McElroy; Murray & Lopez, 1996). There is also a high rate of lifetime suicide attempts (29.2%, compared with 15.9% for major depressive disorder) (Citrome & Goldberg, 2005a) and a lifetime suicide rate of 15.05%, which is nearly double the 8.45% suicide rate among patients with schizophrenia (Simon, 2008, p. 1641).

Prevalence

The lifetime prevalence of bipolar disorder in the general population is 3.7% to 3.9% (Kessler, Berglund, Demler, et al., 2005). There is a movement to consider bipolar disorder as a spectrum disorder that would include mania, hypomania, recurrent brief hypomania, sporadic brief hypomania, and cyclomania (Goodwin, Jacobi, Bittner, et al., 2006). If the prevalence rate includes bipolar spectrum disorders, the rate is 6.4% (Stimmel, 2004). Rates of bipolar disorder are higher among single individuals, those who have never married, or those who are separated, divorced, or widowed (Weissman, Bruce, Leaf, et al., 1991).

Age of Onset

The peak age of onset of first symptoms is 15 to 19 years (Bauer & Pfennig, 2005) with approximately one-third of adults with bipolar disorder having developed the illness as children (Hirschfeld et al., 2006). Anticipation—such as earlier onset, greater severity, and more frequent occurrence among individuals with relatives who have the illness—has been observed in bipolar disorder (Geller, Tillman, Bolhofner, et al., 2006; Grigoroiu-Serbanescu, Wickramaratne, Hodge, et al., 1997). Grigoroiu-Serbanescu et al. found a significantly earlier age of onset of bipolar disorder among children who had parents or aunts or uncles with bipolar disorder. To illustrate, among the parents, the mean age of onset of bipolar disorder was 27.5 years, and among their children who developed bipolar disorder, the mean age of onset was 22.5—5 years earlier than their parents.

There is also *late age onset* bipolar disorder, occurring after age 50. Late-onset bipolar disorder is more common in females, and there are more depressive episodes than episodes of mania. Late-onset mania is often due to medical disorders such as trauma, tumors, multiple sclerosis, strokes, hyperthyroidism, AIDS, and systemic lupus erythematosus (Bauer & Pfennig, 2005). It can also be caused by stimulants such as cocaine or alcohol, by psychotropic medications such as antidepressants or stimulants, and by other medications such as anticholinergics, steroids, and thyroxine (Brooks, Sommer, & Ketter, 2010).

Gender

Bipolar I disorder is equally prevalent in men and women. Bipolar II disorder appears to be more common in women (Bauer & Pfenning, 2005). Some women with bipolar disorder experience seasonal and premenstrual changes in mood and behavior (Choi, Baek, Noh, et al., 2011). Women with bipolar disorder with premenstrual exacerbation have a more severe course—more severe symptoms and more relapses (Dias, Lafer, Russo, et al., 2011). Overall, manic episodes are more common in men and depressive episodes are more common in women. Women with bipolar disorder are at increased risk of developing postpartum mood episodes (Suppes, Kelly, & Perla, 2005). Bipolar disorder with rapid cycling, in which four or more episodes occur in 1 year, is more common in women: 80% to 90% of patients with bipolar disorder with rapid cycling are women (Bauer & Pfennig). Women are also more likely to experience manic switches when receiving treatment with antidepressant medications and are more likely to have comorbid medical and psychiatric disorders (Bauer & Pfennig).

Ethnic and Cultural Factors

The prevalence rates of bipolar disorder are similar across races and ethnicity; however, because individuals with bipolar disorder experience the disorder within a cultural framework that has been constructed from their cultural beliefs, values, and norms, there are differences in symptoms, social functioning, and acceptance of treatment (Warren, 2007).

Differences in severity of the illness, presence of comorbidities, and treatment received also exist among different cultural groups (Gonzalez, Thompson, Escamilla, et al., 2007). For example, in African Americans the severity of bipolar disorder may be greater, and the subtypes of mania—mixed mania, rapid cycling, and mania with psychotic features—are more common than pure mania. African Caribbean patients and African American patients with bipolar disorder are less likely to have experienced a depressive episode before the onset of the first episode of mania and are more likely to present with psychotic symptoms such as hallucinations. Those with mania are more likely to show irritability and suspiciousness (Kennedy, Boydell, van Os, et al., 2004). Despite presenting with symptoms of bipolar disorder, African Americans are frequently misdiagnosed as having schizophrenia (Lawson, 1996; Minsky, Vega, Miskimen, et al., 2003). They are more likely to receive antipsychotics than mood stabilizers, more likely to have more hospitalizations, and more likely to have a higher rate of attempted suicides than Caucasians with bipolar disorder (Kupfer, Frank, Grochocinski, et al., 2005; Segal, Bola, & Watson, 1996; Strakowski, McElroy, Keck, et al., 1996). In the study by Gonzalez et al. (2007), Latino patients had more alcohol abuse comorbidity and received fewer psychiatric medication prescriptions and fewer mental health care appointments than European or African American patients.

Risk Factors and Protective Factors

Factors that have been found to be associated with development of bipolar disorder include family history of mood disorders, instability of circadian rhythms, and changes in social rhythms such as sleeping and eating (Bauer, Juckel, Correll, et al., 2008). Other researchers have identified risk factors such as early lack of attachment and childhood abuse, negative stressful life events (interpersonal conflicts, role transitions, and loss of social support), East to West travel, criticism or overinvolvement by relatives, and use of recreational drugs (Alloy, Abramson, Urosevic, et al., 2005; Duckworth, 2008; Hauser, Pfennig, Ozgurdal, et al., 2007). It has been found that use of marijuana is associated with the onset of bipolar disorder at an earlier age (De Hert, Wampers, Jendricko, et al., 2011). Risk factors associated with bipolar disorder with a chronic course include low self-esteem and sense of mastery, an anxious personality, and childhood exposure to persistent family problems (Angst, Gamma, Rossler, et al., 2011).

Protective factors include abstinence from alcohol and recreational drugs, a structured schedule of sleep, work, and social activities, regular exercise, a healthy diet, and presence of a support system (Duckworth, 2008).

Etiology

Bipolar disorder is attributed to an interaction of genetic vulnerabilities, abnormalities of brain development, temperament and personality traits, childhood maltreatment, and stressful life events (Leverich & Post, 2006; Post, 2007). The process of kindling is also considered to be part of the etiological basis of bipolar disorder.

Genetic Influence

The heritability (the amount of variance due to genetic influence) for bipolar disorder may be as high as 80% to 90% (Kieseppa, Partonen, Haukka, et al., 2004). Among individuals with bipolar disorder, half have a relative with a bipolar disorder. Having one first-degree relative with bipolar disorder confers a risk of about 10% for an individual's developing the disorder (Smoller, Sheidley, & Tsuang, 2008). Having two parents with bipolar disorder increases the risk to 70% (Ketter, 2010). Evidence of the strong genetic influence is seen in a concordance rate for bipolar disorder among identical twins that ranges from 40% to 45% according to Smoller et al. (2008) but may be as high as 80% according to McGuffin, Rijsdijk, Andrew, et al. (2003).

The presence of bipolar disorders in first-degree relatives is also associated with an individual's increased risk of developing major depressive disorder (MDD) and attention deficit-hyperactivity disorder (ADHD) (Smoller et al., 2008). For example, Hillegers, Burger, Wals, et al. (2004), in their prospective study of the risk for developing psychopathology among adolescents who had a parent with bipolar disorder, found that 27% of the offspring (12 to 21 years of age) had a mood disorder and 16% had other psychiatric disorders. Their finding of a strong relationship between stressful life events and the risk for developing mood disorders in the adolescents who were genetically vulnerable supports the theory that stress is part of the etiology of bipolar disorder.

Studies suggest that bipolar disorders result from the effect of a small number of mutant genes (Gilliam, Kandel, & Jessell, 2000). In addition, the genetic liability to develop depression appears to overlap with the genetic vulnerability to experience greater exposure to stressful life events, such as assaults, serious marital problems, divorce, loss of employment, financial problems, and illnesses (Kendler & Karkowski-Shuman, 1997)—genetic influences mold the development of temperament or early personality, and personality modulates individuals' selection of life experiences and environments that increase their potential to encounter stressors (Hillegers et al., 2004). In brief, genes influence the decisions that individuals make that put them in harm's way.

Kindling Theory

Kindling (described in Chapter 13) is believed to be involved in bipolar disorder as well as in MDD and seizure disorders (Post, 2007). It is believed that the response to the first stressful event results in long-lasting changes in the brain, including alterations of brain structures, neuronal systems, neurochemistry, and gene expression (Post, 2007). The first stressful event also sensitizes the brain so that experiencing additional stressful life events increases an individual's vulnerability to developing psychiatric disorders (Deak & Panksepp, 2004; Post, 1992, 2007). Whether kindling occurs depends on the balance between risk factors or pathological factors—such as stress and elevated levels of the stress hormone cortisol—and protective or adaptive factors—such as thyrotropin-releasing hormone (TRH) and brain-derived neurotropic factor (BDNF). For example, BDNF is low in episodes of depression and in mania, and it is normal in treated patients and in patients whose mood is euthymic (Post, 2007). The kindling theory of bipolar disorder supports the use of treatment interventions to reduce stress—such as preventing disruptions of social rhythms—and to increase the availability of BDNF through the use of medications such as lithium, valproate (Depakote), and carbamazepine (Tegretol) (Post, 2007).

Stress Theory

The diathesis-stress model proposes that exposure to stressful life events plays a role in the development of major psychiatric disorders. (See Chapters 9 and 13 for more information on the stress response.) Post and Weiss (1995) suggested that stress is the spark that starts the process of developing a bipolar episode of mania or depression. Patients with bipolar disorder report the presence of a major stressor before the *first* episode of bipolar disorder more often than they do with *recurrent* episodes. Potential causes of stress include stressful life events, goal dysregulation, disruption of social rhythms, and family expressed emotion.

Stressful Life Events

Childhood abuse or trauma is associated with an increased risk of developing bipolar disorder. For example, Goldberg and Garno (2005) found that 51% of patients with bipolar disorder had a history of severe childhood maltreatment. Compared with patients with bipolar disorder without a history of childhood abuse, those with a history of childhood abuse had earlier onset of their illness, a more severe course, faster cycling, more suicide attempts, and more comorbid psychiatric disorders (Leverich, McElroy, Suppes, et al., 2002). The patients who had been abused as children reported more negative life stressors before the onset of their first episode of bipolar illness. Leverich and Post (2006) suggested that early childhood abuse results in long-lasting behavioral and neurobiological consequences that put the child at risk for other negative events in life and for an earlier onset and a more severe course of bipolar disorder. Recently it has been found that the adverse experience in early adolescence of being bullied is associated with increased risk of developing bipolar disorder (Vaughn, Fu, Bender, et al., 2010).

Different adverse life events are associated with depressive episodes and manic episodes of bipolar disorder. Negative life events—such as loss of loved ones, lack of social support, criticism or intrusiveness of family members, negative thinking, and low self-esteem—have been found to be linked to the development of depressive episodes within bipolar disorder, but their role in precipitating mania is less certain (Johnson & Roberts, 1995; Miklowitz & Johnson, 2006). Life events associated with symptoms of mania include events that are related to attaining goals—such as being accepted into a desired college, getting married, or being promoted to a higher position at work—and life events that disrupt social rhythms—such as the birth of a baby, traveling across time zones, or working the night shift (Johnson, Cueller, Ruggero, et al., 2008).

Goal Dysregulation

Individuals with bipolar disorder have increased sensitivity to reward (Meyer, Johnson, & Winters, 2001) such as public recognition and wealth (Johnson, Eisner, & Carver, 2009), which may be due to abnormalities of the dopaminergic reward pathways (Johnson, Ruggero, & Carver, 2005). Johnson et al. (2005) suggested that individuals with bipolar disorder may develop an unrealistic level of self-confidence after attaining a desired goal. This overconfidence may lead them to use more energy in pursuing other goals, resulting, for instance, in the tendency of manic patients to pursue rewards without weighing possible negative consequences (Swann, Dougherty, Pazzaglia, et al., 2004).

Disruption of Social Rhythms

Disruption of social rhythms, which may be due to stressful life events, has an influence on bipolar disorder (Phelps, 2008). Patients with bipolar disorder have been found to have had more social disruptive events in their lives during the months before the onset of bipolar disorder than individuals without bipolar disorder.

Social rhythms are regulated by zeitgerbers ("time givers") (Aschoff, 1981; Ehlers, Kupfer, Frank, et al., 1993), which are factors in the environment that set individuals' circadian clocks, such as the sunrise, the timing of meals and social interactions, tasks related to the family, social demands, the presence of another individual in one's life, or work (Frank, Gonzalez, & Fagiolini, 2006). Social rhythms may be disrupted by zeitstorers ("time disrupters"), which are life events such as getting married, having a new baby in the house, having house guests, going on vacation, flying across time zones, working the night shift, and having marital separations (Frank et al.; Phelps, 2008).

Factors that modulate response to disruptions include coping skills, social support, gender, temperament, and the flexibility of the individual's "biological clock" (i.e., the ability to adapt to time changes) (Frank, 2005, p. 21). Social rhythm disruptions associated with the onset of manic episodes of bipolar disorder are thought to be related to disruption of sleep-wake patterns (Umlauf & Shattell, 2005).

Family Expressed Emotion

Family expressed emotion, a construct that is thought to reflect the attitudes of the family or caregivers toward the patient, encompasses expressed criticism and hostility toward a patient and overinvolvement in the patient's life (Yan, Hammen, Cohen, et al., 2004). High expressed emotion is believed to create a stressful environment, and in the families of patients with bipolar disorder it is associated with increased rates of relapse (Butzlaff & Hooley, 1998). Recent evidence suggests that high levels of expressed emotion may influence the development of depressive episodes but not manic episodes (Yan et al.). In general, depressive episodes appear to be influenced by problems with interpersonal relationships, whereas manic episodes appear to be influenced by variables such as sleep disruptions and changes in daily activities (Cohen, Hammen, Henry, et al., 2004; Malkoff-Swartz, Frank, Anderson, et al., 1998).

Biological Basis

The biological basis of bipolar disorder includes structural, functional, neurochemical, and endocrine abnormalities that are associated with deviations of mood regulation, functioning, and behaviors (Soares, 2003). It is believed that the symptoms of bipolar disorder result from dysfunction in the interaction of the prefrontal-subcortical network with the limbic network (amygdala, anterior cingulate cortex, and insula) (Ellison-Wright & Bullmore, 2010; Haldane & Frangou, 2004; Higgins & George, 2007). Evidence-based data about the biological basis of bipolar disorder provides a foundation to guide psychiatric advanced practice nurses in their assessment, generation of diagnosis, case formulation, and development of a treatment plan. Information about the biological basis can be incorporated into psychoeducation for patients and families about the causes of bipolar disorder, the action of medications, and the effect of psychotherapy and psychosocial interventions.

Abnormalities of Brain Structures

Imaging studies of the brain of patients with bipolar disorder have found abnormalities in the ventricles, prefrontal cortex, subgenual cingulate cortex, medial temporal lobe structures (amygdala, hippocampus, thalamus, and striatum), and cerebellum (Hajek, Carrey, & Alda, 2005). These structures are components of mood-regulating neuronal circuits (Monkul, Malhi, & Soares, 2005). The most consistent structural abnormality found in patients with bipolar disorder is decreased gray matter density of the subgenual area of the prefrontal cortex, specifically a 36% reduction of volume of the left subgenual prefrontal cortex (Hajek et al.). Patients with defects of the subgenual prefrontal cortex have been found to demonstrate abnormal autonomic responses to emotional experiences, decreased ability to experience emotions related to concepts that usually evoke emotion, and an inability to adjust their social behavior based on the likelihood that their behavior will result in punishment or reward (Hajek et al., p. 398). It is thought that the structural abnormalities of this area of the brain and its functioning may underlie the symptoms of pathological guilt and mania (Hajek et al.). Other specific brain abnormalities identified by neuroimaging techniques are presented in Table 14-1.

Abnormalities of Brain Cells: Neurons and Glial Cells

As discussed in Chapter 2, neurons that make up the gray matter of the brain carry and receive messages. Glial cells that make up the white matter of the brain provide support for neurons, supplying them with oxygen and glucose. Glial cells also supply neurons with neurotropins, such as nerve growth factor and BDNF, which are involved in the neuron's survival, in the formation of synapses, and in the process of neurotransmission (Rajkowska, 2006). In addition to these functions, glial cells also modulate the excitatory neurotransmitter glutamate. Deficits in functioning of glial cells may result in lack of modulation of glutamate with resulting overexcitement of neuronal cells by glutamate and cell death (Hajek et al., 2005).

Postmortem examination has shown decreased density of both neurons and glial cells in the prefrontal cortex of patients with bipolar disorder (Rajkowska, 2006; Rajkowska, Halaris, & Selemon, 2001). Abnormalities of neurons are thought to be related to impaired functioning of the neural circuits that regulate somatic symptoms, cognition, and emotions (Rajkowska). Abnormalities of glial cells are seen in a reduction of glial cells in specific frontal brain regions, such as in the anterior cingulate cortex, the subgenual prefrontal cortex, the dorsolateral prefrontal cortex, the orbitofrontal cortex, and the hippocampus (Rajkowska) and in the presence of white matter hyperintensities (WMH) (Altshuler, Bookheimer, Townsend, et al., 2005).

WMH are small white areas in the brain that are made up of glial cells. They occur three times more frequently in patients with bipolar disorder than in normal controls (Altshuler, Curran, Hauser, et al., 1995; Moore, El-Badri, Cousins, et al., 2001). WMH impair cortical functioning and damage brain tissue, and they may indicate disruptions in connections of brain areas (Haznedar, Roversi, Pallanti, et al., 2005). Their cause is unknown, but their presence has been linked to a poorer clinical outcome (Moore, Sheperd, Ecceleston, et al., 2001b). One explanation for WMH, proposed by McCracken, Dewar, and Hunter (2001), suggested that there may be a glial vulnerability to oxidative stress; that is, antioxidant defense enzymes may be lower in patients with bipolar disorder. Moore, El-Badri, Cousins, et al. (2001a) found a correlation between season of birth, illness outcome, and white matter lesions, and they suggested that the lesions may be markers of fetal exposure to a toxin or infection.

TABLE 14-1 BRAIN STRUCTURAL ABNORMALITIES IN BIPOLAR DISORDER AND THEIR RELATIONSHIP TO FUNCTIONING

Brain Structural Abnormalities	Relationship to Brain Functioning
Enlargement of cortical sulci and lateral ventricles (Coyle, Kochunov, Patel, et al., 2006; Elkis, Friedman, Wise, et al., 1995)	Enlargement may indicate prenatal maldevelopment of the brain (Voelbel, Bates, Buckman, et al., 2006).
Larger caudate nuclei (Dupont, Jernigan, Heindel, et al., 1995)	Caudate and putamen are part of the basal ganglia that are involved in the cognitive expression of emotion; enlargement may be involved with impulsivity and impairment of problem-solving and planning (Voelbel et al., 2006).
Reduced volume of subgenual prefrontal cortex	Reduced volume may be involved in abnormal autonomic responses to emotional experiences; may be involved in depression and mania (Hajek, Kopecek, Kozeny, et al., 2009).
Decreased hippocampal volume (Blumberg, Kaufman, Martin, et al., 2003; Hajek et al., 2005). Specific reduction of volume of neurons in hippocampus (Konradi, Zimmerman, Yang, et al., 2011).	Hippocampus is involved in learning and memory and is sensitive to the effects of stress; decreased volume may be linked with impairment of cognitive functioning and symptoms of depression (Ellison-Wright & Bullmore, 2010).
Increased left amygdala volume (Brambilla, Harenski, Nicoletti, et al., 2003); enlargement of the amygdala (Berns & Nemeroff, 2003; Strakowski, DelBello, Sax, et al., 1999); however, a meta-analysis of left and right amygdala volume revealed no change in bipolar disorder (Hajek et al., 2009).	Left amygdala is thought to be involved in processing emotional experiences, such as fear, happiness, and sadness; Involvement of amygdala in bipolar disorder is not known (Arnone, Cavanagh, Gerber, et al., 2009).
Decreased pituitary volumes (Sassi, Nicoletti, Brambilla, et al., 2001)	Decreased volume may be associated with impaired hypothalamic-pituitary-adrenal functioning that is involved in emotional expression and regulation of emotions (Sassi et al., 2001)
Enlargement of the thalamus (Strakowski et al., 1999); however, no difference in the thalamus of patients with bipolar disorder was found by Caetano, Sassi, Brambilla, et al. (2001)	Thalamus is involved in information processing and relaying neuronal activity to the cerebral cortex. Role in bipolar disorder is not clear.
Reduced left anterior cingulate cortex volumes (Sassi et al., 2001)	Left anterior cingulate cortex is involved in emotional expression and regulation of emotions; reduction may be involved in symptoms of depression and impairment of cognition (Beckman, Johansen-Berg, & Rushworth, 2009; Brooks, Wang, Bonner, et al., 2009).
Smaller prefrontal lobe volumes (Berns & Nemeroff, 2003)	Prefrontal lobe is involved in mood, emotional arousal, judgment, and adaptive behaviors. Reduced volume of prefrontal lobe that interacts with the limbic system may underlie affective and psychotic symptoms of bipolar disorder (Strakowski, DelBello, & Adler, 2005).

WMH are not specific to patients with bipolar disorder. They are also found in older adults, especially those with hypertension and cerebrovascular disease and with late-onset bipolar disorder. It is thought that vascular WMH may be linked to late-onset bipolar disorder through the damage that they cause to the frontolimbic circuits that are involved in mania (Zanetti, Cordeiro, & Busatto, 2007).

Abnormalities of Brain Functioning

Computed tomography, magnetic resonance imaging, positron emission tomography, single-photon emission computed tomography, functional magnetic resonance imaging, and magnetic resonance spectroscopy are used to study the relationship between brain structures and brain functioning and other variables such as brain blood flow and glucose metabolism (Mayberg, 2006, p. 219). Brain imaging studies have shown abnormalities of functioning in certain areas of the brains of patients with bipolar disorder, including the frontal lobes, the cingulate gyrus, the caudate, and the orbitofrontal cortex. These areas are involved in regulation of mood and in language and memory (Blumberg, Stern, Martinez, et al., 2000; Blumberg, Stern, Rickets, et al., 1999; Shirtcliff, Vitacco, Graf, et al., 2009). There is reduced activity of the prefrontal and anterior cingulate cortexes during episodes of bipolar disorder and also during remission, and there is persistently increased activity of the amygdala (Haldane & Frangou, 2004).

Abnormalities of brain functioning are also identified by neurological examination and neuropsychological evaluation. On neurological examination, patients with bipolar disorder display a higher rate of soft neurological signs than control subjects, but a lower rate than patients with schizophrenia, suggesting less severe prenatally compromised development of the brain (Torrey & Knable, 2002). (See Chapter 2 for discussion of brain development.) On neuropsychological evaluation, patients with bipolar disorder demonstrate abnormalities in mental processes such as intelligence, psychomotor speed, attention, memory, visual-spatial skills, and executive functioning (Antila, Partonen, Kieseppa, et al., 2009). They also show neurophysiological differences such as increased speed of association between thoughts (the physiology underlying flight of ideas), faster reaction time and rate of speech, and impaired visual processing (Torrey & Knable). On clinical evaluation, patients with bipolar disorder have been found to have impairment of cognitive functioning, especially executive functioning that includes ability to plan, weigh consequences, and shift strategies (Frangou, 2005; Rossi, 2000). These deficits in cognitive function are also present in family members who do not have bipolar disorder, which suggests that there is a genetic heritability of cognitive functioning. It also suggests that deficits of cognitive functioning in bipolar disorder are present before onset of the illness rather than being the result of the illness.

The impairment of the ability of patients with bipolar disorder to plan and weigh consequences has clinical implications for psychiatric advanced practice nurses. In planning interventions that will reduce risk of relapse or recurrence and move patients toward recovery, psychiatric advanced practice nurses need to incorporate interventions that compensate for cognitive impairment (see Chapter 8).

Abnormalities of Brain Chemistry

Anatomical abnormalities in the prefrontal cortex of patients with bipolar disorder are associated with abnormalities of the neurotransmitter systems that are involved in modulating emotions: serotonin, norepinephrine, and dopamine. In considering the possible relationship of specific neurotransmitters to bipolar disorder, it must be kept in mind that many neurotransmitters interact with each other and with other brain chemicals, such as the hormones of the hypothalamic-pituitary-adrenal axis (Seidman, 2006a).

In the past, it was believed that decreased dopamine activity was associated with the depressive phase of bipolar disorder and that increased dopamine activity was associated with the manic phase (Anand & Charney, 2000). It is now thought that there are region-specific alterations of dopamine activity (Cousins, Butts, & Young, 2009). For example, reduced dopamine activity has been found in the reward pathways of the brain during acute mania, suggesting that diminished activity of the dopaminergic system may be involved in the excessive or abnormal pursuit of goals often seen during episodes of mania (Abler, Greenhouse, Ongur, et al., 2008). Patients with bipolar disorder have evidence of a decrease in the levels of both gamma-aminobutyric acid, which inhibits neuronal excitability and activity (Petty, Rush, Davis, et al., 1996), and *N*-acetylaspartic acid, a neurochemical that is needed for healthy neurons (Winsberg, Sachs, Tate, et al., 2000).

Abnormalities of chemistry associated with bipolar disorder also include abnormalities of the neuropeptides that serve as intracellular second messengers (Torrey & Knable, 2002). The second-messenger system—the signal transduction system—carries messages within the cell. Neuropeptides also function as neurotransmitters and influence other neurotransmitters and neurohormones. Neuropeptides that are being studied in relation to depression and bipolar disorder are endorphins, somatostatin, vasopressin, oxytocin, substance P, cholecystokinin, neurotensin, and calcitonin (Torrey & Knable).

Abnormalities of Endocrine Functioning

The relationship between dysfunction of the endocrine system—especially the thyroid gland—and the hypothalamic-pituitary-adrenal axis in bipolar disorder has been studied extensively over time based on the finding that diseases of the thyroid and adrenal glands may produce depression, hyperactivity, or mood elevation.

Hypothyroidism is often accompanied by depressed mood, and *hyperthyroidism* is often accompanied by increased energy and euphoria. Patients with Cushing's disease, in which the adrenal gland secretes excessive cortisol, may experience affective lability, depression, elevated mood, and psychotic symptoms (Price, Goetz, & Lovell, 2010; Torrey & Knable, 2002).

The endocrine system is regulated to some degree by the hypothalamus, which is thought to be involved in bipolar disorder. The hypothalamus is regulated by pituitary, thyroid, adrenal, and sex glands (Torrey & Knable, 2002), and it modulates the functions that are often abnormal in patients with bipolar disorder—sleep, appetite, and sexual drive. The hypothalamus circuit has three phases:

1. First, the hypothalamus secretes TRH.
2. Next, TRH stimulates the pituitary gland to secrete thyroid-stimulating hormone (TSH).
3. Finally, TSH stimulates the thyroid gland to release thyroid hormones.

In patients with bipolar disorder, there may be abnormalities in one or all three phases of the circuit. Moderate to severe mood symptoms of bipolar disorder have been found to be associated with a reduced TSH response to TRH (Larsen, Faber, Christensen, et al., 2004), and about half of patients with rapid-cycling bipolar disorder (four or more episodes in 12 months) are likely to have hypothyroidism (Esposito, Prange, & Golden, 1997).

The hypothalamus also secretes corticotropin-releasing factor, which stimulates the pituitary gland to release adrenocorticotropin; in turn, adrenocorticotropin stimulates the adrenal gland to release cortisol. Patients with depression and bipolar disorder have been found to have abnormalities of this circuit (Torrey & Knable, 2002).

Clinical Presentation

Clinical presentation varies depending on what type of episode (depressed, manic, or mixed) and what phase of the disorder that the patient is experiencing. Phases include prodromal, acute, continuation, and maintenance (Ketter, Wang, & Culver, 2010).

In the prodromal phase, patients do not meet the criteria for a manic episode or a major depressive episode, but they do notice changes in thoughts, feelings, and behaviors (Breit-Gabauer, Berg, Demelbauer, et al., 2010). The time from when the first symptoms occur until a diagnosis of bipolar disorder is determined and treatment is begun may be 5 to 10 years (Baldessarini, Tondo, & Hennen, 2003).

The prodromal phase is followed by the acute phase (Bauer et al., 2008). The acute phase usually lasts 3 to 8 weeks, and the symptoms are syndromal; that is, they meet the criteria for bipolar disorder. Patients are most often seen for evaluation in the acute phase, although some may be seen in prodromal phase.

The continuation phase usually lasts 2 to 6 months, and symptoms may be subsyndromal or absent. The maintenance phase is indefinite, and symptoms are absent or limited to one or two. Patients in continuation phase and maintenance phase are usually seen during monitoring of response to treatment. Continuation and maintenance phases will be discussed in the treatment section.

Prodromal Phase

In sharp contrast to the abundance of research related to the prodromal phase of schizophrenia and to evidence-based preventive interventions, interest in the prodromal phase of bipolar disorder and in identifying preventive interventions is a recent phenomenon (Bauer et al., 2008; Breit-Gabauer et al., 2010). Among adults who are in the prodromal phase of mania, changes include reduced sleep, increased activity, increased talkativeness, euphoria, racing thoughts, irritability or sensitivity, spending of money, and promiscuous sexual behavior. In the prodromal phase of depression, changes include decline in energy and interest in activities and people, difficulty concentrating, sadness, increased need for sleep, and rumination about fears and worries (Breit-Gabauer et al.). In the prodromal phase, patients often present in general medical settings with physical symptoms, such as difficulty sleeping, or with symptoms of depression, anxiety, or substance abuse (Hirschfeld, 2005). They may describe specific problems with functioning—emotional, social, interpersonal, occupational, and financial—or less obvious impairments of functioning such as getting tired very easily, being less sentimental and empathic than others, being less helpful to others, not having a strong purpose in life, and having less control of impulses (Baldassano, 2009; Engstrom, Brandstrom, Sigvardsson, et al., 2004).

Patients often do not identify the changes that they are experiencing as premonitory symptoms of bipolar disorder (Breit-Gabauer et al., 2010). However, the sooner interventions are instituted in the prodromal phase, the more likely it is that a full episode can be prevented (Jackson, Cavanagh, & Scott, 2003). Interventions that can be used to prevent an episode of mania include calming activities (reading, listening to music), regular meals and rest periods, relaxation strategies, talking with friends and relatives, visiting the clinician for adjustment of medication, avoiding changes such as starting new projects, or going on vacation. Interventions that can be used to prevent an episode of depression include visiting the clinician for adjustment of medications, walking or sports, social contact, doing something enjoyable (music, reading, art, or cooking), and limiting intake of caffeine and alcohol (Breit-Gabauer et al., 2010). Prodromal signs also occur before mania relapse and depression relapse (Keltner, Solomon, Ryan, et al., 1996). Approximately two-thirds of patients experience prodromal symptoms before relapse. Prodromal signs of manic and depressive relapse in order of frequency of occurrence are listed in Table 14-2.

Acute Phase

During the acute phase, the patient may exhibit signs of depression, impulsivity, irritability, agitation, and substance use; the patient may also describe insomnia and problems with relationships. Patients often show impairment of executive functioning and strong emotional reactions to successes and rewards that they have achieved (Antila et al., 2009). They may describe a strong interest in achieving greater rewards, such as being more popular or acquiring more wealth (Johnson & Fulford, 2009; Johnson et al., 2009). Patients often do not volunteer a history of past mood disturbances. The psychiatric advanced practice nurse should inquire about any family history of mood disorders and ask if the patient has a history of risk-taking behaviors, suicidal thoughts or attempts, violent behavior toward others or toward property, and psychotic symptoms such as hallucinations and delusions (Hirschfeld et al., 2006). Upon questioning, the patient may give a history of early onset of symptoms, episodes of mania or hypomania, and failure to respond to prescribed medications. Family history may include depressive or bipolar disorder, treatment with medications and electroconvulsive therapy (ECT), and suicidality.

The acute phase can consist of depressive episodes, manic episodes (bipolar I), hypomanic episodes (bipolar II), or mixed episodes.

TABLE 14-2 PRODROMAL SIGNS OF DEPRESSIVE AND MANIC RELAPSE IN ORDER OF FREQUENCY OF OCCURRENCE

Prodromal Signs of Depression	Prodromal Signs of Mania
Mood change	Sleep disturbance
Increased anxiety	Psychotic symptoms
Psychomotor change	Mood change
Appetite change	Psychomotor change
Suicidal ideation	Appetite change
Sleep disturbance	Increased anxiety

Sources: Jackson, Cavanagh, & Scott, 2003; Perry, Tarrier, Morriss, et al., 1999.

Clinical Presentation of Depressive Episodes (Bipolar I and II)

Bipolar disorder is more likely to begin with an episode of depression than with an episode of mania or hypomania; overall, individuals with bipolar disorder have more and longer episodes of depression than episodes of mania (Strakowski & Shelton, 2006). Depressive episodes are characterized by sadness and anhedonia plus at least five other symptoms for most of the day nearly every day for 2 weeks (Ketter, 2010). The depression may be characterized by hopelessness, negativity, suicidal ideation, inability to concentrate and to problem solve, sleep disturbances, loss of energy, decreased self-esteem, guilt, feelings of worthlessness, thought blocking, forgetfulness, obsessional thoughts, and suicidality. Patients experience high levels of distress, disability, and impairment of functioning, including occupational functioning (Judd, Akiskal, Schettler, et al., 2002). The symptoms vary in severity and may include psychosis (Ketter, 2010).

Although depressive symptoms are present in both MDD and bipolar disorder in the depressive phase, the presentation differs. Patients with bipolar disorder in the depressive phase have an earlier onset of mood symptoms, more episodes of depression, a higher rate of melancholic-type depression, and more psychotic symptoms than patients with MDD (Sharma, 2005). Bipolar depression is less likely to be associated with anxiety, tearfulness, and initial insomnia (Mitchell, Goodwin, Johnson, et al., 2008) but more likely to be associated with feelings of worthlessness, anhedonia, restlessness, leaden paralysis, and hypersomnia (Mitchell et al.). While there is considerable overlapping, the symptoms of bipolar disorder and MDD do differ (Table 14-3).

Clinical Presentation of Manic Episodes (Bipolar I)

Bipolar I is characterized by one or more manic episodes or mixed episodes. The onset of mania is often sudden. There are changes in mood, cognition, speech, appearance, and behaviors, and there are often somatic symptoms and changes in hygiene and grooming; there may also be psychotic symptoms (McColm et al., 2006):

- ***Mood.*** The mood may be elated or euphoric, angry, irritable, or hostile and aggressive. The patient may be easily excited, and there may be tearfulness alternating with good humor (Cookson, 2005).
- ***Cognition.*** Thinking is often characterized by grandiose and expansive ideas, racing thoughts, flight of ideas, lack of insight, and delusions that fit the mood (St. John, 2005). Cognitive impairment may be evidenced as distractibility, inability to concentrate, and executive dysfunction (Joska & Stein, 2008).
- ***Speech.*** There may be increased output of speech. Speech may be pressured, and the patient may describe a sense of being connected to the world (Joska & Stein, 2008, p. 464). Patients in the manic phase tend to talk very rapidly, display circumstantiality (including details and asides before eventually reaching the point), and express an inflated view of their abilities, wealth, and status (Cookson, 2005).
- ***Somatic symptoms.*** Somatic symptoms include decreased need for sleep, decreased appetite, excessive energy, and significant weight loss. There may be psychomotor agitation that includes using excessive gestures and hurried, clumsy movements.
- ***Appearance.*** The patient's appearance may seem untidy and neglected. Dress may be inappropriate or overdone

TABLE 14-3 SYMPTOMS OF MAJOR DEPRESSIVE DISORDER AND BIPOLAR DISORDER, DEPRESSIVE PHASE

Major Depressive Disorder	Bipolar Disorder, Depressive Phase
Insomnia, reduced amount of sleep, early morning waking	Hypersomnia and increased daytime napping
Poor appetite; weight loss	Hyperphagia; increased weight gain
Normal or increased activity; restlessness	Psychomotor retardation
Somatic complaints	Feelings of leaden paralysis
Sadness and anhedonia	Marked anhedonia; hopelessness and negativity
Anxiety and tearfulness	Lack of anxiety and tearfulness
Excessive guilt	Psychotic features including hallucinations, delusions, and pathological guilt
Impaired memory and executive functioning	Greater impairment of memory and executive functioning
Symptoms of worthlessness, low self-esteem, and social withdrawal	Symptoms of worthlessness, low self-esteem, and social withdrawal; hostility, violence and suicidal ideation; obsessive thoughts
Melancholic type less frequent	Melancholic type most frequent, with psychotic features more frequent. Symptoms of pathological guilt
No family history of bipolar disorder	Family history of bipolar disorder
Later onset of first depressive episode, after 25 years of age	Early onset of first episode of depression, before 25 years of age

Sources: Hirschfeld, 2005; Mitchell et al., 2008; Parker, Roy, Wilhelm, et al., 2000; Sharma, 2005; St. John, 2005.

and flamboyant (Cookson, 2005). Patients may neglect normal hygiene practices (showering, shaving, combing their hair, brushing their teeth, and changing dirty clothes).

- *Behavior.* Patients with bipolar disorder in the manic phase have increased goal-directed activity. That activity may be directed toward social goals, work accomplishments, or sexual activities. There may be excessive involvement in pleasurable activities that have a risk for adverse results. For example, there may be indiscreet behaviors as a result of diminished social inhibition and impaired judgment such as impulsive, pleasurable, but risky behaviors that are not characteristic of the patient when he or she is not experiencing mania, e.g., lying, buying sprees, gambling, traveling, substance use, social intrusiveness, and sexual indiscretions (Cookson, 2005; Joska & Stein, 2008).
- *Psychotic symptoms.* Psychotic symptoms include grandiose ideas, hallucinations, and delusions (Black & Andreasen, 2011). Hallucinations are usually auditory hallucinations, a voice telling the individual something exciting (Cookson, 2005). Delusions are often beliefs that the individual has supernatural powers (ability to heal people or to fly); that he or she is important and wealthy; and that he or she has a special mission to complete (McColm et al., 2006).

In addition to the presence of significant euphoria, expansiveness, or irritability a diagnosis of manic episode requires three of the following symptoms (or four if the only other symptom is irritability): inflated self-esteem; decreased need for sleep; overtalkativeness; flight of ideas; distractibility; excessive goal-directed activities; psychomotor agitation; or impulsivity for at least a week or a briefer time if hospitalization was required (Black & Andreasen, 2011; Ketter, 2010, p. 12).

Case Study 14-1 illustrates the onset of an episode of mania in a woman with bipolar disorder.

Clinical Presentation of Mixed Episodes (Bipolar I)

A mixed episode is characterized by symptoms that meet the criteria for both manic episode and major depressive episode (except for duration) nearly every day during at least a 1-week period (American Psychiatric Association, 2000, p. 365; Black & Andreasen, 2011; Ketter, 2010). The depressive symptoms tend to occur more often early in the day and the manic symptoms later in the day. The mixed episode must be severe enough to cause impairment of functioning in social or work roles or to require hospitalization. It may be characterized by psychotic symptoms that require hospitalization (American Psychiatric Association, 2000, p. 362; Ketter & Wang, 2010a, 2010b). Mixed episodes may be a combined syndrome; a transitional state in which the patient is moving from one mood pole to the other, such as depression to mania; or ultradian cycling (cycling within a day) (Ketter, 2010). Mixed episodes can evolve from mania or depression and are characterized by extreme distress, irritability, psychomotor agitation, sexual excitement, fatigue, racing thoughts, and anxiety (Lewis, 2004). There may be rapidly alternating moods—such as sadness or irritability, agitation, insomnia, psychotic features, and suicidal ideation. Mixed episodes may last for weeks or for several months. They may remit or evolve into a major depressive episode (American Psychiatric Association, 2000, p. 363).

CASE STUDY 14-1

The Onset of an Episode of Mania in a Woman With Bipolar Disorder

Waiting in the Florida noonday sun for the shuttle bus that will take her from the airport to the hotel where the psychiatric nursing conference is being held, Colleen, a psychiatric nursing student, could not help noticing one of the women who was also waiting for the shuttle. The woman introduces herself as Gretchen, "Fetching Gretchen," she says. She begins to talk in a lively, rapid manner and in a very short time has told everyone waiting at the bus stop that she is 34 years old, owns her own decorating business, has just been dumped by her boyfriend, and has not slept for 2 days. She goes on to say that she has left the cold gray days of Seattle behind and intends to party all night. Still talking, she slides into the seat next to Colleen and insists that Colleen join her that evening for "some fun on the beach." She laughs and says, "From now on, it is going to be thrills, not pills."

Late in the afternoon the next day, Colleen notices a sunburned and exhausted-looking Gretchen shouting at the hotel cashier who has refused to cash her check for $10,000. Gretchen spies Colleen and shouts, "There is my best friend. She will tell you that my check is good. We are going to buy a sailboat together." When the manager says that he is unable to cash the check, Gretchen becomes verbally abusive and threatens to "tear the place apart if you don't cash my check." When Gretchen continues screaming at the manager and pounding on the counter, the manager calls the police.

As Gretchen is being removed by the police, she begs Colleen to help her. The manager asks Colleen, since she is Gretchen's friend, if she will go with her. Colleen explains that she has only just met Gretchen but yes, she will accompany her. Colleen bases her decision on her understanding of the Good Samaritan law. In the hospital emergency room, Colleen provides what information she can, and the ER team manages to elicit from Gretchen that she had been taking lamotrigine (Lamictal) but stopped taking it. They admit Gretchen and treat her for a manic episode.

Questions

1. What factors may have precipitated the episode of mania?
2. What symptoms of mania did Gretchen display?
3. What were safety issues?
4. How is the Good Samaritan law relevant?

Answers to these questions can be found at the end of this chapter.

Clinical Presentation of Hypomanic Episodes (Bipolar II)

Bipolar II is characterized by one or more major depressive episodes and by at least one hypomanic episode. Hypomania differs from mania by degree of functional impairment. In comparison to patients with mania, patients with hypomania are usually able to continue to function at work and in their social relationships. They do not experience psychosis nor require hospitalizations, and the duration of their episodes is shorter, 4 days instead of 7 days (Ketter, 2010).

Hypomania is characterized by a lively, happily euphoric mood; carefree, unrealistic thinking; a witty, joking attitude; and being unaware or uncaring of others' feelings. Patients with hypomania can be full of energy and enthusiasm, but they are not able to pursue their ideas to a goal-directed end and their mood swings to anger and irritation if others criticize their plans. They also have racing thoughts and poor concentration; they use jokes, puns, sarcasm, and needling; they have difficulty following through on projects; and they have no insight into their behaviors. Patients with hypomania may also increase the following activities: smoking, consuming alcohol, or both; engaging in superficial relationships; talking, joking, or teasing; meddling; and making frequent telephone calls or writing letters (St. John, 2005).

Comorbidity

Patients with bipolar disorder have high rates of other psychiatric disorders: Axis I psychiatric disorders, Axis II psychiatric disorders, and suicide. They also have high rates of medical disorders.

Axis I Psychiatric Disorders

Other psychiatric disorders—such as anxiety disorders, affective disorders, and substance use disorders—co-occur in two-thirds of patients with bipolar disorder (Goodwin et al., 2006). Among patients with bipolar disorder and comorbid psychiatric disorders, about 90% will have a co-occurring anxiety disorder, such as panic disorder (Hirschfeld, 2005); 60% will experience alcohol dependence; and 50% will experience drug dependence (Kessler, McGonagle, Zhao, et al., 1994). These comorbid psychiatric disorders are associated with more episodes of bipolar, relapse, readmission to the hospital, poor social outcomes, and slower recovery (Kosten & Kosten, 2004).

Axis II Psychiatric Disorders: Personality Disorders

Among patients with bipolar disorder, 29% to 48% will have at least one co-occurring personality disorder. The most frequent are narcissistic, borderline, antisocial, and obsessive-compulsive personality disorders (Brieger, Ehrt, & Marneros, 2003; Citrome & Goldberg, 2005b). (See Chapter 18 for information on personality disorders.) The comorbidity of one or more personality disorders increases the risk for suicide, impedes response to treatment, and is associated with lower recovery rates (Citrome & Goldberg; Dunayevich, Sax, Keck, et al., 2000).

Suicide

Bipolar disorder has a higher rate of suicide than any other psychiatric disorder (Miklowitz & Johnson, 2006). The risk for suicide is equally high for bipolar I disorder and bipolar II disorder (Novic et al., 2010). Among patients with bipolar disorder, 30% have made at least one suicide attempt (Bauer & Pfennig, 2005). Other researchers say that between 25% and 60% of patients with bipolar disorder will attempt suicide at some time in their lives (Goodwin & Jamison, 1990). Twenty percent of patients with bipolar disorder die by suicide (Bauer & Pfennig). Suicide attempts are more common among younger patients with bipolar disorder, tend to occur in the early phases of their illness and during a depressive phase (Fagiolini, Kupfer, Rucci, et al., 2004; Mitchell & Malhi, 2004), and occur more often among patients who have had a family member die by suicide (Tsai, Kuo, Chen, et al., 2002).

The fact that the risk for suicide is as high among patients with bipolar II disorder as it is among patients with bipolar I disorder has serious clinical implications for psychiatric advanced practice nurses. Nurses must assess for suicidal ideation in patients with bipolar II disorder—which has erroneously been thought to be a milder version because the patient does not experience manic episodes—with the same thoroughness and frequency as they do for patients with bipolar I disorder, and they must institute interventions that target immediate and long-term suicide risk factors. Box 14-2 provides risk factors and protective factors for suicide among patients with bipolar disorder. Note that protective factors are factors that *reduce* the risk of suicide. The level of suicide lethality and presence of protective factors of each patient with bipolar disorder should be evaluated at every clinical visit across all phases of treatment (Sachs, Yan, Swann, et al., 2001). A suicide lethality assessment (Box 14-3) should be done for every patient with a mood disorder at every visit.

Based on the level of lethality and presence of suicide risk factors, appropriate preventive strategies should be initiated. The three strategies that have been found to be effective are

1. Using emergency care procedures, e.g., reducing access to lethal means, such as firearms; preventing isolation; increasing social support; and hospitalization (Sachs et al., 2001)
2. Training the patient in using problem-solving skills
3. Using comprehensive interventions that include problem-solving and skill building to compensate for cognitive, social, emotional, and distress-tolerance deficits (Gray & Otto, 2001)

BOX 14-2 Risk Factors and Protective Factors for Suicide Among Patients With Bipolar Disorder

Risk Factors

- Prior suicide attempt (patients with bipolar disorder and previous suicide attempts are at the highest risk for suicide) (Sachs et al., 2001)
- Presence of symptoms of pervasive insomnia, agitation, and impulsivity (Fawcett, 2001)
- Severe depression with feelings of hopelessness (Ketter, 2010)
- Self-blame and feelings of hopelessness during a depressive episode
- Increased number of stressful life events (Garno, Goldberg, Ramirez, et al., 2005)
- Disruption of social and occupational functioning
- Social isolation
- Recent loss or losses (death of a parent or partner, divorce, loss of a job, and loss of housing)
- Poor response to treatment
- Early age of onset
- High rate of depressive episodes
- History of antidepressant-induced mania
- Co-occurring personality disorders
- Co-occurring panic disorder, other anxiety disorders, and psychosis (Ketter, 2010).
- Family history of suicide
- Comorbid substance abuse (Slama, Bellivier, Henry, et al., 2004), which doubles the risk for suicide (Comtois, Russo, Roy-Byrne, et al., 2004)
- Absence of a reason for living (Ketter, 2010).

Protective Factors

- A moral objection to suicide
- Fear of social disapproval
- Sense of responsibility for the family
- Presence of plans for the future
- A reason for living

Adapted from Torrey & Knable, 2002.

BOX 14-3 Suicide Lethality Assessment

Assessment of Current Status of Suicidality

1. Presence of suicidal ideas or intent, specific thoughts of death or suicide.
2. Presence of a plan to commit suicide and lethality of plan. More detailed plans are associated with higher risk.
3. Access to means for suicide (firearms, medications, or poisons) and the lethality of those means
4. Presence of command hallucinations, other psychotic symptoms, or severe anxiety
5. Presence of alcohol or substance use.
6. Prior history of suicide attempts, a major risk factor for suicide attempts and for death by suicide.
7. Presence of family history of suicide or recent exposure to suicide. Family history of suicide is associated with a four times greater risk of suicide,

Assessment of Factors That Contribute to Suicidal Behavior

In addition to using the suicide lethality assessment form to determine the level of risk for suicide (high, medium, or low), psychiatric advanced practice nurses should remember that suicide risk is estimated by determining the presence or absence of the following:

- Demographic factors; male gender; widowed, divorced, or single status; younger and older age groups; white race; and occupation. (Risk of suicide is highest among physicians and dentists but also increased among nurses, social workers, artists, mathematicians, and scientists [Stack, 2001].)
- High risk factors: presence of a psychiatric disorder (major depressive disorder, bipolar disorder, schizophrenia, and cluster B personality disorders); prior suicide attempts; hopelessness; alcohol abuse; cocaine abuse; and recent loss of an important relationship
- Acute risk factors: anxiety, persistent insomnia, panic attacks, delusions, and sense of hopelessness
- Protective factors: sense of responsibility to family, children in the family, pregnancy, moral objections to suicide, religious beliefs, coping and problem-solving skills, employment, financial stability, and social connectedness)

Adapted from Jacobs, Baldessarini, Conwell, et al. (2006). Practice guideline for the assessment and treatment of patients with suicidal behaviors. In American psychiatric association practice guideline for the assessment and treatment of patients with suicidal behaviors (pp. 1315-1495). Washington, DC: American Psychiatric Publishing, Inc.

Some clinicians—more than half of 267 psychiatrists surveyed—use a verbal or written no-suicide contract in which the patient agrees to abstain from suicide and to inform a relative or care provider of suicidal intent. However, among the psychiatrists using no-suicide contracts, 27% reported that a patient had attempted suicide after agreeing to the no-suicide contract (Kroll, 2000). Chapter 13 contains more information on suicide.

Medical Disorders

About 22% of patients with bipolar disorder have co-occurring medical conditions such as migraine headaches, obesity, diabetes; cardiovascular, respiratory, gastrointestinal, urogenital disorders; multiple sclerosis, HIV infections, and hepatitis C infection (Beyer, Kuchibhatla, Gersing, et al., 2005; McIntyre, Konarski, & Yatham, 2004; Stimmel, 2004). Even higher rates of comorbid medical conditions have been reported. For example, Fenn, Bauer, Altshuler, et al. (2005) found that 81% of the patients with bipolar disorder that they studied had comorbid medical conditions, including coronary heart disease, hypertension, hyperthyroidism, diabetes, or hepatitis. Not only do hypertension and cardiovascular disease occur more frequently among patients with bipolar disorder than among those without bipolar disorder, but their onset is 13 to 14 years earlier (Goldstein, Fagiolini, Houck, et al., 2009).

Patients with bipolar disorder are at increased risk of premature death from medical illnesses in comparison to the general population, cardiovascular disease being responsible for the majority of premature deaths among patients with bipolar disease (Roshanaei-Moghaddam & Katon, 2009). Premature death may be associated with several factors, including smoking, alcohol and substance abuse, poor diet, sedentary lifestyle, obesity, and chronic stress (Roshanaei-Moghaddam & Katon). In addition, clinicians managing the care of patients with bipolar disorder may fail to inquire about medical problems and lifestyle practices. This failure to address medical problems follows the "competing needs theory" (Roshanaei-Moghaddam & Katon, p. 147) whereby clinicians give precedence to problems that require immediate attention and delay addressing less critical problems.

Differential Diagnosis

Bipolar disorder must be differentiated from other psychiatric disorders and from other conditions that can cause disturbed behaviors, psychotic symptoms, depression, mania, or mania-like behavior. Mania may be caused by medical conditions, certain prescribed medications, and substance use (Joska & Stein, 2008). Medical conditions include neurological disorders, such as multiple sclerosis or traumatic brain injury; infectious diseases, such as neurosyphilis and HIV or AIDS; tumors of the central nervous system; endocrine disorders, such as hypothyroidism and hyperthyroidism; diabetes mellitus, hypercortisolemia, and vitamin deficiencies; and inflammatory disorders, such as collagen vascular diseases (dermatomyositis, polyarteritis nodosa, rheumatoid arthritis, scleroderma, and systemic lupus erythematosus). Medications that may cause mania include antidepressants, amantadine, bromocriptine, baclofen, anabolic steroids, corticosteroids, dapsone (sulfone, a topical treatment for acne vulgaris), isoniazid (a drug used to treat tuberculosis), metoclopramide (Reglan), theophylline, and chloroquine (Aralen, used for malaria). Substances associated with the development of mania include alcohol, amphetamines, cocaine, methylphenidate, and pseudoephedrine (e.g., Sudafed, Allegra D, Zyrtec D) (Joska & Stein, 2008, pp. 468-469).

Clues that suggest substance abuse as a cause of mania include older age (over 40 years); no family history of bipolar disorder; lack of a precipitant factor; mood that is more irritable than manic; and fewer psychotic symptoms. Nonpsychiatric causes should be considered when there are symptoms such as impaired memory, confusion, disorientation, abnormal endocrine functioning, and evidence of substance abuse. Common medical conditions that may induce mania include head injuries, cerebrovascular disease, diabetes mellitus, multiple sclerosis, tumors of the central nervous system, and infections such as HIV or syphilis (Joska & Stein, 2011). Table 14-4 provides more information about the differential diagnoses that should be considered.

Treatment

Treatment is based on a comprehensive assessment and a biopsychosocial case formulation. It includes somatic and nonsomatic interventions. Somatic interventions include pharmacotherapy, ECT, repetitive magnetic brain stimulation, vagal nerve stimulation, and the incorporation of omega-3 fatty acids into the diet. Nonsomatic interventions include psychotherapy and psychosocial interventions (Crowe, Whitehead, Wilson, et al., 2010; Hirschfeld et al., 2006).

Assessment

Bipolar disorder is often misdiagnosed, with half of patients with bipolar disorder describing a 5-year lapse between going for treatment and being diagnosed as having bipolar disorder (Hirschfeld, Lewis, & Vornik, 2003).

TABLE 14-4 DIFFERENTIAL DIAGNOSIS OF BIPOLAR I DISORDER

Other Disorder	Differentiating Characteristics
Mood disorder due to medical condition	Mania may be due to head injuries, multiple sclerosis, tumors of the central nervous system, stroke, infections such as HIV or syphilis, Lyme disease, hyperthyroidism, or medications (Joska & Stein, 2011; Keltner & Folks, 2005).
Substance-induced mood disorder	Symptoms are due to effects of a substance, including antidepressant medications (First, Frances, & Pincus, 2002).
Major depressive disorder or dysthymic disorder	Absence of episode of mania, hypomania, mixed mania and depression, and psychotic depression. No family history of manic episodes (Leyton & Barrera, 2010).
Bipolar II disorder	Presence of hypomania and major depressive episodes. Absence of mania or mixed episodes (First et al., 2002).
Borderline personality disorder	Interpersonal relationships are more disturbed. Mood is more labile. Higher levels of impulsiveness and hostility. More suicide attempts (Ketter & Wang, 2010b). More frequent childhood history of abuse. Fear of abandonment (Fiedorowicz & Black, 2010).
Cyclothymic disorder	Repeated periods of hypomanic symptoms that do not meet criteria for a manic episode and repeated periods of depressive symptoms that do not meet criteria for a major depressive disorder.
Psychotic disorders (nonmood)	Psychotic symptoms that occur without mood symptoms.

Others have been found to have a 10-year delay between seeking treatment and receiving a diagnosis of bipolar disorder (Berk, Dodd, Callaly, et al., 2007). Because bipolar disorder is a chronic illness with residual disabilities and high rates of comorbid psychiatric disorders (including substance-related disorders), risk for suicide, and medical illnesses, it is common during the assessment process to find problems on all five axes of the *DSM-IV-TR* (McIntyre et al., 2004). Problems for Axis I (psychiatric disorders), Axis II (personality disorders and mental retardation), and Axis III disorders (general medical conditions) were discussed in the Comorbidity section of this chapter. Information about Axis IV and Axis V follows:

- *Axis IV: Psychosocial and Environmental Problems:* In comparison with the general population, individuals with bipolar disorder have lower rates of employment, a greater number of interpersonal stressors, and more interactions with the criminal justice system (St. John, 2005). They are more likely to be single, defined as never married, separated, divorced, or widowed (Weissman et al., 1991). After age 16 years, patients with bipolar disorder experience more physical and sexual abuse than those without bipolar disorder, possibly because of cognitive deficits, impaired judgment, impulsivity, and high-risk living environments (Coverdale & Turbott, 2000).
- *Axis V: Global Assessment of Functioning:* Among patients with bipolar disorder, only 40% are able to function at the level they achieved before becoming ill; 25% to 35% have partial impairment of functioning; and 25% to 35% have severe impairment of functioning (Bauer, Kirk, Gavin, et al., 2001). Severity of impairment of functioning may be evidenced by a history of failure of intimate relationships, multiple employment terminations, bankruptcy, violence, arrests, or incarceration (Leahy, 2007; Perlis, Ostacher, Patel, et al., 2006). Impaired functioning at work and in managing finances is often associated with problems with housing and transportation (Piterman, Jones, & Castle, 2010).

In writing about assessment and treatment of bipolar disorder, Ketter (2010) said that the diagnosis of bipolar disorders relies on clinical information and that a comprehensive biopsychosocial assessment is crucial for generating an accurate diagnosis and for developing an effective plan of treatment. Psychiatric advanced practice nurses carry out a comprehensive biopsychosocial assessment to gather detailed information about the patient's

- Medical and psychiatric illnesses
- Biological, psychological, and social stressors
- Impulsive acts
- Suicidal ideation or attempts
- Relationship changes or problems
- Work changes or problems
- Financial changes or problems
- Support system and resources (changes or problems)
- Increases or decreases of self-esteem, mood, sleep, energy, and social activities

Because patients with bipolar disorder spend more time in the depressive phase of the illness than in a phase of mood elevation, they may respond to questions about their moods with descriptions of depression; however, patients may not report periods of hypomania or mania because they may be embarrassed by their behaviors during such episodes (Howland, 2006). The psychiatric advanced practice nurse should ask the patient detailed questions about having high levels of energy; being able to go without sleep for long periods of time or having no desire for sleep; excessive spending; and taking on several new projects. They should also ask for collateral information from partners or family members who may be able to describe episodes of elevated mood (Ketter & Wang, 2010b). Because bipolar disorder has a strong genetic influence, a detailed family history of mania or hypomania should also be taken.

A 15-item screening tool for bipolar disorder, the *Mood Disorder Questionnaire (MDQ)* (Hirschfeld, Williams, Spitzer, et al., 2000), can be used to elicit information from patients about their symptoms, family history of bipolar disorder, past diagnoses, and disease severity. Screening for mania can be done using the *Young Mania Rating Scale (YMRS)* (Young, Biggs, Ziegler, et al., 1978). Screening for hypomania can be done using the 32-item self-assessment scale, the *Hypomania Checklist (HCL-32)* (Meyer, Hammelstein, Nilsson, et al., 2007).

A history of response to medications is important in evaluating a patient for bipolar disorder. Patients with bipolar disorder are likely to have had a poor response—e.g., irritability, anxiety, restlessness, agitation, or insomnia—to antidepressant medications (Howland, 2006, p. 11).

Case Formulation

Information obtained (1) during the comprehensive psychiatric evaluation, (2) from a review of records, and (3) by asking partners or family members for collateral information is used to generate a diagnosis that includes the subtype of bipolar disorder, the phase of bipolar disorder (that is, the prodromal, acute, continuation, or maintenance phase), the current clinical status, and features.

Ketter et al. (2010, pp. 69-70) described clinical status as transition points that they called the Five R's:

1. *Response:* Index episode is still present, but there is 50% or greater reduction of symptoms following an intervention. Discontinuation of treatment as soon as response is achieved carries a high risk of relapse.
2. *Remission:* Absence of symptoms following an intervention for 2 months. Discontinuation of treatment carries a risk of relapse.
3. *Recovery:* Absence of symptoms for more that 2 months. Because bipolar disorder is a chronic recurring illness, there is a risk for new episodes.

4. *Relapse:* Index episode returns after response or remission.
5. *Recurrence:* New episode that emerges after recovery.

Features of bipolar disorder include

- Longitudinal course specifiers (with and without interepisode recovery)
- "With seasonal pattern," which is used to describe major depressive episodes in bipolar I disorder and bipolar II disorder
- "With rapid cycling," which can be used with bipolar I disorder and bipolar II disorder. In rapid cycling, there must be four or more mood episodes (any combination of major depressive episode and manic, hypomanic, or mixed episode) in 1 year.

In the process of generating a diagnosis and considering differential diagnoses, it should be remembered that patients with bipolar disorder tend to have a poorer clinical status than patients with unipolar depression and more impairment of family, social, and vocational functioning. They are also likely to have more medical comorbidities, have more psychiatric comorbidities, and make more suicide attempts (Howland, 2006).

Treatment of the Stages of Bipolar Disorder

Treatment in the Prodromal Phase

Because research related to the prodromal phase of bipolar disorder has only recently been instituted, there is little information about the effectiveness of preventive interventions. Trials with medications suggest that valproate (Chang, Dienes, Blasey, et al., 2003) and quetiapine (Seroquel) (DelBello, Adler, Whitsel, et al., 2007) improve prodromal symptoms. Other preventive interventions that have been recommended include omega-3 fatty acids and family-focused therapy (McNamara, Nandagopal, & Strakowski, 2010). Other studies suggest that cognitive therapy and psychoeducation in combination with medication are effective in reducing prodromal symptoms (Colom & Lam, 2005; Zaretsky, Lancee, Miller, et al., 2008). Psychosocial interventions (education, stress management, and regulation of sleep-wake cycles) are thought to be effective in reducing the risk of those subsyndromal symptoms' developing into more severe symptoms of bipolar disorder (Rouget & Aubry, 2007).

Treatment in the Acute Phase

Patients who present for treatment are often in the acute phase, which may be an initial manic episode, an initial depressive episode, a relapse, or a recurrence (Ketter et al., 2010). Acute mania is a medical emergency (Belmaker, 2004). Without prompt treatment, patients may engage in activities that endanger their lives, their marriages, their jobs, the family's finances, and their children's well-being. Patients may need to be protected from risk-taking behaviors and from death by suicide (McColm et al., 2006). A depressive episode may develop suddenly or gradually and is often accompanied by a high risk for suicide (Black & Andreasen, 2011).

The goals of treatment during the acute phase are to

1. Ensure the patient's safety and meet physiological needs
2. Assess and treat acute exacerbations, e.g., reduce symptoms and improve functioning
3. Provide information and support for the patient and family
4. Prevent recurrences

The first step in treatment is to meet the patient's needs for safety, food, fluids, rest, and medical care and to reduce environmental stimuli, such as television, noise, lights, music, the presence of other individuals, and animated conversations. Hospitalization should be considered for patients who are at high risk for suicide, who are severely ill, who are without social support, who demonstrate impaired judgment, and who did not respond well to outpatient treatment during a previous acute phase of bipolar illness (Hirschfeld et al., 2006).

Pharmacotherapy is used to achieve a rapid reduction of symptoms for both manic episodes and major depressive episodes in the acute phase (Ketter et al., 2010). Medications that have been approved for treating the acute phase of manic episodes and depressive episodes are described in the following sections.

Pharmacotherapy for Manic Episodes or Mixed Episodes in the Acute Phase

Pharmacotherapy for manic or mixed episodes includes

- Mood stabilizers
- Antipsychotics
- Atypical antipsychotics, as monotherapy and as augmenting agents
- Benzodiazepines

The first line of treatment for severe manic or mixed episodes is the use of a mood stabilizer in combination with an atypical antipsychotic (Hirschfeld et al., 2006). Benzodiazepines are also used to supplement mood stabilizers and antipsychotics, although caution must be used with benzodiazepines because of their interactions with other drugs.

Mood Stabilizers Used to Treat Manic or Mixed Episodes

Mood stabilizers that have been approved for use include lithium and the anticonvulsants carbamazepine (Tegretol), oxcarbazepine (Trileptal), and valproate (divalproex, a formulation of valproate) Other medications are also being studied as mood stabilizers.

Lithium

Lithium is a naturally occurring alkali metal. John Cade discovered lithium's calming properties in 1949, and it has been used to treat bipolar disorder for more than 50 years. Lithium is effective for treating acute episodes of mania and hypomania and may prevent recurrences of mania and depression and decrease suicidality (Freeman, Wiegland, & Gleneberg, 2004; Keck & McElroy, 2004; Ketter & Wang, 2010d). Its efficacy is comparable to that of divalproex (Bowden, Brugger, Swann, et al., 1994), carbamazepine (Small, Klapper, Milstein, et al., 1991), risperidone (Risperdal) (Segal, Berk, & Brook, 1998), olanzapine (Zyprexa) (Beck, Ichim, & Brook, 1999), and older typical antipsychotics (Garfinkel, Stancer, & Persad, 1980). Lithium acts more slowly than atypical antipsychotics, with 7 to 14 days for onset of action (Keck & McElroy, 2001), and lithium may be less effective than atypical antipsychotics for patients with psychotic mania (Schatzberg, Cole, & DeBattista, 2007).

Lithium is effective (1) for patients with mania that occurs early in the illness without depressive symptoms and (2) when there are no medical comorbidities (Goldberg & Citrome, 2005). It is less effective in mixed episodes, secondary mania, and rapid-cycling bipolar disorder (Ketter & Wang, 2010d). Currently, lithium is the most effective medication in reducing suicidal behaviors (Baldessarini et al., 2003; Ernst & Goldberg, 2004; Schou, 1998). (See Chapter 6 for more information on lithium.)

Anticonvulsants or Antikindling Medications

Anticonvulsants are not strictly mood stabilizers, but they may stabilize symptoms of mania. Common anticonvulsants include carbamazepine, oxcarbazepine, and valproate.

Carbamazepine is effective in acute mania, with onset of antimanic effect in 7 to 10 days (Ketter, Wang, & Post, 2004; Weisler, Keck, Swann, et al., 2005). It is not clear if it is effective for the depressive phase of bipolar disorder (Stahl, 2005). An extended-release formulation (Equetro) has been approved for use in mania and mixed episodes of bipolar disorder (Goldberg & Citrome, 2005). Carbamazepine is also used as an *augmenting* agent with lithium, other anticonvulsants, and atypical antipsychotics. Carbamazepine is used less often as a first-line medication for bipolar disorder because of its side effects and interactions with other medication. Some patients may have only a partial response.

Oxcarbazepine is similar to carbamazepine, but it does not induce blood dyscrasias—such as aplastic anemia or hepatotoxicity—and it does not cause induction of the cytochrome P-450 enzyme system. However, some studies suggest that oxcarbazepine is less effective than carbamazepine in the treatment of acute mania (Ketter, Wang, & Post, 2009) and is more likely than carbamazepine to cause hyponatremia (Goldberg & Citrome, 2005). Oxcarbazepine lacks sufficient evidence for use as monotherapy (Wagner, Kowatch, & Emslie, 2006). A few studies have found oxcarbazepine to be useful as add-on therapy in refractory mania (Mazza, DiNicola, Martinotti, et al., 2007).

Valproate in the form of divalproex has been approved for treatment of manic episodes associated with bipolar disorder (Bowden, 2009) and for acute mania (Goldberg & Citrome, 2005). It has been found to be as effective as lithium in the acute treatment of manic episodes of bipolar disorder or mixed bipolar disorder (Bowden, 2004; Bowden, 2009; Bowden et al., 1994), haloperidol (Haldol) (Bowden, 2009; McElroy, Keck, Stanton, et al., 1996), and olanzapine (Zajecka, Weisler, & Swann, 2000). Divalproex is more effective than lithium for patients with mixed mania, symptoms of irritability and hostility, more episodes (10 or more), comorbid alcohol dependence, and mania with depression (Bowden; Goldberg & Citrome). Divalproex has been found to be effective for patients who do not respond to lithium (Ketter & Wang, 2010b) and for patients with rapid-cycling bipolar disorder (Stahl, 2000). It has been found to be as effective as antipsychotics for patients with psychosis (Tohen, Baker, Altshuler, et al., 2002a).

Although the divalproex formulation of valproate is often prescribed for off-label use in relapse prevention of bipolar disorder, controlled trials have not yet shown its superiority over placebo (Goldberg & Citrome, 2005), and divalproex has been found to be less effective than olanzapine in reducing manic symptoms of patients in remission (Tohen, Baker, Altshuler, et al., 2002a). It should be noted that valproate treatment has been found to be associated with polycystic ovary syndrome (Hirschfeld et al., 2006) and that it has three black box warnings: hepatotoxicity, pancreatitis, and teratogenicity (Lewis, 2004). In 2008, the U.S. Food and Drug Administration (FDA) released an alert regarding the risk of increased suicidal ideation and behavior for patients with epilepsy and psychiatric disorders for 11 anticonvulsants including divalproex. The risk was higher for patients with epilepsy (Ketter & Wang, 2010d).

Mood Stabilizers Being Studied

Mood stabilizers currently being studied are gabapentin (Neurontin), lamotrigene, topiramate (Topamax), and tiagabine (Gabitril).

The effectiveness of *gabapentin* as *monotherapy* for mania or rapid-cycling bipolar disorder is not supported by research (Ketter & Wang, 2010d; Nierenberg et al., 2007); however, it is frequently added to lithium or divalproex when patients have breakthrough symptoms. Gabapentin has been found to be effective in preventing migraine headaches that frequently co-occur with bipolar disorder (Frye, 2004).

Lamotrigine has both mood stabilizing and antidepressant properties and is effective for rapid-cycling bipolar disorder (Fagiolini, 2005). There is no demonstrated efficacy of its use for acute mania (Nierenberg, Ostacher, & Delgado, 2007). Shelton and Calabrese (2004) suggested that it is particularly effective in the acute and prophylactic treatment of depressive episodes in both bipolar I and bipolar II disorders, and it is approved for maintenance treatment of bipolar disorder (Martinez, Marangell, & Martinez, 2008).

Topiramate is not effective for acute mania (Ketter & Wang, 2010b). It may be useful for bipolar disorder that is comorbid with medication-induced weight gain, binge eating, alcohol abuse, and migraine headaches (McElroy & Keck, 2009). When added to lithium or divalproex, it is associated with a decrease of depressive symptoms ("Diagnosis and Pharmacologic Treatment of Bipolar Disorder," 2007).

Tiagabine appears to have anxiolytic properties and it acts by increasing gamma-aminobutyric acid levels. So far, no firm evidence is available to support its use in bipolar disorders (Gajwani, Forsthoff, Muzina, et al., 2005).

Antipsychotics Used to Treat Manic Episodes

In the past, typical antipsychotics—such as chlorpromazine hydrochloride (Thorazine) or haloperidol—were used to treat agitation or psychosis during manic episodes (Ketter & Wang, 2010d). They are used less often now because of their extrapyramidal tract side effects and their potential for causing tardive dyskinesia and depression (Zarate & Tohen, 2004). There is evidence that supports the use of some typical antipsychotics—haloperidol and chlorpromazine—in the treatment of acute mania (Keck & Wang, 2010d). However, currently, atypical antipsychotics are used more often than typical antipsychotics for bipolar disorder both with psychotic symptoms and also in the absence of psychotic symptoms. Through their action on the serotonergic system, atypical antipsychotics produce antidepressant and mood-stabilizing effects. They also enhance dopaminergic transmission in the prefrontal cortex, thus having the potential to improve cognition (Goldberg & Citrome, 2005).

Atypical Antipsychotics as Monotherapy for Manic Episodes

The atypical antipsychotics—olanzapine, risperidone, quetiapine, ziprasidone (Geodon), and aripiprazole (Abilify)—have been approved by the FDA for *monotherapy* in bipolar mania, and reviews of research studies support their efficacy as monotherapy (Keck, Nelson, & McElroy, 2003a; Keck & McElroy, 2009; McIntyre et al., 2004; Strakowski & Shelton, 2006; Yatham, 2005). One of the newer atypical antipsychotics, asenapine (Saphris), has recently been approved for treatment of acute mania of bipolar disorder and for mixed mania (Balaraman & Hardik, 2010; Meltzer, Dritselis, Yasothan, et al., 2009). Another atypical antipsychotic, clozapine (Clozaril), is held in reserve because of its challenging side effects (Ketter & Wang, 2010d) and used when manic symptoms are not responsive to other medications (Marder & Wirshing, 2009).

Atypical Antipsychotics as Augmenting Agents for Manic Episodes

Although monotherapy for acute mania using lithium, divalproex, carbamazepine, olanzapine, risperidone, quetiapine, ziprasidone, aripiprazole, haloperidol, and chlorpromazine has been found to result in a 50% reduction of symptoms in 3- to 4-week trials (McElroy & Keck, 2000), only about 25% of patients achieve remission within that time period. Therefore, combinations of medications are often used (Suppes, Dennehy, Hirschfeld, et al., 2005). Combination therapy has been found to have greater and more rapid efficacy than monotherapy in the treatment of mania (Scherk, Pajonk, & Leucht, 2007). For example, the addition of atypical antipsychotics to mood stabilizers has been found to be more effective than the use of mood stabilizers alone (Smith, Cornelius, Warnock, et al., 2007; Tohen, Chengappa, Suppes, et al., 2002b). Atypical antipsychotics used in combination therapy include

- *Risperidone*—approved for use in combination with mood stabilizers, lithium, or valproate and found to improve their effectiveness (Ketter et al., 2010)
- *Quetiapine*—in combination with lithium or divalproex is approved for acute manic episodes and for maintenance treatment (Ketter & Wang, 2010b, 2010d)
- *Aripiprazole*—approved for combination treatment with lithium or valproate (Ketter & Wang, 2010d)

Benzodiazepines Used to Treat Manic Episodes

There are limited data about the antimanic activity of benzodiazepines. Muzina and Calabrese (2006) noted that their clinical benefit may be due to their ability to provide rapid relief of excitement, insomnia, anxiety, and agitation that often are present with mania. Although there are different opinions about the use of benzodiazepines in acute mania, clonazepam (Klonopin) and lorazepam (Ativan) are often used as adjuncts for agitation to calm patients until mood-stabilizing agents can reduce the effects of mania or hypomania (Fagiolini, 2005); they are also used for comorbid anxiety disorders (such as panic disorder) and for insomnia (Ketter & Wang, 2010b). However, benzodiazepines should be used with caution because of the potential for lethal interactions with alcohol and drugs, development of dependency, and problems with withdrawal (Sheehan & Raj, 2009).

Pharmacotherapy for Depressive Episodes in the Acute Phase

Pharmacotherapy for depressive episodes includes

- Mood stabilizers
- Atypical antipsychotics
- Antidepressants

The American Psychiatric Association Practice Guideline for the treatment of patients with bipolar disorder (Hirschfeld et al., 2006) recommended that the first-line treatment for a depressive episode of bipolar disorder should be lithium or lamotrigine. When an acute depressive episode does not respond to first-line medications, lamotrigine (if lithium was the first-line treatment), bupropion (Wellbutrin), or paroxetine (Paxil) may be added. Different selective serotonin reuptake inhibitors (SSRIs) or venlafaxine (Effexor) can be tried. Depressive episodes with psychotic features may require adjunctive treatment with antipsychotic medications or ECT (Hirschfeld et al., 2006).

The FDA-approved medications for treating acute depression in bipolar disorder are (1) the combination of olanzapine and fluoxetine (Symbyax) and (2) quetiapine (Keck & McElroy, 2009; Wang & Ketter, 2010). The olanzapine and fluoxetine combination has demonstrated effectiveness in reducing depressive symptoms and has been found to be more effective than lamotrigine (Brown, McElroy, Keck, et al., 2006); however, olanzapine is associated with weight gain, sedation, and increased appetite. Quetiapine has been found to be effective in reducing depressive symptoms and also in improving sleep and reducing anxiety symptoms. However, quetiapine is associated with sedation, which may be a problem if it interferes with functioning.

Mood Stabilizers Used to Treat Bipolar Depression

Lamotrigine has been approved for maintenance treatment of bipolar disorder, but it has not been approved for acute bipolar depression. However, because of the troublesome side effects of olanzapine and quetiapine and because of evidence that supports the use of lithium or lamotrigine as monotherapy or in combination with antidepressants, lithium and lamotrigine are frequently used in the treatment of acute bipolar depression (Joska & Stein, 2011). Lithium has been found to be less effective for acute bipolar depression than for acute mania (Wang & Ketter, 2010).

In comparing the efficacy and safety of (1) lamotrigine monotherapy and (2) olanzapine combined with fluoxetine for the treatment of acute bipolar depression, Brown et al. (2006) found that the combination of olanzapine and fluoxetine was associated with a greater reduction of symptoms than lamotrigine monotherapy. However, patients receiving lamotrigine had fewer problems with weight gain, increased appetite, dry mouth, sedation, and elevation of cholesterol and triglyceride levels. Wang and Ketter (2010) suggested that patients with insomnia and who are underweight, anxious, and agitated may benefit more from olanzapine combined with fluoxetine than from lamotrigine.

In contrast to lithium, lamotrigine appears to be more effective for acute bipolar depression than for acute mania. Because it is also effective for long-term use, patients who benefit from lamotrigine for acute bipolar depression may remain on it during maintenance treatment (Wang & Ketter, 2010). There have been small studies that have suggested that divalproex is effective for acute bipolar depression (Muzina, Ganocy, Khalife, et al., 2008; Wang & Ketter, 2010).

Atypical Antipsychotics Used to Treat Bipolar Depression

Bipolar depressive symptoms may also be treated with atypical antipsychotics that are not likely to induce mania (Strakowski & Shelton, 2006). According to Wang & Ketter (2010), quetiapine monotherapy and olanzapine monotherapy have moderate efficacy, and aripiprazole monotherapy and ziprasidone monotherapy lack efficacy. There is insufficient research-generated evidence about the use of risperidone and clozapine for the treatment of acute bipolar depression to evaluate their effectiveness.

Antidepressants Used to Treat Bipolar Depression

The decision to use antidepressants in the treatment of the depressive phase of bipolar disorder must take into consideration (1) the goal of relieving the depression and (2) the risk of precipitating a mood switch to mania or accelerating frequency of episodes (Keck & McElroy, 2009; Wang & Ketter, 2010). All antidepressants have the potential to induce manic or hypomanic episodes (Fagiolini, 2005), with increased risk being associated with a previous antidepressant-induced mania, a family history of bipolar disorder, and exposure to multiple antidepressant trials (Goldberg & Truman, 2003).

In the past, it was thought that the switch rate was 10% to 70%; however, recent research suggests a much lower rate. Post, Altshuler, Frye, et al. (2001) found that among patients with bipolar disorder treated for acute depression with a combination of antidepressants and mood stabilizer, the switch rate was 14% (8% to hypomania and 6% to mania). However, different classes of antidepressants have different rates of risk. For example, the overall switch rate has been reported as 34% for patients receiving tricyclic antidepressants; 12% for those receiving SSRIs; 8% for those receiving monoamine oxidase inhibitors; and 14% for those receiving other agents. Administration of mood stabilizers in combination with antidepressants appears to offer some protection against switching from depression to mania or hypomania (Henry, Sorbara, Lacoste, et al., 2001; Wang & Ketter, 2010). For example, among patients receiving tricyclic antidepressants and no mood stabilizer, 57% switched, whereas among patients receiving tricyclic antidepressants and a mood stabilizer, 26% switched (Bottlender, Rudolf, Strauss, et al., 2001). Post et al. (2001) reviewed switch data for bupropion, sertraline (Zoloft), and venlafaxine added to therapeutic doses of mood stabilizers for bipolar depression and found no significant difference in switch rates among the three medications.

There is controversy over the use of antidepressants for the treatment of acute bipolar depression (Wang & Ketter, 2010), with some researchers pointing to the lack of evidence supporting their effectiveness (Ghaemi, Lenox, & Baldessarini, 2001) and others describing adverse responses such as irritability, anxiety, restlessness, agitation, and insomnia (Grunze, 2005).

Other somatic treatment options for acute bipolar depression include the use of other mood stabilizers, other atypical antipsychotics, adjunctive antidepressants, adjunctive thyroid hormones, sleep deprivation, adjunctive ECT, adjunctive light therapy, adjunctive omega-3 fatty acids, adjunctive vagus nerve stimulation, and adjunctive transcranial magnetic stimulation (Wang & Ketter, 2010). (Some of these adjunctive options are discussed in Chapter 13.)

Treatment in the Continuation Phase

The continuation phase is the time between the acute phase and the maintenance phase (Ketter et al., 2010). It is often considered the time during which patients are receiving treatment for an acute episode as they improve or after they have been discharged from the hospital. It starts with response or remission and ends with recovery or relapse. The duration of the continuation phase is the interval after which an episode might be expected to occur, usually 2 to 6 months after treatment in the acute stage.

Medications that are approved for monotherapy include lithium, lamotrigine, olanzapine, and aripiprazole. Quetiapine is approved as adjunctive treatment with lithium or divalproex. Pharmacotherapy involves continuing full doses of the mood stabilizers and adjuncts that helped the patient to achieve remission. Attempts are made to balance medications to achieve control of symptoms and tolerability of side effects. The goal of treatment in the continuation phase is symptom relief so that the patient can avoid relapse and move toward recovery from the illness (Ketter & Wang, 2010c).

Treatment in the Maintenance Phase

The maintenance phase starts with the recovery, and thus in the beginning there are no symptoms (Ketter et al., 2010). The goals of maintenance therapy are stability of mood, prevention of recurrences, prevention of suicide, and return to full functioning. During the maintenance phase, treatment should include pharmacotherapy, psychotherapy, and psychosocial interventions such as education and stress reduction. Long-term maintenance pharmacotherapy is recommended for patients who have had a severe manic or depressive episode and for those who have had two or more episodes, have a family history of bipolar disorder, or lack social support (American Psychiatric Association, 2002).

Four medications have been approved by the FDA for use as monotherapy for the maintenance phase of bipolar disorder: lithium, lamotrigine, olanzapine, and aripiprazole. Quetiapine has been approved as an adjunctive medication that can be used with lithium or divalproex. Although it has not been approved for maintenance therapy, divalproex is considered to be a frontline choice by many clinicians (Ketter & Wang, 2010b). There is evidence that recurrence rates and suicide rates can be reduced with continued use of lithium or mood stabilizers (Dubovsky, 2005).

Maintenance treatment is used for both episodes of mania and episodes of depression.

Maintenance Treatment for Episodes of Mania

Four monotherapies—lithium, lamotrigine, olanzapine, and aripiprazole—and quetiapine as an adjunctive added to lithium or divalproex are approved for maintenance treatment (Ketter & Wang, 2010e). Evidence supports the use of lithium and valproate. Other medications, such as lamotrigine, carbamazepine, oxcarbazepine, or atypical antipsychotics, may be used. The atypical antipsychotic olanzapine, in the form of the fluoxetine-olanzapine combination Symbyax, is approved for relapse prevention (Strakowski & Shelton, 2006). Aripiprazole, which is approved for relapse prevention and for maintenance monotherapy for adults, is effective for mania and mixed episodes with or without psychotic features and with or without rapid cycling (Ketter & Wang, 2010b). In a review of the effectiveness of anticonvulsant drugs for the maintenance treatment of bipolar disorder, Melvin, Carey, Goodman, et al. (2008) reported that carbamazepine, valproate, and lamotrigine were effective in preventing remission for mania or mixed episodes. During the maintenance phase, psychosocial interventions that address adherence to treatment, lifestyle changes, coping strategies, prevention of recurrences, and interpersonal problems that are related to the illness or the consequences of behaviors during manic episodes may be beneficial (Beynon et al., 2008; Goossens, van Achterberg, & Knoppert-van der Klein, 2007; Hirschfeld, 2009; Rouget & Aubry, 2007). (See Chapter 8 for a description of psychosocial interventions.)

Maintenance Treatment for Episodes of Depression

For patients in the maintenance phase who have had an episode of depression, two medications—lithium and lamotrigine—have been approved for prevention, with lamotrigine having the most potential for preventing relapse of depressive episodes (Hirschfeld et al., 2006). If antidepressants are used for depression, they should be used in combination with antimanic medications to prevent the risks of manic switches or cycle acceleration (Muzina & Calabrese, 2006).

Long-term use of adjunctive antidepressants in patients with bipolar disorder is controversial. Post, Leverich, Altshuler, et al. (2003) found that two-thirds of patients with bipolar disorder who were receiving pharmacotherapy—such as mood stabilizers, antidepressants, benzodiazepines, and antipsychotics—continued to have high levels of residual depressive symptoms that were three times more frequent than symptoms of mania or hypomania. Some patients benefit from long-term use of antidepressants as adjunctive treatment (Ketter & Wang, 2010c). Altshuler, Suppes, Black, et al. (2003) found that patients who discontinued antidepressants within the first 6 months after successful treatment had a shorter time before relapse than those who continued treatment with antidepressants. Those who were continued on antidepressant medications had about half the rate of relapse of those in whom antidepressant medications were discontinued.

In summary, the treatment of bipolar disorder has benefited from a greater awareness of the efficacy of different treatment approaches during different phases of the illness. However, despite the availability of effective pharmacological treatments, ongoing symptoms, relapses, recurrences, and nonresponse to treatment are common problems (Melvin et al., 2008).

Somatic Interventions

Pharmacological Interventions for Comorbid Psychiatric Disorders

As previously discussed, mood stabilizers, antipsychotics, atypical antipsychotics, benzodiazepines, and antidepressants are all pharmacotherapeutic means of stabilizing patients with bipolar disorder. Additionally, patients with bipolar disorder have high rates of comorbid psychiatric disorders—such as personality disorders, panic disorder, and substance-related disorders—that affect response to treatment and course of the bipolar disorder (Keck & McElroy, 2008). For example, comorbid alcohol abuse is associated with higher rates of rapid cycling, greater severity of symptoms, suicidality, aggressiveness, and impulsivity (Leahy, 2007). Pharmacotherapeutic interventions for various comorbid psychiatric disorders can be found in Table 14-5.

Nonpharmacological Somatic Interventions

Electroconvulsive Therapy

ECT is considered to be an effective treatment for depression that has not responded to pharmacotherapy, for psychotic depression, for mania, and for severe suicidality. It has the highest rate of response of any form of antidepressant treatment (Karasu, Gelenberg, Merriam, et al., 2004). (See Chapter 13 for description of ECT.) ECT may be used in bipolar disorder for acute mania and in the depressive phase (Ketter & Wang, 2010d). After relief of an acute depressive episode with ECT, maintenance ECT may be needed for patients with severe bipolar disorder that does not respond to maintenance pharmacotherapy (Hirschfeld et al., 2006). Even with maintenance ECT therapy, 39% of patients relapse in 6 months (Nahas, Lorberbaum, Kozel, et al., 2004). Patients with limited response to ECT often have a co-occurring personality disorder and poor response to other treatment.

Brain Stimulation

Methods of brain stimulation—such as transcranial magnetic stimulation, vagus nerve stimulation, and deep brain stimulation—that are used in the treatment of depression are also being studied for use in bipolar disorder. These treatments are discussed in Chapter 13.

Omega-3 Fatty Acids

The human brain is nearly 60% fat, and fatty acids play a vital role in the building of brain structures, the functioning of the brain, and the process of neurotransmission (Chang, Ke, & Chen, 2009; Peet & Stokes, 2005). Fatty acids within the omega-3 fatty acids—such as eicosapentaenoic acid, docosahexaenoic acid, and the omega-6 fatty acid arachidonic acid—influence brain membranes, enzymes, ion channels, and receptors (Hallahan & Garland, 2005). Omega-3 fatty acids affect neuroplasticity and cell survival through their influence on neurotropic factors, such as BDNF; they also directly affect gene expression. Omega-3 fatty acids, which

TABLE 14-5 PHARMACOTHERAPY FOR COMORBID CONDITIONS OF BIPOLAR DISORDER

Comorbid Disorder	Pharmacotherapy
Social anxiety disorder	SSRIs and topiramate (Mancini, van Ameringen, Pipe, et al., 2002)
Generalized anxiety disorder	Benzodiazepines, paroxetine, and venlafaxine
Panic disorder	TCAs and SSRIs (McIntyre et al., 2004); gabapentin (Perugi, Toni, Frare, et al., 2002)
Obsessive-compulsive disorder	TCAs and SSRIs
Post-traumatic stress disorder	TCAs, SSRIs, and topiramate (Berlant & van Kammen, 2002)
Alcohol abuse	First line: divalproex, topiramate, lithium, psychotherapy, and self-help groups Second line: atypical antipsychotics, gabapentin, and carbamazepine (Sachs, Grossman, Ghaemi, et al., 2002; Zarate & Tohen, 2002)
Substance-related disorders	First line: psychotherapy and self-help groups Second line: carbamazepine, lithium, atypical antipsychotics, and gabapentin (Sachs et al., 2002; Zarate & Tohen, 2002)
Atypical antipsychotic–induced weight gain (Lessig, Shapira, & Murphy, 2001)	Behavioral modification and topiramate (Sachs et al., 2000; Teter, Early, & Gibbs, 2000; Zarate & Tohen, 2002)
Impulse control disorder (explosive temper)	Divalproex (Donovan, Stewart, Nunes, et al., 2000)
Personality disorders	Divalproex for comorbid borderline personality disorder (Frankenburg & Zanarini, 2002) Olanzapine and risperidone for other personality disorders (Zanarini & Frankenburg, 2001)
Migraine headache	Valproate; gabapentin (Frye, 2004)

SRI, selective serotonin reuptake inhibitors; TCA, tricyclic antidepressants.

are found in seafood, fish oil, olive oil, garlic, nuts, and other food items, compete for metabolism with omega-6 fatty acids, which are found in meat and vegetable oils, trans fats, and some processed foods (Stoll, 2001). An optimal ratio of omega-3 fatty acids to omega-6 fatty acids (1:2) contributes to overall health (Owen, Rees, & Parker, 2008; Peet & Stokes, 2005; Stoll, 2001). It has been suggested that the increase in intake of the omega-6 fatty acids relative to the omega-3 fatty acids owing to changes in the American diet may play a role in the increased rate of depressive disorders (Hibbein & Salem, 1995). Patients with depression have lower levels of omega-3 polyunsaturated fatty acids and higher ratios of omega-6 fatty acids to omega-3 fatty acids (Ross, 2007), and the ratio of omega-3 fatty acids to omega-6 fatty acids was found to be a stronger predictor of suicide attempts among a group of patients with depression who had attempted suicide previously than gender, age, and baseline suicidal ideation (Sublette, Hibbeln, Gallalvy, et al., 2006).

There has been a great deal of interest in the link between omega-3 fatty acids and mental health (Laraia, 2005; Stoll, 2001), especially the mood disorders (Owen et al., 2008). Some studies have suggested that omega-3 fatty acids protect against depression, other neuropsychiatric disorders, and suicide (Bourre, 2004; Bourre, 2005; Young & Conquer, 2005). For example, Peet & Horrobin (2001) found a three times greater improvement in depression among patients receiving omega-3 fatty acids in comparison to those receiving placebo. A cross-national comparison of seafood consumption and rates of bipolar disorder demonstrated that there is a relationship between greater seafood consumption and lower prevalence of bipolar disorders. Although the evidence is not conclusive, these data provided support for trials of omega-3 fatty acids for the treatment of bipolar disorder (Noaghiul & Hibbeln, 2003).

While not consistent, the results suggest that omega-3 fatty acids are beneficial for bipolar disorder (Freeman, Hibbeln, Wisner, et al., 2006). For example, in one study of patients with bipolar disorder who received omega-3 fatty acids in addition to standard treatment, there were longer remissions and greater improvement of symptoms (Stoll, Severus, Freeman, et al., 1999). In a later clinical trial, Osher, Bersudsky, and Belmaker (2005) reported that omega-3 supplementation was beneficial for bipolar depression. In a clinical trial reported in 2006, no benefit from omega-3 was found (Keck, Mintz, McElroy, et al., 2006); however, in another trial, omega-3 was associated with improvement of depression and overall functioning (Frangou, Lewis, & McCrone, 2006). The consensus of the subcommittee on omega-3 fatty acids that was assembled by the American Psychiatric Association supported the protective effect of omega-3 in mood disorders and the benefits of its use in unipolar and bipolar disorders (Freeman et al., 2006). There has been no evidence that omega-3 is effective in mania (Owen et al., 2008).

Nonsomatic Treatment: Psychotherapy and Psychosocial Interventions

Psychotherapy

Early studies found that psychotherapy for patients with bipolar disorder enhanced the effect of medications, helped patients and families manage the psychological and environmental stressors that contribute to recurrences, and helped patients deal with the adverse consequences resulting from recurrent episodes (Huxley, Parikh, & Baldessarini, 2000; Torrey & Knable, 2002). These early studies showed that when provided in addition to pharmacotherapy, each mode of psychotherapy was beneficial. Outcomes included increased adherence to medications, fewer hospitalizations, and possible additional benefits—including improved interpersonal and vocational skills, more acceptance of the illness, improved coping, and overall improved quality of life—that were not outcomes of adherence to medication (Huxley et al., 2000).

It is now widely accepted that psychotherapy is effective when used in combination with pharmacotherapy in stabilizing episodes of bipolar disorder, in reducing the length of the episode, and in preventing recurrence of episodes (Miklowitz, Goodwin, Bauer, et al., 2008). The combination of psychotherapy and pharmacotherapy has been found to be more effective than pharmacotherapy alone in preventing relapse (Scott & Gutierrez, 2004).

Psychotherapies frequently used for patients with bipolar disorder include CBT, interpersonal and social rhythm therapy (IPSRT), and family-focused therapy (FFT). Recent studies have shown that specific psychotherapies are more useful in acute phases and recovery phases and that some are more effective for mania and some for depression (Miklowitz, 2008).

Interpersonal Therapy and Cognitive Psychotherapy

Both interpersonal therapy and cognitive therapy have been adapted for use in conjunction with pharmacotherapy for patients with bipolar disorder. They share goals of reducing symptoms, improving functioning, preventing relapse, and decreasing the risk factors for recurrence. Both include an educational component related to bipolar disorder and promotion of adherence to treatment.

Interpersonal Therapy and Social Rhythm Therapy (IPSRT)

Interpersonal therapy was modified as IPSRT for patients with bipolar disorder. Frank, Kupfer, Thase, et al. (2005, p. 998) have said that IPSRT is based on the assumption that stability of interpersonal relationships and regularity of social routines have a protective effect on recurrent mood disorders: they have been found to be associated with a reduction of recurrences. IPSRT, which integrates education, social rhythm therapy, and interpersonal psychotherapy, focuses on addressing interpersonal problem areas, such as grief, bereavement, role transitions, role disputes, and interpersonal skills deficits; it also focuses on stabilizing biological and social rhythms, such as getting up and going to bed at the same time each day, eating at the same time each day, and exercising and engaging in social activities for the same amount of time each day (Frank, Swartz, & Kupfer, 2000; Friedman & Thase, 2007). IPSRT was found to be more effective in reducing the rate of recurrences if it was initiated during the acute phase rather than in the recovery phase. IPSRT has a strong effect on preventing recurrence of depression and a marginally significant effect on reducing suicide attempts (Miklowitz et al., 2008).

Cognitive Behavioral Therapy (CBT)

Cognitive therapy and CBT have been adapted to target cognitive and affective changes in depression and mania by helping patients to manage their bipolar illness. Patients are taught how lifestyle practices and interpersonal interactions affect their cognition and behaviors. They are taught how to change lifestyle practices (such as sleep and exercise) and how to decrease the risk of relapse by reducing psychosocial stressors (Basco, McDonald, Merlock, et al., 2004; Miklowitz, Otto, Frank, et al., 2007). Research studies have shown that CBT not only lessens the rate of relapse among patients with bipolar disorder but also is associated with improved social functioning and coping with bipolar symptoms and with more realistic goal expectations. The greatest benefits were obtained in the first 6 months while receiving therapy and for 6 months after (Lam, Hayward, Watkins, et al., 2005). Miklowitz et al. (2008) said that CBT appears to have a greater impact on depressive symptoms than on manic symptoms.

Family-Focused Therapy (FFT)

FFT, which has been found to help prevent relapse in patients with schizophrenia, was adapted for use with patients with bipolar disorder (Miklowitz & Goldstein, 1997). FFT is based on evidence that high levels of expressed emotion (criticism, hostility, and overinvolvement) by the family toward the patient are associated with increased risk of relapse and poor outcomes for the patient. FFT includes psychoeducation for the family about bipolar disorder and treatment, skills training in effective communication, and training in problem-solving (Miklowitz & Goldstein). Outcome studies suggest that FFT is a useful adjunct to pharmacotherapy for reducing relapses and recurrences of bipolar episodes (Culver & Pratchett, 2010; Rea, Tompson, Miklowitz, et al., 2003).

Response to psychotherapy in conjunction with pharmacotherapy is influenced not only by the phase of the illness (prodromal, acute, continuation, or maintenance) but also by the clinical state (depressive episode or manic episode) and by patient and family characteristics. CBT and group psychoeducation appear to be more effective for patients who are in the maintenance phase rather than in the acute phase or prodromal phase. FFT and IPSRT appear to be effective for patients who are in the acute phase. Psychoeducational programs, CBT, and FFT appear to be more effective for manic episodes than for depressive episodes (Bauer, McBride, Williford, et al., 2006; Colom, Vieta, Martinez-Aran, et al., 2003; Miklowitz et al., 2007), whereas IPSRT appears to be more effective for depression and suicidality (Miklowitz, 2008). FFT is more effective in stabilizing patients' depressive symptoms in families with high levels of conflict (criticism, hostility, marital conflict, parent/patient conflict) than in families with low levels of conflict. IPSRT may be less effective among patients with comorbid medical illness or anxiety disorders (Frank et al., 2005) and among those with borderline personality disorder (Swartz, Pilkonis, Frank, et al., 2005).

Psychotherapy appears to be most effective when used in combination with pharmacotherapy (McIntyre, 2011). Psychotherapy in combination with pharmacotherapy appears to be associated with faster recovery, reduction of relapse rates, and greater gains in relationship functioning and life satisfaction but not in vocational functioning (Miklowitz, 2008). However, even with optimal psychotherapy and pharmacotherapy, 50% to 70% of patients with bipolar disorder experience recurrences (Miklowitz, 2008).

Psychosocial Interventions

Psychosocial interventions target problems that are not modified by pharmacotherapy such as the need for knowledge about bipolar disorder, for more effective coping skills, for relapse prevention planning, and for social support (Beynon et al., 2008). Psychosocial interventions are designed to

- Educate the patient and family about bipolar disorder and the prodromal signs of manic and depressive episodes
- Build patient skills in stress management
- Promote adherence to treatment
- Prevent relapse
- Improve coping skills
- Provide social support
- Improve the attitude of spouse and/or family toward the illness (Huxley et al., 2000)

Psychosocial interventions that have been found to be effective for patients with bipolar disorder include family education, patient education, goal dysregulation interventions, social rhythm therapy, social support, problem-solving therapy, and multicomponent care programs. Psychosocial interventions that are not specific to bipolar disorder but are helpful in many psychiatric disorders can be found in Box 14-4.

Family Education

Family education involves teaching about bipolar disorder, the vulnerability to recurrences, relapse prevention, and the importance of taking medications, avoiding triggers or stressors, and keeping regular sleep-wake cycles. Families are taught about the role of stress caused by high

BOX 14-4 Psychosocial Interventions Not Specific to Bipolar Disorder

Psychosocial interventions that have been found to be helpful in managing psychiatric disorders but are not specific to bipolar disorder include

- Sleep therapy
- Socializing interventions to reduce isolation
- Problem-solving therapy
- Social skills training
- Mood charts
- Exercise
- Writing therapy

See Chapter 8 for more information on psychosocial interventions.

emotional exchanges between the family and patient in increasing the risk for recurrence of mood symptoms. They are taught effective communication skills and problem-solving skills. Family education appears to have a greater impact on depressive symptoms than on manic symptoms (Miklowitz, 2008; Miklowitz, Goodwin, Bauer, et al., 2008).

Patient Education

An educational plan to prevent recurrence must be designed specifically for each patient and should include identification of potential triggers and a plan of action once prodromal signs have been identified.

Stressors that act as triggers include a change in sleep due to working the night shift, staying up late to study or finish a project, or flying across several time zones; marital changes (marriage, separation, divorce, or remarriage with or without children); parenting challenges (children marrying, leaving, or returning home); and other events such as unemployment, failure to be promoted, need to care for aging parents, and financial problems (Frank et al., 2006). The patient's plan to prevent relapse is based on a history of symptoms, circumstances, and triggers that preceded previous manic and depressive relapses.

Education for patients also includes teaching about the illness, treatment options, need for adherence to medications, symptoms of relapse, and factors that contribute to relapse, such as substance abuse, stress, nonadherence to medications, and interruptions of social rhythms (Frank, 2005; Miklowitz & Johnson, 2006). Studies have shown that individual psychoeducation has clear benefits for preventing recurrence of manic episodes but not depressive episodes (Miklowitz, 2008).

Goal Dysregulation Interventions

Manic symptoms are linked to behavioral systems that control emotions, cognition, and behavior before and after goals are gained (Johnson & Fulford, 2009). Changes in behavioral systems associated with working toward achieving a goal and with having achieved the goal are seen in inflated self-esteem, increased talkativeness, flight of ideas, increased goal-directed activity, and increased pursuit of pleasurable activities. One intervention designed to reduce recurrence of mania by focusing on goal dysregulation is the GOALS program (Johnson & Fulford). GOALS is composed of 5 modules:

1. Education (about bipolar disorder)
2. Emotional reactivity to successes (promoting calmness after successes)
3. High goal-setting (reviewing life goals and whether some goals are too ambitious)
4. Increase in confidence after success (monitoring how confidence influences mood)
5. Goal pacing (using goal-pacing strategies, such as working on one goal at a time and limiting the amount of time spent working on a goal)

Preliminary examination of the GOALS program suggests that it may result in reduction of symptoms of mania in patients with bipolar disorder.

Social Rhythm Therapy

It is well known that challenges to the circadian system, such as traveling across time zones or working night shifts, are risk factors for the development of manic episodes of bipolar disorder. However, nonstressful changes in the pattern of daily living such as a weekend vacation or attending a conference are also risk factors (Frank et al., 2006). Social rhythm therapy stabilizes social and circadian rhythms by teaching patients to be consistent in daily activities—sleeping, waking, eating, exercising, working, participating in leisure activities, socializing, and relaxing—and to reduce excessive amounts of work or social activities, such as working long hours to complete a task or prepare for an examination (Frank et al.). Frank reported that "Social rhythm therapy is associated with significantly reduced risk of recurrence of both depression and mania over a 2-year period" (p. 983).

Social Support

Lack of social support among patients with bipolar disorder is associated with more symptoms and greater persistence of symptoms. The presence of social support has been found to be associated with fewer recurrences of depressive episodes of bipolar disorder, although it has less effect in reducing recurrences of manic episodes. Interestingly, the benefits of social support are the same whether the support comes from spouse, family, or friends (Cohen et al., 2004). Psychiatric advanced practice nurses can help patients to strengthen their social support networks by recommending participation in support groups and self-help groups (see Chapter 8 for interventions that promote social support).

Problem-Solving Therapy (PST)

PST focuses on teaching patients constructive problem-solving attitudes and skills that are necessary for successful adaptation to life's challenges and dilemmas (D'Zurilla & Nezu, 2009). (The theoretical foundation and processes of problem-solving therapy are discussed in detail in Chapter 8.) PST has been found to be an effective treatment for depression (Bell & D'Zurilla, 2009; Cuijpers, van Straten, & Warmerdam, 2007), and among older adults, PST has been found to be more effective than supportive therapy in reducing depressive symptoms and disability and in improving executive functioning (Alexopoulos, Raue, & Aredin, 2003).

Multicomponent Care Programs

An example of a multicomponent care program is a group intervention program administered by nurse care managers that provides psychoeducation, monthly telephone calls to each patient to monitor mood symptoms and medication adherence, feedback to mental health care providers treating the patients, and follow-up, outreach, and crisis intervention as needed. After 2 years, it was found that the intervention reduced the severity of mania symptoms and the duration during which mania symptoms were experienced but did not affect depressive symptoms (Simon, Ludman, Bauer, et al., 2006).

To summarize, psychosocial interventions have been found to be effective additions to pharmacotherapy in stabilization and prevention of episodes of bipolar disorder (Miklowitz et al. 2008). Certain components—problem solving, sleep/wake cycle stabilization, cognitive restructuring, mood charting, family communication training, and relapse prevention planning—appear to increase effectiveness of pharmacotherapy (Miklowitz et al.).

Course

The symptoms of bipolar disorder begin before age 18 years in about two-thirds of individuals with the disorder (Perlis, Miyahara, Marangell, et al., 2004). Patients with bipolar disorder often are seen first in primary care settings with depressive symptoms or physical symptoms. It may take years before they are seen in a psychiatric care setting and before they receive a diagnosis of bipolar disorder (Bauer, Unutzer, Pincus, et al., 2002; Berk et al., 2007). Although the first episode of bipolar disorder—manic, hypomanic, mixed, or depressive—may be followed by several years during which the patient is symptom free, recurrence is typical (Post, 2007). Each recurrence increases the risk that another episode will occur and that it will be less responsive to treatment (McIntyre, 2001). Among patients with bipolar disorder, 24% will have a recurrence within 6 months after the episode, 36% within 1 year, about 50% within 2 years, and about 61% within 4 years (Baldassano, 2009). In addition to the problem of recurrence, 70% or more of patients with bipolar disorder experience ongoing subsyndromal symptoms (Altshuler, Post, Black, et al., 2006) and poor functional recovery (Crowe et al., 2010). They also experience a high rate of medical problems, such as migraine headaches, diabetes, obesity, and cardiovascular disease, and a high rate of psychiatric disorders, such as anxiety disorders, substance-related disorders, and suicidal ideation. They may also have disabilities associated with the disorder, such as impairment of cognition and executive functioning that results in interpersonal, social, and vocational problems (Crowe et al.).

If patients with bipolar disorder do not receive treatment or if the disorder is inadequately treated, the episodes may recur more frequently, with a shorter time of being well between the recurrences (Post, 2007). Untreated patients with bipolar disorder may have more than 10 episodes during their lifetime (Swann, Bowden, Calabrese, et al., 1999). Untreated depressive episodes last 6 to 12 months, and untreated manic episodes last 3 to 6 months (Post et al., 2003). Whereas 27% to 42% of patients with bipolar disorder function well after a manic episode, only 28% are able to achieve good occupational outcomes (Gitlin, Swendsen, Heller, et al., 1995).

Although treatment can improve the outcomes for patients with bipolar disorder—including improvement in health, mortality, functioning, and quality of life—many patients are ambivalent about treatment and do not adhere. Other factors that influence the course of bipolar disorder include co-occurring psychiatric disorders and medical disorders, substance abuse, unhealthy lifestyle practices, and inadequate family, vocational, and community support. According to Miklowitz (2008), "Even with optimal psychotherapy and pharmacotherapy, recurrences occur in 50% to 75% of patients in 1 Year" (p. 1417). Symptoms—primarily depressive symptoms—will be present about 50% of the time (Citrome & Goldberg, 2005b), and the risk for suicide remains high (Leverich, Altshuler, Frye, et al., 2003). Among patients who do achieve remission, approximately 50% achieve functional recovery (Haro, Reed, Gonzalez-Pinto, et al., 2011).

Bipolar Disorder in Specific Populations

Children and Adolescents

Bipolar disorder begins before age 18 years in about two-thirds of patients (Perlis et al., 2004) and may present as bipolar disorder with rapid cycling, mixed mania, or psychosis (Fagiolini, 2005). Children and adolescents with bipolar disorder have higher rates of mixed episodes, rapid cycling, and co-occurring ADHD compared to adults with bipolar disorder (DelBello & Chang, 2005).

Epidemiology

Bipolar disorder occurs in approximately 1% of children and adolescents (Keller & Baker, 1991), and the prevalence appears to be increasing in the United States but not internationally (Soutullo, Chang, Diez-Suarez, et al., 2005; Chang et al., 2010). One study found that between

1994-1995 and 2002-2003, there was a 39-fold increase in the number of outpatient pediatric office visits for bipolar disorder in the United States (Moreno, Laje, Blanco, et al., 2007). The increase may be due to greater recognition of a previously under-recognized disorder (Chang et al.). However, another view is presented by Reichart and Nolen (2004), who suggested that early symptoms of bipolar disorder in children—hyperactivity, irritability, temper tantrums, and mood lability—may be interpreted as symptoms of depression or ADHD, treatment of which with antidepressants or stimulants may induce bipolar disorder, a switch into mania, or hypomania. Reichart and Nolen pointed out that the use of stimulants and antidepressants for children is less in Europe, which may account for less medication-induced bipolar disorder there.

Etiology

About 90% of children with bipolar disorder have a family history of mood disorders or substance abuse disorders (Faedda, Baldessarini, Glovinsky, et al., 2004), suggesting a strong genetic influence. A child who has one bipolar parent has a risk factor of 15% to 30% of developing a mood disorder. If both parents have bipolar disorder, the child has a risk factor of 50% to 75% (Koplewicz, 1996; Papolos & Papolos, 2002). The presence of prenatal and perinatal risk factors such as prenatal exposure to drugs or adverse circumstances of birth increases the likelihood of the child's developing pediatric bipolar disorder (Pavuluri, Henry, Nadimpalli, et al., 2006). (See Chapter 3 for prenatal risk factors and the influence of adverse circumstances of birth on the development of psychopathology.)

Higher rates of pediatric bipolar disorder have been found among children who were identified as having a difficult temperament as infants, particularly a difficult temperament that included the inability to inhibit behavioral responses, difficulty with emotional regulation, or difficulty regulating emotional responses and responses to environmental stimuli (West, Schenkel, & Pavuluri, 2008). (See Chapter 1 for discussion of temperament.)

In addition to genetic vulnerability, difficult temperament, and dysfunction of brain circuits, experienced factors are also risk factors for pediatric bipolar disorder. For example, among children experiencing mania, 50% have abused drugs, alcohol, or both. Among adolescents, it appears that stressors have a causal relationship with mood symptoms. For example, chronic stress in the family and in romantic or peer relationships and frequent stressful life events are associated with mood symptoms in adolescents (Kim, Miklowitz, Biuckians, et al., 2007).

Biological Basis

Evidence suggests that dysfunction of the frontolimbic circuitry may be involved in the exaggerated emotional responses and difficulty regulating emotional responses seen in children with bipolar disorder; that is, impairment of circuits that control thinking and emotions may underlie symptoms of pediatric bipolar disorder (Pavuluri & Bogarapu, 2008). For example, researchers found that children with bipolar disorder lagged behind children who did not have any psychiatric disorder in neurocognitive functioning: children with bipolar disorder had lower scores on attention, working memory, executive functioning, and verbal memory, and 3 years later, after treatment for the bipolar disorder, they still had not caught up with the other children (Pavuluri, West, Hill, et al., 2009).

Clinical Presentation

Children

Symptoms in young children (6 years old or younger) include increased energy; bold or demanding behavior; cognitive problems; anxious, fearful, or worried mood; shyness or timidity; and quick temper (Bauer et al., 2008, p. 52). Symptoms in children between 7 years and 12 years include irritable mood, quick temper, oversensitivity, decreased energy or feeling tired, or increased energy and labile mood (Bauer et al.). There may also be mood disturbances (such as hypomania), sleep disturbances (such as insomnia), hyperactivity, giddiness, agitation, belligerence, panic attacks, hostility/aggression, and impulsivity (Citrome & Goldberg, 2005b; Faedda et al., 2004).

Children with mania seldom show a euphoric mood. Instead, they present with a predominantly irritable mood mixed with symptoms of depression; there may also be psychotic symptoms (Brown, 2002-2003). The irritability can be severe, persistent, and aggressive. Outbursts often include a threatening or attacking behavior toward family members, other children, adults, and teachers. In between the outbursts, the children are irritable or angry. Inflated self-esteem or grandiosity may be evidenced by their belief that they have super-powers. They may have trouble falling asleep and sleep less than other children of the same age. Their speech may be rapid and they may demonstrate a flight of ideas. They may start new projects or engage in reckless activities (Chang et al., 2010).

In the depressive phase, children may complain of headaches, muscle aches, and tiredness and may miss school. They may be extremely sensitive to rejection and may talk about running away (Brown, 2002-2003).

Adolescents

Among adolescents, symptoms include depressed mood, irritable mood, decreased energy, crying, guilt and self-reproach, and being withdrawn. Symptoms can also include decreased sleep, garrulousness, problems with anger control, bold and demanding actions (Bauer et al., 2008), hypomania, hyperactivity, agitation, panic attacks, irritability, hostility/aggression, impulsivity, and anxiety (Citrome & Goldberg, 2005b; Faedda et al., 2004).

Adolescents may present with silliness, oppositional behaviors, hostility, racing thoughts, pressured speech, going without sleep, and reckless, thrill-seeking behaviors (Emslie, Mayes, Kennard, et al., 2006). Among older adolescents, the onset of bipolar disorder may be a manic episode, and the pattern of the episodes of mania and depression is similar to that of adults with bipolar disorder (Brown, 2002-2003; Ghaemi & Martin, 2007).

Comorbidity

Children and adolescents diagnosed with bipolar disorder are at increased risk for comorbidities such as self-injurious behaviors, academic problems, conduct disorder, substance use, psychiatric disorders, and suicide (Chang et al., 2010). Comorbid medical disorders that may cause symptoms of mania include thyroid disease, infectious mononucleosis, systemic lupus erythematosus, temporal lobe epilepsy, and anemia. Medications that may cause symptoms of mania include antidepressants, psychostimulants, corticosteroids, antimalarial agents, and thyroxine (Chang et al., p. 394).

Differential Diagnosis

Bipolar disorder in children may be misdiagnosed as depression, anxiety disorders, conduct disorder, and ADHD (Emslie et al., 2006). According to Papolos and Papolos (2002), approximately one-third of children in the United States who are diagnosed with ADHD are actually experiencing an early onset of mania. The symptoms of mania may overlap with the symptoms of ADHD and conduct disorder. Symptoms of bipolar disorder that overlap with symptoms of ADHD include irritable mood, accelerated speech, distractibility, temper tantrums, and increased energy. Symptoms of bipolar disorder that do not overlap include elated mood, grandiosity, flight of ideas, racing thoughts, daredevil activities (jumping off roofs), decreased need for sleep, starting elaborate projects, hypersexuality (usually there is no history of sexual abuse), feelings of guilt or worthlessness, and suicidal ideation (Emslie et al; Chang et al., 2010). An inaccurate diagnosis of ADHD and treatment with a prescribed stimulant can precipitate an early onset of bipolar disorder (Olson & Pacheco, 2005).

Children with ADHD often have learning disabilities, whereas children with bipolar disorder may have above-average verbal and artistic skills (Brown, 2002-2003). In children with bipolar disorder, angry outbursts may last for 4 hours, whereas in children with ADHD, the outbursts are more likely to last 45 minutes or less (Brown, 2002-2003). Currently, approximately 30% of children originally diagnosed with ADHD are later given a diagnosis of bipolar disorder ("Bipolar Disorder in Children," 2007).

Treatment

Assessment and making the correct diagnosis is crucial for helping children and adolescents obtain the appropriate treatment for bipolar disorder. If bipolar disorder is not correctly diagnosed and treated, children and adolescents may develop bipolar disorder with rapid cycling, psychosis, and suicidality (Olson & Pacheco, 2005).

Treatment of bipolar disorder in children and adolescents should include a comprehensive treatment plan that promotes age-appropriate growth and development (Chang et al., 2010) as well as manages the bipolar disorder. Comprehensive treatment for bipolar disorder includes pharmacotherapy, psychotherapy, psychosocial interventions (lifestyle adjustments, reduction of stress, establishing stable sleep patterns, exercise, and adjustments at school that accommodate impairments in attention, executive functioning, working memory, and verbal learning) (Olson & Pacheco, 2005; Reichart & Nolen, 2007), There is evidence that early intervention for children and adolescents may prevent early symptoms of bipolar disorder from progressing to the full syndrome of bipolar disorder (Chang, Howe, Gallelli, et al., 2006).

Pharmacotherapy

Although researchers have published the effectiveness of pharmacotherapy for children and adolescents with bipolar disorder in case studies, open-label trials, and chart reviews, there are few double-blind, placebo-controlled studies (Chang et al., 2010). The guidelines for the treatment of pediatric bipolar disorder of The American Academy of Child and Adolescent Psychiatry endorse the use of lithium, divalproex, and second generation antipsychotics and medications that have FDA approval for the treatment of bipolar disorder in adults (McClellan, Kowatch, & Findling, 2007).

Lithium was the first medication approved by the FDA for treatment of mania in adolescents (Chang et al., 2010). In a review of studies of adolescents with bipolar disorder who received lithium, the response rate varied from 38% to 48% (Wagner & Pliszka, 2009). The FDA has approved risperidone as monotherapy and aripiprazole as monotherapy or as an adjunct to lithium or valproate for acute mania and mixed episodes in children and adolescents ages 10 to 17 years. The response rate for valproate in the form of divalproex was between 53% and 61% (Wagner & Pliszka), but the response rate of extended-release divalproex was 24% (Wagner, Redden, Kowatach, et al., 2009). The response rate of risperidone varied between 59% and 63%, and the response rate of aripiprazole varied between 44.8% and 63.6%. The variations are related to whether patients received a low dose or high dose of the medications (Chang et al., 2010). Psychiatric advanced practice nurses are advised to consult current psychopharmacotherapy textbooks for guidelines in the use of medications for children and adolescents with bipolar disorder.

Drugs to be avoided include beta blockers such as propranolol that can cause depression; caffeine; tricyclic antidepressants; steroids; St. John's wort or Ginkgo biloba; and Sudafed, which may increase norepinephrine and arousal (Brown, 2002-2003, p. 35). The adverse effect of precipitating mania among children with undiagnosed bipolar disorder is more common among children receiving antidepressants than among children receiving stimulant medications. In addition to mania, children with unrecognized bipolar disorder who receive antidepressant medications are at risk for developing suicidal, homicidal, or psychotic behaviors (Faedda et al., 2004).

Psychotherapy and Psychosocial Interventions

Current guidelines for the treatment of bipolar disorder in children and adolescents recommend that all patients receive a combination of medication and psychotherapy (Kowatch, Fristad, Birmaher, et al., 2005). Psychotherapies that are used in the treatment of children and adolescents with bipolar disorder include CBT, interpersonal and social rhythm therapy, and family therapy (Chang et al., 2010).

Psychosocial interventions for children and adolescents with bipolar disorder are similar to those for adults and include developing a relapse prevention plan, education for the family, stress reduction, nutrition, setting regular times for sleep and exercise, and support from other families. One psychosocial intervention, school accommodations, is specific to children and adolescents (Emslie et al., 2006; Reichart & Nolen, 2007).

Accommodations may be made by the school as part of the treatment plan, based on the student's needs. Accommodations include placement in the least-restrictive setting; increased time for assignments and tests; teaching the student how to use organizational strategies; tutoring if the student is absent from school; a behavioral intervention plan; and calling 911 if the student becomes suicidal, homicidal, or delusional (Child and Adolescent Bipolar Foundation, 2004).

Course

The course of bipolar disorder in children is chronic, with cycling patterns that differ from those of adults with bipolar disorder. Prepubertal onset of bipolar disorder is associated with an increased risk of developing rapid-cycling bipolar disorder (four or more episodes in 12 months); ultra-rapid cycling (mood changes within a few days or weeks); and ultradian cycling (four cycles per day) (Emslie et al., 2006). In a 5-year follow-up study of adolescents with bipolar disorder who had received mood stabilizers, 44% had one or more relapses and 20% had made a serious suicide attempt (Strober, Schmidt-Lackner, Freeman, et al., 1995). Risks for poorer outcomes include early age of onset, long duration of illness, mixed episodes, rapid cycling, psychosis, subsyndromal symptoms, comorbid disorders, low socioeconomic status, exposure to negative life events, lack of psychotherapy treatment, poor adherence to medications, and family psychopathology (Birmaher, Axelson, Goldstein, et al., 2009). In brief, although recovery from the first episode is common, many patients will experience recurring symptoms of depression and rapid mood changes, and more than half (62.5%) will have a recurrence following recovery from the first episode (Birmaher et al.).

Older Adults

Often, individuals who appear to develop bipolar disorder late in life may have had symptoms of the disorder earlier that were not recognized. Frequently, older adults with bipolar disorder are diagnosed as having schizophrenia and are treated accordingly (Luggen, 2005). The first episode of late-onset bipolar disorder among older adults usually occurs among those who are in the early to mid 70s (Shulman, 2004). Older adults with bipolar disorder often present with a combination of manic and depressive symptoms or they may appear delirious (Aziz, Lorberg, & Tampi, 2006). They are also likely to have more cognitive impairment than younger patients with bipolar disorder (Depp, Lindamer, Folsom, et al., 2005). Depressive episodes in older adults may be associated with pseudodementia, which means that they have symptoms that are similar to symptoms of dementia, such as distractibility, poor concentration, memory loss, and impaired executive functioning (Brooks, Sommer, & Ketter, 2010). Depression can be differentiated from dementia by its more acute onset of cognitive decline—over weeks rather than years—and by the fact that patients with depression complain of both short-term and long-term memory loss rather than the short-term memory deficits seen in patients with dementia.

Epidemiology

The prevalence of bipolar I disorder in American older adults (ages 65 years and older) is 0.1%, and the prevalence of bipolar II disorder is similar. Bipolar disorder is much less common in older adults than in adults in the 30- to 44-year-old group. Despite the lower prevalence, older adults with bipolar disorder account for 15% of emergency room visits by older adults and 10% of psychiatric hospital admissions (Brooks et al., 2010).

Etiology

Among older adults, certain medical illness, medications, substances, and situations precipitate mania. Medical conditions that increase an individual's likelihood of developing mania include hyperthyroidism, epilepsy, stroke, head injury (often sustained in falls), uremia, and vitamin B_{12} deficiency. Medications associated with increased risk of mania include antidepressants (especially tricyclics), brochodilators, dopamine agonists, and pseudoephedrine (such as Sudafed and Contac Cold, used to treat nasal congestion) (Luggen, 2005). Substances associated with mania include caffeine, alcohol, St. John's wort, and cocaine. Situations associated with increased risk for mania include sleep deprivation, stress, problems with family relationships, changes in social support networks, and increased light exposure (Luggen, 2005).

Clinical Presentation

Older adults with bipolar disorder may present with manic symptoms, hypomanic symptoms, or depression; however, the first episode is more likely to be a depressive episode (Luggen, 2005). Frequent symptoms include confusion, disorientation, irritability, and distractibility. The symptoms may be due to the bipolar disorder or to secondary medical conditions such as delirium, multiple sclerosis, hyperthyroidism, tertiary syphilis, or HIV/AIDS. The symptoms may also be caused by their use of medications—such as the angiotensin-converting enzyme inhibitor captopril (Capoten) or steroids—or by their use of substances such as cocaine and illicit stimulants (Brooks et al., 2010, p. 456). Among adults over the age of 60 years with bipolar disorder, the onset of mania is less likely to be associated with a family history of bipolar disorder and more likely to be due to a medical illness such as cerebrovascular problems, trauma, stroke, multiple sclerosis, hyperthyroidism, AIDS, or systemic lupus erythematosus (Bauer & Pfennig, 2005).

Comorbidity

Bipolar disorder among older adults is accompanied by high rates of comorbid medical and neurological disorders, disabilities, and diminished quality of life (Brooks et al., 2010). For example, among older adults with manic episodes, the rate of co-occurring neurological disorders is 70% and the rate of co-occurring cerebrovascular diseases is 35% (Shulman, 2004). Comorbid medical conditions that must be considered when choosing medications for older patients with bipolar disorder include glaucoma, prostatic hypertrophy, pulmonary diseases, and Parkinson's disease. In addition to comorbid medical and neurological disorders that must be considered in planning treatment, dementia, which is present in 3% of older adults with bipolar disorder, must be considered (Brooks, Hoblyn, Kraemer, et al., 2006).

Differential Diagnosis

Psychiatric disorders that should be ruled out include substance abuse, post-traumatic stress disorder, anxiety, and dementia. If the patient has episodes of mania, infections, medications, and medical illness such as thyroid disorders, cerebrovascular disorders, and cardiovascular disorders must be ruled out (Sherrod, Quinlan-Colwell, Lattimore, et al., 2010).

Treatment

Before deciding on treatment for older adults with bipolar disorder, psychiatric advanced practice nurses should obtain a medical history, physical examination, baseline laboratory tests, and information about the treatment of any co-occurring medical or psychiatric disorders.

Pharmacotherapy

There is a lack of evidenced-based information about pharmacotherapy for older adults with bipolar disorder, which is a population likely to have medical comorbidities, neurological comorbidities, psychiatric comorbidities, and disabilities and to be receiving multiple medications (Brooks et al., 2010). General principles for pharmacotherapy for older adults with bipolar disorder include

- Ongoing monitoring of psychiatric status, medical status, and cognition
- Starting medications at low doses (20% to 50% of the adult dose)
- Gradually increasing the dose if necessary

In addition:

- Target dose should be 25% to 50% of that for young adult patients if the older adult has co-occurring medical or neurological disorders
- Target dose should be 50% of that for young adult patients if the older adult does not have comorbid medical and neurological disorders (adapted from Brooks et al., 2010)

Mood-stabilizing agents are recommended as the first line for treatment of bipolar disorder in older adults (Kennedy, 2008). Aziz et al. (2006) have suggested that valproate (divalproex sodium, valproate sodium, and valproic acid) and lamotrigine may be effective and cause fewer troublesome side effects than lithium. Among older adults, lithium is known to increase the risk of polyuria and polydipsia, which may lead to nocturia and falls. Lamotrigine is well tolerated by older adults and is known to delay the recurrence of bipolar depression, although it is less effective in preventing or delaying recurrence of mania. One of the risks of lamotrigine therapy is the development of Stevens-Johnson syndrome, which occurs in about 0.13% of patients with mood disorders who receive lamotrigine. Atypical antipsychotic medications that are often used for bipolar disorder may, when used for older adults, increase mortality from cardiac and infectious illnesses (Brooks et al., 2010).

Nonpharmacological Therapy

ECT is also effective in treating bipolar disorder in older adults and is the treatment of choice when acuity of symptoms compromises the patient's medical stability (Brooks et al., 2010, p. 483).

Psychotherapy and psychosocial interventions are also used in treating bipolar disorder in older adults. CBT, supportive psychotherapy, and interpersonal psychotherapy have been found to benefit older patients with depression (Alexopoulos, Katz, Reynolds, et al., 2001). Psychosocial interventions include problem-solving therapy, case management, psychoeducation, and visiting nurses (Brooks et al., 2010). (See Chapter 8 for information on psychosocial interventions.)

Course

Bipolar disorder in older adults is associated with a poorer response to treatment, recurrent episodes, higher mortality rates, and higher rates of suicide than in younger patients with bipolar disorder (Aziz et al., 2006).

Key Points

- Bipolar disorder is a recurring, lifelong illness that disrupts patients' lives and causes them and their families great suffering (Bauer & Pfennig, 2005).

- Bipolar I is characterized by one or more manic episodes or mixed episodes usually accompanied by major depressive episodes.
- Bipolar II is characterized by one or more major depressive episodes accompanied by at least one episode of hypomania. There is no history of a manic episode.
- Treatment in the manic phase of bipolar disorder includes mood stabilizers and atypical antipsychotics.
- Treatment in the depressive phase of bipolar disorder includes an olanzapine plus fluoxetine combination and quetiapine monotherapy.
- Bipolar disorder has a severe impact on relationships, parenting, functioning, vocational achievements, and well-being.
- Patients with bipolar disorder tend to have more symptoms, more depression, more unemployment, and more rehospitalizations than patients with other mood disorders.
- Divorce rates are two to three times higher than normal comparison subjects, and vocational status is twice as likely to deteriorate.
- For many patients, the time lag between onset of symptoms, correct diagnosis, and treatment is 5 to 10 years (Sachs, Printz, Kahn, et al., 2000), and even when patients do receive treatment, many do not receive appropriate treatment with mood stabilizers (Blanco, Laje, Olfson, et al., 2002).
- Challenging issues in managing the care of patients with bipolar disorder are reducing recurrences, managing co-occurring medical and psychiatric disorders, preventing suicide, and accessing support and services to assist patients in compensating for the disabilities associated with their illness.
- A biopsychosocial approach to preventing recurrences in bipolar disorder includes meeting the patient's needs; structuring activities of work, sleep, and exercise; promoting healthy lifestyle practices; monitoring medications; facilitating adherence to treatment; and providing education for the patient and family.
- Lack of treatment or inappropriate treatment increases the patient's and family's suffering, adds to health-care costs, and results in achievement of complete remission in less than half of patients with bipolar disorder (Goldberg & Harrow, 2004).

Resources

Organizations

National Alliance on Mental Illness (NAMI)
www.nami.org
Mental Health America
www.nmha.org
Depression and Bipolar Support Alliance
www.dbsalliance.org
Child and Adolescent Bipolar Foundation
www.bpkids.org
Juvenile Bipolar Research Foundation
www.jbrf.org

Manuals

Life Chart Manual for Recurrent Affective Illness (can be ordered from NDMDA at www.ndmda.org)

Books

Jamison, K. R. (1996). *An unquiet mind: A memoir of moods and madness.* New York: Random House.

Goodwin, F. K., & Jamison, K. R. (1990). *Manic-depressive illness.* New York: Oxford University Press.

Thompson, T. (1995). *The beast: A reckoning with depression.* New York: G. P. Putnam's Sons.

Torrey, E. F., & Knable, M. B. (2002). *Surviving manic depression: A manual on bipolar disorder for patients, families and providers.* New York: Basic Books.

McManamy, J. (2006). *Living well with depression and bipolar disorder: What your doctor doesn't tell you.* New York: Collins.

Duke, P., & Hockman, G. (1992). *A brilliant madness: Living with manic-depressive illness.* New York: Bantam Books.

Movies

Figgis, M. (Director). (1993). *Mr. Jones* [Motion picture]. United States: TriStar Pictures.

Stillman, W. (Director). (1998). *The last days of disco* [Motion picture]. United States: Gramercy Pictures.

Cates, G. (Director). (1990). *Call me Anna* [TV Motion picture].

Richardson, T. (Director). (1994). *Blue sky* [Motion picture]. United States: Orion Pictures.

Gilroy, T. (Director). (2007). *Michael Clayton* [Motion picture]. United States: Warner Brothers.

SOURCE: WEDDING, BOYD, & NIEMIEC, 2010, PP. 56-58.

References

Abler, B., Greenhouse, I., Ongur, D., et al. (2008). Abnormal reward system activation in mania. *Neuropsychopharmacology, 33*(9), 2217-2227.

Alexopoulos, G. S., Katz, I. R., Reynolds, C. F. 3rd, et al. (2001). The expert consensus guideline series: Pharmacotherapy of depressive disorders in older patients. *Postgraduate Medicine (Spec No Pharmacotherapy)*, 1-86.

Alexopoulos, G. S., Raue, P., & Aredin, P. (2003). Problem-solving therapy versus supportive therapy in geriatric major depression with executive dysfunction. *American Journal of Geriatric Psychiatry, 11*(1), 46-52.

Alloy, L. B., Abramson, L. Y., Urosevic, S., et al. (2005). The psychosocial context of bipolar disorder: Environmental, cognitive, and developmental risk factors. *Clinical Psychology Review, 25*(8), 1043-1075.

Altshuler, L. I., Bookheimer, S. Y., Townsend, J., et al. (2005). Blunted activation in orbitofronatal cortex during mania: A functional magnetic resonance imaging study. *Biological Psychiatry, 58*, 763-769.

Altshuler, L., Curran, J. G., Hauser, P., et al. (1995). T2 hyperintensities in bipolar disorder: Magnetic resonance imaging comparison and literature meta-analysis. *American Journal of Psychiatry, 152*, 1139-1144.

Altshuler, L. L., Post, R. M., Black, D. O., et al. (2006). Subsyndromal depressive symptoms are associated with functional impairment in patients with bipolar disorders: Results of a large, multisite study. *Journal of Clinical Psychiatry, 67*, 1551-1560.

Altshuler, L., Suppes, T., Black, D., et al. (2003). Impact of antidepressant discontinuation after acute bipolar depression remission on rates of depressive relapse at 1-year follow-up. *American Journal of Psychiatry, 160*, 1252-1262.

American Psychiatric Association (2000). *Diagnostic and statistical manual of mental disorders* (4th ed., text rev.). Washington, DC: American Psychiatric Publishing, Inc.

American Psychiatric Association. (2002). Practice guideline for the treatment of patients with bipolar disorder (revision). *American Journal of Psychiatry, 159*(Suppl), 1-50.

Anand, A., & Charney, D. S. (2000). Abnormalities in catecholamines and pathophysiology of bipolar disorder. In J. C. Soares & S. Gershon (Eds.),

Bipolar disorders: Basic mechanisms and therapeutic implications (pp. 59-94). New York: Marcel Dekker.

Angst, J., Gamma, A., Rossler, W., et al. (2011). Childhood adversity and chronicity of mood disorders. *European Archives of Psychiatry and Clinical Neuroscience, 261*(1), 21-27.

Antila, M., Partonen, T., Kieseppa, T., et al. (2009). Cognitive functioning of bipolar I patients and relatives from families with or without schizophrenia or schizoaffective disorder. *Journal of Affective Disorders, 116*(1-2), 70-79.

Arnone, D., Cavanagh, J., Gerber, D., et al. (2009). Magnetic resonance imaging studies in bipolar disorder and schizophrenia: Meta-analysis. *The British Journal of Psychiatry, 195,* 194-201.

Aschoff, J. (1981). *Handbook of behavioral neurobiology* (Vol. 4. Biological Rhythms). New York: Plenum Press.

Aziz, R., Lorberg, B., & Tampi, R. (2006). Treatments for late-life bipolar disorder. *The American Journal of Geriatric Pharmacotherapy, 4*(4), 347-364.

Balaraman, R., & Hardik, G. (2010). Asenapine, a new sublingual atypical antipsychotic. *Journal of Pharmacology and Pharmacotherapeutics, 8*(1), 60-61.

Baldassano, C. F. (2009). Promoting wellness in patients with bipolar disorder: Strategies to move beyond maintaining stability and minimizing adverse events in effective long-term management. *Supplement to Current Psychiatry, October,* S12-S22. Retrieved from: www.currentpsychiatry.com

Baldessarini, R. J., Tondo, L., & Hennen, J. (2003). Lithium treatment and suicide risk in major affective disorders: Update and new findings. *Journal of Clinical Psychiatry, 64*(Suppl 5), 44-52.

Basco, M. R., McDonald, N., Merlock, M. C., et al. (2004). A cognitive behavioral approach to treatment of bipolar I disorder. In J. H. Wright (Ed.), *Cognitive behavioral therapy* (pp. 25-53). Washington, DC: American Psychiatric Publishing, Inc.

Bauer, M., Juckel, G., Correll, C. U., et al. (2008). Diagnosis and treatment in the early illness phase of bipolar disorders. *European Archives of Psychiatry and Clinical Neuroscience, 258*(Suppl 5), 50-54.

Bauer, M. S., Kirk, G. F., Gavin, C., et al. (2001). Determinants of functional outcome and healthcare costs in bipolar disorder: A high-intensity follow-up study. *Journal of Affective Disorders, 65,* 231-241.

Bauer, M. S., McBride, L., Williford, W. O., et al. (2006). Collaborative care for bipolar disorder: Part II. Impact on clinical outcomes, function, and costs. *Psychiatry Services, 57,* 937-945.

Bauer, M., & Pfennig, A. (2005). Epidemiology of bipolar disorders. *Epilepsia, 46*(Suppl 4), 8-13.

Bauer, M., Unutzer, J., Pincus, H. A., et al. (2002). Bipolar disorder. *Mental Health Services Research, 4,* 225-229.

Beckmann, M., Johansen-Berg, H., & Rushworth, M. F. (2009). Connectivity-based parcellation of human cingulate cortex and its relation to functional specialization. *Journal of Neuroscience, 29,* 1175-1190.

Bell, A. C., & D'Zurilla, T. J. (2009). Problem-solving therapy for depression: A meta-analysis. *Clinical Psychology Review, 29,* 348-353.

Belmaker, R. H. (2004). Medical progress: Bipolar disorder. *The New England Journal of Medicine, 351*(5), 476-486.

Berk, M., Dodd, S., Callaly, P., et al. (2007). History of illness prior to a diagnosis of bipolar disorder or schizoaffective disorder. *Affective Disorders, 103*(1), 181-186.

Berk, M., Ichim, L., & Brook, S. (1999). Olanzapine (Zyprexa) compared to lithium in mania: A double-blind randomized controlled trial. *International Clinical Psychopharmacology, 14,* 339-343.

Berlant, J., & van Kammen, D. P. (2002). Open-label topiramate as primary or adjunctive therapy in chronic civilian posttraumatic stress disorder: A preliminary report. *Journal of Clinical Psychiatry, 63,* 15-20.

Berns, G. S., & Nemeroff, C. B. (2003). The neurobiology of bipolar disorder. *American Journal of Medical Genetics. Part C, Seminars in Medical Genetics, 123C,* 76-84.

Beyer, J., Kuchibhatla, M., Gersing, K., et al. (2005). Medical comorbidity in a bipolar outpatient clinical population. *Neuropsychopharmacology, 30*(2), 401-404.

Beynon, S., Soares-Weiser, K., Woolacott, N., et al. (2008). Psychosocial interventions for the prevention of relapse in bipolar disorder: Systematic review of controlled trials. *British Journal of Psychiatry, 192,* 5-11.

Bipolar disorder in children. (2007). *Harvard Mental Health Letter, 23*(11), 1-3.

Birmaher, B., Axelson, D., Goldstein, B., et al. (2009). Four-year longitudinal course of children and adolescents with bipolar spectrum disorders: The course and outcome of bipolar youth (COBY) study. *American Journal of Psychiatry, 166,* 795-804.

Black, E. W., & Andreasen, N. C. (2011). *Introductory textbook of psychiatry* (5th ed.). Washington, DC: American Psychiatric Publishing, Inc.

Blanco, C., Laje, G., Olfson, M., et al. (2002). Trends in the treatment of bipolar disorder by out-patient psychiatrists. *American Journal of Psychiatry, 159,* 1005-1010.

Blumberg, H. P., Kaufman, J., Martin, A., et al. (2003). Amygdala and hippocampal volumes in adolescents and adults with bipolar disorder. *Archives of General Psychiatry, 60*(12), 1201-1208.

Blumberg, H. P., Stern, E., Martinez, D., et al. (2000). Increased anterior cingulate and caudate activity in bipolar mania. *Biological Psychiatry, 48*(11), 1045-1052.

Blumberg, H. P., Stern, E., Ricketts, S., et al. (1999). Rostral and orbital-prefrontal cortex dysfunction in the manic state of bipolar disorder. *American Journal of Psychiatry, 156,* 1986-1988.

Bottlender, R., Rudolf, D., Strauss, A., et al. (2001). Mood-stabilizers reduce the risk of developing antidepressant-induced maniform states in acute treatment of bipolar I depressed patients. *Journal of Affective Disorders, 63,* 79-83.

Bourre, J. M. (2004). The role of nutritional factors on the structure and function of the brain: An update on dietary requirements. *Revue Neurologique, 160*(8-9), 767-792.

Bourre, J. M. (2005). Omega-3 fatty acids in psychiatry. *Médecine Sciences: M/S, 21*(2), 216-221.

Bowden, C. L. (2004). Valproate. In A. F. Schatzberg & C. B. Nemeroff (Eds.), *Textbook of psychopharmacology* (3rd ed.) (pp. 567-579). Washington, DC: American Psychiatric Publishing, Inc.

Bowden, C. L. (2009). Valproate. In A. F. Schatzberg & C. B. Nemeroff (Eds.), *Textbook of psychopharmacology* (4th ed.) (pp. 719-734). Washington, DC: American Psychiatric Publishing, Inc.

Bowden, C. L., Brugger, A. M., Swann, A. C., et al. (1994). Efficacy of divalproex vs lithium and placebo in the treatment of mania. *Journal of the American Medical Association, 271,* 918-924.

Brambilla, P., Harenski, K., Nicoletti, M., et al. (2003). MRI investigation of temporal lobe structures in bipolar patients. *Journal of Psychiatric Research, 37*(4), 287-295.

Breit-Gabauer, B., Berg, A., Demelbauer, S., et al. (2010). Prodromes and coping strategies in patients with bipolar disorder. *Verhaltenstherapie, 20,* 183-191.

Brieger, P., Ehrt, U., & Marneros, A. (2003). Frequency of comorbid personality disorders in bipolar and unipolar affective disorders. *Comprehensive Psychiatry, 44*(1), 28-34.

Brooks, J. O., Hoblyn, J. C., Kraemer, H. C., et al. (2006). Factors associated with psychiatric hospitalization of individuals diagnoses with dementia and comorbid bipolar disorder. *Journal of Geriatric Psychiatry and Neurology, 19,* 72-77.

Brooks, J. O., Sommer, B. R., & Ketter, T. A. (2010). Management of bipolar disorders in older adults. In T. A. Ketter (Ed.), *Handbook of diagnosis and treatment of bipolar disorders* (pp. 453-497). Washington, DC: American Psychiatric Publishing, Inc.

Brooks, J. O., Wang, P. W., Bonner, J. C., et al. (2009). Decreased prefrontal, anterior cingulate, insula, and ventral striatal metabolism in medication-free depressed outpatients with bipolar disorder. *Journal of Psychiatric Research, 43,* 181-188.

Brown, A. B. (2002-2003). Why is bipolar disorder often under-diagnosed in children. *NARSAD Research Newsletter, Winter, 14*(4), 31-36.

Brown, E. B., McElroy, S. L., Keck, P. E., Jr., et al. (2006). A 7-week, randomized, double-blind trial of olanzapine (Zyprexa)/fluoxetine combination versus lamotrigine in the treatment of bipolar I depression. *Journal of Clinical Psychiatry, 67,* 1024-1033.

Butzlaff, R. L., & Hooley, J. M. (1998). Expressed emotion and psychiatric relapse: A meta-analysis. *Archives of General Psychiatry, 55,* 547-552.

Caetano, S. C., Sassi, R., Brambilla, P., et al. (2001). MRI study of thalamic volumes in bipolar and unipolar and healthy individuals. *Psychiatric Research, 108*(3), 161-168.

Calabrese, J. R., Keck, P. E., Jr., MacFadden, W., et al. (2005). A randomized, double-blind, placebo-controlled trial of quetiapine in the treatment of bipolar I or II depression. *American Journal of Psychiatry, 162*, 1351-1360.

Calabrese, J. R., Shelton, M. D., Bowden, C. L., et al. (2001). Bipolar rapid cycling: Focus on depression as its hallmark. *Journal of Clinical Psychiatry, 62*(Suppl 14), 34-41.

Chang, C. Y., Ke, D. S., & Chen, J. Y. (2009). Essential fatty acids and human brain. *Acta Neurologica Taiwanica, 18*(4), 231-241.

Chang, K. D., Dienes, K., Blasey, C., et al. (2003). Divalproex monotherapy in the treatment of bipolar offspring with mood and behavioral disorders and at least mild affective symptoms. *Journal of Clinical Psychiatry, 64*(8), 936-942.

Chang, K., Howe, M., Gallelli, K., et al. (2006). Prevention of pediatric bipolar disorder: Integration of neurobiological and psychosocial processes. *Annals of the New York Academy of Sciences, 1094*, 235-247.

Chang, K. D., Singh, M. K., Wang, P. W., et al. (2010). Management of bipolar disorder in children and adolescents. In T. A. Ketter (Ed.), *Handbook of diagnosis and treatment of bipolar disorders* (pp. 389-424). Washington, DC: American Psychiatric Publishing, Inc.

Child and Adolescent Bipolar Foundation (CABF). (2004). *About early-onset bipolar disorder.* Retrieved from http://www.bpkids.org/learning/about.htm

Choi, J., Baek, J. H., Noh, J., et al. (2011). Association of seasonality and premenstrual symptoms in bipolar I and bipolar II disorders. *Journal of Affective Disorders, 129*(1-3), 313-316.

Citrome, L., & Goldberg, J. F. (2005a). Bipolar disorder is a potentially fatal disease. *Postgraduate Medicine Online, 117*(2), 1-6

Citrome, L., & Goldberg, J. F. (2005b). The many faces of bipolar disorder. *Postgraduate Medicine Online, 117*(2), 1-12.

Cohen, A., Hammen, C., Henry, R., et al. (2004). Effects of stress and social support on recurrence in bipolar disorder. *Journal of Affective Disorders, 82*, 143-147.

Colom, F., & Lam, D. (2005). Psychoeducation: Improving outcomes in bipolar disorder. *European Psychiatry, 20*, 359-364.

Colom, F., Vieta, E., Martinez-Aran, A., et al. (2003). A randomized trial on the efficacy of group psychoeducation in prophylaxis of recurrences in bipolar patients whose disease is in remission. *Archives of General Psychiatry, 60*, 402-407.

Comtois, K. A., Russo, J. E., Roy-Byrne, P., et al. (2004). Clinicians' assessments of bipolar disorder and substance abuse as predictors of suicidal behavior in acutely hospitalized psychiatric inpatients. *Biological Psychiatry, 56*(10), 757-763.

Cookson, J. (2005). Toward a clinical understanding of bipolar disorders: Classification and presentation. *Epilepsia, 46*(Suppl 4), 3-7.

Cousins, D. A., Butts, K., & Young, A. H. (2009). The role of dopamine in bipolar disorder. *Bipolar Disorders, 11*, 787-806.

Coverdale, J. H., & Turbott, S. H. (2000). Sexual and physical abuse of chronically ill psychiatric outpatients compared with a matched sample of medical outpatients. *Journal of Nervous & Mental Disease, 188*(7), 440-445.

Coyle, T. R., Kochunov, D., Patel, R. D., et al. (2006). Cortical sulci and bipolar disorders. *Brain Imaging, 17*, 1739-1742.

Crowe, M., Whitehead, L., Wilson, L., et al. (2010). Disorder-specific psychosocial interventions for bipolar disorder: A systematic review of the evidence for mental health nursing practice. *International Journal of Nursing Studies, 47*, 896-908.

Cuijpers, P., van Straten, A., & Warmerdam, L. (2007). Problem solving therapies for depression: A meta-analysis. *European Psychiatry, 22*, 9-15.

Culver, J. L., & Pratchett, L. C. (2010). Adjunctive psychosocial interventions in the management of bipolar disorders. In T. A. Ketter (Ed.), *Handbook of diagnosis and treatment of bipolar disorders* (pp. 661-676). Washington, DC: American Psychiatric Publishing, Inc.

Deak, T., & Panksepp, J. (2004). Stress, sleep, and sexuality in psychiatric disorders. In J. Panksepp (Ed.), *Textbook of biological psychiatry* (pp. 111-143). Hoboken, NJ: Wiley-Liss, Inc.

De Hert, M., Wampers, M., Jendricko, T., et al. (2011). Effects of cannabis use on age of onset in schizophrenia and bipolar disorder. *Schizophrenia Research, 126*(1-3), 270-276.

DelBello, M. P., Adler, C. M., Whitsel, R. M., et al. (2007). A 12-week single-blind trial of quetiapine for the treatment of mood symptoms in adolescents at high risk for developing bipolar I disorder. *Journal of Clinical Psychiatry, 68*(5), 789-795.

DelBello, M. P., & Chang, K. D. (2005). Editorial: Bipolar disorder in children and adolescents: Are we approaching the final frontier? *Bipolar Disorders, 7*, 479-482.

Depp, C. A., Lindamer, L. A., Folsom, D. P., et al. (2005). Differences in clinical features and mental health service use in bipolar disorder across the lifespan. *American Journal of Geriatric Psychiatry, 13*, 290-298.

Diagnosis and Pharmacologic Treatment of Bipolar Disorder (2007). *Psychiatric Nurse Counseling Points, 1*(4), 3-11.

Dias, R. S., Lafer, B., Russo, C., et al. (2011). Longitudinal follow-up of bipolar disorder in women with premenstrual exacerbation: Findings from STEP-BD. *American Journal of Psychiatry, 168*(4), 386-394.

Dilsaver, S. C. (2011). An estimated economic burden of bipolar I and II disorders in the United States: 2009. *Journal of Affective Disorders, 129* (1-3), 79-83.

Donovan, S. J., Stewart, J. W., Nunes, E. V., et al. (2000). Divalproex treatment for youth with explosive temper and mood lability: A double-blind, placebo-controlled crossover design. *American Journal of Psychiatry, 157*, 818-820.

Dubovsky, S. (2005). *Clinical guide to psychotropic medications.* New York: W. W. Norton & Company.

Duckworth, K. (2008). *Understanding bipolar disorder and recovery.* Arlington, VA: National Alliance on Mental Illness.

Dunayevich, E., Sax, K. W., Keck, P. E., Jr., et al. (2000). Twelve-month outcome in bipolar patients with and without personality disorders. *Journal of Clinical Psychiatry, 61*, 134-139.

Dupont, R. M., Jernigan, T. L., Heindel, W., et al. (1995). Magnetic resonance imaging and mood disorders: Localization of white matter and other subcortical abnormalities. *Archives of General Psychiatry, 52*, 747-755.

D'Zurilla, T. J., & Nezu, A. M. (2009). Problem-solving therapy. In K. S. Dobson (Ed.), *Handbook of cognitive-behavioral therapies* (3rd ed.). New York: Guilford Press.

Ehlers, C. L., Kupfer, D. J., Frank, E., et al. (1993). Biological rhythms and depression: The role of Zeitgebers and Zeitstoreres. *Depression, 1*, 285-293.

Elkis, H., Friedman, L., Wise, A., et al. (1995). Meta-analyses of studies of ventricular enlargement and cortical sulcal prominence in mood disorders: Comparisons with controls or patients with schizophrenia. *Archives of General Psychiatry, 52*, 735-746.

Ellison-Wright, I., & Bullmore, E. (2010). Anatomy of bipolar disorder and schizophrenia: A meta-analysis. *Schizophrenia Research, 117*, 1-12.

Emslie, G. J., Mayes, T. L., Kennard, B. D., et al. (2006). Pediatric mood disorders. In D. J. Stein, D. J. Kupfer, & A. F. Schatzberg (Eds.), *The American psychiatric publishing textbook of mood disorders* (pp. 573-601). Washington, DC: American Psychiatric Publishing, Inc.

Engstrom, C., Brandstrom, S., Sigvardsson, S., et al. (2004). Bipolar disorder 1. Temperament and character. *Journal of Affective Disorders, 82*(1), 131-134.

Ernst, C. L., & Goldberg, J. F. (2004). Anti-suicide properties of psychotropic drugs: A critical review. *Harvard Review of Psychiatry, 12*(1), 14-41.

Esposito, S., Prange, A. J., & Golden, R. N. (1997). The thyroid axis and mood disorders: Overview and future prospects. *Psychopharmacology Bulletin, 33*, 205-217.

Faedda, G. L., Baldessarini, R. J., Glovinsky, I. P., et al. (2004). Pediatric bipolar disorder: Phenomenology and course of illness. *Bipolar Disorders, 6*(4), 305-313.

Fagiolini, A. (2005). Battling bipolar disorder: Therapeutic approaches. *Clinical Advisor, March*, 11-20.

Fagiolini, A., Kupfer, D. J., Rucci, P., et al. (2004). Suicide attempts and ideation in patients with bipolar I disorder. *Journal of Clinical Psychiatry, 65*(4), 509-514.

Fawcett, J. (2001). Treating impulsivity and anxiety in the suicidal patient. *Annals of the New York Academy of Sciences, 932*, 14-102.

Fenn, H. H., Bauer, M. S., Altshuler, L., et al. (2005). Medical comorbidity and health-related quality of life in bipolar disorder across the adult age span. *Journal of Affective Disorders, 86*(1), 47-60.

Fiedorowicz, J. G., & Black, D. W. (2010). Borderline, bipolar, or both? Frame your diagnosis on the patient history. *Current Psychiatry Online, 9*(1). Retrieved from http://www.currentpsychiatry.com/

First, M. B., Frances, A., & Pincus, H. A. (2002). *DSM-IV-TR handbook of differential diagnosis*. Washington, DC: American Psychiatric Publishing, Inc.

Frangou, S. (2005). The Maudsley bipolar disorder project. *Epilepsia, 46*(Suppl 4), 19-25.

Frangou, S., Lewis, M., & McCrone, P. (2006). Efficacy of ethyl-eicosapentaenoic acid in bipolar depression: Randomized double-blind placebo-controlled study. *British Journal of Psychiatry, 188*, 46-50.

Frank, E. (2005). *Treating bipolar disorder: A clinician's guide to interpersonal and social rhythm therapy*. New York: Guilford Press.

Frank, E., Gonzalez, J. M., & Fagiolini, A. (2006). The importance of routine for preventing recurrence in bipolar disorder. *American Journal of Psychiatry, 163*(6), 981-985.

Frank, E., Kupfer, D. J., Thase, M. E., et al. (2005). Two-year outcomes for interpersonal and social rhythm therapy in individuals with bipolar I disorder. *Archives of General Psychiatry, 62*, 996-1004.

Frank, E., Swartz, H. A., & Kupfer, D. J. (2000). Interpersonal and social rhythm therapy: Managing the chaos of bipolar disorder. *Biological Psychiatry, 48*, 593-604.

Frankenburg, F. R., & Zanarini, M. C. (2002). Divalproex sodium treatment of women with borderline personality disorder and bipolar II disorder: A double-blind placebo-controlled trial. *Journal of Clinical Psychiatry, 63*, 442-446.

Freeman, M. P., Hibbeln, J. R., Wisner, K. L., et al. (2006). Omega-3 fatty acids: Evidence basis for treatment and future research in psychiatry. *Journal of Clinical Psychiatry, 67*(12), 1954-1967.

Freeman, M. P., Wiegand, C., & Gleneberg, A. J. (2004). Lithium. In A. F. Schatzberg & C. B. Nemeroff (Eds.), *Textbook of psychopharmacology* (3rd ed.) (pp. 547-565). Washington, DC: American Psychiatric Publishing, Inc.

Friedman, E. S., & Thase, M. E. (2007). Depression-focused psychotherapies. In *Gabbard's treatments of psychiatric disorders* (4th ed.) (pp. 409-431). Washington, DC: American Psychiatric Publishing, Inc.

Frye, M. A. (2004). Gabapentin. In A. F. Schatzberg & C. B. Nemeroff (Eds.), *Textbook of psychopharmacology* (3rd ed.) (pp. 607-613). Washington, DC: American Psychiatric Publishing, Inc.

Frye, M. A., & Salloum, I. M. (2006). Bipolar disorder and comorbid alcoholisms: Prevalence rate and treatment considerations. *Bipolar Disorders, 8*(6), 677-685.

Gajwani, P. L., Forsthoff, A., Muzina, D., et al. (2005). Antiepileptic drugs in mood-disordered patients. *Epilepsia, 46*(Suppl 4), 38-44.

Garfinkel, P. E., Stancer, H. C., & Persad, E. (1980). A comparison of haloperidol, lithium and their combination in the treatment of mania. *Journal of Affective Disorders, 2*, 279-288.

Garno, J. L., Goldberg, J. F., Ramirez, P. M., et al. (2005). Impact of childhood abuse on the clinical course of bipolar disorder. *The British Journal of Psychiatry, 186*, 121-125.

Geller, B., Tillman, R., Bolhofner, K., et al. (2006). Controlled, blindly rated, direct-interview family study of a prepubertal and early-adolescent bipolar I disorder phenotype. *Archives of General Psychiatry, 63*, 1130-1138.

Ghaemi, S. N., Lenox, M. S., & Baldessarini, R. J. (2001). Effectiveness and safety of long-term antidepressant treatment of bipolar disorder. *Journal of Clinical Psychiatry, 62*, 565-569.

Ghaemi, S. N., & Martin, A. (2007). Defining the boundaries of childhood bipolar disorder. *American Journal of Psychiatry, 164*(2), 185-188.

Gilliam, T. C., Kandel, E. R., & Jessell, T. M. (2000). Genes and behavior. In E. R. Kandel, J. H. Schwartz, & T. M. Jessell (Eds.), *Principles of neural science* (4th ed.) (pp. 36-66). New York: McGraw-Hill.

Gitlin, M. S., Swendsen, J., Heller, T. L., et al. (1995). Relapse and impairment in bipolar disorder. *American Journal of Psychiatry, 152*, 1635-1640.

Goldberg, J. F., & Citrome, L. (2005). Latest therapies for bipolar disorder. *Postgraduate Medicine Online, 117*(2), 1-11.

Goldberg, J. F., & Garno, J. L. (2005). Development of posttraumatic stress disorder in adult bipolar patients with histories of severe childhood abuse. *Journal of Psychiatric Research, 39*, 595-601.

Goldberg, J., & Harrow, M. (2004). Consistency of remission and outcome in bipolar and unipolar mood disorders: A 10-year prospective follow-up. *Journal of Affective Disorders, 81*(2), 123-131.

Goldberg, J., & Truman, C. (2003). Antidepressant-induced mania: An overview of current controversies. *Bipolar Disorders, 5*(6), 407-420.

Goldstein, B., Fagiolini, A., Houck, P., et al. (2009). Cardiovascular disease and hypertension among adults with bipolar I disorder in the United States. *Bipolar Disorders, 11*(6), 657-662.

Gonzalez, J. M., Thompson, P., Escamilla, M., et al. (2007). Treatment characteristics and illness burden among European Americans, African Americans, and Latinos in the first 2,000 patients of the systematic treatment enhancement program for bipolar disorder. *Psychopharmacology Bulletin, 40*(1), 31-46.

Goodwin, F. K., & Jamison, K. R. (1990). *Manic-depressive illness*. New York: Oxford University Press.

Goodwin, R. D., Jacobi, F., Bittner, A., et al. (2006). Epidemiology of mood disorders. In D. J. Stein, D. J. Kupfer, & A. F. Schatzberg (Eds.), *The American psychiatric publishing textbook of mood disorders* (pp. 33-54). Washington, DC: American Psychiatric Publishing, Inc.

Goossens, P. J. J., van Achterberg, T., & Knoppert-van der Klein, E. A. M. (2007). Nursing processes used in the treatment of patients with bipolar disorder. *International Journal of Mental Health Nursing, 16*, 168-177.

Gray, S. M., & Otto, M. W. (2001). Psychosocial approaches to suicide prevention: Applications to patients with bipolar disorder. *Journal of Clinical Psychiatry, 62*(Suppl 25), 56-64.

Grigoroiu-Serbanescu, M., Wickramaratne, P. J., Hodge, S. E., et al. (1997). Genetic anticipation and imprinting in bipolar illness. *The British Journal of Psychiatry, 170*(2), 162-166.

Grunze, H. (2005). Re-evaluating therapies for bipolar depression. *Journal of Clinical Psychiatry, 66*(Suppl 5), 17-25.

Hajek, T., Carrey, N., & Alda, M. (2005). Neuroanatomical abnormalities as risk factors for bipolar disorder. *Bipolar Disorders, 7*, 393-403.

Hajek, T., Kopecek, M., Kozeny, J., et al. (2009). Amygdala volumes in mood disorders—meta-analysis of magnetic resonance volumetry studies. *Journal of Affective Disorders, 115*, 395-410.

Haldane, M., & Frangou, S. (2004). New insights help define the pathophysiology of bipolar affective disorder: Neuroimaging and neuropathology findings. *Progress in Neuro-Psychopharmacology & Biological Psychiatry, 28*(6), 943-960.

Hallahan, B., & Garland, M. (2005). Essential fatty acids and mental health. *British Journal of Psychiatry, 186*, 275-277.

Haro, J. M., Reed, C., Gonzalez-Pinto, A., et al. EMBLEM Advisory Board. (2011). 2-Year course of bipolar disorder type I patients in outpatient care: Factors associated with remission and functional recovery. *European Neuropsychopharmacology, 21*(4), 287-293.

Hauser, M., Pfennig, A., Ozgurdal, S., et al. (2006). Early recognition of bipolar disorder. *European Psychiatry, 22*(2), 92-98.

Haznedar, M. M., Roversi, F., Pallanti, S., et al. (2005). Fronto-thalamo-striatal gray and white matter volumes and anisotropy of their connections in bipolar spectrum illnesses. *Biological Psychiatry, 57*, 733-742.

Henry, C., Sorbara, F., Lacoste, J., et al. (2001). Antidepressant-induced mania in bipolar patients: Identification of risk factors. *Journal of Clinical Psychiatry, 62*, 249-255.

Hibbein, J. R., & Salem, N., Jr. (1995). Dietary polyunsaturated fatty acids and depression: When cholesterol does not satisfy. *American Journal of Clinical Nutrition, 62*, 1-9.

Higgins, E. S., & George, M. S. (2007). *The neuroscience of clinical psychiatry: The pathophysiology of behavior and mental illness*. Philadelphia: Wolters Kluwer-Lippincott Williams & Wilkins.

Hillegers, M. H., Burger, H. T., Wals, M., et al. (2004). Impact of stressful life events, familial loading and their interaction on the onset of mood disorders: Study in a high risk cohort of adolescent off-spring of parents with bipolar disorder. *The British Journal of Psychiatry, 185*, 97-101.

Hirschfeld, R. M. (2005). Identifying bipolar disorder: The importance of differentiating bipolar disorder from unipolar depression. *Consultant (Supplement), 45*(14), S5-S10.

Hirschfeld, R. M. A. (2009). Making efficacious choices: The integration of pharmacotherapy and nonpharmacologic approaches to the treatment of patients with bipolar disorder. *Supplement to Current Psychiatry, October*, S6-S11. Retrieved from www.currentpsychiatry.com

Hirschfeld, R. M. A., Bowden, C. L., & Gitlin, M. J. et al. (2006). Practice guideline for the treatment of patients with bipolar disorder. In *American psychiatric association practice guidelines for the treatment of psychiatric disorders: Compendium 2006* (pp. 851-932). Washington, DC: American Psychiatric Publishing, Inc.

Hirschfeld, R. M., Lewis, L., & Vornik, L. A. (2003). Perceptions and impact of bipolar disorder: How far have we really come? Results of the National Depressive and Manic-Depressive Association 2000 survey of individuals with bipolar disorder. *Journal of Clinical Psychiatry, 64*, 161-174.

Hirschfeld, R. M., Williams, J. B., Spitzer, R. L., et al. (2000). Development and validation of a screening instrument for bipolar spectrum disorder: The Mood Disorder Questionnaire. *American Journal of Psychiatry, 157*, 1873-1875.

Howland, R. H. (2006). Challenges in the diagnosis & treatment of bipolar depression: Part 1: Assessment. *Journal of Psychosocial Nursing, 44*(4), 9-12.

Huxley, N. A., Parikh, S. V., & Baldessarini, R. J. (2000). Effectiveness of psychosocial treatments in bipolar disorder: State of the evidence. *Harvard Review of Psychiatry, 8*, 126-140.

Jackson, A., Cavanagh, J., & Scott, J. (2003). A systematic review of manic and depressive prodromes. *Journal of Affective Disorders, 74*, 209-217.

Jacobs, D. G., Baldessarini, R. J., Conwell, Y., et al. (2006). Practice guideline for the assessment and treatment of patients with suicidal behaviors. In *American psychiatric association practice guidelines for the treatment of psychiatric disorders: Compendium 2006* (pp. 1315-1495). Washington, DC: American Psychiatric Publishing, Inc.

Johnson, S. L., Cueller, A. K., Ruggero, C., et al. (2008). Life events as predictors of mania and depression in bipolar I disorder. *Journal of Abnormal Psychology, 117*(3), 268-277.

Johnson, S. L., Eisner, L. R., & Carver, C. S. (2009). Elevated expectancies among persons diagnosed with bipolar disorder. *British Journal of Clinical Psychology, 48*(Pt 2), 217-222.

Johnson, S. L., & Fulford, D. (2009). Preventing mania: A preliminary examination of the GOALS program. *Behavior Therapy, 40*, 103-113.

Johnson, S. L., & Roberts, J. E. (1995). Life events and bipolar disorder: Implications from biological theories. *American Journal of Psychiatry, 146*, 435-443.

Johnson, S. L., Ruggero, C., & Carver, C. (2005). Cognitive, behavioral and affective responses to reward: Links with hypomanic vulnerability. *Journal of Social and Clinical Psychology, 24*, 894-906.

Joska, J. A., & Stein, D. J. (2008). Mood disorders. In R. E. Hales, S. C. Yudofsky, & G. O. Gabbard (Eds.), *The American psychiatric publishing textbook of psychiatry* (5th ed.) (pp. 457-503). Washington, DC: American Psychiatric Publishing, Inc.

Joska, J. A., & Stein, D. J. (2011). Mood disorders. In R. E. Hales, S. C. Yudofsky, & G. O. Gabbard (Eds.), *Essentials of psychiatry* (3rd ed.) (pp. 151-183). Washington, DC: American Psychiatric Publishing, Inc.

Judd, L. L., & Akiskal, H. S. (2002). The prevalence and disability of bipolar spectrum disorders in the U.S. population: Re-analysis of the ECA database taking into account sub-threshold cases. *Journal of Affective Disorders, 73*(1-2), 123-131.

Judd, L. L., Akiskal, H. S., Schettler, P. J., et al. (2002). The long-term natural history of the weekly symptomatic status of bipolar I disorder. *Archives of General Psychiatry, 59*, 530-537.

Karasu, T. B., Gelenberg, A., Merriam, A., et al. (2004). Practice guidelines for the treatment of patients with major depressive disorder, 2nd ed. In *American psychiatric association practice guidelines for the treatment of psychiatric disorders: Compendium 2004* (pp. 441-523). Washington, DC: American Psychiatric Publishing, Inc.

Keck, P. E., & McElroy, S. L. (2001). Definition, evaluation, and management of treatment refractory mania. *Psychopharmacology Bulletin, 35*, 130-148.

Keck, P. E., & McElroy, S. L. (2004). Treatment of bipolar disorder. In A. F. Schatzberg & C. B. Nemeroff (Eds.), *Textbook of psychopharmacology* (3rd ed.) (pp. 865-883). Washington, DC: American Psychiatric Publishing, Inc.

Keck, P. E., & McElroy, S. L. (2006). Lithium and mood stabilizers. In D. J. Stein, D. J. Kupfer, & A. F. Schatzberg (Eds.), *The American psychiatric publishing textbook of mood disorders* (pp. 281-290). Washington, DC: American Psychiatric Publishing, Inc.

Keck, P. E., & McElroy, S. L. (2008). Lithium and mood stabilizers. In D. J. Stein, D. J. Kupfer, & A. F. Schatzberg (Eds.). *The American psychiatric publishing textbook of mood disorders* (pp. 281-289). Washington, DC: American Psychiatric Publishing, Inc.

Keck, P. E., & McElroy, S. L. (2009). Treatment of bipolar disorder. In A. F. Schatzberg & C. B. Nemeroff (Eds.), *The American psychiatric publishing textbook of psychopharmacology* (4th ed.) (pp. 1113-1133). Washington, DC: American Psychiatric Publishing, Inc.

Keck, P. E., Jr., McElroy, S. L., Strakowski, S. M., et al. (1998). 12-month outcome of patients with bipolar disorder following hospitalization for a manic or mixed episode. *American Journal of Psychiatry, 155*(5), 646-652.

Keck, P. E., Jr., Mintz, J., McElroy, S. L., et al. (2006). Double-blind, randomized, placebo-controlled trials of ethyl-eicosapentanoate in the treatment of bipolar depression and rapid cycling bipolar disorder. *Biological Psychiatry, 60*, 1020-1022.

Keck, P. E., Jr., Nelson, E. B., & McElroy, S. L. (2003). Advances in the pharmacologic treatment of bipolar depression. *Biological Psychiatry, 53*(8), 671-679.

Keller, M. B., & Baker, L. (1991). Bipolar disorder: Epidemiology, course, diagnosis, and treatment. *Bulletin of Menninger Clinic, 55*, 172-181.

Keltner, G. I., Solomon, D. A., Ryan, C. E., et al. (1996). Prodromal and residual symptoms in bipolar 1 disorder. *Comprehensive Psychiatry, 37*(5), 362-367.

Keltner, N. L., & Folks, D. G. (2005). *Psychotropic drugs* (4th ed.). St. Louis: Elsevier Mosby.

Kendler, K. S., & Karkowski-Shuman, L. (1997). Stressful life events and genetic liability to major depression: Genetic control of exposure to the environment. *Psychological Medicine, 27*(3), 539-647.

Kennedy, G. L. (2008). Bipolar disorder in late life: Mania. *Primary Psychiatry, 13*, 28-33.

Kennedy, N., Boydell, J., van Os, J., et al. (2004). Ethnic differences in first clinical presentation of bipolar disorder: Results from an epidemiological study. *Journal of Affective Disorders, 83*(2-3), 161-168.

Kessler, R. C., Berglund, P., Demler, O., et al. (2005). Lifetime prevalence and age-of-onset distributions of DSM-IV disorders in the National Comorbidity Survey Replication. *Archives of General Psychiatry, 62*(6), 593-602.

Kessler, R. C., McGonagle, K. A., Zhao, S., et al. (1994). Lifetime and 12-month prevalence of DSM-III-R psychiatric disorders in the United States: Results from the National Comorbidity Survey. *Archives of General Psychiatry, 51*, 8-19.

Ketter, T. A. (2010). Principles of assessment and treatment of bipolar disorders. In T. A. Ketter (Ed.), *Handbook of diagnosis and treatment of bipolar disorders* (pp. 1-9). Washington, DC: American Psychiatric Publishing, Inc.

Ketter, T. A., & Wang, P. W. (2010a). DSM-IV-TR diagnosis of bipolar disorders. In T. A. Ketter (Ed.), *Handbook of diagnosis and treatment of bipolar disorders* (pp. 11-37). Washington, DC: American Psychiatric Publishing, Inc.

Ketter, T. A., & Wang, P. W. (2010b). Addressing clinical diagnostic challenges in bipolar disorders. In T. A. Ketter (Ed.), *Handbook of diagnosis and treatment of bipolar disorders* (pp. 39-68). Washington, DC: American Psychiatric Publishing, Inc.

Ketter, T. A., & Wang, P. W. (2010c). Overview of pharmacotherapy for bipolar disorders. In T. A. Ketter (Ed.), *Handbook of diagnosis and treatment of bipolar disorders* (pp. 83-106). Washington, DC: American Psychiatric Publishing, Inc.

Ketter, T. A., & Wang, P. W. (2010d). Management of acute manic and mixed episodes in bipolar disorders. In T. A. Ketter (Ed.), *Handbook of diagnosis and treatment of bipolar disorders* (pp. 107-164). Washington, DC: American Psychiatric Publishing, Inc.

Ketter, T. A., & Wang, P. W. (2010e). Longer-term management of bipolar disorders. In T. A. Kettler (Ed.), *Handbook of diagnosis and treatment of bipolar disorders* (pp. 251-330). Washington, DC: American Psychiatric Publishing, Inc.

Ketter, T. A, & Wang, P. W. (2010f). Management of rapid-cycling bipolar disorders. In T. A. Ketter (Ed.), *Handbook of diagnosis and treatment of bipolar disorders* (pp. 331-387). Washington, DC: American Psychiatric Publishing, Inc.

Ketter, T. A., Wang, P. W., & Culver, J. L. (2010). Multiphase treatment strategy for bipolar disorders. In T. A. Ketter (Ed.), *Handbook of diagnosis and treatment of bipolar disorders* (pp. 69-81). Washington, DC: American Psychiatric Publishing, Inc.

Ketter, T. A., Wang, P. W., & Post, R. M. (2004). Carbamazepine and oxcarbazepine. In A. F. Schatzberg & C. B. Nemeroff (Eds.), *Textbook of psychopharmacology* (3rd ed.) (pp. 581-606). Washington, DC: American Psychiatric Publishing, Inc.

Ketter, T. A., Wang, P. W., & Post, R. M. (2009). Carbamazepine and oxcarbazepine. In A. F. Schatzberg & C. B. Nemeroff (Eds.), *Textbook of psychopharmacology* (4th ed.) (pp. 735-756). Washington, DC: American Psychiatric Publishing, Inc.

Kieseppa, T., Partonen, T., Haukka, J., et al. (2004). High concordance of bipolar I disorder in a nationwide sample of twins. *American Journal of Psychiatry, 161*, 1814-1821.

Kim, E. Y., Miklowitz, D. J., Biuckians, A., et al. (2007). Life stress and course of early-onset bipolar disorder. *Journal of Affective Disorders, 99*(1-3), 37-44.

Konradi, C., Zimmerman, E. I., Yang, C. K., et al. (2011). Hippocampal interneurons in bipolar disorder. *Archives of General Psychiatry, 68*(4), 340-350.

Koplewicz, H. S. (1996). *It's nobody's fault: New hope and help for difficult children and their parents.* New York: Times Books.

Kosten, R. R., & Kosten, T. A. (2004). New medication strategies for comorbid substance use and bipolar affective disorders. *Biological Psychiatry, 56*, 771-777.

Kowatch, R. A., Fristad, M., Birmaher, B., et al. (2005). Treatment guidelines for children and adolescents with bipolar disorder. *Journal of American Academy of Child and Adolescent Psychiatry, 44*, 213-235.

Kramlinger, K. G., & Post, R. M. (1996). Ultra-rapid and ultradian cycling in bipolar affective illness. *British Journal of Psychiatry, 168*, 314-323.

Kroll, J. (2000). Use of no-suicide contracts by psychiatrists in Minnesota. *American Journal of Psychiatry, 157*, 1684-1686.

Kupfer, D. J., Frank, E., Grochocinski, F. J., et al. (2005). African-American participants in a bipolar disorder registry: Clinical and treatment characteristics. *Bipolar Disorders, 7*(1), 82-88.

Lam, D. H., Hayward, P., Watkins, E. R., et al. (2005). Relapse prevention in patients with bipolar disorder: Cognitive therapy outcome after 2 years. *The American Journal of Psychiatry, 162*(2), 324-329.

Laraia, M. T. (2005). Omega-3 fatty acids: A "fish story" for mental health. *APNA News, 17*(4), 10-11, 16.

Larsen, J. K., Faber, J., Christensen, E. M., et al. (2004). Relationship between mood and TSH response to TRH stimulation in bipolar affective disorder. *Psychoneuroendocrinology, 29*, 917-924.

Lawson, W. B. (1996). Clinical issues in the pharmacotherapy of African-Americans. *Psychopharmacological Bulletin, 32*, 275-281.

Leahy, R. L. (2007). Bipolar disorder: Causes, contexts, and treatments. *Journal of Clinical Psychology: In Session, 63*(5), 417-424.

Lessig, M., Shapira, N., & Murphy, T. (2001). Topiramate for reversing atypical antipsychotic weight gain. *Journal of the American Academy of Child and Adolescent Psychiatry, 40*, 1364.

Leverich, G. S., Altshuler, L. L., Frye, M. A., et al. (2003). Factors associated with suicide attempts in 648 patients with bipolar disorder in the Stanley Foundation Bipolar Network. *Journal of Clinical Psychiatry, 64*(5), 506-515.

Leverich, G. S., McElroy, S. L., Suppes, T., et al. (2002). Early physical and sexual abuse associated with an adverse course of bipolar illness. *Biological Psychiatry, 51*, 288-297.

Leverich, G. S., & Post, R. M. (2006). Course of bipolar illness after history of childhood trauma. *Lancet, 367*(9516), 1040-1042.

Lewis, F. T. (2004). Demystifying the disease state: Understanding diagnosis and treatment across the bipolar spectrum. *Journal of the American Psychiatric Nurses Association, 10*(S3), S6-S15.

Leyton, F., & Barrera, A. (2010). Bipolar depression and unipolar depression; Differential diagnosis in clinical practice. *Revista Medica de Chile, 138*(6), 773-779.

Luggen, A. S. (2005). Bipolar disorder: An uncommon illness? Recognizing and caring for the elderly person with bipolar disorder. *Geriatric Nursing, 26*(5), 326-329.

Malkoff-Schwartz, S., Frank, E., Anderson, B., et al. (1998). Stressful life events and social rhythm disruption in the onset of manic and depressive bipolar episodes: A preliminary investigation. *Archives of General Psychiatry, 55*, 702-707.

Mancini, C., van Ameringen, M., Pipe, B., et al. (2002, December). Topiramate in the treatment of generalized social phobia: An open trial. Poster presentation at the 41st meeting of the American College of Neuropsychopharmacology, San Juan, Puerto Rico.

Marder, S. R., & Wirshing, D. A. (2009). Clozapine. In A. F. Schatzberg & C. B. Nemeroff (Eds.), *The American psychiatric publishing textbook of psychopharmacology* (4th ed.) (pp. 555-571). Washington, DC: American Psychiatric Publishing, Inc.

Martinez, M., Marangell, L. B., & Martinez, J. M. (2008). Psychopharmacology. In R. E. Hales, S. C. Yudofsky, & G. O. Gabbard (Eds.), *The American psychiatric publishing textbook of psychiatry* (5th ed.) (pp. 1053-1131). Washington, DC: American Psychiatric Publishing, Inc.

Mayberg, H. S. (2006). Brain imaging. In D. J. Stein, D. J. Kupfer, & A. F. Schatzberg (Eds.), *The American psychiatric publishing textbook of mood disorders* (pp. 219-234). Washington, DC: American Psychiatric Publishing, Inc.

Mazza, M., DiNicola, M., Martinotti, G., et al. (2007). Oxcarbazepine in bipolar disorder: A critical review of the literature. *Expert Opinion on Pharmacotherapy, 8*(5), 649-656.

McClellan, J., Kowatch, R., & Findling, R. L. (2007). Practice parameter for the assessment and treatment of children and adolescents with bipolar disorder. *Journal of American Academy of Child and Adolescent Psychiatry, 46*, 107-125.

McColm, R., Brown, J., & Anderson, J. (2006). Nursing interventions for the management of patients with mania. *Nursing Standard, 20*(17), 46-49.

McCracken, E., Dewar, D., & Hunter, A. J. (2001). White matter damage following systemic injection of the mitochondrial inhibitor 3-nitropropionic acid in rat. *Brain Research, 892*, 329-335.

McElroy, S. L., & Keck, P. E., Jr. (2000). Pharmacologic agents for the treatment of acute bipolar mania. *Biological Psychiatry, 48*(6), 539-557.

McElroy, S. L., & Keck, P. E., Jr. (2009). Topiramate. In A. F. Schatzberg & C. B. Nemeroff (Eds.), *The American psychiatric publishing textbook of psychopharmacology* (4th ed.) (pp. 795-807). Washington, DC: American Psychiatric Publishing, Inc.

McElroy, S., Keck, P. E., Jr., Stanton, S. P., et al. (1996). A randomized comparison of divalproex oral loading versus haloperidol in the initial treatment of acute psychotic mania. *Journal of Clinical Psychiatry, 57*, 142-146.

McGuffin, P., Rijsdijk, F., Andrew, M., et al. (2003). The heritability of bipolar affective disorder and the genetic relationship to unipolar depression. *Archives of General Psychiatry, 60*, 497-502.

McIntyre, R. S. (2011). Long-term treatment of bipolar disorders in adults. *Journal of Clinical Psychiatry, 72*(2).e06.February.

McIntyre, R. S., Konarski, J. Z., & Yatham, L. N. (2004). Comorbidity in bipolar disorder: A framework for rational treatment selection. *Human Psychopharmacology, 19*, 369-386.

McNamara, R. K., Nandagopal, J. J., & Strakowski, S. M. (2010). Preventive strategies for early-onset bipolar disorder: Towards a clinical staging model. *CNS Drugs, 24*(12), 983-996.

Meltzer, H. Y., Dritselis, A., Yasothan, U., et al. (2009). Asenapine. *Nature Reviews Drug Discovery, 8*, 843-844.

Melvin, C. L., Carey, T. S., Goodman, F., et al. (2008). Effectiveness of antiepileptic drugs for the treatment of bipolar disorder: Findings from a systematic review. *Journal of Psychiatric Practice, 14*(Suppl 1), 9-14.

Meyer, B., Johnson, S. L., & Winters, R. (2001). Responsiveness to threat and incentive in bipolar disorder: Relations of the BIS/BAS scales with symptoms. *Journal of Psychopathology and Behavior Assessment, 23*, 133-143.

Meyer, T. D., Hammelstein, P., Nilsson, L., et al. (2007). The hypomania checklist (HCL-32): Its factorial structure and association to indices of impairment in German and Swedish non-clinical samples. *Science Direct-Comprehensive Psychiatry, 48*(1), 79-87.

Miklowitz, D. J. (2008). Adjunctive psychotherapy for bipolar disorder: State of the Evidence. *American Journal of Psychiatry, 165*, 1408-1419.

Miklowitz, D. J., & Goldstein, M. J. (1997). *Bipolar disorder: A family focused treatment approach.* New York: Guilford Press.

Miklowitz, D. J., Goodwin, G. M., Bauer, M. S., et al. (2008). Common and specific elements of psychosocial treatments for bipolar disorder: A survey of clinicians participating in randomized trials. *Journal of Psychiatric Practice, 14*(2), 77-85.

Miklowitz, D. J., & Johnson, S. L. (2006). The psychopathology and treatment of bipolar disorder. *Annual Review of Clinical Psychology, 2*, 199-234.

Miklowitz, D. J., Otto, M. W., Frank, E., et al. (2007). Psychosocial treatments for bipolar depression. *Archives of General Psychiatry, 64*, 419-427.

Minsky, S., Vega, W., Miskimen, T., et al. (2003). Diagnostic patterns in Latino, African American and European American psychiatric patients. *Archives of General Psychiatry, 60*(6), 637-644.

Mitchell, P. B., Goodwin, G. M., Johnson, G. F., et al. (2008). Diagnostic guidelines for bipolar depression: A probabilistic approach. *Bipolar Disorders, 10*(1 Pt 2), 144-152.

Mitchell, P. B., & Malhi, G. S. (2004). Bipolar depression: Phenomenological overview and clinical characteristics. *Bipolar Disorders, 6*, 530-539.

Monkul, E. S., Malhi, G. S., & Soares, J. C. (2005). Anatomical MRI abnormalities in bipolar disorder: Do they exist and do they progress? *Australian and New Zealand Journal of Psychiatry, 39*, 222-226.

Moore, P. B., El-Badri, S. M., Cousins, D., et al. (2001a). White matter lesions and season of birth of patients with bipolar affective disorder. *American Journal of Psychiatry, 158*(9), 1521-1525.

Moore, P. B., Shepherd, D. J., Eccleston, D., et al. (2001b). Cerebral white matter lesions in bipolar affective disorder: Relationship to outcome. *The British Journal of Psychiatry, 178*, 172-176.

Moreno, C., Laje, G., Blanco, C., et al. (2007). National trends in the outpatient diagnosis and treatment of bipolar disorder in youths. *Archives of General Psychiatry, 64*(9), 1032-1039.

Murray, C. J. L., & Lopez, A. D. (1996). *The global burden of disease: Summary.* Cambridge, MA: Harvard University Press.

Muzina, D. J., & Calabrese, J. R. (2006). Guidelines for the treatment of bipolar disorder. In D. J. Stein, D. J. Kupfer, & A. F. Schatzberg (Eds.), *The American psychiatric publishing textbook of mood disorders* (pp. 463-483). Washington, DC: American Psychiatric Publishing, Inc.

Muzina, D. J., Ganocy, S., Khalife, S., et al. (2008, May). A double-blind, placebo-controlled study of divalproex extended release in newly diagnosed mood stabilizer naive patients with acute bipolar depression (9NR3-028). In New Research Abstracts of the 161st Annual Meeting of the American Psychiatric Association, Washington, DC, p. 101.

Nahas, Z., Lorberbaum, J. P., Kozel, F. A., et al. (2004). Somatic treatments in psychiatry. In J. Panksepp (Ed.), *Textbook of biological psychiatry* (pp. 521-548). Hoboken, NJ: John Wiley & Sons, Inc.

National Diabetes Fact Sheet. (2011). Alexandria, VA: American Diabetes Association.

Nierenberg, A. A., Ostacher, M. J., & Delgado, P. L. (2007). Antidepressant and anti-manic medications. In G. O. Gabbard (Ed.), *Gabbard's treatments of psychiatric disorders* (4th ed.) (pp. 385-407). Washington, DC: American Psychiatric Publishing, Inc.

Noaghiul, S., & Hibbeln, J. R. (2003). Cross-national comparisons of seafood consumption and rates of bipolar disorders. *The American Journal of Psychiatry, 1609*(12), 2222-2227.

Novick, D. M., Swartz, H. A., & Frank, E. (2010). Suicide attempts in bipolar I and bipolar II disorder: A review and meta-analysis of the evidence. *Bipolar Disorders, 12*, 1-9.

Olson, P., & Pacheco, M. R. (2005). Bipolar disorder in school-age children. *The Journal of School Nursing, 21*(3), 152-157.

Osher, Y., Bersudsky, W., & Belmaker, R. H. (2005). Omega-3 eicosapentaenoic acid in bipolar depression: Report of a small open-label study. *Journal of Clinical Psychiatry, 66*(6), 726-729

Owen, C., Rees, A., & Parker, G. (2008). The role of fatty acids in the development and treatment of mood disorders. *Current Opinion in Psychiatry, 21*, 19-24.

Papolos, D. F., & Papolos, J. (2002). *The bipolar child.* New York: Broadway Books.

Parker, G., Roy, K., Wilhelm, K., et al. (2000). The nature of bipolar depression: Implications for the definition of melancholia. *Journal of Affective Disorders, 59*, 217-234.

Pavuluri, M., & Bogarapu, S. (2008). Brain model for pediatric bipolar disorder. *Biological Child Psychiatry, Recent Trends and Development. Advances in Biological Psychiatry, 24*, 39-52.

Pavuluri, M., Henry, D. B., Nadimpalli, S. S., et al. (2006). Biological risk factors in pediatric bipolar disorder. *Biological Psychiatry, 60*, 936-941.

Pavuluri, M., West, A., Hill, S., et al. (2009). Neurocognitive function in pediatric bipolar disorder: 3-year follow-up shows cognitive development lagging behind healthy youth. *Journal of the American Academy of Child & Adolescent Psychiatry, 48*(3), 299-307.

Peet, M., & Horrobin, D. F. (2001). A dose-ranging study of ethyl-eicosapentaenoic acid in treatment-unresponsive depression. *Journal of Psychopharmacology, 15*(Suppl), A12.

Peet, M., & Stokes, C. (2005). Omega-3 fatty acids in the treatment of psychiatric disorders. *Drugs, 65*(8), 1051-1059.

Perlis, R. H., Miyahara, S., Marangell, L. B., et al. (2004). Long-term implications of early onset in bipolar disorder: Data from the first 1000 participants in the systematic treatment enhancement program for bipolar disorder (STEP-BD). *Biological Psychiatry, 55*, 875-881.

Perlis, R. H., Ostacher, M. J., Patel, J. K., et al. (2006). Predictors of recurrence in bipolar disorder: Primary outcomes from the systematic treatment enhancement program for bipolar disorder (STEP-BD). *American Journal of Psychiatry, 163*(2), 217-224.

Perry, A., Tarrier, N., Morriss, R., et al. (1999). Randomized controlled trial of efficacy of teaching patients with bipolar disorder to identify early symptoms of relapse and obtain treatment. *British Medical Journal, 318*, 149-153.

Perugi, G., Toni, C., Frare, F., et al. (2002). Effectiveness of adjunctive gabapentin in resistant bipolar disorder: Is it due to anxious-alcohol abuse comorbidity? *Journal of Clinical Psychopharmacology, 22*, 584-591.

Petty, F., Rush, A. J., Davis, J. M., et al. (1996). Plasma GABA predicts acute response to divalproex in mania. *Biological Psychiatry, 39*, 278-284.

Phelps, J. (2008). The biologic basis of bipolar disorder. Retrieved from www.psycheducation.org. Retrieved July 10, 2011.

Piterman, L., Jones, K. M., & Castle, D. J. (2010). Bipolar disorder in general practice: Challenges and opportunities. *The Medical Journal of Australia, 193*(4), S14-S17.

Post, R. M. (1992). Transduction of psychosocial stress into neurobiology of recurrent affective disorder. *American Journal of Psychiatry, 149*, 999-1010.

Post, R. M. (2007). Kindling and sensitization as models for affective episode recurrence, cyclicity, and tolerance phenomena. *Neuroscience & Biobehavioral Reviews, 31*(6), 858-873.

Post, R. M., Altshuler, L. L., Frye, M. A., et al. (2001). Rate of switch in bipolar patients prospectively treated with second-generation antidepressants as augmentation to mood stabilizers. *Bipolar Disorders, 3*, 259-265.

Post, R. M., Leverich, G. S., Altshuler, L. L., et al. (2003). An overview of recent findings of the Stanley Foundation Bipolar Network (Part 1). *Bipolar Disorders, 5*(5), 310-319.

Post, R. M., & Weiss, R. R. B. (1995). The neurobiology of treatment-resistant mood disorders. In F. E. Bloom and D. J. Kupfer (Eds.), *Psychopharmacology: The fourth generation of progress* (pp. 1155-1170). New York: Raven Press.

Price, T. R. P., Goetz, K. L., & Lovell, M. R. (2010). Neuropsychiatric aspects of brain tumors. In S. C. Yudofsky & R. E. Hales (Eds.), *Essentials of neuropsychiatry and behavioral neurosciences* (2nd ed.) (pp. 323-347). Washington, DC: American Psychiatric Publishing, Inc.

Rabasseda, X. (2010). A report from the 4th Biennial Conference of the International Society of Bipolar Disorder (March 17-20, 2010 - Sao Paulo, Brazil). *Drugs Today, 46*(6), 433-466.

Rajkowska, G. (2006). Anatomical pathology. In D. J. Stein, D. J. Kupfer, & A. F. Schatzberg (Eds.), *The American psychiatric publishing textbook of mood disorders* (pp. 179-195). Washington, DC: American Psychiatric Publishing, Inc.

Rajkowska, G., Halaris, A., & Selemon, L. D. (2001). Reductions in neuronal and glial density characterize the dorsolateral prefrontal cortex in bipolar disorder. *Biological Psychiatry, 49*, 741-752.

Rea, M. M., Tompson, M. C., Miklowitz, D. J., et al. (2003). Family focused treatment versus individual treatment for bipolar disorders. *Journal of Consulting and Clinical Psychology, 71*(3), 482-492.

Reichart, C. G., & Nolen, W. A. (2004). Earlier onset of bipolar disorder in children by antidepressants or stimulants? A hypothesis. *Journal of Affective Disorders, 78*, 81-84.

Reichart, C. G., & Nolen, W. A. (2007). Diagnosis and treatment of bipolar disorder in children. *Nederlands Tijdschrift voor Geneeskunde, 151*(11), 630-634.

Roshanaei-Moghaddam, B., & Katon, W. (2009). Premature mortality from general medical illnesses among persons with bipolar disorder: A review. *Psychiatric Services, 60*(2), 147-156.

Ross, B. M. (2007). Omega-3 fatty acid deficiency in major depressive disorder is caused by the interaction between diet and a genetically determined abnormality in phospholipids metabolism. *Medical Hypotheses, 68*, 515-524.

Rossi, A. (2000). Cognitive functioning in euthymic bipolar patients. *Journal of Psychiatric Research, 34,* 333-339.

Rouget, B. W., & Aubry, J-M. (2007). Efficacy of psychoeducational approaches on bipolar disorders: A review of the literature. *Journal of Affective Disorders, 98*(1-2), 11-27.

Sachs, G., Grossman, F., Ghaemi, S. N., et al. (2002). Combination of a mood stabilizer with risperidone or haloperidol for treatment of acute mania: A double-blind, placebo-controlled comparison of efficacy and safety. *American Journal of Psychiatry, 159,* 1146-1154.

Sachs, G. S., Printz, D. J., Kahn, D. A., et al. (2000). The expert consensus guidelines series: Medication treatment of bipolar disorder. *Postgraduate Medicine, 108*(special no), 1-104.

Sachs, G. S., Yan, L. J., Swann, A. C., et al. (2001). Integration of suicide prevention into outpatient management of bipolar disorder. *Journal of Clinical Psychiatry, 62*(Suppl 25), 3-11.

Sassi, R. B., Nicoletti, M., Brambilla, P., et al. (2001). Decreased pituitary volume in patients with bipolar disorder. *Biological Psychiatry, 50*(4), 271-280.

Schatzberg, A. F., Cole, J. O., & DeBattista, C. (2007). *Manual of clinical psychopharmacology* (6th ed.). Washington, DC: American Psychiatric Publishing, Inc.

Scherk, H., Pajonk, F. G., & Leucht, S. (2007). Second-generation antipsychotic agents in the treatment of acute mania: A systematic review and meta-analysis of randomized controlled trials. *Archives of General Psychiatry, 64,* 442-455.

Schneck, C. D., Miklowitz, D. J., Calabrese, J. R., et al. (2004). Phenomenology of rapid-cycling bipolar disorder: Data from the first 500 participants in the Systematic Treatment Enhancement Program. *The American Journal of Psychiatry, 161*(10), 1902-1908.

Schou, M. (1998). The effect of prophylactic lithium treatment on mortality and suicidal behavior: A review for clinicians. *Journal of Affective Disorders, 50,* 253-259.

Scott, J., & Gutierrez, M. J. (2004). The current status of psychological treatments in bipolar disorders: A systematic review of relapse prevention. *Bipolar Disorder, 6,* 498-503.

Segal, J., Berk, M., & Brook, S. (1998). Risperidone compared with both lithium and haloperidol in mania: A double-blind randomized controlled trial. *Clinical Neuropharmacology, 21,* 176-180.

Segal, S. P., Bola, J., & Watson, M. (1996). Race, quality of care, and antipsychotic prescribing practices in psychiatric emergency services. *Psychiatric Services, 47,* 282-286.

Seidman, S. N. (2006a). Psychoneuroendocrinology of mood disorders. In D. J. Stein, D. J. Kupfer, & A. F. Schatzberg (Eds.), *The American psychiatric publishing textbook of mood disorders* (pp. 117-130). Washington, DC: American Psychiatric Publishing, Inc.

Seidman, S. N. (2006b). Targeting peptide and hormonal systems. In D. J. Stein, D. J. Kupfer, & A. F. Schatzberg (Eds.), *The American psychiatric publishing textbook of mood disorders* (pp. 305-316). Washington, DC: American Psychiatric Publishing, Inc.

Sharma, V. (2005). *Misdiagnosed bipolar disorder.* Presentation at 54th annual meeting of the Canadian Psychiatric Association. Available at http://www.medscape.com/viewarticle/491491.

Sheehan, D. V., & Raj, B. A. (2009). Benzodiazepines. In A. F. Schatzberg & C. B. Nemeroff (Eds.), *The American psychiatric publishing textbook of psychopharmacology* (4th ed.) (pp. 465-486). Washington, DC: American Psychiatric Publishing, Inc.

Shelton, M. D., & Calabrese, J. R. (2004). Lamotrigine. In A. F. Schatzberg & C. B. Nemeroff (Eds.), *Textbook of psychopharmacology* (3rd ed.) (pp. 615-626). Washington, DC: American Psychiatric Publishing, Inc.

Sherrod, T., Quinlan-Colwell, A., Lattimore, T. B., et al. (2010). Older adults with bipolar disorder: Guidelines for primary care providers. *Journal of Gerontological Nursing, 36*(5), 20-27.

Shirtcliff, E. A., Vitacco, M. J., Graf, A. R., et al. (2009). Neurobiology of empathy and callousness: Implications for the development of antisocial behavior. *Behavior, Science, and The Law, 27,* 137-171.

Shulman, K. (2004). Mania in old age: A neuropsychiatric syndrome. *Geriatrics and Aging, 7,* 34-37.

Simon, G. E., Ludman, E., Bauer, M. S., et al. (2006). Long-term effectiveness and cost of a systematic care program for bipolar disorder. *Archives of General Psychiatry, 63,* 500-508.

Simon, R. I. (2008). Suicide. In R. E. Hales, S. C. Yudofsky, & G. O. Gabbard (Eds.). *The American psychiatric publishing textbook of psychiatry* (5th ed.) (pp. 1637-1654). Washington, DC: American Psychiatric Publishing, Inc.

Slama, F., Bellivier, F., Henry, C., et al. (2004). Bipolar patients with suicidal behavior: Toward the identification of a clinical subgroup. *Journal of Clinical Psychiatry, 65*(8), 227-244.

Small, J. G., Klapper, M. H., & Milstein, V., et al. (1991). Carbamazepine compared with lithium in the treatment of mania. *Archives of General Psychiatry, 48,* 915-921.

Smith, L. A., Cornelius, V., Warnock, A., et al. (2007). Acute bipolar mania: A systematic review and meta-analysis of co-therapy vs. monotherapy. *Acta Psychiatrica Scandinavica, 115*(1), 12-20.

Smoller, J. W., Sheidley, B. R., & Tsuang, M. T. (2008). *Psychiatric genetics: Applications in clinical practice.* Washington, DC: American Psychiatric Publishing, Inc.

Soares, J. C. (2003). Contributions from brain imaging to the elucidation of pathophysiology of bipolar disorder. *International Journal of Neuropsychopharmacology, 6*(2), 171-180.

Soutullo, C. A., Chang, K. D., Diez-Suarez, A., et al. (2005). Bipolar disorder in children and adolescents: International perspective on epidemiology and phenomenology. *Bipolar Disorders, 7,* 497-506.

Stack, S. (2001). Occupation and suicide. *Social Science Quarterly, 82,* 384-396.

Stahl, S. M. (2000). *Essential psychopharmacology: Neuroscientific basis and practical applications.* Cambridge, UK: Cambridge University Press.

Stahl, S. M. (2005). *Essential psychopharmacology: The prescriber's guide.* Cambridge, UK: Cambridge University Press.

Stimmel, G. L. (2004). The economic burden of bipolar disorder. *Psychiatric Services, 55*(2), 117-118.

St. John, D. D. (2005). Bipolar disorder: Diagnosing a devastating illness. *Clinical Advisor, March,* 3-10.

Stoll, A. L. (2001). *The omega-3 connection: The ground-breaking antidepression diet and brain program.* New York: Simon & Schuster.

Stoll, A. L., Severus, E., Freeman, M. P., et al. (1999). Omega-3 fatty acids in bipolar disorder. *Archives of General Psychiatry, 56,* 407-412.

Strakowski, S. M., DelBello, M. P., & Adler, C. M. (2005). The functional neuroanatomy of bipolar disorder: A review of neuroimaging findings. *Molecular Psychiatry, 10,* 105-116.

Strakowski, S. M., DelBello, M. P., Sax, K. W., et al. (1999). Brain magnetic resonance imaging of structural abnormalities in bipolar disorder. *Archives of General Psychiatry, 56*(3), 254-260.

Strakowski, S. M., McElroy, S. L., Keck, P. E., Jr., et al. (1996). Racial influence on diagnosis in psychotic mania. *Journal of Affective Disorders, 39,* 157-162.

Strakowski, S. M., & Shelton, R. C. (2006). Antipsychotic medications. In D. J. Stein, D. J. Kupfer, & A. F. Schatzberg (Eds.), *The American psychiatric publishing textbook of mood disorders* (pp. 291-303). Washington, DC: American Psychiatric Publishing, Inc.

Strober, M., Schmidt-Lackner, S., Freeman, R., et al. (1995). Recovery and relapse in adolescents with bipolar affective illness: A five-year naturalistic prospective follow-up. *Journal of American Academy of Child and Adolescent Psychiatry, 34,* 724-731.

Sublette, M. E., Hibbeln, J. R., Gallalvy, H., et al. (2006). Omega-3 polyunsaturated essential fatty acid status as a predictor of future suicide risk. *American Journal of Psychiatry, 163,* 1100-1102.

Suppes, T., Dennehy, E. B., Hirschfeld, R. M. A., et al. (2005). The Texas implementation of medication algorithms: Update to the algorithms for the treatment of bipolar I disorder. *Journal of Clinical Psychiatry, 66,* 870-886.

Suppes, T., Kelly, D. I., & Perla, J. M. (2005). Challenges in the management of bipolar depression. *Journal of Clinical Psychiatry, 66*(Suppl 5), 11-16.

Swann, A. C., Bowden, C. L., Calabrese, J. R., et al. (1999). Differential effects of number of previous episodes of affective disorder on response to lithium or divalproex in acute mania. *American Journal of Psychiatry, 156,* 1264-1266.

Swann, A. C., Dougherty, D. M., Pazzaglia, P. J., et al. (2004). Impulsivity: A link between bipolar disorder and substance abuse. *Bipolar Disorder, 6,* 204-212.

Swartz, H. A., Pilkonis, P. A., Frank E., et al. (2005). Acute treatment outcomes in patients with bipolar I disorder and co-morbid borderline personality disorder receiving medication and psychotherapy. *Bipolar Disorders, 7,* 192-197.

Teter, C., Early, J., & Gibbs, C. (2000). Treatment of affective disorder and obesity with topiramate. *Annals of Pharmacotherapy, 34,* 1262-1265.

Tohen, M., Baker, R. W., Altshuler, L. L., et al. (2002a). Olanzapine (Zyprexa) versus divalproex in the treatment of acute mania. *American Journal of Psychiatry, 159*(6), 1011-1017.

Tohen, M., Chengappa, K. N., Suppes, T. S., et al. (2002b). Efficacy of olanzapine (Zyprexa) in combination with valproate or lithium in the treatment of mania in patients partially non-responsive to valproate or lithium monotherapy. *Archives of General Psychiatry, 59,* 62-69.

Tohen, M., Hennen, J., Zarate, C. M., Jr., et al. (2000). Two-year recovery in 219 cases of first episode major affective disorder with psychotic features. *American Journal of Psychiatry, 157,* 220-228.

Tondo, L., Baldessarini, R. J., Hennen, J., et al. (1998). Lithium maintenance treatment of depression and mania in bipolar I and bipolar II disorders. *American Journal of Psychiatry, 155,* 638-645.

Torrey, E. F., & Knable, M. B. (2002). *Surviving manic depression: A manual on bipolar disorder for patients, families and providers.* New York: Basic Books.

Tsai, S. Y., Kuo, C. J., Chen, C. C., et al. (2002). Risk factors for completed suicide in bipolar disorder. *Journal of Clinical Psychiatry, 63*(6), 469-476.

Umlauf, M. G., & Shattell, M. (2005). The ecology of bipolar disorder: The importance of sleep. *Issues in Mental Health Nursing, 26,* 699-720.

Vaughn, M. G., Fu, Q., Bender, K., et al. (2010). Psychiatric correlates of bullying in the United States: Findings from a national sample. *The Psychiatric Quarterly, 81*(3), 183-195.

Vieta, E., Calabrese, J. R., Hennen, J., et al. (2004). Comparison of rapid-cycling and non-rapid-cycling bipolar 1 manic patients during treatment with olanzapine (Zyprexa): Analysis of pooled data. *Journal of Clinical Psychiatry, 65,* 1420-1428.

Voelbel, G. T., Bates, M. E., Buckman, J., et al. (2006). Caudate nucleus volume and cognitive performance: Are they related to childhood psychopathology? *Biological Psychiatry, 60*(4), 942-950.

Wagner, K. D., Kowatch, R. A., & Emslie, G. J. (2006). A double-blind, randomized, placebo-controlled trial of oxcarbazepine in the treatment of bipolar disorder in children and adolescents. *American Journal of Psychiatry, 163,* 1179-1186.

Wagner, K. D., & Pliszka, S. R. (2009). Treatment of child and adolescent disorders. In A. F. Schatzberg & C. B. Nemeroff (Eds.), *The American psychiatric publishing textbook of psychopharmacology* (4th ed.) (pp. 1309-1371). Washington, DC: American Psychiatric Publishing, Inc.

Wagner, K. D., Redden, L., Kowatach, R. A., et al. (2009). A double-blind, randomized, placebo-controlled trial of divalproex extended-release in the treatment of bipolar disorder in children and adolescents. *Journal of American Academy of Child and Adolescent Psychiatry, 48,* 519-532.

Wang, P. O., & Ketter, T. A. (2010). Management of acute major depressive episodes in bipolar disorders. In T. A. Ketter (Ed.), *Handbook of diagnosis and treatment of bipolar disorders* (pp. 165-250). Washington, DC: American Psychiatric Publishing, Inc.

Warren, B. J. (2007). Cultural aspects of bipolar disorder: Interpersonal meaning for clients & psychiatric nurses. *Journal of Psychosocial Nursing and Mental Health Services, 45*(7), 32-37.

Wedding, D., Boyd, M. A., & Niemiec, R. M. (2010). *Movies and mental illness 3: Using films to understand psychopathology* (3rd ed.). Cambridge, MA: Hogrefe Publishers.

Weisler, R. H., Keck, P. E., Jr., Swann, A. C., et al. (2005). Extended-release carbamazepine capsules as monotherapy for acute mania in bipolar disorder: A multicenter, randomized, double-blind, placebo-controlled trial. *Journal of Clinical Psychiatry, 66,* 323-330.

Weissman, M. M., Bruce, L. M., Leaf, P. J., et al. (1991). Affective disorders. In L. N. Robins & D. A. Regier (Eds.), *Psychiatric disorders in America: The epidemiologic catchment area study* (pp. 53-80). New York: Free Press.

West, A. E., Schenkel, L. S., & Pavuluri, M. N. (2008). Early childhood temperament in pediatric bipolar disorder and attention deficit hyperactivity disorder. *Journal of Clinical Psychology, 64*(4), 402-421.

Winsberg, M. E., Sachs, N., & Tate, D. L. (2000). Decreased dorsolateral prefrontal N-acetyl aspartate in bipolar disorder. *Biological Psychiatry, 47,* 475-481.

Yan, L. J., Hammen, C., Cohen, A. N., et al. (2004). Expressed emotion versus relationship quality variables in the prediction of recurrence in bipolar patients. *Journal of Affective Disorders, 83,* 199-206.

Yatham, L. M. (2005). Atypical antipsychotics for bipolar disorder. *Psychiatric Clinics of North America, 28,* 325-347.

Young, G., & Conquer, J. (2005). Omega-3 fatty acids and neuropsychiatric disorders. *Reproduction, Nutrition, Development, 45*(1), 1-28.

Young, R. C., Biggs, J. T., Ziegler, V. E., et al. (1978). A rating scale for mania: Reliability, validity, and sensitivity. *British Journal of Psychiatry, 133,* 429-435.

Zajecka, J. M., Weisler, R., & Swann, A. C. (2000, December). *Divalproex sodium versus olanzapine (Zyprexa) for the treatment of acute mania in bipolar disorder.* Poster abstracts from the American College of Neuropsychopharmacology annual meeting, Nashville, TN.

Zanarini, M., & Frankenburg, F. (2001). Olanzapine (Zyprexa) treatment of female borderline personality disorder patients: A double-blind, placebo-controlled pilot study. *Journal of Clinical Psychiatry, 62,* 849-854.

Zanetti, M., Cordeiro, Q., & Busatto, G. (2007). Late onset bipolar disorder associated with white matter hyperintensities: A pathophysiological hypothesis. *Progress in Neuro-Psychopharmacology & Biological Psychiatry, 31*(2), 551-556.

Zarate, C., & Tohen, M. (2002). Bipolar disorder and comorbid axis I disorders: Diagnosis and management. In L. Yatham, V. Kusumakar, & S. Kutcher (Eds.), *Bipolar disorder: A clinician's guide to biological treatments* (pp. 115-138). New York: Brunner-Routledge.

Zarate, C. A., Jr., & Tohen, M. (2004). Double-blind comparison of the continued use of antipsychotic treatment versus its discontinuation in remitted manic patients. *American Journal of Psychiatry, 161,* 169-171.

Zaretsky, A., Lancee, W., Miller, C., et al. (2008). Is cognitive-behavioural therapy more effective than psychoeducation in bipolar disorder? *Canadian Journal of Psychiatry, 53,* 441-448.

Answers to Case Study 14-1 Questions

1. Major life stressor (being dumped by boyfriend), sleep deprivation, flying across time zones, nonadherence to medications, and large amounts of exposure to sunlight are possible precipitators of mania.
2. Gretchen displayed judgment as manifested in indiscriminate self-disclosure; rapid, pressured speech; rhyming of words; expansive mood; financial irresponsibility; irritability; anger; and abusive behaviors.
3. Safety issues include but are not limited to danger to the patient's physical health (dehydration, sunburn, sleep deprivation, and exhaustion); injury to the patient's dignity and self-identity; and threats to the patient's financial status, professional reputation, and legal status.
4. The Good Samaritan law (Good Samaritan Doctrine) refers to a Good Samaritan as one who provides aid to an injured stranger on a voluntary basis. If the stranger is conscious, then the Samaritan should ask for permission to help. Colleen had been asked by Gretchen to help her. All states in the United States have some form of Good Samaritan law that prevents a rescuer who has voluntarily helped a person in distress from being sued for wrongdoing, and most offer immunity to Good Samaritans.

UNIT VI

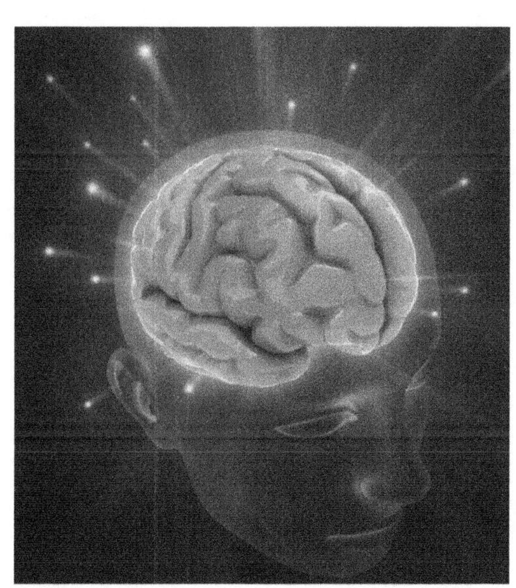

Psychiatric Disorders: Thought Disorders

CHAPTER 15

Schizophrenia

Lora Humphrey Beebe, PhD, PMHNP-BC

Approximately 1.9 million Americans suffer from schizophrenia (American Psychiatric Association, 2000a). Schizophrenia is the most chronic and disabling of the severe mental disorders, causing psychotic symptoms, social withdrawal, and bizarre behavior. Symptoms of schizophrenia affect multiple areas of functioning, including language, cognition, perception, attention, emotions, initiative, use of language, and social interaction. The description, diagnosis, treatment, and support of patients with this devastating illness have challenged clinicians and families for hundreds of years.

From its earliest descriptions, schizophrenia has been characterized as a disease of neurocognition. In the late 1800s, Emil Kraepelin believed that schizophrenia was a disease of the brain, characterized by irreversible decline (dementia) and early onset (praecox). Kraepelin identified two symptom types common to all dementia praecox patients: bizarre thoughts and avolition (Snowden, 2009a). In contrast to symptom description, Eugene Bleuler in the same era sought to explain schizophrenia in psychodynamic terms. Bleuler is credited with making the critical observation that the disorder did not always end in a state of dementia. Bleuler identified the following four primary symptoms of schizophrenia, known as "the four As": flattened Affect, Ambivalence, Autism, and loosening of Associations (Sadock and Sadock, 2007).

Later, Kurt Schneider contributed descriptions of so-called first-rank symptoms. First-rank symptoms include hallucinations, delusions, thought broadcasting, and thought insertion; because they represent additions to "normal" experience, they are commonly referred to as *positive* symptoms. Schneider emphasized that while first-rank symptoms were easily detectable, second-rank symptoms such as avolition were critical to accurate diagnosis (Snowden, 2009a). Schneiderian criteria, more than any others, have come to be associated with a schizophrenia diagnosis today.

Today, in the United States, schizophrenia is most commonly diagnosed using the criteria presented in the *Diagnostic and Statistical Manual of Mental Disorders*, fourth edition, text revision (*DSM-IV-TR*) (American Psychiatric Association, 2000a). The *DSM-IV-TR* defines schizophrenia as a disturbance (1) lasting at least 6 months (if untreated), (2) not due to substance use or a general medical condition such as a brain tumor, and (3) in which two or more of the following symptoms are present for at least 1 month: delusions or hallucinations, disorganized speech, disorganized or catatonic behavior, or negative symptoms (defined as affects and behaviors that are lacking). See Table 15-1 for *DSM-IV-TR* diagnostic criteria for schizophrenia.

The *DSM-IV-TR* goes on to define the following five subtypes of schizophrenia:

- Paranoid, in which delusions and hallucinations are the predominant symptoms
- Catatonic, in which motor symptoms are predominant
- Disorganized, in which disorganized speech and behavior or inappropriate affect are predominant
- Residual, in which there is absence of prominent positive symptoms but continuing evidence of disturbance through less severe positive symptoms or through negative symptoms
- Undifferentiated, in which none of the above symptom clusters are predominant (American Psychiatric Association, 2000a)

There are no specific treatment strategies for any subtype, with the exception of the use of benzodiazepines for catatonia (American Psychiatric Association, 2004a).

Epidemiology

The absence of objective diagnostic criteria, the lack of a single unique diagnostic feature of schizophrenia, and frequent difficulties obtaining accurate historical information create diagnostic challenges for practitioners and contribute to variable incidence rates (Eaton, Hall, Macdonald, et al.,

TABLE 15-1 ***DSM-IV-TR* DIAGNOSTIC CRITERIA FOR SCHIZOPHRENIA**

Criteria	Manifestation
A: Characteristic symptoms: • Delusions • Hallucinations • Disorganized speech • Grossly disorganized or catatonic behavior • Negative symptoms	Two or more, each present for a significant portion of time during a 1-month period (or less if successfully treated).*
B. Social/occupational dysfunction: • Interpersonal • Academic • Social • Occupational	For a significant portion of the time since onset of the disturbance, one or more major areas of functioning are markedly below the level achieved prior to onset. If onset is in childhood/adolescence, failure to achieve expected level of achievement in one or more areas.
C. Duration: • At least 6 months • Must include at least 1 month of symptoms (or less if successfully treated) that meet Criterion A and may include periods of prodromal or residual symptoms	During prodromal or residual period, signs of disturbance may be manifested by only negative symptoms or by two or more Criterion A symptoms present in an attenuated form.
D. Schizoaffective disorder and mood disorder exclusion: • Schizoaffective disorder and mood disorder have been ruled out	Because of either of the following: 1. No major depressive, manic, or mixed episodes have occurred concurrently with active-phase symptoms. 2. If mood episodes have occurred during active-phase symptoms, their total duration has been brief relative to the duration of the active and residual periods.
E. Substance/general medical condition exclusion: • Substance use and general medical causes of symptoms have been ruled out	The disturbance is not due to the direct physiological effects of a substance or a general medical condition.
F. Relationship to pervasive developmental disorder: • Autistic or other pervasive developmental disorder(s)	If there is a history of autistic disorder or another pervasive developmental disorder, the additional diagnosis of schizophrenia is made only if prominent delusions or hallucinations have also been present for at least 1 month (less if successfully treated).

*Note: Only one Criterion A symptom is required if delusions are bizarre or if hallucinations consist of (1) a voice keeping up a running commentary on the individual's behavior or thoughts or (2) two or more voices conversing with each other.

Adapted from American Psychiatric Association. (2000a). Diagnostic and statistical manual of mental disorders (4th ed., text rev.) (pp. 274-287). Washington, DC: American Psychiatric Association.

2007). Although medical descriptions of schizophrenia have been consistent for at least the past 200 years (Tandon, Keshavan, & Nasrallah, 2008), community surveys may overestimate rates due to false-positives (Anthony, Folstein, & Romanoski, 1985; Regier, Kaelber, Rae, et al., 1998), while studies based on service provision might underestimate rates if affected individuals fail to seek treatment (Tandon et al., 2008).

Based on these differences in description and approach, current estimates of the incidence of schizophrenia vary across studies. A meta-analysis of 55 studies from 33 countries reported a median incidence of 15.2/100,000/year (McGrath, Saha, Welham, et al., 2004). In the United States, the incidence of schizophrenia is 7.2 per 1000 (McGrath et al.).

Prevalence is a function of both incidence and illness duration. However, recovery rates vary, and the definition of schizophrenia remission is as yet unclear (Andreasen, Carpenter, Kane, et al., 2005; Leucht & Lasser, 2006; van Os, Burns, Cavallaro, et al., 2006). The present knowledge of schizophrenia is insufficient to produce a cure, and the average affected individual can expect to live with schizophrenia for approximately 30 years (Tandon et al., 2008). Approximately 2.2 million people in the United States currently have a diagnosis of schizophrenia, and approximately 100,000 are diagnosed in a given year. Based on a meta-analysis of 67 studies worldwide, median point, period (up to 1 year), and lifetime prevalence rates were estimated at 4.6, 3.3, and 4.0 per 1000, respectively (Saha, Chant, Welham, et al., 2005). These rates of illness are probably influenced by both biological and social mechanisms of disease.

Cultural factors also affect diagnosis, course, and treatment of schizophrenia (Karno & Jenkins, 1993). While scholars debate the precise definition of "culture," it is classically considered to be a pattern of meaning that is historically and symbolically transmitted. Culture categorizes knowledge and influences attitudes (Olafsdottir & Pescosolido, 2009). Individuals with schizophrenia are embedded in cultures whose impact on beliefs, opinions, and attitudes shape not only their own help-seeking behavior, but also the mental health system's responses to them.

Compared with Caucasians, African Americans—especially men—are more likely to be diagnosed with schizophrenia and less likely to be diagnosed with an affective disorder (Baker & Bell, 1999; Rayburn &

Stonecypher, 1996). African Americans with schizophrenia are less likely to be diagnosed with a comorbid anxiety or mood disorder (Delahanty, Ram, Postrado, et al., 2001; Dixon, Green-Paden, Delahanty, et al., 2001). The source of these differences may include actual variability among cultural groups, but evidence exists for disparities in symptom interpretation, help-seeking, and treatment referral, reflecting cultural bias by clinicians (Cuffe, Waller, Cuccaro, et al., 1995; Klinkenberg & Calsyn, 1997) as well as lack of research samples of minorities, possible bias in assessment tools, and researcher lack of attention to controls for variables such as socioeconomic status, urbanicity, and educational level (Neighbors, Jackson, Campbell, et al., 1989; Somervell, Leaf, Weissman, et al., 1989). Because of the cultural implications of stigma, the lack of public understanding of schizophrenia, and the use of legal coercion to control behavior, understanding of cultural context is especially important for clinicians treating individuals with schizophrenia. Clinicians should also remain mindful of unacknowledged cultural bias of a personal nature.

Etiology

The complexity of schizophrenia and the multitude of factors influencing the course of illness and treatment responses have resulted in numerous models to explain the disease. Two proposed models are biological basis and environmental factors.

Biological Basis

Biological theories of schizophrenia etiology include genetics, biochemical alterations, neuropathology, neural circuitry deficits, and brain metabolism dysfunction.

Genetics

The genetic basis of schizophrenia has long been documented (Kallman, 1946). A seminal series of adoption and twin studies elucidated the following heritability patterns:

- Schizophrenia risk in an individual is higher than in the general population by approximately 12 times if the disease is present in one biological parent and by approximately 40 times if present in both biological parents; the risk remains when the child is raised by adoptive parents (Heston, 1966).
- Concordance in monozygotic twins is over three times greater than in dizygotic twins (Gottesman, McGuffin, & Farmer, 1987; Sullivan, Cendler, & Neale, 2003).

Heritability is estimated based on twin concordance rates and refers to the proportion of illness risk in the general population accounted for by both genetic effects and genetic-environmental interactions. The proportion of schizophrenia risk related to these factors is estimated at approximately 80% (Cannon, Kaprio, Lonnqvist, et al., 1998; Cardno, Marshall, Coid, et al., 1999; Sullivan et al., 2003). The 20-year search for specific susceptibility genes, using either linkage studies (attempting to identify regions where chromosomal abnormalities exist) or association studies (attempting to detect relationships between gene variation and schizophrenia risk), has been disappointing (Tosato and Lasalvia, 2009).

Linkage studies in schizophrenia most often note abnormalities on the following three chromosomes: X, 22q11, and 1q42/11q14 (Blackwood, Fordyce, Walker, et al., 2001; DeLisi, Friedrich, Wahlstrom, et al., 1994; Williams, O'Donnovan, & Owen, 2006). Two meta-analyses of over 30 genome-wide examinations (Badner & Gershon, 2002; Lewis, Levinson, Wise, et al., 2003) revealed a total of 400 genes linked to schizophrenia—approximately one-quarter of all known genes (Tandon et al., 2008). In addition to this lack of specificity and sensitivity, linkage analysis is limited by lack of power because the number of available subjects in current samples is limited (Moldin, 1997; Risch & Merinkangas, 1996).

Association studies compare variations in specific gene sequences among individuals with and without schizophrenia; variations that occur at significantly greater frequency in individuals with schizophrenia are thought to increase susceptibility to the disease. A number of the genetic associations that have been reported are supported by variable evidence. Genes currently considered promising include *NRG1* (neuroregulin), *DED1-4* (dopamine receptors D1–D4), and *GRM3* (metabotropic glutamate receptor) (Chubb, Bradshaw, Soares, et al., 2008; Duan, Martinez, Sanders, et al., 2007; Hanninen, Katila, Saarela, et al., 2008; Lewandowski, 2007; Li & He, 2007; Munafo, Atwood, & Flint, 2008; Nicodemus, Kolachana, Vakkalanka, et al., 2007; Schwab, Plummer, Albus, et al., 2008; Talkowski, Kirov, Bamne, et al., 2008; Tan, Wang, Gold, et al., 2007). Unfortunately, even these so-called promising genes have not been consistently identified across studies (Tosato & Lasalvia, 2009).

Disrupted-in-schizophrenia 1 (*DISC1*) is a gene that has demonstrated an association with schizophrenia as well as bipolar disorder, major depression, autism, and Asperger's syndrome. *DISC1* functions as a common hub for many proteins acting along several pathways (Camargo, Collura, Rain, et al., 2007), suggesting that disruption of *DISC1*-involved *pathways* rather than disruption of *DISC1* itself contributes to schizophrenia etiology (Hennah, Thomson, Peltonen, et al., 2006). Three genes involved in *DISC1* intracellular pathways that are significantly associated with schizophrenia are *PDE4B*, *PDE4D*, and *NDEL1*.

In summary, a conclusively identified gene variant that increases schizophrenia risk remains elusive. At present, the dominant paradigm characterizes schizophrenia as a heterogeneous disease with multiple genetic variants, each contributing only a small portion of susceptibility for development of the disorder (Chakravarti, 1999).

Biochemical Alterations

A number of neurochemical explanations for schizophrenia and its associated symptoms have been advanced. The most common and well known is the dopamine hypothesis, which states that psychotic symptoms result from excess dopaminergic activity in the brain, usually in the mesocortical and mesolimbic tracts. These neural pathways connect the ventral tegmentum to the cerebral cortex and limbic system, respectively. The dopamine hypothesis rests on two observations:

1. The most effective medications for managing psychotic symptoms have antagonist action on the dopamine type 2 (D2) receptor.
2. Drugs that increase dopaminergic activity (e.g., amphetamine and cocaine) are psychotomimetic (Sadock and Sadock, 2007).

A majority of recent studies confirm that dopamine dysregulation is intrinsic to schizophrenia (rather than being a medication side effect) and pre-dates the first psychotic episode (Perez-Costas, Melendez-Ferro, & Roberts, 2010). Unfortunately, the dopamine hypothesis does not address the mechanism by which increased dopamine activity occurs. Thus, it remains unknown whether excess dopamine activity is best explained by an excess of dopamine levels, increased dopamine sensitivity, high numbers of dopamine receptors, some combination of these, or another factor that is as yet unknown.

Based on the effectiveness of clozapine and other second generation antipsychotics (SGAs) with serotonin antagonist effects on both positive and negative symptoms of schizophrenia, it is hypothesized that serotonin excess causes these symptom clusters. The inhibitory amino acid neurotransmitter gamma-aminobutyric acid (GABA) has been implicated in schizophrenia because some individuals with the disease experience a loss of GABAergic neurons in the hippocampus. Because GABA regulates dopamine activity, the loss of GABAergic neurons could lead to hyperactivity of dopaminergic neurons (Sadock & Sadock, 2007).

Neuropathology

Neuropathological processes in schizophrenia consist of structural defects in multiple areas. Three-dimensional imaging studies have shown consistent gray matter reductions in the anterior cingulate, bilateral frontal lobe, hippocampus, and amygdala (Ashburner & Friston, 2000; Ellison-Wright & Bullmore, 2009; Segall, Turner, van Erp, et al., 2009). Many individuals with schizophrenia also have enlargement of the third ventricles (Wexler, Zhu, Bell, et al., 2009). Less consistently found are volume reductions, metabolic disturbances, and asymmetry in the thalamus (Buchsbaum, Someya, Teng, et al., 1996; Gur, Maany, Mozley, et al., 1998; Konick & Friedman, 2001). Wexler et al. recently reported that more-impaired individuals with schizophrenia had reductions in white matter volume and enlargement of the lateral ventricle, changes that were not present in less-impaired individuals with the disease.

These alterations may be related to deficits in numbers of cells (Kreczmanski, Heinsen, Mantua, et al., 2007), abnormalities in synaptic organization (Perez-Costas et al., 2010), or both. Reductions in glial cell density (Beasley, Chana, Honavar, et al., 2005) and reduced density of calbindin-expressing neurons (Chance, Walker, & Crow, 2005) have been reported in temporal lobe gray matter in schizophrenia, but studies of temporal lobe white matter alterations are inconclusive (Lee, Yoshida, Kubicki, et al., 2009). Glial cell deficits are also often present in prefrontal gray matter (Starke, Uylings, Sanz-Arigita, et al., 2004). Reductions in glial cell density may reflect deficits in astrocytes or oligodendrites (Beasley, Honavar, Everell, et al., 2009).

Longitudinal studies have shown the aforementioned changes to be progressive throughout the course of schizophrenia (Hulshoff Pol & Kahn, 2008). Factors implicated in these processes include cannabis abuse (Rais, Cahn, van Haren, et al., 2008), psychotropic medications (van Haren, Hulshoff Pol, Schnack, et al., 2007), stress (Pariante, Dazzan, Danese, et al., 2005), or the neurotoxic effects of psychotic states (Cahn, Rais, Stigter, et al., 2008). At present, the etiology of such deficits remains unknown.

Neural Circuitry Deficits

Neural circuitry deficits are particularly important as possible explanations for the memory alterations observed in individuals with schizophrenia. Working memory is mediated by a cortical network activated by the dorsolateral prefrontal cortex (Kim, Tura, Potkin, et al., 2010). Two problematic patterns occur in individuals with schizophrenia—hypoactivation and hyperactivation of a variety of cortical and subcortical regions. Hypoactivation of the dorsolateral prefrontal cortex suggests problems mobilizing neural resources for memory tasks (Barch, Sheline, Csernansky, et al., 2003; Perlstein, Dixit, Carter, et al., 2003). In contrast, a pattern of hyperactivation has also been observed, indicating that individuals with schizophrenia devote greater cortical resources than the general population to perform similar tasks, despite the fact that they are less accurate and require more time than the general population to complete the same task (Callicott, Bertolino, Mattay, et al., 2000; Manoach, Press, Thangaraj, et al., 1999).

Brain Metabolism Dysfunction

Recent studies indicate the presence of mitochondrial dysfunction—including reduced mitochondrial density and volume (Kung & Roberts, 1999; Uranova, Orlovskaya, Vikhreva, et al., 2001)—as well as defective mitochondrial energy production in individuals with schizophrenia (Maurer, Zierz, & Moller, 2001; Prabakaran, Swatton, Ryan, et al., 2004). These alterations are associated with oxidative stress, which has been found to induce cell damage (Wang, Shao, Sun, et al., 2009).

Environmental Basis

Because schizophrenia clusters in families, investigators have entertained causative hypotheses related to environmental exposures and family interaction patterns (Bateson, Jackson, Haley, et al., 1956; Lidz, Cornelison, Fleck, et al., 1965). A variety of environmental factors have been implicated in schizophrenia etiology and its geographical and demographical incidence variation (Kirkbride, Fearon, Morgan, et al., 2006; McGrath et al., 2004). Environmental conditions include both biological and psychosocial risk factors spanning the period before birth through young adulthood (Maki, Veijola, Jones, et al., 2005).

A meta-analysis (McGrath et al., 2004) reported a significantly higher risk for schizophrenia in males, in those living in urban rather than rural environments, and in individuals with a personal or family history of migration. Recent studies have clarified that this higher risk stems from both (1) the tendency of individuals with schizophrenia to congregate in inner cities (Dohrenwend, Levav, Shrout, et al., 1992) and (2) an *additional* association between urban birth and upbringing (until age 15) and an increased risk for developing schizophrenia (Kirkbride et al., 2006). This increased risk for schizophrenia with increasing time spent in urban settings before age 15 lends support to a causal factor related to urban living. Although this factor or factors remain unknown, likely candidates include higher rates of cannabis and other substance use in urban settings, high social stress, low social connectedness, poverty, and environmental toxins associated with urbanicity (Tandon et al., 2008).

The relative risk of developing schizophrenia has been documented as 2.7 times greater than in the general population for first-generation immigrants and 4.5 times greater than in the general population for second-generation immigrants. Proposed explanations include the socially isolated status of immigrants, discrimination (Boydell, van Os, McKenzie, et al., 2001; Cooper, Morgan, Byrne, et al., 2008), or biological explanations such as vitamin D deficiency (Dealberto, 2007); however, a specific factor associated with immigration status remains to be identified. A significantly higher prevalence of schizophrenia has been observed in more-developed as opposed to less-developed countries, as well as among individuals of lower as opposed to higher socioeconomic status (Saha et al., 2005). Table 15-2 shows environmental events associated with schizophrenia.

TABLE 15-2 ENVIRONMENTAL EVENTS ASSOCIATED WITH SCHIZOPHRENIA

Time Period	Event	Association	Mechanism	References
Conception	Paternal age greater than 60 years	Doubles the risk of schizophrenia	Unknown, but may be due to impaired spermatogenesis and resultant mutation(s)	Byrne, Agerbo, Ewald, et al., 2003; Cheng, Ko, Chen, et al., 2008; Malaspina, Harlap, Fennig, et al., 2001; Perrin, Brown, & Malaspina, 2007; Wohl & Gorwood, 2007
First trimester	Severe maternal nutritional deficiency Severe maternal stress	Increased risk of developing schizophrenia	Stress sensitization with resultant hyperdopaminergia	Khashan, Abel, McNamee, et al., 2008; Koenig, Elmer, Shepard, et al., 2005; Lipska, Jaskiw, & Weinberger, 1993; St. Clair, Xu, Wang, et al., 2005; Susser, Neugebauer, Hoek, et al., 1996; Yuii, Suzuki, & Kurachi, 2007
First trimester and early second trimester	Maternal influenza, rubella, or toxoplasmosis	Increased risk of developing schizophrenia	Unknown, but may involve suboptimal immune response, elevated maternal antibody titers, or both	Ashdown, Dumont, Ng, et al., 2006; Brown, Cohen, Harkavy-Friedman, et al., 2001; Brown, Scheafer, & Quesenberry, 2002; Goldberg & Gomar, 2009; Mednick, Machon, Huttunen, et al., 1988; Meyer, Yee, & Feldon, 2007; Penner & Brown, 2007
Birthing process	Complicated delivery	Doubles the risk of schizophrenia	Hypoxia	Byrne, Agerbo, Bennedsen, et al., 2007; Cannon, Jones, & Murray, 2002b; Geddes & Lawrie, 1995
Birth	During late winter or early spring	5%–10% greater likelihood of schizophrenia	Unknown, but may be related to prenatal maternal infection	Davies, Welham, Chant, et al., 2003; McGrath & Welham, 1999; Torrey, Miller, Rawlings, et al., 1997
Childhood	Trauma Head injury Parental separation or death Infection Urban rearing Migration	Increased risk for schizophrenia	Unknown	Dalman, Alleback, Gunnell, et al., 2008; David & Prince, 2005; Morgan & Fisher, 2007; Read, van Os, Morrison, et al., 2005; Wilcox & Nasrallah, 1987
Adolescence	Cannabis use Social adversity Stressful life events	Increased risk for schizophrenia	Unknown	Allardyce & Boydell, 2006; Barnes, Mutsatsa, Hutton, et al., 2006; Degenhardt & Hall, 2006; Harrison, 2004; Moore, Zammit, Lingford-Hughes, et al., 2007; Norman & Malla, 1993; Semple, McIntosh, & Lawrie, 2005

A number of other objective signs—including delay in language and poor social adjustment in childhood or adolescence—have been linked to schizophrenia, but whether these are true risk factors or early disease symptoms remains unknown (Cannon, Caspi, Moffitt, et al., 2002a; Cornblatt, Obuchowski, Roberts, et al., 1999; Fish, Marcus, Hans, et al., 1992; Jones, Rodgers, Murray, et al., 1994; Keshavan, Diwadkar, Montrose, et al., 2005; Walker & Lewine, 1990).

No environmental risk factor has thus far been shown to be sufficient or necessary to cause schizophrenia. While biological and environmental influences are clearly important, specific risks and the mechanisms of causation remain a mystery. It is possible that there may be no one schizophrenia with a single etiology, but rather multiple pathways to disease (Tosato & Lasalvia, 2009).

Clinical Presentation

The symptoms of schizophrenia have been divided into positive, negative, and cognitive types. Additional clinical features include disorganized thoughts or behaviors, motor symptoms, neurological signs, and comorbid mood and anxiety symptoms.

Positive Symptoms

Positive (or Schneiderian) first-rank symptoms involve additions to normal experiences and consist of hallucinations and delusions. Although delusions of control, thought broadcasting, and thought insertion are traditionally associated with schizophrenia, the most common delusions are those of reference or persecution. While hallucinations may involve any of the senses, auditory hallucinations are by far the most common. Voices conversing among themselves or commenting on the individual's behavior are considered characteristic, but threatening or accusatory auditory hallucinations are more common (Tandon, Nasrallah, & Keshavan, 2009).

Negative Symptoms

Negative symptoms refer to affects and behaviors that are lacking in individuals with schizophrenia. They include a flat or blunted affect, thought blocking, poverty of speech, avolition, and social withdrawal. Negative symptoms may be further conceptualized as primary or secondary. Primary negative symptoms are intrinsic to schizophrenia itself, whereas secondary negative symptoms reflect external factors such as depression or medication side effects (Kirkpatrick, Fenton, Carpenter, et al., 2006). The pathophysiology of negative symptoms is not well understood (Keshavan, Tandon, Boutros, et al., 2008); they remain difficult to treat and produce significant disability in patients with the disorder (Stahl & Buckley, 2007). Table 15-3 compares positive and negative symptoms.

TABLE 15-3 COMPARISON OF POSITIVE AND NEGATIVE SYMPTOMS OF SCHIZOPHRENIA

Positive Symptoms	Negative symptoms
• "Additions" to normal experiences • Delusions (most commonly of reference or persecution) • Hallucinations (most commonly auditory, and of a threatening or accusatory nature)	• "Absent" affects, behaviors, or both • Flat or blunted affect • Thought blocking • Poverty of speech • Avolition • Social withdrawal

Cognitive Symptoms

Cognitive symptoms include memory and attention deficits, language difficulties, and problems with executive functioning. Problems with executive functioning are evidenced by difficulties in ordering sequential behaviors, establishing goal-directed plans, staying on task when interrupted, monitoring personal behavior, and associating knowledge with required responses. Current literature indicates that cognitive impairment of some magnitude is all but universal in individuals with schizophrenia (Keefe, Eesley, & Poe, 2005). The cognitive impairments in schizophrenia include deficits specific to episodic memory (Ranganath, Minzenberg, & Ragland, 2008), verbal fluency (Henry & Crawford, 2005), attention (Fioravanti, Carlone, & Vitale, 2005), processing speed (Dickinson, Ramsey, & Gold, 2007), and executive functioning (Reichenberg & Harvey, 2007). Cognitive deficits are present throughout the disease course (Woodberry, Guiliano, & Seidman, 2008), although they can be improved somewhat with antipsychotic treatment (Keefe, Bilder, & Davis, 2007). The presence of cognitive impairment is associated with poorer outcomes, especially in social and vocational areas (Bowie, Leung, & Reichenberg, 2008; van Winkel, Myin-Germeys, & De Hert, 2007).

Disorganization

Disorganization can be categorized into formal thought disorder, derailment, poverty of speech, or behavioral disorganization. Formal thought disorder describes a lack of progressive goal-directed thought processes and includes both derailment and poverty of speech. Derailment is a pattern of speech in which an individual's ideas slip off track onto another unrelated or obliquely related topic; derailment is also known as "loosening of associations." Poverty of speech is the inability to start or take part in a conversation, particularly small talk. Behavioral disorganization ranges from inappropriate affect to attire inappropriate to the season/activity, and it often accompanies formal thought disorder. Both behavioral disorganization and formal thought disorder are more pronounced during illness exacerbations; their presence is associated with poor outcomes (Tandon et al., 2009).

Motor Symptoms

Motor symptoms are common in individuals with schizophrenia and include simple slowing of psychomotor activity (Morrens, Hulstijn, & Sabbe, 2007), isolated posturing (Morrens, Hulstijn, Lewi, et al., 2006), and states of catatonia (Ungvari, Coggins, Leung, et al., 2007). Catatonic symptoms, although rarely observed in today's clinical practice (Stompe, Ortwein-Soboda, & Ritter, 2002), involve echolalia, echopraxia, waxy flexibility, and automatic obedience (Weder, Muralee, Penland, et al., 2008).

Neurological Signs

Neurological signs are divided into hard signs and soft signs. Hard signs indicate impaired reflex, sensory, or motor functioning and are localized to a particular brain region. Hard signs include hypoalgesia, impaired olfactory functioning, and oculomotor abnormalities (Tandon et al., 2009). Soft signs, deficits that do not implicate a specific brain area, include grimacing, increased blink rates, problems sequencing motor tasks (Walker & Green, 1982), asterognosis (Tucker, Campion, & Silberforth, 1975), or difficulties with smooth alternating movements (Ho, Mola, & Andreasen, 2004).

Comorbid Mood and Anxiety Symptoms

Significant depressive symptoms are a problem for most individuals with schizophrenia at some point during their illness. Mood symptoms can occur at any time but are more pronounced during acute psychoses and are more severe in individuals with co-occurring substance abuse disorders (Potvin, Ali, & Stip, 2007; Siris & Bench, 2003). Whereas anxiety symptoms are often significant early in schizophrenia (Chapman, 1966), anxiety later in the disease is commonly treated as a comorbid disease rather than a symptom of schizophrenia. The most common anxiety disorders diagnosed in individuals with schizophrenia are social phobia, obsessive-compulsive disorder, and panic disorder: all are associated with a poorer prognosis (Ciapparelli, Paggani, & Marazziti, 2007; Muller, Koen, Soraya, et al., 2004).

Diagnosis and Prognosis

No single symptom is diagnostic and no laboratory test confirms a diagnosis of schizophrenia. There is wide variability in symptom expression, affect, and level of functioning both among individuals with schizophrenia and within the same individual over time. Good prognostic indicators include late onset, the presence of precipitating factor(s), acute onset, high premorbid function, mood symptoms, being married rather than single, a family history of mood disorders, a good support system, and positive symptoms. Indicators of a poor prognosis include early onset, the absence of precipitating factor(s), insidious onset, poor premorbid function, withdrawn or autistic symptoms, being single, divorced or widowed, a family history of schizophrenia, a poor support system, negative or neurological signs or symptoms, a history of prenatal trauma, no remissions in a 3-year period, multiple relapses, and a history of assaultiveness.

Individuals with schizophrenia are faced with multiple barriers to the achievement of optimal health. Their health barriers include (1) negative symptoms, such as apathy and poor concentration, (2) sedative effects of medication, (3) poverty, and (4) lack of access to health education and programs. In addition, the symptoms of their disease negatively affect their social functioning, with the result that many of those with schizophrenia are isolated and lack social supports. In addition to providing psychiatric care and monitoring, psychiatric advanced practice nurses assess physical and psychological risk factors, monitor medication responses, and provide health promotion. Health promotion for individuals with schizophrenia includes psychosocial treatments to prevent relapse (e.g., education on the importance of treatment adherence) and to promote recovery (e.g., involving family members in treatment when possible).

In contrast to cure, recovery in patients with schizophrenia connotes relative success in several domains in spite of the relapse vulnerability associated with schizophrenia. Recovery domains include socialization, symptoms, and community functioning (Bellack, 2006). Good outcomes are accomplished through experiences and processes that contribute to both emotional and physical healing, in addition to positive changes in attitudes, feelings, and self esteem (Liberman & Kopelowicz, 2005; Loveland, Weaver-Randall, & Corrigan, 2005). Recovery is fostered through treatments targeted at symptom management and by additional attention to fostering engagement in work and community life. Outcomes associated with recovery include independent living, work or school involvement, symptom reductions, and having friends (Anthony, 2000; Liberman, Kopelowicz, Ventura, et al., 2005).

Differential Diagnosis

Whereas psychotic symptoms are the cardinal sign of schizophrenia, a number of physical and psychiatric disorders also result in psychotic symptoms. When psychotic symptoms are the result of a general medical condition, the diagnosis is psychotic disorder due to a general medical condition. Factors such as age of onset and the association of physical and psychotic symptoms in time may be helpful in making this distinction. Among the many medical conditions with associated psychotic symptoms are cerebral tumors, Cushing's syndrome, and vascular dementia.

When psychotic symptoms are the result of substance use, the diagnosis is substance-induced psychotic disorder. This diagnosis requires a careful history as to the timing of symptoms and substances used. Collateral information is frequently helpful in this regard. The most common substances associated with psychotic symptoms are cannabis and cocaine (Nunes & Broderick, 2007; Shapiro & Buckley-Hunter, 2010).

The presence of mood symptoms in both schizophrenia and schizoaffective disorder presents diagnostic challenges. Schizoaffective disorder is the diagnosis when mood symptoms co-occur with psychotic symptoms, along with at least a 2-week period of psychotic symptoms in the *absence* of mood symptoms, and when mood symptoms are present for a significant portion of the total illness duration (Kane, 2010).

The differentiation between schizophrenia and schizophreniform disorder is one of duration. In contrast to schizophrenia, schizophreniform disorder lasts less than 6 months and is not associated with functional decline (American Psychiatric Association, 2000b).

The current classification of schizophrenia is under worldwide review for the *Diagnostic and Statistical Manual of Mental Disorders,* fifth edition (*DSM-V*), scheduled for release in 2012. One paradigm shift under consideration is a change from categorical (all or nothing) diagnoses to dimensional diagnoses that describe a range of symptoms along a continuum. Contributing to this shift is the notion that common psychiatric illnesses may not be discrete entities, but rather symptom clusters within pathophysiological families. For example, schizophrenia and autism are known to result from common background variants (genetic deletions or mutations) in association with deleterious mutations and environmental insults. It is possible that the common variants contribute small increments of risk in an additive manner and that, depending on the presence of certain additional mutations or environmental conditions, different symptoms of differing severity are expressed. Hence, it may be beneficial to describe disorders more broadly in terms of classes such as "psychotic disorders." Clinicians would then assess patients along a spectrum including typical symptoms, atypical symptoms, behavioral tendencies, interpersonal relationships, and associated features (Kupfer, 2009). As part of societal conceptualizations of mental illness, this debate has important implications for psychiatric advanced practice nurses and for the nursing care of patients with schizophrenia (Snowden, 2009b).

Comorbidity

Management issues include promoting health, managing comorbid health problems (obesity, smoking), caring for women who are pregnant, treating substance abuse, identifying risk for suicide, and promoting adherence to treatment.

Physical Health Promotion

In addition to their chronic psychiatric illness, individuals with schizophrenia are at increased risk for a number of physical health problems across the life span. They have higher mortality and morbidity rates than the general population, only one-fourth of which is explained by their higher rates of suicide and accidents (Saha, Chant, & McGrath, 2007). Mortality rates for individuals with schizophrenia are approximately double those of the general population, and their life spans are 15 to 20 years shorter (Auquier, Lancon, Rouillon, et al., 2007). This excess mortality is attributed not only to the shorter life span associated with an increased prevalence of several medical conditions (diabetes and cardiovascular disease, for example), but also to high rates of risk factors in schizophrenia, including obesity, smoking, sedentary lifestyle, and poor diet (Newcomer & Hennekens, 2007). In addition, cardiovascular diseases are often not diagnosed or are diagnosed later in individuals with schizophrenia than in the general population owing to inadequate reporting of symptoms or poor access to care (Leucht, Burkhard, & Henderson, 2007). Finally, individuals with schizophrenia experience higher rates of treatment complications than the general population owing to the interactions of psychiatric and medical treatments (Daumit, Pronovost, & Anthony, 2006).

Managing Comorbid Health Problems

Comorbid health problems occurring across the life span include obesity, smoking, and substance abuse disorders. Other health-related problems include pregnancy, suicide, and adherence to treatment.

Individuals with schizophrenia have many risk factors that lead to increased morbidity and mortality, such as taking medications that are associated with weight gain, poor diet, sedentary lifestyle, and lack of access to medical care. The rates of obesity (Meyer, Nasrallah, McEvoy, et al., 2005), dyslipidemia (Casey, 2004), glucose dysregulation (Brambilia, Guastalla, Guerrini, et al., 1976; Holden, 1995; Holden & Mooney, 1994; Richter, 1957), and type II diabetes (Dixon, Weiden, Delahanty, et al., 2000; Mukherjee, 1995; Mukherjee, Decina, Bocola, et al., 1996) are higher in individuals with schizophrenia than in the general population and combine to increase their risk for cardiovascular disease approximately 12-fold over that of the general population. Cardiovascular disease contributes the greatest number of excess deaths in women with schizophrenia, whereas suicide contributes the greatest number of excess deaths among men with the disease (Goff, Cather, & Evins, 2005).

Obesity

Excess visceral fat (as opposed to subcutaneous fat) increases the circulatory workload, leading to an increased likelihood of type II diabetes, hypertension, and elevated triglycerides. These medical conditions, which are common among individuals with schizophrenia, ultimately increase cardiovascular mortality and morbidity (Van Gaal, 2006).

Hence, abdominal obesity is a key modifiable factor known to contribute to the health risks of those with schizophrenia. The Clinical Antipsychotic Trials of Intervention Effectiveness (CATIE) schizophrenia study found that 76.35% of women and 35.5% of men were abdominally obese at baseline (Meyer et al., 2005).

The problem of weight gain among those prescribed SGAs is well known. The FDA lists weight gain as a class effect of this group of medications, although research to date indicates some variability in expected weight gain among the different SGAs. While the FDA classifies a mere 7% increase in weight over baseline as an adverse event (Mitchell & Malone, 2006), 40% to 80% of patients on any antipsychotic (SGAs or FGAs) have weight gain that exceeds ideal body weight by 20% or more (Masand, Blackburn, Ganguli, et al., 1999; Umbricht, Pollack, & Kane, 1994). Obesity rates (by weight classification, body mass index [BMI], or waist circumference) among individuals with schizophrenia range from 40% to 62% and are especially high in women (Allison, Fontaine, Heo, et al., 1999; Centorrino, Baldessarini, Kando, et al., 1994; Kendrick, 1996; Silverstone, Smith, & Goodall, 1988; Stedman & Welham, 1993).

The precise mechanism of weight gain associated with antipsychotic medications is unknown (American Psychiatric Association, 2004b; Peet, 2004). Weight gain occurs when more energy is consumed than expended, and it may be due to increased intake, reduced expenditure, or both. Hunger and satiety may be altered in individuals taking antipsychotic medications owing to binding of these medications with histamine H1 as well as with serotonin, dopamine, and norepinephrine receptors (Kaur & Kulkarni, 2003).

The diets of individuals with schizophrenia are higher in fat and lower in fiber than those of individuals with no mental illness. Recent studies have documented that individuals with schizophrenia consume more saturated fat (Ryan, Collins, & Thakore, 2003) and refined sugar (Stokes & Peet, 2003) than healthy individuals. Poor diet in this group is associated with poverty and unstable living conditions, as is the frequent consumption of fast food (Masand, 1999). Furthermore, individuals with schizophrenia may not understand the relationships between weight and diet, or they may not understand how to improve their eating habits (Dixon, 2003).

Individuals with schizophrenia are less active and less aerobically fit than the general population (Beebe, 2006a; Beebe, Tian, Morris, et al., 2005; Daumit, Goldberg, Anthony, et al., 2005). This state of affairs is particularly troubling because physical inactivity is one of the most prevalent risk factors for the development of obesity and cardiovascular disease (United States Department of Health and Human Services, 2010). Factors contributing to reduced physical activity and exercise in individuals with schizophrenia include negative symptoms; lack of access to fitness information, facilities, or equipment; and the sedative effects of medications.

Assessments

Psychiatric advanced practice nurses are in an excellent position to provide monitoring for physical health risks associated with schizophrenia. Their scope of practice includes a number of health-promotion activities with the potential to positively impact physical health outcomes. A number of physical assessment and monitoring procedures are recommended in this group.

Because of their obesity risks, patients with schizophrenia require careful baseline assessment and ongoing monitoring of physical health parameters. The American Diabetes Association (ADA), in collaboration with the American Psychiatric Association (APA), the American Association of Clinical Endocrinologists (AACE), and the North American Association for the Study of Obesity (NAASO) (ADA/APA/AACE/NAASO, 2004) recommended the following baseline assessments for individuals with schizophrenia: (1) family history, including history of cardiovascular disease, hypertension, diabetes, obesity, and dyslipidemias, and (2) measurement of height and weight to calculate BMI. These measurements should be done with patients in light-weight clothing and stocking feet, using the same scale each time.

BMI is an accepted measure of obesity and is calculated as the ratio of weight to height, using the formula BMI = weight in kilograms/height in meters^2. Centers for Disease Control and Prevention (2010) guidelines define those with a BMI between 25 and 29.9 as overweight, and those with a BMI greater than 30 as obese.

Waist circumference is the primary procedure for identification of abdominal obesity. Waist circumference is measured with the patient unclothed. A flexible tape measure is positioned horizontally halfway between the lower rib cage and the superior anterior iliac crest in women, and at the level of the umbilicus in men (National Heart Lung and Blood Institute, 2010). The National Cholesterol Education Panel III (2002) defines abdominal obesity as a waist circumference greater than 40 inches in men and greater than 35 inches in women.

Additional recommended baseline assessments include blood pressure, fasting glucose panels, and fasting lipid panels. High-risk individuals for whom medical referrals should be obtained include those with blood pressures above 130/85, fasting glucose panels greater than 110 mg/dL, triglycerides greater than 150 mg/dL, or high-density lipoprotein greater than 40 in men and greater than 50 in women (National Cholesterol Education Panel, 2002).

Monitoring

Recommended ongoing monitoring includes weighing the patient monthly for the first 3 months and quarterly thereafter. Blood pressure, fasting glucose, and lipid measurements are recommended at baseline, at 3 months, and annually thereafter (ADA/APA/AACE/NAASO, 2004). Clinical status may necessitate more frequent monitoring for some individuals—for example, more frequent weighing for patients prescribed olanzapine or clozapine, as weight gain from these medications has been documented to continue for up to 1 year (McEvoy, 2002). In addition, patients with extensive family history of risk or who are nonadherent with dietary or activity recommendations may need more frequent monitoring or a referral for specialty management of diabetes or other medical conditions.

Medication Choices

The most important treatment choice that psychiatric advanced practice nurses make with regard to weight implications for individuals with schizophrenia is the choice of antipsychotic medication. (See Table 15-6 for a comparison of the risks for weight gain, diabetes, and lipid elevation among SGAs.) To minimize risks, one might begin with ziprasidone or aripiprazole in drug-naive patients. However, for a variety of reasons, many patients seen in practice settings will already have been prescribed another FGA or SGA with a less favorable weight-gain profile.

If weight gain exceeds 5% of baseline or glucose control or lipid profile shows negative changes, a switch to a medication with a more desirable profile should be considered (Van Gaal, 2006). Switching should be undertaken on an outpatient basis after symptoms have been stable for at least 3 months, or sooner if side effects are of major clinical concern (Ganguli, 2002). Psychiatric advanced practice nurses must evaluate the potential problem of further weight gain and its associated risks against a possible period of psychiatric instability when making this determination, as medication switching is associated with significantly increased risk of hospitalization and a 25% increase in annual health care costs for the year in which the switch occurs (Faries, Ascher-Svanum, Nyhuis, et al., 2009).

The three commonly used switching techniques for oral antipsychotic medications are

1. *Immediate:* discontinue the first medication and immediately start the new medication at full dose
2. *Cross-taper:* gradually taper the first medication, while simultaneously titrating the new medication
3. *Individual taper:* while continuing the same dose of first medication, start the new medication and gradually titrate to the recommended dose; after the new medication is at full dose, taper off the first medication

Each of these techniques has disadvantages—for instance, whereas tapers are more complex for patients to manage, abrupt discontinuation of antipsychotic medication has been associated with withdrawal dyskinesia and rebound cholinergic effects (Masand, 2005). Two studies examined the three specific strategies for switching between SGAs. Switching was well tolerated, with similar rates of adverse events with the three methods and no increases in extrapyramidal symptoms in any group (Casey, Carson, Saha, et al., 2003a; Weiden, Simpson, Potkin, et al., 2003). However, patients in research studies generally have greatly increased contact with study staff and more monitoring than is realistic in most clinical practice settings, and these supports may have contributed to the research outcomes observed. Thus, whenever switching is conducted, clinicians would be wise to include patient and family education, more frequent monitoring, and titration of new medication to optimum dose prior to discontinuation of the first medication.

Adjunctive Medications

Metformin reduces serum glucose by reducing hepatic glucose production and reducing intestinal absorption of glucose. It is recommended as an adjunct to diet and exercise to reduce serum glucose in patients with type II diabetes mellitus and for the management of antipsychotic-induced weight gain. The initial adult dose is 500 mg bid or 850 mg once daily with food. Dose may be increased by 500 mg weekly (if bid dosing) or 850 mg every 2 weeks (if once-daily dosing) to a maximum of 2000 mg/day. Common side effects include diarrhea, nausea, vomiting, and abdominal distention. Metformin is contraindicated in the presence of renal disease. Individuals taking medications known to produce hyperglycemia (e.g., calcium channel blockers, corticosteroids, diuretics, oral contraceptives, phenothiazines, phenytoin, or thyroid preparations) must have their glucose levels monitored closely.

The use of metformin in individuals with schizophrenia was investigated in five randomized controlled trials, with four of the five studies indicating beneficial effects on weight (Baptista, Martinez, Lacruz, et al., 2006; Baptista, Rangel, Fernandez, et al., 2007; Klein, Cottingham, Sorter, et al., 2006; Wu, Zhao, Guo, et al., 2008a; Wu, Zhao, Jin, et al., 2008b). Patients receiving metformin along with making lifestyle changes experienced the best outcomes.

Topiramate is an anticonvulsant that is occasionally prescribed off-label for management of obesity and also for alcohol abuse, eating disorders, and smoking cessation. As an official treatment of epilepsy, topiramate is initiated at 25 to 50 mg/day and increased by 25 to 50 mg/week to a maximum of 400 mg/day in divided doses in adults. Two randomized controlled trials of topiramate in overweight individuals with schizophrenia taking olanzapine (Nickel, Nickel, Muehlbacher, et al., 2005), risperidone, quetiapine, or clozapine (Ko, Joe, Jung, et al., 2005) reported weight loss. Side effects of topiramate include dizziness, fatigue, and anorexia. Alcohol may potentiate central nervous system depression with topiramate, and carbamazepine may reduce topiramate levels. Topiramate may reduce the effectiveness of oral contraceptives and reduce plasma concentrations of digitalis and lithium. Dosage should be reduced by 50% in individuals with renal disease.

The small improvements in weight control with the use of metformin and topiramate must be evaluated against the increased complexity of treatment and monitoring regimens, the potential side effects of the additional medications, the possibility of drug interactions, and financial considerations (American Psychiatric Association, 2009).

Lifestyle Interventions

Commonly recommended lifestyle interventions to achieve weight loss include dietary changes, physical exercise, or both. All studies of diet and exercise in individuals with schizophrenia showed small weight reductions (Beebe et al., 2005; Brown & Chen, 2006; Mitchell & Malone, 2006; Wu, Wang, Bai, et al., 2007; Wu et al., 2008a). These findings should not be underestimated, because weight loss as low as 5% to 10% of body weight has been shown to reduce obesity-related disorders (Blackburn, 1995; Kanders & Blackburn, 1992; Knowler, Barrett-Connor, Fowler, et al., 2002) and improve glucose levels, glucose tolerance test results, and blood pressure in obese adults (Chan, Rimm, Colditz, et al., 1994; Daly, Solomon, & Manson, 1996).

Two studies examined nutritional education interventions for outpatients with schizophrenia. Littrell, Hilligoss, Kirshner, et al. (2003) provided a weekly psychoeducational class that focused on dietary guidelines, appropriate portion sizes, and the importance of a healthy diet to 35 outpatients with schizophrenia for 4 months, then compared weight change to a control group of 35 outpatients with schizophrenia receiving standard care. At both 4 and 6 months, a statistically significant weight difference was observed between the two groups, with the intervention group exhibiting greater weight loss. Likewise, Evans, Newton, and Higgins (2005) provided 29 outpatients with schizophrenia with six 1-hour nutritional education classes over a 6-month period, and compared them to 22 controls receiving standard care. All subjects entered the study on commencement of treatment with olanzapine. The experimental group had significantly less weight gain than controls at both 3 and 6 months; however 13% of those in the experimental group still gained more than 7% of their baseline weight (compared to 64% of controls). This study highlights the serious issue of weight gain (especially when medications such as olanzapine are used) and the need for aggressive management of patients for whom this medication is chosen.

Psychiatric advanced practice nurses should plan simple diet teaching, taking into account the cognitive limitations of patients with schizophrenia in memory and attention. The use of concrete examples, repetition, reminders, and positive reinforcement is desirable to offset these difficulties. Patients should be frequently reminded to strive for a goal of consuming five servings of fruit and vegetables per day, reducing fat and salt intake by limiting fast food and salty snacks, and limiting foods containing refined sugar such as baked goods and sweets. In addition, individuals with schizophrenia have been shown to benefit from education regarding proper portion control (Littrell et al., 2003). For some patients, the use of diet soda to replace high-calorie soda or juice, and reminders to drink 6 to 8 glasses of water daily, would also be helpful in managing intake and satiety.

A few small studies have consistently documented both psychiatric health improvements (e.g., reduced depression and anxiety) (Acil, Dogan, & Dogan, 2008; Chamove, 1986; Gimino & Levin, 1984; Pelham, Campagna, Ritvo, et al., 1993) and physical health improvements (e.g., increased flexibility, weight loss, or reduced BMI) (Beebe et al., 2005; Centorrino, Wurtman, Duca, et al., 2006; Chen, Chen, & Huang, 2009; Fogarty, Happell, & Pininkahana, 2004; Kwon, Choi, Bahk, et al., 2006; Pendlebury, Haddad, & Dursun, 2005; Vreeland, Minsk, Menza, et al., 2003) associated with exercise in individuals with schizophrenia. The most serious and consistent problem in this group of studies was motivating individuals with schizophrenia to attend and adhere to exercise (Ball, Coons, & Buchanan, 2001; Centorrino et al.; Chen et al.; Kwon et al.; Pelham et al.; Pendlebury et al.; Vreeland et al.). Archie, Wilson, Osborne, et al. (2003) provided free access to a fitness facility to 20 outpatients with schizophrenia for 6 months and monitored their exercise behavior. Dropout rates were 40% after 4 months, 70% after 5 months, and 90% after 6 months. These rates compare unfavorably with general population exercise cessation (50% after 6 months). The main reason given for dropout by individuals with schizophrenia was lack of motivation. Menza, Vreeland, Minsky, et al. (2004) tested a 1-year weight control program of counseling and exercise for schizophrenia outpatients. Weight and BMI decreased significantly in those receiving the program, but only 66% of subjects completed the program, and average attendance was less than 70%. Beebe, Smith, Burk, et al. (2010b) recently evaluated a motivational intervention designed to improve exercise attitudes and behavior, documenting significant increases in self-efficacy for exercise postintervention.

After medical clearance for exercise is obtained, psychiatric advanced practice nurses should first focus on motivation. One aspect of motivation is the concept of self-efficacy, which includes confidence in one's ability to perform the behavior along with expectation of benefits from the behavior (Bandura, 1995). Clinicians should assess the patient's confidence level in his or her ability to perform the exercises from the outset. Interventions to increase confidence include education, appropriate equipment (for example, verifying that the patient has adequate footwear if walking is recommended), memory prompts of earlier physical competence, and discussion of other activities in which the patient is proficient (Beebe, 2006b). Walking is the most popular form of exercise for individuals with schizophrenia, but they often require assistance to plan systematic exercise sessions (Dixon, 2003). For maximum health benefit, patients need 30 minutes of moderate exercise at least five times a week (Cormac & Ferriter, 2006). When possible, either treatment staff or a buddy should participate in exercises with patients, as this motivates participation and increases social interaction. Positive reinforcement, problem-solving of exercise barriers, and periodic booster sessions enhance adherence (Green et al., 2000). Patients must also be educated about the strong evidence for physical, mental, and social benefits of exercise. Pointing out observed improvements as the exercise program continues will reinforce patients' awareness of their progress and enhance exercise adherence.

Smoking

Approximately 70% to 80% of individuals with schizophrenia smoke; most consume more than 20 cigarettes a day. Individuals with schizophrenia are five times more likely to smoke than the general population (deLeon & Diaz, 2005). Smoking reduces plasma levels of many FGAs and SGAs, including haloperidol, olanzapine, and clozapine, by approximately one-third through enzyme induction of cytochrome-P450. Plasma levels of risperidone, aripiprazole, quetiapine, and ziprasidone are metabolized through cytochrome-P2D6 and cytochrome-YP3A and thus are unaffected by smoking (Winterer, 2010).

Treatment

Smoking cessation treatments include nicotine replacement, bupropion, and psychosocial approaches. Several studies have shown that nicotine replacement therapy with or without additional behavioral interventions significantly improves the chances of smoking reduction or cessation in individuals with schizophrenia (Evins, Cather, Deckersbach, et al., 2005; Evins, Cather, Culhane, et al., 2007; Fatemi, Stary, Hatsukami, et al., 2005; George, Vessicchio, Saccok, et al., 2008), but rates of relapse were significant, suggesting that clinicians wishing to support these behaviors in the long term need to consider extending pharmacological treatment and providing continuous and active psychosocial support (American Psychiatric Association, 2009).

Bupropion is a norepinephrine dopamine reuptake inhibitor FDA approved for nicotine addiction. It should be initiated 1 to 2 weeks before smoking is discontinued at a dosage of 150 mg daily and increased to 150 bid after 3 days (maximum dose 300 mg/day). Common side effects include dry mouth, constipation, dizziness, and headache. Bupropion can be fatal in combination with monoamine oxidase inhibitors and should not be used with thioridazine, because bupropion may interfere with thioridazine metabolism, resulting in increased thioridazine levels and potentially fatal cardiac arrhythmias. The dosage should be reduced in patients with renal or hepatic disease and in the elderly (Stahl, 2009). Recently an FDA black box warning was added advising of potential serious symptoms, including changes in behavior, hostility, agitation, depression, suicidal ideation, and suicidal attempts in patients prescribed bupropion (United States Food and Drug Administration, 2009); therefore, it should be used with caution in individuals with schizophrenia. Although the FDA has approved varenicline (Chantix) for treatment of smoking cessation, it has not been randomly studied in individuals with schizophrenia (American Psychiatric Association, 2009).

Substance Abuse Disorders

A comorbid substance abuse disorder is present in 20% to 65% of individuals with schizophrenia (Barbee, Clark, Crapanzano, et al., 1989; Mueser, Yarnold, & Bellack, 1992). Alcohol, nicotine, and cannabis are the most common drugs of abuse. In individuals with schizophrenia, substance abuse is associated with male gender, single marital status, less education, early onset of schizophrenia, more frequent and longer hospitalizations, worse psychotic symptoms, more gray matter volume deficits, poor treatment adherence, depression, suicide, violence, legal problems, incarceration, family burden, housing instability, and increased risk for HIV and hepatitis C (Drake, Osher, Noordsy, et al., 1990; Drake, Osher, & Wallach, 1989; Kivlahan, Heiman, Wright, et al., 1990; Mathalon, Pfefferbaum, Limk, et al., 2003; Rosenberg, Goodman, Osher, et al., 2001).

Assessment

Psychiatric advanced practice nurses should be constantly vigilant in substance abuse assessments in patients with schizophrenia. When possible, collateral information should be obtained to verify patient report, and screening with an objective instrument such as the four-item *CAGE questionnaire* (Ewing, 1984) should be considered. The CAGE questionnaire was originally designed to identify potential alcohol dependence but can be adapted for other substances of abuse. CAGE is an acronym for the four items:

1. Have you ever felt you should **C**ut down on your drinking?
2. Have people **A**nnoyed you by criticizing your drinking?
3. Have you ever felt bad or **G**uilty about your drinking?
4. Have you ever had a drink first thing in the morning to steady your nerves or get rid of a hangover (**E**ye-opener)?

Any positive response should be followed up by an open-ended question, allowing the patient to elaborate (Isaacson & Schorling, 1999). Each *yes* answer scores 1 point, and *no* answers are scored as 0. A score of 2 or more should be followed by a targeted diagnostic interview to confirm the diagnosis of a substance abuse disorder. The CAGE questionnaire has demonstrated high test-retest reliability (0.80 to 0.95) and adequate correlations with other screening instruments (0.48 to 0.70). In psychiatric patients specifically, sensitivity for alcohol use disorders (individuals with the disease who test as positive) is 0.71, and specificity (individuals without the disease who test as negative) is 0.90. The questionnaire is less specific in women and college students, and it is not recommended as a screening instrument for heavy/hazardous alcohol consumption (Dhalla & Kopec, 2007).

Treatment

Psychiatric advanced practice nurses should assess the lifetime history of all substances used, including amount, pattern, and circumstances of use. Urine or blood toxicology screening and liver function studies will assist in interpreting subjective reports of use. In addition, substance-related symptoms must be carefully differentiated from psychotic symptoms. Finally, substance abuse treatment should ideally be integrated with a multidisciplinary team, including assertive outreach, family intervention, case management, rehabilitation, and medication management.

Because their receptor profiles may result in reduced cravings (Soyka, 1996; Wilkins, 1997), SGAs are recommended for individuals with schizophrenia with comorbid substance abuse (Falkai, Wobrock, Lieberman, et al., 2005). Among the SGAs, there is evidence for the superiority of oral clozapine, olanzapine, and quetiapine (Wobrock & Soyka, 2009). One randomized controlled trial showed long-acting risperidone microspheres to be associated with less drug use, longer time to first drug use, and better substance abuse treatment compliance in individuals with schizophrenia compared with FGAs (Rubio, Martinez, & Ponce, 2006).

A few studies have examined the use of naltrexone, a long-acting opioid receptor antagonist, for individuals with schizophrenia with comorbid alcohol abuse and have reported reduced cravings and reduced alcohol consumption (Batki, Dimmock, Wade, et al., 2007; Maxwell & Shinderman, 2000; Petrakis, O'Malley, Rounsaville, et al., 2004). Naltrexone is a mu-opioid receptor antagonist that is FDA approved for alcohol dependence. The drug acts by blocking mu-opioid receptors, preventing alcohol from binding there and thereby preventing pleasurable effects. The usual adult dose is 50 mg/day by mouth. Common side effects include nausea, vomiting, and anorexia, and the medication is contraindicated in acute hepatitis or liver failure (Stahl, 2009). Because disulfiram may induce psychosis and accelerate antipsychotic metabolism, its use in schizophrenia is controversial (Wobrock & Soyka, 2009).

Pregnancy

The care of a woman with schizophrenia of childbearing age or pregnant is complex and requires attention to both prenatal care and psychiatric management. Available data to guide medication choices come from animal studies and case reports of uncontrolled human exposure (Table 15-4). Risks are known to be highest in the first trimester. Data indicate a relatively low risk of fetal harm with SGAs (American Academy of Pediatrics, 2000; Cohen & Rosenbaum, 1998; Gold, 2000). One case report showed that olanzapine did not increase fetal harm (Goldstein, Corbin, & Fung, 2000). Clozapine has been associated with gestational diabetes but not fetal harm (Dickson & Hogg, 1998) (see Table 15-6). On the other hand, adjunctive medications such as mood stabilizers and benzodiazepines are associated with serious fetal malformations and behavioral effects. For example, lithium is associated with a two to three times increased risk of major birth defects including Ebstein's anomaly, and lorazepam and other benzodiazepines are associated with birth defects. Both medications are assigned to pregnancy category D, indicating positive evidence of risk to the human fetus (American Academy of Pediatrics, 2000; Ernst & Goldberg, 2002; Gold, 2000; Stahl, 2009).

TABLE 15-4 PREGNANCY CATEGORIES FOR ANTIPSYCHOTIC MEDICATIONS

Medication	Pregnancy Category
Clozapine	B
Olanzapine	C
Risperidone	C
Quetiapine	C
Ziprasidone	C
Aripiprazole	C
Thioridazine	C
Perphenazine	C
Haloperidol	C

Note. Category B = animal studies do not show adverse effects, no controlled studies in humans; Category C = some animal studies show adverse effects, no controlled studies in humans.

Psychiatric advanced practice nurses must be vigilant in assessing sexual activity and addressing appropriate means of birth control in women of childbearing potential. If a pregnancy occurs, clinicians should make every effort to assist patients in obtaining and complying with prenatal care, understanding the risks of fetal harm and the possibility of a poor pregnancy outcome owing to uncontrolled psychiatric illness, and making informed decisions about their care. Additional issues during pregnancy may involve smoking cessation, the management of comorbid substance abuse, and the reduction of obesity.

Suicide

Suicide is the leading cause of premature death in individuals with schizophrenia. Some risks for suicide are identical in individuals with schizophrenia and in the U.S. general population: male gender, Caucasian ethnicity, single marital status, social isolation, a family history of suicide, unemployment, previous suicide attempt, substance use, depression, and adverse life events. Suicide risks specific to schizophrenia include young age at onset, high socioeconomic status, high intelligence, high aspirations, chronic course (American Psychiatric Association, 2004), greater insight, and higher premorbid achievement (Melle, Johannson, & Friis, 2006). Approximately 33% of individuals with schizophrenia attempt suicide at least once, and 5% die by suicide (Tandon et al., 2009). Protective factors associated with lower suicide rates in individuals with schizophrenia include family support, social connectedness, and treatment with clozapine (Hennen & Baldessarini, 2005; Meltzer et al., 2003).

Assessment

A complete suicide assessment includes not only risk factors and protective factors, but also a frank discussion of quality of life and reasons for living, along with suicidal thoughts, behavior, or intent. Psychiatric advanced practice nurses are encouraged to ask directly about the presence of suicidal thoughts, plans, and intent. American Psychiatric Association (2003) guidelines state that direct discussion of suicidality does not increase its severity (Williams, Noel, Cordes, et al., 2002) and may actually be beneficial as it provides opportunities for expression of feelings and problem-solving (Gould, Marrocco, Kleinman, et al., 2005). Based on the outcomes of this assessment, psychiatric advanced practice nurses should increase patient contact, limit access to means of self-harm, set up crisis plans (Rudd, Mandrusiak, & Joiner, 2006), and consider inpatient hospitalization if safety cannot be ensured.

Treatment

Mobilization of the patient's support system and communication with other members of the health care team are essential (Meerwijk, vanMeijel, van den Bout, et al., 2010). Follow-up care may include antidepressant medication, antipsychotic medication dose adjustments, psychotherapy, or other supports, depending on the specific situation.

Clozapine has been shown to exert a protective effect in individuals with schizophrenia with suicidal ideation (Meltzer et al., 2003; Meltzer & Okayli, 1995; Walker, Lanza, Arellano, et al., 1997) and may be considered for this group of patients. The mechanism of this protective effect remains unclear but is hypothesized to relate to clozapine's effect on depressive symptoms (Saunders & Hawton, 2009).

Adherence to Treatment

The rates of adherence to antipsychotic medications for individuals with schizophrenia range from 11% to 80% with average rates of 50%, depending on measures used and definitions of adherence (Dolder, Lacro, Dunn, et al., 2002; Dolder, Lacro, & Jeste, 2003; Lacro, Dunn, Dolder, et al., 2002; Weiden & Olfson, 1995). Although many clinicians and researchers believed that adherence to psychiatric medications would improve owing to the more favorable side effect profile of SGAs than the previously used FGAs, research has not confirmed this (Dolder et al.). Antipsychotic medication adherence in patients with schizophrenia is believed by some to diminish over time (Weiden, Aquila, & Standard, 1996)—a critical issue, considering that schizophrenia necessitates lifelong treatment.

The low levels of adherence to medications prescribed for chronic physical illnesses such as asthma, diabetes, and hypertension are well known (Byerly, Fisher, Whatley, et al., 2005; Keith & Kane, 2003; Nakonezny & Byerly, 2005; Puschner, Born, Giessler, et al., 2005), making it reasonable to conclude that adherence to medications prescribed for physical illnesses might also be problematic for individuals with schizophrenia.

Measures

Measures of medication adherence include self-report, clinician assessments, blood or urine levels, monitoring of prescription refill rates, pill counts, and electronic monitoring. Self-report is the most commonly used method and the most likely to overestimate adherence (Ascher-Svanum, Zhu, Faries, et al., 2006; Velligan, Lam, Ereshefsky, et al., 2003). Blood and urine level tests are not available for all psychiatric medications and are poorly accepted by patients. In addition, they provide information on adherence for a time frame of only a few days (Frangou, Sachpazidis, Stassinakis, et al., 2005). Pharmacy refill rate monitoring can pose logistical problems or be incomplete if patients use multiple pharmacies or change pharmacies. Furthermore, pharmacy refill records provide information about medications filled, not taken. Pill counts and electronic monitoring have proven acceptable to patients, but both are labor intensive for clinicians and neither guarantees that missing medications were actually ingested (Nakonezny & Byerly, 2005).

Interventions

Interventions to improve adherence include problem-solving and motivation, behavioral strategies, and psychoeducation (Kane, 2006). Motivational interventions are designed to increase adherence behavior by focusing on the role of medications in reducing symptoms and rehospitalizations. Problem-solving techniques are used to assist in overcoming adherence barriers—such as forgetfulness or disorganization—with concrete suggestions, such as placing medications in a prominent location or tying medication administration to an established routine. Behavioral strategies include positive reinforcement and the provision of cues such as calendars for marking off doses as they are taken. Psychoeducation involves didactic sharing of information about the disease and management of schizophrenia.

Four studies have examined psychosocial interventions for psychiatric medication adherence in individuals with schizophrenia. Kemp et al. (1998) tested compliance therapy, a manualized series of four to six individual sessions, combining cognitive and educational content. Forty-three individuals with schizophrenia receiving compliance therapy as inpatients had significantly higher psychiatric medication adherence by clinician report at 18-month outpatient follow-up. A limitation of this study is the use of clinician ratings of adherence, which have been shown to dramatically overestimate adherence (Byerly et al., 2005). Because not all clinician raters were blinded, the possibility of rater bias exists. Two studies (Azrin & Teicher, 1998; Razali, Hasanah, Khan, et al., 2000) used family intervention with behavioral components, and both reported significantly higher psychiatric medication adherence compared to control groups.

Finally, Frangou et al. (2005) demonstrated that adherence monitoring in itself, without any other intervention, may significantly increase medication-taking behavior.

Only two studies have addressed nonpsychiatric medication adherence in individuals with schizophrenia. Pratt, Mueser, Driscoll, et al. (2006) reported average pill count adherence of 57% for psychiatric medications and 64% for nonpsychiatric medications. In contrast, Piette, Heisler, Ganoczy, et al. (2007) examined the percentage of medication prescription doses filled, out of the total doses of psychiatric and nonpsychiatric medications ordered, for 1686 outpatients. Participants were significantly ($P < .001$) more likely to have poor adherence (defined as a medication possession ratio of less than 80%) to nonpsychiatric medications than to psychiatric medications.

Taken together, these studies highlight a complicated set of factors affecting medication adherence in individuals with schizophrenia. The picture is further obscured by the use of a variety of measures and definitions of adherence. Because participants must agree to participate in studies and cooperate with study requirements, it is likely that study participants exhibit higher than average levels of adherence (Frangou et al., 2005; Gray, Wykes, & Gournay, 2002). Furthermore, no ideal adherence measure exists; all of the available measures are subject to conscious manipulation. Also troubling is the dearth of information on adherence to nonpsychiatric medications, and whether adherence interventions affect nonpsychiatric medication–taking behaviors.

As part of prudent practice, adherence should be assessed in patients who are defined as partial medication responders (individuals who experience ongoing hallucinations or delusions). Clinicians should first verify that an adequate trial of antipsychotic medication has taken place. An adequate trial is defined as an optimum medication dose with good patient adherence (at least 80% of prescribed doses are ingested) for 4 to 6 weeks (American Psychiatric Association, 2004a). Reasons for nonadherence vary and include personal factors, system factors, and illness factors (Heinssen, 2002). Personal factors include attitudes toward illness, response to medication side effects, and lack of transportation. System factors include the provision of care by multiple practitioners at multiple sites, complex medication regimens, and insurance policies that limit treatment options. Illness factors include psychotic symptoms that inhibit insight into the illness and the need for medication, memory impairments, and dual diagnoses. Clinicians must tailor medication adherence interventions to individual needs, keeping in mind that the importance of therapeutic alliance in fostering adherence.

In conclusion, a multitude of factors contribute to the challenge of management of individuals with schizophrenia. Psychiatric advanced practice nurses must consider cultural contributions to illness attitudes and responses while providing assessment, monitoring, and care that takes into account a number of additional risks known to be associated with schizophrenia. These additional risks include higher rates of suicide, substance abuse, and smoking than in the general population.

In addition to the psychotherapy, pharmacotherapy, and psychosocial interventions that have been presented, psychiatric advanced practice nurses also incorporate education and referrals into managing the care of patients with schizophrenia across the life span.

Patient Education

Psychoeducation constitutes a large portion of quality care for individuals with schizophrenia and their families. Patients and families have indicated the following areas of need: general information about the disease, symptom coping strategies, and communication and social relationships (Gumus, 2008). Specific information on medication side effects, monitoring, and health promotion activities should be tailored to individual patients and families. Patients and families may benefit from referrals for a variety of activities designed to provide support, education, and resources.

Referral Options

Multiple options exist for individuals with schizophrenia and their families wishing to take part in self-help activities. Three programs include the National Alliance on Mental Illness (NAMI); Recovery International; and the GROW international health movement. Participation in such programs has been associated with increased social networks, improved coping, and improved quality of life (Davidson, Chinman, Kloos, et al., 1999; Raiff, 1984) (see Chapter 8 for a description of NAMI, Recovery International, and GROW).

Treatment

The first step in schizophrenia treatment is a thorough assessment. A schizophrenia assessment includes both psychiatric and medical history, verification of diagnostic criteria, and a suicide/violence assessment. Considering the nature of schizophrenia and its effect on cognition, collateral information is helpful to verify the history. Recommended assessments for patients with schizophrenia may be found in Table 15-5.

Psychotherapy

Since the advent of the SGAs, expert clinicians and researchers have understandably increased their focus on educating psychiatric advanced practice nurses in the nuances of medication management for individuals with schizophrenia. Unfortunately, limiting the focus of schizophrenia management to medication alone is a disservice to patients, as medications alone do not completely address many of the deficits of this disease. While the SGAs have

TABLE 15-5 **RECOMMENDED ASSESSMENTS FOR INDIVIDUALS WITH SCHIZOPHRENIA**

Assessment	Baseline	Follow-up
Vital signs[a]	Pulse, blood pressure, and temperature	As clinically indicated and especially when titrating medication dosage
Height, weight[b]	BMI and waist circumference	Every visit for 6 months and at least quarterly thereafter
Hematology	Complete blood count	When clinically indicated
Blood chemistry	Electrolytes, blood urea nitrogen, creatinine, liver function studies, and thyroid function studies	Annually and as clinically indicated
Infectious diseases	Syphilis, hepatitis C, and HIV	When clinically indicated
Pregnancy	In women of childbearing potential	If clinically indicated
Toxicology	Drug screen and heavy metal screen	If clinically indicated
Brain imaging	Electroencephalogram, computed tomography, or magnetic resonance imagery of head	If clinically indicated
Diabetes screening[c]	Family history, sedentary lifestyle, ethnicity, vascular disease, fasting glucose, hemoglobin A1C[d]	Fasting glucose or hemoglobin A1C at baseline, 4 months after initiating new treatment, and at least annually thereafter
Hyperlipidemia screening	Lipid panel	At baseline, at 3 months, and annually thereafter
QTc prolongation[e]	Electrocardiogram and potassium level	Before treatment with thioridazine, ziprasidone, or clozapine, and as clinically indicated in the presence of cardiac risk factors
Hyperprolactinemia[f]	Symptom screening and prolactin level	As clinically indicated
Extrapyramidal symptoms	Clinical assessment	Weekly during acute treatment, at each visit during stable phase
Tardive dyskinesia[g]	Abnormal involuntary movement scale (AIMS)	Every 6 months if on FGAs and every year if on SGAs. For high-risk patients, assess every 3 months if on FGAs and every 6 months if on SGAs
Cataracts	Clinical history to assess for changes in distance vision or blurred vision, ocular examination with slit-lamp examination for patients treated with FGAs associated with cataracts (e.g., chlorpromazine)	Annually, ocular examination every 2 years for patients under age 40 and every year if over age 40

[a]Frequency of monitoring is influenced by history, pre-existing conditions, and other medications.
[b]Except for patients with BMI below 18.5, an increase of 1 BMI point requires intervention.
[c]Ethnicities at risk for diabetes include African Americans, Hispanics, Native Americans, Asians, and Pacific Islanders. In patients of these ethnicities, hypertension (blood pressure greater than 130/85), high density lipoprotein level less than 40 mg/dL in men or less than 50 mg/dL in women, triglycerides greater than 150 mg/dL, and/or fasting glucose greater than 110 mg/dL require medical consultation (National Cholesterol Education Panel, 2002).
[d]A hemoglobin A1C between 5.7 and 6.4 constitutes prediabetes and requires diet and exercise counseling about reducing risk. A hemoglobin A1C above 6.4 is diagnostic of diabetes and requires a medical consultation (American Diabetes Association, 2010).
[e]Cardiac risk factors include known heart disease, history of syncope, family history of sudden death, or prolonged QTc.
[f]Symptom screening for hyperprolactinemia includes changes in libido, menstrual changes, and galactorrhea in women or changes in libido or erectile or ejaculatory function in men.
[g]High risk for tardive dyskinesia includes elderly individuals, those with a history of acute dystonia, clinically significant extrapyramidal symptoms, or akathisia.
BMI, body mass index; FGA, first generation antipsychotic; SGA, second generation antipsychotic.
Source: American Psychiatric Association. (2004a). Practice guidelines for the treatment of patients with schizophrenia (2nd ed.). Washington, DC: American Psychiatric Association.

provided a step forward in positive symptom control and enhancement of some cognitive functions, up to 60% of fully treatment-adherent individuals with schizophrenia continue to experience ongoing positive or negative symptoms (Turkington, Dudley, Warman, et al., 2004). Even among those individuals who respond well to medication, many struggle with social functioning deficits, have difficulty with activities of daily living, lack productivity, and suffer a reduced quality of life. Because of the far-reaching deficits and multifactorial complexity associated with schizophrenia, numerous psychotherapy and psychosocial treatments have been proposed.

Psychotherapy modalities used for patients with schizophrenia include cognitive behavioral therapy (CBT). (See Chapter 7 for a description of CBT.)

Cognitive Behavioral Therapy (CBT)

CBT is based on Aaron Beck's cognitive theory of depression, which states that the cognitions of depressed individuals are characterized by cognitive distortions reflecting dysfunctional beliefs and assumptions. Beck theorized that patients can learn to actively modify faulty cognitions to experience relief. The goal is to change the way patients think by encouraging them to gather and evaluate evidence in support of their beliefs. Once cognitive distortions have been examined in light of the evidence, the patient is encouraged to form alternative interpretations (Alford & Beck, 1997).

The cognitive deficits of individuals with schizophrenia in information processing, especially frontal lobe functioning, are well known (Sharma & Harvey, 2000). A number of studies have examined CBT as a psychosocial treatment for individuals with schizophrenia to enhance coping and reduce symptoms that do not respond to medications. CBT has been shown to be effective in reducing general symptoms (Gumley, Karatzias, & Power, 2006; Haddock & Lewis, 2005) and positive symptoms (Pfammatter, Junghan, & Brenner, 2006) and in faster improvement of both positive and negative symptoms when provided early in the disease (Gumley et al.; Turkington, Sensky, Scott, et al., 2008). The effects of CBT on rehospitalization (Gumley et al.; Startup, Jackson, & Bendix, 2004) and social and occupational functioning (Bechdolf, Kohn, & Knost, 2005; Temple & Ho, 2005) are inconsistent. Pilling, Bebbington, Kuipers, et al. (2002a) reviewed eight randomized controlled trials and reported that patients receiving CBT had significant improvements in overall symptoms, depression, and negative symptoms as compared to controls receiving supportive services ranging from professional emotional support to peer befriending. Effects persisted for up to 9 months in three of the studies reviewed.

Many different CBT-type therapies exist: more than 20 different schools of therapy have been labeled either cognitive behavioral therapy or cognitive therapy. While CBT encompasses a wide variety of treatment approaches and therapy techniques, the key elements of successful programs include establishment of the therapeutic alliance prior to the use of CBT, psychoeducation regarding the nature of the illness, stress reduction techniques, use of CBT to assist in coping with psychotic symptoms not managed with medications, and a focus on relapse prevention. During CBT interventions, individuals with schizophrenia are encouraged to reframe psychotic symptoms as coping attempts, rather than as signs that the individual is crazy or weak. The problem-solving process is used to identify new coping strategies and reinforce their use. Coping strategies may involve cognitive processes such as distraction or positive self-talk, or behavioral processes such as exercising or taking a walk. Homework consists of practicing techniques and reporting on results. CBT is typically provided in outpatient settings on an individual or group basis and varies from six sessions to more than 20 (Pilling et al., 2002a; Wykes, Steel, Everitt, et al., 2008).

Psychiatric advanced practice nurses may use CBT principles in interactions to assist individuals with schizophrenia to begin to identify and change cognitive distortions. The interaction below illustrates how a nurse might use CBT concepts in a one-to-one intervention to assist an outpatient in preparing for an interview for a supervised apartment:

Patient: *I don't think I can do that interview.*

Nurse: *What seems to be the trouble?*

Patient: *I'm nervous; I'll get confused and forget what to say.*

Nurse: *It's O.K. to be nervous at first. Let's talk about things that might help. What things have you done that have helped when you've been nervous in the past?*

Patient: *I know how to do deep breathing.*

Nurse: *That's an important skill. Deep breathing is a good way to cope with nervousness. Can you think of other things that help, if you had trouble remembering what to do?*

Patient: *Not really.*

Nurse: *Practicing in advance, or writing down a list helps some people remember. Which of these things would you like to try?*

Patient: *I think a list might help.*

Nurse: *I would be happy to help you work up a reminder list. It's also important to think differently about this interview. Everyone gets nervous when doing something new, but we have made a good plan to help you. What might work to help you remember to do the things we have talked about?*

Patient: *Can I ask my dad to remind me?*

Nurse: *Yes, your dad knows that people need extra help sometimes. I will talk with him about our plan before we go for your apartment interview.*

Patient: *O.K. I think that will work.*

In addition to using CBT concepts, the graduate-level psychiatric advanced practice nurse is trained to provide CBT to groups or individuals in a variety of settings. Ongoing supervision in the techniques of group therapy from a colleague with knowledge and experience of this modality assists the psychiatric advanced practice nurse to maintain and increase self-awareness through examination of feelings, behaviors, and interventions used in the group. Many psychiatric advanced practice nurses choose to pursue additional expertise through attendance at workshops and training seminars or by independent review of the many texts and manuals available. Details on obtaining such expertise are available through the National Association of Cognitive Behavioral Therapists (www.nacbt.org).

Pharmacotherapy

Antipsychotic medications are the mainstay of schizophrenia treatment. They have been divided into the categories of typical (first generation) and atypical (second generation) on the basis of their mechanism of action.

First Generation Antipsychotics (FGAs)

The older antipsychotic medications, known as typical or first generation antipsychotics (FGAs), include perphenazine (Trilafon), thioridazine (Mellaril), and chlorpromazine (Thorazine). These medications act primarily to block dopamine receptors and increase dopamine destruction; this mechanism of action is thought to explain the effectiveness of these medications in reducing the positive symptoms of schizophrenia.

Second Generation Antipsychotics (SGAs)

During the past 20 years, additional atypical, or second generation, antipsychotic medications were introduced, resulting in major changes in prescribing patterns for the control of the symptoms of schizophrenia. Clozapine (Clozaril) was the first of these medications. It was followed by risperidone (Risperdal), olanzapine (Zyprexa), and quetiapine (Seroquel). Ziprasidone (Geodon) and aripiprazole (Abilify) are the most recent introductions.

All of the SGAs have an antagonist function against serotonin as well as dopamine (Carnahan, Lund, & Perry, 2001). Although FGAs are still prescribed, SGAs are generally the treatment of choice based on side-effect profile and improvements in negative symptoms. The primary advantages of SGAs over FGAs were originally thought to be control of positive symptoms and reductions in negative and cognitive symptoms (Green, Marder, Glynn, et al., 2002). However, the National Institute of Mental Health (NIMH) Clinical Antipsychotic Trial for Intervention Effectiveness (CATIE) study suggested a reconsideration of perphenazine and other FGAs (except haloperidol [Haldol], which has significantly greater extrapyramidal side effects [EPSs] and a less robust clinical response) (Leucht, Corves, & Arbter, 2009). A recent study with over 11 years of follow-up showed decreased rates of mortality with perphenazine than with other FGAs and SGAs, with outcomes second only to those with clozapine (Tiihonen, Lonnqvist, Wahlbeck, et al., 2009). SGAs carry a different side effect profile than FGAs, with fewer extrapyramidal symptoms and less risk of tardive dyskinesia (TD) but a greater incidence of weight gain and glucose dysregulation. Also, most SGAs are considerably more expensive than FGAs. Nevertheless, the Texas Medication Algorithm Project (TMAP) (Box 15-1) recommends SGAs as first-line treatment for schizophrenia (Argo, Crismon, Miller, et al., 2008).

The choice of which SGA to prescribe is based primarily on side-effect profile and individual efficacy. The use of certain SGAs has been implicated in increased rates of glucose dysregulation, obesity, and diabetes mellitus in individuals with schizophrenia (Green, Patel, Goisman, et al., 2000). There are no consistent data showing that any one SGA is superior to another in symptom control. Table 15-6 presents dosage information, side effects, and monitoring requirements for the most commonly used SGAs.

BOX 15-1 The Texas Medication Algorithm Project

The TMAP project began in 1995 and consisted of a collaboration between Texas Universities and the Texas Department of Mental Health and Mental Retardation. Practitioners, patients, families, and administrators contributed to the manual, which provides recommendations for clinical management as well as medication selection for both first episode and multiepisode schizophrenia. The manual is based on expert recommendations gleaned from available evidence as well as from the application of the algorithms in public mental health systems and may be found at http://www.dshs.state.tx.us/mhprograms/TMAPover.shtm

Clozapine

Mechanism of Action and Dosage

Clozapine, the first of the SGAs, revolutionized the treatment of patients with refractory schizophrenia. Clozapine is the only SGA with high anticholinergic activity. It is a muscarinergic agonist and exhibits α_1, α_2, β, and dopamine antagonism (Eschweller, Vartels, Langle, et al., 2002). A number of studies have demonstrated the effectiveness of clozapine in individuals with schizophrenia who have responded unsatisfactorily to other medications (Breier, Buchanan, Irish, et al., 1993; Conley, Love, Kelly, et al., 1999; Essock, Hargreaves, Covell, et al., 1996; Kane, Honigfeld, Singer, et al., 1998; Meltzer, Alphs, Green, et al., 2003; Shopsin, Klein, Aaronson, et al., 1979). In all these studies, clozapine significantly reduced psychotic symptoms, relapse rates, and hospitalization episodes in both newly diagnosed and chronically ill individuals with schizophrenia.

The American Psychiatric Association (2004a) recommends that individuals with schizophrenia receive a trial of clozapine if they (1) have no response to a 6-week trial of two other antipsychotic medications or (2) have persistent suicidal ideation or hostility/aggression. The clozapine trial should last at least 3 months. Clozapine may be initiated at 12.5 mg twice a day and increased by not more than 50 mg/day until the target dose is reached. The maximum dosage of clozapine is 900 mg/day. Doses above 300 mg/day should be divided, and dosage of 450 mg/day should be adjusted weekly. Generally, response is most robust at doses of at least 300 mg/day.

Side Effects

The most common side effects of clozapine are sedation, weight gain, and hypersalivation, which are at their worst during the initial phase of treatment (Safferman, Lieberman, Kane, et al., 1991). In addition, clozapine is associated with a dosage-related risk of seizures. Unfortunately, the use of clozapine is also associated with a 1.3% incidence of potentially fatal agranulocytosis, defined as a granulocyte count less than 500/mm^3 (Janicak, Davis, Preskorn, et al., 1993). This risk is highest during the first 6 months of treatment and appears to peak in the third month of use. The most common cause of

TABLE 15-6 SECOND GENERATION ANTIPSYCHOTIC MEDICATIONS APPROVED FOR SCHIZOPHRENIA MAINTENANCE

Medication	Dosage Range	Side-Effect Profile	Special Monitoring	Drug Interactions, Contraindications, and Comments
Clozapine	300–450 mg/day orally in divided doses	Sedation, weight gain, hypersalivation, agranulocytosis	Weekly blood counts; report symptoms of infections	Avoid carbamazepine due to white blood cell count reductions Respiratory/cardiac arrest has been reported with benzodiazepines Dilantin and smoking may reduce clozapine level Cimetidine, fluvoxamine, paroxetine, and erythromycin increase clozapine level
Risperidone	4–8 mg/day orally once daily or divided Long-acting microspheres 25–50 mg intramuscularly every 2 weeks	Weight gain, sedation, orthostatic hypotension, glucose dysregulation	Fasting blood glucose/lipid monitoring; nutritional and exercise counseling	Fluoxetine and paroxetine may increase risperidone to toxic level
Olanzapine	10–20 mg/day orally or intramuscularly once daily	Weight gain, glucose dysregulation, sedation, dose-related extrapyramidal symptoms	Fasting blood glucose monitoring; nutritional and exercise counseling	Smoking reduces olanzapine level Women have higher olanzapine level than men at equivalent doses
Quetiapine	400–800 mg/day orally once daily or divided	Sedation, orthostatic hypotension, constipation	Monitor for sedation; check weight, fasting blood glucose, and lipids	Use caution in liver disease Phenytoin reduces quetiapine level Contraindicated in long QT syndrome, QTc interval greater than 500, history of recent myocardial infarction, arrhythmia, or heart failure
Ziprasidone	40–200 mg/day orally in divided doses or 10–20 mg intramuscularly for acute agitation	Sedation, rhinitis, muscle weakness; may prolong QT interval	Cautious use in obesity, diabetes, history of myocardial infarction or congestive heart failure Report syncope, dizziness, palpitations Monitor electrolytes and electrocardiogram	Avoid use of diuretics, calcium channel blockers, beta blockers, or digoxin
Aripiprazole	10–30 mg/day orally once daily	Headache, anxiety, insomnia	Cautious use in cardiovascular disease or seizures	Carbamazepine increases level Fluoxetine and paroxetine reduce level

this condition is the destruction of autologous granulocytes by drug-induced antibodies (Young, 1994). Other drug classes associated with agranulocytosis include analgesics, anticonvulsants, antibiotics, and cardiovascular agents. The most common symptom of agranulocytosis is fever (Oyen, Claessens, Raemaekers, et al., 1992). The condition is usually reversible if treatment is instituted immediately. Treatment includes discontinuing the causal medication and providing antibiotic therapy and granulocyte-macrophage colony stimulating factor if needed (Schauwecker, 2002).

Monitoring

American Psychiatric Association (2004a) guidelines specify that the white blood cell (WBC) count should be checked:

- Before starting clozapine
- Each week for the first 6 months
- Every 2 weeks thereafter for the duration of treatment
- Weekly for 1 month after discontinuation

Practitioners should advise patients to report tachycardia and sedation during dose titration (Meltzer, 1992; Meltzer, Burnett, Bastani, et al., 1990; Safferman et al., 1991), as well as any symptoms of infection such as sore throat, fever, weakness, or lethargy. Table 15-7 summarizes other American Psychiatric Association recommendations.

Risperidone

Mechanism of Action and Dosage

Risperidone acts by blocking postsynaptic dopamine, serotonin, α_1-adrenergic, α_2-adrenergic, and histamine (H1) receptors (Reeves, Mack, & Beddingfield, 2002). In addition, risperidone has potent serotonin 5-HT_{2a} and moderate dopamine D2 antagonistic activity (Spina, Avenoso, Scordo, et al., 2002). Risperidone has been shown to improve symptoms and reduce length of hospitalization in individuals with refractory schizophrenia (Dinakar, Sobel, Bopp, et al., 2002) and to reduce relapse in outpatients with schizophrenia (Csernansky, Mahmoud, & Brenner, 2002). Some early investigators concluded that risperidone was more effective than FGAs for negative symptoms (Chouinard, Jones, Remington, et al., 1993; Marder, Davis, & Chouinard, 1997;

TABLE 15-7 AMERICAN PSYCHIATRIC ASSOCIATION GUIDELINES FOR PATIENTS TAKING CLOZAPINE

Clinical Situation			Action
WHITE BLOOD CELL (WBC) COUNT	AND/ OR	ABSOLUTE NEUTROPHIL COUNT (ANC)	
Less than 2000 mm^3	Or	Less than 1000 mm^3	Stop clozapine immediately Perform WBC count with differential daily Consider bone marrow aspiration Consider protective isolation Do NOT resume clozapine
2000–3000 mm^3	Or	1000–1500 mm^3	Stop clozapine immediately Perform WBC count with differential daily Monitor for symptoms of infection Resume clozapine when infection absent, WBC is greater than 3000, and ANC is greater than 1500
Initially 3000–3500 mm^3 but falls to 3000 in 3 weeks or less	And	1500 mm^3	Repeat WBC with differential twice a week until WBC greater than 3500

Source: American Psychiatric Association. (2004a). Practice guidelines for the treatment of patients with schizophrenia *(2nd ed.). Washington, DC: American Psychiatric Association.*

Marder & Meibach, 1994); however, a later study comparing risperidone to low-dose haloperidol did not support this view (Green et al., 2002).

The most effective dosage appears to be 4 to 8 mg/day. Although a single daily dose is permissible, elderly individuals or others experiencing orthostatic hypotension may benefit from twice-daily dosing.

Side Effects

The most commonly reported side effects of risperidone include drowsiness, orthostatic hypotension, and weight gain. Compared with other SGAs, risperidone has a higher risk of associated increases in serum prolactin levels. Effects of hyperprolactinemia may include breast tenderness and enlargement, decreased sexual interest in both sexes, menstrual cycle disruptions in women (Pollack, Reiter, & Hammerness, 1992), and retrograde ejaculation in men (Chouinard et al., 1993). Although the risk is lower than with FGAs, risperidone has also been associated with dosage-related increases in EPSs, such as dystonia and akathisia (Chouinard et al., 1993; Marder & Meiback, 1994; Peuskens, 1995).

Paliperidone and Risperdal Consta

Paliperidone, approved by the Food and Drug Administration (FDA) in 2006, is the major active metabolite of risperidone in an extended-release formulation. Side effects and efficacy are similar to those of risperidone, and the relative advantages or disadvantages compared to risperidone remain unknown (American Psychiatric Association, 2009). Risperdal Consta consists of microspheres delivered intramuscularly and released over time. The usual dosage is 25 to 50 mg intramuscularly every 2 weeks.

Olanzapine

Mechanism of Action and Dosage

The FDA approved olanzapine in 1996. Like risperidone, it exhibits antagonist action against dopamine and serotonin. Olanzapine has significant inhibitor activity on dopamine D1, D2, D3, and D4 receptors; serotonin 5-HT$_{2a}$ and 5-HT$_{2c}$ receptors; histamine H1 receptors; and α_1-adrenergic and muscarinic M1, M2, M3, M5 receptors; it also has a moderate affinity for serotonin 5-HT$_{2a}$, 5-HT$_{2c}$, and 5-HT$_3$ receptors (Kroeze, Hufeisen, Popadak, et al., 2003; Lykouras, Agelopoulos, & Tzavellas, 2002). Olanzapine has been shown to be superior to haloperidol for negative symptoms of schizophrenia and as effective as haloperidol for positive symptoms (Beasley, Tollefson, Tran, et al., 1996; Davis & Chen, 2001; Kinon, Milton, & Stouffer, 1999; Tollefson, Beasely, Tran, et al., 1997; Tollefson, Sanger, Lu, et al., 1998). Improvement in neurocognitive symptoms with olanzapine compared to haloperidol has been shown relatively consistently across studies (Bilder, Goldman, Volvaka, et al., 2002; Keefe, Seidman, Christensen, et al., 2004; Purdon, Jones, Stip, et al., 2000; Smith, Infante, Singh, et al., 2001). In addition, olanzapine has been effectively used to treat TD associated with other agents (Lykouras et al., 2002).

Olanzapine may be given orally at 10 mg/day (5 mg/day for elderly patients) in a single dose and increased by 5 mg/day until the therapeutic dose of 10 to 20 mg daily is reached. Olanzapine is also available in an orally disintegrating formulation (Zyprexa Zydis) that is dosed in the same manner. In addition, olanzapine may be administered intramuscularly for agitation associated with schizophrenia (daily dosage range 2.5 to 10 mg).

Side Effects

The most common side effects of olanzapine are sedation and weight gain. Weight gain is significant and can be up to 1 pound a week for a year (McEvoy, 2002). Koller and Doraiswamy (2002) reviewed published reports of hyperglycemia in patients treated with olanzapine and concluded that the medication may precipitate diabetes in vulnerable individuals. Furthermore, the onset of hyperglycemia may be rapid and severe and is not dosage dependent—that is, the severity of hyperglycemia is not reduced as duration of olanzapine therapy increases. Time to hyperglycemia was 6 months or less in 73% of patients. These results suggest a causal relationship between olanzapine and development or worsening of diabetes.

Quetiapine

Mechanism of Action and Dosage

Quetiapine is a weak dopamine antagonist that interacts with dopamine D1 and D2 receptors, serotonin 5-HT_{1a}, 5-HT_{2a}, 5-HT_{2c}, and 5-HT_6 receptors, histamine H1 receptors, and α_1-, α_2-, and α_{2c}-adrenergic receptors (Kroeze et al., 2003; Margolese, Chouinard, Beauclair, et al., 2002). It occupies fewer serotonin receptors than other SGAs and does not saturate the receptors, even at high doses (Remington & Kapur, 1999). Clinical trials have demonstrated quetiapine's effectiveness for treatment of psychosis (Emsley, Raniwalla, Bailey, et al., 2000; King, Link, & Kowalcyk, 1998; Peuskens & Link, 1997). However, one study noted that the medication appeared to be more effective in a less ill population (Goren & Levin, 1998). In a 3-year study, Margolese et al. (2002) reported that therapeutic tolerance necessitated continued dosage increases to control symptoms, ending with a mean 86.6% dosage increase over the course of the study. In addition, 6 of 23 patients maintained on quetiapine monotherapy required rehospitalization because of psychotic relapse. These authors concluded that quetiapine remains a promising option for combination antipsychotic polytherapy in monotherapy-resistant patients. Two studies have documented quetiapine's beneficial effects on neurocognition as compared to FGAs (Purdon, Mala, Labelle, et al., 2001; Velligan, Newcomer, Pultz, et al., 2002).

Effective doses range from 400 to 800 mg and may be administered once daily or divided (Borison, Arvanitis, & Miller, 1996).

Side Effects

The most common side effects of quetiapine are drowsiness, constipation, and hypotension.

Ziprasidone

Mechanism of Action and Dosage

Ziprasidone is a serotonin 5-HT_{2a}, dopamine D2, and α_1-adrenergic inhibitor with a greater affinity for 5-HT_{2a} receptors than for D2 receptors. It is the only SGA that is a partial agonist at 5-HT_{1a} receptor sites, an antagonist at 5-HT_{1d} receptor sites, and an inhibitor of norepinephrine and serotonin reuptake (Rosenquist, Walker, & Ghaemi, 2002). This inhibition of norepinephrine and serotonin reuptake means that ziprasidone has the potential for antidepressant and antianxiety activity in addition to antipsychotic effects (Stimmel, Gutierrez, & Lee, 2002). In clinical trials, ziprasidone has been shown to be effective in reducing positive and negative symptoms of schizophrenia (Hirsch, Kissling, Bauml, et al., 2002). In addition, it was associated with significantly lower emergent movement disorders than haloperidol (Hirsch et al.). Ziprasidone is also available in an intramuscular formulation that is effective in acute agitation in schizophrenic relapse (Daniel, Potkin, Reeves, et al., 2001; Lesem, Zajecka, Swift, et al., 2001).

Oral doses of ziprasidone may be initiated at 40 mg/day and then titrated to a maximum of 200 mg/day in divided doses (Carnahan et al., 2001). The usual dosage is 10 to 20 mg intramuscularly.

Side Effects

The most common side effects of ziprasidone are somnolence, rhinitis, and muscle weakness (Carnahan et al., 2001).

Initial concerns about the effect of ziprasidone on the QTc interval led to extensive evaluation of ziprasidone's cardiovascular effects on the QTc interval. The QTc interval is measured from the beginning of the Q wave to the end of the T wave on electrocardiogram. It represents the duration of electrical systole (Goldschlager & Goldman, 1989). QTc prolongation can lead to syncope, the ventricular arrhythmia Torsades de pointes, and sudden death. Most cases of Torsades de pointes occur in patients with QTc intervals greater than 500 to 700 milliseconds. In placebo-controlled trials (Stimmel et al., 2002), a ziprasidone dose of 160 mg/day increased the QTc interval by 10 milliseconds over placebo. Of 2,988 patients in the trial, 3 had a QTc interval of 500 milliseconds or greater; ziprasidone was not implicated in any of these cases.

Torsades de pointes is more likely to occur in patients with multiple risk factors for QTc prolongation. Risk factors include medications that increase the QTc interval (e.g., potassium channel blockers), hypokalemia, hypomagnesemia, bradycardia, and syncope. Women are also at greater risk than men. If several of these risk factors for QTc prolongation are present, olanzapine is the SGA of choice because it has the lowest risk of QTc prolongation (Carnahan et al., 2001).

Monitoring

Patients should receive a baseline electrocardiogram and electrolytes and have monthly follow-up electrocardiograms for the initial 6 to 12 months when receiving ziprasidone. Patients should be advised to report syncopal episodes promptly.

Aripiprazole

Mechanism of Action and Dosage

Aripiprazole was approved in 2002. It has partial agonist activity at dopamine D2 and D3 and serotonin 5-HT_{1a} and 5-HT_{2a} receptors (Burris, Molski, Xu, et al., 2002; Jordan, Koprivica, Chen, et al., 2002). In addition, aripiprazole moderately inhibits serotonin reuptake (Millan, 2000; Shapiro, Renock, Arrington, et al., 2003). Aripiprazole has been demonstrated to improve the number and severity of both positive and negative symptoms in clinical trials

(Fleischhacker, McQuade, & Marcus, 2009; Kane, Crandall, & Marcus, 2007; Tandon, Marcus, & Stork, 2006).

The recommended dose of aripiprazole is 10 to 30 mg/day in a single dose with or without food. Higher doses have not been shown to be more effective in clinical trials. Patients require 2 weeks to achieve adequate plasma concentrations of this medication.

Side Effects

The most commonly reported side effects of aripiprazole include agitation, nausea, and insomnia. Similar to other SGAs, the potential for EPSs is small with aripiprazole (Yeung, Carson, Saha, et al., 2001). In addition, aripiprazole is associated with minimal increases in body weight and serum cholesterol and is unlikely to be associated with increased prolactin levels or prolongation of the QTc interval (Stip & Tourjman, 2010).

Asenapine

Mechanism of Action and Dosage

The most recent addition to the SGA arsenal is asenapine (Saphris). Asenapine was recently approved, but only for *acute* treatment of schizophrenia in adults. Like most other SGAs, asenapine is an antagonist at dopamine D2 receptors with greater binding affinity at serotonin 5-HT_{2a} receptors and almost no affinity for muscarinic receptors. Asenapine has been shown superior to placebo for both positive and negative symptoms in a 6-week placebo-controlled trial (Potkin, Cohen, & Panagides, 2007).

Asenapine is dosed at 5 mg sublingually twice daily (tablets should not be swallowed). Patients must avoid food and drink for 10 minutes following administration. Asenapine should not be used in combination with central nervous system depressants or alcohol and may potentiate the effects of antihypertensive medications through α_1-adrenergic antagonism.

Side Effects

The most frequently reported side effects of asenapine are drowsiness, nausea, anxiety, and agitation. In a 52-week study, 14.7% of asenapine-treated patients experienced weight gain greater than 7% of body weight. Asenapine should be used with caution in individuals with a history of leukopenia or neutropenia, as well as those with cardiac arrhythmias and seizures.

Comparison of FGAs and SGAs

Generally, extrapyramidal symptoms are greater with risperidone and olanzapine and less with quetiapine and aripiprazole. Weight gain appears to be substantial with olanzapine and clozapine, moderate with risperidone and quetiapine, and least with ziprasidone and aripiprazole. Rates of diabetes mellitus induction are highest with olanzapine and clozapine and lowest with ziprasidone and aripiprazole (Lieberman, Stroup, & McEvoy, 2005).

A recent meta-analysis of 150 double-blind studies including 21,533 individuals with schizophrenia compared FGAs and SGAs. For overall efficacy, the SGAs clozapine, olanzapine, and risperidone were significantly better than FGAs. The other SGAs were no more efficacious than FGAs. All SGAs except aripiprazole and ziprasidone were likely to be associated with weight gain (Leucht et al., 2009). Table 15-8 compares common side effects of antipsychotic medications.

The costs of most SGAs are significantly higher than those of the FGAs. Cost may be an important consideration in individuals with schizophrenia, many of whom are unemployed and uninsured. Among the SGAs, ziprasidone is the least expensive per dose, costing approximately 40% less than olanzapine, the most expensive. Although clozapine is recommended for treatment of individuals who have been unresponsive to other medications, the necessary laboratory tests greatly increase the cost of using this medication. Further, many individuals with schizophrenia are unwilling or unable to comply with the required laboratory monitoring. If it is expected that relatively high doses will be necessary to maintain stability, ziprasidone should be considered because it can be prescribed for the same cost regardless of daily dosage. A low dose of risperidone is another economical regimen.

Extrapyramidal Symptoms

EPSs occur in approximately 60% of patients treated with antipsychotic medications (Ayd, 1961; Casey, 1991; Chakos, Mayerhoff, Loebel, et al., 1992). These side effects have been divided into acute and chronic types (American Psychiatric Association, 2004a). Acute EPSs include medication-induced parkinsonism, dystonia, akathisia, and neuroleptic malignant syndrome (NMS). These side effects occur within the first days or weeks of treatment, are dose dependent, and are reversible if the medication is reduced or discontinued. The primary chronic EPS is TD, which occurs after months or years of medication exposure and may be irreversible even if medication is discontinued.

Medication-Induced Parkinsonism

The symptoms of medication-induced parkinsonism include bradykinesia, tremor, rigidity, and akinesia. The first clinical consideration is to distinguish these symptoms from negative symptoms. Parkinsonian side effects, unlike negative symptoms, usually respond to a reduction in antipsychotic medication or to the addition of an anticholinergic antiparkinsonian medication, such as trihexyphenidyl (Artane) or benztropine (Cogentin).

Trihexyphenidyl is a synthetic antispasmodic with a direct inhibiting effect on the parasympathetic nervous system, as well as relaxant effects on smooth muscle. It is prescribed at 6 to 10 mg/day in divided doses and is best given without food. Common side effects include dry mouth, nausea, blurred vision, and dizziness and are often more common in elderly individuals. Patients receiving trihexyphenidyl

TABLE 15-8 COMPARISON OF COMMON SIDE EFFECTS OF ANTIPSYCHOTIC MEDICATIONS

Medication	Increased Prolactin Level	Hypotension	Sedation	Glucose Abnormalities	Increased Qtc Interval	Extrapyramidal Symptoms	Lipid Abnormalities	Weight Gain	Anticholinergic Effects
Clozapine	Negligible	High	High	High	Negligible	Low	High	High	High
Risperidone	High	Moderate	Low	Moderate	Low	Moderate	Moderate	Moderate	Negligible
Olanzapine	Low	Low	Low	High	Low	Low	High	High	Moderate
Quetiapine	Low	Moderate	High	Moderate	Low	Low	Moderate	Moderate	Low
Ziprasidone	Low	Low	Low	Low	Moderate	Low	Low	Low	Low
Aripiprazole	Low	Low	Moderate	Low	Low	Low	Low	Low	Low
Thioridazine	Moderate	Moderate	Moderate	Low	High	Low	Low	Low	Moderate
Perphenazine	Moderate	Low	Low	Low	Negligible	Moderate	Low	Low	Negligible
Haloperidol	High	Negligible	Moderate	Negligible	Negligible	High	Negligible	Low	Negligible

Adapted from Stimmel et al., 2002; APA, 2004a.

should be monitored for increased intraocular pressure at regular intervals, as closed-angle glaucoma has been reported with this medication.

Benztropine is an anticholinergic and antihistamine. It is prescribed at 1 to 2 mg twice or three times daily. Common side effects include dry month, blurred vision, and urinary retention. Patients prescribed benztropine along with phenothiazines, haloperidol, or tricyclic antidepressants should be instructed to promptly report gastrointestinal complaints, fever, or heat intolerance, as the administration of these medications concomitantly has been associated with paralytic ileus and hyperthermia, which have been fatal in some individuals. Benztropine is also associated with glaucoma.

Dystonia

Dystonia involves the spastic contraction of muscle groups, most commonly in the neck, eyes, and torso. It occurs in approximately 10% of patients on initiation of antipsychotic therapy. The contractions are sudden, dramatic, and frightening to the patient. However, dystonia responds quickly to intramuscular administration of benztropine (1 to 2 mg) or diphenhydramine (50 mg). American Psychiatric Association (2004a) guidelines recommend oral maintenance anticholinergic antiparkinsonian medications for patients who have experienced dystonia in the past.

Akathisia

Akathisia, which is sensations of restlessness, pacing, and an inability to sit still, occurs in up to 30% of patients treated with antipsychotic medication (Braude, Barnes, & Gore, 1983; Van Putten & May, 1978). This increased motor activity must be differentiated from the agitation accompanying psychosis. Akathisia may respond to a reduction in antipsychotic medication or to the addition of trihexyphenidyl, benztropine, or lorazepam (Lima, Soares-Weiser, Bacaltchuk, et al., 2002).

Lorazepam is a benzodiazepine anxiolytic and central nervous system depressant. Usual dosage ranges from 2 to 3 mg/day in divided doses. Common side effects of lorazepam include drowsiness and muscle weakness. Lorazepam is contraindicated in patients with glaucoma. Dosage should be reduced by 50% for elderly patients, and all patients should be counseled about the risk of physical and psychological dependence. Lorazepam is not recommended for long-term use and should not be prescribed to women of childbearing potential or pregnant women owing to an increased risk of congenital malformations if the fetus is exposed during the first trimester.

Neuroleptic Malignant Syndrome (NMS)

NMS is a rare but potentially fatal form of acute EPS. It appears to be a reaction to acute dopamine depletion and has been reported with use of virtually all dopamine D2 receptor antagonists, including risperidone (Reeves et al., 2002), clozapine (Bottlender, Jager, Hofschuster, et al., 2002), and ziprasidone (Yang & McNeely, 2002). Estimates of the incidence of NMS range from 0.5% to 2.4% (Reeves et al.). An increased dose of a neuroleptic, abrupt withdrawal of dopamine agonists, dehydration, electrolyte imbalance, and concurrent use of lithium and tricyclic antidepressants can trigger NMS, although it may occur at any time during antipsychotic treatment (Lappa, Podesta, Capelli, et al., 2002).

The classic presentation of NMS includes fever, skeletal muscle rigidity, altered mental status, and autonomic dysfunction. Creatine phosphokinase and WBC counts are usually elevated (Reeves et al., 2002). Complications such as rhabdomyolysis, disseminated intravascular coagulation, and renal failure result in death in 20% of cases (Lappa et al., 2002). Treatment of NMS is extensive, and hospitalization is required. After immediate discontinuation of the offending agent, dopamine agonists are given to reverse receptor blockade. Dantrolene sodium is used to reduce fever and muscle rigidity (Caroff, Mann, & Keck, 1998). Urine alkalinization with high volumes of crystalloids may prevent renal failure (Lappa et al.); however, hemodialysis is sometimes required (Yang & McNeely, 2002). Recovery may take several weeks. Fully recovered patients may be retreated cautiously with antipsychotic medications (using an agent other than the precipitant), gradual dose increases, and frequent monitoring (Rosebush, Stewart, & Gelenberg, 1989).

Tardive Dyskinesia (TD)

TD, a movement disorder associated with chronic neuroleptic treatment and advanced age, has long been a concern in patients receiving antipsychotic medications. Although there is less of a risk than with FGAs, a number of studies have implicated SGAs such as risperidone, olanzapine, and ziprasidone in the disorder (Rosenquist et al., 2002; Terezhalmy, Riley, & Moore, 2002). In spite of the reduced risk with SGAs, the disabling and irreversible effects of this disorder warrant continued clinical vigilance.

Prolonged treatment with antipsychotic medications increases dopamine metabolism. This process of dopamine metabolism generates free radicals (Terezhalmy et al., 2002). Excessive production of free radicals destabilizes the neuronal membrane in the extrapyramidal system, which regulates repetitive, rhythmical activities, both voluntary and involuntary (Taylor, 2002). TD is characterized by involuntary rapid, writhing movements that affect the orofacial region in 75% of cases, the limbs in 50% of cases, and the trunk in 25% of cases. Puckering, lip smacking, chewing, and jaw clenching are common. Tongue protrusion and lip licking also appear as the condition progresses (Terezhalmy et al.). Treatment involves stopping the offending agent if possible. Providers should strive to identify and prescribe the lowest dose of antipsychotic medication needed to control symptoms and should reevaluate the dose at least annually.

Patients receiving antipsychotic medication for more than 1 month must be evaluated at least every 3 months for side effects, including acute and chronic EPSs. One option for evaluation of such movements is the Abnormal Involuntary Movement Scale (AIMS) (Guy, 1976). The AIMS is a 12-item scale designed to record the occurrence of dyskinesias in patients receiving antipsychotic medication (Table 15-9). The examiner rates facial and oral movements (items 1 through 4), extremity and trunk movements (items 5 through 7), global judgments (items 8 through 10), and dental status (items 11 through 14). The scale and examination procedure are public domain and may be copied (American Psychiatric Association, 2000b).

Schooler and Kane (1982) suggested that TD be diagnosed when the following three criteria are met:

1. At least 3 months' cumulative antipsychotic medication exposure
2. Absence of other problems that could cause the abnormal movements (e.g., problems with teeth or dentures)
3. Movements of at least mild severity in two different body areas, or movements of at least moderate severity in one area

If symptoms of TD are identified, the antipsychotic medication dosage may be gradually decreased by up to 50% over a period of 12 weeks. Such an approach often leads to diminution or remission of symptoms. However, if medication exposure continues after TD develops, the likelihood of reversibility is diminished. Some cases persist even after medication is completely discontinued. If medication reduction or discontinuation does not improve symptoms within 1 year, a switch to an SGA with minimal extrapyramidal activity (clozapine or risperidone) may be desirable (Lykouras et al., 2002). Lieberman, Saltz, Johns, et al. (1991) reviewed eight studies and reported improvement in 43% of patients with TD after switching to clozapine. The use of vitamin E has been shown to reduce risk for development of TD (Adler, Rotrosen, Edson, et al., 1999; Soares & McGrath, 2001), and American Psychiatric Association (2004a) guidelines suggest 400 to 800 IU as daily prophylaxis for patients at risk.

Adjunctive Medications

Adjunctive medications are often prescribed to individuals with schizophrenia for a variety of comorbid conditions. For example, antidepressants may be considered for comorbid

TABLE 15-9 THE ABNORMAL INVOLUNTARY MOVEMENT SCALE

Location	Description	Rating (0–4)
Facial and oral	1. Muscles of facial expression (forehead, eyebrows, periorbital area, cheeks): Frowning, blinking, smiling, grimacing	
	2. Lips and perioral area: Puckering, pouting, smacking	
	3. Jaw: Biting, clenching, chewing, mouth opening, lateral movement	
	4. Tongue (rate only increases in movement both in and out of mouth, not inability to sustain movement): Darting in and out of mouth	
Extremities	5. Upper (arms, wrists, hands, fingers): Choreic movements (i.e., rapid, objectively purposeless, irregular, spontaneous), athetoid movements (i.e., slow, irregular, complex, serpentine) DO NOT INCLUDE tremor (i.e., repetitive, regular, rhythmic)	
	6. Lower legs (knees, ankles, toes): e.g., lateral knee movement, foot tapping, heel dropping, foot squirming, inversion and eversion of foot	
Trunk	7. Neck, shoulders, hips: e.g., rocking, twisting, squirming, pelvic gyrations	
Global judgments	8. Severity of abnormal movements overall	
	9. Incapacitation due to abnormal movements	
	10. Patient's awareness of abnormal movements. Rate only patient's report: No awareness = 0 Aware, no distress = 1 Aware, mild distress = 2 Aware, moderate distress = 3 Aware, severe distress = 4	
Dental status	11. Current problems with teeth and/or dentures	Yes/no
	12. Are dentures usually worn?	Yes/no
	13. Does the patient have edentia?	Yes/no
	14. Do movements disappear in sleep?	Yes/no

Note: 0 = none, 1 = minimal (may be extreme normal), 2 = mild, 3= moderate, 4 = severe

Source: Guy, W. (1976). Assessment manual for psychopharmacology—revised (DHEW Publication No. ADM 76-338, pp. 534-537). Rockville, MD: U.S. Department of Health, Education, and Welfare, Public Health Service, Alcohol, Drug Abuse, and Mental Health Administration, NIMH Psychopharmacology Research Branch, Division of Extramural Research Programs.

major depression or obsessive-compulsive disorder (Reznik & Sirota, 2000), although careful monitoring is required because some antidepressants increase the risk of psychotic symptom exacerbations (Kemp, Kirov, Everitt, et al., 1998). Benzodiazepines (usually lorazepam 2 to 4 mg orally three to four times daily as needed) (Lee, Schwartz, & Hallmayer, 2000) have been used successfully to treat catatonia, anxiety, and agitation. Potential drug interactions must be monitored carefully.

Pharmacological Treatment Response

Ten to thirty percent of individuals with schizophrenia have little or no response to medications and another 30% have a partial response, defined as ongoing hallucinations and delusions. Partial response may be due to suboptimal dosing or nonadherence. Practitioners should first verify that an adequate trial (2 to 4 weeks) was conducted and that the patient was approximately 80% adherent to the dosing schedule during that time period. After several such trials with different medications, prescribers may consider augmentation with

- A second antipsychotic, for example, aripiprazole (Friedman, Ault, & Powchik, 1997; Henderson & Goff, 1996; Mowerman & Siris, 1996; Stahl, 2009). (See dosage range in Table 15-6.)
- An anticonvulsant, for example, lithium (usual dosage range 900 to 1200 mg/day) or valproic acid (usual dosage range 500 to 1000 mg/day) (Casey, Daniel, Wassef, et al., 2003b; Dose, Hellweg, Yassouridis, et al., 1998; Hesslinger, Normann, Langosch, et al., 1999; Stahl, 2009).
- A benzodiazepine, for example, lorazepam (usual dosage range 2 to 6 mg/day) (Stahl, 2009; Walkowitz & Pickar, 1991).

Psychosocial Interventions

Psychosocial treatments are designed to reduce stressful life events and enhance coping efforts. Psychiatric clinicians have long observed how various types of stress can precipitate both the onset and relapse of schizophrenia (Ishiguro, Okuyama, Toru, et al., 2000). Once antipsychotic medication is initiated and the dosage titrated for maximum benefit, individuals with schizophrenia are in the best position to benefit from a number of psychosocial treatments of value in promoting stability and community functioning. The American Psychiatric Association (2004a, 2009) recommends the provision of psychosocial interventions such as family therapy, social skills training (SST), vocational rehabilitation, and assertive community treatment (ACT). (See Chapter 7 for a description of family therapy and Chapter 8 for additional psychosocial interventions.)

Family Therapy

Family therapy is one of the most longstanding, best-researched, and most successful of the psychosocial treatments for schizophrenia. Family therapy was developed in the early 1950s as an adjunct to individual and group psychotherapy. It is based on the premise that psychiatric difficulties are related to current social interactions, especially those of the family unit. The World Schizophrenia Fellowship (1998) identified the following key elements of effective family interventions for schizophrenia: duration of at least 9 months, mutually agreed-upon goals, resolution of family conflict, provision of education on disease course and relapse prevention, development of specific crisis plans, improvement in family communication, training in problem-solving techniques, and expanding family social support networks. Family therapy programs that include these key elements have strong empirical support.

Over 30 randomized controlled trials have demonstrated family therapy's effectiveness in improving symptoms, reducing relapse, and fostering positive outcomes (Murray-Swank & Dixon, 2004). These effects are among the most consistent and substantial of *any* mental health treatment. In particular, the effect in reducing relapse rates has been consistently replicated in spite of the fact that studies used differing definitions of relapse, ranging from simple rehospitalization to increased symptoms using a variety of patient, family, and provider rating scales. Relapse rates for individuals with schizophrenia who were provided family therapy have been documented to be on average 40% less than those of individuals receiving either medication alone, or medication and individual therapy (Dyck, Hendryx, & Short, 2002). Studies of family interventions have shown reduced hospitalization rates, improved patient-family relationships (Bebbington, Kuipers, & Garety, 2002; Magliano, Fiorillo, & Nakabgibem, 2006; Pfammater et al., 2006), improved medication adherence (Pilling, Bebbington, Kuipers, et al., 2002a, 2000b), and improved social functioning (Chien, Chan, & Morrissey, 2005; Li & Arthur, 2005; Magliano et al., 2006), but barriers to its implementation exist.

Although family therapy is time-efficient and cost-effective, as has been well documented, it is rarely offered to community-dwelling individuals with schizophrenia. In a follow-up survey of 719 individuals with schizophrenia receiving care in two states in the United States, Lehman and Steinwachs (1998, 2003) reported that only about one-third of outpatients with schizophrenia were offered family therapy. Barriers to the provision of family therapy include lack of qualified providers and lack of clinician training, as well as resource, time, and reimbursement issues. Families may be reluctant to engage in the therapy process owing to stigmatization, or they may lack reliable transportation. At times, the demands of caring for their ill family member may leave families little time or interest to engage in therapy themselves. Many mental health providers lack knowledge regarding the benefits of family therapy. On the other hand, the advantages of family therapy are that it provides an opportunity to assess and work for health change at the system level, enabling families to be of optimal support and assistance to their ill loved ones.

Psychiatric advanced practice nurses wishing to offer family therapy have a variety of options for doing so, based on their levels of education and expertise. Psychiatric nurses with master's level preparation have the practical and theoretical knowledge base as well as experience to provide family therapy to those with schizophrenia. In addition, psychiatric advanced practice nurses providing family therapy function within a framework of ongoing professional supervision to maintain standards of care. Within a family therapy framework, psychiatric advanced practice nurses use a variety of theories to tailor assessment, goal setting, interventions, and evaluation to the families of individuals with schizophrenia, with the goal of improving family communication and functioning. Strategies for increasing access to this evidence-based treatment modality include educating both providers and families regarding its benefits, increasing the flexibility of therapy programs, and providing family therapy at more accessible sites such as patient homes. Psychiatric advanced practice nurses can incorporate into their practice many of the key elements of family therapy, such as education, conflict resolution, and crisis management.

Social Skills Training (SST)

SST is based on the social skills model proposed by Morrison & Bellack (1984), which breaks social functioning into three key elements:

1. Receiving skills, which involve social perception
2. Processing skills, which involve social cognition
3. Expressive skills, which involve behavioral responses

Receiving skills include the correct interpretation of vocal and affective cues, verbal information, and the context of the interaction. Processing skills (also known as social problem-solving) involve analysis of the present situation in light of past experience to plan an appropriate response. Expressive skills include the integration of verbal expression with suitable nonverbal behaviors, such as gestures, posture, and facial expressions.

Social skills deficits of various levels are widely present in individuals with schizophrenia. These deficits are relatively unchanging and medication resistant. They interfere not only with performance of life roles but also with treatment engagement, limiting individuals from obtaining the full benefit of other psychosocial treatments. A comprehensive body of research has validated the social skills model (Kurtz & Mueser, 2008).

A review of the literature on the specific content of SST available to individuals with schizophrenia reveals that various skills have been targeted, including social, financial, communication, and problem-solving skills. Individuals with schizophrenia typically require assistance with the acquisition of skills such as conversing, preparing food, shopping, and using public transportation. Although the content and duration of SST programs vary, all of the programs break target behaviors into smaller tasks. For example, a complex skill such as making friends is divided into manageable steps. The first step teaches the use of introductory remarks, followed by more specific questions, and finally, sharing of personal information. Nonverbal behaviors, gestures, tones of voice, and mannerisms are likewise broken down, and reminders such as "make eye contact," "nod your head," and so on are used. Other SST techniques include modeling, behavioral rehearsal, corrective feedback, positive reinforcement, and homework assignments (Kopelowicz, Kreyenbuhl, & Buchanan, 2006). Frequent repetition and handouts are used to cope with the attention and executive functioning deficits that are common in individuals with schizophrenia. Most SST is done in small groups meeting two or three times a week for 6 months to 2 years, depending on the program type and number of skills addressed.

Research studies have examined patient outcomes following the provision of SST. Social skills groups have been documented to exert positive effects on specific skills, with learning maintained for up to 12 months and skills generalizing from training settings to everyday life (Kurtz & Mueser, 2008; Liberman & Kopelowicz, 2002). Pfammatter et al. (2006) conducted a meta-analysis of randomized controlled trials and concluded that SST produces large effects on skill development, with smaller effects observed for social functioning, assertiveness, and overall psychopathology. More recently, Kurtz and Mueser conducted a meta-analysis of 22 studies including 1,521 participants in randomized controlled trials and concluded that SST produced large effects on content; moderate effects on performance of social and daily life skills, negative symptoms, and community functioning; and small effects on relapse rates.

The psychiatric advanced practice nurse may provide SST as part of individual and group psychotherapy. The psychiatric advanced practice nurse may independently plan, form, conduct, and evaluate social skills groups in the hospital or community setting. When planning such groups, the advanced practice nurse should take advantage of available training manuals, such as that of the UCLA Social and Independent Living Skills Program (Liberman, Wallace, Blackwell, et al., 1993). Issues that may be pertinent in the decision to offer SST include the patients' level of symptoms, the number of interested patients, clinician expertise with modalities, availability of supervision, or time and space constraints of the treatment setting. Advantages of individual sessions are the opportunity for one-on-one intervention (which ensures that the desired behavior is demonstrated properly), more time for individual assessment than is possible in a group, and the ability to engage an individual who might be reluctant to participate in a group setting. The primary advantages of group intervention are reduced costs and the additional benefits of interaction among group members. SST can also be provided in individual patient homes. The advantages of this method are an opportunity to engage family members, assess family environment, and observe family interactions directly.

Vocational Rehabilitation

The competitive employment level of individuals with schizophrenia rarely reaches 15%; when employed, individuals with schizophrenia work fewer hours and earn only two-thirds of the national average hourly rate (Gold, Meisler, Santos, et al., 2006). The goal of vocational rehabilitation is the improvement of work outcomes and primarily involves direct assistance in finding and keeping employment (Mueser, Drake, & Bond, 1997). Vocational rehabilitation provides a variety of support services on a continuum from cognitive and skills assessments, to supported employment, to advocacy in obtaining and maintaining competitive employment. Among a wide variety of programs that have been developed are vocational skills training, job placement, transitional employment, supported employment, vocational counseling, and vocational education.

A long-term body of literature has associated employment with a number of positive outcomes in schizophrenia. Employment has been associated with increased social contact, reduced positive and negative symptom severity, reduced hospitalizations, higher self-esteem, reduced health-care costs, better clinician assessments of functioning, and improved quality of life (Bond, Resnick, & Drake, 2001; Cook, Leff, Blyler, et al., 2005; Krupa, 2004). Factors associated with improved vocational outcomes include an emphasis on patient preferences, rapid job placement, ongoing support, a focus on problem-solving, and support and education for employers and coworkers.

Vocational rehabilitation counselors possess specialized knowledge and skills in the assessment of patient interests, strengths, vocational knowledge, and motivation as well as the individualized provision of a wide variety of educational, motivational, and supportive services. Their comprehensive assessment includes a variety of work-related areas including psychological, physical, and special equipment needs. They also are able to support and educate the coworkers and employers of individuals with schizophrenia in order to assist them in providing a flexible, supportive workplace environment. The key elements of vocational rehabilitation services include individualized job development for each patient, rapid placement, ongoing support, and an integration of mental health and vocational services (Lehman, Dickerson, Dixon, et al., 2004).

When assisting patients who are receiving vocational rehabilitation services, psychiatric advanced practice nurses take a primarily collaborative role, working with other health-care team members to move the patient toward identified vocational goals. In addition, psychiatric advanced practice nurses have adjunct roles including the provision of medication management, psychotherapy, coping skills interventions, and crisis intervention, all of which may assist the patient in meeting vocational goals. Psychiatric advanced practice nurses may make independent referrals for specific patients with vocational needs and should contact their local mental health center for program and referral information.

Assertive Community Treatment (ACT)

ACT teams were developed at the height of deinstitutionalization in the mid-1970s. As large numbers of seriously mentally ill individuals exited long-term hospital care, it became apparent that communities were poorly equipped to provide for their needs in a number of life areas. Traditional community mental health centers were inadequate to coordinate the broad range of supports needed, including medical care, housing, and socialization needs. As a result, many patients went through the revolving door of repeated short-term hospitalizations. ACT teams were introduced with the primary goal of preventing hospitalization and promoting housing stability, based on the assumption that outcomes are improved when support is provided directly in the community. Rather than a clinical intervention, ACT teams provide a framework for organizing services to successfully integrate at-risk individuals with severe mental illnesses into the community (Shean, 2009).

The key element of ACT programs is the assignment of high-risk individuals to a multidisciplinary team (psychiatrist, master's-prepared mental health clinician, bachelor's-prepared nurses, and case managers) that delivers around-the-clock care whenever and wherever the patient experiences a need. The team is responsible for 24-hour-a day community care, including treatment, transportation, rehabilitation, socialization, and support services. Teams meet daily to review and update treatment goals. One of the primary defining factors of an ACT team is a patient-to-staff ratio of not more than 10:1. The most positive outcomes are observed when fidelity to these program components is high.

The most consistent effect of ACT is a reduction of time spent in the hospital. Studies in the United States, Australia, and Sweden have demonstrated the effectiveness of ACT teams in reducing length of hospitalizations and symptoms (Latimer, 2005; Rosenheck & Dennis, 2001; Test & Stein, 1980). ACT has been shown to be more beneficial than case management in reducing hospital admissions and lengths of stay, improving employment outcomes and patient satisfaction (Latimer, 2005), and reducing homelessness (Coldwell & Bender, 2007). ACT patients are more likely to participate in other psychosocial treatments and have improved quality of life and social functioning (Bond, Drake, Mueser, et al., 2001). In addition to a focus on community reintegration, the strengths of ACT teams include their flexibility and the unlimited access to care that they provide.

Unfortunately, ACT is another psychosocial program with limited implementation. At present, ACT is offered to only about 20% of regular service users (i.e., those who respond poorly to services and are frequently hospitalized). The reasons for this are numerous. Expensive labor-intensive services such as ACT programs are unlikely to be adopted in understaffed and underfunded community sites. The lack of insurance parity continues to limit service offerings, and funding for clinician training (which would help ensure program fidelity) is minimal. Program fidelity is a critical component of ACT intervention, as high fidelity to the original model has been associated with improved patient outcomes (Bond et al., 2001; Burns, Catty, Dash, et al., 2007). If available, ACT programs should be considered by psychiatric advanced practice nurses for individuals with chronic symptoms who are poor responders, high users of services, or both.

The psychiatric advanced practice nurse brings additional resources to the ACT team by virtue of a broader scope of practice. Psychiatric advanced practice nurses are qualified to offer many proven psychosocial treatments to ACT team patients. In addition, psychiatric advanced practice nurses are qualified to prescribe and monitor adherence to and effects of psychiatric medications. Finally, psychiatric advanced practice nurses provide leadership as graduate-prepared ACT team members and offer resources to other staff members.

Psychiatric advanced practice nurses now have access to a variety of proven psychosocial treatments for their patients with schizophrenia. It is unlikely that any two patients with this illness would require the same complement of treatments, or even that a single individual with schizophrenia would require the same psychosocial treatments at different stages of illness. In addition to selecting the most appropriate psychosocial treatments, psychiatric advanced practice nurses also must make decisions about delivery method, either in a group setting or individually. The current literature indicates that clinicians should consider providing family therapy, SST, and education in group settings. In contrast, vocational rehabilitation assessments, job placements, and education for job performance—along with medication management follow-up—are often done individually owing to variability in symptoms, skill levels, and service needs.

Delivery Methods for Psychosocial Interventions

Considering the documented high relapse rate in nonadherent patients with schizophrenia, adherence to pharmacological treatment is important. Poor adherence is strongly linked to hospital readmission, which accounts for a majority of the nearly $50 billion annual cost of treatment for schizophrenia. A large body of research shows that problem-solving interventions effectively foster adherence and reduce hospitalization in individuals with schizophrenia. Unfortunately, these interventions are expensive and are unlikely to be adopted by overburdened service delivery systems. Moreover, communities that have problem-solving programs generally offer them only to a small group of the most severely ill individuals owing to financial and personnel constraints. This situation creates a need for effective, accessible, and economical delivery methods for problem-solving interventions for outpatients with schizophrenia.

Telephone Intervention

One cost-effective and time-efficient way to provide a variety of services is through telephone intervention. Weekly telephone intervention can be added to usual care for schizophrenia at an average cost of less than $240.00 per participant per year (Salzer, Tunner, & Charney, 2004). Based on decades of research on behavioral problem-solving interventions for patients with schizophrenia, researchers developed a telephone intervention program known as Telephone Intervention–Problem Solving for Schizophrenia (TIPS).

TIPS is a manualized outpatient intervention provided by community mental health clinicians designed to support problem-solving in response to a variety of everyday problems. The use of the problem-solving process compensates for a variety of cognitive deficits often present in schizophrenia that interfere with effective daily coping. TIPS is designed to foster problem-solving, offer coping alternatives, suggest reminders so that patients remember to use these alternatives, and assess the effectiveness of these coping efforts. Effective use of problem-solving may reduce stress, reduce symptoms, and improve community functioning for individuals with schizophrenia (Beebe, 2001).

TIPS is offered to stable outpatients on a weekly basis. TIPS is scheduled for a specific day and time according to patient preference (morning, afternoon, or evening) and is initiated by the clinician. The initial TIPS session is used to instruct the patient about the treatment and how problem-solving may help him or her. The clinician presents each step in the problem-solving process with a brief explanation and a more detailed handout. During this initial session, the clinician discusses how reduced memory and concentration make it hard to cope with everyday problems and explains how the problem-solving process can help everyone. Then the clinician and patient establish a day and time for the weekly TIPS call, and the clinician answers any questions.

TIPS includes seven protocol items to be addressed during each call. Five protocol items address specific problems in community living identified by individuals with schizophrenia (Beebe, 2002); examples include

- Protocol Item 1: Taking medications as prescribed.
- Protocol Item 2: Attending scheduled follow-up appointments.
- Protocol Item 3: Dealing with symptoms of schizophrenia.

- Protocol Item 4: Abstaining from alcohol and other drugs.
- Protocol Item 5: Dealing with interpersonal problems.

Protocol items 6 and 7 provide an opportunity for patients to identify any areas about which they need information or education, and anything else they wish to discuss that was not covered in previous items.

The clinician concludes by thanking the patient for his or her time and reminding the patient of the date and time of the next TIPS call. A section from the TIPS manual is included in Box 15-2 as an example of how to explain the problem-solving process.

The observed benefits of TIPS include reduced readmission rates, reduced lengths of rehospitalization, and statistically significant increases in psychiatric medication adherence (Beebe, 2001; Beebe, Smith, Crye, et al., 2008). Psychiatric advanced practice nurses desiring to offer TIPS to outpatients with schizophrenia should consider the educational preparation and experience of those who will provide the intervention. In the TIPS studies (Beebe, 2001; Beebe & Tian, 2004; Beebe et al., 2008; Beebe, Smith, Bennett, et al., 2010a), TIPS was provided by either a nurse with a bachelor's degree or a nurse with a master's degree. Hence, the responses observed may not be comparable. The use of an intervention protocol has the additional benefit of ensuring consistency of assessments and interventions.

A common difficulty in TIPS studies was making telephone contact. Participants required an average of three calls before contact was made. Thus, clinicians need to plan for repeated attempts to contact patients. Offering telephone intervention during evening hours may increase the likelihood of contact. In TIPS studies, calls in which contact was made averaged 5 to 8 minutes in length, but some calls lasted up to 20 minutes. It would be prudent to consider whether calls should be time limited, and if so, what is a reasonable time limit per call. If calls are time limited, provisions need to be made for situations in which patients may wish to talk for longer than the time allotted. Such plans might include face-to-face appointments or emergency evaluations. In TIPS studies, face-to-face follow-up appointments were made in less than 1% of interventions; in every case, the problem was assistance in obtaining prescribed medications (Beebe, 2001; Beebe & Tian, 2004; Beebe et al., 2008).

TIPS is documented in a similar manner as a face-to-face encounter. The loss of visual and nonverbal cues must be compensated for by greater attention to voice tone, quality, and pauses during speech. Clinicians must be attentive to and document verbal cues such as drawn-out sentences, throat clearings, and lengthy silences.

To date, researchers and clinicians have provided over 850 telephone interventions to over 70 community-dwelling individuals with schizophrenia (Beebe, 2001; Beebe & Tian, 2004; Beebe et al., 2008; Beebe et al., 2010a). No TIPS study participant experienced worsening symptoms as a result of telephone intervention, nor were any suicidal, homicidal, psychiatric, or other emergencies identified in the course of the TIPS interventions (Beebe, 2001; Beebe & Tian, 2004; Beebe et al., 2008; Beebe et al., 2010a; Salzer et al., 2004). Nevertheless, owing to the seriousness of this safety issue, the slim chance of suicidal or homicidal thoughts must be considered and a response prepared. Plans for dispatching emergency personnel or police to the scene must be in place in the event that a patient voices symptoms that indicate immediate danger to self or others. The TIPS provider should have a telephone line other than the TIPS line set aside for this use.

In summary, preliminary studies have consistently identified trends toward fewer hospitalizations, longer community survival, and improved medication adherence in patients receiving a variety of psychosocial interventions combined with optimal medication dosages. Clinicians must choose from this menu of interventions based on a number of patient, illness, and system factors, providing for safety, emergency evaluations, or face-to-face interventions if necessary. Such activities will allow psychosocial interventions to contribute their full potential as adjunctive treatments.

Case Study 15-1 illustrates a patient with schizophrenic symptoms.

BOX 15-2 Excerpt from Telephone Intervention Problem Solving (TIPS) Manual

The Problem Solving Process

Stressors are life events (such as interpersonal conflict) or internal processes (such as hallucinations) that are perceived as stressful by the person experiencing them. Coping is a response to perceived stress that involves behavioral and cognitive processes. Examples of behavioral processes include exercising, moving to a less stimulating location, or listening to music. Examples of cognitive processes include thought stopping techniques, reading, or talking to a support person. The ability of persons with schizophrenia to use specific cognitive or behavioral strategies to manage stressful events is limited by impairments in problem solving ability. Improving the problem solving ability of persons with schizophrenia has been shown to be related to successful community functioning and reduced time in the hospital. Researchers believe that regular use of problem solving can protect against relapse in persons with schizophrenia. The provision of TIPS involves helping clients respond to everyday problems by guiding them through the steps of the problem-solving process, as follows:

- Identify the problem
- Generate solutions
- Discuss solutions
- Select a solution

Source: Beebe, L. H. (2005). Telephone Intervention Problem Solving (TIPS) for persons with schizophrenia. Directions in Psychiatric Nursing, *11(9), 103-112.*

CASE STUDY 15-1

A Patient With Schizophrenic Symptoms

Ming is a 24-year-old Asian American female only child who comes to you for outpatient follow-up after a recent psychiatric hospitalization. Ming was born in the United States of a Chinese woman who immigrated at age 15 and an American man who she met in college. There is no known family history of schizophrenia. Ming's parents (with whom she lives) report that she was a high achiever throughout her elementary and high school years, but her functioning deteriorated after she left home at age 18 to attend college in another state. She became convinced that one of her professors was involved in a plot with the student organizations on campus to discredit and humiliate her. Over the course of 2 months, she refused to attend courses or eat, believing the cafeteria food was poisoned. She slept little, being constantly vigilant for attack by "people trying to ruin my life." She did not develop any friendships or attend any social functions. She denies alcohol use; however, she reported that during this period she could only sleep after smoking marijuana, which she did approximately 5 nights a week. She denies marijuana or other drug use since leaving college.

She eventually left college and returned home, where her symptoms lessened without treatment; during this time, she worked stocking the shelves at her mother's Asian grocery store and spent her free time alone or with her parents. However, at age 20, she again became extremely mistrustful of others, this time her parents. She withdrew from them, refusing to leave her room for meals or to bathe, accusing her parents of "being in league with the devil" and "spying on me for information." Her parents consulted her primary care physician, who recommended a psychiatrist who subsequently hospitalized Ming and prescribed olanzapine. Olanzapine reduced her symptoms, but she gained 15 pounds in the first 3 months and refused to continue the medication. Around this time, Ming took up smoking "to help me slim down" and currently smokes one pack of cigarettes a day. She was switched to risperidone with fair results; she returned to her job at her mother's store and resumed attending church with her parents, but remains socially isolated and guarded.

The most recent hospitalization (her fourth in 4 years) was brought on by stress associated with the remodeling of her mother's store and the presence of workmen there. Ming became convinced she was involved in a love affair with one of the workmen and pregnant with his child. She feared that her prescribed medication would harm the baby and discontinued it. After she followed the workman home and threatened suicide if he did not admit his paternity and agree to "help me raise your child," the police were called and she was involuntarily hospitalized. Records from the hospital indicate that the delusions faded after an increase in her risperidone dosage, but she refused participation in most unit activities.

On assessment today she is a 5'5", 170-pound Asian American female appearing her stated age, BP 128/75, pulse 80 and regular, with no known allergies. Her cranial nerve tests and extraocular movements are intact, reflexes 2+ bilaterally, and she correctly identifies a pen and a pair of eyeglasses with her eyes closed. She is dressed in clean but wrinkled clothing appropriate to the season, except for a stocking cap she refuses to remove, stating "it helps keep my thoughts inside my head where they belong." She appears restless, crossing and uncrossing her legs and picking at her fingernails; eye contact is poor. Although she answers all questions, her answers are vague and she does not initiate any verbalizations. She exhibits occasional thought blocking, and she denies substance use and suicidal or homicidal ideation at this time. She admits to mild paranoia regarding "people reading my thoughts: that's why I wear this hat" and is alert and oriented to time, place, person, and situation. You estimate her to be of above-average intelligence; her memory appears good but her insight is limited. She relates the reason for her hospitalization, "I had a misunderstanding with one of mom's workmen at the store; it's no big deal."

Questions

1. Write a concise case formulation of Ming's *DSM-IV-TR* diagnosis and how she meets diagnostic criteria.
2. Provide a list of at least three other diagnoses that you considered and why they were ruled out.
3. List immediate assessments including historical information, laboratory or other tests, and collateral information needed.
4. What immediate medication recommendations would you make? Be sure to include rationale and medication education.
5. Describe your plans to enhance medication adherence.
6. List appropriate treatments and plans to maintain safety in view of recent suicide threats.
7. What psychosocial interventions are needed, and with what goals?
8. What health promotion activities are needed?

Answers to these questions can be found at the end of this chapter.

Course

Schizophrenia is usually diagnosed in adolescence or early adulthood. Premorbid symptoms occurring in childhood, often only recognized in hindsight, include nonspecific social, cognitive, or motor dysfunctions (Schenkel & Silverstein, 2004). Abnormalities include motor delays, social isolation, poor academic performance, or emotional detachment.

Schizophrenia is often preceded by a prodromal period, which may last only weeks but usually lasts between 2 and 5 years (Beiser, Erickson, Fleming, et al., 1993). The prodromal period represents a definite change from premorbid functioning, is clearly identified as problematic, and continues until the emergence of psychotic symptoms. The prodrome is associated with severe impairment and nonspecific symptoms such as sleep disturbance, poor concentration, and social withdrawal (Schultze-Lutter, 2009; Yung & McGorry, 1996).

Later in the prodrome, positive symptoms such as perceptual abnormalities, suspiciousness, and ideas of reference emerge (Woods, Tandy, & McGlashan, 2001). For example, individuals in the prodromal period may believe they have special gifts, such as the ability to communicate with inanimate objects. The first psychotic episode may be insidious or acute and heralds the onset of schizophrenia, which typically occurs between the ages of 15 and 45 years.

The psychotic phase of the illness has three distinct phases:

- *Acute:* florid psychosis—for example, delusions, hallucinations, thought disorder
- *Recovery:* the 6- to 18-month period following the acute psychosis
- *Stable:* a period when negative and residual symptoms typically remain but are less severe (American Psychiatric Association, 2009)

The first 5 years after the first episode are known as the "early course" and may be associated with additional deterioration, which tapers off by 5 to 10 years after diagnosis (Lieberman, Perkins, Belger, et al., 2001). Long-term outcomes vary from recovery to incapacitation. Of those with schizophrenia, 10% to 15% have no further episodes, most have exacerbations and remissions throughout their lifetime, and 10% to 15% are chronically and severely psychotic (Hogarty, Baldessarini, Tohen, et al., 1994).

The classic course of schizophrenia is one of symptom exacerbations and remissions. Although the positive symptoms of schizophrenia appear to plateau within 5 to 10 years of diagnosis, negative symptoms become more pronounced as the disease progresses; thus, individuals with schizophrenia become increasingly socially disabled over time. Pronounced negative symptoms, poor social support, and social withdrawal are indicators of a poor outcome, with cognitive deficits being more predictive of poor community functioning than symptom level (Cutler, 2002).

Men with schizophrenia have a younger age at onset, poorer premorbid history, more negative symptoms, and a poorer course than women with the disease. Women with schizophrenia have more affective symptoms, more positive symptoms, and a better disease course (defined as fewer hospitalizations and less substance abuse) than men. Women have more rapid responses to medications, have more improvement regardless of stage of illness, and require lower medication doses than men with schizophrenia. However, women with schizophrenia have more dystonia, parkinsonism, akathisia, and TD than men and experience higher medication-related prolactin elevations (Kelly, Conley, & Tamminga, 1999; Leung & Chue, 2000).

Key Points

- Schizophrenia is the most chronic and disabling of the severe mental disorders, affecting multiple areas of functioning, with an exacerbating and remitting course; at present, there is no known cure.
- Theories of schizophrenia etiology include a variety of biological anomalies, environmental conditions, and family interaction patterns.
- Symptoms are divided into positive, negative, and cognitive types; other characteristics include disorganization, mood symptoms, motor symptoms, and neurological signs.
- A schizophrenia assessment includes psychiatric and medical history, verification of diagnostic criteria, and a suicide/violence assessment.
- Antipsychotic medications are the mainstay of schizophrenia treatment.
- Antipsychotic medications have been divided into the categories of typical and atypical on the basis of similarities in mechanism of action.
- Antipsychotic medication side effects include both acute and chronic extrapyramidal symptoms.
- Psychosocial treatments include family therapy, social skills training (SST), vocational rehabilitation, cognitive behavioral therapy (CBT), and the services of an assertive community treatment (ACT) team.
- Management issues include physical health promotion, adherence, culture, suicide, substance abuse, smoking, patient education, and self-help referrals.

Resources

Movies

Grazer, B. (Producer), & Howard, R. (Director). (2001). *A beautiful mind* [Motion picture]. United States: Universal Studios and Dreamworks.

It portrays the suffering and losses associated with having schizophrenia. It also shows the role of newer treatment approaches in promoting recovery.

Greco, J. (Director). (2006). *Canvas* [Motion picture]. United States: Rebellion Pictures.

It portrays schizophrenia with paranoid features.

Madden, J. (Director). (2005). *Proof* [Motion picture]. United States: Miramax Pictures.

It shows impact of schizophrenia on family.

SOURCE: WEDDING, BOYD, & NIEMIEC, 2010.

References

Acil, A. A., Dogan, S., & Dogan, O. (2008). The effects of physical exercises to mental state and quality of life in patients with schizophrenia. *Journal of Psychiatric and Mental Health Nursing, 15,* 808-815.

Adler, L. A., Rotrosen, J., Edson, R., et al. (1999). Veterans affairs cooperative study # 394 study group. Vitamin E for tardive dyskinesia. *Archives of General Psychiatry, 56,* 836-845.

Alford, B. A., & Beck, A. T. (1997). *The integrative power of cognitive therapy.* New York: Guilford Press.

Allardyce, J., & Boydell, J. (2006). Review: The wider social environment and schizophrenia. *Schizophrenia Bulletin, 32,* 592-598.

Allison, D. B., Fontaine, K. R., Heo, M., et al. (1999). The distribution of body mass index among individuals with and without schizophrenia. *Journal of Clinical Psychiatry, 60,* 215-220.

American Academy of Pediatrics. (2000). Use of psychoactive medication during pregnancy and possible effects on the fetus and newborn. *Pediatrics, 105,* 880-887.

American Diabetes Association. (2010). American Diabetes Association standards of medical care in diabetes. *Diabetes Care, 33*(Suppl 1), S4-S10.

American Diabetes Association, American Psychiatric Association, American Association of Clinical Endocrinologists, North American Association for the Study of Obesity. (2004). Consensus development conference on antipsychotic drugs and obesity and diabetes. *Diabetes Care, 27,* 596-601.

American Psychiatric Association. (2000a). *Diagnostic and statistical manual of mental disorders* (4th ed., text rev.) (pp. 274-287). Washington, DC: American Psychiatric Publishing, Inc.

American Psychiatric Association. (2000b). *Handbook of psychiatric measures.* Washington, DC: American Psychiatric Publishing, Inc.

American Psychiatric Association. (2003). *Practice guidelines for the assessment and treatment of patients with suicidal behaviors.* Washington, DC: American Psychiatric Publishing, Inc.

American Psychiatric Association. (2004a). *Practice guidelines for the treatment of patients with schizophrenia* (2nd ed.). Washington, DC: American Psychiatric Publishing, Inc.

American Psychiatric Association. (2004b). Consensus statement on antipsychotic drugs and obesity and diabetes. *Diabetes Care, 27*(2), 596-601.

American Psychiatric Association. (2009). *Guideline watch: Practice guideline for the treatment of patients with schizophrenia.* Washington, DC: American Psychiatric Association.

Andreasen, N. C., Carpenter, W. T., Jr., Kane, J. M., et al. (2005). Remission in schizophrenia: Proposed criteria and rationale for consensus. *American Journal of Psychiatry, 162*(3), 441-449.

Anthony, J. C., Folstein, M., & Romanoski, A. J. (1985). Comparison of the Lay diagnostic interview schedule and a standardized psychiatric diagnosis. *Archives of General Psychiatry, 42,* 667-675.

Anthony, W. (2000). A recovery-oriented service system: Setting some system level standards. *Psychiatric Rehabilitation Journal, 24,* 159-175.

Archie, W., Wilson, J. H., Osborne, S., et al. (2003). Pilot study: Access to fitness facility and exercise levels in olanzapine-treated patients. *Canadian Journal of Psychiatry, 48*(9), 628-632.

Argo, T. R., Crismon, M. L., Miller, A. L., et al. (2008). *Texas Medication Algorithm Project Procedural manual: Schizophrenia algorithm.* Austin, TX: The Texas Department of State Health Services.

Ascher-Svanum, H., Zhu, B., Faries, D., et al. (2006). A prospective study of risk factors for nonadherence with antipsychotic medication in the treatment of schizophrenia. *Journal of Clinical Psychiatry, 67,* 1114-1123.

Ashburner, J., & Friston, K. J. (2000). Voxel-based morphometry—the methods. *Neuroimage, 11,* 805-821.

Ashdown, H., Dumont, Y., Ng, M., et al. (2006). The role of cytokines in mediating effects of prenatal infection in the fetus: Implications for schizophrenia. *Molecular Psychiatry, 11,* 47-55.

Auquier, P., Lancon, C., Rouillon, F., et al. (2007). Mortality in schizophrenia. *Pharmacoepidemiology and Drug Safety, 16,* 1308-1312.

Ayd, F. J. (1961). A survey of drug induced extrapyramidal reactions. *Journal of the American Medical Association, 75,* 1054-1060.

Azrin, N. H., & Teicher, G. (1998). Evaluation of an instructional program for improving medication compliance for chronically mentally ill outpatients. *Behavioral Research and Therapy, 36,* 849-861.

Badner, J. A., & Gershon, E. S. (2002). Meta-analysis of whole-genome linkage scans of bipolar disorder and schizophrenia. *Medical Psychiatry, 7,* 405-411.

Baker, F. M., & Bell, C. C. (1999). Issues in the psychiatric treatment of African Americans. *Psychiatric Services, 50,* 362-368.

Ball, M. P., Coons, V. B., & Buchanan, R. W. (2001). A program for treating olanzapine related weight gain. *Psychiatric Services, 52*(7), 967-969.

Bandura, A. (1995). *Self-efficacy in changing societies.* New York: Cambridge University Press.

Baptista, T., Martinez, J., Lacruz, A., et al. (2006). Metformin for prevention of weight gain and insulin resistance with olanzapine: A double-blind placebo-controlled trial. *Canadian Journal of Psychiatry, 51,* 192-196.

Baptista, T., Rangel, N., Fernandez, V., et al. (2007). Metformin as an adjunctive treatment to control body weight and metabolic dysfunction during olanzapine administration: A multicentric, double-blind, placebo-controlled trial. *Schizophrenia Research, 93,* 99-108.

Barbee, J. G., Clark, P. D., Crapanzano, M. S., et al. (1989). Alcohol and substance abuse among schizophrenic patients presenting to an emergency psychiatric service. *Journal of Nervous and Mental Disease, 177,* 400-407.

Barch, D. M., Sheline, Y. I., Csernansky, J. G., et al. (2003). Working memory and prefrontal cortex dysfunction: Specificity to schizophrenia, compared with major depression. *Biological Psychiatry, 53*(5), 376-384.

Barnes, T. R. E., Mutsatsa, S. H., Hutton, S. B., et al. (2006). Comorbid substance abuse and age of onset of schizophrenia. *British Journal of Psychiatry, 188,* 237-242.

Bateson, G., Jackson, D., Haley, J., et al. (1956). Towards a theory of schizophrenia. *Behavioral Science, 1,* 251-264.

Batki, S. L., Dimmock, J. A., Wade, M., et al. (2007). Monitored naltrexone without counseling for alcohol abuse/dependence in schizophrenia spectrum disorders. *American Journal of Addiction, 16*(4), 253-259.

Beasley, C. L., Chana, C., Honavar, M., et al. (2005). Evidence for altered neuronal organization within the planum temporale in major psychotic disorders. *Schizophrenia Research, 73,* 69-78.

Beasley, C. L., Honavar, M., Everell, J. P., et al. (2009). Two dimensional assessment of cytoarchitecture in the superior temporal white matter in schizophrenia, major depressive disorder and bipolar disorder. *Schizophrenia Research, 115,* 156-162.

Beasley, C. M., Jr., Tollefson, G., Tran, P., et al. (1996). Olanzapine versus placebo and haloperidol: Acute phase results of the North American double-blind olanzapine trial. *Neuropsychopharmacology, 14,* 111-123.

Bebbington, P., Kuipers, E., & Garety, P. (2002). Long-term community care through an assertive continuous treatment team. In C. A. Tammaniga & S. Schulz (Eds.), *Advances in neuropsychiatry and psychopharmacology* (Vol. 1: Schizophrenia Research) (pp. 239-246). New York: Raven Press.

Bechdolf, A., Kohn, D., & Knost, B. (2005). A randomized comparison of group cognitive behavioral therapy and group psychoeducation in acute patients with schizophrenia: Outcome at 24 months. *Acta Psychiatrica Scandanavica, 112,* 173-179.

Beebe, L. H. (2001). Community nursing support for schizophrenic clients. *Archives of Psychiatric Nursing, 15*(5), 214-222.

Beebe, L. H. (2002). Problems in community living identified by persons with schizophrenia. *Journal of Psychosocial Nursing and Mental Health Services, 40*(2), 38-46.

Beebe, L. H. (2005). Telephone Intervention Problem Solving (TIPS) for persons with schizophrenia. *Directions in Psychiatric Nursing, 11*(9), 103-112.

Beebe, L. H. (2006a). Describing the health parameters of outpatients with schizophrenia. *Applied Nursing Research, 19,* 43-47.

Beebe, L. H. (2006b). Walking tall: A person with schizophrenia on a journey to better health. *Journal of Psychosocial Nursing, 44*(6), 53-55.

Beebe, L. H., Smith, K., Bennett, C., et al. (2010a). Keeping in touch. *Journal of Psychosocial Nursing and Mental Health Services, 48*(4), 31-37.

Beebe, L. H., Smith, K., Burk, R., et al. (2010b). Effect of a motivational group intervention on exercise self-efficacy and outcome expectations for exercise in schizophrenia spectrum disorders. *Journal of the American Psychiatric Nurses' Association, 16*(2), 105-113.

Beebe, L. H., Smith, K., Crye, C., et al. (2008). Telenursing intervention increases psychiatric medication adherence in schizophrenia outpatients. *Journal of the American Psychiatric Nurses Association, 14*(3), 217-224.

Beebe, L. H., & Tian, L. (2004). TIPS: Telephone Intervention-Problem Solving for persons with schizophrenia. *Issues in Mental Health Nursing, 25*(3), 317-329.

Beebe, L. H., Tian, L., Morris, N., et al. (2005). Effects of exercise on mental and physical health parameters of persons with schizophrenia. *Issues in Mental Health Nursing, 26*(6), 661-676.

Beiser, M., Erickson, D., Fleming, J. A., et al. (1993). Estimating the onset of psychiatric illness. *American Journal of Psychiatry, 150,* 1349-1354.

Bellack, A. S. (2006). Scientific and consumer models of recovery in schizophrenia: Concordance, contrasts and implications. *Schizophrenia Bulletin, 32,* 432-442.

Bilder, R. M., Goldman, R. S., Volvaka, J., et al. (2002). Neurocognitive effects of clozapine, olanzapine, risperidone and haloperidol in patients with chronic schizophrenia or schizoaffective disorder. *American Journal of Psychiatry, 159,* 1018-1028.

Blackburn, G. L. (1995). Effect of degree of weight loss on health benefits. *Obesity Research, 3*(Suppl 2), 211S-216S.

Blackwood, D. H., Fordyce, A., Walker, M. T., et al. (2001). Schizophrenia and affective disorders: Cosegregation with a translocation at chromosome 1q42 that directly disrupts brain-expressed genes clinical and P300 findings in a family. *American Journal of Human Genetics, 69,* 428-433.

Bond, G. R., Drake, R., Mueser, K., et al. (2001). Assertive community treatment for people with severe mental illness: Critical ingredients and impact on patients. *Disease Management and Health Outcomes, 9,* 141-159.

Bond, G. R., Resnick, S. G., & Drake, R. E. (2001). Does competitive employment improve non-vocational outcomes for people with severe mental illness? *Journal of Consulting and Clinical Psychology, 69,* 489-501.

Borison, R. L., Arvanitis, L. A., & Miller, B. G. (1996). Multiple fixed doses of "Seroquel" (quetiapine) in patients with acute exacerbation of schizophrenia: A comparison with haloperidol and placebo. *Biological Psychiatry, 42,* 33-46.

Bottlender, R., Jager, M., Hofschuster, E., et al. (2002). Neuroleptic malignant syndrome due to atypical neuroleptics: Three episodes in one patient. *Pharmacopsychiatry, 35,* 119-121.

Bowie, C. R., Leung, W. W., & Reichenberg, A. (2008). Predicting schizophrenia patients' real-world behavior with specific neuropsychological and functional capacity measures. *Biological Psychiatry, 63,* 505-511.

Boydell, J., van Os, J., McKenzie, K., et al. (2001). Incidence of schizophrenia in ethnic minorities in London, ecological study into interactions with the environment. *British Medical Journal, 323,* 1336-1338.

Brambilia, F., Guastalla, A., Guerrini, A., et al. (1976). Glucose insulin metabolism in chronic schizophrenia. *Diseases of the Nervous System, 37*(2), 98-103.

Braude, W. M., Barnes, T. R. E., & Gore, S. M. (1983). Clinical characteristics of akathisia: A systematic investigation of acute psychiatric inpatient admissions. *British Journal of Psychiatry, 143,* 139-150.

Breier, B. A., Buchanan, R. W., Irish, D., et al. (1993). Clozapine treatment of outpatients with schizophrenia: Outcome and long-term response pattern. *Hospital and Community Psychiatry, 44,* 1145-1149.

Brown, S., & Chen, K. (2006). A randomized controlled trial of a brief health promotion intervention in a population with serious mental illness. *Journal of Mental Health, 15,* 543-549.

Brown, A. S., Cohen, P., Harkavy-Friedman, J., et al. (2001). Prenatal rubella, premorbid abnormalities, and adult schizophrenia. *Biological Psychiatry, 49,* 473-486.

Brown, A. S., Scheafer, C. A., & Quesenberry, C. P. (2002). Maternal exposure to toxoplasmosis and risk of schizophrenia in adult offspring. *American Journal of Psychiatry, 162,* 767-773.

Buchsbaum, M. S., Someya, T., Teng, C. Y., et al. (1996). PET and MRI of the thalamus in never-medicated patients with schizophrenia. *American Journal of Psychiatry, 153,* 191-199.

Burns, T., Catty, J., Dash, M., et al. (2007). Use of intensive case management to reduce time in hospital in people with severe mental illness: Systematic review and meta-regression. *British Medical Journal, 335,* 336.

Burris, K. D., Molski, T. E., Xu, C., et al. (2002). Aripiprazole: A novel antipsychotic is a high-affinity partial agonist at human dopamine D2 receptors. *Journal of Pharmacology and Experimental Therapeutics, 302,* 281-289.

Byerly, M., Fisher, R., Whatley, K., et al. (2005). A comparison of electronic monitoring vs. clinician rating of antipsychotic adherence in outpatients with schizophrenia. *Psychiatry Research, 133*(2-3), 129-133.

Byrne, M., Agerbo, E., Bennedsen, B., et al. (2007). Obstetric conditions and risk of first admission with schizophrenia: A Danish national register-based study. *Schizophrenia Research, 97,* 51-59.

Byrne, M., Agerbo, E., Ewald, H., et al. (2003). Parental age and risk of schizophrenia: A case-controlled study. *Archives of General Psychiatry, 60,* 673-678.

Cahn, W., Rais, M., Stigter, F. P., et al. (2008). Psychosis and brain volume changes during the first five years of schizophrenia. *European Neuropsychopharmacology, 19,* 147-151.

Callicott, J. H., Bertolino, A., Mattay, V. S., et al. (2000). Physiological dysfunction of the dorsolateral prefrontal cortex in schizophrenia revisited. *Cerebral Cortex, 10*(11), 1078-1092.

Camargo, L. M., Collura, V. I., Rain, J. C., et al. (2007). Disrupted in schizophrenia 1 interactome: Evidence for the close connectivity of risk genes and a potential synaptic basis for schizophrenia. *Molecular Psychiatry, 12*(1), 74-86.

Cannon, M., Caspi, A., Moffitt, T. E., et al. (2002a). Evidence for early childhood, pan-development impairment specific to schizophreniform disorder: Results from a longitudinal birth cohort. *Archives of General Psychiatry, 59,* 449-456.

Cannon, M., Jones, P. B., & Murray, R. M. (2002b). Obstetrical complications and schizophrenia: Historical and meta-analytic review. *American Journal of Psychiatry, 159,* 1080-1092.

Cannon, T. D., Kaprio, J., Lonnqvist, J., et al. (1998). The genetic epidemiology of schizophrenia in a Finnish twin cohort: A population-based modeling study. *Archives of General Psychiatry, 55,* 67-74.

Cardno, A. G., Marshall, E. J., Coid, B., et al. (1999). Heritability estimates for psychotic disorders: The Maudsley twin psychosis series. *Archives of General Psychiatry, 56,* 162-168.

Carnahan, R. M., Lund, B. C., & Perry, P. J. (2001). Ziprasidone, a new atypical antipsychotic drug. *Pharmacotherapy, 21,* 717-730.

Caroff, S. N., Mann, S. C., & Keck, P. E. (1998). Specific treatment of the neuroleptic malignant syndrome. *Biological Psychiatry, 44,* 378-381.

Casey, D. E. (1991). Neuroleptic induced extrapyramidal syndromes and tardive dyskinesia. *Schizophrenia Research, 4,* 109-120.

Casey, D. E. (2004). Dyslipidemia and atypical antipsychotic drugs. *Journal of Clinical Psychiatry, 65*(Suppl 18), 27-35.

Casey, D. E., Carson, W. H., Saha, A. R., et al. (2003). Switching patients to aripiprazole from other antipsychotic agents: A multicenter randomized study. *Psychopharmacology, 166,* 391-399.

Casey, D. E., Daniel, D. G., Wassef, A. A., et al. (2003b). Effect of divalproex combined with olanzapine in patients with an acute exacerbation of schizophrenia. *Neuropsychopharmacology, 28,* 182-192.

Centers for Disease Control and Prevention. (2010). Defining overweight and obesity. Retrieved from http://www.cdc.gov/obesity/defining.html

Centorrino, F., Baldessarini, R. J., Kando, J. C., et al. (1994). Clozapine and metabolites: Concentrations in serum and clinical findings during treatment of chronically psychotic patients. *Journal of Clinical Psychopharmacology, 14,* 119-125.

Centorrino, F., Wurtman, J. J., Duca, K. A., et al. (2006). Weight loss in overweight patients maintained on atypical antipsychotic agents. *International Journal of Obesity, 30,* 1011-1016.

Chakos, M. H., Mayerhoff, D. I., Loebel, A. D., et al. (1992). Incidence and correlates of acute extrapyramidal symptoms in first episode schizophrenia. *Psychopharmacology Bulletin, 28,* 81-86.

Chakravarti, A. (1999). Population genetics: Making sense out of sequence. *Nature Genetics, 21*(Suppl 1), 56-60.

Chamove, A. S. (1986). Positive short-term effects of activity on behavior in chronic schizophrenic patients. *British Journal of Clinical Psychology, 25,* 125-133.

Chan, J. M., Rimm, E. B., Colditz, G. A., et al. (1994). Obesity, fat distribution, and weight gain as risk factors for clinical diabetes in men. *Diabetes Care, 17,* 961-969.

Chance, S. A., Walker, M., & Crow, T. J. (2005). Reduced density of calbindin-immunoreactive interneurons in the planum temporale in schizophrenia. *Brain Research, 1046,* 32-37.

Chapman, J. (1966). The early symptoms of schizophrenia. *British Journal of Psychiatry, 112,* 225-251.

Chen, C. K., Chen, Y. C., & Huang, Y. S. (2009). Effects of a 10-week weight control program on obese patients with schizophrenia or schizoaffective disorder: A 12-month follow up. *Psychiatry and Clinical Neuroscience, 63*(1), 17-22.

Cheng, J. Y., Ko, J. S., Chen, R. Y., et al. (2008). Meta-regression analysis using latitude as moderator of paternal age related schizophrenia risk. *Schizophrenia Research, 99*, 71-76.

Chien, W. T., Chan, S., & Morrissey, J. (2005). Effectiveness of a mutual support group for families of patients with schizophrenia. *Journal of Advanced Nursing, 51*, 595-605.

Chouinard, G., Jones, B., Remington, G., et al. (1993). A Canadian multicenter placebo controlled study of fixed doses of risperidone and haloperidol in the treatment of chronic schizophrenic patients. *Journal of Clinical Psychopharmacology, 13*, 25-49.

Chubb, J. E., Bradshaw, D. C., Soares, D. C., et al. (2008). The DISC locus in psychiatric illness. *Molecular Psychiatry, 13*, 36-64.

Ciapparelli, A., Paggani, R., & Marazziti, D. (2007). Comorbidity with axis I anxiety disorders in remitted psychotic patients, 1 year after hospitalization. *CNS Spectrums, 12*, 913-919.

Cohen, L. S., & Rosenbaum, J. F. (1998). Psychotropic drug use during pregnancy: Weighing the risks. *Journal of Clinical Psychiatry, 59*(Suppl 2), 18-28.

Coldwell, C. M., & Bender, W. S. (2007). The effectiveness of assertive community treatment for homeless populations with severe mental illness: A meta-analysis. *American Journal of Psychiatry, 164*, 393-399.

Conley, R. R., Love, R. C., Kelly, D. L., et al. (1999). Rehospitalization rates of patients recently discharged on a regimen of risperidone or clozapine. *American Journal of Psychiatry, 156*, 863-868.

Cook, J. A., Leff, H. S., Blyler, C. R., et al. (2005). Results of a multisite randomized trial of supported employment interventions for individuals with severe mental illness. *Archives of General Psychiatry, 62*, 502-512.

Cooper, C., Morgan, C., Byrne, M., et al. (2008). Perceptions of disadvantage, ethnicity and psychosis. *British Journal of Psychiatry, 192*, 185-190.

Cormac, I., & Ferriter, M. (2006). The physical health care of psychiatric patients in adult mental health services. *The Mental Health Review, 11*(1), 21-26.

Cornblatt, B., Obuchowski, M., Roberts, S., et al. (1999). Cognitive and behavioral precursors of schizophrenia. *Developmental Psychopathology, 11*, 487-508.

Csernansky, J. G., Mahmoud, R., & Brenner, R. (2002). Risperidone reduced the risk of relapse in outpatient schizophrenia and schizoaffective disorder. *Evidence-Based Mental Health, 5*, 77.

Cuffe, S. P., Waller, J. L., Cuccaro, M. L., et al. (1995). Race and gender differences in the treatment of psychiatric disorders in young adolescents. *Journal of the American Academy of Child and Adolescent Psychiatry, 34*, 1536-1543.

Cutler, A. J. (2002, May). Optimizing management of schizophrenia: Bridging the gap between clinical research and real-world clinical practice. *Advances in the Treatment of Psychosis: Minimizing the Burden of Disease.* Symposium conducted at the meeting of the American Psychiatric Association, Philadelphia.

Dalman, C., Alleback, P., Gunnell, D., et al. (2008). Infections in the CNS during childhood and the risk of subsequent psychotic illness: A cohort study of more than one million Swedish subjects. *American Journal of Psychiatry, 165*, 59-65.

Daly, P. A., Solomon, C. G., & Manson, J. E. (Eds.). (1996). *Risk modification in the obese patient.* New York: Oxford University Press.

Daniel, D. G., Potkin, S. G., Reeves, K. R., et al. (2001). Intramuscular (IM) ziprasidone 20 mg is effective in reducing acute agitation associated with psychosis: A double-blind randomized trial. *Psychopharmacology, 155*, 128-134.

Daumit, G. L., Goldberg, R. W., Anthony, C., et al. (2005). Physical activity patterns in adults with severe mental illness. *Journal of Nervous and Mental Disease, 193*, 541-545.

Daumit, G., Pronovost, P. J., & Anthony, C. B. (2006). Adverse events during medical and surgical hospitalizations for persons with schizophrenia. *Archives of General Psychiatry, 63*, 267-272.

David, A. S., & Prince, M. (2005). Psychosis following head injury: A critical review. *Journal of Neurology and Neurosurgical Psychiatry, 76*(Suppl 1), 453-460.

Davidson, L., Chinman, M., Kloos, B., et al. (1999). Peer support among individuals with severe mental illness: A review of the evidence. *Clinical Psychology: Science and Practice, 6*, 165-187.

Davies, G., Welham, J., Chant, D., et al. (2003). A systematic review and meta-analysis of northern hemisphere season of birth studies in schizophrenia. *Schizophrenia Bulletin, 29*, 587-593.

Davis, J. M., & Chen, N. (2001). The effects of olanzapine on the 5 dimensions of schizophrenia derived by factor analysis: Combined results of the North American and international trials. *Journal of Clinical Psychiatry, 62*, 757-771.

Dealberto, M. J. (2007). Why are immigrants at increased risk for psychosis? Vitamin D insufficiency, epigenetic mechanisms, or both? *Medical Hypotheses, 68*, 259-267.

Degenhardt, L., & Hall, W. (2006). Is cannabis use a contributory cause of psychosis? *Canadian Journal of Psychiatry, 51*, 566-574.

Delahanty, J., Ram, R., Postrado, L., et al. (2001). Differences in rates of depression in schizophrenia by race. *Schizophrenia Bulletin, 27*, 29-38.

deLeon, J., & Diaz, E. J. (2005). Meta-analysis of worldwide studies demonstrates an association between schizophrenia and tobacco smoking behaviors. *Schizophrenia Research, 76*, 135-157.

DeLisi, L. E., Friedrich, U., Wahlstrom, J., et al. (1994). Schizophrenia and sex chromosome anomalies. *Schizophrenia Bulletin, 20*, 495-505.

Dhalla, S., & Kopec, J. A. (2007). The CAGE questionnaire for alcohol misuse: A review of reliability and validity studies. *Clinical and Investigational Medicine, 30*(1), 33-41.

Dickinson, D., Ramsey, M. E., & Gold, J. M. (2007). Overlooking the obvious: A meta-analytic comparison of digit symbol coding tasks and other cognitive measures in schizophrenia. *Archives of General Psychiatry, 64*, 532-542.

Dickson, R. A., & Hogg, L. (1998). Pregnancy of a patient treated with olanzapine. *Psychiatric Services, 49*, 1081-1083.

Dinakar, H. S., Sobel, R. N., Bopp, J. H., et al. (2002). Efficacy of olanzapine and risperidone for treatment of refractory schizophrenia among long-stay state hospital patients. *Psychiatric Services, 53*, 755-777.

Dixon, L. B. (2003). Diabetes and mental illness: Factors to keep in mind. *Consultant, 43*(3), 337-348.

Dixon, L., Green-Paden, L., Delahanty, J., et al. (2001). Variables associated with disparities in treatment of patients with schizophrenia and comorbid mood and anxiety disorders. *Psychiatric Services, 52*, 1216-1222.

Dixon, L., Weiden, P., Delahanty, J., et al. (2000). Prevalence and correlates of diabetes in national schizophrenia samples. *Schizophrenia Bulletin, 26*, 903-912.

Dohrenwend, B. P., Levav, I., Shrout, P. E., et al. (1992). Socioeconomic status, psychiatric disorders and causation-selection issue. *Science, 255*, 946-952.

Dolder, C. R., Lacro, J. P., Dunn, L. B., et al. (2002). Antipsychotic medication adherence: Is there a difference between typical and atypical agents? *American Journal of Psychiatry, 159*, 103-108.

Dolder, C. R., Lacro, J. P., & Jeste, D. V. (2003). Adherence to antipsychotic and nonpsychiatric medications in middle aged and older patients with psychotic disorders. *Psychosomatic Medicine, 65*, 156-162.

Dose, M., Hellweg, R., Yassouridis, A., et al. (1998). Combined treatment of schizophrenia psychoses with haloperidol and valproate. *Pharmacopsychiatry, 31*, 122-125.

Drake, R. E., Osher, F. C., Noordsy, D. L., et al. (1990). Diagnosis of alcohol use disorders in schizophrenia. *Schizophrenia Bulletin, 16*, 57-67.

Drake, R. E., Osher, F. C., & Wallach, M. A. (1989). Alcohol use and abuse in schizophrenia: A prospective community study. *Journal of Nervous and Mental Disease, 177*, 408-414.

Duan, J., Martinez, M., Sanders, A. R., et al. (2007). DTNBP1 and schizophrenia: Association evidence in the 3′ end of the gene. *Human Heredity, 64*, 97-106.

Dyck, D. G., Hendryx, M. S., & Short, R. A. (2002). Service use among patients with schizophrenia in psycho educational multiple-family group treatment. *Psychiatric Services, 53*, 749-754.

Eaton, W. W., Hall, A. J., Macdonold, R., et al. (2007). Case identification in psychiatric epidemiology: A review. *International Research in Psychiatry, 19*, 497-507.

Ellison-Wright, E., & Bullmore, E. (2009). Anatomy of bipolar disorder and schizophrenia: A meta-analysis. *Schizophrenia Research, 117*, 1-12.

Emsley, R. A., Raniwalla, J., Bailey, P. J., et al. (2000). A comparison of the effects of quetiapine and haloperidol in schizophrenia patients with a history of and demonstrated partial response to conventional antipsychotic treatment. *International Clinical Psychopharmacology, 15,* 121-131.

Ernst, C. L., & Goldberg, J. F. (2002). The reproductive safety profile of mood stabilizers, atypical antipsychotics and broad spectrum psychotropic. *Journal of Clinical Psychiatry, 63*(Suppl 4), 42-55.

Eschweller, G. W., Bartels, M., Langle, G., et al. (2002). Heart rate variability in the ECG trace of routine EEGs: Fast monitoring for the anticholinergic effects of clozapine and olanzapine? *Pharmacopsychiatry, 35,* 96-100.

Essock, S. M., Hargreaves, W. A., Covell, N. H., et al. (1996). Clozapine's effectiveness for patients in state hospitals: Results from a randomized trial. *Psychopharmacology Bulletin, 32,* 683-697.

Evans, S., Newton, R., & Higgins, S. (2005). Nutritional intervention to prevent weight gain in inpatients commenced on Olanzapine: A randomized controlled trial. *Australian and New Zealand Journal of Psychiatry, 39,* 479-486.

Evins, A. E., Cather, C., Culhane, M. A., et al. (2007). A 12-week double-blind placebo-controlled study of bupropion SR added to high-dose dual nicotine replacement therapy for smoking cessation or reduction in schizophrenia. *Journal of Clinical Psychopharmacology, 27,* 380-386.

Evins, A. E., Cather, C., Deckersbach, T., et al. (2005). A double-blind placebo-controlled trial of bupropion SR for smoking cessation in schizophrenia. *Journal of Clinical Psychopharmacology, 25,* 218-225.

Ewing, J. A. (1984). Detecting alcoholism: The CAGE questionnaire. *Journal of the American Medical Association,* 252, 1905-1907.

Falkai, P., Wobrock, T., Lieberman, J., et al. (2005). World Federation of Societies of Biological Psychiatry (WFSBP) guidelines for biological treatment of schizophrenia, part I: Acute treatment of schizophrenia. *World Journal of Biological Psychiatry, 6*(3), 132-191.

Faries, D. E., Ascher-Svanum, H., Nyhuis, A. W., et al. (2009). Clinical and economic ramifications of switching antipsychotics in the treatment of schizophrenia. *BMC Psychiatry, 9*(54), 1-9.

Fatemi, S. H., Stary, J. M., Hatsukami, D. K., et al. (2005). A double-blind placebo-controlled crossover trial of bupropion in smoking reduction in schizophrenia. *Schizophrenia Research, 76,* 353-356.

Fioravanti, M., Carlone, O., & Vitale, B. (2005). A meta-analysis of cognitive deficits in adults with a diagnosis of schizophrenia. *Neurological Review, 15,* 73-95.

Fish, B., Marcus, J., Hans, S. L., et al. (1992). Infants at risk for schizophrenia: Sequelae of a genetic neurointegrative defect. A review and replication analysis of pandysmaturation in the Jerusalem Infant Development Study. *Archives of General Psychiatry, 49,* 221-235.

Fleischhacker, W. W., McQuade, R. D., & Marcus, R. N. (2009). A double-blind randomized comparative study of aripiprazole and olanzapine in patients with schizophrenia. *Biological Psychiatry, 65,* 510-517.

Fogarty, M., Happell, B., & Pininkahana, J. (2004). The benefits of an exercise program for people with schizophrenia: A pilot study. *Psychiatric Rehabilitation Journal, 28*(2), 173-176.

Frangou, S., Sachpazidis, B. A., Stassinakis, A., et al. (2005). Telemonitoring of medication adherence in patients with schizophrenia. *Telemedicine and E-health, 11*(6), 675-683.

Friedman, J., Ault, K., & Powchik, P. (1997). Pimozide augmentation for the treatment of schizophrenic patients who are partial responders to clozapine. *Biological Psychiatry, 42,* 522-523.

Ganguli, R. (2002). Rationale and strategies for switching antipsychotics. *American Journal of Health and Systems Pharmacology, 59,* S22-S26.

Geddes, J. R., & Lawrie, S. M. (1995). Obstetric complications and schizophrenia: A meta-analysis. *British Journal of Psychiatry, 167,* 786-793.

George, T. P., Vessicchio, J. C., Saccok, A., et al. (2008). A placebo controlled trial of bupropion combined with nicotine patch for smoking cessation in schizophrenia. *Biological Psychiatry, 63,* 1092-1096.

Gimino, F. A., & Levin, S. J. (1984). The effects of aerobic exercise on perceived self-image in post-hospitalized schizophrenic patients. *Medicine and Science in Sports and Exercise, 16,* 139.

Goff, D. C, Cather, C., & Evins, A. E. (2005). Medical morbidity in schizophrenia guidelines for psychiatrists. *Journal of Clinical Psychiatry, 66,* 183-194.

Gold, L. H. (2000). Use of psychotropic medication during pregnancy: Risk management guidelines. *Psychiatric Annals, 30,* 421-432.

Gold, P. B., Meisler, N., Santos, A. B., et al. (2006). Randomized trial of supported employment integrated with assertive community treatment for rural adults with mental illness. *Schizophrenia Bulletin, 32*(2), 378-395.

Goldberg, T. E., & Gomar, J. J. (2009). Targeting cognition in schizophrenia research: From etiology to treatment. *American Journal of Psychiatry, 166*(6), 631-644.

Goldschlager, N., & Goldman, M. J. (1989). *Principles of clinical electrocardiography* (13th ed.). Norwalk, CT: Appleton and Lange.

Goldstein, D. J., Corbin, L. A., & Fung, M. C. (2000). Olanzapine exposed pregnancies and lactation: Early experience. *Journal of Clinical Psychopharmacology, 20,* 399-403.

Goren, J. L., & Levin, G. M. (1998). Quetiapine: An atypical antipsychotic. *Pharmacotherapy, 18,* 1183-1194.

Gottesman, I. I., McGuffin, P., & Farmer, A. F. (1987). Clinical genetics as clues to the "real" genetics of schizophrenia. *Schizophrenia Bulletin, 13,* 23-47.

Gould, M. S., Marrocco, F. A., Kleinman, M., et al. (2005). Evaluating iatrogenic risk of youth suicide screening programs: A randomized controlled trial. *Journal of the American Medical Association, 293,* 1635-1643.

Gray, R., Wykes, T., & Gournay, K. (2002). From compliance to concordance: A review of literature on interventions to enhance compliance with antipsychotic medication. *Journal of Psychiatric and Mental Health Nursing, 9*(3), 277-284.

Green, A. I., Patel, J. K., Goisman, R. M., et al. (2000). Weight gain from novel antipsychotic drugs: Need for action. *General Hospital Psychiatry, 22,* 224-235.

Green, M. F., Marder, S. R., Glynn, S. M., et al. (2002). The neurocognitive effects of low dose haloperidol: A 2-year comparison with risperidone. *Biological Psychiatry, 51,* 972-978.

Gumley, A., Karatzias, A., & Power, K. (2006). Early intervention for relapse in schizophrenia: Impact of cognitive behavioral therapy on negative beliefs about psychosis and self-esteem. *British Journal of Clinical Psychology, 45,* 247-260.

Gumus, A. B. (2008). Health education needs of patients with schizophrenia and their families. *Archives of Psychiatric Nursing, 22*(3), 156-165.

Gur, R. E., Maany, V., Mozley, P. D., et al. (1998). Subcortical MRI volumes in neuroleptic naïve and treated patients with schizophrenia. *American Journal of Psychiatry, 155,* 1711-1717.

Guy, W. (1976). *Assessment manual for psychopharmacology—revised* (DHEW Publication No. ADM 76-338, pp. 534-537). Rockville, MD: U.S. Department of Health, Education, and Welfare, Public Health Service, Alcohol, Drug Abuse, and Mental Health Administration, NIMH Psychopharmacology Research Branch, Division of Extramural Research Programs.

Haddock, G., & Lewis, S. (2005). Psychological interventions in early psychosis. *Schizophrenia Bulletin, 31,* 697-704.

Hanninen, K., Katila, H., Saarela, M., et al. (2008). Interleukin-1 beta gene polymorphism and its interactions with neuroregulin-1 gene polymorphism are associated with schizophrenia. *European Archives of Psychiatry and Clinical Neuroscience, 258,* 10-15.

Harrison, G. (2004). Trajectories of psychosis: Towards a new social biology of schizophrenia. *Epidemiological Psychiatry Society, 13,* 152-157.

Heinssen, R. K. (2002). Improving medication compliance of a patient with schizophrenia through collaborative behavioral therapy. *Psychiatric Services, 53*(3), 255-257.

Henderson, D. C., & Goff, D. C. (1996). Risperidone as an adjunct to clozapine therapy in chronic schizophrenics. *Journal of Clinical Psychiatry, 57,* 395-397.

Hennah, W., Thomson, P., Peltonen, L., et al. (2006). Genes and schizophrenia: Beyond schizophrenia: The role of DISC1 in major mental illness. *Schizophrenia Bulletin, 32*(3), 409-416.

Hennen, J., & Baldessarini, R. J. (2005). Suicidal risk during treatment with clozapine: A meta-analysis. *Schizophrenia Research, 73,* 139-145.

Henry, J. D., & Crawford, J. R. (2005). A meta-analytic review of verbal fluency deficits in schizophrenia relative to other neurocognitive deficits. *Cognitive Neuropsychiatry, 10,* 1-33.

Hesslinger, B., Normann, C., Langosch, J. M., et al. (1999). Effects of carbamazepine and valproate on haldoperidol plasma levels and on psychopathologic outcomes in schizophrenic patients. *Journal of Clinical Psychopharmacology, 19*, 310-315.

Heston, L. L. (1966). Psychiatric disorders in the foster home reared children of schizophrenic mothers. *British Journal of Psychiatry, 112*, 819-825.

Hirsch, S. R., Kissling, W., Bauml, J., et al. (2002). A 28-week comparison of ziprasidone and haloperidol in outpatients with stable schizophrenia. *Journal of Clinical Psychiatry, 63*, 516-523.

Ho, B. C., Mola, C., & Andreasen, N. C. (2004). Cerebellar dysfunction in neuroleptic naïve schizophrenic patients. *Biological Psychiatry, 55*, 1146-1153.

Hogarty, J. D., Baldessarini, R. J., Tohen, M., et al. (1994). One hundred years of schizophrenia: A meta-analysis of the outcome literature. *American Journal of Psychiatry, 151*, 1409-1416.

Holden, R. J. (1995). Schizophrenia, suicide and the serotonin story. *Medical Hypotheses, 44*, 379-391.

Holden, R. J., & Mooney, P. A. (1994). Schizophrenia is a diabetic brain state: An elucidation of impaired neurometabolism. *Medical Hypotheses, 43*, 420-435.

Hulshoff Pol, H. E., & Kahn, R. S. (2008). What happens after the first episode? A review of progressive brain changes in chronically ill patients with schizophrenia. *Schizophrenia Bulletin, 34*(2), 354-366.

Isaacson, J. H., & Schorling, J. B. (1999). Screening for alcohol problems in primary care. *Medical Clinics of North America, 83*(6), 1547-1563.

Ishiguro, H., Okuyama, Y., Toru, M., et al. (2000). Mutation and association analysis of the 5′ region of the dopamine D3 receptor gene in schizophrenia patients: Identification of the Ala38Thr polymorphism and suggested association between DRD3 haplotypes and schizophrenia. *Molecular Psychiatry, 5*(4), 433-438.

Janicak, P. G., Davis, J. M., Preskorn, S. H., et al. (1993). *Principles and practice of psychopharmacotherapy.* Baltimore: Williams and Wilkins.

Jones, P., Rodgers, B., Murray, R., et al. (1994). Child developmental risk factors for adult schizophrenia in the British 1946 birth cohort. *Lancet, 344*, 1398-1402.

Jordan, S., Koprivica, V., Chen, R., et al. (2002). The antipsychotic aripiprazole is a potent, partial agonist at the human 5-HT1A receptor. *European Journal of Pharmacology, 441*, 137-140.

Kallman, F. J. (1946). The genetic theory of schizophrenia: An analysis of 691 schizophrenic twin index families. *American Journal of Psychiatry, 103*, 309-322.

Kanders, B. S., & Blackburn, G. L. (1992). Health consequences of therapeutic weight loss: Reducing primary risk factors. In T. A. Wadden & T. B. Van Itallie (Eds.), *The treatment of the seriously obese patient* (pp. 213-230). New York: Guilford Press.

Kane, J. M. (2006). Review of treatments that can ameliorate nonadherence in patients with schizophrenia. *Journal of Clinical Psychiatry, 67*(Suppl 5), 9-14.

Kane, J. M. (2010). The differential diagnosis of schizoaffective disorder. *Journal of Clinical Psychiatry, 12*, 33.

Kane, J. M., Crandall, D. T., & Marcus, R. N. (2007). Symptomatic remission in schizophrenia patients treated with aripiprazole or haloperidol for up to 52 weeks. *Schizophrenia Research, 95*, 143-150.

Kane, J., Honigfeld, G., Singer, J., et al. (1998). Clozapine for the treatment resistant schizophrenia: A double-blind comparison with chlorpromazine. *Archives of General Psychiatry, 45*, 789-796.

Karno, M., & Jenkins, J. H. (1993). Cross cultural issues in the course and treatment of schizophrenia. *Psychiatric Clinics of North America, 16*, 339-350.

Kaur, G., & Kulkarni, S. K. (2003). Involvement of normal physiological mechanisms in mediation of satiety by polyherbal antiobesity preparation, OB-200G, in female mice. *Methods and Findings in Clinical Pharmacology, 25*(1), 33-39.

Keefe, R. S., Bilder, R. M., & Davis, S. M. (2007). Neurocognitive effects of antipsychotic medications in patients with schizophrenia in the CATIE trial. *Archives of General Psychiatry, 64*, 633-647.

Keefe, R. S., Eesley, C. E., & Poe, M. P. (2005). Defining a cognitive function decrement in schizophrenia? *Biologic Psychiatry, 57*, 688-691.

Keefe, R. S., Seidman, L. J., Christensen, B. K., et al.; HGDH research group. (2004). Comparative effect of atypical and conventional antipsychotic drugs on neurocognition in first-episode psychosis: A randomized double-blind trial of olanzapine versus haloperidol. *American Journal of Psychiatry, 161*, 985-995.

Keith, S. J., & Kane, J. M. (2003). Partial compliance and patient consequences in schizophrenia: Our patients can do better. *Journal of Clinical Psychiatry, 64*, 1308-1315.

Kelly, D. L., Conley, R. R., & Tamminga, C. A. (1999). Differential olanzapine plasma concentrations by sex in a fixed dose study. *Schizophrenia Research, 40*, 101-104.

Kemp, R., Kirov, G., Everitt, B., et al. (1998). Randomized controlled trial of compliance therapy: 18-month follow-up. *British Journal of Psychiatry, 172*, 413-419.

Kendrick, T. (1996). Cardiovascular and respiratory risk factors and symptoms among general practice patients with long term mental illness. *British Journal of Psychiatry, 169*, 733-739.

Keshavan, M. S., Diwadkar, V. A., Montrose, D. M., et al. (2005). Premorbid indicators and risk for schizophrenia: A selective review and update. *Schizophrenia Research, 79*, 45-57.

Keshavan, M. S., Tandon, R., Boutros, N., et al. (2008). Schizophrenia, "just the facts": What we know in 2008 Part 3. Neurobiology. *Schizophrenia Research, 106*, 89-107.

Khashan, A. S., Abel, K. M., McNamee, R., et al. (2008). Higher risk of offspring schizophrenia following antenatal exposure to serious adverse life events. *Archives of General Psychiatry, 65*, 146-152.

Kim, M. A., Tura, E., Potkin, S. G., et al. (2010). Working memory circuitry in schizophrenia shows widespread cortical inefficiency and compensation. *Schizophrenia Research, 117*, 42-51.

King, D. J., Link, C. G. G., & Kowalcyk, B. (1998). A comparison of BID and TID dose regimens of quetiapine in the treatment of schizophrenia. *Psychopharmacology, 137*, 139-146.

Kinon, B. J., Milton, D. R., & Stouffer, V. L. (1999, May). *Effect of chronic olanzapine treatment on the course of presumptive TD.* Paper presented at the meeting of the American Psychiatric Association, Washington, DC.

Kirkbride, J. B., Fearon, P., Morgan, C., et al. (2006). Heterogeneity in incidence rates of schizophrenia and other psychotic syndromes: Findings from the 3-center Aetiology and Ethnicity in Schizophrenia and Related Psychosis (AeSOP) study. *Archives of General Psychiatry, 63*, 250-258.

Kirkpatrick, B., Fenton, W. S., Carpenter, W. T., Jr., et al. (2006). The NIMH-MATRICS consensus statement on negative symptoms. *Schizophrenia Bulletin, 32*, 214-219.

Kivlahan, D. R., Heiman, J. R., Wright, R. C., et al. (1990). Treatment cost and rehospitalization in schizophrenic outpatients with a history of substance abuse. *Hospital and Community Psychiatry, 42*, 609-614.

Klein, D. J., Cottingham, E. M., Sorter, M., et al. (2006). A randomized double-blind placebo-controlled trial of metformin treatment of weight gain associated with initiation of atypical antipsychotic therapy in children and adolescents. *American Journal of Psychiatry, 163*, 2072-2079.

Klinkenberg, W. D., & Calsyn, R. J. (1997). The moderating effects of race on return visits to the psychiatric emergency room. *Psychiatric Services, 48*, 942-945.

Knowler, W. C., Barrett-Connor, E., Fowler, S. E., et al. (2002). Reduction in the incidence of type II diabetes with lifestyle intervention or metformin. *The New England Journal of Medicine, 346*, 393-403.

Ko, Y. H., Joe, S. H., Jung, I. K., et al. (2005). Topiramate as an adjuvant treatment with atypical antipsychotics in schizophrenia patients experiencing weight gain. *Clinical Neuropharmacology, 28*, 169-175.

Koenig, J. I., Elmer, G. I., Shepard, P. D., et al. (2005). Prenatal exposure to a repeated variable stress paradigm elicits behavioral and neuroendocrinological changes in the adult offspring: Potential relevance to schizophrenia. *Behavioral Brain Research, 156*, 251-256.

Koller, E. A., & Doraiswamy, P. M. (2002). Olanzapine-induced diabetes mellitus. *Pharmacotherapy, 22*, 841-852.

Konick, L. C., & Friedman, L. (2001). Meta-analysis of thalamic size in schizophrenia. *Biological Psychiatry, 49*, 28-39.

Kopelowicz, A., Kreyenbuhl, J., & Buchanan, R. (2006). Recent advances in social skills training for schizophrenia. *Schizophrenia Bulletin, 32*, s12-s23.

Kreczmanski, P., Heinsen, H., Mantua, V., et al. (2007). Volume, neuronal density and total neuron number in five subcortical regions in schizophrenia. *Brain, 130*, 678-692.

Kroeze, W. K., Hufeisen, S. J., Popadak, B. A., et al. (2003). H1-histamine receptor affinity predicts short-term weight gain for typical and atypical antipsychotic drugs. *Neuropsychopharmacology, 28,* 519-526.

Krupa, T. (2004). Employment, recovery and schizophrenia: Integrating health and disorder at work. *Psychiatric Rehabilitation Journal, 28,* 8-15.

Kung, L., & Roberts, R. C. (1999). Mitochondrial pathology in human schizophrenic striatum: A post mortem ultrastructural study. *Synapse, 31,* 67-75.

Kupfer, D. J. (2009, March). *Diagnostic spectra: Assessing the validity of disorder groupings.* Presented at the 2009 annual meeting of the American Psychopathological Association, New York.

Kurtz, M. M., & Mueser, K. T. (2008). A meta-analysis of controlled research on social skills training for schizophrenia. *Journal of Consulting and Clinical Psychology, 76,* 491-504.

Kwon, J. S., Choi, J. S., Bahk, W. M., et al. (2006). Weight management program for treatment-emergent weight gain in Olanzapine-treated patients with schizophrenia or schizoaffective disorder: A 12-week randomized controlled clinical trial. *Journal of Clinical Psychiatry, 67*(4), 547-553.

Lacro, J. P., Dunn, L. B., Dolder, C. R., et al. (2002). Prevalence of and risk factors for medication non-adherence in patients with schizophrenia: A comprehensive review of recent literature. *Journal of Clinical Psychiatry, 63*(10), 892-909.

Lappa, A., Podesta, M., Capelli, O., et al. (2002). Successful treatment of a complicated case of NMS. *Intensive Care Medicine, 28,* 976-977.

Latimer, E. (2005). Economic considerations associated with assertive community treatment and supported employment for people with severe mental illness. *Journal of Psychiatry and Neuroscience, 30,* 355-359.

Lee, J. W., Schwartz, D. L., & Hallmayer, J. (2000). Catatonia in a psychiatric intensive care facility: Incidence and response to benzodiazepines. *Annals of Clinical Psychiatry, 12,* 89-96.

Lee, K., Yoshida, T., Kubicki, M., et al. (2009). Increased diffusivity in superior temporal gyrus in patients with schizophrenia a diffusion tensor imaging study. *Schizophrenia Research, 108,* 33-40.

Lehman, A. F., Dickerson, F. B., Dixon, L. B., et al. (2004). The schizophrenia patient outcomes research team (PORT): Updated treatment recommendations. *Schizophrenia Bulletin, 30,* 193-217.

Lehman, A., & Steinwachs, D. (1998). Patterns of usual care for schizophrenia: Initial results from the Schizophrenia patient outcomes research team (PORT) survey. *Schizophrenia Bulletin, 24*(1), 11-20.

Lehman, A., & Steinwachs, D. (2003). Evidence-based psychosocial treatment practices in schizophrenia: Lessons from the patient outcomes research team (PORT) project. *Journal of the American Academy of Psychoanalysis and Dynamic Psychiatry, 31*(1), 141-154.

Lesem, M. D., Zajecka, J. M., Swift, R. H., et al. (2001). Intramuscular ziprasidone 2 mg versus 10 mg in the short-term management of agitated psychotic patients. *Journal of Clinical Psychiatry, 62,* 12-18.

Leucht, S., Burkhard, T., & Henderson, J. (2007). Physical illness and schizophrenia: A review of literature. *Acta Psychiatrica Scandanavica, 116,* 317-333.

Leucht, S., Corves, C., & Arbter, D. (2009). Second generation versus first generation antipsychotic drugs for schizophrenia: A meta-analysis. *Lancet, 373,* 31-41.

Leucht, S., & Lasser, R. (2006). The concepts of remission and recovery in schizophrenia. *Pharmacopsychiatry, 39*(5), 161-170.

Leung, A., & Chue, P. (2000). Sex differences in schizophrenia, a review of literature. *Acta Psychiatrica Scandanavica Suppl, 401,* 3-38.

Lewandowski, K. E. (2007). Relationship of catechol-O-methyltransferase to schizophrenia and its correlates; evidence for associations and complex interactions. *Harvard Reviews in Psychiatry, 15,* 233-244.

Lewis, C. M., Levinson, D. F., Wise, L. H., et al. (2003). Genome scan meta-analysis of schizophrenia and bipolar disorder, part II; schizophrenia. *American Journal of Human Genetics, 73,* 34-48.

Li, D., & He, I. (2007). Association study between the dystrobrevin binding protein I gene (DTNBP1) and schizophrenia: A meta-analysis. *Schizophrenia Research, 96,* 112-118.

Li, Z., & Arthur, D. (2005). Family education for people with schizophrenia in Beijing, China: Randomized controlled trial. *British Journal of Psychiatry, 187,* 339-345.

Liberman, R. P., & Kopelowicz, A. (2002). Recovery from schizophrenia: A challenge for the 21st century. *International Review of Psychiatry, 14,* 245-255.

Liberman, R. P., & Kopelowicz, A. (2005). Recovery from schizophrenia: A recovery-based definition. In R. O. Ralph & P. W. Corrigan (Eds.), *Recovery in mental illness* (pp. 101-129). Washington, DC: American Psychological Association.

Liberman, R. P., Kopelowicz, A., Ventura, J., et al. (2005). Operational criteria and factors related to recovery from schizophrenia. In L. Davidson, C. Harding, & L. Spanol (Eds.), *Recovery from severe mental illnesses: Research evidence and implications for practice* (Vol. 1) (pp. 260-292). Boston: Center for Psychiatric Rehabilitation.

Liberman, R. P., Wallace, C. J., Blackwell, G., et al. (1993). Innovations in skills training for the seriously mentally ill: The UCLA Social and Independent Living Skills Modules. *Innovations and Research, 2,* 43-60.

Lidz, T., Cornelison, A., Fleck, S., et al. (1965). The intrafamilial environment of schizophrenia patients, II. Marital schism and marital skew. *American Journal of Psychiatry, 114,* 241-248.

Lieberman, J. A., Perkins, D., Belger, A., et al. (2001). The early stages of schizophrenia; speculations on pathogenesis, pathophysiology and therapeutic approaches. *Biological Psychiatry, 50,* 884-897.

Lieberman, J. A., Saltz, B. L., Johns, C. A., et al. (1991). The effects of clozapine on tardive dyskinesia. *British Journal of Psychiatry, 158,* 503-510.

Lieberman, J. A., Stroup, S., & McEvoy, J. P.; Clinical Antipsychotic Trials of Intervention Effectiveness (CATIE) Investigators. (2005). Effectiveness of antipsychotic drugs in patients with chronic schizophrenia. *The New England Journal of Medicine, 353,* 1209-1223.

Lima, A. R., Soares-Weiser, K., Bacaltchuk, J., et al. (2002). Benzodiazepines for neuroleptic induced acute akathisia. *The Cochrane Database of Systemic Reviews,* (1). CD001950.

Lipska, B. K., Jaskiw, G. E., & Weinberger, D. R. (1993). Postpubertal emergence of hyperresponsiveness to stress and to amphetamine after neonatal excitotoxic hippocampal damage: A potential animal model of schizophrenia. *Neuropsychopharmacology, 9,* 67-75.

Littrell, K. H., Hilligoss, N. M., Kirshner, C. D., et al. (2003). The effects of an educational intervention on antipsychotic induced weight gain. *Journal of Nursing Scholarship, 35*(3), 237-241.

Loveland, D., Weaver-Randall, K., & Corrigan, P. W. (2005). Research methods for exploring and assessing recovery. In R. O. Ralph & P. W. Corrigan (Eds.), *Recovery in mental illness* (pp. 101-129). Washington, DC: American Psychological Association.

Lykouras, L., Agelopoulos, E., & Tzavellas, E. (2002). Improvement of TD following switch from neuroleptics to olanzapine. *Progress in Neuro-Psychopharmacology and Biological Psychiatry, 26,* 815-817.

Magliano, L., Fiorillo, A., & Nakabgibem, C. (2006). Family psycho educational interventions for schizophrenia in routine settings: Impact on patients' clinical status and social functioning and on relatives' burden and resources. *Epidemiological Psychiatry and Society, 15,* 219-227.

Maki, P., Veijola, J., Jones, P. B., et al. (2005). Predictors of schizophrenia: A review. *British Medical Bulletin, 73/74,* 1-15.

Malaspina, D., Harlap, S., Fennig, S., et al. (2001). Advancing paternal age and the risk of schizophrenia. *Archives of General Psychiatry, 58,* 361-367.

Manoach, D. S., Press, D. Z., Thangaraj, V., et al. (1999). Schizophrenic subjects activate dorsolateral prefrontal cortex during a working memory task as measured by fMRI. *Biological Psychiatry, 45*(9), 1128-1137.

Marder, S. R., Davis, J. M., & Chouinard, G. (1997). The effects of risperidone on the five dimensions of schizophrenia derived by factor analysis: Combined results of the North American trials. *Journal of Clinical Psychiatry, 58,* 538-546.

Marder, S. R., & Meibach, R. C. (1994). Risperidone in the treatment of schizophrenia. *American Journal of Psychiatry, 151,* 825-835.

Margolese, H. C., Chouinard, G., Beauclair, L., et al. (2002). Therapeutic tolerance and rebound psychosis during quetiapine maintenance immunotherapy in patients with schizophrenia and schizoaffective disorder. *Journal of Clinical Psychopharmacology, 22,* 347-352.

Masand, P. (1999). *Weight gain and antipsychotic medications.* Memphis, TN: Physicians Postgraduate Press.

Masand, P. S. (2005). Review of pharmacologic strategies for switching to atypical antipsychotics. *Primary Care Companion-Journal of Clinical Psychiatry, 7*(3), 121-129.

Masand, P. S., Blackburn, G. L., Ganguli, R., et al. (1999). Weight gain associated with the use of antipsychotic medications. *Journal of Clinical Psychiatry,* Audiograph series, 2.

Mathalon, D. H., Pfefferbaum, A., Limk, O., et al. (2003). Compounded brain volume deficits in schizophrenia-alcoholism comorbidity. *Archives of General Psychiatry, 60,* 245-252.

Maurer, I., Zierz, S., & Moller, H. (2001). Evidence for a mitochondrial oxidative phosphorylation defect in brains from patients with schizophrenia. *Schizophrenia Research, 48,* 125-136.

Maxwell, S., & Shinderman, M. S. (2000). Use of naltrexone in the treatment of alcohol use disorders in patients with concomitant major mental illness. *Journal of Addiction Disorders, 19*(3), 61-69.

McEvoy, J. P. (2002, May). The impact of safety and tolerability on patients' satisfaction with therapy. In D. O. Perkins (Chair), *Challenges and Opportunities in the Management of Psychotic Disorders.* Symposium presented at the meeting of the American Psychiatric Association, Philadelphia.

McGrath, J., Saha, S., Welham, J., et al. (2004). A systematic review of the incidence of schizophrenia: The distribution of rates and the influence of sex, urbanicity, migrant status and methodology. *BMC Medicine, 2,* 13.

McGrath, J. J., & Welham, J. L. (1999). Season of birth and schizophrenia: A systematic review and meta-analysis of data from the Southern Hemisphere. *Schizophrenia Research, 35,* 237-242.

Mednick, S. A., Machon, R. A., Huttunen, M. O., et al. (1988). Adult schizophrenia following exposure to an influenza epidemic. *Archives of General Psychiatry, 45,* 189-192.

Meerwijk, E. L., vanMeijel, B., van den Bout, J., et al. (2010). Development and evaluation of a guideline for nursing care of suicidal patients with schizophrenia. *Perspectives in Psychiatric Care, 46*(1), 65-73.

Melle, I., Johannson, J. O., & Friis, O. (2006). Early detection of the first episode of schizophrenia and suicidal behavior. *American Journal of Psychiatry, 163,* 800-804.

Meltzer, H. Y. (1992). Treatment of the neuroleptic nonresponsive schizophrenic patient. *Schizophrenia Bulletin, 18,* 515-542.

Meltzer, H. Y., Alphs, L., Green, A. L., et al. (2003). Clozapine treatment for suicidality in schizophrenia: International suicide prevention trial (InterSePT). *Archives of General Psychiatry, 60,* 82-91.

Meltzer, H. Y., Burnett, S., Bastani, B., et al. (1990). Effects of six months of clozapine treatment on the quality of life of chronic schizophrenic patients. *Hospital and Community Psychiatry, 41,* 892-897.

Meltzer, H. Y., & Okayli, G. (1995). Reduction of suicidality during clozapine treatment of neuroleptic resistant schizophrenia: Impact on risk benefit assessment. *American Journal of Psychiatry, 152,* 183-190.

Menza, M., Vreeland, B., Minsky, S., et al. (2004). Managing atypical antipsychotic associated weight gain: 12-month data on a multimodal weight control program. *Journal of Clinical Psychiatry, 65*(4), 471-477.

Meyer, J. M., Nasrallah, H. A., McEvoy, J. P., et al. (2005). The Clinical Antipsychotic Trials of Intervention Effectiveness (CATIE) schizophrenia trial: Clinical comparison of subgroups with and without the metabolic syndrome. *Schizophrenia Research, 80,* 9-18.

Meyer, U., Yee, B. K., & Feldon, J. (2007). The neurodevelopment impact of prenatal infections at different times in pregnancy: The earlier the worse. *Neuroscientist, 13,* 241-266.

Millan, M. J. (2000). Improving the treatment of schizophrenia: Focus on serotonin (5-HT)1A receptors. *Journal of Pharmacology and Experimental Therapeutics, 295,* 853-861.

Mitchell, A. J., & Malone, D. (2006). Physical health and schizophrenia. *Current Opinions in Psychiatry, 19,* 432-437.

Moldin, S. O. (1997). The maddening hunt for madness genes. *Nature Genetics, 17,* 127-129.

Moore, T. H. M., Zammit, S., Lingford-Hughes, A., et al. (2007). Cannabis use and risk of psychotic or affective mental health outcomes: A systematic review. *Lancet, 370,* 319-328.

Morgan, C., & Fisher, H. (2007). Environment and schizophrenia; Environmental factors in schizophrenia: Childhood trauma—A critical review. *Schizophrenia Bulletin, 33,* 3-10.

Morrens, M., Hulstijn, W., Lewi, P. J., et al. (2006). Stereotypy in schizophrenia. *Schizophrenia Research, 84,* 397-404.

Morrens, M., Hulstijn, W., & Sabbe, B. (2007). Psychomotor slowing in schizophrenia. *Schizophrenia Bulletin, 33,* 1038-1053.

Morrison, R. L., & Bellack, A. S. (1984). Social skills training. In A. S. Bellack (Ed.), *Schizophrenia: Treatment, management, and rehabilitation* (pp. 247-279). Orlando, FL: Grune and Stratton, Inc.

Mowerman, S., & Siris, S. G. (1996). Adjunctive loxapine in a clozapine resistant cohort of schizophrenic patients. *Annals of Clinical Psychiatry, 8*(4), 193-197.

Mueser, K. T., Drake, R. E., & Bond, G. R. (1997). Recent advances in psychiatric rehabilitation for patients with severe mental illness. *Harvard Review of Psychiatry, 5,* 123-137.

Mueser, K. T., Yarnold, P. R., & Bellack, A. S. (1992). Diagnostic and demographic correlates of substance abuse in schizophrenia and major affective disorders. *Acta Psychiatrica Scandanavica, 85,* 48-55.

Mukherjee, S. (1995). High prevalence of type II diabetes in schizophrenic patients. *Schizophrenia Research, 15,* 195.

Mukherjee, S., Decina, P., Bocola, V., et al. (1996). Diabetes mellitus in schizophrenic patients. *Comprehensive Psychiatry, 37,* 66-73.

Muller, J. E., Koen, L., & Soraya, S. (2004). Anxiety disorders and schizophrenia. *Current Psychiatry Reports, 6,* 255-261.

Munafo, M. R., Atwood, A. S., & Flint, J. (2008). Neuregulin I genotype and schizophrenia. *Schizophrenia Bulletin, 34,* 9-12.

Murray-Swank, A. B., & Dixon, L. (2004). Family psychoeducation as an evidence-based practice. *CNS Spectrums, 9*(12), 905-912.

Nakonezny, P. A., & Byerly, M. J. (2005). Electronically monitored adherence in outpatients with schizophrenia or schizoaffective disorder: A comparison of first vs. second-generation antipsychotics. *Schizophrenia Research, 82*(1), 107-114.

National Cholesterol Education Panel. (2002). Third report of the National Cholesterol Education Program Expert Panel on Detection, Evaluation and Treatment of High Blood Cholesterol in Adults (Adult Treatment Panel III). Final report. *Circulation, 106,* 3143-3421.

National Heart Lung and Blood Institute. (2010). Aim for a healthy weight. Retrieved from http://www.nhlbi.nih.gov/health/public/heart/obesity/lose_wt/risk.htm

Neighbors, H. W., Jackson, J. S., Campbell, L., et al. (1989). The influence of racial factors on psychiatric diagnosis: A review and suggestions for research. *Community Mental Health Journal, 25,* 301-311.

Newcomer, J. W., & Hennekens, C. H. (2007). Severe mental illness and risk of cardiovascular disease. *Journal of the American Medical Association, 298,* 1794-1796.

Nickel, M. K., Nickel, C., Muehlbacher, M., et al. (2005). Influence of topiramate on olanzapine-related adiposity in women: A random, double-blind, placebo-controlled study. *Journal of Clinical Psychopharmacology, 25,* 211-217.

Nicodemus, K. K., Kolachana, B. S., Vakkalanka, R., et al. (2007). Evidence for statistical epistasis between catechol-O-methyltransferase (COMT) and polymorphisms in RGS4, G72, GRM3, and DISC1: Influence on risk of schizophrenia. *Human Genetics, 120,* 889-906.

Norman, R. M., & Malla, A. K. (1993). Stressful life events and schizophrenia. I: A review of the research. *British Journal of Psychiatry, 162,* 161-166.

Nunes, J. V., & Broderick, P. A. (2007). Novel research translates to clinical cases of schizophrenia and cocaine psychosis. *Neuropsychiatric Disorders and Treatment, 3*(4), 475-485.

Olafsdottir, S., & Pescosolido, B. (2009). Drawing the line: The cultural cartography of utilization recommendations for mental health problems. *Journal of Health and Social Behavior, 50,* 228-244.

Oyen, W. J., Claessens, R. A., Raemaekers, J. M., et al. (1992). Diagnosing infection in febrile granulocytopenic patients with indium-III-labeled human immunoglobulin. *Journal of Clinical Oncology, 10,* 61-68.

Pariante, C. M., Dazzan, P., Danese, A., et al. (2005). Increased pituitary volume in antipsychotic free and antipsychotic treated patients of the AESOP first onset psychosis study. *Neuropsychopharmacology, 30*(10), 1923-1931.

Peet, M. (2004). Diet, diabetes and schizophrenia: Review and hypothesis. *British Journal of Psychiatry Suppl, 47,* s102-s105.

Pelham, T. W., Campagna, P. D., Ritvo, P. G., et al. (1993). The effects of exercise therapy on clients in a psychiatric rehabilitation program. *Psychosocial Rehabilitation Journal, 16,* 75-84.

Pendlebury, J., Haddad, P., & Dursun, S. (2005). Evaluation of a behavioral weight management programme for patients with severe mental illness: 3 year results. *Human Psychopharmacology, 20,* 447-448.

Penner, J. D., & Brown, A. S. (2007). Prenatal infections and nutritional factors and risk of schizophrenia. *Expert Reviews in Neurotherapeutics, 7,* 797-805.

Perez-Costas, E., Melendez-Ferro, M., & Roberts, R. (2010). Basal ganglia pathology in schizophrenia: Dopamine connections and anomalies. *Journal of Neurochemistry, 10,* 1-16.

Perlstein, W. M., Dixit, N. K., Carter, C. S., et al. (2003). Prefrontal cortex dysfunction mediates deficits in working memory and prepotent responding in schizophrenia. *Biological Psychiatry, 53*(1), 25-38.

Perrin, M. C., Brown, A. S., & Malaspina, D. (2007). Aberrant epigenetic regulation could explain the relationship of paternal age to schizophrenia. *Schizophrenia Bulletin, 33,* 1270-1273.

Petrakis, H., O'Malley, S., Rounsaville, B., et al. (2004). Naltrexone augmentation of neuroleptic treatment in alcohol abusing patients with schizophrenia. *Psychopharmacology, 172*(3), 291-297.

Peuskens, J. (1995). Risperidone in the treatment of patients with chronic schizophrenia: A multinational, multicentre, double blind, parallel group study versus haloperidol. *British Journal of Psychiatry, 166,* 712-726.

Peuskens, J., & Link, C. G. (1997). A comparison of quetiapine and chlorpromazine in the treatment of schizophrenia. *Acta Psychiatrica Scandanavica, 96,* 265-273.

Pfammatter, M., Junghan, U. M., & Brenner, H. D. (2006). Efficacy of psychological therapy in schizophrenia: Conclusions from meta-analyses. *Schizophrenia Bulletin, 32*(Suppl 1), s4-s68.

Piette, J. D., Heisler, M., Ganoczy, D., et al. (2007). Differential medication adherence among patients with schizophrenia and comorbid diabetes and hypertension. *Psychiatric Services, 58,* 207-212.

Pilling, S., Bebbington, P., Kuipers, E., et al. (2002a). Psychological treatments in schizophrenia I: Meta-analysis of family intervention and cognitive behavior therapy. *Psychological Medicine, 32,* 763-782.

Pilling, S., Bebbington, P., Kuipers, E., et al. (2002b). Psychological treatment in schizophrenia II: Meta-analysis of randomized controlled trials of social skills training and cognitive remediation. *Psychological Medicine, 32,* 783-791.

Pollock, M. H., Reiter, S., & Hammerness, P. (1992). Genitourinary and sexual adverse effects of psychotropic medications. *International Journal of Psychiatric Medicine, 22,* 305-327.

Potkin, S. G., Cohen, M., & Panagides, J. (2007). Efficacy and tolerability of asenapine in acute schizophrenia: A placebo- and risperidone-controlled trial. *Journal of Clinical Psychiatry, 68*(10), 1492-1500.

Potvin, S., Ali, A., & Stip, E. (2007). Meta-analysis of depressive symptoms in dual diagnosis schizophrenia. *Australian New Zealand Psychiatry, 41,* 792-799.

Prabakaran, S., Swatton, J. E., Ryan, M. M., et al. (2004). Mitochondrial dysfunction in schizophrenia: Evidence for compromised brain metabolism and oxidative stress. *Molecular Psychiatry, 9,* 684-697.

Pratt, S. I., Mueser, K. T., Driscoll, M., et al. (2006). Medication nonadherence in older people with serious mental illness: Prevalence and correlates. *Psychiatric Rehabilitation Journal, 29*(4), 299-310.

Purdon, S. E., Jones, B. D., Stip, E., et al; Canadian collaborative group for research in schizophrenia. (2000). Neuropsychological change in early phase schizophrenia during 12 months of treatment with olanzapine, risperidone or haloperidol. *Archives of General Psychiatry, 57,* 249-258.

Purdon, S. E., Mala, A., Labelle, A., et al. (2001). Neurological change in patients with schizophrenia after treatment with quetiapine or haloperidol. *Journal of Psychiatry and Neuroscience, 26,* 137-149.

Puschner, B., Born, A., Giessler, A., et al. (2005). Effects of interventions to improve compliance with antipsychotic medication in people suffering from schizophrenia: Results of recent reviews. *Psychiatry Research, 32*(2), 62-67.

Raiff, N. (1984). Some health-related outcomes of self-help participation. Recovery Inc. as a case example of a self-help organization in mental health. In A. Gartner & E. Reissman (Eds.), *The self-help revolution* (pp. 183-193). New York: Human Sciences Press.

Rais, M., Cahn, W., van Haren, N. E., et al. (2008). Excessive brain volume loss over time in cannabis-using first-episode schizophrenia patients. *American Journal of Psychiatry, 165*(4), 490-496.

Ranganath, C., Minzenberg, M. J., & Ragland, D. J. (2008). The cognitive neuroscience of memory function and dysfunction in schizophrenia. *Biological Psychiatry, 64,* 18-25.

Rayburn, T. M., & Stonecypher, J. F. (1996). Diagnostic differences related to age and race of involuntarily committed psychiatric patients. *Psychological Reports, 79,* 881-882.

Razali, S. M., Hasanah, C. I., Khan, A., et al. (2000). Psychosocial interventions for schizophrenia. *Journal of Mental Health, 9,* 283-289.

Read, J., van Os, J., Morrison, A. P., et al. (2005). Childhood trauma, psychosis and schizophrenia: A literature review with theoretical and clinical implications. *Acta Psychiatrica Scandanavica, 112,* 330-350.

Reeves, R. R., Mack, J. E., & Beddingfield, J. J. (2002). Neurotoxic syndrome associated with risperidone and fluvoxamine. *Annals of Pharmacotherapy, 36,* 440-443.

Regier, D. A., Kaelber, C. T., Rae, D. S., et al. (1998). Limitations of diagnostic criteria and assessment instruments for mental disorders: Implications for research and policy. *Archives of General Psychiatry, 55,* 109-115.

Reichenberg, A., & Harvey, P. D. (2007). Neuropsychological impairments in schizophrenia: Integration of performance-based and brain imaging findings. *Psychological Bulletin, 133,* 833-858.

Remington, G., & Kapur, S. (1999). D2 and 5-HT2 receptor effects of antipsychotics: Bridging basic and clinical findings using PET. *Journal of Clinical Psychiatry, 60*(Suppl 10), 15-19.

Reznik, I., & Sirota, P. (2000). An open study of fluvoxamine augmentation of neuroleptics in schizophrenia with obsessive and compulsive symptoms. *Clinical Neuropharmacology, 23,* 157-160.

Richter, D. (1957). Biochemical aspects of schizophrenia. In D. Richter (Ed.), *Schizophrenia: Somatic aspects.* London: Pergamon Press.

Risch, N., & Merinkangas, K. (1996). The future of genetic studies of complex human diseases. *Science, 273,* 1516-1517.

Rosebush, P. I., Stewart, T. D., & Gelenberg, A. J. (1989). 20 neuroleptic challenges after neuroleptic malignant syndrome in 15 patients. *Journal of Clinical Psychiatry, 50,* 295-298.

Rosenberg, S. D., Goodman, L. A., Osher, F. L., et al. (2001). Prevalence of HIV, hepatitis B and hepatitis C in people with serious mental illness. *American Journal of Public Health, 91,* 31-37.

Rosenheck, R., & Dennis, D. (2001). Time limited assertive community treatment for homeless persons with severe mental illness. *Archives of General Psychiatry, 58,* 1073-1080.

Rosenquist, K. J., Walker, S. S., & Ghaemi, S. N. (2002). Tardive dyskinesia and ziprasidone. *American Journal of Psychiatry, 159,* 1436.

Rubio, G., Martinez, I., & Ponce, G. (2006). Long-acting injectible risperidone compared with zuclopenthixol in the treatment of schizophrenia with substance abuse comorbidity. *Canadian Journal of Psychiatry, 51*(8), 531-539.

Rudd, M. D., Mandrusiak, M., & Joiner, T. E., Jr. (2006). The case against no-suicide contracts: The commitment to treatment statement as a practice alternative. *Journal of Clinical Psychology, 62,* 243-251.

Ryan, M. C., Collins, P., & Thakore, J. H. (2003). Impaired fasting glucose tolerance in first episode, drug naïve patients with schizophrenia. *American Journal of Psychiatry, 160*(2), 284-289.

Sadock, B. J., & Sadock, V. A. (2007). *Kaplan and Sadock's synopsis of psychiatry* (10th ed.). Philadelphia: Lippincott, Williams and Wilkins.

Safferman, A., Lieberman, J. A., Kane, J. M., et al. (1991). Update on the clinical efficacy and side effects of clozapine. *Schizophrenia Bulletin, 17,* 247-261.

Saha, S., Chant, D., & McGrath, J. (2007). A systematic review of mortality in schizophrenia is the differential mortality gap worsening over time. *Archives of General Psychiatry, 64,* 1123-1131.

Saha, S., Chant, D., Welham, J., et al. (2005). A systematic review of the prevalence of schizophrenia. *PloS Medicine, 2,* 413-433.

Salzer, M. S., Tunner, T., & Charney, N. J. (2004). A low-cost, telephone intervention to enhance schizophrenia treatment: A demonstration study. *Schizophrenia Research, 66,* 75-76.

Saunders, K. E., & Hawton, K. (2009). The role of psychopharmacology in suicide prevention. *Epidemiologia e Psichiatrica Sociale, 18*(3), 172-178.

Schauwecker, D. S. (2002). Imaging infection in patients with agranulocytosis. *Journal of Nuclear Medicine, 43,* 925-927.

Schenkel, L. S., & Silverstein, S. M. (2004). Dimensions of premorbid functioning in schizophrenia: A review of neuromotor, cognitive, social and behavioral domains. *Genetic, Social and General Psychological Monographs, 130,* 241-270.

Schooler, N. R., & Kane, J. M. (1982). Research diagnoses for tardive dyskinesia. *Archives of General Psychiatry, 39,* 486-487.

Schultze-Lutter, F. (2009). Subjective symptoms of schizophrenia in research and the clinic: The basic symptom concept. *Schizophrenia Bulletin, 35,* 5-8.

Schwab, S. G., Plummer, C., Albus, M., et al. (2008). DNA sequence variants in the metabotropic glutamate receptor 3 and risk in schizophrenia: An association study. *Psychiatric Genetics, 18,* 25-30.

Segall, J. M., Turner, J. A., van Erp, T. G., et al. (2009). Voxel-based morphometric multisite collaborative study on schizophrenia. *Schizophrenia Bulletin, 35,* 82-95.

Semple, D. M., McIntosh, A. M., & Lawrie, S. M. (2005). Cannabis as a risk factor for psychosis: Systematic review. *Journal of Psychopharmacology, 19,* 187-194.

Shapiro, D. A., Renock, S., Arrington, E., et al. (2003). Aripiprazole, a novel atypical antipsychotic drug with a unique and robust pharmacology. *Neuropsychopharmacology, 28*(8), 1400-1411.

Shapiro, G. K., & Buckley-Hunter, L. (2010). What every adolescent needs to know: Cannabis can cause psychosis. *Journal of Psychosomatic Research, 6,* 533-539.

Sharma, T., & Harvey, P. D. (2000). Cognitive enhancement as a treatment strategy in schizophrenia. In T. Sharma & P. Harvey (Eds.), *Cognition in schizophrenia. Impairments, importance and treatment strategies* (pp. 286-302). New York: Oxford University Press.

Shean, G. D. (2009). Evidence-based psychosocial practices and recovery from schizophrenia. *Psychiatry, 72*(4), 307-320.

Shopsin, N. B., Klein, H., Aaronson, M., et al. (1979). Clozapine, chlorpromazine and placebo in newly hospitalized, acutely schizophrenic patients: A controlled, double-blind comparison. *Archives of General Psychiatry, 36,* 657-664.

Silverstone, T., Smith, G., & Goodall, E. (1988). Prevalence of obesity in patients receiving depot antipsychotics. *British Journal of Psychology, 153,* 214-217.

Siris, S. G., & Bench, C. (2003). Depression and schizophrenia. In S. R. Hirsch & D. R. Weinberger (Eds.), *Schizophrenia* (2nd ed.). Malden, MA: Blackwell Publishing.

Smith, R. C., Infante, M., Singh, A., et al. (2001). The effects of olanzapine on neurocognitive function in medication-refractory schizophrenia. *International Journal of Neuropsychopharmacology, 4,* 239-250.

Snowden, A. (2009a). Classification of schizophrenia. Part one: The enduring existence of madness. *British Journal of Nursing, 18*(19), 1176-1180.

Snowden, A. (2009b). Classification of schizophrenia. Part 2: The nonsense of mental health illness. *British Journal of Nursing, 18*(20), 1228-1232.

Soares, K. V., & McGrath, J. J. (2001). Vitamin E for neuroleptic-induced tardive dyskinesia. *The Cochrane Database of Systematic Reviews,* (4). CD000209.

Somervell, P. D., Leaf, P. J., Weissman, M. M., et al. (1989). The prevalence of major depression in black and white adults in 5 US communities. *American Journal of Epidemiology, 130,* 725-735.

Soyka, M. (1996). Dual diagnosis in patients with schizophrenia. Issues in Pharmacological treatments. *CNS Drugs, 5,* 414-425.

Spina, E., Avenoso, A., Scordo, M. G., et al. (2002). Inhibition of risperidone metabolism by fluoxetine in patients with schizophrenia: A clinically relevant pharmacokinetic drug interaction. *Journal of Clinical Psychopharmacology, 22,* 419-423.

Stahl, S. M. (2009). *The prescriber's guide: Stahl's essential psychopharmacology.* New York: Cambridge University Press.

Stahl, S. M., & Buckley, P. F. (2007). Negative symptoms of schizophrenia: A problem that will not go away. *Acta Psychiatrica Scandanavica, 115,* 4-11.

Starke, A. K., Uylings, H. B., Sanz-Arigita, E., et al. (2004). Glial cell loss in the anterior cingulate cortex, a subregion of the prefrontal cortex in subjects with schizophrenia. *American Journal of Psychiatry, 161,* 882-888.

Startup, M., Jackson, M. C., & Bendix, S. (2004). North Wales randomized controlled trial of cognitive behavioral therapy for acute schizophrenia spectrum disorders. Outcomes at 6 and 12 months. *Psychological Medicine, 34,* 413-422.

St. Clair, D., Xu, M., Wang, P., et al. (2005). Rates of adult schizophrenia following prenatal exposure to the Chinese famine of 1959-1961. *Journal of the American Medical Association, 294,* 557-562.

Stedman, T., & Welham, J. (1993). The distribution of adipose tissue in female inpatients receiving psychotropic drugs. *British Journal of Psychiatry, 162,* 249-250.

Stimmel, G. L., Gutierrez, M. A., & Lee, V. (2002). Ziprasidone: An atypical antipsychotic drug for the treatment of schizophrenia. *Clinical Therapeutics, 24*(1), 21-37.

Stip, E., & Tourjman, V. (2010). Aripiprazole in schizophrenia and schizoaffective disorder: A review. *Clinical Therapeutics, 32*(Suppl A), S3-S20.

Stokes, C., & Peet, M. (2003). Dietary sugar and polyunsaturated fatty acid consumption as predictors of severity of schizophrenia symptoms. *Nutrition and Neuroscience, 7*(4), 247-249.

Stompe, T., Ortwein-Soboda, G., & Ritter, K. (2002). Are we witnessing the disappearance of catatonic schizophrenia? *Comprehensive Psychiatry, 43,* 167-174.

Sullivan, P. F., Cendler, K. S., & Neale, M. C. (2003). Schizophrenia as a complex trait: Evidence from a meta-analysis of twin studies. *Archives of General Psychiatry, 60,* 1187-1192.

Susser, E., Neugebauer, R., Hoek, H. W., et al. (1996). Schizophrenia after prenatal famine. Further evidence. *Archives of General Psychiatry, 53,* 25-31.

Talkowski, M. E., Kirov, G., Bamne, M., et al. (2008). A network of dopaminergic gene variations implicated as risk factors for schizophrenia. *Human Molecular Genetics, 17,* 747-758.

Tan, W., Wang, Y., Gold, B., et al. (2007). Molecular cloning of a brain-specific, developmentally regulated neuregulin 1 (NRG1) isoform and identification of a functional promoter variant associated with schizophrenia. *Journal of Biological Chemistry, 282,* 24343-24351.

Tandon, R., Marcus, R. N., & Stork, E. G. (2006). A prospective, multicenter, randomized, parallel group, open-label study of aripiprazole in the management of patients with schizophrenia or schizoaffective disorder in generally psychiatry practice: Broad Effectiveness Trial with Aripiprazole (BETA). *Schizophrenia Research, 84,* 77-89.

Tandon, R., Keshavan, M. S., & Nasrallah, H. A. (2008). Schizophrenia, "just the facts": What we know in 2008. Epidemiology and etiology. *Schizophrenia Research, 102,* 1-18.

Tandon, R., Nasrallah, H. A., & Keshavan, M. S. (2009). Schizophrenia, "just the facts" 4. Clinical features and conceptualization. *Schizophrenia Research, 110,* 1-23.

Taylor, J. (2002). Development of a screening tool to assess risk of tardive dyskinesia. *British Journal of Nursing, 11,* 374-378.

Temple, S., & Ho, B. C. (2005). Cognitive therapy for persistent psychosis in schizophrenia: A case-controlled clinical trial. *Schizophrenia Research, 74,* 195-199.

Terezhalmy, G. T., Riley, C., & Moore, W. S. (2002). Tardive dyskinesia. *Quintessence International, 33,* 326-327.

Test, M. A., & Stein, L: I. (1980). Alternative to mental hospital treatment-III Social Cost. *Archives of General Psychiatry, 37,* 409-412.

Tiihonen, J., Lonnqvist, J., Wahlbeck, K., et al. (2009). 11-year follow-up of mortality in patients with schizophrenia: A population-based cohort study (FIN11study). *Lancet, 374*(9690), 620-627.

Tollefson, G. D., Beasley, C. M., Tran, P. V., et al. (1997). Olanzapine versus haloperidol in the treatment of schizophrenia and schizoaffective and schizophreniform disorders: Results of an international collaborative trial. *American Journal of Psychiatry, 154,* 457-465.

Tollefson, G. D., Sanger, T. M., Lu, Y., et al. (1998). Depressive signs and symptoms in schizophrenia: A prospective blinded trial of olanzapine and haloperidol. *Archives of General Psychiatry, 55,* 250-258.

Torrey, E. F., Miller, J., Rawlings, R., et al. (1997). Seasonality of birth in schizophrenia and bipolar disorder: A review of the literature. *Schizophrenia Research, 28,* 1-38.

Tosato, S., & Lasalvia, A. (2009). The contribution of epidemiology to defining the most appropriate approach to genetic research on schizophrenia. *Epidemiology and Social Psychiatry, 18*(2), 81-90.

Tucker, G. J., Campion, E. W., & Silberforth, P. M. (1975). Sensorimotor function and cognitive disturbance in schizophrenia. *American Journal of Psychiatry, 132,* 17-21.

Turkington, D., Dudley, R., Warman, D. M., et al. (2004). Cognitive behavioral therapy for schizophrenia: A review. *Journal of Psychiatric Practice, 10*(1), 5-16.

Turkington, D., Sensky, T., Scott, J., et al. (2008). A randomized controlled trial of cognitive behavioral therapy for persistent symptoms in schizophrenia: A 5-year follow-up. *Schizophrenia Research, 98,* 1-7.

Umbricht, D. S., Pollack, S., & Kane, J. M. (1994). Clozapine and weight gain. *Journal of Clinical Psychiatry, 55*(Suppl B), 157-160.

Ungvari, G. S., Coggins, W., Leung, S. K., et al. (2007). Schizophrenia with prominent catatonic features ('catatonic schizophrenia'). II. Factor analysis of the catatonic syndrome. *Progress in Neuro-psychopharmacology & Biological Psychiatry, 31,* 462-468.

United States Department of Health and Human Services. (2010). The benefits of physical activity. Retrieved from http://www.cdc.gov/physicalactivity/everyone/health/index.html

United States Food and Drug Administration. (2009). Chantix and Zyban to get boxed warning on serious mental health events. Retrieved from http://www.fda.gov/ForConsumers/ConsumerUpdates/ucm170356.htm

Uranova, N., Orlovskaya, D., Vikhreva, D., et al. (2001). Electron microscopy of oligodendroglia in severe mental illness. *Brain Research Bulletin, 55*(5), 597-610.

Van Gaal, L. F. (2006). Long-term health considerations in schizophrenia: Metabolic effects and the role of abdominal adiposity. *European Neuropsychopharmacology, 16*(Suppl 3), S142-S 148.

Van Haren, N. E., Hulshoff Pol, H. E., Schnack, H. G., et al. (2007). Focal gray matter changes in schizophrenia across the course of the illness: A five-year follow-up study. *Neuropsychopharmacology, 32*(10), 2057-2066.

Van Os, J., Burns, T., Cavallaro, R., et al. (2006). Standardized remission criteria in schizophrenia. *Acta Psychiatrica Scandanavica, 113*(2), 91-95.

Van Putten, T., & May, P. R. A. (1978). "Akinetic depression" in schizophrenia. *Archives of General Psychiatry, 35,* 1101-1107.

van Winkel, R., Myin-Germeys, I., & De Hert, M. (2007). The association between cognition and functional outcome in first episode patients with schizophrenia: Mystery solved. *Acta Psychiatrica Scandanavica, 116,* 119-124.

Velligan, D. I., Lam, F., Ereshefsky, L., et al. (2003). Psychopharmacology, perspectives on medication adherence and atypical antipsychotic medications. *Psychiatric Services, 54,* 665-667.

Velligan, D. I., Newcomer, J., Pultz, J., et al. (2002). Does cognitive function improve with quetiapine in comparison to haloperidol? *Schizophrenia Research, 53,* 239-248.

Vreeland, B., Minsk, S., Menza, M., et al. (2003). A program for managing weight gain associated with atypical antipsychotics. *Psychiatric Services, 54*(8), 1155-1157.

Walker, A. M., Lanza, I. L., Arellano, F., et al. (1997). Mortality in current and former users of clozapine. *Epidemiology, 8,* 671-677.

Walker, E., & Green, M. (1982). Soft signs of neurological dysfunction in schizophrenia. *Biological Psychiatry, 17,* 381-386.

Walker, E., & Lewine, R. J. (1990). Prediction of adult-onset schizophrenia from childhood home movies of the patients. *American Journal of Psychiatry, 147,* 1052-1056.

Walkowitz, O. M., & Pickar, D. (1991). Benzodiazepines in the treatment of schizophrenia: A review and reappraisal. *American Journal of Psychiatry, 148,* 714-726.

Wang, J. F., Shao, C., Sun, X., et al. (2009). Increased oxidative stress in the anterior cingulate cortex of subjects with bipolar disorder and schizophrenia. *Bipolar Disorders, 11,* 523-529.

Weder, N., Muralee, S., Penland, H., et al. (2008). Catatonia: A review. *Annals of Clinical Psychiatry, 20,* 97-107.

Wedding, D., Boyd, M. A., & Niemiec, R. M. (2010). *Movies and mental illness 3: Using films to understand psychopathology* (3rd ed.) (pp. 128-131). Cambridge, MA: Hogrefe.

Weiden, P., Aquila, R., & Standard, J. (1996). Atypical antipsychotic drugs and long term outcome in schizophrenia. *Journal of Clinical Psychiatry, 57*(Suppl 11), 53-60.

Weiden, P. J., & Olfson, M. (1995). Cost of relapse in schizophrenia. *Schizophrenia Bulletin, 21,* 419-429.

Weiden, P. J., Simpson, G. M., Potkin, G. G., et al. (2003). Effectiveness of switching to ziprasidone for stable but symptomatic outpatients with schizophrenia. *Journal of Clinical Psychiatry, 64,* 58

Wexler, B. E., Zhu, H., Bell, M. D., et al. (2009). Neuropsychological near normality and brain structure abnormality in schizophrenia. *American Journal of Psychiatry, 166*(2), 189-195.

Wilcox, J. A., & Nasrallah, H. A. (1987). Childhood head trauma and psychosis. *Psychiatry Research, 21,* 303-306.

Wilkins, J. N. (1997). Pharmacotherapy of schizophrenia patients with comorbid substance abuse. *Schizophrenia Bulletin, 23*(2), 1215-1228.

Williams, J. W., Jr., Noel, P. H., Cordes, J. A., et al. (2002). Is this patient clinically depressed? *Journal of the American Medical Association, 287,* 1160-1170.

Williams, N. M., O'Donnovan, M. C., & Owen, M. J. (2006). Chromosomal 22 deletion syndrome and schizophrenia. *International Reviews in Neurobiology, 73,* 1-27.

Winterer, G. (2010). Why do patients with schizophrenia smoke? *Current Opinion in Psychiatry, 23,* 112-119.

Wobrock, T., & Soyka, M. (2009). Pharmacotherapy of patients with schizophrenia and substance abuse. *Expert Opinion in Pharmacotherapy, 10*(3), 353-367.

Wohl, M., & Gorwood, P. (2007). Paternal ages below of above 35 years old are associated with a different risk of schizophrenia in the offspring. *European Psychiatry, 22,* 22-26.

Woodberry, K. A., Guiliano, A. J., & Seidman, I. J. (2008). Premorbid IQ in schizophrenia: A meta-analytic review. *American Journal of Psychiatry, 165,* 579-587.

Woods, S. W., Tandy, M., & McGlashan, T. H. (2001). The "prodromal" patient: Both symptomatic and at-risk. *CNS Spectrums, 6,* 223-232.

World Schizophrenia Fellowship. (1998). *Families as Partners in care: A document developed to launch a strategy for the implementation of programs of family training, education, and support.* Toronto, Ontario, Canada: World Schizophrenia Fellowship.

Wu, M. K., Wang, C. K., Bai, Y. M., et al. (2007). Outcomes of obese clozapine-treated in patients with schizophrenia placed on a 6-month diet and physical activity program. *Psychiatric Services, 58,* 544-550.

Wu, R. R., Zhao, J. P., Guo, X. F., et al. (2008a). Metformin addition attenuates olanzapine-induced weight gain in drug-naïve first-episode schizophrenia patients: A double-blind, placebo-controlled study. *American Journal of Psychiatry, 165,* 352-358.

Wu, R. R., Zhao, J. P., Jin, H., et al. (2008b). Lifestyle intervention and metformin for treatment of antipsychotic-induced weight gain: A randomized controlled trial. *Journal of the American Medical Association, 299,* 185-193.

Wykes, T., Steel, C., Everitt, B., et al. (2008). Cognitive behavioral therapy for schizophrenia: Effect sizes, clinical models, and methodological rigor. *Schizophrenia Bulletin, 34,* 523-537.

Yang, S., & McNeely, M. J. (2002). Rhabdomyolysis, pancreatitis and hyperglycemia with ziprasidone. *American Journal of Psychiatry, 159,* 1435.

Yeung, P. P., Carson, W. H., Saha, A. R., et al. (2001). Efficacy of aripiprazole, a novel antipsychotic, in schizophrenia and schizoaffective disorder: Results of a placebo-controlled trial with risperidone. *European Neuropsychopharmacology, 3*(Suppl 11), S241.

Young, N. S. (1994). Agranulocytosis. *Journal of the American Medical Association, 271,* 935-938.

Yuii, K., Suzuki, M., & Kurachi, M. (2007). Stress sensitization in schizophrenia. *Annals of the New York Academy of Sciences, USA, 1113,* 276-290.

Yung, A. R., & McGorry, P. D. (1996). The initial prodrome in psychosis: Descriptive and qualitative aspects. *Australian and New Zealand Journal of Psychiatry, 30,* 587-599.

Answers to Case Study 15-1 Questions

1. Meets diagnostic criteria for schizophrenia, paranoid type.
2. Rule out:
   - Substance-induced psychotic disorder. Ruled out by symptoms in the absence of marijuana use (abstinence by report [need collateral information] and abstinence while in hospital).
   - Psychotic disorder due to a general medical condition. Ruled out by history, physical, labs, and computed tomography.
   - Mood disorder with psychotic features. Ruled out because mood symptoms are not prominent and psychotic symptoms occur when mood symptoms are not present.
   - Schizoaffective disorder. Ruled out because no mood episode is current with active schizophrenia symptoms, and mood symptoms are brief compared to total duration of disturbance.
3. Immediate assessment: history, vital signs, height, weight, abdominal circumference, complete blood count, electrolyte levels, infectious diseases panel, pregnancy test, drug screen, fasting blood glucose, lipid panel, electrocardiogram, prolactin level, extrapyramidal symptom assessment, and tardive dyskinesia assessment.
4. Restart risperidone since she had a positive response to it historically. Dosage range is 4–8 mg PO. Side effects are weight gain, sedation, orthostatic hypotension, and glucose dysregulation. Monitoring includes fasting blood glucose, lipid monitoring, and nutrition and exercise counseling. Also could consider Risperidal Consta in view of past noncompliance with oral medications.
5. Education about the importance of adherence to maintaining stability and reducing hospitalization. Carefully question about side effects that could influence adherence (e.g., weight gain), work as a team to manage side effects in a manner satisfactory to patient. Monitor adherence by asking directly, seeking collateral information from the family if possible. Enlist the help of family in adherence monitoring and consider telephone follow-up calls between face-to-face visits.
6. Assess risk factors and protective factors, discuss quality of life and reasons for living, and directly ask about the presence of suicidal thoughts, plans, and intent. Increase patient contact, limit access to means of self-harm, set up crisis plans (i.e., safety contract, provide number for mobile crisis), consider antidepressant medication and, as a last resort, inpatient hospitalization.
7. Psychosocial interventions include individual and family therapy, cognitive behavioral therapy (CBT), social skills training (SST), patient education, and referrals for Assertive Community Treatment (ACT) and self-help groups.
   - Immediate individual and family therapy
     - Short-term goal: increased trust in provider
     - Long-term goal: attendance and participation in groups
   - After these goals are met, consider SST and/or CBT
     - Short-term goal for SST: successful role-play of specific social skills, for example, small talk
     - Long-term goal for SST: development of new friendships
     - Short-term goal for CBT: verbalize relationship between thoughts, feelings, and behavior
     - Long-term goal for CBT: analysis of effect of thoughts on feelings and behaviors
   - Consider referral to ACT program if available
     - Short-term goal: housing stability
     - Long-term goal: reduction of hospitalization
   - Follow-up assessments (in addition to weekly meetings for SST, CBT, and ACT team activities):
     - First month after discharge: telephone follow-up twice a week and face-to-face meetings weekly
     - Second month after discharge: telephone follow-up at least weekly and at least one face-to-face meeting
     - Every 3 months thereafter: telephone follow-up as needed and face-to-face assessment every 3 months
   - Patient education: adherence, expected medication side effects, when to see the provider, emergency plans, neuroleptic malignant syndrome symptoms, diet teaching (as appropriate for cultural group)
   - Referrals: possible referrals for self-help groups for patient and family: Recovery International and National Alliance on Mental Illness.
8. Health promotion activities include a physiological assessment, a discussion of birth control options, consideration of cultural values, and information about smoking cessation:
   - Physiological assessment:
     - Assess motivation and interest in a fitness program in consultation with the primary care provider (as appropriate for cultural group)
     - Assess for obesity: family history including history of cardiovascular disease, hypertension, diabetes, obesity, and dyslipidemias
     - Obtain measurement of height and weight to calculate BMI (as appropriate for cultural group)
   - Birth control: Assess level of sexual activity and patient preference as to birth control method, including importance of notifying the provider immediately of missed menses and the pros and cons of psychiatric medications if pregnancy occurs. Gynecologist referral for preventive care and check-ups.
   - Culture: One cultural characteristic of Asian individuals is the importance of family, particularly great respect for one's parents and other elders. In keeping with this, include the patient's parents in treatment plans and decisions if she desires.
   - Smoking cessation: Assess smoking behavior by self-report and parental report, assess readiness and interest in smoking cessation, and teach short- and long-term health effects of nicotine use and effect of smoking on effectiveness of psychiatric medications. When patient expresses desire/readiness, explore smoking cessation treatments including nicotine replacement, bupropion, and psychosocial approaches. Assess effect of treatment via self-report and parental report of smoking behavior and possible by physical health assessments, e.g., chest x-ray.

CHAPTER 16

Dementia and Delirium

Eris F. Perese, APRN-PMH

Dementia and delirium are cognitive disorders. Patients with dementia and delirium have symptoms of impaired memory and problems with abstract thinking and judgment. Whereas dementia is characterized by many cognitive deficits in addition to impairment of memory with an insidious onset, often *over many years*, delirium is characterized by a disturbance of consciousness and a change in cognition that develops *over a short time*, usually hours to days (Weiner, Garrett, & Bret, 2009). Delirium can often be a symptom of dementia, but patients with delirium do not necessarily have dementia. Table 16-1 presents the differential diagnosis of dementia and delirium.

Some impairment of cognitive functioning is common as individuals grow older. Therefore, the symptoms of dementia must be differentiated from those of normal aging and of mild cognitive impairment (Weiner et al., 2009).

Normal Aging and Cognitive Changes

Older adults often complain of forgetting people's names, losing their keys, and forgetting telephone numbers, but their vocabulary, memory for general information, and memory of historical or personal events usually remains intact (Petersen, Smith, Kokmen, et al., 1992; Weiner et al., 2009). Memory problems have been found to increase with age. For example, among older adults between the ages of 65 and 69, only 4% have been found to have moderate to severe memory problems, but among those 85 years old or older, 36% have moderate to severe memory problems (Federal Interagency Forum on Aging Related Statistics, 2000).

Normal aging is associated with a decline in memory performance, cognitive speed, learning of new material, recalling details, visuospatial functioning, ability to find the right word, and executive functioning (Weiner et al., 2009). Memory performance depends on both crystallized intelligence and fluid intelligence. *Crystallized intelligence* embodies the learning, knowledge, and skills that are acquired over a lifetime. Crystallized intelligence increases up to the age of 60 or 70 years and may not decline until after 85 years (Christensen, 2001); crystallized verbal abilities, such as vocabulary and sight-reading, do not deteriorate with age (Weiner et al.). *Fluid intelligence* involves one's current ability to reason, problem-solve, and deal with complex information. It peaks in early adulthood and then gradually declines (Serwach, 2008).

Problems with remembering as individuals age appear to be due to a widening focus of attention that makes it more difficult to hold one fact, such as a name or a telephone number. Older people take in more information from a situation and then are able to combine it with their comparatively greater stored general knowledge (Reistad-Long, 2008; Sorrel, 2008).

Whereas younger individuals use one side of the brain's prefrontal cortex in carrying out new memory tasks, older adults use both sides. They use more neuronal circuits to process the information to be learned (Persson, Sylvester, Nelson, et al., 2004).

However, changes in brain functioning are not the same for all aging individuals. Genetic factors account for approximately 50% of cognitive variability in older adults (Spar & LaRue, 2006). Poor health—such as with decreased lung functioning, atrial fibrillation, and cardiovascular disease—is associated with a more rapid cognitive decline. Other factors associated with more rapid cognitive decline include lower levels of education, fewer mentally stimulating activities, and less physical exercise. The presence of depression more than doubles the risk of a transition from normal aging to a greater cognitive decline known as mild cognitive impairment (MCI), which will be discussed in the next section (Geda, Knopman, Mrazek, et al., 2006).

There are also protective factors for cognitive function. Maintenance of cognitive function in older adults is associated with having achieved a high school education or greater, having at least a ninth grade literacy level, being employed or volunteering, engaging in moderately vigorous

TABLE 16-1 DIFFERENTIAL DIAGNOSIS OF DELIRIUM AND DEMENTIA

Feature	Delirium	Dementia
Onset of symptoms	Abrupt	Gradual
Course	Fluctuating course over the course of the day	Slow progressive deterioration. In dementia with Lewy bodies, there will be fluctuation of cognition.
Duration	Weeks	Years
Sleep	Disrupted	Normal
Speech	Rapid, incoherent	Trouble finding words, slow
Perceptions	Illusions and visual hallucinations	Normal in early stages

exercise, having social support and good health (absence of diabetes, hypertension, and depression), having one glass of alcohol a day, and not smoking (Yaffee, Fiocco, Linquist, et al., 2009). For example, the Maastricht Aging Study showed that middle-age and older adults who routinely engaged in intellectual, social, and physical activities had a decreased rate of cognitive decline (Bosma, van Boxtel, Ponds, et al., 2002).

Mild Cognitive Impairment (MCI)

Dementia is thought to be preceded by a preclinical stage of decline in cognition that is different from that of normal aging (Backman, 2008; Flicker, Ferris, & Reisberg, 1991; Larrieu, Letenneur, Orgogozo, et al., 2002). This state of early changes in cognition is frequently called *mild cognitive impairment*. MCI is a cognitive decline that is greater than that expected for the patient's age and educational level but that does not interfere with functioning (Bourgeois, Seaman, & Servis, 2008). Geda, Negash, and Petersen (2009, p. 173) referred to MCI as "the gray zone" between normal cognitive aging and early dementia. The main predictors for transitioning from normal cognition to MCI are having anxiety or depression, increased systolic blood pressure, a history of past high levels of alcohol intake, and a history of smoking (Cherbuin, Reglade-Meslin, Kumar, et al., 2009).

Patients with MCI have deterioration of memory performances that can be identified using screening tools or a report of decline by the patient or others. This deterioration of memory represents early pathological changes of the hippocampus with resulting impairment of functioning (Knopman, 2010). In addition to cognitive problems, approximately 10% to 25% of patients with MCI have symptoms of dysphoria (depression and anguish), irritability, apathy, anxiety, and agitation (Apostolova & Cummings, 2010). Activities of daily living are not impaired, and other functioning is usually not impaired or only minimally impaired (Palmer, Backman, Winblad, et al., 2008; Winblad, Palmer, Kivipelto, et al., 2004).

Epidemiology

Prevalence

Prevalence of MCI without dementia using strict criteria (memory deficits, but no impairment of other cognitive functioning and no impairment of activities of daily living) ranges from 3% to 19% of adults older than 65 years (Gauthier, Reisberg, Zaudig, et al., 2006).

Risk Factors

Risk factors for the development of MCI include older age, lower level of education completed, presence of apolipoprotein E (*APOE*) *e4* allele (Boyle, Buchman, Wilson, et al., 2010), low performance on cognitive tests, cortical atrophy, infarcts in the brain, depression, and African American race (Lopez, Jagust, Dulberg, et al., 2003). Midlife hypertension and hypercholesterolemia are believed to increase the risk of MCI (Kivipelto, Helkala, Hänninen, et al., 2001). Lack of exercise may be a risk factor. For example, recently, it has been reported that moderate exercise in late life was associated with a 32% reduced risk for the development of MCI (Geda, Roberts, Knopman, et al., 2010).

Etiology and Biological Basis

MCI is thought to be due to many causes—degenerative disorders such as Alzheimer's disease (AD); vascular, metabolic, or medical disorders; traumatic events; psychiatric disorders such as depression and substance abuse; and response to medications such as antihistamines (Spar & LaRue, 2006; Winblad et al., 2004). The neuropathology of MCI involves changes in the medial temporal lobe and hippocampus and a decrease of overall brain volume that are similar to the early changes seen with dementia of Alzheimer's type (Knopman, 2010).

Clinical Presentation

Older adults often present with complaints of memory problems, such as difficulty remembering recent events and future commitments. Sometimes a family member has noticed memory problems and has urged the patient to seek treatment. The patient's general cognitive functioning is normal, and there is usually no difficulty in carrying out normal activities of living (Geda et al., 2009).

Treatment

Although there is no treatment that can prevent the progression of MCI to dementia, acetylcholinesterase inhibitors may delay it (Saykin, Wishart, Rabin, et al., 2004); for instance, donepezil (Aricept) was found to reduce the risk of MCI's progressing to AD for the first 18 months of a trial study (Petersen, Thomas, Grundman, et al., 2005), and controlling risk factors—such as hypertension, diabetes, atrial fibrillation, and low folate levels—may help prevent conversion of MCI to vascular dementia (VaD) (Ravaglia, Forti, Maioli, et al., 2006).

Course

Although MCI may be a transitional period between normal aging and dementia for some individuals, other individuals with MCI do not develop dementia. Some remain stable, and some recover (Winblad et al., 2004); however, more than half develop dementia within 5 years (Bourgeois et al., 2008). Risk for progressing to dementia is related to greater severity of memory impairment at baseline and the presence of comorbid depression, the combination of which doubles the risk (Modrego & Ferrández, 2004). Transitioning to AD is greater among those with MCI whose symptoms include olfactory deficits (impaired ability to identify odors); memory impairment plus impairment of other cognitive areas such as language, attention, visuospatial functioning, and executive functioning; and an informant's reporting of impairment of functioning (Devanand, Liu, Tabert, et al., 2008; Knopman, 2010; Tabert, Manley, Liu, et al., 2006). Most conversion to AD occurs within 3 years of development of symptoms of MCI (Devanand et al.).

However, in addition to the risk conferred by MCI, the majority of older adults have some type of brain pathology (Bachman 2008; Schneider, Arvanitakis, Bang, et al., 2007). In a study that followed older adults with a mean age of 88 until their death and then examined their brains on autopsy, Schneider et al. found that whereas the brains of older adults without dementia had evidence of one type of brain pathology such as AD, vascular disease, Parkinson's disease, or Lewy body disease, the brains of older adults with dementia had two or more types of pathology. They concluded that the greater the number of brain pathologies, the greater the risk for developing dementia (Schneider et al.).

PART ONE: Dementia

Introduction

Dementia is a syndrome that occurs primarily among older adults and is caused by neurodegenerative processes, trauma, strokes, immunological processes, and infections (Korczyn, 2009). The key feature is impairment of cognitive functioning, particularly memory.

Dementia and Subtypes of Dementia

Dementia is often categorized as cortical or subcortical (Weiner et al., 2009) and by subtypes.

Cortical and Subcortical Dementias

Cortical dementias involve the cortex of the brain and are characterized by prominent memory impairment, such as problems with recall and recognition; language deficits; apraxia; agnosia; visuospatial deficits; personality changes; and difficulties with judgment (Weiner et al., 2009). Cortical dementias include dementia of Alzheimer's type, frontotemporal dementia (FTD) (an example of which is Pick's disease), dementia due to Creutzfeldt-Jakob disease, and dementia due to chronic subdural hematoma (Bourgeois et al., 2008).

Subcortical dementias involve areas below the cortex, e.g., the thalamus, basal ganglia, and brainstem. Subcortical dementias include dementia due to HIV, Parkinson's disease, Huntington's disease, Wilson's disease, and multiple sclerosis. Symptoms include greater impairment of recall and memory, decreased verbal fluency, bradyphrenia (slowed thinking), depressed mood, affective lability, apathy, difficulty concentrating, and deficits in social judgment. There are more motor signs than in cortical dementias (Bourgeois et al., 2008; Doody, Garivlova, Sano, et al., 1998; Geldmacher & Whitehouse, 1997).

Some dementias have both cortical and subcortical characteristics. The most common of these are vascular dementia (multi-infarct dementia and post-stroke dementia), mixed dementia (AD and vascular dementia), dementia with Lewy bodies (DLB), and dementia due to trauma (Lipton & Rubin, 2009).

Dementia Subtypes

Although dementia also occurs as part of other disorders (such as Parkinson's disease, systemic lupus erythematosus, and multiple sclerosis), as a sequela to infectious diseases (such as Creutzfeldt-Jakob disease, syphilis, and HIV), and as a result of trauma and alcohol abuse (Ngandu, 2006), the four major subtypes of dementia are considered to be

1. Alzheimer's disease
2. Vascular dementia
3. Dementia with Lewy bodies
4. Frontotemporal dementia

The symptoms and behaviors of the different subtypes of dementia may be similar, but each type is characterized by specifics of age of onset, symptoms that require different approaches and treatments, course, and duration (Yuhas, McGowan, Fontaine, et al., 2006). This chapter discusses characteristics of all dementias first and then covers the characteristics of the individual subtypes.

All Types of Dementia

Dementia is associated with an acquired impairment of cognitive functioning (Weiner, 2009) and is America's third most costly health condition (following cancer and heart disease) (Breitner & Albert, 2009). The impairment of cognition is severe enough to cause limitations of memory, self-care, and family, social, and occupational functioning (Bossen, 2009; Ngandu, 2006). The initial symptoms of impaired cognitive functioning are followed by changes in affect, personality, and behavior that are disruptive to patients and their families, negatively affect their quality of life, and may even endanger their safety (Yuhas et al., 2006).

Dementia affects patients' quality of life through its effect on their cognitive, interpersonal, vocational, and social functioning; through its effect on their autonomy; and through its effect on their ability to be independent. Dementia increases their vulnerability for accidents related to water, fire, or electrical hazards; for falls; for getting lost; for developing physical health problems and psychiatric problems; and for emotional, physical, and financial abuse (Bossen, 2009; Savva & Brayne, 2009).

Dementia also affects the family of patients with the illness. The primary care providers are often spouses or adult children who, without knowledge or preparation, must deal with the responsibility of caring for someone with the cognitive, emotional, and behavioral problems associated with dementia. Caregivers of patients with dementia often feel overwhelmed and physically threatened by aggressive behavior. In comparison to noncaregivers, they experience higher rates of biopsychosocial health problems—hypertension, loss of sleep, poor diet, anxiety, depression, and loneliness (Beach, Schulz, Yee, et al., 2000; Gallagher-Thompson, Lonergan, Holland, et al., 2009). Often they must reduce their hours of employment, their time spent with their children, and their social activities. They suffer financial losses, are unable to save for retirement or their children's college education, and are at risk for earlier death. The impact on children in the family is seen in less time for the caregiver to participate in the children's school and other activities, less financial resources for their present education, and fewer resources for their college education (Beach, Schulz, Williamson, et al., 2005; Reyes & Shi, 2006).

Dementia's impact on society is most evident in its cost, which includes costs for direct care, costs for treatment of medical comorbid conditions, and lost productivity of patients and their care providers. Eighty percent of patients with dementia receive informal care, usually from family members. Among these care providers, 60% have to reduce their work hours; 42% report being late for work because of caregiving responsibilities; and 39% take sick leave. Some are forced to take early retirement to provide full-time care for a family member with dementia (Savva & Brayne, 2009).

Epidemiology

Prevalence

Dementia affects about 1% of the population under 65 years of age. The prevalence doubles every 5 years after the age of 55 years (Savva & Brayne, 2009), and at age 85 years and older, the prevalence is 50% (Avramopoulos, 2009). AD accounts for the majority of cases of dementia, 60% to 75% of all cases (Fratiglioni, Launer, Andersen, et al., 2000a; Qiu, Kivipelto, & von Strauss, 2009; Yuhas et al., 2006).

Age of Onset

Dementia is described as early-onset dementia (EOD) (sometimes called presenile dementia) when the onset is before age 65 years (sometimes early onset is defined as before 60 years of age) and as late-onset dementia (LOD) when the onset occurs after age 65 years (Alzheimer's Association, 2006; McMurtray, Clark, Christine, et al., 2006). LODs include AD, DLB, and parkinsonian disorder with dementia (McMurtray et al.).

EODs include AD, FTD, VaD, cerebral vasculitis, Parkinson's disease (in which dementia can also have a late onset), Huntington's disease, progressive supranuclear palsy, multiple sclerosis, amyotropic lateral sclerosis, traumatic brain injury, HIV, chronic alcoholism, chronic drug abuse, and brain tumors (Arciniegas & Dubovsky, 2007; Sampson, Warren, & Rossor, 2004; Werner, Stein-Shvachman, & Korczyn, 2009). EOD also occurs frequently among adults with Down's syndrome (Arciniegas & Dubovsky). Some of the symptoms of EOD are similar to those of LOD, such as memory loss, depression, and anxiety. Symptoms in EOD not commonly present in LOD include delusions and hallucinations, aggressive behavior, difficulties in finding the right words, and problems with concentration (Hasse, 2005; Werner et al., 2009). Patients with EOD face loss of independence and changes in their roles as employee, breadwinner, and parent that affect their sense of self-esteem and worth. Their illness may require caregiving by young adults in the family and may severely affect the family's financial security (Werner et al.). Patients with EOD have an increased mortality risk in comparison to individuals of similar age without EOD and in comparison to patients with LOD (Koedam, Pijnenburg, Deeg, et al., 2008).

Projected Increase in Prevalence

As the population ages, the number of individuals with dementia is anticipated to increase in both developed and developing countries: Korczyn (2009) estimated that the number of individuals with dementia will double every 20 years. It is estimated that the prevalence of dementia will quadruple in the next 50 years if nothing is done to decrease the incidence of dementia (i.e., the development of new cases) (Brookmeyer, Gray, & Kawas, 1998). Some researchers have described the potential increase in dementia as the biggest health-care challenge of the 21st century (Avramopoulos, 2009); others have called it a dementia epidemic (Korczyn & Vakhapova, 2007). These projections are fueling the urgency to identify modifiable risk factors in order to prevent cognitive decline and delay the onset of dementia (Korczyn & Vakhapova; Lautenschlager, Almeida, & Flicker, 2003). According to Korczyn and Vakhapova, "Because the prevalence of dementia doubles every 5 years, delay in the onset of dementia by five years is equivalent to a reduction of the prevalence by half in any given age group" (p. 3). They pointed out that prevention is based on understanding the etiology of dementia (genetic influence, infectious processes, vascular lesions, trauma, and degenerative processes) and on reducing the risk factors and increasing the protective factors associated with the development of dementia.

In the past, risk and protective factors have been identified primarily from retrospective studies that indicated the prevalence of certain factors among those who later develop dementia or who do not. More recent studies have obtained baseline measures of risk and protective factors and then followed the individuals forward for 20 years to determine which individuals develop dementia.

Risk Factors

Some risk factors for the development of dementia can be modified and some cannot. The primary risk factor for dementia—advanced age—cannot be modified. The incidence of dementia is higher in women, and this risk factor also cannot be changed (Savva & Brayne, 2009). Genetic influences, such as having the apolipoprotein gene with the e4 allele (*APOE e4*), which increases vulnerability for the development of AD, cannot be changed; however, the vulnerability conferred by the *APOE e4* gene may be influenced by other factors such as high cholesterol levels (Savva & Brayne). Other risk factors include events, conditions, or lifestyle practices that are present in middle adulthood—years before the onset of dementia—and risk factors that occur in old age, some of which are modifiable (Lee, Back, Kim, et al., 2010; Savva & Brayne).

Risk Factors for Dementia That Occur at Middle Age

Risk factors for the development of dementia that occur at middle age include physical trauma to the head, untreated hypertension, diabetes mellitus, high total cholesterol, obesity, smoking, coronary artery disease, depression, low level of education, and physical, mental, and social inactivity (Korczyn, 2009; Savva & Brayne, 2009). Other risk factors include exposure to medications with anticholinergic properties (which further deplete acetylcholine), surgery with general anesthesia, environmental factors such as poverty, and lack of social support.

Trauma to the Head

Each year in the United States, there are 1.1 million emergency room visits for traumatic brain injuries (Centers for Diseases Control and Prevention, 2007); however, the actual number of traumatic brain injuries is likely much higher because individuals with mild cases are not usually taken to the emergency room (Bigler, 2009; Langlois, Marr, Mitchko, et al., 2005). For example, concussion is a frequent occurrence in sports, and most individuals recover within days; however, among individuals with repetitive concussions, 17% develop traumatic encephalopathy (Roberts, Allsop, & Bruton, 1990). Even in patients who have appeared to recover from a trauma to the head, the injury to the brain is a vulnerability factor that increases the risk of their developing dementia later in life (McKee, Cantu, Nowinski, et al., 2009; Plassman, Havlik, Steffens, et al., 2000; Starkstein & Jorge, 2005), especially when there are additional risk factors such as genetic vulnerability, diabetes, cardiovascular disease, other head injuries, and drug and alcohol abuse (Bigler).

It has long been known that repeated injury to the brain experienced in boxing is associated with progressive neurological deterioration and dementia, a condition called dementia pugilistica (McKee et al., 2009, p. 709). It is now known that brain injuries may be incurred in other sports, such as soccer (in which players "head" the ball or experience concussions from contact with other players or goal posts) (Koutures & Gregory, 2010). Jordan, Green, Galanty, et al. (1996) found that chronic encephalopathy in soccer players was associated with acute head injuries encountered during play (hitting each other's heads or the goal posts) rather than with "heading the ball." However, in an earlier study examining soccer players who were over 65 years old, Sortland and Tysvaer (1989) found that cerebral atrophy was present in one-third of the soccer players and that it occurred more frequently among the players who were the most frequent "headers." Although studies of soccer players and later development of dementia are inconclusive, it is hypothesized that their head injuries may result in chronic traumatic encephalopathy (Barnett & Curran, 2003).

Chronic traumatic encephalopathy results in atrophy of the cerebral hemispheres and development of neurofibrillary tangles and tangles of astrocytes (glial cells), and it is manifested in deterioration of memory and ability to concentrate, headaches, confusion, and disorientation. There may be progression to poor judgment, lack of insight, and dementia. The risk for developing dementia following head trauma increases with the severity of the trauma (Plassman et al., 2000). In another study, head trauma has been found to be associated with increased risk of developing a specific type of dementia, frontotemporal dementia (Rosso, Landweer, Houterman, et al., 2003b).

Hypertension

Hypertension has been found to be associated with increased risk of dementia (Peters, 2009). Untreated hypertension in middle-age men is associated with an increased risk for dementia in late life (Launer, Ross, Petrovitch, et al., 2000). In an early study, treatment of hypertension in older adults was associated with a 50% reduction in the incidence of dementia (Forette, Seux, Staessen, et al., 1998). Other studies have supported these earlier findings and have suggested that treatment of hypertension reduces the risk of developing VaD and possibly the risk of cognitive impairment due to other causes (Aronow & Frishman, 2006).

Diabetes

Diabetes is associated with an increased risk of both VaD and neurodegenerative dementia, and it is thought that midlife diabetes may play a role in AD. Even borderline diabetes or impaired glucose tolerance is associated with increased risk of dementia and AD in very old individuals (Xu, Qiu, Winblad, et al., 2007).

Obesity

Midlife obesity and even being overweight has been found to increase the risk for developing dementia (Whitmer, Gunderson, Quesenberry, et al., 2007). Obesity in combination with high blood pressure and high total cholesterol increases the risk of developing dementia by six times (Ngandu, 2006).

Cigarette Smoking

Midlife smoking has been found to be associated with a higher risk in later life of cognitive impairment (Galanis, Petrovitch, Launer, et al., 1997) and dementia (Reitz, den Heijer, van Duijn, et al., 2007). Exposure to secondhand smoke is also a risk factor. For example, older adults who have been exposed to 25 years or more of secondhand smoke are at increased risk of developing cognitive impairment and dementia (Barnes, Haight, Mehta, et al., 2010).

Physical Inactivity

Physical inactivity has been found to double the risk for dementia and AD (Abbott, White, Ross, et al., 2004; Kivipelto, Rovio, Ngandu, et al., 2008). For example, engagement twice weekly in physical leisure activities such as walking or dancing during youth and midlife was associated with a 50% lower risk for developing dementia later in life and a 60% lower risk for developing AD. The protective effect was stronger for individuals who were *APOE e4* carriers (Rovio, Kareholt, Helkala, et al., 2005).

High Cholesterol

Higher levels of cholesterol at midlife are associated with an increased risk of developing AD at age 65 or older (Anstey, Lipnicki, & Low, 2008). Individuals with high cholesterol levels and the *APOE e4* allele are at greater risk for developing AD than are those with the *APOE e4* allele without elevated cholesterol and those with high cholesterol alone (Kivipelto, Helkala, Laakso, et al., 2002). Reports on the use of statins that are used to reduce hypercholesterolemia are conflicting (Breitner & Albert, 2009). Rea, Breitner, Psaty, et al. (2005) reported that there is no difference in development of dementia between those who use statin drugs and those who do not. However, Li, Larson, Sonnen, et al. (2007) found on autopsy that use of statin was associated with reduced neurofibrillary changes.

Depression

Biringer, Mykletun, Dahl, et al. (2005) suggested that depression may be a prodromal symptom of dementia. Other researchers have considered depression to be a risk factor for cognitive decline and the development of cognitive impairment (Chodosh, Kado, Seeman, et al., 2007). It has been found that individuals who have experienced depression at some time during their life have twice the risk of developing dementia later in life in comparison to those without a prior history of depression (Gellis, McClive-Reed, & Brown, 2009; Ownby, Crocco, Acevedo, et al., 2006).

Protective Factors for Dementia That Occur at Middle Age

Factors associated with lower risk of developing dementia include educational achievement, Mediterranean diet, more mental activity, greater physical activity, and moderate use of alcohol. It is thought that the use of certain medications—antihypertensives, folic acid, vitamin B_{12}, and antioxidants—may reduce the risk of developing dementia (Korczyn & Vakhapova, 2007). Some researchers are studying the possibility that antihistamines may be protective against the development of dementia (Doody et al., 2008).

Higher Education

Higher levels of educational achievement are associated with maintenance of cognitive functioning and a lower risk of developing dementia (Farmer, Kittner, Rae, et al., 1995). This may be due to greater acquired brain reserve or to healthier lifestyle practices (Ngandu, 2006). Breitner and Albert (2009) said that the process of attaining higher levels of education may generate more synaptic connections, which provide more ways to process information. Among individuals who did not achieve high levels of education, complex work with data and with people has been found to be associated with lower risks for developing dementia, suggesting that the complexity of the work may offset less education (Karp, Andel, Parker, et al., 2009).

Cognitive/Brain Reserve

The concept of brain reserve (Valenzuela, 2008, p. 296) underlies the principle of "use it or lose it" as applied to maintaining optimal brain functioning and preventing dementia. At first, the term "brain reserve" was used to describe the finding that, on postmortem examination, some individuals with high levels of AD pathology who had not developed dementia had double the number of large pyramidal neurons in the cerebral cortex. It was concluded that these individuals might have started with more neurons and thus had more reserve to use. A more recent interpretation of brain reserve suggests that individuals who have acquired a range of cognitive strategies for solving complex problems have greater flexibility of brain functioning and a greater number of neural pathways that they can use in cognition. When some areas of the brain are damaged, they are able to use alternative brain networks.

Valenzuela (2008, p. 297) suggested that brain reserve is represented by "proxies"—level of education achieved, complexity of life occupations, diversity and frequency of social interactions, and cognitive challenges of past and present leisure activities—throughout life.

When the presence of these proxies was measured, it was found that a higher number of proxies was associated with lower rates of cognitive decline and a reduced rate of hippocampal atrophy. A meta-analysis of studies of complex mental activities and risk of dementia reported a risk reduction of 46% for high mental activity levels compared with low activity levels (Valenzuela & Sachdev, 2006). Valenzuela, Breakspear, and Sachdev (2007) suggested that clinical dementia may be thought of as a balance of network compensation versus disease process.

Diet

Among the U.S. population, individuals who adhere to a Mediterranean diet (Box 16-1) have a lower risk of developing dementia (Mitrou, Kipnis, Thiebaut, et al., 2007; Scarmeas, Stern, Tang, et al., 2006). It is proposed that the unsaturated fatty acids in the diet are involved in keeping nerve cell membranes and synaptic connections plastic, or better able to process information (Qiu et al., 2009). A moderate intake of polyunsaturated fats such as olive oil, avocados, and nuts at midlife is associated with a decreased risk of developing dementia later in life, whereas, a moderate intake of saturated fats such as butter, red meat, and eggs is associated with increased risk of developing dementia, especially among individuals who are *APOE e4* carriers (Laitinen, Ngandu, Rovio, et al., 2006). Similarly, high consumption of fatty fish, more than twice a week, has been found to be associated with reduced incidence of dementia overall and of AD among individuals who do not have the *APOE e4* allele (Huang, Zandi, Tucker, et al., 2005). High consumption of vegetables, particularly green leafy vegetables, has been found to be associated with a slower rate of cognitive decline (Morris, Evans, Tangney, et al., 2006). Morris et al. wrote, "The decrease in rate for persons who consumed greater than two vegetable servings per day was equivalent to about 5 years of younger age" (p. 1374). High consumption of fruit and vegetable juices, at least three times a week, has been found to be associated with a decreased risk of AD (Dai, Borenstein, Wu, et al., 2006). Midlife consumption of coffee has been found to be associated with lower incidence of dementia and AD in later life.

BOX 16-1 The Mediterranean Diet

The Mediterranean diet consists of

- Daily intake of fruits, vegetables, whole-grain breads, cereals, beans, nuts, seeds, unsaturated fatty acids such as olive oil, and low to moderate amounts of low-fat cheese and yogurt
- Weekly intake of fish and poultry and up to 4 eggs
- Intake of saturated fatty acids and meat should be limited to a few times per month.

Among the U.S. population, individuals who adhere to a Mediterranean diet have a lower risk of developing dementia.

Sources: Mitrou et al., 2007; Scarmeas et al., 2006.

The lowest risk was among those who drank three to four cups a day (Eskelinen, Ngandu, Tuomilehto, et al., 2009). No reduction of risk has been found among tea drinkers (Dai et al.). Taking supplements does not seem to have the same protective effect as eating a healthy diet (Donini, Felice, & Cannella, 2007).

Mental Activity

Intellectually challenging activities have been found to be associated with reduced risk of dementia (Carlson, Helms, Steffens, et al., 2008; Patterson, Feightner, Garcia, et al., 2007). There is some evidence that cognitive training may delay cognitive decline (Willis, Tennstedt, Marsiske, et al., 2006). In a 28-year prospective study of dementia, greater cognitive activity at midlife (age 50 years) was associated with a 26% reduction of dementia. In a subgroup of individuals with an *APOE e4* allele, there was a 30% reduction (Carlson et al., 2008). It was intermediate cognitive activity—home hobbies, home and family activities, club activities (parties and games), and visiting with family and friends—rather than novel information-processing activities—studying for courses, reading to master new information, or extra work—that was most strongly associated with reduced dementia risk. Even passive activities (going to the movies, watching television, doing crossword puzzles, and reading) were associated with reduced dementia risk.

Physical Activity

Recently, physical exercise at midlife such as gardening, walking, or participating in sports has been found to be associated with reduced risk for developing dementia, in comparison with engaging in hardly any exercise (Andel, Crowe, Pedersen, et al., 2008).

Moderate Use of Alcohol

Individuals who use alcohol moderately in midlife have lower rates of dementia than those who never drink alcohol and those who drink alcohol frequently (Anstey, Mack, & Cherbuin, 2009; Ngandu, 2006). Binge drinking has been found to be associated with increased risk of dementia (Jarvenpaa, Rinne, Koskenvuo, et al., 2005).

Risk Factors for Dementia That Occur at Old Age

In addition to advanced age and health problems such as cardiovascular disease and a history of bypass surgery (Barnes, Covinsky, Whitmer, et al., 2009) factors associated with cognitive decline in older adults include stress and depression (Brummel-Smith, 2007); smoking (Ott, Andersen, Dewey, et al., 2004); social isolation and loneliness (Wilson, Krueger, Arnold, et al., 2007b); and use of medications with anticholinergic properties (Nebes, Pollock, Meltzer, et al., 2005).

Stress

It is known that the brain responds to increased levels of stress with increased production of cortisol and that sustained higher levels of cortisol are associated with the development of osteoporosis, diabetes, and vascular disease and with increased risk for cognitive impairment and dementia

(Ball, Berch, Helmers, et al., 2002), but not all individuals respond to stress in the same way. Some individuals are more prone to experiencing psychological distress, such as worry, tension, angry feelings, and belief that they are unable to solve their problems. Older adults who are more highly prone to distress have higher rates of cognitive decline, MCI, and dementia than older adults who tend not to be prone to distress (Wilson, Arnold, Schneider, et al., 2007a; Wilson, Bennett, Mendes de Leon, et al., 2005; Wilson, Schneider, Boyle, et al., 2007d). For example, the rate of cognitive decline has been found to be 30% greater among those more prone to distress.

Cigarette Smoking

Current smoking was associated with higher rates of cognitive decline among both men and women. Higher rates of cognitive decline were found among older adults with and without a family history of dementia (Ott et al., 2004).

Depression

Depression is known to be associated with the development of dementia (Berger, Fratiglioni, Forsell, et al., 1999; Green, Cupples, Kurz, et al., 2003; Yaffe, Blackwell, Gore, et al., 1999), and it is known that depression is associated with chronic elevation of cortisol, which is believed to kill brain cells in the hippocampal area. There is some evidence that depression is associated with structural brain changes, such as loss of neurons in the hippocampal area.

Head Injuries

There is evidence that head injuries among older adults (ages 70 years or older), such as injuries sustained during falls, are associated with earlier onset of dementia, with the effect greater among those who carry the *APOE e4* allele (Luukinen, Veramo, Herala, et al., 2005).

Social Isolation and Loneliness

Social isolation (having a small social network, being unmarried, or having limited participation in social activities with others) has been found to be associated with cognitive decline and increased risk for developing dementia (Wilson et al., 2007b). Wilson et al. also found that loneliness (feeling disconnected from others or not having social contacts) among older adults (those 80 to 85 years of age) was associated with cognitive decline and increased risk of developing dementia. Loneliness has been found to be associated with an increased risk for AD, one of the subcategories of dementia (Wilson et al., 2007b). The researchers suggested that loneliness may compromise neural systems underlying cognition and memory.

Medications With Anticholinergic Properties

Among older adults, an association has been found between impairment of cognitive functioning, including memory and learning, and use of medications with anticholinergic effects (Nebes et al., 2005). Continuous use over a 1-year period has been found to be associated with a decrease in cognitive functioning (Dumas, Hancur-Bucci, Naylor, et al., 2008). In a recent 4-year prospective study of older adults living in the community, it was found that 7.5% of them were taking at least one drug with anticholinergic properties—antidepressants, digestive antispasmodics, genitourinary antispasmodics, antihistamines, anxiolytics, cardiovascular medications, antiepileptics, antipsychotics, antiasthmatics, and anti-Parkinson drugs (Carriere, Fourrier-Reglat, Dartigues, et al., 2009). Carriere et al. found that older adults taking anticholinergic drugs are at increased risk for cognitive decline and dementia and that discontinuing the anticholinergic medications resulted in a reduction of the risk.

Protective Factors for Dementia That Occur at Older Age

Among older adults (those over 65 years of age), factors that have been found to be associated with a decreased risk of developing dementia include dietary patterns, alcohol consumption, physical exercise, leisure activities (mental and social activities), and social support.

Dietary Patterns

According to Scarmeas et al. (2006), following a Mediterranean diet can reduce the risk among older adults of developing dementia by 40%. Similar findings were reported in a study of older adults who were regular consumers of fish, omega-3 oils, fruits, and vegetables. They were found to have lower rates of dementia, including AD. The reduced risks were greater among those who did not carry the *APOE e4* allele that is associated with increased risk for developing AD (Barberger-Gateau, Raffaitin, Letenneur, et al., 2007). The authors suggested that the beneficial effect of fish consumption may be due to its high content of omega-3 polyunsaturated fatty acids, which are a component of neuron membranes and are believed to have anti-inflammatory properties. The beneficial effect of fruits and vegetables may be due to their antioxidant properties.

Alcohol Consumption

In a prospective 3-year study of 3,777 residents 65 years old or older in France, it was found that drinking three to four standard glasses of wine per day was associated with an 80% reduced risk of developing dementia and a 75% reduced risk of developing AD (Orgogozo, Dartigues, Lafont, et al., 1997). Luchsinger (2004) found that drinking three servings of wine daily was associated with a lower rate of developing AD, but only among older adults without the *APOE e4* allele. Mukamal, Kuller, Fitzpatrick, et al. (2003) found that, compared to abstaining, drinking one to six drinks weekly of any alcoholic beverage was associated with decreased risk of dementia; however, heavy alcohol consumption was associated with increased risk of dementia, particularly among men with the *APOE e4* allele. A meta-analysis found that light to moderate alcohol intake among older adults was associated with a 25% to 28% reduction in risk for developing dementia, AD, and VaD (Anstey et al., 2009). Anstey et al. (p. 553) suggested that the benefit of light to moderate alcohol intake may be due to alcohol's effects of increasing high-density cholesterol, increasing cerebral blood flow, decreasing blood coagulation, increasing antithrombotic activity, and increasing insulin sensitivity.

Physical Activity

Some researchers have not found physical activities to be associated with reduced risk for dementia (Verghese, Lipton, Katz, et al., 2003). However, in a prospective study of 9,008 adults over the age of 65 years, Laurin, Verreault, Lindsay, et al. (2001) found that moderate-intensity physical activity (exercise engaged in three times a week at the level of walking) and high-intensity physical activity (exercise engaged in three times a week at a level greater than walking) were associated with a reduced rate for cognitive impairment and dementia, particularly in women; among older adults (70 to 89 years of age), exercise improved cognitive functioning (Williamson, Espeland, Kritchevsky, et al., 2009). Fabel and Kempermann (2008) said that exercise regulates adult hippocampal neurogenesis (birth of new cells in the hippocampus). They believed that exercise within the context of cognitive challenges may be the most beneficial.

Cognitively Stimulating Activities

The protective effect of complex mental activity is evident among older adults (Fratiglioni, Wang, Ericsson, et al., 2000b; Scarmeas, Levy, Tang, et al., 2001; Verghese et al., 2003). Frequent engagement in cognitively stimulating activities—activities that involved information processing such as reading the newspaper, listening to the radio, viewing television, reading books, playing cards, doing crossword puzzles, and going to museums—has been found to be associated with a reduced risk for developing AD (Wilson, Mendes de Leon, Barnes, et al., 2002). The more frequently an individual participates in cognitively stimulating activities, the greater the reduction of risk for developing AD.

Leisure Activities

Among older adults (those over age 65 years), a higher level of participation in leisure activities has been found to be associated with reduced rates of dementia. Leisure activities included knitting; music; walking for pleasure; visiting friends or relatives or being visited by them; physical conditioning; going to movies, restaurants, or sporting events; reading magazines, newspapers, or books; watching television or listening to the radio; volunteering; playing card games or bingo; going to a club or center; going to classes; and going to a place of worship. A stronger association was found between the leisure activities that involved social interactions—visiting friends or relatives, going to movies or restaurants, and walking for pleasure—and reduced risk of developing AD. There was also a cumulative effect: participation in more leisure activities was associated with greater reduction of risk (Scarmeas et al., 2001).

Combined Effects of Physical, Mental, and Social Activities

Among older adults (those over age 75 years), those who engaged in mental, physical, and social activities have been found to have a lower rate of developing dementia than those who do not. Those who engaged in leisure activities—reading, playing board games, playing musical instruments, and dancing—4 days a week were found to have a lower risk for developing dementia, both AD and VaD, and a lower rate of decline in memory than those who engaged in leisure activities only once a week or not at all (Verghese et al., 2003). Those who engaged in all three types of activities had the lowest rate of developing dementia (Karp, Paillard-Borg, Want, et al., 2006).

Social Networks

Researchers have found that among older adults (those age 75 years or older), the presence of rich social networks—being married or living with someone, having children and having daily contacts with them, and having relatives and friends and having satisfying contacts with them—is associated with a decreased risk of developing dementia (Bennett, Schneider, Tang, et al., 2006; Wang, Karp, Winblad, et al., 2002).

Evidence-Supported Preventive Interventions

Flicker (2009) made the point that many of the studies of interventions that have been found to be associated with decreased incidence of dementia are based on observations rather than on random controlled trials and therefore lack strong evidence. However, Breitner and Albert (2009) said that there is strong evidence that some activities are associated with preventing or delaying cognitive decline and dementia. Four factors have been found to be independently predictive of maintenance of cognitive functioning: high levels of physical activity, high levels of mental activity, high levels of social engagement, and control of vascular risk factors (smoking, hypertension, high cholesterol, and diabetes) (Hendrie, Albert, Butters, et al., 2006; Whitaker, Sidney, Selby, et al., 2005).

- *Physical activity.* Higher levels of physical activity have been found to be associated with maintaining cognitive functioning (Weuve, Kang, Manson, et al., 2004) and delaying the onset of AD (Podewils, Guallar, Kuller, et al., 2005). A later study found that among older adults, exercise has been found to improve cognition, attention, and executive functioning (Erickson, Colcombe, Wadhwa, et al., 2007).
- *Mental activity.* It has been known for a number of years that a higher level of education predicts maintenance of cognition and decreased risk of dementia (Farmer et al., 1995). Now, studies of older adults have shown that a higher number of hours spent in ongoing intellectual activities—reading books, going to lectures, and playing board games—is associated with decreased risk of cognitive decline and development of dementia (Verghese et al., 2003; Wilson, Scherr, Schneider, et al., 2007c).

- ***Social engagement.*** Social engagement encompasses individuals' social networks and sense of self-efficacy and self-worth (Breitner & Albert, 2009). Social engagement has been reported to have a positive effect on maintaining cognitive functioning and delaying onset of AD (Karp et al., 2006; Saczynski, Pfeifer, Masaki, et al., 2006). It is thought that social engagement buffers the impact of stressors in life and thus reduces the adverse effect of stress hormones, such as cortisol, on the brain (Breitner & Albert).
- ***Control of vascular risk factors.*** Vascular disease has an impact on cognition, and the presence of vascular risk factors—hypertension, hypercholesterolemia, diabetes, heart disease, and current smoking—increases the risk of developing AD (Newman, Fitzpatrick, Lopez, et al., 2005; Schneider, Arvanitakis, Bang, et al., 2007). It is believed that treatment to reduce vascular risk factors may be effective in reducing risk for cognitive decline, VaD, and AD (Peila, White, Masaki, et al., 2006).

The risk of cognitive decline is reduced further when two or more of these protective factors are present (Karp et al., 2006).

Etiology

Dementia is thought to be due to brain pathologies such as AD and other disorders (Savva & Brayne, 2009) but it is influenced by genetic vulnerabilities, the effect of lifelong molding of the brain, and the effect of exposure to risk factors that have adverse effects on the brain and its functioning (Ngandu, 2006; Rabins, 2007). Symptoms of dementia can be caused by medical disorders and infections, neurological disorders, nutritional disorders, space-occupying lesions, and substances such as medications and other chemicals (Spar & LaRue, 2006). Dementia is the end-stage of several pathophysiological processes (Kivipelto & Solomon, 2009), processes that have occurred over many years (Barnes, 2011). Etiology of each subtype of dementia is discussed later.

Clinical Presentation

In the early stage of dementia, changes of cognitive functioning—particularly memory—are greater than would be expected due to age. In addition, more than 80% of patients with dementia have behavioral-psychological symptoms (Lyketsos, Lopez, Jones, et al., 2002) and impairment of functioning (Knopman, Boeve, & Peterson, 2003). There are often symptoms of psychological distress related to patients' awareness of the illness. Apathy, irritability, anxiety, and depression are common symptoms (Aalten, de Vugt, Jaspers, et al., 2005a). There may be changes in weight and appetite (Aalten et al.). Impairment of functioning may be evidenced as problems in remembering appointments, writing checks, paying bills on time, shopping alone, using the telephone, and driving (Bossen, 2009). Gait problems such as difficulty in walking, slower walking, and falls are frequent occurrences and often precede symptoms of impaired cognitive functioning (Ramakers, Visser, Aalten, et al., 2007). A list of features common to all dementias (AD, VaD, DLB, and FTD) can be found in Box 16-2.

Differential Diagnosis

Dementia can be caused by medical conditions, neurological conditions, psychiatric disorders, health problems, and medications.

- ***Medical conditions:*** liver/kidney failure; toxins; hypothyroidism; vitamin B_{12} deficiency; vitamin B_6 deficiency (pellagra); infectious diseases (bacterial, fungal, viral, and prion); autoimmune diseases, such as multiple sclerosis and lupus; and delirium

BOX 16-2 Features Common to All Dementias

1. *Multiple cognitive deficits.* These include anterograde memory impairment (the inability to store, retain, or recall new knowledge); retrograde memory impairment (the loss of memories); aphasia (impaired ability to speak, write, or comprehend the meaning of spoken or written words); apraxia (impaired ability to perform purposeful acts); and agnosia (loss of ability to recognize familiar objects).
2. *Disturbances in executive functioning.* These cause impairment of role functioning and that is a significant decline from previous functioning.
3. *Difficulty with multitasking.*
4. *Apathy and withdrawal.* These may be linked to patients' thinking that they cannot understand the environment or to a feeling of being overwhelmed.
5. *Emotional disinhibition,* such as uncontrollable laughing or crying.
6. *Anxiety and fearfulness* that occur with cognitive decline. Some patients fear losing their minds, and many fear new situations or complex situations.
7. *Sleep disturbances.* Daytime sleepiness may be due to nighttime insomnia or to the lack of interesting activities or boredom. Insomnia in patients with dementia may be caused by depression, lack of exercise during the day, caffeine in tea or coffee, or theophylline used for pulmonary disease.
8. *Decreased self-awareness.* Patients are less aware of how their behavior affects others; e.g., poor hygiene, inappropriate sexual activity, eating from others' plates, and eating nonfood items.
9. *Agitation.* This is manifested in pacing, hitting, kicking, verbal abuse, and screaming.
10. *Psychotic symptoms.* These include delusions, such as the belief that someone is stealing their things or that there is a stranger living in their home (phantom boarder syndrome); or hallucinations, such as hearing the voices of family members who have died or visual hallucinations.

Sources: Bourgeois et al., 2008; Tractenberg, Weiner, Patterson, et al., 2002; Weiner et al., 2009.

- Neurological conditions: hypoxia, poisoning due to lead or other heavy metals, trauma, tumors, and Parkinson's disease
- *Psychiatric disorders:* anxiety, depression, mania, and psychosis
- *Health problems:* fecal impaction, loss of vision, or loss of hearing
- *Medications:* corticosteroids, sedatives, and medications with anticholinergic properties (Carriere et al., 2009)

Comorbidity

A frequently quoted early study reported that patients with dementia had the same number of comorbid illnesses as patients without dementia (Schubert, Boustani, Callahan, et al., 2006). Other studies have found that patients with dementia have more comorbid illnesses than patients without dementia (Gellis et al., 2009; Hill, Futterman, Duttagupta, et al., 2002) and that medical comorbidities are associated with decreased cognitive functioning, decreased ability for self-care, greater impairment of mobility, and more problems with incontinence (Doraiswamy, Leon, Cummings, et al., 2002). Medical illnesses and psychiatric disorders are frequent comorbidities of dementia.

Medical Illnesses

Commonly occurring medical illnesses include cerebrovascular disease, congestive heart failure, chronic pulmonary disease, diabetes, peripheral vascular disease, myocardial infarction, malignancy, renal disease, complications of diabetes, and peptic ulcer disease (Hill et al., 2002). Oral health problems are also common; poor oral health has been found to be associated with malnutrition and pneumonia and accounts for death in a large number of patients with severe dementia (Chen, Lamberg, Chen, et al., 2006).

In a study of patients with advanced dementia in nursing homes, the most frequently occurring health problems included skin disorders (95%); nutritional/hydration problems (85%); gastrointestinal problems (80%); genitourinary/gynecological problems (73%); pain (63%); and pressure ulcers (61%). About half of the residents had arthritis, fall-related problems, heart disease, hypertension, and oncological disorders (Black, Finucane, Baker, et al., 2006).

Psychiatric Disorders

Commonly occurring psychiatric disorders include depression and anxiety disorders. Comorbid depression in patients with dementia is associated with a shorter life span, diminished quality of life, greater caregiver burden and distress, and higher rates of out-of-home placement for care (Gellis et al., 2009). Comorbid anxiety among patients with dementia is associated with an increase of behavioral problems, such as agitation, wandering, verbal threats, physical abuse, and aggressiveness (Smith, Samus, Steele, et al., 2008).

Treatment

Treatment is directed at treating the cause of the dementia, if modifiable, and at improving cognitive, behavioral, and functional impairments caused by the disorder (Arciniegas & Dubovsky, 2007). Treatment is based on a comprehensive evaluation.

Assessment for All Dementias

In addition to a comprehensive psychiatric evaluation, assessment includes evaluation of medical and neurological causes of cognitive impairment (Weiner et al., 2009); functioning and behaviors; capacity of caregivers; and patient's environment (Fletcher, 2008). (See Chapter 4 for discussion of the psychiatric interview and comprehensive psychiatric assessment.) Some symptoms of dementia are not stable. For example, changes in consciousness occur in 80% to 90% of patients with DLB (Byrne, Lennox, Lowe, et al., 1989), in 40% of patients with VaD, and in 20% of patients with AD (Kolbeinsson & Jonsson, 1993). Therefore, fluctuations in confusion and consciousness should also be evaluated (Walker, Ayre, Cummings, et al., 2000).

Assessment of patients presenting with cognitive impairment includes a review of medical, neurological, and psychiatric disorders; neurodevelopment; social development; substance use; and family illnesses; a review of medical records; information about medications currently prescribed and any relation to changes in cognition; and information about use of over-the-counter drugs and herbs. During the assessment process, the psychiatric advanced practice nurse should begin to think of dementias that are progressive and irreversible, such as AD; degenerative dementias; dementias that can be stopped but not reversed, such as VaD; dementias that might be reversed, such as dementias due to infections, trauma, or substance-related disorders; and dementias that may be due to medical conditions, medications/substances, or depression (Arciniegas & Dubovsky, 2007). Suggested laboratory assessments for individuals with all types of dementia are listed in Box 16-3. Mental status examination, functional assessment, behavioral assessment, and fluctuation assessment are used to determine the presence and type of dementia.

Mental Status Examination

The mental status examination provides information about level of alertness, ability to cooperate, mood, thought content, psychomotor activity, judgment, insight, presence of psychotic symptoms such as hallucinations or delusions, and cognitive functioning. Cognitive functioning among older adults can be evaluated by using the following scales:

- *Mini-Mental State Examination* (Folstein, Folstein, & McHugh, 1975). This is an 11-item scale that can be used to measure orientation, recall, language, attention, and visuoconstruction, e.g., ability to draw the face of a clock with hands set for ten after eleven.

BOX 16-3 Laboratory Evaluation for All Dementias

Laboratory tests are done to identify illnesses that are known to cause dementia. Tests include

- Blood chemistries—electrolytes, blood urea nitrogen, creatinine, glucose
- Complete blood cell count and differential
- Blood glucose
- Homocysteine
- Lipid profile
- Thyroid profile
- Vitamin B_{12} and folate levels
- Tests for syphilis
- Test for HIV antibodies, as indicated by history
- Urinalysis and urine toxicology
- Electrocardiogram
- Chest x-ray

Sources: Bourgeois et al., 2008; Lipton & Rubin, 2009.

- *Dementia Rating Scale (DRS)* (Mattis, 1976) and *DRS2* (Jurica, Leitten, & Mattis, 2002). These scales provide a global measurement of cognitive impairment based on measures of functioning in five cognitive areas: attention, initiation and perseveration, visuoconstruction, conceptualization, and memory.
- *Animal Naming Task* (Duff-Canning, Leach, Stuss, et al., 2004). This scale asks patients to name as many animals as possible within 60 seconds. If the patient identifies less than 14 animals in 60 seconds it suggests early stages of dementia or development of cognitive impairment. It is brief and capable of detecting moderate to severe dementia.
- *Clock Drawing Test (CDT)* (Tuokko, Hadjistavropoulos, Miller, et al., 1995). The CDT measures cognitive functions that correlate with executive-control functions (Royall, Mulroy, Chiodo, et al., 1999). The patient is asked to draw the face of a clock and to put in the time that the examiner has asked to be included. The CDT requires that the patient use multiple cognitive processes including hearing and understanding the verbal instructions, being able to draw a representation of a clock, planning how to place the hands of the clock, and visuospatial and visual-motor skills. Performance on the CDT is not related to age or level of education and has been found to be sensitive to the presence of mild dementia and cognitive decline (Rush, First, & Blacker, 2008). The CDT is brief and can detect moderate to severe dementia (Shulman, 2000).
- *Mini-cog* (Borson, Scanlan, Brush, et al., 2000). This is a combination of a three-word learning and recall test and clock drawing that takes approximately 3 minutes to administer. First, the patient is asked to listen carefully to the three unrelated words that the examiner will use and to remember the three words. Next, the patient is asked to draw a clock and position the hands at the time the examiner requests. Then, the patient is asked to repeat the three words. Recalling all three words is indicative of no dementia. Recalling only one or two words indicates possible dementia. Abnormalities on the clock drawing indicate the presence of dementia (Carolan Doerflinger, 2007). The Mini-cog is a brief test for discriminating individuals with dementia and can be used in a diverse population, including patients with low levels of education and non-English speakers. It is able to detect moderate to severe dementia.
- *Saint Louis University Mental Status Examination (SLUMS)* (Morley & Tumosa, 2002; Tariq, Tumosa, Chibnall, et al., 2006). The SLUMS asks patients to perform tasks such as doing simple math computations, naming animals, recalling facts, and drawing the hands on a clock. It can identify patients with mild cognitive problems. The SLUMS, which is free and currently used at many Veterans Administration hospitals, is available at http://medschool.slu.edu/agingsuccessfully/pdfsurveys/slumsexam_05.pdf

Functional Assessment

The *Functional Activities Questionnaire (FAQ)* (Pfeffer, Kurosaki, Harrah, et al., 1982) can detect dementia with sensitivity and specificity. It is also used in monitoring the progression of functional decline.

Behavioral Assessment

Behavioral symptoms include paranoid and delusional ideation, hallucinations, aggressiveness, anxiety, disruptions of daily rhythms, and behaviors that are troublesome for caregivers. The *Behavioral Pathology in AD Rating Scale (BEHAVE-AD)* (Reisberg, Borenstein, Salob, et al., 1987) is designed to measure these behaviors. It has 25 items divided into seven categories: paranoid and delusional ideation, hallucinations, activity disturbances, aggressiveness, diurnal rhythm disturbances, affective disturbances, and anxiety and phobias. It is useful in identifying specific behavior disturbances and can be used to measure response to treatment (Rush et al., 2008).

Fluctuation Assessment

The *Clinician Assessment of Fluctuation* scale consists of two questions that the clinician asks an informant (someone who knows the patient well) a series of questions regarding the frequency and duration of fluctuating confusion and impaired consciousness during the past month. The *One Day Fluctuation Assessment Scale* measures an informant's observations during the day preceding the interview; the informant is instructed to observe and note any patient behaviors that are associated with changes in confusion such as falls, drowsiness, lack of attention, disorganized thinking, altered level of consciousness, or problems with communication (Walker et al., 2000, p. 252).

Interventions for Physiological, Psychological, and Behavioral Symptoms

Treatment for patients with dementia involves managing the physiological, psychological, and behavioral symptoms that are common features of dementia (Lyketsos, Steinberg, Tschanz, et al., 2000).

- **Physiological problems** include sensory loss (smell, taste, vision, spatial, and hearing), oral health problems, infections, eating difficulties, constipation, incontinence, impairment of motor functioning, and pain.
- **Psychological symptoms** include attention, concentration, memory and cognitive impairments, deficits of executive functioning, apathy, anxiety, fear, depression, mania, agitation, suspiciousness, and sometimes psychosis (Bourgeois, Seaman, & Servis, 2011; Yaari, Tariot, & Richards, 2009).
- **Behavioral symptoms** include hoarding and hiding things, withdrawal, restlessness, agitation, wandering, screaming, aggression, assaultiveness, evening agitation (sundowning), and disinhibited social and sexual behavior (Ferman, Smith, & Melom, 2005; Mace & Rabins, 2006; Bourgeois et al., 2011).

Treatment of specific dementias will be discussed later in the chapter with each subtype of dementia. Over time, the treatment of specific dementias becomes more similar than different, and therefore issues in treatment and psychotherapeutic, pharmacological, and psychosocial interventions that are applicable to patients with all dementias will be discussed in this section. This section will also discuss managing specific symptoms associated with dementia and managing advanced dementia.

Psychotherapy

Psychotherapy for patients with dementia is based on the belief that patients' behaviors are adaptive responses to the experience of memory loss and cognitive decline and to stressors such as changes in living situation, problems related to memory impairment, anxiety, restriction of activities such as driving, and loss of life roles, self-identity, and autonomy, rather than being the direct result of brain pathology (Bryden, 2002), and that patients' behaviors occur within a social and environmental context (Kasl-Godley & Gatz, 2000). Different models of psychotherapy—family therapy, supportive therapy, and cognitive behavioral therapy (CBT)—are effective for different phases of dementia (early, middle, and advanced) (Bryden, 2002; Junaid & Hegde, 2007). The majority of patients with dementia experience anxiety in the early and middle phases of the illness, in association with a decrease in patients' independence and increased risk of placement in a nursing home (Kraus, Sesignourel, Balasubramanyam, et al., 2008). Therefore, one of the goals of psychotherapy in the early and middle phases is to reduce anxiety. Other goals of psychotherapy are to help patients to accept themselves as they are, facilitate social interaction and communication, and provide opportunities for reminiscence about past accomplishments (Greene, Ingram, & Johnson, 1993). Family therapy in the early phase of dementia may help patients and families to adjust to patients' impairments and changes in family and social activities (Arciniegas & Dubovsky, 2007; Bourgeois & Hickey, 2009; Hepple, 2004). Family therapy that includes psychoeducation has been found to be effective in the early phase of dementia (Pinquart & Sorensen, 2006). Supportive psychotherapy, which focuses on strengthening patients' self-esteem, adaptive skills, and functioning through the use of empathy, instillation of hope, inspiration, reassurance, suggestion, persuasion, counseling, and re-education is beneficial in the early and middle phases of dementia (Junaid & Hegde, 2007, p. 19). Supportive psychotherapy helps patients in dealing with their grief and losses (Bourgeois et al., 2011). CBT has been modified for patients with dementia in the early and middle phases to include a caregiver or other collateral person and focuses on education, awareness training, breathing exercises, coping skills, and use of positive self-statements (Kraus et al., 2008). One example of modified CBT is the intervention *Peaceful Mind,* which includes self-awareness training, use of calming thoughts, sleep hygiene, and behavioral activation. Patients and collaterals who received this intervention reported improvement in patients' anxiety, depression, and distress, and improvement of family communication (Paukert, Calleo, & Kraus-Schuman, 2010). In addition to the use of CBT to reduce anxiety and distress and to assist in meeting patients' needs (Lenze, Pollock, Shear, et al., 2003), it is used in the late phase of dementia to modify behaviors such as wandering (Hepple, 2004).

Pharmacotherapy

Pharmacotherapy is used for patients with dementia to maintain their cognitive functioning or prevent a decline; to manage behavioral problems such as agitation, aggression, or psychotic symptoms that occur among nearly all patients with dementia during some stage of their illness; and to manage co-occurring depression and anxiety. Cognitive enhancers (cholinesterase inhibitors and memantine [Namenda]), antipsychotics, antidepressants, benzodiazepines, and anticonvulsants are frequently used to manage the symptoms of dementia (Yaari et al., 2009). In general, low doses of medications are used and the dose is increased slowly.

Cognitive Enhancers

Cognitive enhancers are agents that improve cognitive functioning by delaying neuropathological changes within the brain or by altering brain chemistry to improve functioning (Brown, 2009).

Cholinesterase Inhibitors

Disturbances of acetylcholine neurotransmission, especially in the hippocampus and cerebral cortex, are associated with dementia. Based on this finding, medications that increase the level of available acetylcholine in the brain have been developed to increase its availability for synaptic transmission of information and to improve cognitive functioning (Brown, 2009). Cholinesterase inhibitors should be used early in the course of dementia to reduce the rate of cognitive decline (Blennow, de Leon, & Zetterberg, 2006). They may also be used to manage psychotic symptoms (Rao & Lyketos, 1998).

Four medications have been approved for use: tacrine (Cognex); donepezil; rivastigmine (Exelon, Exelon patch); and galantamine (Razadyne). Tacrine is not used very often because of its hepatotoxicity, its drug interactions, and the need for dosing four times a day (Brown, 2009). Donepezil is approved for mild, moderate, and severe AD and has been found to be effective for other dementias. Rivastigmine is approved for mild to moderate dementia of Alzheimer's type. Galantamine is approved for mild to moderate dementia of Alzheimer's type (Brown). Donepezil, rivastigmine, and galantamine have resulted in improved cognitive functioning, with similar efficacy (Farlow & Boustani, 2009). However, Jones (2003) pointed out that there are a significant number of patients who do not respond to cholinesterase inhibitors.

Memantine

Memantine is a cognitive enhancer that acts on the glutamatergic system, which stimulates nerve cells. It is a glutamate *N*-methyl-D-aspartate (NMDA) receptor antagonist. (The NMDA receptor is involved in memory.) It is believed that memantine protects neurons from too much stimulation and slows cognitive decline (Black & Andreasen, 2011). It has shown modest effect in improving cognitive, functional, and behavioral symptoms (Herrmann, Li, & Lanctot, 2011). Memantine in combination with an acetylcholinesterase inhibitor improves cognition, agitation, aggression, irritability, and appetite (Cummings, Schneider, Tariot, et al., 2006).

Antipsychotic Medications

Antipsychotic medications are used for symptoms of paranoid thinking, hallucinations, delirium, and agitation (Bourgeois et al., 2011). The atypical antipsychotics are used more often than the typical antipsychotics such as haloperidol (Haldol), which has moderate efficacy in decreasing aggression but is less effective in reducing agitation (Lonergan, Luxenberg, & Colford, 2002). The side effects of haloperidol include extrapyramidal side effects (EPSs), such as parkinsonian symptoms, dystonias, akathisia, cardiac effects, dry mouth, confusion, tardive dyskinesia, and neuroleptic malignant syndrome; these EPSs limit its use for older adults (Roose, Pollock, & Devanand, 2009).

The atypical antipsychotics that are used most often are risperidone (Risperdal), olanzapine (Zyprexa), quetiapine (Seroquel), aripiprazole (Abilify), and ziprasidone (Geodon). Risperidone has been found to be more effective than placebo for treatment of physical threats, violence, agitation, and nonparanoid delusions (Rabinowitz, Katz, DeDeyn, et al., 2004). It has been found to be more effective than haloperidol in managing aggression, sexual advances, pacing, wandering, hoarding, and verbal and physical repetitive activities (Suh, Son, Ju, et al., 2006). It has also been reported to be effective for sleep disturbances (Duran, Greenspan, Diago, et al., 2005). However, it may cause EPS and tardive dyskinesia in elderly patients. Olanzapine has been found to be associated with improvement of agitation, aggression, hallucinations, and delusions. However, it is also associated with sedation, postural instability, and weight gain (Wood, Cummings, Hsu, et al., 2000). Quetiapine was not found to be more effective than placebo for agitation, but it does have sedative effects (Ballard, Margallo-Lana, Juszczak, et al., 2005). There is insufficient information about the use of ziprasidone and aripiprazole for dementia (Yaari, Tariot, & Richards, 2009). The use of clozapine (Clozaril) is limited by its risk for agranulocytosis and side effect of orthostatic hypotension, which increases the risk for falls among older adults (Roose et al., 2009). However, it is used when psychotic symptoms do not respond to other mediations, in Parkinson's disease with dementia, and in DLB (Keys & DeWald, 2005).

To summarize the information about the use of atypical antipsychotics for dementia, a 2006 meta-analysis of the use of atypical antipsychotics in 5,000 patients with dementia found that the overall response rate was 48% to 65%, in comparison to a response rate of 30% to 48% for placebo. The average benefit of medication over placebo was 18% (Schneider, Dagerman, & Insel, 2006b). Olanzapine and risperidone were found to have superior efficacy, but side effects must be considered. There was lack of evidence for or against quetiapine. Following the warning from the U.S. Food and Drug Administration (FDA) in 2005 that use of atypical antipsychotics for dementia was associated with increased mortality, there has been a decrease in their use (Kales, Zivin, Kim, et al., 2011).

Antidepressant Medications

Antidepressant medications are used for comorbid depressive disorders, symptoms of depression and anxiety, sleep disturbances, and agitation (Bourgeois et al., 2011). Among the selective serotonin reuptake inhibitors (SSRIs), citalopram (Celexa) has been found to be effective for depression, agitation, and psychotic symptoms (Sink, Holden, & Yaffe, 2005). It has been found to be as effective as risperidone for agitation and psychotic symptoms (Pollock, Mulsant, Rosen, et al., 2007).

The antidepressant trazodone (Desyrel) is a mixed serotonergic agonist-antagonist (Golden, Dawkins, & Nicholas, 2009). It has been found to be associated with improvement of irritability, anxiety, restlessness, depression, and sleep disruptions (Yaari et al., 2009). However, others have reported no benefits (Teri, Logsdon, Peskind, et al., 2000). Trazodone has been found to be helpful when used as an add-on medication when antipsychotics or other medications are not controlling disruptive behavior (Salzman & Tariot, 2009).

Benzodiazepines

Benzodiazepines have adverse effects on learning and memory. They also have side effects of ataxia, confusion, anterograde amnesia, and sedation and increase the risk of falls (Yaari et al., 2009). They should be used only in low doses for short-term crises or for management of agitated or anxious behaviors if antipsychotics or other medications are not effective (Roose et al., 2009).

Anticonvulsant Medications

Studies of the use of one of the classes of anticonvulsant medications, the valproates—divalproex sodium (Depakote), valproate sodium (Depacon), and valproic acid (Depakene)—for agitation associated with dementia are inconclusive (Roose et al., 2009). At this time, there is insufficient evidence to support the use of anticonvulsant medications for treatment of dementia (Alexopoulos, Streim, Carpenter, et al., 2004).

In summarizing pharmacotherapy for dementia, Yarri et al. (2009) said, "Clinical trials in this patient group show that the overall treatment effect for drugs that 'work' is about 20%, which is nearly the same rate as the likelihood of significant side effects" (p. 296). They recommended the use of nonpharmacological interventions when possible.

Psychosocial Interventions

Psychosocial interventions are provided for patients with dementia to promote health, independence, pleasure, and a sense of self-identity and well-being (Smith, Kolanowski, Buettner, et al., 2009). Psychosocial interventions can be categorized as communication techniques, behavioral interventions, environmental modification, and education of caregivers (Yuhas et al., 2006). Psychosocial strategies include meeting patients' basic needs and the needs of their families or caregivers; helping patients to maintain maximum functioning, such as self-care; and facilitating patients' participation in mental, physical, and social activities (Gellis et al., 2009).

The rationale for psychiatric advanced practice nurses' use of psychosocial interventions in the care of patients with dementia is provided by two theories: the *Need-Driven Dementia-Compromised Behavior (NDB)* model (Algase, Beck, Kolanowski, et al., 1996) and the *Lawton and Nahemow's Competence Press Model* (Lawton & Nahemow, 1973).

The *NDB* model proposes that disruptive symptoms of dementia—such as wandering, loud vocalizations, passivity, or aggression—result from the interaction of existing patient factors (neurological changes, cognitive abilities, functioning abilities, coping strengths, and personality traits) with the physical and social environment (Kovach, Noonan, Schlidt, et al., 2005). The interaction produces need-driven behaviors (Smith et al., 2009), which are patients' behavioral responses to unmet physical, emotional, psychological, and social needs. Frequently unmet needs include

- Relief of pain, depression, or anxiety
- Safety
- Assistance with self-care
- Daytime activities to relieve boredom and loneliness
- Social interaction (nursing home residents with dementia who lacked the ability to initiate activities or social interactions sat for hours with little stimulation or activity provided for them: they had nothing to do for 60% to 80% of their waking hours) (Buettner, 1999)
- Exercise
- Sense of self-identity
- Contact with the outside world (Scholzel-Dorenbos, Meeuwsen, Olde Rikkert, et al., 2010).

There is evidence that psychosocial interventions that address patients' unmet needs—needs that they may not be able to communicate and are expressed in disruptive behaviors—are effective in reducing irritability, verbal agitation, and physical aggression (Hilgeman, Burgio, & Allen, 2009). Conversely, the consequences of unmet needs include escalation of behavioral symptoms, decreased quality of life, and placement in institutions (Scholzel-Dorenbos et al., 2010).

The *Lawton and Nahemow's Competence Press model* proposes that it is the environment that maintains, supports, and stimulates individuals. Individuals' ability to interact with their environment, meet the demands of their environment, and control their environment decreases as their cognitive capabilities decline, and they experience distress when they are less able to control their environment. Based on this theory, the environment must be modified for patients with dementia to facilitate their interactions with their environment and to maximize their control of their environment.

Psychosocial Interventions for Patients

Psychosocial interventions include those that are included in the care of all patients, those that are provided in response to symptoms and disruptive behaviors, those that target specific identity domains, and those that are provided for family or caregivers.

Psychosocial interventions that are included in the care of all patients with dementia are

- Providing a safe, comfortable environment
- Providing visual cues
- Establishing a regular schedule for daily activities
- Using simple language
- Avoiding confrontation (Lyketsos, Colenda, Beck, et al., 2006)

Specific psychosocial interventions for individual patients are often selected by staff or caregivers based on patients' symptoms and disruptive behaviors (Yaari et al., 2009). (Specific interventions for symptoms and behaviors will be discussed later.) Another approach to selecting interventions is based on evidence that patients with dementia, even patients in the middle to late stages of AD, exhibit a sense of self-identity and are able to recall domains of self-identity, such as their role in the family. Five domains of self-identity have been identified by patients, family, and staff as being important:

1. Family and social role (such as being a spouse, partner, parent, or grandparent)
2. Occupation (such as homemaker, teacher, nurse, salesman, or mechanic)
3. Achievements and traits (such as academic achievement, professional accomplishments, volunteer activities, or being a resourceful person)
4. Leisure activities and hobbies (such as music of a specific era, reading, telling stories, or religious or spiritual activities)
5. Heritage (such as family customs and achievements, place of birth, or success of a relative) (Cohen-Mansfield, Golander, & Arnheim, 2000).

It has been found that in comparison to a control group of patients with dementia who received standard treatment, patients who received interventions related to their strongest role identity showed greater improvement in pleasure, interest, and activities and a decrease in agitation and disorientation (Cohen-Mansfield, Parpura-Gill, & Golander, 2006).

Psychosocial Interventions for Caregivers

Caregivers' unmet needs include their physical and mental health problems; information about dementia, respite care, and financial assistance; help in creating safe living environments; and help with household chores. According to Fletcher (2008), interventions that should be provided for all families and caregivers include support, education about the illness, and information about resources, such as the book *The 36-hour Day,* 4th edition: *A Family Guide to Caring for People with Alzheimer Disease, Other Dementias, and Memory Loss in Later Life* (Mace & Rabins, 2006).

Psychosocial Interventions for Specific Symptoms and Behaviors

Symptoms of dementia can be divided into disturbances of ability for self-care; difficulties with communication and cognition; sleep disruptions; affective and psychotic symptoms; and disruptive behavioral symptoms. Disruptive behavioral symptoms exist in 67% to 82% of patients with dementia in the community (Tractenberg, Weiner, & Thal, 2002) and 90% of patients with dementia in nursing homes (Yuhas et al., 2006).

Self-Care and Activities of Daily Living

Learning related to habitual behaviors involves a different process than cognitive/memory learning, and patients with dementia may retain learning related to habitual behaviors longer than cognitive learning. Therefore, using patients' usual routines for eating, sleeping, bathing/showering, dressing, exercising, performing chores, socializing, and engaging in leisure activities will help patients to stay involved in self-care and meaningful activities longer.

Activities of Self-Care

The activities of self-care that are most often problematic among patients with dementia are dressing, toileting, bathing, and eating (Grigaitis, 2006). To simplify dressing, it is helpful to limit choices and to place the clothes ready for the patient in the order in which they should be put on. To manage toileting and continence, patients should be directed to void every 2 to 3 hours. Showers may be less stressful than tub baths, and bedbaths or towel baths may be used as the illness progresses (Grigaitis). To encourage eating, it is helpful to reduce distractions around food and to use calorie-dense foods and foods that patients can eat with their fingers. Foods high in antioxidants—blueberries, strawberries, purple grape juice, and spinach—are believed to have neuroprotective value.

Mental and Physical Exercises

Jigsaw puzzles, card games, word games, and reading can be used early in the illness. Physical exercise or staying physically active has been found to reduce risk of falls; improve energy, sleep, and mood; maintain regular bowel functioning; and promote a sense of belonging and purpose (Ferman et al., 2005). Examples of physical activity include walking, dancing, folding laundry, raking leaves, sweeping, dusting, making beds, and clearing and setting the table. Fabel and Kempermann (2008) have noted that exercise regulates adult hippocampal neurogenesis (the production of new neurons in the hippocampus) by signaling to the brain that there are new opportunities and that new neurons are needed. They theorized that it is physical activity in the context of cognitive challenges (and not just any exercise) that brings about changes in the brain.

Communication and Cognition

As dementia progresses, patients may have increased difficulty communicating. They may be unable to find the right words and have difficulty organizing their thoughts. There may be loss of ability to reason or follow explanations. It is helpful to speak slowly, calmly, and quietly and to avoid questioning patients to find out if they remember something or recognize someone. It is helpful to use reassurance and comforting techniques, such as reminiscence therapy, rather than trying to reorient them to reality. Reminiscence therapy has been found to increase social interaction, self-care, and sense of well-being (Douglas, James, & Ballard, 2004). Use of nonthreatening, nonverbal communication—tone of voice, posture, facial expression, and pointing—is a successful strategy. Other helpful communication strategies include

- Addressing the patient by name
- Facing the patient when speaking
- Using short sentences with one question or statement
- Not arguing or reasoning (avoid using the word "don't" because it may be interpreted as a reprimand)

- Avoiding saying "no" and instead use redirection and distraction
- Forming questions so that patient can respond "yes" or "no"
- Breaking tasks down into small steps
- Explaining what is going to happen
- Responding to what patients are communicating (not just the words)
- Having patients wear eyeglasses and hearing aids if needed
- Reducing background noise (Ferman et al., 2005; Mace & Rabins, 2006; Yuhas et al., 2006)

Sleep Disruptions

Many older adults have sleep problems, but older adults with dementia have more sleep problems and more severe sleep problems (Ancoli-Israel, 2005; Ferman et al., 2005). For example, it has been found that among older adults with AD living in the community, 35% have problems with sleep—trouble falling asleep, fragmented sleep, and increased daytime napping—and the incidence and severity of sleep problems are even greater among older adults with dementia living in institutions (Aalten et al., 2005a; Deschenes & McCurry, 2009; Shub, Darvishi, & Kunik, 2009). Patients with dementia spend more time in lighter stages of sleep with less low-wave stages of sleep, rapid eye movement sleep, and total sleep time (Ancoli-Israel, 2005; Vitiello & Borson, 2001). These changes are evidenced in sleep fragmentation, more arousals, and daytime sleepiness and napping (Shub et al.).

Sleep and circadian regulation of sleep are modulated by centers in the brain—the hypothalamus, reticular activating system, suprachiasmatic nucleus (a group of neurons located at the base of the hypothalamus that control the pineal gland's production of melatonin)—and the pineal gland. It is believed that sleep disturbances in dementia are due to brain changes, namely a reduction of neurons in the suprachiasmatic nucleus (Deschenes & McCurry, 2009). Neurons in this area promote sleep. They inhibit the arousal system by reducing the level of acetylcholine and norepinephrine, which are involved in attention and arousal. The medication donepezil, which increases the level of acetylcholine during the night as well as during the day, has been found to be associated with exacerbation of sleep disorders, including insomnia and nightmares, among some patients (Martorana, Esposito, & Koch, 2010).

Pharmacotherapy for sleep disturbances carries the risk of decreased cognitive functioning, increased incidence of falls, and increased risk of death (Glass, Lanctot, Hermann, et al., 2005). Psychosocial interventions—such as light therapy, exercise, and sleep hygiene—are safe, effective adjuncts for treatment of insomnia. Light therapy has been found to be effective in reducing nighttime awakenings and total time awake at night (Box 16-4) (McCurry, Gibbons, Logsdon, et al., 2005; Sloane, Williams, & Mitchell, 2007).

> **BOX 16-4 Light Therapy**
>
> Light therapy requires 30 to 90 minutes of exposure to a light source of sufficient luminosity to affect circadian phase shift, such as specialized light equipment known as light boxes. Patients must face the light source with their eyes open and be approximately 2 to 3 feet from it. Because light must fall on the retina to affect the circadian system, Shub et al. (2009) have suggested putting the light box on top of the television set or developing other activities to keep patients seated and looking at the light box. Another approach that compared the use of ceiling-mounted light illumination (bright light) systems with standard lighting found that bright light exposure all day was associated with significant improvements in total nighttime sleep. Shub et al. (p. 24) made the point that the cost of a light box ($130.00) is equivalent to a 1-month's supply of zolpidem (Ambien).

Exercise has been found to improve sleep among patients with dementia and also to improve independent functioning, health, and depression (McCurry et al.; Teri, Gibbons, McCurry, et al., 2003). Exercise should start with walking, with a goal of 30 minutes of walking a day. Other exercises, such as balance and flexibility training, can be added to the walking. There is evidence that improving sleep hygiene in patients with dementia is helpful in reducing sleep and nighttime disturbances (McCurry et al.). See Chapter 8 for a discussion of sleep hygiene.

Affective and Psychotic Symptoms

Almost all patients with dementia will experience psychiatric symptoms during the course of their illness (Aalten, van Valen, Clare, et al., 2005b). The most frequent symptoms are apathy, depression, and agitation. For example, approximately 32% of patients with dementia experience depression (Lyketsos et al., 2002). Depression is likely to be manifested as confusion and problems with concentration, delusions, hallucinations, and behavioral symptoms (Weiner et al., 2009). Treatment includes nonpharmacological interventions, such as social support and exercise, and pharmacotherapy, such as the use of SSRI antidepressant medications (Steinberg & Lyketsos, 2009).

Other psychiatric symptoms include disinhibition, delusions, hallucinations, and aggression (Lyketsos et al., 2002). Delusions and hallucinations are different from those seen in patients with schizophrenia. Delusions tend to be simple, such as a belief that someone has stolen something from them. Hallucinations are more likely to be visual rather than auditory, e.g., seeing relatives who have died. Sometimes delusions and hallucinations are mild and require no treatment (Steinberg & Lyketsos, 2009). Patients may respond to nonpharmacological treatment, such as reassurance that they are safe, redirection, distraction, and use of reminiscence therapy. The use of antipsychotic medications must be considered in relation to the risks, which include increased risk of cerebrovascular events and death

(Steinberg & Lyketsos). Psychiatric advanced practice nurses should monitor the response of patients receiving antipsychotic medications, and the medications should be discontinued if there is no clinical improvement (Sink et al., 2005).

Disruptive Behavioral Symptoms

Behavioral changes are common in patients with dementia. At first, these individuals may be anxious and repeat the same questions. Later, they may engage in behaviors that are impulsive, inappropriate, or disruptive. Managing disruptive symptoms reduces the strain on caregivers, reduces the need for care outside of the home, thus reducing societal costs, and improves the quality of life for patients with dementia and for their families. Agitation, vocally disruptive behavior, wandering, and aggression are common behavioral symptoms; new strategies for coping with these symptoms include *Simple Pleasures* and the *Namaste program,* which are discussed later.

Agitation

Agitation occurs in high rates among patients in long-term care settings (Steinberg & Lyketsos, 2009). Agitation can be expressed through irritability, anger, and motor movements such as pacing or wandering (Grigaitis, 2006). Behaviors associated with agitation include restless behaviors, aggressive behaviors, and vocal or verbal behaviors.

Sundowning is a term that has been used to describe increases in confusion and agitated behaviors that occur among patients with dementia in the afternoon and evening hours (Bachman & Rabins, 2006). It occurs in approximately 25% of patients and is more frequent in those in the advanced stage of the illness (Little, Satlin, Sunderland, et al., 1995). Sundowning may be due to a disruption of circadian rhythm that is related to a phase delay in changes in body temperature (Volicer, Harper, Manning, et al., 2001).

Cohen-Mansfield (2007) found that 26% of patients with dementia in nursing homes showed a gradual increase of confusion, restlessness, and agitation that peaked at around 4 p.m., with a decrease after that for most patients. Patients with more severe impairments experienced increased agitation that continued into the evening hours. The following strategies can be used to lessen nighttime agitation:

- Maintain regular times for going to bed.
- Limit napping during the day.
- Take the patient outside during the day for exposure to natural light.
- Keep the patient active during the day.
- Promote abstinence from alcohol.
- Limit coffee and caffeine-containing foods to early in the day, with none after noon.
- Provide a light snack such as warm milk and crackers at bedtime.
- Avoid upsetting activities near bedtime (Ferman et al., 2005; Mace & Rabins, 2006).

Vocally Disruptive Behavior

Vocally disruptive behavior is a term that encompasses screaming, abusive language, moaning, and repetitive, inappropriate requests (McMinn & Draper, 2005). It occurs in 25% of patients in the community and 50% of patients in inpatient facilities (Leonard, Tinetti, Allore, et al., 2006). Vocally disruptive behavior causes emotional distress and feelings of powerlessness and anger among caregivers and staff in nursing homes or assisted living facilities and makes other patients anxious and agitated.

Vocally disruptive behavior tends to occur more frequently among patients with more severe dementia, patients with greater dependency, and patients experiencing hallucinations and delusions. It has also been found to occur frequently among patients who are depressed, experiencing pain, thirsty, or uncomfortable. It is associated with being left alone, a lack of support from social networks, and sensory impairments (McMinn & Draper, 2005).

Treatment of vocally disruptive behavior is very difficult. Risperidone appears to be the most effective of the pharmacological agents. Psychosocial interventions that correct sensory deprivation (eyeglasses and hearing aids) and that alleviate social isolation, unmet needs, and pain have been found to be associated with reduction of vocally disruptive behaviors (Ayslon, Gum, Feliciano, et al., 2006; Lindgren & Hallberg, 1992). Strategies that have been used with some success include talking to the patient or reading to the patient; talking about what the patient did in the past (hobbies, food, holidays); music; and showing family videotapes. McMinn and Draper (2005) have suggested that multiple interventions be used, such as reducing environmental stimuli, using nonverbal communication, relieving discomfort, meeting basic needs, and providing frequent orientation cues.

Wandering

Wandering occurs in approximately 50% of older adults with dementia living in the community and in a larger number—with estimates as high as 100%—of older adults with dementia in residential care settings. Wandering is a dangerous behavior (Yao & Algase, 2006). The mortality rate for patients with dementia who are missing for 24 hours is 40% (Hermans, Htay, & McShane, 2007; Koester & Stooksbury, 1995). Patients with the greatest cognitive impairment are the most likely to wander (Yao & Algase). Their wandering may be an expression of restlessness or boredom, but it may also be an expression of fear, loneliness, confusion, or unmet needs. Treatment of wandering involves identifying and addressing the underlying causes, such as having unmet needs for food, fluids, use of the bathroom, or warmth or coolness. Strategies for managing wandering include those focusing on patient care and those directed at modifying the environment. Interventions related to patient care include

- Arranging for daily walks or exercise
- Allowing patients to wander in a safe place, such as fenced yard

- Keeping patients busy with activities, e.g., involving them in daily chores to reduce restlessness and boredom
- Providing patients with a "wanderer's cart" (Smith et al., 2009, p. 26)
- Enrolling patients in Alzheimer's Association's *Safe Return* program by calling 1-800-272-3900
- Having patients wear identification bracelets, carry identification cards, and have identification sewn into their clothing (Ferman et al., 2005; Mace & Rabins, 2006)

Changes in the environment to reduce wandering include making the environment safe and also making the environment appealing, comforting, and interesting. Yao and Algase (2006) found that engaging environments were associated with a decrease in wandering behaviors and proposed that environments have features that engage people through both cognitive and emotional paths. Emotional paths—known as "approach and stay" or "avoid and leave"—are processed more rapidly and independently than cognitive ones by patients with dementia: their emotional response to the environment is stronger and quicker. Modifying the environment to make it safe involves installing gates at stairs, locks high on doors, knobs that cannot be turned easily, and motion monitors; securing sharp, poisonous, or inflammable items; and removing car keys and weapons. Modifying the environment to send the emotional signal of "approach and stay" involves making the environment engaging by creating a stimulating, warm, embellished, welcoming, and colorful environment with opportunities for engaging in novel activities. The environment must promote a sense of coziness, comfort, attachment, and familiarity such as a home setting or a nature setting (not an institutional setting).

Aggression

Aggression is another manifestation of agitation. Aggressive behaviors include pushing, spitting, grabbing, kicking, hitting, biting, and assaultive behaviors. Aggression may be an expression of fear, frustration, depression, helplessness, anger, or anticipation of pain such as with medical procedures. Among patients with dementia in nursing homes, the factors that have been found to predict aggression are depression, delusions, hallucinations, and constipation (Leonard et al., 2006).

Leonard et al. (2006) pointed out that two of the risk factors—depression, which is the strongest predictor of aggression, and constipation—can be modified. Episodes of aggression may be triggered when patients with dementia become frustrated or fearful or have a catastrophic reaction to an occurrence, such as being scolded, having an encounter with an irritable caregiver, being questioned, or being asked to do something that is beyond them. Fatigue can increase risk for combativeness.

Strategies for managing aggression include being pleasant, calm, and reassuring; reducing loud noises and clutter; limiting television time and number of visitors; and including exercise and chores in daily activities to reduce restlessness. Short-term treatment for aggressive behavior includes the use of lorazepam (Ativan) or low-dose antipsychotics. Long-term treatment includes low-dose antipsychotics, carbamazepine (Tegretol) or valproic acid, propranolol (Inderal), SSRIs, or buspirone (Buspar) (Weigel, Purselle, D'Orio, et al., 2009).

Strategies for Treatment of Behavioral Symptoms

One of the first steps in managing behavioral symptoms is to try to find the cause of the behavior (pain, loneliness, fear, frustration, thirst, or constipation) and (1) correct the cause or (2) respond to the emotion behind the behavior, such as responding to the fear of losing a loved one by reassuring patients that their loved ones are safe. Another step is to decrease triggers in the environment by reducing shadows in rooms (reduces fear and paranoia); removing mirrors, stuffed animals, and dolls that may stimulate illusions, delusions, or hallucinations; limiting contact with strangers; and providing dependable, routine, structured activities such as walks and crafts. Reorienting patients through the use of calendars, clocks, pictures, and colors in the environment is helpful. Strategies such as redirection of patients' activities and use of soothing music and scents such as lavender and *Melissa* balm (lemon balm) are also helpful.

Another strategy is called *validate, join, and distract.* First, caregivers try to understand why the behavior is taking place. Caregivers validate the emotion behind the behavior (such as missing their family) by letting the individual know that they recognize the feeling behind the behavior. The caregiver joins the patient by looking at pictures of the family and then distracts the individual with an activity that will meet the emotional need (loneliness) that caused the behavior. The strategy of validating, joining, and distracting is believed to be more effective with individuals in the early or middle stages of dementia (Ferman et al., 2005; Grigaitis, 2006).

An intervention called *Simple Pleasures* (Colling & Buettner, 2002) consists of sensorimotor interventions that are designed to increase interesting, pleasurable activities among nonactive patients and to increase opportunities for social interactions (Smith et al., 2009). There are over 80 identified therapeutic interventions that Smith et al. have placed in the following categories:

- Adventure-based (wheelchair biking)
- Life roles (cooking, gardening in raised beds, decorating things)
- Physical-based (exercises, tether balloon, early morning walks, pushing carts of games or finger foods, manipulating soft items such as felt butterflies filled with soft material, opening purses or tool boxes and taking out the items and then replacing them, and putting items into fishing baskets)

- Cognitive-based (games, guessing the cost of items such as in the game *The Price is Right*)
- Psychosocial club–based (bird watching, bowling, cars, needlecrafts, music, art, and sports)
- Nurturing (caring for animals or birds)

Colling & Buettner (2002) found that the use of Simple Pleasures reduced wandering, vocalization, boredom, and passivity. The intervention resulted in more family visits, and families said that they appreciated having activities that they could do with their relatives during visits.

The Namaste program was developed to maintain quality of life for patients with advanced or late-stage dementia (Simard, 2007). Activities are planned to be related to patients' life experiences and their sense of self-identity. The program provides gentle touch, a pleasant environment, meaningful activities, music, and aromatherapy (Nguyen & Paton, 2008). For example, aromatherapy using lavender and *Melissa* balm has been found to reduce agitation among patients in the late stage of dementia (Douglas et al., 2004; Lin, Chang, Ng, et al., 2007). Family members who are encouraged to massage their family members' hands or feet and to talk with them report that they like knowing what they can do to comfort their relatives (Volicer & Simard, 2009).

Managing Advanced Dementia

During the late stage of dementia, the symptoms of the four subtypes of dementia are similar. In addition to symptoms of earlier stages—cognitive impairment, spatial disorientation, personality changes, aphasia, apraxia, confusion, agitation, and sleep disturbances—patients in the late stage of dementia frequently have resistiveness to care, incontinence, eating difficulties, motor impairment, infections, and seizures; they may also be bedridden and dependent on others for care (Volicer & Simard, 2009). The goals of care in the late stage of dementia are maintenance of quality of life, dignity, and comfort. These goals require medical care, treatment of behavioral symptoms, and meaningful, comforting activities in a pleasant, safe environment (Volicer, 2007).

Treatment of Comorbid Medical Issues of Advanced Dementia

Comorbid medical conditions that occur frequently among patients with late-stage dementia include cerebrovascular disease, congestive heart failure, pulmonary disease, and diabetes. Cerebrovascular disease and congestive heart failure occur more than twice as frequently among patients with dementia as they do in patients without dementia (Hill et al., 2002). Volicer and Simard (2009) identified the most common secondary conditions among patients with late-stage dementia as infections, pressure ulcers, eating difficulties, aspiration, constipation, pain, and seizures; they identified the most frequent causes of death as pneumonia, renal failure, and dehydration.

Infections, Aspiration, and Eating Difficulties

Infections of the urinary tract, upper respiratory tract, lower respiratory tract, skin, intestinal tract, and eye are the most common infections in patients with late-stage dementia.

Avoiding the use of indwelling catheters may prevent urinary tract infections. Swallowing difficulties create a risk for aspiration and hence respiratory tract infections and pneumonia. Care in feeding and using thicker liquids rather than thin liquids may reduce risk of aspiration (Morris & Volicer, 2001). Risk for pneumonia may be further reduced with the use of pneumococcal vaccinations (Wagner, Popp, Posch, et al., 2003). Pneumococcal disease is 4.4 times greater among patients in long-term-care facilities than among older adults living in the community (Volicer & Simard, 2009). Because periodontal disease and dental plaque are risk factors for pneumonia, oral care has the potential to reduce the risk of pneumonia (Yoneyama, Yoshida, Ohrui, et al., 2002).

Constipation

Constipation occurs in half of nursing home residents. It may be due to a decrease in the neurons in the autonomic nervous system, medication side effects, and lack of exercise such as walking daily (Volicer & Simard, 2009). It is usually treated with two high-fiber meals each day. Volicer and Simard (p. 337) say that the use of psyllium (Fiberall, Metamucil), sorbitol (Glucitol), lactulose (Cephulac, Enulose), or polyethylene glycol (MiraLAX) is effective in managing constipation and reduces the need for enemas, which are often very disturbing for patients with dementia. Volicer, Lane, Panke, et al. (2005) pointed out that sorbitol is as effective as other approaches and less expensive.

Pressure Ulcers

Among patients with late-stage dementia in nursing homes, 14.7% have pressure ulcers. Ten percent of those admitted from a hospital to a nursing home already have pressure ulcers, whereas 4.7% of those admitted from home have pressure ulcers (Mitchell, Kiely, & Hamel, 2004). Pressure ulcers tend to occur in the sacrum, trochanters, and heels and are related to being chairbound or bedridden, being underweight, or having fecal incontinence (Volicer & Simard, 2009). They are associated with infections and increased risk of death (Redeling, Lee, & Sorvillo, 2005).

Pain

Among patients with late-stage dementia in nursing homes, 63% have pain (Black et al., 2006). Pain may result in sleep disturbances, depression, weight loss, agitation, and confusion (Herr & Mobily, 1991). Pain may be manifested in behavioral changes such as restless body movements, crying, oral vocalizations, resisting care, and facial grimacing (Volicer & Simard, 2009). Treatment of pain includes meeting the patient's needs such as thirst, hunger, coldness, or loneliness; using applications of heat and cold; positioning; and mild exercise. Pharmacotherapy includes the use of acetaminophen, oral morphine, and fentanyl skin patches (Volicer & Simard).

Seizures

Dementia is associated with a sixfold increased risk of developing seizures. The rate increases with the severity of the illness (Volicer & Simard, 2009). Seizures are treated with antiepileptic drugs (Mendez & Lim, 2003). However, Volicer and Simard cautioned that antiepileptic medication may cause problems with walking and may increase the risk for falls.

Hospice Care

The use of Hospice for patients with late-stage dementia is limited because of the Hospice Eligibility Criteria requirement that patients have a life expectancy of 6 months or less (Volicer & Simard, 2009). In addition, patients must have had at least one of the following in the last 12 months: aspiration pneumonia; pyelonephritis or other upper urinary tract infection; septicemia; decubitus ulcers, multiple, stage 3-4; fever, recurrent after antibiotics; inability to maintain sufficient fluid and calorie intake; and 10% weight loss during the previous 6 months.

Course

For some dementias, such as AD, the dementia is irreversible. For other dementias—such as those due to medical conditions, medications, infections, or vitamin deficiencies—the symptoms may be stopped or reversed to varying degrees (Weiner et al., 2009). The average length of life after establishment of a diagnosis of an irreversible dementia is 3 to 10 years. It is 10 years for individuals who develop dementia in their late 60s; 5.4 years for those who develop dementia in their 70s; 4.3 years for those who develop it in their 80s; and 3.8 years for those who develop it in their 90s (Savva & Brayne, 2009). Many patients are able to be maintained in their homes with care provided by their families (Savva & Brayne, 2009), but patients with severely regressed behaviors and those who are suicidal, violent, or psychotic may need to be admitted to a psychiatric inpatient unit (Bourgeois et al., 2011).

Working With Families and Caregivers

Caregivers and families should be monitored for biopsychosocial health problems during the patient's life and after the patient's death. Because family caregivers are at increased risk of medical and psychiatric disorders (Schulz & Martire, 2004), they should be offered information about how to protect their health. They should be told that problem-solving, coping, social support, emotional support, and religion have been found to be protective for caregivers (Roth, Mittelman, Clay, et al., 2005). For example, frequent attendance at religious services has been found to lessen depression and complicated grief among caregivers (Hebert, Dang, & Schulz, 2007).

Psychosocial Education

Education includes teaching specific skills and interventions that have been found to be helpful for family caregivers. These skills include behavioral management, treatment of depression, anger management, and lowering stress (Huang, Shyu, Chen, et al., 2003). Psychiatric advanced practice nurses may use the *Savvy Caregiver Program* (Hepburn, Lewis, Sherman, et al., 2003), which provides intervention training tools to teach the caregiver and the family. Families should be informed that patients' financial capabilities may be impaired very early on, even in the mild stage of AD. They should receive information on trust and estate arrangements; delegating financial decision-making powers; providing increased supervision of existing financial activities; and protecting patients and families from fraud schemes (Martin, Griffith, Belue, et al., 2008).

Education also includes teaching the family and caregivers how to modify the patient's environment. In addition to the environmental modifications described previously for patients with dementia who wander, certain modifications to the home environment can facilitate adaptive behaviors and promote safety (Calkins, 2004). They include the installation of grab-bars near the bathtub or shower, roll-in showers, and toilet seat risers. Structural modifications include widening doorways to accommodate wheelchairs or walkers, leveling walkways or building ramps, and fencing in walking areas in the yard (Burgio, Schmid, & Johnson, 2008). Warner and Warner (1996) provided specific suggestions for making the home safe for patients with AD. Some of their suggestions include securing windows and sliding doors; putting safety plugs in electrical outlets; removing extension cords, small tables, glass shelves, low stools, and scatter rugs; disconnecting the garbage disposal; using night lights; lowering the hot water setting to prevent burns; removing toxic substances; and locking up guns, sharp knives, power tools, car keys, liquor, matches, and medications.

Bereavement

Caregivers who have been caring for a family member with dementia for a long time may not be prepared for death (Hebert, Dang, & Schulz, 2006). In fact, complicated grief has been found to develop in 20% of caregivers after the death of the person they were caring for (Schulz, Boerner, Shear, et al., 2006). Caregivers and families should be offered bereavement support (Volicer & Simard, 2009).

Subtypes of Dementia

The characteristics, epidemiology, etiology, biological basis, clinical presentation, treatment, and course of the four major subtypes of dementia—Alzheimer's disease, vascular dementia, dementia with Lewy bodies, and frontotemporal dementia—will be discussed in the following section.

Alzheimer's Disease (AD)

Dr. Alois Alzheimer described a disease over 100 years ago that later became known as Alzheimer's disease (Mauer, 2006). He noted that the patient had progressive cognitive impairment, focal symptoms, hallucinations, delusions, and psychosocial incompetence. At autopsy, he found plaques, neurofibrillary tangles, and arteriosclerotic changes in the brain—the defining pathology of AD.

AD is a slow, progressive neuropsychiatric disorder that often begins with periods of memory impairment. Patients show early deficits in several cognitive functions, including memory, executive functioning, perceptual speed, verbal ability, visuospatial ability, and attention (Apostolova & Cummings, 2010; Backman, Jones, Berger, et al., 2005). Cognitive functioning declines slowly, and the diagnosis of AD is considered when impairments in memory and other cognitive functioning are severe enough to impact social or vocational functioning (Ngandu, 2006). Later symptoms include confusion, changes in behavior, sleep-wake disturbances, and changes in motor activity and activities of daily living (bathing, dressing, eating, and toileting) (Apostolova & Cummings).

Epidemiology

AD accounts for 50% to 70% of all cases of dementia (Malaspina, Corcoran, Schobel, et al., 2010). The cost of caring for patients with AD in the United States is approximately $100 billion annually (Geldmacher, 2009; Khachaturian Snyder, Doody, et al. 2009), which does not include the unpaid health care provided by family, friends, and neighbors. In the United States in 2009, nearly 11 million people provided 12.5 billion hours of unpaid care for patients with AD and other dementias. That care is valued at $144 billion a year (Alzheimer's Association, 2011). Thus, the 1-year cost of caring for individuals with AD is nearly $250 billion. Caregiving often carries a cost to the health of the caregiver; for instance, caregivers of patients with AD have a 63% higher risk of death than noncaregivers of the same age (Qiu et al., 2009).

Prevalence

Among the general population, prevalence of AD is 0.6% in males and 0.8% in females age 65; 11% in males and 14% in females age 85; 21% in males and 25% in females age 90; and 36% in males and 41% in females age 95 (American Psychiatric Association, 2000, p. 156). There are approximately 5 million people in the United States with AD (Geldmacher, 2009). Hebert, Scherr, Bienias, et al. (2003) predicted that there will be a sharp increase in the incidence of AD around 2030 when all the baby boomers will be over age 65, and by 2050 there will be 13.2 million people with AD in the United States. Among these, 8 million—approximately 60%—will be over 85 years of age. The anticipated tidal wave of AD and other dementias challenges psychiatric advanced practice nurses to develop ways to prevent or delay the onset, to manage the care of patients with AD, and to support their caregivers (Barnes, 2011).

Onset

The preclinical stage of AD is thought to last 10 years or longer (Amieva, Le Goff, Millet, et al., 2008; Korczyn, 2009). For example, Amieva et al. found that older adults who later developed AD had significant cognitive changes in semantic cognition and conceptual cognition 12 years before the diagnosis of AD was made. These cognitive impairments became more global, with problems with memory and symptoms of depression. Two years later, there was a decline in activities of daily living. Thus, the preclinical stage, in which there are already changes in the brain, starts more than a decade before the symptoms meet the criteria for a diagnosis of AD. Recent evidence suggests that the preclinical stage may cover several decades. A study of cognition in children between the ages of 11 and 16 years who have two risk factors for AD—a family history of AD and the *APOE e4* allele—found that, although they tested within the mean on cognitive testing, their performance was lower relative to other groups. These findings suggest that cognitive functioning may be impaired as early as childhood in individuals who will later develop AD (Bloss, Delis, Salmon, et al., 2008).

Risk Factors

Some risk factors for the development of AD are not modifiable, but others can be modified to reduce the incidence or delay the onset of AD. Risk factors for the development of AD that cannot be modified include advanced age, female gender, and ethnicity. For example, African Americans have twice the risk of developing AD as Caucasians, and individuals with Hispanic ethnicity are at one and one-half the risk (Alzheimer's Association, 2011). Other nonmodifiable risk factors include genetic vulnerability (genetic abnormalities of chromosomes 1, 6, 12, 14, and 21); Down's syndrome (individuals with Down's syndrome are at increased risk of developing AD, often by age 40, because they carry an extra copy of the *APP* gene [Tsuang & Bird, 2002]); and being the mother of a child with Down's syndrome (Alzheimer's Association).

Modifiable risk factors include cigarette smoking, heavy alcohol intake, midlife medical conditions (high blood pressure, obesity, diabetes, and cerebrovascular lesions), depression, head trauma, and lifestyle practices such as diet, physical and mental inactivity, and social isolation (Bassil & Grossberg, 2010; Geldmacher, 2009; Qiu et al., 2009).

- Among older adults, *current smoking* is a risk factor for the development of AD (Cataldo, Prochaska, & Glantz, 2010; Peters, Poulter, Warner, et al., 2008; Weih, Wiltfang, & Kornhuber, 2007). Their risk for developing AD is higher than that of older adults who have never smoked (Anstey, von Sanden, Salim, et al., 2007). *Heavy alcohol intake* (defined as more than two drinks a day [Harwood, Kalechstein, Barker, et al., 2010]) in midlife is a risk factor for the development of AD

(Weih et al., 2007). *Midlife hypertension*, especially untreated midlife hypertension, was found to be associated with increased risk of development of AD in late life (Qiu et al., 2009). Some studies have shown that use of antihypertensive medications is protective against the development of dementia and AD. For example, Aronow and Frishman (2006) found that treating hypertension provides protection against the development of both VaD and AD. Midlife high total cholesterol levels have been found to be associated with increased risk of AD later in life (Anstey et al., 2008; Kivipelto et al., 2002).

Depressive symptoms among older adults are associated with increased risk for AD (Luchsinger, Honig, Tang, et al., 2008).

- *Head injury* in early adult life is a risk factor for later development of AD and other dementias (Jellinger, Paulus, Wrocklage, et al., 2001). The risk for developing AD increases with the severity of the head injury (Plassman et al., 2000).
- There is some evidence that *lack of intellectually challenging activities* in midlife is associated with increased risk of AD later in life. For example, individuals who watch more television during the middle years have been found to have an increased risk of developing AD in comparison to those who watch less (Lindstrom, Fritsch, Petot, et al., 2005).

Protective Factors

Factors that may protect against the development of AD include a higher level of education; being married; maintaining regular physical activity (walking 15 minutes a day); engaging in cognitive, social and mental activities; having a rich social network; adhering to a healthy diet; and drinking a moderate amount of alcohol (Ngandu, 2006; Qiu et al., 2009; Weih et al., 2007). A high level of leisure activities—such as reading, visiting friends or relatives, going to the movies or out to eat, and walking for pleasure or going on trips—was found to be associated with a decreased risk of developing AD (Fratiglioni, Paillard-Borg, & Winblad, 2004; Scarmeas et al., 2001), as has participation in intellectually stimulating activities (Wilson et al., 2002).

Diet may also play a role in preventing the development of AD (Barnes, 2011; Luchsinger & Mayeux, 2004). Research studies have demonstrated an association between adherence to a Mediterranean diet and reduction of risk of developing AD (Scarmeas et al., 2006). Scarmeas et al. found that in comparison to the subjects who had the lowest level of adherence to the Mediterranean diet, those with moderate adherence had 15% to 21% less risk for developing AD, and those with high adherence to the Mediterranean diet had a 30% to 40% less risk for developing AD. Light to moderate alcohol drinking in late life has been found to reduce risk of developing AD (Anstey et al., 2009). Bassil and Grossberg (2010, p. 23) said that clinicians can reduce the risk of their patients' developing AD by supporting their mental, physical, and social health.

Etiology

The etiology of AD includes environmental influences, lifestyle practices, history of head trauma, and genetic vulnerability (Black & Andreasen, 2011; Malaspina et al., 2010). The overall heritability of AD is 58% (Smoller, Sheidley, & Tsuang, 2008), but genetic influences differ according to age of onset. AD is categorized as either early onset—at age 60 years or younger—or late onset—at older than age 60 years (McQueen & Blacker, 2008; National Institute on Aging, 2011).

Early-Onset Alzheimer's Disease

Early onset is more likely to be familial, to be rapidly progressive, to have temporal and parietal lobe features such as dysphasia and dyspraxia (Malaspina et al., 2010), and to follow an autosomal dominant inheritance pattern (McQueen & Blacker, p. 180). It is caused by mutations (permanent abnormal changes) in certain genes such as the amyloid precursor protein gene and the two presenilin genes, but these genes do not account for all of the cases of early-onset AD (Avramopoulos, 2009; Tanzi, Kovacs, & Kim, 1996).

Genes that have been found to be involved in early-onset AD include

1. The amyloid precursor protein (*APP*) gene on chromosome 21, which is associated with a mean age of onset of 51.5 years.
2. The *presenilin 1* gene on chromosome 14, which is associated with a mean age of onset of 44.1 years.
3. The *presenilin 2* gene on chromosome 1, which is associated with a mean age of onset of 57.1 years (McQueen & Blacker, 2008; Patterson et al., 2007).

If a parent has one of these genetic mutations, his or her child has a 50% chance of inheriting the mutated gene and developing early-onset AD (National Institute on Aging, 2011). However, mutation of these genes accounts for less than 2% of all cases of AD (Cedazo-Minguez & Cowburn, 2001; Spar & LaRue, 2006; Tsuang & Bird, 2002).

Late-Onset Alzheimer's Disease

Late-onset AD is the more common form of AD, accounting for 95% of all cases of AD (Avramopoulos, 2009). It is believed that the development of late-onset AD is influenced by the interaction of genetic risk factors—such as the presence of the *APOE e4* allele and the sortilin-related sorting receptor 1 (*SORL1*) gene—and factors such as head trauma, lack of mental and physical exercise, lower educational achievement, and a diet high in saturated fats (Apostolova & Cummings, 2010; Rosenberg, 2009). For example, researchers in Sweden found that physical inactivity, alcohol drinking, and smoking increased the risk of dementia among *APOE e4* carriers (Kivipelto et al., 2008). The theory of interaction of genetic and environment influences is also supported by research that has found that the concordance rate for late-onset AD among identical twins is approximately 60%, which is considered to be a moderate heritability (not high and not low) (Gatz, Fratiglioni, Johansson, et al., 2005). Thus, other factors play a role in the development of AD.

The *APOE e4* allele, which is located on chromosome 19 and has been confirmed as a genetic risk factor for late-onset AD (Hsiung & Sadovnick, 2007), is involved in metabolism of cholesterol and triglycerides and in beta-amyloid formation. It is synthesized and secreted by glial cells (astrocytes and microglia), and its production is increased in response to injury to the brain (Cedazo-Minguez & Cowburn, 2001). It has an effect on neurofibrillary tangle formation of tau protein, neuronal cell death, oxidative stress, synaptic plasticity, and dysfunctions in lipid homeostasis and cholinergic signaling (Bourgeois et al., 2008; Cedazo-Minguez & Cowburn).

There are three alleles of the *APOE* gene that influence the risk of late-onset AD.

1. *APOE e2* allele, which is found in 7% to 8% of the general population, may provide some protection against AD. It is also associated with decreased risk for cardiovascular disease and increased longevity.
2. *APOE e3* allele, which is found in 77% to 78% of the general population, plays a neutral role, neither increasing nor decreasing risk.
3. *APOE e4* allele, which is found in 14% to 16% of the general population, is associated with increased risk for late-onset AD. It is also associated with increased risk for cardiovascular disease, LBD, and frontal lobe dementia (Smith, 2000); with cognitive deficits in normal aging (overall cognitive functioning, memory, and executive functioning) (Small, Rosnick, Fratiglioni, et al., 2004); and with decreased longevity (McQueen & Blacker, 2008, p. 185). The association between the *APOE e4* allele and AD is stronger among women than men and diminishes with age. The fact that the *APOE e4* gene is present in only 50% of individuals who develop AD indicates that having the *APOE e4* allele does not mean that a person will develop AD, but it does increase the risk of his or her developing AD and the risk of earlier onset of AD (McQueen & Blacker).

SORL1 has recently been found to be associated with late-onset AD (Rogaeva, Meng, Lee, et al., 2007). *SORL1* is involved in amyloid precursor protein processing and transportation. Abnormalities of *SORL1* are associated with increased levels of beta-amyloid in the brain (Patterson, Feightner, Garcia, et al., 2007).

Biological Basis

Structural changes in AD include global cerebral atrophy (but with atrophy occurring to a greater extent in the temporal areas, parietal areas, and association areas), enlarged ventricles, and enlarged sulci (Geldmacher, 2009). In early-onset dementia, there is atrophy of the precuneus, which is the posterior medial portion of the parietal lobe. The percuneus is involved in spatially guided behavior and in complex cognitive functions. A smaller precuneus is associated with impaired visuospatial functioning; this correlates with the complaints of visuospatial problems and apraxia (inability to carry out motor functions although there is no loss of motor functioning), which occur more often in early-onset AD than do complaints of memory decline (Karas, Scheltens, Rombouts, et al., 2007). In late-onset AD, one of the first areas to be affected is the hippocampus (responsible for learning and memory). Hippocampal volume is already diminished in the predementia stage of MCI and in the presymptomatic stage of AD. There is also atrophy of the amygdala and cerebral cortex. The key pathological features of AD are neuritic plaques and neurofibrillary tangles (Davis, Lah, & Levey, 2009; Geldmacher, 2009). Postmortem examination of the brains of individuals with AD show brain atrophy, neuritic plaques, neurofibrillary tangles, and synaptic loss (Avramopoulos, 2009).

Neuritic Plaques

Neuritic plaques are microscopic and *extracellular.* They consist of a core amyloid (an abnormal proteinaceous material) mixed with branches of dying nerve cells. The core is surrounded by immune-activated microglia and reactive astrocytes. Neuritic plaque density is highest in the hippocampus, but neuritic plaques are also distributed in the cortex, entorhinal area (associated with smell), amygdala, and cerebral vessels of patients with AD, and the density increases as the disease progresses (Avramopoulos, 2009; Felician & Sandson, 1999; Geldmacher, 2009).

Neurofibrillary Tangles

Neurofibrillary tangles are *intracellular,* occupying large areas within the cell bodies of affected neurons, particularly neurons that communicate within and between the hemispheres. Neurofibrillary tangles contain hyperphosphorylated tau proteins and extracellular amyloid plaques that contain deposits of beta-amyloid (Avramopoulos, 2009). Neurofibrillary tangles are found throughout the cerebral cortex and the limbic system (Geldmacher, 2009).

Synaptic Loss

In AD, there is widespread loss of synaptic connections in the cortex of the brain. The deep layers of the temporal lobe and the hippocampus, which are areas of the brain involved in memory, have the greatest amount of loss of synaptic connections. In addition to loss of connections, there is loss of neurons that produce the neurotransmitters acetylcholine, norepinephrine, and serotonin (Geldmacher, 2009). According to Davis et al. (2009), failed neurotransmission at cholinergic synapses in the neocortex and hippocampus is a key factor in AD.

Clinical Presentation

Clinical presentation is usually of a gradual onset, and patients experience continuing cognitive decline that is most evident in memory deficits (Bourgeois et al., 2008;

Geldmacher, 2009). The deficits in cognition are due to loss of neurons and synaptic dysfunctioning, particularly in the hippocampus, limbic system, and polymodal association centers of the brain (Geldmacher).

Clinical presentation of AD is often discussed in terms of symptoms present in each stage of AD (mild, moderate, and advanced/late). Box 16-5 provides a list of symptoms of mild, moderate, and advanced stages of AD. Clinical presentation can also be discussed in terms of early-onset AD and late-onset AD.

BOX 16-5 Symptoms in Mild, Moderate, and Advanced Stages of Alzheimer's Disease

Mild Stage of Alzheimer's Disease

- Memory loss; patient misplaces objects; spatial disorientation
- Language problems; problems finding words; frequent repeating
- Mood swings
- Personality change
- Apathy
- Problems with judgment
- Reduced ability to plan or organize
- Problem with functioning at work or in social situations is noted by family or coworkers
- Preference for sweets
- Decreased ability to identify the smell of things

Moderate Stage of Alzheimer's Disease (worsening of previous symptoms)

- Increased memory loss; reduced memory of personal history
- Disoriented to time and place
- Impaired ability to do mental arithmetic and problems with abstract thinking
- Decreased ability to do complex tasks, such as paying bills or planning a dinner for guests
- Wandering
- Agitation
- Confusion; mood subdued or withdrawn
- Aggression; violent behavior
- Hallucinations (usually visual)
- Delusions: Capgras syndrome, e.g., familiar people are believed to be imposters; persecutory (theft and jealousy) (Rao & Lyketsos, 1998)

Advanced Stage of Alzheimer's Disease (worsening of previous symptoms)

- Problems walking
- May forget name of spouse or caregiver
- Problems eating, dressing self, and toileting
- Increasing suspiciousness
- Increasing psychotic symptoms
- Incontinence
- Inability to communicate
- Impaired swallowing
- Bedridden
- Death is usually from infection or pneumonia

Sources: Alzheimer's Association, 2010; Geldmacher, 2009.

Clinical Presentation in Early-Onset Alzheimer's Disease

Early-onset AD is characterized by losing of items, forgetfulness, confusion, personality changes, poor judgment, difficulty carrying out common tasks, problems with communication and language, social withdrawal, visuospatial problems, and apraxia. One of the most common symptoms is impairment of executive functioning (Balasa, Gelpi, Antonell, et al., 2011). There may be more psychiatric symptoms, such as depression and functional impairment, in patients with early-onset DA than in patients with late-onset AD. A family history of psychiatric disorders (such as schizophrenia, alcoholism, and completed suicide) is two-and-a-half times more common among patients with early-onset AD than among patients with late-onset AD (Devi, Williamson, Massoud, et al., 2004).

Clinical Presentation in Late-Onset Alzheimer's Disease

Early signs and symptoms of late-onset AD include loss of ability to identify smells, amnesia and cognitive symptoms, poor insight, spatial disorientation (e.g., the patient wanders aimlessly), apraxia, impaired ability for self-care, and inability to drive, work, or manage money.

Olfactory Dysfunction

Olfactory dysfunction, particularly impaired ability to identify odors such as orange or lemon, strawberry, cloves, leather, menthol, smoke, soap, and lilac, has been found to be present early on in patients with AD (Duff, McCaffrey, & Solomon, 2002; Luzzi, Snowden, Neary, et al., 2007; Tabert, Liu, Doty, et al., 2005).

Devanand et al. (2008) found that the presence of an olfactory identification deficit predicted which patients with MCI were at risk for developing AD. They suggested that an olfactory identification deficit reflects early AD pathology in the entorhinal cortex of the brain, which receives both direct olfactory input (odors) from the olfactory bulb and information from the brain's association areas, and transmits the information to the hippocampus, where memory and learning take place (p. 877). They stated that studies have shown that "neurofibrillary tangles begin in transentorhinal cortex and progress though limbic areas to neocortex" (p. 877). Thus, the first pathology of AD starts in the entorhinal cortex, moves on to the limbic area, and then to the cerebral cortex.

Wilson, Arnold, Schneider, et al. (2009) found that the presence of olfactory impairment among older adults without symptoms of MCI or AD was associated with later development of prodromal symptoms of both conditions. According to Duff et al. (2002), using a test such as the *Pocket Smell Test* (Sensonics, Inc.) or the *University of Pennsylvania Smell Identification Test (UPSIT)* (Doty, Shaman, & Dann, 1984) can be helpful in identifying which patients with MCI are transitioning to AD and in differentiating among AD, VaD, and major depressive disorder.

Cognitive Symptoms

In the early stage of AD, the following cognitive symptoms are frequently present:

- **Memory loss:** Short-term memory loss and difficulty learning new material (Geldmacher, 2009).
- **Language problems:** Problems finding words and frequent repeating. Language becomes vague, and that vagueness creates problems in communicating with others (Geldmacher, 2009).
- **Executive dysfunction:** Problems with executive functioning—judgment, problem-solving, planning, and abstract thinking. Impaired executive functioning is manifested in difficulty preparing meals, not persisting in completing tasks, and socially inappropriate behavior. Impairment of executive functioning is often the transition point from MCI to early dementia (Geldmacher, 2009).
- **Decreased capability of functioning in fiscal tasks:** In comparison to a control group of older adults without dementia, patients with mild AD had a 20% decrease in capability to carry out financial tasks (13% of the patients with mild AD were classified as capable and 87% were classified as marginally capable or incapable). Impairment was evident in bill-paying, checkbook and bank statement management, and ability to recognize mail fraud, telephone fraud, or exploitive scams. Progression of decreased fiscal capability is rapid. One year later, the patients with AD had a 30% decreased capability to carry out financial tasks, with only 9% classified as capable (Martin et al., 2008).

Orientation Problems

Patients misplace objects and have problems with time and space. Patients get lost in familiar settings and may even be unable to locate rooms, such as the bathroom (Geldmacher, 2009).

Apraxia

Patients experience *ideomotor apraxia*, which is the difficulty in translating an idea into spatial action, e.g., problems using eating utensils or buttons and zippers. They also experience *limb-kinetic apraxia*, which are problems positioning the body or limbs, e.g., putting arms in sleeves or getting out of a car (Geldmacher, 2009).

Visual Functioning

Patients have impairment of ability to recognize objects or faces. They have problems with depth perception, perception of movement or contrast, and directing or shifting attention. These abilities are essential for driving a car (Geldmacher, 2009).

Noncognitive and Behavioral Symptoms

Although cognitive symptoms are the most prominent and earliest of the symptoms of AD, noncognitive and behavioral symptoms may also be present (Geldmacher, 2009). As the disease progresses, noncognitive and behavioral symptoms often present more challenges to caregivers than cognitive symptoms (Geldmacher, 2009). Noncognitive and behavioral symptoms of AD include

- **Mood swings:** Approximately 20% of patients with AD have depressive symptoms (Aalten, de Vugt, Lousberg, et al., 2003; Zubenko, Zubenko, McPherson, et al., 2003).
- **Anxiety:** Anxiety is present in 25% of patients with AD who have moderate cognitive impairment (Porter, Buxton, Fairbanks, et al., 2003). Anxiety is manifested as catastrophic reactions (intense emotional outbursts of short duration), tears, and aggressive behaviors usually in response to a stressor, such as the caregiver bathing them or not letting them do something that they want to do (Geldmacher, 2009).
- **Apathy:** Apathy is evidenced as loss of motivation, reduced emotional expression, social withdrawal, and mood changes. Apathy is common in early stages of AD and occurs in 25% to 50% of patients (Geldmacher, 2009).
- **Agitation:** Agitation is reported in 50% to 60% of patients with AD (Geldmacher, 2009). Agitation may be spontaneous, occurring without a trigger. One example of agitation includes sundowning, which occurs in approximately 25% of patients with AD in the advanced stage of the illness (Little et al., 1995). Sundowning is now considered to be a composite of behaviors, including wandering, loud vocalizations, maladaptive behaviors, and physical aggression (Bliwise, 2004). Disinhibited agitation is a chronic form of agitation that has no trigger and is characterized by intrusiveness, restlessness, and aggressive manic-like symptoms.
- **Sleep disturbances:** Sleep disturbances occur in 25% to 35% of patients with AD. They parallel the severity of the dementia and are often the factor that precipitates placement of the patient in an institution (Vecchierini, 2010).
- **Behavioral changes:** Behavioral changes include withdrawal, wandering, pacing, and restlessness (Geldmacher, 2009).
- **Disinhibition:** Disinhibition is evidenced as uncharacteristic use of profanity, inappropriate sexual behavior, socially intrusive behavior, agitation, hostility, resistiveness, and oppositional behaviors. Disinhibition reflects impaired functioning of the frontal lobe (Geldmacher, 2009).
- **Motor slowing, gait disturbances:** In the early stage of AD, patients walk more slowly and with a shorter stride than older adults without AD (Nadkarni, Mawji, McIlroy, et al., 2009).
- **Personality changes:** Personality changes include becoming withdrawn, becoming suspicious of others, reacting with angry outbursts, and changes in attention to hygiene (Mace & Rabins, 2006).

- **Psychosis:** The presence of psychosis occurs later in the AD process. About 41% of patients with AD experience delusions, and 36% experience hallucinations at some point of their illness (Steinberg & Lyketsos, 2009). Delusions are often paranoid, and patients may accuse others of stealing their things, of infidelity, and of persecuting them. They may believe that family members are imposters, that where they are living is not their real home, or that they have been abandoned (Geldmacher, 2009; McKeith, Fairbairn, Perry, et al., 1992a). Delusions are very distressful symptoms for family caregivers to manage (Steinberg & Lyketsos). Hallucinations are usually visual and occur in 20% of patients with AD (McKeith et al.). They are often hallucinations of deceased relatives, of intruders (the phantom boarder syndrome), or of animals (Geldmacher & Whitehouse, 1996). Auditory hallucinations occur less often, and olfactory and tactile hallucinations are rare (Swearer, 1994).

Treatment

Treatment can be divided into interventions for cognitive symptoms, interventions for neuropsychiatric disruptive symptoms, and interventions for the specific behavioral symptoms of AD. Data obtained with a comprehensive psychiatric assessment provides the basis for treatment decisions.

Assessment

A clinical history is first obtained *from the patient* regarding his or her cognitive functioning, medical history, and social history. Then, history of the patient's cognitive functioning and behaviors is obtained *from the family* (Bourgeois et al., 2008). The following data should be obtained:

- History of functioning (work, social, and driving), memory loss, psychiatric history, family psychiatric history, and history of dementias
- History of medical conditions associated with increased risk of dementia: hypertension, diabetes mellitus, hyperlipidemia, Parkinson's disease, multiple sclerosis, cerebrovascular accident
- Medications
- Social history: social support, living situation, insurance, personal relationships
- History of agitation, violence, paranoia, neglect, or abuse
- Cognitive assessment: mini-mental status examination (score of 24 or less with clinical findings suggests dementia), clock drawing, and category generation (e.g., name as many animals as possible in 1 minute, naming 14 or less is suggestive of dementia)
- Physical assessment: hearing, vision, gait (often slower than normal for age), nutrition, weight loss or gain, dehydration
- Laboratory tests: electrolytes, liver enzymes, glucose, complete blood cell count, blood urea nitrogen, thyroid profile, vitamin B_{12}, and folate (Bourgeois et al., 2008; Geldmacher, 2009)

Interventions for Cognitive Symptoms

Pharmacotherapy is the main intervention for treatment of cognitive symptoms. Three cholinesterase inhibitors are used:

- *Donepezil* is approved for mild, moderate, and severe AD. When used early in the illness, donepezil has been found to improve cognitive functioning, activities of daily living, and global functioning (Gauthier, Lopez, Waldemar, et al., 2010; Winblad, Wimo, Engedal, et al., 2006).
- *Rivastigmine* is approved for mild to moderate dementia of Alzheimer's type. When used early in the illness, rivastigmine has been found to improve cognitive functioning (Cummings & Winblad, 2007). When rivastigmine was augmented with fluoxetine (Prozac), recipients had greater improvement of activities of daily living and global functioning than those who received rivastigmine alone or placebo (Mowla, Mosavinasab, Haghshenas, et al., 2007).
- *Galantamine* is approved for mild to moderate dementia of Alzheimer's type (Brown, 2009). Galantamine is a cholinesterase inhibitor that also acts at nicotinergic receptors (responsible for memory and alertness). It is believed that it enhances acetylcholine release (Raskind, Peskind, Wessel, et al., 2000). When used early in the illness, it improves cognition, behavior, and global functioning, including activities of daily living (Prvulovic, Hampel, & Pantel, 2010; Winblad et al., 2006). Seltzer (2010) found that galantamine was associated with improvement of cognitive functioning but not with improvement of behavioral symptoms.

There is general agreement that treatment with these three cholinesterase inhibitors is appropriate for mild and moderate stages of AD. They increase the availability of acetylcholine in the synaptic cleft and have been found to have modest effects on cognition, functioning, and behavior (Apostolova & Cummings, 2010; Farlow & Boustani, 2009). In addition to keeping more acetylcholine available in the synaptic cleft, cholinesterase inhibitors may have a neuroprotective function for the neurons in the hippocampus (Hashimoto, Kazui, Matsumoto, et al., 2005). Among patients with severe AD, donepezil has been found to result in symptomatic benefits in cognition, global functioning, and activities of daily living (Winblad, Black, Homma, et al., 2009).

There is some evidence that long-term treatment with cholinesterase inhibitors (for 3 to 5 years) is beneficial (Seltzer, 2007). However, in a 36-week prospective observational study of 938 patients with mild to moderate AD who were receiving donepezil, galantamine, or rivastigmine, the researchers reported that no significant improvement in cognition, activities of daily living, or symptoms of AD was found. They did make the point that in studying patients in clinical practice (in comparison to clinical trials), the dose of medications may have been lower, the length of treatment may have been shorter, and the patients may have had more comorbid illnesses (Santoro, Siviero, Minicuci, 2010).

Other medications being studied for treating cognitive symptoms of AD include NMDA receptor antagonists, antihistamines, and monoamine oxidase inhibitor type B.

- *NMDA receptor antagonist.* Memantine, an NMDA receptor antagonist, is approved for treatment of moderate to severe AD (Apostolova & Cummings, 2010). Memantine modulates activity of glutamate (Reisberg, Doody, Stoffler, et al., 2003) and is believed to have neuroprotective effects (Hartmann & Mobius, 2003). When added to donepezil, memantine has been found to increase the benefits of donepezil with resulting improvement in functioning, cognition, behavior and global change (McKeage, 2010). The combination of memantine with any of the three approved cholinesterase inhibitors is considered to be the gold standard of treatment for moderate to severe AD and possibly for mild to moderate AD as well (Patel & Grossberg, 2011).
- *Antihistamine medications.* Research has shown that latrepirdine (Dimebon), a nonselective antihistamine drug, improves the clinical course of patients with mild to moderate AD. Patients receiving latrepirdine showed improvement in cognitive functioning, memory, ability to perform tasks of daily living, and behaviors. The improvements continued and lasted over time (Doody et al., 2008).
- *Monoamine oxidase inhibitor type B.* Selegiline (Eldepryl) is used for its antioxidant properties. It has a positive effect on cognition and behavior. A tyramine-restricted diet is not required at doses up to 10 mg a day. It is contraindicated for patients receiving SSRIs, tricyclic antidepressants, meperidine (Demerol), or opioids.

Interventions for Neuropsychiatric Disruptive Symptoms

Patients with neuropsychiatric symptoms should be assessed for physical health problems, such as urinary tract infections or dental infections, as possible causes of the symptoms. Pain has also been found to be the cause of neuropsychiatric disturbances (Ballard, Corbett, Chitramohan, et al., 2009).

The first line of treatment of neuropsychiatric disruptive symptoms is the use of psychosocial interventions, such as those discussed earlier for treatment of dementia. Reminiscence therapy, personalized music, nonconfrontational and enjoyable social interactions, walking, and aromatherapy have been found to be effective in reducing disruptive symptoms (Yaari et al., 2009). For example, aromatherapy using lavender oils or *Melissa* oil (lemon balm) has been found to reduce agitation (Ballard, O'Brien, Reichelt, et al., 2002). Psychosocial interventions have been found to reduce agitation overall and to reduce the specific behavior of shouting (Cohen-Mansfield, Libin, & Marx, 2007; Cohen-Mansfield & Werner, 1997).

If there is a high risk of danger for the patient or others or a high level of distress, pharmacotherapy may be considered the first line of treatment (Ballard et al., 2009). Salzman & Tariot (2009) have reminded clinicians that "No drugs have been approved by the FDA for the treatment of persisting psychosis, agitation or aggression associated with dementia" (p. 1201). However, antipsychotic medications are usually considered to be the first choice for agitation and psychotic symptoms. Because of the side effects—such as akathisia, parkinsonian symptoms, tardive dyskinesia, sedation, postural hypotension, and increased risk for falling—of conventional antipsychotics (e.g., haloperidol), atypical antipsychotics are used more frequently (Yaari et al., 2009).

In 2005, the FDA issued a warning about a significant increase in mortality among patients with AD who were treated with atypical antipsychotics; mortality was most often from infections and cerebrovascular causes (Steinberg & Lyketsos, 2009). In nursing homes, the Omnibus Budget Reconciliation Act of 1987 regulates use of antipsychotics; for instance, there must be clear documentation of clinical indications and considerations of alternative interventions (American Psychiatric Association, 1997). With regard to risk of cerebrovascular accidents and death in patients with dementia treated with atypical antipsychotics, Schneider, Dagerman, and Insel (2005) reviewed the evidence and concluded that there was a significant increase in mortality, and they found no difference among the different atypical antipsychotics. Patients at higher risk for developing stroke are those with hypertension, diabetes, and atrial fibrillation (Bullock, 2005; Sink et al., 2005). Ballard et al. (2009, p. 535) recommended that the use of atypical antipsychotics be limited to short-term treatment (6 to 12 weeks) for severe physical aggression or severe psychotic symptoms.

Interventions for Specific Behavioral Symptoms of Alzheimer's Disease

Specific behavioral symptoms of AD include depression with agitation, agitation and aggression, paranoia, and psychosis.

Depression With Agitation

- For depression with agitation or aggression, the antidepressant medication citalopram has been found to be as effective as the atypical antipsychotic risperidone (Pollock et al., 2002).
- For depression with psychotic symptoms or for treatment of psychosis, the atypical antipsychotics risperidone, quetiapine, olanzapine, aripiprazole, and ziprasidone are helpful (Apostolova & Cummings, 2010).

Agitation and Aggression

- Agitation occurs in 40% to 60% of patients with AD in institutions (Margallo-Lana, Swann, O'Brien, et al., 2001).

- Physical aggression occurs in 11% to 46% of patients with dementia living in the community and in 31% to 42% of patients with dementia in institutional settings (Cohen-Mansfield, Werner, Watson, et al., 1995).
- For mild symptoms, behavioral modification—such as structured activities, redirection, and reassurance—may be effective.
- When nonpharmacological interventions are not successful, atypical antipsychotics and SSRIs may be used (Apostolova & Cummings, 2010). Risperidone has the best evidence for treatment of agitation/aggression, and there is some evidence for success with aripiprazole. There is no clear evidence of the effectiveness of other atypical antipsychotics (Schneider et al., 2006b).
- There is little evidence of effectiveness of long-term use of atypical antipsychotics for the treatment of agitation or aggression (Schneider, Tariot, Dagerman, et al., 2006c).

Paranoid Thinking and Psychosis

- Psychosocial interventions, such as distraction, reassurance of the patient's safety, and reminiscence therapy, are tried first to reduce the distress associated with paranoid thinking and psychosis.
- Atypical antipsychotics such as risperidone, olanzapine, quetiapine, ziprasidone, and aripiprazole may be used to manage symptoms of paranoid thinking and psychosis. Note that olanzapine and quetiapine have sedative properties, but olanzapine may cause gait disturbances and weight gain.

Summary of the Use of Atypical Antipsychotics

Based on a meta-analysis of 15 placebo-controlled trials of atypical antipsychotic medications used for patients with dementia, Schneider et al. (2006b) found that the response rate was 48% to 65% in comparison to a response rate to placebo of 30% to 48%. Adverse effects of the atypical antipsychotics included sleepiness, falls, edema, extrapyramidal tract symptoms, and urinary tract infections. For responders, the overall treatment effect is about 20% (i.e., atypical antipsychotics may be only about 20% more effective than placebo) (Yaari et al., 2009).

Course

Most patients who develop AD have MCI or predementia symptoms of cognitive decline before converting to AD. The course of AD is progressive, with symptoms becoming more severe, with greater impairment of functioning, and with increased dependence on others for care. The average life span after diagnosis of AD is 6 to 9 years (Korczyn, 2009). Shorter survival time is associated with earlier onset, older age, male gender, Caucasian race, lower levels of education, presence of comorbidities such as hypertension or diabetes, poorer cognitive functioning, physical disabilities, disruptive behavioral symptoms, falls, and wandering (Larson, Shadlen, Want, et al., 2004; Qiu et al., 2009).

Dementia With Lewy Bodies (DLB)

In 1984, Kosaka and colleagues identified DLB as a type of dementia that is different from AD (Kosaka, Yashimura, Ikeda, et al.). On examining the brains at autopsy of patients with dementia, they found that some of the brains had Lewy bodies instead of the plaques and neurofibrillary tangles usually seen in the brains of patients with AD (Neef & Walling, 2006). A decade later, in 1996, the key features of DLB were agreed upon at the First International Workshop of the Consortium on Dementia with Lewy Bodies (McKeith, Galaski, Kosaka, et al., 1996). It is now accepted that DLB is a distinct syndrome. Some of the symptoms are specific and some overlap with AD and with Parkinson's disease with dementia. It is crucial that psychiatric advanced practice nurses be able to make the correct diagnosis because the treatment, prognosis, and response to pharmacotherapy of patients with DLB are different than those of patients with Parkinson's disease or of patients with AD. For example, patients with DLB are at risk of *severe adverse reactions to antipsychotic medications,* including a twofold to threefold increase in mortality (Neef & Walling), and patients with DLB have a better response to cholinesterase inhibitors (McKeith, Del Ser, Spano, et al., 2000).

DLB is a neurodegenerative dementia that is characterized by (1) a progressive cognitive decline that is severe enough to limit social and work functioning and by (2) two of the following symptoms: fluctuating cognition that is sometimes called "pseudodelirium" (Neef & Walling, 2006, p. 1225); visual hallucinations; and parkinsonian symptoms (McKeith, Perry, Fairbairn, et al., 1992b). Additional features of DLB include daytime sleeping for longer than 2 hours; staring into space for long periods; disorganized speech (Ferman, Smith, Boeve, et al., 2004; Geser, Wenning, Poewe, et al., 2005); repeated falls; syncope; depression; sensitivity to antipsychotic medications (McKeith et al.); rapid eye movement sleep behavior disorder (Geser et al.); and sundowning (Carr, 2006). In contrast to patients with AD, short-term memory may be good in patients with Lewy body dementia (Yuhas et al., 2006).

Epidemiology and Prevalence

DLB is the second most common cause of neurodegenerative dementia among older adults, after AD (Geser et al., 2005; Josif & Graham, 2008). Prevalence is 0 to 5% of general population (Zaccai, McCracken, & Brayne, 2005). It accounts for about 15% to 20% of all late-onset dementias (Apostolova & Cummings, 2010). However, postmortem studies have shown that 40% of the brains of patients with dementia had sufficient cortical Lewy bodies to be diagnosed as DLB, suggesting that the diagnosis of DLB is often missed (Galvin, Pollack, & Morris, 2006). The age of onset is 75 to 80 years of age, and it is more common in males.

Etiology

Among patients with LBD, approximately half have a relative with dementia or memory problems (Woodruff, Graff-Radford, Ferman, et al., 2006). It appears that genetic factors influence the development of DLB, but no genetic abnormalities have been identified at this time (Lippa, Duda, Grossman, et al., 2007).

Biological Basis

Microscopic Abnormalities

There are distinctive microscopic abnormalities inside neurons that are called *Lewy bodies*. The Lewy bodies contain a protein called alpha-synuclein, which functions as a modulator of synaptic neurotransmission and synaptic vesicle transport. It plays a role in neuronal plasticity (Jellinger, 2003). Lewy bodies are found in subcortical areas of the brain (amygdala and limbic structures), in the cortical areas of the brain (frontotemporal, insular, and cingulate cortexes), and in the brainstem (Neef & Walling, 2006). In DLB there may also be the amyloid plaques that are seen in AD, but there are not usually the neurofibrillary tangles that are associated with AD (Geldmacher, 2004; Tarawneh & Galvin, 2009). Both the acetylcholine neurotransmitter system and the dopamine system are involved in DLB. There is also believed to be an imbalance of the serotonergic system (Bowen, Procter, Mann, et al., 2008).

Structural and Functional Abnormalities

Patients with DLB have brain atrophy similar to that found in AD, but less severe. The structures of the limbic system—the amygdala, hypothalamus, and basal forebrain—and areas of the cortex—the cingulate cortex, entorhinal area, and temporal cortex—are most often involved. There is less involvement of the hippocampus, and this lack of involvement may account for less severe memory impairment in patients with DLB in comparison to patients with AD. There is impairment of functioning of temporoparietal and occipital brain areas in DLB; there are also abnormalities of the dopamine transport function in DLB, which do not occur in AD (O'Brien, Colloby, Fenwick, et al., 2004; Tarawneh & Galvin, 2009).

Clinical Presentation

Clinical presentation frequently includes a progressive decline of cognitive functioning, fluctuation in cognition, and psychotic symptoms such as visual hallucinations. There may be a history of frequent falls and sleep disturbances, and parkinsonian symptoms may be present (Tarawneh & Galvin, 2009).

Decline in Cognitive Functioning

The cognitive impairment of patients with DLB differs from that of patients with AD. The early signs of cognitive dysfunction in patients with DLB are impairment of executive functioning, such as planning and initiating appropriate behaviors; motor slowness; and apathy (Geldmacher, 2004). Verbal skills are not impaired. Patients with DLB may not have memory impairment early in the disease. They have better recall of information than patients with AD; however, as the disease progresses, they have difficulty in retrieving information. Patients with DLB have difficulty with visuospatial functioning; for instance, they have difficulty getting around in their homes. Early in the course of the disease, they have difficulty with visual perceptive tasks and visual counting, and they often do poorly on the clock drawing test.

Fluctuation of Cognition

Fluctuation of cognition is an important clinical symptom that occurs in 80% to 90% of patients with DLB (Apostolova & Cummings, 2010; McKeith et al., 1996), in comparison to 40% of patients with VaD and 20% of patients with AD (Kolbeinsson & Jonsson, 1993). Fluctuation of cognition in DLB may resemble delirium, but without a precipitating cause (Ferman et al., 2004). Fluctuations include transient changes in cognition, functional abilities, and arousal (Ferman et al.). Fluctuations of cognition and functioning include both periods of behavioral confusion, inattention, and incoherent speech and periods of cognitive awareness and ability to carry out tasks. Fluctuations of arousal are manifested as hypersomnolence, daytime drowsiness and lethargy, daytime sleeping, and staring into space for long periods of time (McKeith et al.).

Ferman et al. (2004) suggested that fluctuations in cognition be evaluated by asking about drowsiness and lethargy during the day; daytime sleep of 2 hours or more; staring into space for long periods of time; and periods when the patient's thoughts seem unclear, disorganized, or not logical. Three or four of these signs of fluctuation of cognition have been found to be experienced by 63% of patients with DLB, but only 12% of patients with AD and only 0.5% of older adults without dementia experience these same signs (Ferman et al.). Fluctuation of cognition, functional abilities, and arousal can also be assessed using scales such as the *Clinician Assessment of Fluctuation* and *One Day Fluctuation Assessment Scale* (Walker et al., 2000).

Psychiatric Symptoms: Hallucinations, Delusions, Depression, and Anxiety

Occurrence of hallucinations and delusions early in the course of the disease is a strong indicator of DLB (Litvan, MacIntyre, Goetz, et al., 1998). Visual hallucinations occur in 80% of patients with DLB and tend to occur more frequently in the evening (Apostolova & Cummings, 2010; Neef & Walling, 2006). The hallucinations are usually benign and often are of people or animals. The figures or animals in the hallucinations are smaller than normal size. The visual hallucinations cause fear in some patients but are usually not distressful to the patient (Yuhas et al., 2006). Auditory hallucinations accompany visual hallucinations in approximately half of patients with DLB but rarely occur without visual hallucinations (Apostolova & Cummings; Tarawneh & Galvin, 2009).

Delusions occur more frequently in patients with DLB than in patients with AD. They occur in 65% of patients with DLB over the course of the illness (Tarawneh & Galvin, 2009). They are usually delusions of misidentification, such as mistaking images for real people; Capgras syndrome (believing that familiar relatives have been replaced by strangers); or mistaking their own reflection in a mirror for another person. There may also be paranoid delusions, such as of theft and infidelity, or they may have a delusion of there being a stranger in the house (Apostolova & Cummings, 2010).

Depression is more common in patients with DLB than in patients with AD, occurring in 50% of patients with DLB (Tarawneh & Galvin, 2009). Anxiety occurs in approximately 84% of patients with DLB. Symptoms of apathy, agitation, and aggression are common, but euphoria and disinhibition are not (Del Ser, McKeith, Anand, et al., 2000).

Sleep Disruptions

Sleep disturbances occur early in the disease process and may be present before other symptoms. Patients with DLB have vivid dreams and often vocalize or move about during the dream and may act out the dream (Josif & Graham, 2008).

Extrapyramidal Symptoms

Patients with DLB experience extrapyramidal tract symptoms that include rigidity, resting tremor, and gait disturbances (Apostolova & Cummings, 2010). However, in the early stage, patients with DLB do not usually experience the more severe postural instability, cogwheel rigidity, and dystonia that are seen in Parkinson's disease. The occurrence of frequent falls seems to be related to their inability to prevent the fall if they trip or are bumped (Yuhas et al., 2006). Some patients with DLB experience restless leg syndrome and may describe a pulling or crawling sensation in the legs.

Other extrapyramidal symptoms include depression and dysfunction of the autonomic nervous system with syncope, postural instability, transient loss of consciousness, orthostatic hypotension, constipation, fainting, and swallowing difficulties. Urinary incontinence may occur early in the course of the DLB (Geser et al., 2005).

Differential Diagnosis

Differential diagnoses of DLB include AD, Parkinson's disease, and medical disorders.

- *AD*. Women are more likely to have AD and men are more likely to have DLB. Patients with DLB have more psychiatric symptoms and are assessed as having greater impairment of functioning (Rippon & Marder, 2005). Early visuospatial impairment and visuoconstructional dysfunction—such as seen on the clock drawing test or figure copying test—is more common in DLB than AD. Preservation of short-term memory and ability to name items is greater in patients with DLB (Geser et al., 2005).
- ***Parkinson's disease.*** If motor symptoms begin more than a year before dementia, the diagnosis of Parkinson's disease dementia should be considered. However, if cognitive symptoms start before the motor symptoms or if the motor symptoms and cognitive symptoms start within the same year, the diagnosis of DLB should be considered (Apostolova & Cummings, 2010).
- ***Medical disorders.*** Laboratory tests are done to rule out other causes of dementia, such as vitamin B_{12} deficiency and hypothyroidism (Lippa et al., 2007).

Comorbidity

Parkinson's disease occurs in approximately 75% of patients with DLB.

Treatment

Treatment for DLB includes pharmacotherapy and nonpharmacological/psychosocial interventions.

Pharmacotherapy

No drug has been approved by the FDA for the treatment of DLB (Geldmacher, 2004). However, studies have been done on the use of antipsychotic drugs, dopaminergic therapy, and cholinesterase inhibitors to treat DLB symptoms.

- ***Antipsychotic drugs.*** Patients with DLB have an increased sensitivity to antipsychotic medications (McKeith et al., 1992a), with 81% experiencing extrapyramidal symptoms such as sedation, confusion, severe rigidity, and neuroleptic malignant syndrome. Therefore, the use of antipsychotic medications is not recommended for patients with DLB (Apostolova & Cummings, 2010). Cautious use of atypical antipsychotics in low doses is sometimes tried, with close observation for cognitive symptoms (Swanberg & Cummings, 2002).
- ***Dopaminergic therapy.*** Some patients with DLB with parkinsonian symptoms respond to levodopa-carbidopa (Sinemet). Overall, they do not respond as well as patients with Parkinson's disease with dementia. Side effects include visual hallucinations, delusions, orthostatic hypotension, and gastrointestinal upset (Fernandez, Wu, & Ott, 2003; Mosimann & McKeith, 2003).
- ***Cholinesterase inhibitors.*** Some patients with DLB benefit from cholinesterase inhibitors with an improvement of cognitive symptoms, such as alertness, memory, attention, and executive functioning (McKeith et al., 2000; Wesnes, McKeith, Ferrara, et al., 2002). Other symptoms—hallucinations, paranoid delusions, daytime sleepiness, apathy, aggression, and agitation—have also been found to improve (Fernandez et al., 2003; Simard & van Reekum, 2004).

Nonpharmacological and Psychosocial Interventions

Nonpharmacological interventions or psychosocial interventions are the same as for other dementias. The focus is on changing factors that trigger problematic behaviors such as agitation, aggressiveness, depression, neglect of hygiene, and wandering (Tarawneh & Galvin, 2009).

Course

The most frequent symptoms seen on initial evaluation of patients with DLB are fluctuating cognition, visual hallucinations, and vivid dreams. Other early symptoms include psychiatric symptoms and alterations of consciousness. Symptoms due to impairment of the autonomic nervous system—such as orthostatic hypotension and constipation—occur later. Progression of the symptoms of DLB is more rapid than the progression of symptoms in patients with AD (Geser et al., 2005). Survival rate has been found to be about 8 years (Geldmacher, 2004). Early studies reported that the survival rate of patients with DLB was shorter than that of patients with AD (Lippa, Smith, & Swearer, 1994), but in a follow-up study of 114 patients with dementia, no difference in length of survival was found between patients with DLB and those with AD (Walker, Allen, Shergill, et al., 2000).

Vascular Dementia (VaD)

VaD is the third most frequently occurring dementia among older adults (Apostolova & Cummings, 2010). It is a group of syndromes related to different vascular changes and includes arteriosclerotic dementia, multi-infarct dementia, and post-stroke dementia. Post-stroke dementia occurs in one-third of people over age 65 who have had a stroke (Esiri, Nagy, Smith, et al., 1999). The syndromes within vascular dementia have different clinical presentations and different underlying pathologies (Jellinger, 2008). They are often associated with heart disease, hypertension, alcohol abuse, and stroke. To the extent that vascular changes are preventable, VaD is also preventable (Szoeke, Campbell, Chiu, et al., 2009).

Epidemiology

VaD accounts for 8% to 15% of all dementias (Jellinger, 2008). VaD occurs more frequently in males. It has a more abrupt onset than AD and causes more gait disturbance, mood swings, decreased executive functioning, and parkinsonian symptoms. Vascular lesions often coexist with AD; for example, 25% to 80% of patients with dementia have both AD and vascular pathology.

VaD may have a rapid onset as a consequence of a stroke or transient ischemic attack. Like other dementias, it is characterized by impairment of memory, executive functioning, and physical abilities (Yuhas et al., 2006). In contrast to AD, in which all areas of the brain may be affected, VaD affects only distinct parts of the brain, and thus some abilities are left intact. In contrast to patients with AD and DLB, patients with VaD may have a better understanding of what is happening to them (Yuhas et al.).

Etiology

No clear genetic risk factor for developing VaD has been found at this time (Szoeke et al., 2009). Advancing age and factors associated with aging such as folic acid deficiency, hypertension, diabetes mellitus, hyperlipidemia, atrial fibrillation, decreased physical activity, obesity, cumulative effects of smoking, and previous use of oral contraceptives increase the likelihood of vascular events that are associated with the development of dementia (Korczyn, 2002; Szoeke et al.). Large lesions, such as those due to pathology of large vessels, can cause focal damage, and specific symptoms of dementia are related to the area damaged. Diffuse damage may be due to hypertension's effect on small vessels.

Biological Basis

Pathology of VaD is heterogeneous. There may be infarcts in several areas of the brain, including the cortical and subcortical areas, basal ganglia, thalamus, temporal lobe, white matter, or brainstem (Jellinger, 2008). There may also be diffuse vascular lesions or ischemic lesions.

VaD pathology affects different brain areas and neuronal networks. The cognitive impairment of VaD is consistent with disturbed cortical and subcortical circuits that support cognition, memory, and behavior (Jellinger, 2008). There is evidence of abnormalities of the cholinergic and serotonergic neurotransmitter systems; the findings of disruptions of the cholinergic system support the use of cholinesterase inhibitors. There is some evidence of abnormalities of dopamine, glutamate, and gamma-aminobutyric acid systems (Szoeke et al., 2009).

Clinical Presentation

Symptoms of anxiety, depression, confusion, and wandering are common. Approximately 70% of patients with VaD have symptoms of anxiety and 20% have symptoms of depression (Ballard, Neill, O'Brien, et al., 2000), and major depressive disorder is a frequent comorbid disorder in post-stroke patients with dementia (Yuhas et al., 2006).

Apathy, irritability, and aggressive behaviors may also be present. The apathy, depression, and agitation associated with VaD are more severe than those seen in AD. Cognitive deficits often include impairment of executive functioning. There may be problems with memory, attention, and language, such as naming things (Apostolova & Cummings, 2010). Slowing of motor functioning and physical disabilities may be present.

Treatment

Treatment for VaD includes an initial assessment, preventive interventions, pharmacotherapy, and nonpharmacological/psychosocial interventions.

Assessment

Assessment should include a family history and the patient's history of hypertension, smoking, lipid profile, diabetes, arrhythmias, and presence of cardiovascular or peripheral vascular disease. A history of a stepwise progress of changes is characteristic of multi-infarct dementia. In addition to memory problems, there may be changes in cognition, such as attention, speed of information processing, and executive functioning. Patients may have better recall than patients with AD but may have poor verbal fluency (Szoeke et al., 2009). The occurrence of symptoms of depression and anxiety is greater in vascular dementia than in AD.

Preventive Interventions

Preventing strokes in patients who have a high risk of experiencing a stroke is a primary step in reducing the incidence of VaD (Goldstein, 2006). Preventive interventions include lifestyle changes to a low-fat diet, supplementation with folate and B vitamins, and smoking cessation; treatment of diabetes, hypertension, and hyperlipidemia; and use of aspirin for prophylaxis. Cardiovascular risk factors are treated to delay the progress of the dementia and to prevent the development of vascular comorbidities. As stated previously, atypical antipsychotics increase the risk of stroke and death in older patients with dementia and should be avoided (Bullock, 2005; Sink et al., 2005).

Pharmacotherapy

Treatment with cholinesterase inhibitors has been found to be associated with small but statistically significant improvement of cognitive functioning (Roman, Salloway, Black, et al., 2010). They are also effective in treating apathy (Roth, Flashman, & McAllister, 2007). Patients receiving memantine have been found to have some improvement of cognition but not of functioning (McShane, Areosa, & Minadaran, 2006).

Nonpharmacological and Psychosocial Interventions

Psychosocial interventions that were discussed under treatment of dementia are appropriate for patients with VaD. Support for families and caregivers, provision of information about community resources, and referrals for assistance are important components of treatment.

Course

Patients with vascular cognitive impairment are at high risk of developing dementia (Wentzel, Rockwood, McKnight, et al., 2001). In a 5-year study of patients with vascular cognitive impairment without dementia at baseline, all had developed VaD after 5 years (Wentzel et al.). The life expectancy of patients with VaD is shorter than that of patients with AD and is related to the underlying vascular disorder and comorbid conditions (Szoeke et al., 2009).

Frontotemporal Dementia (FTD)

FTD refers to a group of neurological disorders (Lipton & Boxer, 2009) that result from atrophy of the frontal and anterior temporal lobes of the brain (Apostolova & Cummings, 2010). Although many terms are used for this group of disorders, the preferred term for clinical use is frontotemporal dementia (Arvanitakis, 2010). FTD, which typically occurs between 50 and 60 years of age, is the most common cause of presenile dementia (dementia occurring before age 65 years) (Merrilees & Ketelle, 2010). It accounts for approximately 10% to 20% of all dementia cases (Miller, Boone, Mishkin, et al., 1998). It is a slowly progressing dementia with behavioral or language disturbances and changes in personality but with memory and spatial orientation usually remaining intact in the early stage (Arvanitakis, 2010). Frequently used categories of FTD include frontotemporal dementia with behavioral variant, frontotemporal dementia with language variant, frontotemporal lobar degeneration (used interchangeablely with FTD), Pick's disease, and frontotemporal dementia with motor neuron disease (Arvanitakis, 2010; Mitsuyama & Inoue, 2009). Information on these categories of FTD can be found in Box 16-6.

Epidemiology

The onset of FTD is subtle and insidious, and it is likely to occur among adults in their 50s (Lipton & Boxer, 2009). The mean age of onset of FTD is 52.5 years, and it is more common in males (Arvanitakis, 2010). Risk factors for FTD include the risk factors for dementia that were discussed earlier and also a history of head trauma, especially head trauma with loss of consciousness that suggests a severe head trauma (Rosso et al., 2003b). There is a suggestion that thyroid disease may be a risk factor. For example, Rosso et al. found that thyroid abnormalities occurred in 38% of patients with FTD.

Etiology

In a study of 250 patients with FTD, it was found that 43% of the patients had a family member with dementia (Rosso, Kaat, Baks, et al., 2003a). However, in approximately 60% of cases of FTD, there is no family history of FTD (Rosso et al., 2003b). These cases are called sporadic or nonfamilial FTD, and other individuals in the family are not at increased risk of developing FTD (Memory and Aging Center, University of California at San Francisco, 2010a).

Genetic Influences

Research related to FTD suggests the presence of mutations on chromosome 17 with mutations of the protein tau gene and the progranulin gene (Baker, Mackenzie, Pickering-Brown, et al., 2006; Gijselinck, Van Broeckhoven, & Cruts, 2008). Tau is a microtubule-associated protein that is involved in transporting nutrients and molecules within cells. In neurons, it transports nutrients and molecules

BOX 16-6 Subtypes of Frontotemporal Dementia

Frontotemporal Dementia With Behavioral Variant

FTD with behavioral variant is associated with structural abnormalities of the right frontotemporal lobes (Mychack, Kramer, Boone, et al., 2001). It is characterized by

- Impairment of executive, social, and interpersonal functioning
- Presence of apathy, disinhibition, and sexually inappropriate behaviors
- Changes in personality, self-care, and hygiene
- Impaired judgment
- Poor insight into consequences of actions
- Repetitive and compulsive behaviors such as hyperorality; patients may eat large amounts of food at a time and may have carbohydrate cravings; patients may engage in compulsive hoarding (Lipton & Boxer, 2009)
- Inappropriate social behavior

Frontotemporal Dementia With Language Variant (Semantic Dementia and Progressive Nonfluent Aphasia)

Semantic Dementia

Semantic dementia is caused by progressive degeneration of the anterior temporal lobes (Lipton & Boxer). It is manifested as severe difficulty in naming things and in understanding the meaning of words. Deficits of functioning of the left temporal lobe are associated with difficulty describing how something works. Deficits of functioning of the right temporal lobe are associated with difficulty recognizing faces and with changes in behavior similar to those of FTD with behavioral variant (Lipton & Boxer).

Progressive Nonfluent Aphasia

Progressive nonfluent aphasia involves word-finding difficulty, lack of grammatical elements (verbs, articles, pronouns, prepositions), and phonemic paraphasias such as using words related to the word that cannot be retrieved (e.g., "forks" for "knives"). Functional and behavioral impairment does not usually occur until late in the disorder (Lipton & Boxer).

Frontotemporal Lobar Degeneration (FTLD)

The term FTLD is sometimes used interchangeably with the term FTD (Mitsuyama & Inoue, 2009), and the symptoms are the same as those of FTD with Behavioral Variant.

FTLD tends to occur in younger patients (those younger than age 65 years). Lack of insight is a key feature (Lipton & Boxer). There is gradual progression of the disease, and survival is approximately 6 years (Lipton & Boxer).

Pick's Disease

In Pick's disease, there is shrinking of the frontal and temporal anterior lobes of the brain with neuronal loss, swollen neurons, and spherical tau inclusions (Pick bodies) in the neurons (Lantos & Cairns, 2001; Lipton & Boxer, 2009). Symptoms include

- Changes in behavior (socially inappropriate behaviors, lack of social tact, agitation)
- Neglect of personal hygiene
- Repetitive or compulsive behaviors
- Changes in food preferences and eating habits
- Changes in personality, with patients becoming more impulsive, disinhibited, bored, and apathetic
- Decreased energy and motivation
- Lack of empathy and loss of insight into the behaviors of self or others
- Increased interest in sex

Patients may have problems with language, such as difficulty making or understanding speech. The disease progresses steadily and often rapidly. Survival is approximately 6 years from diagnosis.

Frontotemporal Dementia With Motor Neuron Disease (MND)

FTD with MND is characterized by dementia, loss of motor strength, and diminished muscle mass similar to that seen in amyotrophic lateral sclerosis. It is believed to be the most heritable form of frontotemporal lobe dementia (Goldman, Farmer, Wood, et al., 2005). Symptoms include

- Personality changes
- Impairment of judgment
- Lack of inhibition
- Loss of memory
- Reduction in abstract thinking and ability to make calculations
- Anomia (problems with finding the right word) that progresses to mutism
- Muscle wasting in the face and upper extremities that progresses to bulbar palsy (Mitsuyama & Inoue, 2009)

The occurrence of MND has been found to be high in Western New Guinea, the Kii Peninsula of Japan, and the island of Guam (Lerner & Riley, 2010). Age of onset ranges from 38 to 78 years, and the average age of onset is 55.5 years. Survival time of FTD with MND is shorter than that of other dementias. Death usually occurs within 2 to 5 years of diagnosis and is often due to progressive bulbar palsy (Mitsuyama & Inoue).

along the axon and is believed to play a role in memory formation and storage. When the neuron's transport system is damaged, there is loss of dendritic and synaptic functioning and eventually cell death. Tau also plays a role in motor neuron disorders (MNDs), which include amyotropic lateral sclerosis (ALS), progressive motor dystrophy, primary lateral sclerosis, and progressive bulbar palsy (Lillo & Hodges, 2009). Tau pathology, which is known to be involved in AD, dementia pugilistica, Down's syndrome, and muscular dystrophy, has recently been found to be involved in some forms of FTD (Arvanitakis, 2010; Arvanitakis & Wszolek, 2001).

Progranulin is a growth factor that is believed to be involved in neuronal survival. It is also involved in abnormal metabolism of a ubiquitinated protein, TAR DNA binding protein-43 (TDP-43), which creates ubiquitin-positive inclusions (bodies) that have been found in the hippocampus and spinal cord of some patients with some forms of FTD and in those with ALS (Arvanitakis, 2010; Zhang, Xu, Dickey et al., 2007). Although the pathophysiology of FTD is not well understood at this time, it is believed that two forms of tau pathology are involved in FTD: (1) tau-positive FTD and (2) tau-negative ubiquitin-positive FTD.

Tau-Positive FTD

Tau-positive FTD is associated with Pick's disease, which is characterized by Pick bodies (tau-positive round neuronal inclusions) in the brain.

Tau-Negative Ubiquitin-Positive FTD

In tau-negative ubiquitin-positive FTD, which is due to mutations of the progranulin gene, there is an absence of tau pathology, but there is often a presence of ubiquitinated inclusions. In tau-negative ubiquitin-positive FTD, there is loss of neurons in the cerebral cortex, gliosis (proliferation of astrocytes that represent healing after an injury in the central nervous system), and microvacuolation (spaces or cavities within a cell) (Lillo & Hodges, 2009). Tau-negative ubiquitin-positive FTD is often a familial disorder. Ubiquitin is also involved in MNDs and in the combination of FTD and the MND ALS (Lantos & Cairns, 2001). For example it has been found that 10% of patients with FTD develop ALS and 30% of patients with ALS have mild cognitive impairment (Raaphorst, Grupstra, Linssen, et al., 2010). Some researchers believe that there is a continuum between FTD and MNDs and that the MNDs represent a multisytem disorder with cognitive and behavioral changes that may over time reach the criteria for FTD (Lillo & Hodges).

Biological Basis

In FTD, there are changes in brain structures and brain functioning as well as changes at the cell level. There is severe atrophy of the frontal lobe and the anterior temporal lobe and enlargement of the lateral ventricles (Arvanitakis, 2010). Initially, there is impaired functioning of the frontal lobe and the anterior temporal lobe that progresses to include impaired functioning of other areas of the temporal lobe and of the parietal lobe (Arvanitakis). There are deficits of the serotonin and dopamine neurotransmitter systems but not of the acetylcholine system (Huey, Putnam, & Grafman, 2006). At the cellular level, pathological findings include round Pick bodies (tau-positive round inclusions) in the neurons, ubiquitin-positive inclusions, and gliosis (Arvanitakis). Changes of brain structures, brain functioning, and neurotransmitter systems underlie the cognitive, behavioral, and motor symptoms of FTD.

Clinical Presentation

The earliest signs of FTD are social withdrawal and disinhibition (Miller, Cummings, Villanueva-Meyer, et al., 1991). Patients with FTD may show symptoms of apathy (lack of motivation and spontaneous ideas), perseveration (buying, collecting, and hoarding), depression, anxiety, sleep disturbances, and psychosis (paranoid delusions, agitation, hallucinations [visual more common]) (Caselli & Yaari, 2007-2008, p. 492). Lack of awareness of their impairments and the effect of their behaviors on others occurs more frequently among patients with FTD than among patients with other dementias (Aalten et al., 2005b). Patients with FTD are likely to have problems with language, behavior, and motor activity, such as parkinsonian symptoms (Lipton & Boxer, 2009). There are two main forms of clinical presentation: (1) behavioral symptoms with personality changes and (2) problems with language. Memory and spatial skills are usually not affected (Carr, 2006).

Behavioral Symptoms With Personality Changes

Early signs of FTD are often lack of attention to activities of daily living and lack of interest in social activities. Other symptoms include loss of attention to personal hygiene; inappropriate sexual behaviors (exposing themselves or fondling their genitals); changes in personality, such as indifference, apathy, or inflexible ideas; loss of insight; repetitive behaviors, such as asking the same question over and over; inappropriate social behavior, such as lack of tact, inappropriate remarks, lack of empathy, and loss of insight into the behaviors of self and others; an increased interest in sexual activity (demanding frequent sexual activity); lack of awareness of the consequences of behaviors; and restlessness, pacing, and aggression (Apostolova & Cummings, 2010; Arvanitakis, 2010; Mace & Rabins, 2006; Rosness, Haugen, Passant, et al., 2008; Yuhas et al., 2006).

Problems With Language

Language problems are less common than behavioral symptoms. Early problems include problems with expression and naming items and difficulty with the meaning of words. There is also agrammatism (inability to speak grammatically because of brain injury or disease, usually evidenced as simplified sentence structure); alexia (inability to understand written words); and agraphia (loss of ability to write due to injury to the language center). There may be fluent aphasia, which is the loss of the meaning of words that results in empty speech, and poor comprehension (Arvanitakis, 2010).

During the early stages of FTD, there may be no impairment of memory or spatial skills. Patients' memories are intact and they do not lose their way, as occurs in AD. Later symptoms include impairments of memory and speech (Yuhas et al., 2006), hyperorality (putting inappropriate objects in the mouth), compulsive consumption of the same food or sweets, and consumption of nonedible items such as soap (Apostolova & Cummings, 2010). There may be aggressive or dangerous behaviors. No treatment has been found to slow the progression of the disease (Caselli & Yaari, 2007-2008).

Differential Diagnosis

FTD shares many characteristics with other dementias, such as gradual onset and slow decline from a previous level of functioning. FTD is similar to neurodegenerative dementias of AD and DLB, Creutzfeldt-Jakob disease, and Huntington's disease; however,

- In AD, there is more likely to be early problems with memory.
- In DLB, there is more likely to be visual hallucinations, fluctuations of cognition, and sleep disruptions.
- In Creutzfeldt-Jakob disease, there is more likely to be a very rapid progression of decline and occurrence of motor signs, ataxia, and personality changes.
- In Huntington's disease, there is likely to be motor impairment, chorea, and a family history of the disease.

Other disorders that must be considered include brain tumors and infections, schizophrenia, multiple sclerosis, head trauma, autoimmune diseases such as lupus, and alcohol and drug use (Arvanitakis, 2010).

In the late stage of FTD, symptoms are similar to those of other neurodegenerative dementias and include aphasia, weight loss, parkinsonian symptoms, impairment of mobility, and dependence on others for care (Arvanitakis, 2010).

Treatment

Treatment of FTD requires a biopsychosocial approach to caring for the patient and for the care providers (Arvanitakis, 2010). There is no medication or treatment for FTD at this time (Caselli & Yaari, 2007-2008).

Pharmacotherapy is used for management of difficult behaviors. For example, low doses of atypical antipsychotics are used for aggressive or inappropriate behaviors. Risperidone has been found to be helpful in controlling problematic behaviors, and the sedative effects of quetiapine have been found to be helpful with sleep problems (Arvanitakis, 2010). SSRIs have been found to provide relief from compulsive behaviors, depression, disinhibition, and carbohydrate craving, thus reducing caregiver burden (Moretti, Torre, Antonello, et al., 2003); however, there is lack of consensus over the benefits of SSRIs, with some researchers reporting no improvement of behavioral symptoms and worsening of cognitive functioning (Deakin, Rahman, Nestor, et al., 2004) and others reporting improvement of behavioral symptoms but not of cognitive symptoms (Huey et al., 2006). Trazodone hydrochloride has been found to be effective for irritability, agitation, depressive symptoms, and eating disorders (Lebert, Stekke, Hasenbrocks, et al., 2004). Moclobemide (Auronix, Manerix), a monoamine oxidase type A inhibitor, has been found to improve mood, behavior, and speech (Adler, Teufel, & Drach, 2003). Use of acetylcholinesterase inhibitors is controversial, with some researchers reporting benefits (Moretti, Torre, Antonello, et al., 2004) and others reporting that behavioral symptoms became worse (Mendez, Shapira, McMurtray, et al., 2007).

Other therapeutic interventions include maintaining the patient's autonomy, dignity, and social interactions to the extent possible; providing a structured daily schedule to reduce confusion and anger; and arranging the environment to promote as much independent activity as possible. Safety issues that must be addressed include falls, burns, being around swimming pools, driving, and access to guns or other weapons (Caselli & Yaari, 2007-2008). Tips for managing problems encountered with patients with FTD include suggestions for communicating (use matter-of-fact responses and distraction); personal hygiene (follow a routine for bathing and dressing); sleep disruptions (follow sleep hygiene practices); compulsive eating (lock food cupboards and liquor cabinets); household chores (break them down into small steps); uncontrollable shopping (limit access to credit cards and checking accounts); wandering (use locks and motion detectors); driving; and managing finances (intervene to prevent adverse or tragic consequences) (Memory and Aging Center, University of California at San Francisco, 2010b). Because of the early age of onset (before eligibility for retirement), the patient's inability to work, and the need for family members to reduce their work hours in order to provide care for the patient, there may be challenging financial problems for the patient and family. In 2008, the Social Security Administration included FTD in the Compassionate Allowance Program, which speeds application for social security disability (http://www.socialsecurity.gov/compassionateallowances) (Arvanitakis, 2010).

Course

During the course of FTD, patients may have episodes of abrupt changes in cognition or behavior that may be associated with an infection (such as a urinary tract infection or pneumonia), an injury, or an error in medications. They may suddenly become more confused or agitated, develop an unsteady gait, experience falls, have problems with incontinence, and demonstrate slurred speech and increasing sleepiness (Caselli & Yaari, 2007-2008, p. 494). FTD progresses to death more rapidly than AD, with a mean survival of 6 years (Rascovsky, Salmon, Lipton, et al., 2005). Shorter duration is associated with a positive family history of FTD and older age of onset (Chiu, Kaat, Seelaar, et al., 2010) and with the presence of motor neuron disease (Arvanitakis, 2010).

Ten percent of patients with FTD develop the MND ALS (Raaphorst et al., 2010). In patients with both FTD and MND, the progression of the dementia is rapid, with a combination of language problems, behavioral problems, and psychotic symptoms (Lillo & Hodges, 2009). Overall, the life expectancy is shorter than among patients with FTD without MND (Hu, Seelar, Josephs, et al., 2009), As the disease progresses, patients become mute and bedbound, and some may need 24-hour care either at home or in an institutional setting (Arvanitakis, 2010).

Dementia due to Other Causes

Dementia due to other causes accounts for less than 15% of all dementias (Zamrini & Quiceno, 2009).

Central Nervous System Causes

Dementia may be due to disorders that affect the central nervous system, including genetic disorders and infections. Genetic disorders include Huntington's disease, Wilson's disease, and porphyria. Infections include encephalitis that may be due to a virus, bacterium, prion, parasite, or fungus (Zamrini & Quiceno, 2009).

Human Immunodeficiency Virus and Hepatitis C

HIV is the most common infectious cause of dementia in individuals under 40 years of age (Zamrini & Quiceno, 2009). Mild cognitive impairment may occur without dementia in approximately one-third of individuals with HIV. Early symptoms include forgetfulness, decreased attention/concentration, slowed thinking, and mild tremor. Treatment of HIV with antiretroviral therapy can control the disease and reduce the patient's risk of developing HIV-associated dementia (Zamrini & Quiceno). However, dementia may develop secondary to HIV complications, such as with other infections. Another virus commonly associated with cognitive impairment is the hepatitis C virus: approximately 30% of patients with hepatitis C virus infection develop cognitive impairment with problems with recalling everyday information (Zamrini & Quiceno).

Prion Diseases

Prion diseases, or transmissible spongiform encephalopathies (TSEs), are a family of rare progressive neurodegenerative disorders that affect both humans and animals. They are distinguished by long incubation periods, characteristic spongiform changes associated with neuronal loss, and a failure to induce an inflammatory response. The causative agent of TSEs is believed to be a prion, which is an abnormal, transmissible agent that is able to induce abnormal folding of normal cellular prion proteins in the brain, leading to brain damage and the characteristic signs and symptoms of the disease. Prion diseases are rare, occurring at a rate of one per 1 million people in a year (Zamrini & Quiceno, 2009). Symptoms of dementia, ataxia, and psychiatric symptoms are frequent with prion diseases, and 88% of patients will have extrapyramidal symptoms. Prion diseases are usually rapidly progressive and always fatal. They include Creutzfeldt-Jakob disease (CJD), new variant Creutzfeldt-Jakob disease (nvCJD), Gerstmann-Straussler-Scheinker disease (GSS), familial and sporadic fatal insomnia (FFI), and kuru. Most cases of TSE are sporadic, 15% are inherited, and a few—such as iatrogenic CJD, kuru, and nvCJD—are acquired through exposure to infected material (Zamrini & Quiceno).

Creutzfeldt-Jakob Disease

Creutzfeldt-Jakob Disease (CJD) is the most common form of prion disorder (Collins, McLean, & Masters, 2001). CJD is not related to mad cow disease (bovine spongiform encephalopathy [BSE]). It occurs usually between 45 and 75 years of age, and it may be a sporadic form; a familial inherited form, which accounts for about 15% of all cases and is caused by mutations, insertions, or deletions in the prion gene on chromosome 20; or an iatrogenic form transmitted by exposure to contaminated items such as intracerebral electrodes, grafts of dura mater, corneal transplants, and human-derived growth hormone (Black & Andreasen, 2011; Knight & Will, 2004). Its pathology consists of vacuolations and spongeosis that involve the axons and dendrites of neurons. Vacuoles can be seen in the cerebellum, white matter, basal ganglia, and brainstem. Spongeosis is found in the occipital, temporal, and parietal cortexes. Prodromal symptoms occur in one-third of patients and include fatigue, headache, insomnia, malaise, and depression. Later symptoms include blurred vision, speech impairment, changes in walking (e.g., stumbling and falling), muscle twitching, hallucinations, personality changes, delirium or dementia, blindness, mutism, profound confusion, seizures, and rapidly progressing dementia (Black & Andreasen; Knight & Will). The median duration of the illness is 4 months, with about 66% of patients dying within 2 years (Knight & Will).

New Variation of CJD (nvCJD)

nvCJD is related to mad cow disease. It is the human variant of BSE and is acquired through a cow-to-human species switch. The direct means of transmission is believed to be through eating BSE-contaminated meat products. Secondary means of transmission is through blood, plasma, organ transplants, corneal transplants, and the use of surgical instruments that have been contaminated by contact with a patient with nvCJD (sterilization does not destroy the agent that causes BSE) (Thomas & Roos, 2010). It is more common in younger individuals, with an average age of onset of 27 years (Malaspina et al., 2010). The incubation period may be as long as 12 years (Thomas & Roos). In nvCJD, prion amyloid plaques are seen (Ironside & Bell, 1996). Early symptoms are agitation, aggression, anxiety, insomnia, headaches, depression, pain, numbness, ataxia, and hallucinations (Malaspina, et al.). Later symptoms include chorea, cognitive impairment, paranoia, incontinence, seizures, bulbar palsy, and dementia (Heath, Cooper, Murray, et al., 2011; Thomas & Roos). There is rapid progression from onset of symptoms to disability to death; mean survival is 14 months (Knight & Will, 2004). Treatment is symptomatic and supportive. There is ongoing research for effective treatment (Zamrini & Quiceno, 2009).

Gerstmann-Straussler-Scheinker disease (GSS)

GSS is an unusual variant of a Creutzfeldt-Jakob type. It is thought to be caused by a genetic mutation on chromosome 20 (Collins et al., 2001). It has a similar appearance to Creutzfeldt-Jakob but is very rare and has an earlier onset of symptoms. Onset is in the 40s but may be as young as age 25, and survival time ranges from 3 months to 13 years with a mean of 5 to 6 years. Early symptoms include memory impairment, gait unsteadiness, intention tremor, spasticity, and weakness of the limbs. Later symptoms include learning difficulties, problems in processing information, irritability, aggressiveness, emotional lability, and slowly progressive cerebellar ataxia (Collins et al.). GSS appears to be an inherited form of a Creutzfeldt-Jakob type disease, affecting only certain families (several have been identified throughout the world).

Familial and Sporadic Fatal Insomnia (FFI)

FFI, a very rare, genetically determined prion disease, is associated with degeneration of the thalamus, which controls sleep. Symptoms include a profound disruption of the normal sleep-wake cycle with nocturnal insomnia, abnormalities of endocrine functioning, impairment of cognition, panic attacks, and visual and auditory hallucinations (Collins et al., 2001). Symptoms progress to total insomnia, dementia, motor symptoms of ataxia, dysphagia (difficulty swallowing), dysarthria (difficulty speaking), tremor and myoclonus, and coma (Malaspina et al., 2010).

Kuru

Found in New Guinea, Kuru is one of the prion diseases. Because the disease primarily affects the cerebellum, the first symptoms are unsteady gait, tremors, and slurred speech. Dementia is minimal. Symptoms progress to inabilty to stand or eat and to coma. Patients die 6 months to 1 year after the appearance of the first symptoms. There were epidemic levels of kuru in 1950 to 1960 when the disease was caused by ritualistic cannibalism by mothers and children. Now that cannibalism has been eradicated, kuru has almost disappeared (National Institute of Neurological Disorders and Stroke, 2010).

Non-Central Nervous System Causes

Dementia can also result from diseases that primarily affect organs outside the central nervous system, such as with multiple sclerosis and systemic lupus erythematosus.

- *Multiple sclerosis* is a chronic neurological disease. Approximately half of patients with multiple sclerosis will develop cognitive impairment, e.g., memory impairment and slower processing of information (Bobholz & Rao, 2003); among these, 20% to 30% will develop severe dementia (Schulz, Kopp, Kunkel, et al., 2006).
- *Systemic lupus erythematosus* is an autoimmune disease that affects multiple organs, including the central nervous system. Half or more of patients with systemic lupus erythematosus will have some psychiatric symptoms at some point during their illness, such as anxiety disorders, cognitive dysfunction, mood disorder, and psychosis (Berlit, 2007).

Dementia Related to Nutritional Deficiencies, Head Trauma, and Exposure to Toxins

Beriberi, caused by a thiamin deficiency (vitamin B_1), is characterized by apathy, fatigue, irritability, depression, and poor concentration. Pellagra, which results from niacin deficiency, is characterized by confusion, clouding of consciousness, and dementia (Zamrini & Quiceno, 2009). Head injuries may result in proximal dementia or distal dementia. In proximal dementia, which is less common than distal dementia, patients do not return to normal functioning after the head injury. In distal dementia, it is believed that the trauma to the brain—such as to the temporal lobe and frontal lobe, which are particularly vulnerable to trauma—creates a neuropathological vulnerability that is expressed later in life as dementia (Bigler, 2009). The longer the period of amnesia or coma following the injury, the greater the likelihood of atrophy of the brain and the likelihood of developing dementia. Dementia may also occur as a result of exposure to alcohol; ionizing radiation; and heavy metals, such as lead, mercury, arsenic, manganese, and bismuth.

Key Points

- Dementia has an adverse impact on patients, their families, health-care services, and society.
- Preventing or delaying the onset of dementia requires addressing known risk factors that occur in middle age.
- Mild cognitive impairment is an intermediary stage between cognitive changes of normal aging and Alzheimer's disease.
- Alzheimer's disease is the most common cause of dementia in people over the age of 65 years.
- Dementia with Lewy bodies, the second most commonly occurring dementia, is characterized by fluctuating consciousness and visual hallucinations.
- Vascular dementia is a group of syndromes related to different vascular changes and includes arteriosclerotic dementia, multi-infarct dementia, and post-stroke dementia.

- Frontotemporal dementia, which is an early-onset dementia (with onset in the 50s), is characterized by apathy, withdrawal, disinhibition, and changes in personality.
- Symptoms common to all subtypes of dementia include apathy, agitation, hyperactive behaviors, affective symptoms, and psychotic symptoms.
- Disruptive behavioral symptoms may be a patients' way of expressing unmet needs.
- Treatment for dementias is comprehensive and includes pharmacotherapy and nonpharmacological interventions.
- Dementia caregiving is stressful and increases the caregiver's vulnerability to physical and mental health problems.

Resources

Organizations

Lewy Body Dementia Association
PO Box 451429
Atlanta, GA 31145-9429
lbda@lbda.org; http://www.lewybodydementia.org
Tel 404-935-6444; 800-LEWYSOS (539-9767)
Fax 480-422-5434

Lewy Body Association
http://www.lewybodydementia.org

Alzheimer's Association
225 North Michigan Avenue, 17th Floor
Chicago, IL 60601-7633
Tel 312-335-8700; TDD 312-335-5886
Fax 866-699-1246
http://alz.org/findchapter.asp\; info@alz.org; http://www.alz.org

ADEducation and Referral (ADEAR) Centre
PO Box 8250
Silver Spring, MD 20907-7633
800-272-3900
www.alzheimers.nia.nih.gov

National Institute on Aging Information Center
PO Box 8057
Gaithersburg, MD 20898-8057
800-222-2225
www.nia.nih.gov

Association for Frontotemporal Dementias (AFTD)
1616 Walnut Street, Suite 1100
Philadelphia, PA 19103
267-514-7221
http://www.FTD-Picks.org

Creutzfeldt-Jakob Disease (CJD) Foundation, Inc.
PO Box 5312
Akron, OH 44334
800-659-1991
http://www.cjdfoundation.org

www.ConsultGeriRn.org
www.GeroNurse.online.org

Books

Mace, N. L., & Rabins, P. V. (2006). *The 36-hour day: A family guide to caring for people with Alzheimer disease, other dementias, and memory loss in later life* (4th ed.). Baltimore: The Johns Hopkins Press.

Movies

Beresford, B. (Director). (1989). *Driving Miss Daisy* [Motion picture]. United States: Warner Brothers.

An older woman develops AD and eventually needs to be moved to a nursing home (Wedding, Boyd, Niemiec, 2010, p. 148).

Gilbert, B. (Producer), & Rydell, M. (Director). (1981). *On Golden Pond* [Motion picture]. United States.

An older couple suffers as the husband develops dementia (Wedding, Boyd, Niemiec, 2010, p. 290).

Bleckner, J. (Director), & Bell, D. (Producer). (1985). *Do you remember love?* [TV movie]. United States.

A portrayal of a woman developing AD (Wedding, Boyd, Niemiec, 2010, p. 289).

PART TWO: Delirium

Delirium is an acute brain disorder and a potentially lethal condition (Bourgeois et al., 2008; Samuels & Evers, 2002). It is characterized by impairment of consciousness (sudden changes in level of consciousness), reduced ability to focus or maintain attention, rapid changes in cognition (memory and judgment), and fluctuations in mental status throughout the day. Key features are impairment of attention, sleep-wake disturbances, and changes in motor activity: either increased motor activity, such as agitation, or decreased activity, such as immobility (Weiner et al., 2009). The symptoms that are required to meet the criteria of the *Diagnostic and Statistical Manual of Mental Disorders*, 4th ed., Text Revision (*DSM-IV-TR*) (American Psychiatric Association, 2000) for a diagnosis of delirium include

1. An altered state of consciousness and a change in cognition (memory, orientation, or language disturbance)
2. A rapid onset (hours to days)
3. Fluctuation of symptoms during the day
4. Evidence that the disturbance is the result of a general medical condition (Trzepacz & Meagher, 2010)

Delirium indicates impairment in brain functioning. It is associated with increased functional impairments and mortality, if not treated; it may also be associated with new and permanent cognitive deficits after recovery because of pathological processes that occur in the brain during delirium. For example, among patients with AD, having an episode of delirium has been found to result in a three times faster rate of cognitive decline in comparison to those who did not have delirium (Fong, Jones, Shi, et al., 2009).

Adverse effects of delirium include increased morbidity and mortality. Different rates of increased mortality associated with delirium have been reported. Leslie, Zhang, Holford, et al. (2005) reported an increased rate of 62% at 1-year follow-up of hospitalized elderly patients with delirium, and Curyto, Johnson, TenHave, et al. (2001) reported an increased rate of 75% at 3-year follow-up of elderly patients with delirium compared to similar patients without delirium. Risk of death is reduced when delirium is identified and treated (Trzepacz & Meagher, 2010).

Other adverse effects associated with delirium include increased length of hospitalization; reduced ability to be independent; increased rate of institutionalization; continued symptoms of inattention, disorientation, and poor memory; and distressful memories of experiencing delirium (Gaudreau & Gagnon, 2005; Trzepacz & Meagher, 2010; Warshaw & Mechlin, 2009). There is also increased risk of emergence of dementia after the delirium is resolved. Emergence of dementia after delirium is more likely to occur in older patients and has not been found among patients with delirium in the 35- to 45-year age group (Trzepacz & Meagher).

Epidemiology

Delirium, which is characterized by an acute fluctuating change in mental status, is often unrecognized, and as many as 70% of cases may go undiagnosed (Samuels & Evers, 2002). Delirium is a common condition among patients seen in emergency departments. In one study of older adults who were seen in the emergency room, 8.3% had delirium that was primarily of the hypoactive psychomotor subtype, and in 76% of the instances, the emergency staff did not recognize delirium (Han, Zimmerman, Cutler, et al., 2009). The prevalence of delirium among older hospitalized patients is 56% (Michaud, Bula, Berney, et al., 2007). Among patients who have had hip surgery, the prevalence of delirium has been found to be 35% to 65%, and among older adults in intensive care units, the rate has been found to be 70% to 87% (Tanios, Epstein, & Teres, 2004). Among nursing home residents older than 65 years of age, the rate of delirium has been reported to be 60% (Fann, 2000).

Delirium may also occur in patients with dementia. Fick, Agostini, and Inouye (2002) found that 22% of older adults with dementia living in the community had delirium and that 89% of older adults with dementia in the hospital had delirium. Delirium also occurs among children with fevers and patients who are terminally ill. Delirium occurs in 18% to 30% of burn patients and in 13% to 67% of patients who have had cardiac surgery (Hilty, Seritan, Bourgeois, et al., 2007, p. 150). Among patients seen in the emergency room, 10% to 14% already have delirium (Naughton, Moran, Kadah, et al., 1995).

Risk Factors

There are risk factors that increase the likelihood of an individual's experiencing delirium, but risk factors *are not* causes (Trzepacz & Meagher, 2010). Risk factors for the development of delirium include advanced age, genetic vulnerability, underlying brain pathology, vulnerability due to underlying medical conditions, and precipitating factors (Bourgeois et al., 2008; Han et al., 2009).

Advanced Age

As individuals age, the brain undergoes structural, functional, and neurochemical changes. In addition, older individuals are more likely to have cognitive impairment and changes in metabolism of medications; they also tend to have more medical conditions and tend to be receiving multiple medications. These factors may contribute to the two to three times more frequent occurrence of delirium in older adults with dementia, especially those with AD and VaD (Trzepacz & Meagher, 2010).

Genetic Vulnerability

It has recently been found that there is an increased risk for the development of delirium among patients who are carriers of the *APOE e4* allele (van Munster, Korevaar, Zwinderman, et al., 2009).

Underlying Brain Pathology and Medical Conditions That Increase Vulnerability

The risk factor of underlying brain pathology includes existing brain disorders such as cognitive impairment, AD, VaD, depression, cerebrovascular accidents, and head trauma. Underlying medical conditions include hypertension, diabetes, cancer, and severe chronic illnesses. Nutritional factors, such as a low level of thiamin (which plays a role in the functioning of cholinergic neurons), are risk factors for the development of delirium. A low level of serum albumin, which is involved in controlling availability of drugs, is also a risk factor for delirium (Trzepacz & Meagher, 2010). Other risk factors include withdrawal from drugs in patients with substance dependency (Trzepacz & Meagher; van Munster et al., 2009).

Precipitating Factors

Precipitating factors can be medications, the patient's physical condition or disabilities, the presence of cognitive impairment (such as difficulties with executive functioning), sleep deprivation, and environmental factors such as social isolation, strange environment, relocation, stress, or use of restraints (Bourgeois et al., 2008; Hilty et al., 2007; Trzepacz & Meagher, 2010). Medications that increase the risk of precipitating delirium include

- Benzodiazepines such as diazepam (Valium) and lorazepam
- Medications with anticholinergic effects, such as antihistamines
- Psychotropics
- Opiates
- Corticosteroids
- Muscle relaxants
- Nonsteroidal anti-inflammatory drugs such as aspirin, ibuprofen, and naproxen
- Antacids

- Over-the-counter cold and flu remedies (Brown & Stoudemire, 1998; Ferrario, 2008)

Among medications, lorazepam has been found to precipitate the transition of patients in the intensive care unit to delirium (Pandharipande, Shintani, Peterson, et al., 2006). Patients in the intensive care unit receiving midazolam (Versed) and fentanyl have been found to be at higher risk of developing delirium than patients not receiving these medications. Meperidine may be associated with increased risk of delirium (Adunsky, Levy, Mizrahi, et al., 2002).

Other factors that precipitate or trigger the development of delirium include pain; dehydration; sleep deprivation; visual and hearing impairment; absence of orienting cues, such as clocks and calendars; being restrained; and having an indwelling bladder catheter (Bourgeois et al., 2008; Hilty et al., 2007; Weinhouse, Schwab, Watson, et al., 2009).

Etiology

Approximately 56% of patients with delirium have one identifiable cause, but the remaining 44% have two or more causes (Bourgeois et al., 2008; Francis, Martin, & Kapoor, 1990; Trzepacz & Meagher, 2010). Causes include the following:

- Dehydration
- Heatstroke
- Hypoxia
- Pain
- Medications: sedating or analgesic medications; opioids; stimulants; steroids
- Polypharmacy
- Drug intoxication
- Myocardial infarction
- Infections: malaria, urinary tract infection, pneumonia, syphilis, HIV
- Stroke
- Head injury
- Brain tumors
- Seizures
- Disrupted sleep
- Withdrawal from alcohol or drugs (Fick & Mion, 2008; Hilty et al., 2007; Trzepacz & Meagher, 2010; Warshaw & Mechlin, 2009)

Biological Basis

Delirium is associated with pathology of certain brain structures and the pathways that link them. These structures include the right prefrontal cortex, which processes new experiences; the right parietal cortex, which sustains attention and awareness of the environment; the basal ganglia, which is involved in controlling voluntary movement; and the thalamus, which filters and integrates information (Trzepacz & Meagher, 2010). Abnormalities of neurotransmitters include acetylcholine, which is involved in sleep-wake cycles, learning, memory, and attention; dopamine, which is involved in attention, mood, perception, and executive functioning; and melatonin, which is involved in sleep-wake cycles. Low levels of acetylcholine and melatonin and high levels of dopamine have been found in patients with delirium (Bourgeois et al., 2008; Shigeta, Yasui, Nimura, et al., 2001).

Clinical Presentation

The subtypes of delirium are hyperactive, hypoactive, and mixed (Yang, Marcantonio, Inouye, et al., 2009).

In the *hyperactive* subtype, patients are restless, agitated, and hypervigilant. They may have rapid speech and are irritable and combative. Patients with hyperactive delirium are likely to be startled at a noise, pick at the bedclothes, and try to remove tubes. They may have psychotic symptoms.

In the *hypoactive* subtype, patients tend to have slowed speech and movements, apathy, lethargy, sleepiness, and reduced alertness. They often appear withdrawn, lethargic, or depressed. They may describe psychotic symptoms when they are asked (Bourgeois et al., 2008; Fick & Mion, 2008; Warshaw & Mechlin, 2009). Hypoactive delirium in hospitalized patients is often mistaken for depression (Pun & Ely, 2007; Trzepacz & Meagher, 2010).

Mixed delirium has features of both hyperactive delirium and hypoactive delirium. The mixed type of delirium is the most common type, followed by the hypoactive type (Peterson, Pun, Dittus, et al., 2006). Hypoactive delirium and mixed delirium have a poorer prognosis, greater severity, and higher rates of death (Pun & Ely, 2007; Warshaw & Mechlin, 2009).

More than half of patients who develop delirium have prodromal symptoms, such as clouding of consciousness, inattention, disorientation, and perceptual disturbances. It has been found that 4 days before the development of delirium, there are often symptoms of cognitive disturbances and psychobehavioral disturbances; 3 days before, there are symptoms of memory disturbances, anxiety, disorientation, and disturbances of sleep-wake cycles; and 2 days before, there is increased anxiety and disorientation and calling for help (Duppils & Wikblad, 2004; Trzepacz & Meagher, 2010). For other patients, there may be a rapid onset of symptoms with changes in attention, arousal, sleep patterns, mood, personality, cognition, behavior, and motor activity (Hilty et al., 2007). Case Study 16-1 describes the onset and treatment of delirium in an older adult.

In a medical setting, such as the intensive care unit, patients may have hallucinations or delusions, and referrals for a psychiatric consultation are often requested for psychosis, depression, noncompliance with treatment, or unruly behavior (Bourgeois et al., 2008). Common clinical presentations include disturbance of consciousness and attention, sudden changes in cognitive functioning,

CASE STUDY 16-1

Onset and Treatment of Delirium in an Older Adult

Shirley Keen is a 92-year-old Irish American widow. Her husband died in his late 70s and her only son was killed in Vietnam. She worked all her life as a homemaker and, until recently, had gone to Mass every day. She enjoyed the Rosary and Altar Society at her church but did not socialize outside of that. Her life had centered around taking care of her home and her husband. They had enjoyed watching TV and listening to the radio. After his death, she lived alone and received food each day from Meals on Wheels. Her only other regular social contact was a weekly visit from the Parish nurse, who helped in arranging for volunteers from the church to take Mrs. Keen to medical appointments.

Her routine continued unchanged until, at age 89 while clearing the dishes off the table, she suffered a fall that resulted in a broken hip. The hip was repaired surgically and she went to a rehabilitation facility. After a month of therapy, her balance and weight-bearing status were still poor. Based on her overall frail health and limited mobility owing to osteoarthritis, she was admitted to the assisted living portion of the facility, where she was able to get around using a walker. A year ago, when she went from using a walker to using a wheelchair, she was transferred to the skilled nursing unit.

In the skilled nursing unit she was able to propel herself to the TV lounge and occasionally looked at the donated travel magazines. Her hearing loss progressed but she refused to have a hearing aid. As in the past, she did not socialize much. Cognitively she remained oriented to self, staff, and surroundings but not to time.

On Nov. 16th, the night nurse noted that Mrs. Keen was awake frequently during the night, which was unusual for her. The next day, the evening nurse reported that Mrs. Keen was confused and agitated. She was asking to go home, saying she had to take care of the baby. She was afebrile and did not complain of pain. Appetite was unaffected and no change in elimination had been noted by the aides. The following day, she manifested increased confusion and agitation in the late afternoon and evening. She asked repeatedly for a phone book, saying she had to get out of this place.

The physician was notified and ordered a urine culture and a temporary hold on her scheduled Lortab. She was to continue on acetaminophen for her arthritis pain. The urine culture was obtained by catheterization and sent the following morning. There was no significant improvement in her confusion after 48 hours of withholding the narcotic pain medicine.

On Nov. 21st, the morning lab report showed a urinary tract infection (concentration of greater than 100,000 *E. coli*, which suggests treatment with TMP/sulfa). The first dose of antibiotic medication was given at 10:00 a.m. During the afternoon and evening of that day, there were no requests to leave and there was no agitation. The evening nurse reported that after giving her the second dose, she asked the patient "Are you starting to feel better?" Mrs. Keen seemed back in control as she reminded the nurse, "My other ear is better if you want me to hear what you are saying."

Questions

1. What factors increased Mrs. Keen's risk for developing delirium?
2. What interventions might be used to prevent the occurrence of another episode of delirium?

Answers to these questions can be found at the end of this chapter.

Source: Kerry L. Perese, APRN-WHNP

fluctuating levels of consciousness, disturbances of psychomotor state, mood and anxiety symptoms, and delirium superimposed on dementia.

Disturbance of Consciousness and Attention

One of the key features of delirium is difficulty in sustaining attention. Ability to sustain attention can be tested by reading a list of letters at the rate of 1 per second and asking patients to raise their hands when they hear the letter specified by the clinician. Adults who are not ill will be able to identify the letter most of the time. Patients with delirium will tend to miss the letter.

Sudden Changes in Cognitive Functioning

Short-term memory is usually impaired in patients with delirium, and patients are often disoriented to time and place but not to person. There may be impairment of executive functioning, and they may demonstrate loose association or tangentiality. They often experience misperceptions such as illusions, e.g., they misinterpret visual, tactile, or auditory stimuli. Hallucinations tend to be visual hallucinations, although there may be tactile or olfactory hallucinations. There may be delusions, which are fixed false beliefs, but the delusions are not as organized as they are in other psychotic disorders and they tend to have themes of danger in the environment or persecution (Hilty et al., 2007; Trzepacz & Meagher, 2010).

Fluctuating Levels of Consciousness

Some but not all patients with delirium will have lucid periods during the day (Hilty et al., 2007). The average duration of delirium episodes is 3 to 13 days (Bourgeois et al., 2008).

Disturbances of Psychomotor State

Disturbances of psychomotor activity include hyperactivity—in which patients jump at noises, pick at the linens and tubes, and are tremulous and easily agitated—and hypoactivity—in which patients are lethargic, are sleepy, and have decreased physical activity.

Mood and Anxiety Symptoms

Patients with delirium may demonstrate fear, anger, depression, apathy, anxiety, and euphoria (Gleason, 2003). There may be thoughts of suicide or thoughts of death. The emotions are often noncongruent, are out of the patient's control, and fluctuate rapidly, within minutes (Trzepacz & Meagher, 2010).

Delirium Superimposed on Dementia

The prevalence of delirium in patients with dementia ranges from 22% of older adults (ages 65 and older) living in the community to 89% of older hospitalized patients, and it is associated with increased risk of poor outcomes, prolonged hospitalization, further cognitive and physical decline, nursing home placement, and death (Fick et al., 2002). Patients with delirium superimposed on dementia are more likely to have the hypoactive type of delirium. Factors associated with delirium superimposed on dementia include urinary tract infections, fecal impaction or urinary retention, surgery, immobility, stress, bereavement (such as death of a spouse), change in living arrangements, and severe pain. Medications such as benzodiazepines, anticholinergic medications (Cogentin), sedative-hypnotics, narcotics, antihistamines (Benadryl), antipsychotics, and cardiovascular drugs are also associated with delirium superimposed on dementia (Fick et al., 2002; Fick & Mion, 2008).

Interventions for patients with delirium superimposed on dementia are nonpharmacological and include many strategies: family support; orienting communication (repeatedly telling the patients where they are, the day, and the reason why they are there); adequate hydration; orienting supports, such as hearing aids, eyeglasses, clocks, calendars, and pictures; removal of restraints; decreasing environmental stimuli, such as noise and lights; and providing a familiar caregiver, someone to sit with the patient at all times (Fick et al., 2002).

Differential Diagnosis

Medical conditions that may cause delirium include

- Withdrawal from alcohol, barbiturates, and sedative-hypnotics
- Infections, such as meningitis, encephalitis, brain abscesses, and syphilis
- Trauma, such as head injuries, severe burns, or heatstroke
- Disorders of the central nervous system, such as seizures and tumors
- Hypoxia related to anemia, carbon monoxide poisoning, or cardiac failure
- Endocrine disorders
- Vitamin B_{12} deficiencies and niacin and thiamin deficiencies
- Toxins such as medications, pesticides, solvents, over-the-counter medications, and drugs
- Metabolic disorders, such as renal failure, hepatic failure, electrolyte disturbance, acidosis, and alkalosis (adapted from Hilty et al., 2007, p. 151)

Psychiatric conditions that may cause symptoms similar to delirium include substance-related disorders, mood disorders, and psychotic disorders. However, the symptoms in these disorders do not wax and wane over the course of the day, and there is no diurnal variation. The differential diagnosis that is considered most frequently is dementia.

Treatment

Delirium may present with multiple symptoms—cognitive, affective, sleep disturbances, problems with language, psychomotor changes, delusions, and hallucinations—that may fluctuate rapidly. Thus, delirium requires a comprehensive biopsychosocial approach to assessment and treatment (Bourgeois et al., 2011; Trzepacz & Meagher, 2010).

Assessment

Information relating to duration of the delirium, existing disorders, medications, sleep, and behavior can be obtained from the family and nursing staff. Cognitive testing includes asking the patient to draw a clock face and to place the hands at a certain time (10 minutes after 11 o'clock is the most difficult); asking the patient to name objects; and asking the patient to write a sentence. Screening tests include the *Mini-Mental State Examination* (Folstein et al., 1975); the *Delirium Rating Scale (DRS)* (Trzepacz, Baker, & Greenhouse, 1988), which can differentiate delirium from schizophrenia, dementia, and depression; and the *Confusion Assessment Method (CAM)* (Inouye, van Dyck, Alessi, et al., 1990).

The *DRS* (Trzepacz et al., 1988) is a 10-item clinician-rated scale that can be used to measure the severity of delirium and its response to treatment. The *Delirium Rating Scale-R-98* is a modified version of the original *DRS*. It has 16 items and provides for evaluation of language impairment, thought process abnormalities, and degrees of symptom intensity that are not included in the original scale (Rush et al., 2008).

The *CAM* is a nine-item clinician-rated scale that obtains information from an informant, such as a caregiver. The answers are used to determine the presence of critical features of delirium, including acute onset and fluctuating course, inattention, disorganized thinking, disorientation, memory impairment, perceptual disturbances, agitation or psychomotor retardation, disturbance of sleep-wake cycle, and altered level of consciousness (Rush et al., 2008; Waszynski, 2007). There is also a short version of the *CAM* that involves identifying four features of delirium:

- *Feature one* is acute onset or fluctuating course; e.g., an acute change from the patient's baseline mental status or behavior.

- *Feature two* involves questions about the patient's inattention; e.g., difficulty in focusing attention or being easily distracted.
- *Feature three* involves the patient's thinking; e.g., disorganized, incoherent, or rambling thoughts and sudden switching from one topic to another.
- *Feature four* involves the patient's level of consciousness; e.g., hypervigilant, lethargic, drowsy, easily aroused, difficult to arouse, stuporous, or in a coma.

Positive responses to features one and two and either three or four suggest delirium. Patients with dementia without delirium will not have features one, two, or four (Waszynski, 2007).

Laboratory tests include complete blood cell count, electrolytes, blood urea nitrogen, creatinine, glucose, calcium, pulse oximetry or arterial blood gas, urinalysis, drug screen, liver function test with serum albumin, cultures, HIV screening, and cerebrospinal fluid examination if meningitis or encephalitis is suspected. Other tests include chest x-ray, electrocardiogram, brain imaging, and electroencephalogram. Electroencephalogram in patients with delirium shows generalized slowing (Bourgeois et al., 2008).

Treatment Interventions

The goals of treatment are to prevent the development of delirium and to reverse existing delirium in order to reduce the high risk of associated morbidity and death (Bourgeois et al., 2008). Treatment interventions include prevention strategies; interventions for managing episodes; creating a therapeutic environment; providing psychosocial support; and pharmacotherapy (Trzepacz & Meagher, 2010).

Prevention

Delirium is a predictor of prolonged cognitive impairment, functional decline, worsening of dementia, increased rates of discharge to long-term care facilities, higher death rates, and higher costs of care (Holroyd-Leduc, Khandwala, & Sink, 2010; Pandharipande, Cotton, Shintani, et al., 2008; Pun & Ely, 2007). For example, it has been estimated that delirium directly increases hospital costs by 40% (Milbrandt, Deppen, Harrison, et al., 2004). Prevention of delirium is crucial to reduce (1) the risk of the patient's experiencing the distress of delirium and (2) the long-term consequences of experiencing delirium. Prevention can take place in the preoperative period or the postoperative period.

Prevention in the Preoperative Period

Older adults (ages 65 or older) account for approximately 43% of surgical patients in the United States and have more hospital-acquired delirium than younger patients. However, advanced age is not the only risk factor (Warshaw & Mechlin, 2009). During the preoperative evaluation, the patient's risk for development of delirium can be determined by assessing four factors: visual and hearing impairment, cognitive impairment, severity of illness, and dehydration (Inouye, Viscoli, Horwitz, et al., 1993). Inouye et al. found that among patients with three or four of these factors, 83% later developed delirium. Hospital-generated risk factors include use of physical restraints, malnutrition, use of a bladder catheter, and addition of more than three new medications (Holroyd-Leduc et al., 2010). If the patient is determined to be at high risk, the following two strategies may be instituted:

- Reduce exposure to benzodiazepines and drugs that increase risk of delirium.
- Ask the patient's family to arrange to have someone stay with the patient at all times during hospitalization. It has been found that having a family member present to reorient and reassure the patient reduces the need for sedation and restraints (Warshaw & Mechlin, 2009).

Prevention in the Postoperative Period

All critically ill patients in intensive care units are considered to be at risk for developing delirium (Warshaw & Mechlin, 2009). Delirium has been found to develop in 20% to 50% of patients in the intensive care unit who are not receiving mechanical ventilation, and the incidence increases to 60% to 80% among those receiving mechanical ventilation (Pun & Ely, 2007). Delirium in the intensive care unit is associated with an increased rate of reintubation of patients, 10 additional days in the hospital, and higher rates of death in the intensive care unit and in the hospital (Pun & Ely, 2007). Each additional day of delirium is associated with increased risk of death.

Talking with patients frequently and reorienting them to place, time, and situation (why they are there) is effective in preventing delirium during the postoperative period. Other interventions include encouraging patients to wear their eyeglasses and hearing aids as soon as possible; replacing fluids to prevent dehydration; facilitating mobility, e.g., getting patients out of bed and encouraging them to do range-of-motion exercises; minimizing use of restraints and Foley catheters; using strategies to reduce sleep disturbances (dimming the lights and reducing noise); and having a family member sit with the patient (Warshaw & Mechlin, 2009).

These interventions and others are included in multicomponent intervention programs that are used in the postoperative period to prevent the development of delirium (Holroyd-Leduc et al., 2010, p. 466). Multicomponent intervention programs are designed to target cognitive impairment, functional impairment, social isolation, fluid and electrolyte imbalances, high-risk medications, pain, impaired vision and hearing, malnutrition, sleep deprivation, and use of catheters (Holroyd-Leduc et al.). Multicomponent intervention programs include interventions such as

- Repeatedly orienting patients to place, time, and situation
- Using clocks and calendars to orient patients

- Getting patients out of bed as soon as possible
- Treating dehydration
- Discontinuation of benzodiazepine, anticholinergic, and antihistamine medications
- Having standing orders for use of pain medication
- Encouraging patients to use eyeglasses and hearing aids
- Providing assistance with eating
- Removing urinary catheters by the second postoperative day
- Using sleep hygiene strategies to treat sleep deprivation
- Having someone familiar sit with patients (Vidan, Sanchez, Alonso, et al., 2009)

Although the results were not consistent for three multicomponent intervention programs, there was a reduction of delirium of patients admitted to the hospital for hip fractures. One program demonstrated a reduction of hospital stay, and one study demonstrated a reduction of in-hospital deaths. The multicomponent intervention programs also appear to reduce medical complications and pressure ulcers, urinary tract infections, sleeping problems, and falls (Holroyd-Leduc et al., 2010).

In a study that examined the use of a multicomponent program (similar to the ones previously described) to prevent delirium among older adults with medical illnesses (e.g., with infectious diseases and heart failure) who had been admitted to the hospital, it was found that the intervention was associated with a reduced rate of delirium. Other benefits included lower rates of functional decline, less use of physical restraints, and more ambulation of the patients (Vidan et al., 2009). Thus, it appears that multicomponent intervention programs have the potential to prevent delirium.

Management of a Delirium Episode

When patients develop delirium, the goal of treatment is to shorten the duration and lessen the severity. The most important step is to remove the cause by

- Treating cerebral ischemia; hypoxia, infection, acute intoxication, and acute withdrawal from alcohol (delirium tremens); acute hyperthyroidism (thyroid storm); infections; and fecal impactions
- Removing catheters
- Reducing medications
- Providing pain relief
- Treating dehydration
- Promoting sleep by using sleep hygiene strategies (see Chapter 8)

Creating a Therapeutic Environment

Creating a therapeutic environment for patients with delirium involves

- Ensuring their safety and the safety of family members or friends who are sitting with them
- Maintaining optimal levels of environmental stimulation
- Preventing falls, wandering, and physical harm due to confusion, fluid imbalance, or aggression
- Using orienting strategies such as clocks, calendars, family pictures, and a list of names of staff written in large letters
- Providing patients with their eyeglasses and hearing aids as needed

Psychosocial Support

Support from family, friends, or neighbors is crucial in management of delirium (Bourgeois et al., 2011). Family members and caregivers should sit with patients at all times. They should repeatedly reorient and reassure patients. Patients who have recovered from delirium say that the constant presence of a relative, a clock that they could see, and reorientation by the staff helped them to regain a sense of control (Schofield, 1997). Although these interventions are effective in reducing the incidence of delirium, they are not as effective in treating delirium or decreasing the time spent in delirium (Warshaw & Mechlin, 2009). Therefore, prevention of delirium is crucial.

Pharmacotherapy

Pharmacotherapy for delirium includes the use of antipsychotic medications and cholinesterase inhibitors. Pharmacotherapy may also be used to help with withdrawal delirium, which occurs when patients are experiencing withdrawal from a drug or medication.

Antipsychotic Medications

Because dopamine levels are elevated in delirium, dopamine-receptor antagonists are often used. Haloperidol is frequently used to reduce symptoms of delirium. However, haloperidol has side effects that may limit its use among older adults: it prolongs the QTc interval, and its use is associated with the development of extrapyramidal symptoms (Warshaw & Mechlin, 2009).

Among the atypical antipsychotic medications, olanzapine and risperidone have been found to be effective (Trzepacz & Meagher, 2010). Open-label studies of quetiapine and aripiprazole suggest that they are effective in reducing the symptoms of delirium (Trzepacz & Meagher). In a recent study, it was found that neither haloperidol nor ziprasidone was effective in reducing the duration of delirium among patients with delirium who were on mechanical ventilation in intensive care units (Girard, Pandharipande, Carson, et al., 2010). In trial studies, dexmedetomidine (Precedex), a selective α_2-adrenoceptor agonist that has been approved for sedation in the intensive care unit setting, has been found to be associated with reduced incidence of delirium (Maldonado, VanDerStarre, & Wysong, 2003).

Cholinesterase Inhibitors

Delirium that is nonresponsive to haloperidol or atypical antipsychotics may respond to rivastigmine (Kalisvaart, Boelaarts, de Jonghe, et al., 2004).

Pharmacotherapy of Withdrawal Delirium

Delirium can result from withdrawal from both alcohol and sedative-hypnotics. Delirium develops 48 to 72 hours after discontinuation of alcohol or sedative-hypnotics; symptoms peak after 4 days, although they can last up to 2 weeks. In alcohol withdrawal, there are symptoms of tremulousness, tachycardia, hypertension, and hyperthermia. Some patients experiencing alcohol withdrawal develop alcohol withdrawal delirium, known as *delirium tremens*. Symptoms that predict the development of delirium tremens include seizures, elevated blood pressure, and elevated temperature (Monte, Rabunal, Casariego, et al., 2009). Delirium tremens is a life-threatening medical emergency. Symptoms include fever, disorientation, perceptual disturbances, hallucinations, agitation, confusion, and delirium. Treatment, which should be undertaken in a medical intensive care unit, includes the use of physical restraints, supportive measures, and the use of benzodiazepines with a long half-life such as diazepam or chlordiazepoxide (Librium). The cholinesterase inhibitors donepezil, rivastigmine, and galantamine may be used. For patients who cannot tolerate typical antipsychotics, some of the newer atypical antipsychotics are being used (Trzepacz & Meagher, 2010).

Course

The initial phase of delirium may be a period of either subclinical delirium or prodromal symptoms of delirium, which include restlessness, anxiety, irritability, distractibility, or sleep disturbance. These early symptoms may progress to delirium in 1 to 3 days. The duration of delirium varies from less than 1 week to 2 months, but usually an episode of delirium resolves in 10 to 12 days (Gleason, 2003). Older patients tend to have longer episodes of delirium. The majority of patients recover, but untreated delirium may progress to stupor, coma, seizures, and death (Trzepacz, Breitbart, Franklin, et al., 2006). The mortality rate for older hospitalized patients with delirium ranges from 22% to 76% (approximately 80% of patients with terminal illnesses develop delirium shortly before death) (Trzepacz et al., 2006). Among patients with delirium tremens, the mortality rate is 35% for untreated patients and 5% to 15% for treated patients (Weigel et al., 2009).

Key Points

- Delirium is a neuropsychiatric disorder that affects thinking, perception, language, and sleep.
- Delirium is associated with increased morbidity and mortality.
- Patients at high risk for delirium include those with advanced age, genetic vulnerability, underlying brain pathology, and co-occurring health problems.
- Prevention of delirium is essential.
- Delirium is under-recognized and undertreated.
- Identification and treatment of delirium reduces adverse sequential effects.
- Multicomponent interventions are effective in prevention of delirium.

Resources

Movie

Brackett, C. (Producer) & Wilder, B. (Director). (1945). *The lost weekend* [Motion picture]. United States: Paramount Pictures.

This film provides an example of delirium tremens. (Wedding, Boyd, Niemiec, 2010, p. 263).

References

Aalten, P., de Vugt, M. D., Jaspers, N., et al. (2005a). The course of neuropsychiatric symptoms in dementia. Part I: Findings from the two-year longitudinal Maasbed study. *International Journal of Geriatric Psychiatry, 20,* 523-530.

Aalten, P., de Vugt, M. D., Lousberg, R., et al. (2003). Behavioral problems in dementia: A factor analysis of the neuropsychiatric inventory. *Dementia & Geriatric Cognitive Disorders, 15*(2), 99-105.

Aalten, P., van Valen, E., Clare, L., et al. (2005b). Awareness in dementia: A review of clinical correlates. *Aging & Mental Health, 9*(5), 414-422.

Abbott, R. D., White, L. R., Ross, G. W., et al. (2004). Walking and dementia in physically capable elderly men. *Journal of the American Medical Association, 292,* 1447-1453.

Adler, G., Teufel, M., & Drach, L. M. (2003). Pharmacological treatment of frontotemporal dementia: Treatment response to the MAO-A inhibitor moclobemide. *International Journal of Geriatric Psychiatry, 18,* 653-655.

Adunsky, A., Levy, R., Mizrahi, E., et al. (2002). Exposure to opioid analgesia in cognitively impaired and delirious elderly hip fracture patients. *Archives of Gerontology and Geriatrics, 35,* 245-251.

Alexopoulos, G. S., Streim, J., Carpenter, D., et al. (2004). Using antipsychotic agents in older patients. Expert Consensus Panel for Using Antipsychotic Drugs in Older Patients. *Journal of Clinical Psychiatry, 65*(Suppl 2), 5-99.

Algase, D. L., Beck, C., Kolanowski, A., et al. (1996). Need-driven dementia-Compromised behavior: An alternative view of disruptive behavior. *American Journal of Alzheimer's Disease,* 11(6), 10-19.

Alzheimer's Association. (2006). *Early onset dementia: A national challenge, a future crisis.* Retrieved from http://www.alz.org/documents/national

Alzheimer's Association. (2010). *Stages of Alzheimer's.* Retrieved from http://www.alz.org/alzheimers_disease_stages_of_alzhemers.asp. Retrieved 6/12/2010.

Alzheimer's Association. (2011). *Alzheimer's disease facts & figures.* Retrieved from http://www.alz.org/alzheimers_disease_facts_and_figures.asp

American Psychiatric Association. (1997). Practice guideline for the treatment of patients with Alzheimer's disease and other dementias of late life. *American Journal of Psychiatry, 154*(5 Suppl), 1-39.

American Psychiatric Association. (2000). *Diagnostic and statistical manual of mental disorders* (4th ed., text rev.). Washington, DC: American Psychiatric Publishing, Inc.

Amieva, H., Le Goff, M., Millet, X., et al. (2008). Prodromal Alzheimer's disease: Successive emergence of the clinical symptoms. *Annals of Neurology, 64,* 492-498.

Ancoli-Israel, S. (2005). Sleep disturbances among patients with dementia. *Clinical Geriatrics, 12*(12), 13-16.

Andel, R., Crowe, M., Pedersen, N. L., et al. (2008). Physical exercise at midlife and risk of dementia three decades later: A population-based study of Swedish twins. *The Journals of Gerontology. Series A, Biological Sciences and Medical Sciences, 63*(1), 62-66.

Anstey, K. J., Lipnicki, D. M., & Low, L-F. (2008). Cholesterol as a risk factor for dementia and cognitive decline: A systematic review of prospective studies with meta-analysis. *American Journal of Geriatric Psychiatry, 16*(5), 343-354.

Anstey, K. J., Mack, H. A., & Cherbuin, N. (2009). Alcohol consumption as a risk factor for dementia and cognitive decline: Meta-analysis of prospective studies. *American Journal of Geriatric Psychiatry, 17*(7), 542-555.

Anstey, K. J., von Sanden, C., Salim, A., et al. (2007). Smoking as a risk factor for dementia and cognitive decline: A meta-analysis of prospective studies. *American Journal of Epidemiology, 166,* 367-378.

Apostolova, L. G., & Cummings, J. L. (2010). Neuropsychiatric aspects of Alzheimer's disease and other dementing illnesses. In S. C. Yudofsky & R. E. Hales (Eds.), *Essentials of neuropsychiatry and behavioral neurosciences* (2nd ed.) (pp. 409-432). Washington, DC: American Psychiatric Publishing, Inc.

Arciniegas, D. B., & Dubovsky, S. (2007). Dementia due to other general medical conditions and dementia due to multiple etiologies. In G. O. Gabbard (Ed.), *Gabbard's treatments of psychiatric disorders* (4th ed.) (pp. 159-178). Washington, DC: American Psychiatric Publishing, Inc.

Aronow, W. S., & Frishman, W. H. (2006). Effects of antihypertensive drug treatment on cognitive function and the risk of dementia. *Clinical Geriatrics, 14*(11), 25-28.

Arvanitakis, Z. (2010). Update on frontotemporal dementia. *The Neurologist, 16*(1), 16-22.

Arvanitakis, Z., & Wszolek, Z. K. (2001). Recent advances in the understanding of tau protein and movement disorders. *Current Opinion in Neurology, 14,* 491-497.

Avramopoulos, D. (2009). Genetics of Alzheimer's disease: Recent advances. *Genome Medicine, 1*(3), 34.

Ayalon, L., Gum, A. M., Feliciano, L., et al. (2006). Effectiveness of non-pharmacological interventions for the management of neuropsychiatric symptoms in patients with dementia: A systematic review. *Archives of Internal Medicine, 166*(20), 2182-2188.

Bachman, D., & Rabins, P. (2006). "Sundowning" and other temporally associated agitation states in dementia patients. *Annual Review of Medicine, 57,* 499-511.

Backman, L. (2008). Memory and cognition in preclinical dementia: What we know and what we do not know. *Canadian Journal of Psychiatry, 53*(6), 354-360.

Backman, L., Jones, S., Berger, A. K., et al. (2005). Cognitive impairment in preclinical Alzheimer's disease: A meta-analysis. *Neuropsychology, 19*(4), 520-531.

Baker, M., Mackenzie, J. R., Pickering-Brown, S. M., et al. (2006). Mutations in progranulin cause tau-negative frontotemporal dementia linked to chromosome 17. *Nature, 24,* 916-919.

Balasa, M., Gelpi, E., Antonell, A., et al.; Neurological Tissue Bank/University of Barcelona/Hospital Clínic NTB/UB/HC Collaborative Group. (2011). Clinical features and APOE genotype of pathologically proven early-onset Alzheimer disease. *Neurology, 76*(20), 1720-1725.

Ball, K., Berch, D. B., Helmers, K. F., et al. (2002). Effects of cognitive training interventions with older adults: A randomized controlled trial. *Journal of the American Medical Association, 288*(18), 271-281.

Ballard, C., Corbett, A., Chitramohan, R., et al. (2009). Management of agitation and aggression associated with Alzheimer's disease: Controversies and possible solutions. *Current Opinion in Psychiatry, 22,* 532-540.

Ballard, C., Margallo-Lana, M., Juszczak, E., et al. (2005). Quetiapine and rivastigmine and cognitive decline in Alzheimer's disease: Randomised double blind placebo controlled trial. *British Medical Journal, 330*(7496), 874.

Ballard, C., Neill, D., O'Brien, J., et al. (2000). Anxiety, depression and psychosis in vascular dementia: Prevalence and associations. *Journal of Affective Disorders, 59,* 97-106.

Ballard, C., O'Brien, J. T., Reichelt, K., et al. (2002). Aromatherapy as a safe and effective treatment for the management of agitation in severe dementia: The results of a double-blind placebo-controlled trial with Melissa. *Journal of Clinical Psychiatry, 63,* 553-558.

Barberger-Gateau, P., Raffaitin, C., Letenneur, L., et al. (2007). Dietary patterns and risk of dementia: The Three-City cohort study. *Neurology, 69,* 1921-1930.

Barnes, D. E. (2011). The Mediterranean diet: Good for the heart=good for the brain. *American Neurological Association, 69*(2), 226-228.

Barnes, D. E., Covinsky, K. E., Whitmer, R. A., et al. (2009). Predicting risk of dementia in older adults: The late-life dementia risk index. *Neurology, 73,* 173-179.

Barnes, E. E., Haight, T. J., Mehta, K. M., et al. (2010). Second hand smoke, vascular disease, and dementia incidence: Findings from the cardiovascular health cognition study. *American Journal of Epidemiology, 171*(3), 292-302.

Barnett, C., & Curran, V. (2003). Dementia in footballers. *International Journal of Geriatric Psychiatry, 18,* 86-90.

Bassil, N., & Grossberg, G. T. (2010). Medical, dietary, and lifestyle choices may promote healthy brain aging. *General Psychiatry, 9*(6), 23-36.

Beach, S. R., Schulz, R., Williamson, G. M., et al. (2005). Risk factors for potentially harmful informal caregiver behavior. *Journal of American Geriatric Society, 53,* 255-261.

Beach, S. R., Schulz, R., Yee, J. L., et al. (2000). Negative and positive health effects of caring for a disabled spouse: Longitudinal findings from the Caregiver Health Effects Study. *Psychological Aging, 15,* 259-271.

Bennett, D. A., Schneider, J. A., Tang, Y., et al. (2006). The effect of social networks on the relations between Alzheimer's disease pathology and level of cognitive function in old people: A longitudinal cohort study. *Lancet Neurology, 5*(5), 406-412.

Berger, A. K., Fratiglioni, L., Forsell, Y., et al. (1999). The occurrence of depressive symptoms in the preclinical phase of Alzheimer's disease. *Neurology, 53,* 1998-2001.

Berlit, P. (2007). Neuropsychiatric disease in collagen vascular diseases and vasculitis. *Journal of Neurology, 254*(Suppl 21), 1187-1189.

Bigler, E. D. (2009). Traumatic brain injury. In M. F. Weiner & A. M. Lipton (Eds.), *The American psychiatric publishing textbook of Alzheimer disease and other dementias* (pp. 229-246). Washington, DC: American Psychiatric Publishing, Inc.

Biringer, E., Mykletun, A., Dahl, A., et al. (2005). The association between depression, anxiety, and cognitive function in the elderly general population—the Hordaland Health Study. *International Journal of Geriatric Psychiatry, 20,* 989-997.

Black, B. S., Finucane, T., Baker, A., et al. (2006). Health problems and correlates of pain in nursing home residents with advanced dementia. *Alzheimer Disease and Associated Disorders, 20*(4), 283-290.

Black, D. W., & Andreasen, N. C. (2011). *Introductory textbook of psychiatry* (5th ed.). Washington, DC: American Psychiatric Publishing, Inc.

Blennow, K., de Leon, M. J., & Zetterberg, H. (2006). Alzheimer's disease. *Lancet, 368,* 387-403.

Bliwise, D. L. (2004). Sleep disorders in Alzheimer's disease and other dementias. *Clinical Cornerstone, 7*(Suppl 1A), 16-28.

Bloss, C. S., Delis, D. C., Salmon, D. P., et al. (2008). Decreased cognition in children with risk factors for Alzheimer's disease. *Biological Psychiatry, 64,* 904-906.

Bobholz, J. A., & Rao, S. M. (2003). Cognitive dysfunction in MS: A review of recent developments. *Current Opinions in Neurology, 16,* 283-288.

Borson, S., Scanlan, J., Brush, M., et al. (2000). The Mini-Cog: A cognitive "vital signs" measure for dementia screening in multilingual elderly. *International Journal of Geriatric Psychiatry, 15*(11), 1021-1027.

Bosma, H., van Boxtel, M. P. J., Ponds, R. W. H. M., et al. (2002). Engaged lifestyle and cognitive function in middle and old-aged non-demented persons: A reciprocal association? *Zeitschrift fur Gerontologic und Geriatrie, 35,* 575-581.

Bossen, A. L. (2009). Needs of people with early-stage Alzheimer's disease. *Journal of Gerontological Nursing, 35*(3), 8-15.

Bourgeois, J. A., Seaman, J. S., & Servis, M. E. (2008). Delirium, dementia and amnestic and other cognitive disorders. In R. E. Hales, S. C. Yudofsky, & G. O. Gabbard (Eds.), *The American psychiatric publishing textbook of psychiatry* (5th ed.) (pp. 303-363). Washington, DC: American Psychiatric Publishing, Inc.

Bourgeois, J. A., Seaman, J. S., & Servis, M. E. (2011). Delirium, dementia, and amnestic and other cognitive disorders. In R. E. Hales, S. C. Yudofsky, & G. O. Gabbard (Eds.), *Essentials of psychiatry* (3rd ed.) (pp. 41-82). Washington, DC: American Psychiatric Publishing, Inc.

Bourgeois, M. S., & Hickey, E. M. (Eds.) (2009). *Dementia: From diagnosis to management: A functional approach.* New York: Taylor & Francis.

Bowen, D. M., Procter, A. W., Mann, M. A., et al. (2008). Imbalance of a serotonergic system in frontotemporal dementia: Implication for pharmacotherapy. *Psychopharmacology, 196,* 603-610.

Boyle, P. A., Buchman, A. S., Wilson, R. S., et al. (2010). The APOE epsilon 4 allele is associated with incident mild cognitive impairment among community-dwelling older persons. *Neuroepidemiology, 34*(1), 43-49.

Breitner, J. C. S., & Albert, M. S. (2009). Prevention of dementia and cognitive decline. In M. F. Weiner & A. M. Lipton (Eds.), *The American psychiatric publishing textbook of Alzheimer disease and other dementias* (pp. 443-466). Washington, DC: American Psychiatric Publishing, Inc.

Brookmeyer, R., Gray, S., & Kawas, C. (1998). Projections of Alzheimer's disease in the United States and the public health impact of delaying disease onset. *American Journal of Public Health, 88*(4), 1337-1342.

Brown, F. W. (2009). Cognitive enhancers. In A. F. Schatzberg & C. B. Nemeroff (Eds.), *The American psychiatric publishing textbook of psychopharmacology* (4th ed.) (pp. 811-820). Washington: DC: American Psychiatric Publishing, Inc.

Brown, T. M., & Stoudemire, A. (1998). *Psychiatric side effects of prescription and over-the-counter medications.* Washington, DC: American Psychiatric Publishing, Inc.

Brummell-Smith, K. (2007). Optimal aging, part II: Evidence-based practical steps to achieve it. *Annals of Long-term Care, 15*(12), 32-40.

Bryden, C. (2002). A person-centred approach to counseling, psychotherapy and rehabilitation of people diagnosed with dementia in the early stages. *Dementia, 1*(2), 141-156.

Buettner, L. L. (1999). Simple pleasures: A multilevel sensorimotor intervention for nursing home residents with dementia. *American Journal of Alzheimer's Disease and Other Dementias, 14*(1), 18-24.

Bullock, R. (2005). Treatment of behavioural and psychiatric symptoms in dementia: Implications of recent safety warnings. *Current Medical Research Opinions, 21*, 1-10.

Burgio, L. D., Schmid, B., & Johnson, M. N. (2008). Assessment and interventions for caregiver's distress. In K. Laidlaw & B. G. Knight (Eds.), *The handbook of emotional disorders in late life: Assessment and treatment* (pp. 403-419). Oxford, UK: Oxford University Press.

Byrne, E. J., Lennox, G., Lowe, J., et al. (1989). Diffuse Lewy body disease: Clinical features in 15 cases. *Journal of Neurology, Neurosurgery & Psychiatry, 52*, 709-717.

Calkins, M. P. (2004). Articulating environmental press. *Alzheimer's Care Quarterly, 5*, 165-172.

Carlson, M. C., Helms, M. J., Steffens, D. C., et al. (2008). Midlife activity predicts risk of dementia in older male twin pairs. *Alzheimer's & Dementia, 4*(5), 324-331.

Carolan Doerflinger, M. C. (2007). How to try this: The Mini-Cog. *American Journal of Nursing, 107*(12), 62-71.

Carriere, I., Fourrier-Reglat, A., Dartigues, J-F, et al. (2009). Drugs with anticholinergic properties, cognitive decline, and dementia in an elderly general population. *Archives of Internal Medicine, 169*(14), 1317-1324.

Caselli, R. J., & Yaari, R. (2007-2008). Medical management of frontotemporal dementia. *American Journal of Alzheimer's Disease and Other Dementias, 22*(6), 489-498.

Cataldo, J. K., Prochaska, J. J., & Glantz, S. A. (2010). Cigarette smoking is a risk factor for Alzheimer's: An analysis controlling for tobacco industry affiliation. *Journal of Alzheimer's Disease, 19*(2), 465-480.

Cedazo-Minguez, A., & Cowburn, R. F. (2001). Apolipoprotein E: A major piece in the Alzheimer's disease puzzle. *Journal of Cellular and Molecular Medicine, 5*(3), 254-266.

Centers for Diseases Control and Prevention. (2007). Rates of hospitalization related to traumatic brain injury—nine states, 2003. *MMWR Morbidity Mortality Weekly Report, 56*, 167-170.

Chen, J. H., Lamberg, J. L., Chen, Y. C., et al. (2006). Occurrence and treatment of suspected pneumonia in long-term care residents dying with advanced dementia. *Journal of American Geriatric Society, 54*, 290-295.

Cherbuin, N., Reglade-Meslin, C., Kumar, R., et al. (2009). Risk factors of transition from normal cognition to mild cognitive disorder: The PATH through life study. *Dementia and Geriatric Cognitive Disorders, 28*, 47-55.

Chiu, W., Kaat, L. D., Seelaar, H., et al. (2010). Survival in progressive supranuclear palsy and frontotemporal dementia. *Journal of Neurology, Neurosurgery & Psychiatry, 81*(4), 441-445.

Chodosh, J., Kado, D. M., Seeman, T. E., et al. (2007). Depressive symptoms as a predictor of cognitive decline: MacArthur Studies of successful aging. *American Journal of Geriatric Psychiatry, 15*(5), 406-415.

Christensen, H. (2001). What cognitive changes can be expected with normal ageing? *Australian and New Zealand Journal of Psychiatry, 35*, 768-775.

Cohen-Mansfield, J. (2007). Temporal patterns of agitation in dementia. *American Journal of Geriatric Psychiatry, 15*(5), 395-405.

Cohen-Mansfield, J., Golander, H., & Arnheim, G. (2000). Self-identity in older persons suffering from dementia: Preliminary results. *Social Science & Medicine, 51*, 381-394.

Cohen-Mansfield, J., Libin A., & Marx, M. S. (2007). Nonpharmacological treatment of agitation: A controlled trial of systematic individualized intervention. *The Journals of Gerontology. Series A, Biological Sciences and Medical Sciences, 62*(8), 908-916.

Cohen-Mansfield, J., Parpura-Gill, A., & Golander, H. (2006). Utilization of self-identity roles for designing interventions for persons. *The Journals of Gerontology. Series B, Psychological Sciences and Social Sciences, 61*(4), P202-P212.

Cohen-Mansfield, J., & Werner, P. (1997). Management of verbally disruptive behaviors in nursing home residents. *The Journals of Gerontology. Series A, Biological Sciences and Medical Sciences, 52*(6), M369-M377.

Cohen-Mansfield, J., Werner, P., Watson, V., et al. (1995). Agitation among elderly persons at adult day-care centers: The experiences of relatives and staff members. *International Psychogeriatrics, 7*(3), 447-458.

Colling, K. B., & Buettner, L. L. (2002). Simple Pleasures: Interventions from the need-driven dementia-compromised behavior model. *Journal of Gerontological Nursing, 28*(10), 16-20.

Collins, S., McLean, C. A., Masters, C. L., et al. (2001). Gerstmann-Sträussler-Scheinker syndrome, fatal familial insomnia, and kuru: A review of these less common human transmissible spongiform encephalopathies. *Journal of Clinical Neuroscience, 8*(5), 387-397.

Cummings, J., Schneider, E., Tariot, P., et al. (2006). Behavioral effects of memantine in Alzheimer disease patients receiving donepezil treatment. *Neurology, 67*, 57-63.

Cummings, J., & Winblad, B. (2007). A rivastigmine patch for the treatment of Alzheimer's disease and Parkinson's disease dementia. *Expert Review of Neurotherapeutics, 7*(11), 1457-1463.

Curyto, K. J., Johnson, J., TenHave, T., et al. (2001). Survival of hospitalized elderly patients with delirium: A prospective study. *American Journal of Geriatric Psychiatry, 9*(2), 141-147.

Dai, Q., Borenstein, A. R., Wu, Y., et al. (2006). Fruit and vegetable juices and Alzheimer's disease: The Kame Project. *American Journal of Medicine, 119*, 751-759.

Davis, A. A., Lah, J. J., & Levey, A. I. (2009). Neurobiology of Alzheimer's disease. In F. Schatzberg & C. B. Nemeroff (Eds.), *The American psychiatric publishing textbook of psychopharmacology* (4th ed.) (pp. 987-1003). Washington, DC: American Psychiatric Publishing, Inc.

Deakin, J. B., Rahman, S., Nestor, P. J., et al. (2004). Paroxetine does not improve symptoms and impairs cognition in frontotemporal dementia: A double-blind randomized controlled trial. *Psychopharmacology, 172*, 400-408.

Del Ser, T., McKeith, I., Anand, R., et al. (2000). Dementia with Lewy bodies: Findings from an international multicentre study. *International Journal of Geriatric Psychiatry, 15*, 1034-1045.

Deschenes, C. L., & McCurry, S. M. (2009). Current treatments for sleep disturbances in individuals with dementia. *Current Psychiatry Reports, 11*(1), 20-26.

Devanand, D. P., Liu, X., Tabert, M. H., et al. (2008). Combining early markers strongly predicts conversion from mild cognitive impairment to Alzheimer's disease. *Biological Psychiatry, 64*, 871-879.

Devi, G., Williamson, J., Massoud, F., et al. (2004). A comparison of family history of psychiatric disorders among patients with early- and late-onset Alzheimer's disease. *Journal of Neuropsychiatry and Clinical Neuroscience, 16*(1), 57-62.

Donini, L., Felice, M., & Cannella, C. (2007). Nutritional status determinants and cognition in the elderly. *Archives of Gerontology and Geriatrics, 44*(Suppl 1), 143-153.

Doody, R. S., Garivlova, S. I., Sano, M., et al. (2008). Effects of dimebon on cognition, activities of daily living, behaviour and global function in patients with mild-to-moderate Alzheimer's disease: A randomized, double-blind, placebo-controlled study. *Lancet, 372(9634)*, 207-215.

Doraiswamy, P. M., Leon, J., Cummings, J. L., et al. (2002). Prevalence and impact of medical comorbidity in Alzheimer's disease. *The Journals of Gerontology. Series A, Biological Sciences and Medical Sciences, 57A*, M173-M177.

Doty, R. L., Shaman, P., & Dann, M. (1984). Development of the University of Pennsylvania Smell Identification Test: A standardized microencapsulated test of olfactory function. *Physiological Behavior, 32,* 489-502.

Douglas, S., James, I., & Ballard, C. (2004). Non-pharmacological interventions in dementia. *Advances in Psychiatric Treatment, 10,* 171-179.

Duff, K., McCaffrey, R. J., & Solomon, G. S. (2002). The Pocket Smell Test: successfully discriminating probable Alzheimer's dementia from vascular dementia and major depression. *Journal of Neuropsychiatry and Clinical Neuroscience, 14*(2), 197-201.

Duff-Canning, S. E., Leach, L., Stuss, D., et al. (2004). Diagnostic utility of abbreviated fluency measures in Alzheimer's disease and vascular dementia. *Neurology, 62,* 556-562.

Dumas, J., Hancur-Bucci, C., Naylor, M., et al. (2008). Estradiol interacts with the cholinergic system to affect verbal memory in postmenopausal women: Evidence of the critical period hypothesis. *Hormones & Behavior, 53*(1), 159-169.

Duppils, G. S., & Wikblad, K. (2004). Delirium: Behavioural changes before and during the prodromal phase. *Journal of Clinical Nursing, 13*(5), 609-616.

Duran, J. C., Greenspan, A., Diago, J. I., et al. (2005). Evaluation of risperidone in the treatment of behavioral and psychological symptoms and sleep disturbances associated with dementia. *International Psychogeriatrics, 17,* 591-605.

Erickson, K. I., Colcombe, S. J., Wadhwa, R., et al. (2007). Training-induced functional activation changes in dual-task processing: An FMRI study. *Cerebral Cortex, 17,* 192-204.

Esiri, M. M., Nagy, Z., Smith, M. Z., et al. (1999). Cerebrovascular disease and threshold for dementia in the early stages of Alzheimer's disease. *Lancet, 354,* 919-920.

Eskelinen, M. H., Ngandu, T., Tuomilehto, J., et al. (2009). Midlife coffee and tea drinking and the risk of late-life dementia: A population-based CAIDE study. *Journal of Alzheimer's Disease, 16*(1), 85-91.

Fabel, K., & Kempermann, G. (2008). Physical activity and the regulation of neurogenesis in the adult and aging brain. *NeuroMolecular Medicine, 10*(2), 59-66.

Fann, J. R. (2000). The epidemiology of delirium: A review of studies and methodological issues. *Seminar of Clinical Neuropsychiatry, 5,* 86-92.

Farlow, M. R., & Boustani, M. (2009). Pharmacological treatment of Alzheimer disease and mild cognitive impairment. In M. F. Weiner & A. M. Lipton (Eds.), *The American psychiatric publishing textbook of Alzheimer disease and other dementias* (pp. 317-331). Washington, DC: American Psychiatric Publishing, Inc.

Farmer, M. E., Kittner, S. J., Rae, D. S., et al. (1995). Education and change in cognitive function: The Epidemiologic Catchment Area Study. *Annals of Epidemiology, 5,* 1-7.

Federal Interagency Forum on Aging Related Statistics: Older Americans. (2000). *Key indicators of well-being.* Washington, DC: Government Printing Office.

Felician, O., & Sandson, T. A. (1999). The neurobiology and pharmacotherapy of Alzheimer's disease. *Journal of Neuropsychiatry and Clinical Neurosciences, 11*(1), 19-31.

Ferman, T. J., Smith, G. E., Boeve, B. F., et al. (2004). DLB fluctuations: Specific features that reliably differentiate DLB from Alzheimer's disease and normal aging. *Neurology, 62,* 181-187.

Ferman, T. J., Smith, G. E., & Melom, B. (2005). *Understanding behavioral changes in dementia.* Lewy Body Association, Inc. Retrieved from www.lewybodydementia.org

Fernandez, H. H., Wu, C. K., & Ott, B. R. (2003). Pharmacotherapy of dementia with Lewy bodies. *Expert Opinion Pharmacotherapy, 4,* 2027-2037.

Ferrario, C. G. (2008). Geropharmacology: A primer for advanced practice acute care and critical care nurses, Part II. *AACN Advanced Critical Care, 19*(2), 134-151.

Fick, D. M., Agostini, J. V., & Inouye, S. K. (2002). Delirium superimposed on dementia: A systematic review. *Journal of American Geriatrics Society, 50,* 1723-1732.

Fick, D. M., & Mion, L. C. (2008). Delirium superimposed on dementia. *American Journal of Nursing, 108*(1), 52-60.

Fletcher, K. (2008). Nursing standard of practice protocol: Recognition and management of dementia. *Hartford Institute for Geriatric Nursing.* Retrieved from http://www.consultgerirn.org/topics/dementia/want_to_know_more. Retrieved 6/17/2008.

Flicker, C., Ferris, S. H., & Reisberg, B. (1991). Mild cognitive impairment in the elderly predictors of dementia. *Neurology, 41,* 1006-1009.

Flicker, L. (2009). Life style interventions to reduce the risk of dementia. *Maturitas, 63,* 319-322.

Folstein, M. F., Folstein, S. E., & McHugh, P. R. (1975). Mini-mental state. *Journal of Psychiatric Research, 12,* 189-198.

Fong, T. G., Jones, R. N., Shi, P., et al. (2009). Delirium accelerates cognitive decline in Alzheimer disease. *Neurology, 72*(18), 1570-1575.

Forette, F., Seux, M., Staessen, J., et al. (1998). Prevention of dementia in a randomised double-blind, placebo-controlled Systolic Hypertension in Europe (Syst-Eur) trial. *Lancet, 352,* 1347-1351.

Francis, J., Martin, D., & Kapoor, W. N. (1990). A prospective study of delirium in hospitalized elderly. *Journal of American Medical Association, 263,* 1097-1101.

Fratiglioni, L., Launer, L. J., Andersen, K., et al. (2000a). Incidence of dementia and major subtypes in Europe: A collaborative study of population-based cohorts. *Neurologic Diseases in the Elderly Research Group Neurology, 54*(11 Suppl 5), S10-S15.

Fratiglioni, L., Paillard-Borg, S., & Winblad, B. (2004). An active and socially integrated lifestyle in late life might protect against dementia. *Lancet Neurology, 3,* 259-266.

Fratiglioni, L., Wang, H. S., Ericsson, K., et al. (2000b). Influence of social network on occurrence of dementia: A community-based longitudinal study. *Lancet, 355,* 1315-1319.

Galanis, D. J., Petrovitch, H., Launer, L. J., et al. (1997). Smoking history in middle age and subsequent cognitive performance in elderly Japanese-American men. The Honolulu-Asia Aging Study. *American Journal of Epidemiology, 145*(6), 507-515.

Gallagher-Thompson, D., Lonergan, K. H., Holland, J., et al. (2009). Supporting family caregivers. In M. F. Weiner & A. M. Lipton (Eds.), *The American psychiatric publishing textbook of Alzheimer disease and other dementias* (pp. 353-366). Washington, DC: American Psychiatric Publishing, Inc.

Galvin, J. E., Pollack, J., & Morris, J. C. (2006). Clinical phenotype of Parkinson disease dementia. *Neurology, 67,* 1605-1611.

Gatz, M., Fratiglioni, L., Johansson, B., et al. (2005). Complete ascertainment of dementia in the Swedish Twin Registry: The HARMONY Study. *Neurobiological Aging, 26,* 439-447.

Gaudreau, J. D., & Gagnon, P. (2005). Psychogenic drugs and delirium pathogenesis: The central role of the thalamus. *Medical Hypotheses, 64,* 471-475.

Gauthier, S., Lopez, O. L., Waldemar, G., et al. (2010). Effects of donepezil on activities of daily living: Integrated analysis of patient data from studies in mild, moderate and severe Alzheimer's disease. *International Psychogeriatrics, 22*(6), 973-983.

Gauthier, S., Reisberg, B., Zaudig, M., et al. (2006). Mild cognitive impairment. International Psychogeriatric Association Expert Conference on mild cognitive impairment. *Lancet, 367*(9518), 1262-1270.

Geda, Y. E., Knopman, D. S., Mrazek, D. A., et al. (2006). Depression, apolipoprotein E genotype, and the incidence of mild cognitive impairment: A prospective cohort study. *Archives of Neurology, 63,* 435-440.

Geda, Y. E., Negash, S., & Petersen, R. C. (2009). Mild cognitive impairment. In M. F. Weiner & A. M. Lipton (Eds.), *The American psychiatric publishing textbook of Alzheimer disease and other dementias* (pp. 173-180). Washington, DC: American Psychiatric Publishing, Inc.

Geda, Y. E., Roberts, R. O., Knopman, D. S., et al. (2010). Physical exercise, aging and mild cognitive impairment. *Archives of Neurology, 67*(1), 80-86.

Geldmacher, D. S. (2004). Dementia with Lewy bodies: Diagnosis and clinical approach. *Cleveland Clinic Journal of Medicine, 71*(10), 789-800.

Geldmacher, D. S. (2009). Alzheimer disease. In M. F. Weiner & A. M. Lipton (Eds.), *The American psychiatric publishing textbook of Alzheimer disease and other dementias* (pp. 255-272). Washington, DC: American Psychiatric Publishing, Inc.

Geldmacher, D. S., & Whitehouse, P. J. (1996). Evaluation of dementia. *The New England Journal of Medicine, 335*(5), 330-336.

Geldmacher, D. S., & Whitehouse, P. J., Jr. (1997). Differential diagnosis of Alzheimer's disease. *Neurology, 48*(5 Suppl 6), S2-S9.

Gellis, Z. D., McClive-Reed, K. P., & Brown, E. L. (2009). Treatments for depression in older persons with dementia. *Annals of Long-term Care, 179*(2), 29-36.

Geser, F., Wenning, G., Poewe, W., et al. (2005). How to diagnose dementia with Lewy bodies: State of the art. *Movement Disorders, 20*(Suppl 12), S11-S20.

Gijselinck, I., Van Broeckhoven, C., & Cruts, M. (2008). Granulin mutations associated with frontotemporal lobar degeneration and related disorders: An update. *Human Mutation, 29*, 1373-1386.

Girard, T. D., Pandharipande, P. P., Carson, S. S., et al. (2010). Feasibility, efficacy, and safety of antipsychotics for intensive care unit delirium: The MIND randomized, placebo-controlled trial. *Critical Care Medicine, 38*(2), 428-437.

Glass, J., Lanctot, M., Herrmann, N., et al. (2005). Sedative hypnotics in older people with insomnia: Meta-analysis of risks and benefits. *British Medical Journal, 331*(7525), 1169.

Gleason, O. C. (2003). Delirium. *American Family Physician, 67*(5), 1027-1034.

Golden, R. N., Dawkins, K., & Nicholas, L. (2009). Trazodone and nefazodone. In A. F. Schatzberg & C. B. Nemeroff (Eds.), *The American psychiatric publishing textbook of psychopharmacology* (4th ed.) (pp. 403-414). Washington, DC: American Psychiatric Publishing, Inc.

Goldman, J. S., Farmer, J. M., Wood, E. M., et al. (2005). Comparison of family histories in FTLD subtypes and related tauopathies. *Neurology, 65*, 1817-1819.

Goldstein, L. (2006). Primary prevention of ischemic stroke: A guideline. *Stroke, 37*, 1583-1633.

Green, R. C., Cupples, A., Kurz, A., et al. (2003). Depression as a risk factor for Alzheimer disease. *Archives of Neurology, 60*, 753-759.

Greene, J. A., Ingram, T. A., Johnson, W., et al. (1993). Group psychotherapy for patients with dementia. *Southern Medical Journal, 86*(9), 1033-1035.

Grigaitis, M. M. (2006). Non-pharmacological interventions for use in dementia. *Barrow Quarterly, 22*(1), 15-18.

Han, J. H., Zimmerman, E. E., Cutler, N., et al. (2009). Delirium in older emergency department patients: Recognition, risk factors, and psychomotor subtypes. *Academy of Emergency Medicine, 16*(3), 193-200.

Hartmann, S., & Mobius, H. J. (2003). Tolerability of memantine in combination with cholinesterase inhibitors in dementia therapy. *International Clinical Psychopharmacology, 18*, 81-85.

Harwood, D. G., Kalechstein, A., Barker, W. W., et al. (2010). The effect of alcohol and tobacco consumption, and apolipoprotein E genotype, on the age of onset in Alzheimer's disease. *International Journal of Geriatric Psychiatry, 25*(5), 511-518.

Hashimoto, M., Kazui, H., Matsumoto, K., et al. (2005). Does donepezil treatment slow the progression of hippocampal atrophy in patients with Alzheimer's diseases. *American Journal of Psychiatry, 162*, 676-682.

Hasse, T. (2005). *Early-onset dementia: The needs of younger people with dementia in Ireland.* Retrieved from http://www.alzheimer.le.pdf/earlyOnsetDementia.pdf (accessed December 1, 2007).

Heath, C. A., Cooper, S. A., Murray, K., et al. (2011). Diagnosing variant Creutzfeldt-Jakob disease: A retrospective analysis of the first 150 cases in the UK. *Journal of Neurology, Neurosurgery and Psychiatry, 82*, 646-651.

Hebert, L. E., Scherr, P. A., Bienias, J. L., et al. (2003). Alzheimer disease in the US population: Prevalence estimates using the 2000 census. *Archives of Neurology, 60*, 1119-1122.

Hebert, R. S., Dang, Q., & Schulz, R. (2006). Preparedness for the death of a loved one and mental health in bereaved caregivers of patients with dementia: Finding from the REACH study. *Journal of Palliative Medicine, 9*, 683-693.

Hebert, R. S., Dang, Q., & Schulz, R. (2007). Religious beliefs and practices are associated with better mental health in family caregivers of patients with dementia: Findings from the REACH study. *American Journal of Geriatric Psychiatry, 15*, 292-300.

Hendrie, H. C., Albert, M. S., Butters, M. A., et al. (2006). The NIH Cognitive and Emotional Health Project: Report of the Critical Evaluation Study Committee. *Alzheimer's Dementia, 2*, 12-32.

Hepburn, K. W., Lewis, M., Sherman, C. W., et al. (2003). The savvy caregiver program: Developing a transportable dementia family caregiver training program. *Gerontologist, 43*, 908-915.

Hepple, J. (2004). Psychotherapies with older people: An overview. *Advances in Psychiatric Treatment, 10*, 371-377.

Hermans, D. G., Htay, U. H., & McShane, R. (2007). Non-pharmacological interventions for wandering of people with dementia in the domestic setting. *The Cochrane Database of Systematic Reviews*, (1). doi:10-1002/14651558.CD005994.pub2.

Herr, K. A., & Mobily, P. R. (1991). Pain assessment in the elderly: Clinical considerations. *Journal of Gerontological Nursing, 17*, 12-19.

Herrmann, N., Li, A., & Lanctot, K. (2011). Memantine in dementia; A review of current practice. *Expert Opinion in Pharmacotherapy, 12*(5), 787-800.

Hilgeman, M. M., Burgio, L. D., & Allen, R. S. (2009). Behavioral and environmental management. In M. F. Weiner & A. M. Lipton (Eds.), *The American psychiatric publishing textbook of Alzheimer disease and other dementias* (pp. 301-316). Washington, DC: American Psychiatric Publishing, Inc.

Hill, J. W., Futterman, R., Duttagupta, S., et al. (2002). Alzheimer's disease and related dementias increase costs of comorbidities in managed Medicare. *Neurology, 58*, 62-70.

Hilty, D. M., Seritan, A. L., Bourgeois, J. A., et al. (2007). Delirium due to a general medical condition, delirium due to multiple etiologies, and delirium not otherwise specified. In G. O. Gabbard (Ed.), *Gabbard's treatment of psychiatric disorders* (4th ed.) (pp. 145-157). Washington, DC: American Psychiatric Publishing, Inc.

Holroyd-Leduc, J. M., Khandwala, F., & Sink, K. M. (2010). How can delirium best be prevented and managed in older patients in hospital? *CMAJ: Canadian Medical Association Journal, 182*(5), 465-470.

Hsiung, G. Y., & Sadovnick, A. D. (2007). Genetics and dementia: Risk factors, diagnosis, and management. *Alzheimer's & Dementia, 3*(4), 418-427.

Hu, W. T., Seelaar, H., Josephs, K., et al. (2009). Survival profiles of patients with frontotemporal dementia and motor neuron disease. *Archives of Neurology, 66*(1), 1359-1364.

Huang, H. L., Shyu, Y. I., Chen, M. C., et al. (2003). A pilot study on a home-based caregiver training program for improving caregiver self-efficacy and decreasing the behavioral problems of elders with dementia in Taiwan. *International Journal of Geriatric Psychiatry, 18*, 337-345.

Huang, T. L., Zandi, P. P., Tucker, K. L., et al. (2005). Benefits of fatty fish on dementia risk are stronger for those without APOE episilon 4. *Neurology, 65*, 1409-1414.

Huey, E. D., Putnam, K. T., & Grafman, J. (2006). A systematic review of neurotransmitter deficits and treatments in frontotemporal dementia. *Neurology, 66*, 17-22.

Inouye, S. K., van Dyck, C. H., Alessi, C. A., et al. (1990). Clarifying confusion: The confusion assessment method. A new method for detection of delirium. *Annals of Internal Medicine, 113*(12), 941-948.

Inouye, S. K., Viscoli, C. M., Horwitz, R. I., et al. (1993). A predictive model for delirium in hospitalized elderly medical patients based on admission characteristics. *Annals of Internal Medicine, 119*, 474-481.

Ironside, J., & Bell, J. (1996). Pathology of prion diseases. In J. Collinge & M. Palmer (Eds.), *Prion diseases* (pp. 57-88). Oxford, UK: Oxford University Press.

Jarvenpaa, T., Rinne, J. O., Koskenvuo, M., et al. (2005). Binge drinking in midlife and dementia risk. *Epidemiology, 16*(6), 766-771.

Jellinger, K. A. (2003). Neuropathological spectrum of synucleinopathies. *Movement Disorders, 18*(Suppl 6), S2-S12.

Jellinger, K. A. (2008). Morphologic diagnosis of "vascular dementia"—A critical update. *Journal of the Neurological Sciences, 270*, 1-12.

Jellinger, K. A., Paulus, W., Wrocklage, C., et al. (2001). Effects of closed traumatic brain injury and genetic factors on the development of Alzheimer's disease. *European Journal of Neurology, 8*(6), 707-710.

Jones, R. W. (2003). Have cholinergic therapies reached their clinical boundary in Alzheimer's disease? *International Journal of Geriatric Psychiatry, 18*, S7-S13.

Jordan, S. E., Green, G. A., Galanty, H. L., et al. (1996). Acute and chronic brain injury in United States National Soccer players. *American Journal of Sports Medicine, 24*(2), 205-210.

Josif, S., & Graham, K. (2008). The diagnosis and treatment of dementia with Lewy bodies. *Journal of the American Academy of Physicians Assistants, 21*(15), 22-25.

Junaid, O., & Hegde, S. (2007). Supportive psychotherapy in dementia. *Advances in Psychiatric Treatment, 13,* 17-23.

Jurica, P. J., Leitten, C. L., & Mattis, S. (2002). *Dementia Rating Scale 2: Professional Manual.* Lutz, FL: Psychological Assessment Resources.

Kales, H. C., Zivin, K., Kim, H. M., et al. (2011). Trends in antipsychotic use in dementia 1999-2007. *Archives of General Psychiatry, 68*(2), 190-197.

Kalisvaart, C. J., Boelaarts, L., de Jonghe, J. F., et al. (2004). Successful treatment of three elderly patients suffering from prolonged delirium using the cholinesterase inhibitor rivastigmine. *Nederlands Tijdschrift voor Geneeskunde, 148,* 1501-1504.

Karas, G., Scheltens, P., Rombouts, S., et al. (2007). Precuneus atrophy in early-onset Alzheimer's disease: A morphometric structural MRI study. *Neuroradiology, 49*(12), 967-976.

Karp, A., Andel, R., Parker, M. G., et al. (2009). Mentally stimulating activities at work during midlife and dementia risk after age 75: Follow-up study from the Kungsholmen Project. *American Journal of Geriatric Psychiatry, 17*(3), 227-236.

Karp, A., Paillard-Borg, S., Wang, H-X, et al. (2006). Mental, physical and social components in leisure activities equally contribute to decrease dementia risk. *Dementia and Geriatric Cognitive Disorders, 21,* 65-73.

Kasl-Godley, J., & Gatz, M. (2000). Psychosocial interventions for individuals with dementia: An integration of theory, therapy, and a clinical understanding of dementia. *Clinical Psychology Review, 20*(6), 755-782.

Keys, M. A., & DeWald, C. (2005). Clinical perspective on choice of atypical antipsychotics in elderly patients with dementia, part II. *Annals of Long-Term Care: Clinical Care and Aging, 13*(3), 30-38.

Khachaturian, Z. S., Snyder, P. J., Doody, R., et al. (2009). A roadmap for the prevention of dementia II: Leon Thal symposium 2008. *Alzheimer's & Dementia, 5,* 85-92.

Kivipelto, M., Helkala, E. L., Hänninen, T., et al. (2001). Midlife vascular risk factors and late-life mild cognitive impairment: A population-based study. *Neurology, 56*(12), 1683-1689.

Kivipelto, M., Helkala, E. L., Laakso, M. P., et al. (2002). Apolipoprotein E epsilon4 allele, elevated midlife total cholesterol level and high midlife systolic blood pressure are independent risk factors for late-life Alzheimer disease. *Annals of Internal Medicine, 137,* 149-155.

Kivipelto, M., Rovio, S., Ngandu, T., et al. (2008). Apolipoprotein E epsilon4 magnifies lifestyle risks for dementia: A population-based study. *Journal of Cellular & Molecular Medicine, 12*(68), 2762-2771.

Kivipelto, M., & Solomon, A. (2009). Preventive neurology: On the way from knowledge to action. *Neurology, 73,* 168-169.

Knight, R. S. G., & Will, R. G. (2004). Prion diseases. *Journal of Neurology, Neurosurgery, and Psychiatry, 75*(Suppl 1), 136-142.

Knopman, D. S. (2010). Mild cognitive impairment and on to dementia: Down the slippery slope but faster. *Neurology, 74*(12), 942-944.

Knopman, D. S., Boeve, B. F., & Peterson, R. C. (2003). Essentials of the proper diagnoses of mild cognitive impairment, dementia, and major subtypes of dementia. *Mayo Clinic Proceedings, 78,* 1290-1308.

Koedam, E., Pijnenburg, Y., Deeg, D., et al. (2008). Early-onset dementia is associated with higher mortality. *Dementia and Geriatric Cognitive Disorders, 26,* 147-152.

Koester R. J., & Stooksbury, D. E. (1995). Behavioral profile of possible Alzheimer's patients in Virginia search and rescue incidents. *Wild Environmental Medicine, 6,* 34-43.

Kolbeinsson, H., & Jonsson, A. (1993). Delirium and dementia in acute medical admissions of elderly patients in Iceland. *Acta Psychiatrica Scandinavica, 87,* 123-127.

Korczyn, A. D. (2002). The complex nosological concept of vascular dementia. *Journal of Neurological Science, 203-204,* 3-6.

Korczyn, A. D. (2009). Is dementia preventable? *Dialogues in Clinical Neuroscience, 11*(2), 213-216.

Korczyn, A. D., & Vakhapova, V. (2007). The prevention of the dementia epidemic. *Journal of the Neurological Sciences, 257,* 2-4.

Kosaka, K., Yoshimura, M., Ikeda, K., et al. (1984). Diffuse type of Lewy body disease: Progressive dementia with abundant cortical Lewy bodies and senile changes of varying degree—a new disease? *Clinical Neuropathology, 3,* 185-192.

Koutures, C. G., & Gregory, A. J. M. (2010). Clinical report—injuries in youth soccer. *American Academy of Pediatrics, 125*(2), 410-414.

Kovach, C. R., Noonan, P. E., Schlidt, M., et al. (2005). A model of consequences of need-driven, dementia-compromised behavior. *Journal of Nursing Scholarship, 37*(2), 134-140.

Kraus, C. A., Seignourel, P., Balasubramanyam, V., et al. (2008). Cognitive-behavioral treatment for anxiety in patients with dementia: Two case studies. *Journal of Psychiatric Practice, 14*(3), 186-192.

Laitinen, M. H., Ngandu, T., Rovio, S., et al. (2006). Fat intake at midline midlife and risk of dementia and Alzheimer's disease: A population-based study. *Dementia and Geriatric Cognitive Disorders, 22,* 99-107.

Langlois, J. A., Marr, A., Mitchko, J., et al. (2005). Tracking the silent epidemic and education the public: CDC's traumatic brain injury-associated activities under the TBI Act of 1996 and the Children's Health Act of 2000. *Journal of Head Trauma Rehabilitation, 20,* 196-204.

Lantos, P. L., & Cairns, N. J. (2001). Neuropathology. In J. R. Hodges (Ed.), *Early-onset dementia* (pp. 227-262). New York: Oxford University Press.

Larrieu, S., Letenneur, L., Orgogozo, J. M., et al. (2002). Incidence and outcome of mild cognitive impairment in a population-based prospective cohort. *Neurology, 59,* 1594-1599.

Larson, E. B., Shadlen, M. F., Want, L., et al. (2004). Survival after initial diagnosis of Alzheimer's disease. *Annals of Internal Medicine, 140,* 501-509.

Launer, I. J., Ross, G. W., Petrovitch, H., et al. (2000). Midlife blood pressure and dementia: The Honolulu-Asia aging study. *Neurobiological Aging, 21,* 49-55.

Laurin, D., Verreault, R., Lindsay, J., et al. (2001). Physical activity and risk of cognitive impairment and dementia in elderly persons. *Archives of Neurology, 58,* 498-504.

Lautenschlager, N. T., Almeida, O. P., & Flicker, L. (2003). Preventing dementia: Why we should focus on health promotion now. *International Psychogeriatrics, 15,* 111-119.

Lawton, M. P., & Nahemow, L. E. (1973). Ecology and the aging process. In C. Eisdorfer & M. M. Lawton (Eds.), *The psychology of adult development and aging* (pp. 612-674). Washington, DC: American Psychological Association.

Lebert, F., Stekke, W., Hasenbrocks, C., et al. (2004). Frontotemporal dementia: A randomized, controlled trial with trazodone. *Dementia and Geriatric Cognitive Disorders, 17,* 355-359.

Lee, Y., Back, J. H., Kim, J., et al. (2010). Systematic review of health behavioral risks and cognitive health in older adults. *International Psychogeriatrics, 22*(2), 174-187.

Lenze, E. J., Pollock, B. G., Shear, M. K., et al. (2003). Treatment considerations for anxiety in the elderly. *CNS Spectrums, 8*(12 Suppl 3), 6-13.

Leonard, R., Tinetti, M. E., Allore, H. G., et al. (2006). Potentially modifiable resident characteristics that are associated with physical or verbal aggression among nursing home residents with dementia. *Archives of Internal Medicine, 166,* 1295-1300.

Lerner, A. J., & Riley, D. (2010). Neuropsychiatric aspects of dementias associated with motor dysfunction. In S. C. Yudofsky & R. E. Hales (Eds.), *Essentials of neuropsychiatry and behavioral neurosciences* (2nd ed.) (pp. 387-407). Washington, DC: American Psychiatric Publishing, Inc.

Leslie, D. L., Zhang, Y., Holford, T. R., et al. (2005). Premature death associated with delirium at 1-year follow-up. *Archives of Internal Medicine, 165,* 1657-1662.

Li, G., Larson, E. B., Sonnen, J. A., et al. (2007). Statin therapy is associated with reduced neuropathologic changes of Alzheimer disease. *Neurology, 69,* 878-885.

Lillo, P., & Hodges, J. R. (2009). Frontotemporal dementia and motor neuron disease: Overlapping clinic-pathological disorders. *Journal of Clinical Neuroscience, 16*(9), 1131 doi:10.1016/j.jocn.2009.03.005.

Lin, P. W., Chang, W. C., Ng, B. F., et al. (2007). Efficacy of aromatherapy (Lavandula angustifolia) as an intervention for agitated behaviours in Chinese older persons with dementia: A cross-over randomized trial. *International Journal of Geriatric Psychiatry, 22,* 405-410.

Lindgren, C., & Hallberg, I. R. (1992). Diagnostic reasoning in the care of a vocally disruptive severely demented patient. *Scandinavian Journal of Caring Sciences, 6*(2), 97-103.

Lindstrom, H. A., Fritsch, T., Petot, G., et al. (2005). The relationship between television viewing in midlife and the development of Alzheimer's disease in a case-control study. *Brain and Cognition, 58,* 157-165.

Lippa, C. F., Duda, J. E., Grossman, M., et al. (2007). DLB and PDD boundary issues: Diagnosis, treatment, molecular pathology and biomarkers. *Neurology, 68,* 812-819.

Lippa, C. F., Smith, T. W., & Swearer, J. M. (1994). Alzheimer's disease and Lewy body disease: A comparative clinicopathological study. *Annals of Neurology, 35,* 81-88.

Lipton, A. M., & Boxer, A. (2009). Frontotemporal dementia. In M. F. Weiner & M. Lipton (Eds.), *The American psychiatric publishing textbook of Alzheimer disease and other dementias* (pp. 219-227). Washington, DC: American Psychiatric Publishing, Inc.

Lipton, A. M., & Rubin, C. D. (2009). Medical evaluation and diagnosis. In M. F. Weiner & A. M. Lipton (Eds.), *The American psychiatric publishing textbook of Alzheimer disease and other dementias* (pp. 71-84). Washington, DC: American Psychiatric Publishing, Inc.

Little, J. T., Satlin, A., Sunderland, T., et al. (1995). Sundown syndrome in severely demented patients with probable Alzheimer's disease. *Journal of Geriatric Psychiatry and Neurology, 8,* 103-106.

Litvan, I., MacIntyre, A., Goetz, C. G., et al. (1998). Accuracy of the clinical diagnosis of Lewy Body disease, Parkinson disease, and dementia with Lewy bodies: A clinicopathologic study. *Archives of Neurology, 55,* 969-998.

Lonergan, E., Luxenberg, J., & Colford, J. (2002). Haloperidol for agitation in dementia. *The Cochrane Database Systematic Review,* (2). CD002852.

Lopez, O. L., Jagust, W. J., Dulberg, C., et al. (2003). Risk factors for mild cognitive impairment in the Cardiovascular Health Study Cognition Study. *Archives of Neurology, 60,* 1394-1399.

Luchsinger, J. A. (2004). Alcohol intake and risk of Alzheimer's disease. *Journal of American Geriatric Society, 52,* 540-546.

Luchsinger, J. A., Honig, L. S., Tang, M. S., et al. (2008). Depressive symptoms, vascular risk factors, and Alzheimer's disease. *International Journal of Geriatric Psychiatry, 23*(9), 922-928.

Luchsinger, J. A., & Mayeux, R. (2004). Dietary factors and Alzheimer's disease. *Lancet Neurology, 3,* 579-587.

Luukinen, H., Veramo, P., Herala, M., et al. (2005). Fall-related brain injuries and the risk of dementia in elderly people: A population-based study. *European Journal of Neurology, 12*(2), 86-92.

Luzzi, S., Snowden, J. S., Neary, D., et al. (2007). Distinct patterns of olfactory impairment in Alzheimer's disease, semantic dementia, frontotemporal dementia, and corticobasal degeneration. *Neuropsycholiga, 45,* 1823-1831.

Lyketsos, C. G., Colenda, C. C., Beck, C., et al. (2006). Position statement of the American Association for Geriatric Psychiatry regarding principles of care for patients with dementia resulting from Alzheimer disease. *American Journal of Geriatric Psychiatry, 14,* 51-57.

Lyketsos, C. G., Lopez, O., Jones, B., et al. (2002). Prevalence of neuropsychiatric symptoms in dementia and mild cognitive impairment: Results from the cardiovascular health study. *Journal of the American Medical Association, 23,* 1475-1483.

Lyketsos, C. G., Steinberg, M., Tschanz, J. T., et al. (2000). Mental and behavioral disturbances in dementia: Findings from the Cache County Study on Memory in Aging. *American Journal of Psychiatry, 157,* 708-714.

Mace, N. L., & Rabins, P. V. (2006). *The 36-hour day: A family guide to caring for people with Alzheimer disease, other dementias, and memory loss in later life* (4th ed.). Baltimore: The Johns Hopkins Press.

Malaspina, D., Corcoran, C., Schobel, S., et al. (2010). Epidemiological and genetic aspects of neuropsychiatric disorders. In S. C. Yudofsky & R. E. Hales (Eds.), *Essentials of neuropsychiatry and behavioral neurosciences* (pp. 95-147). Washington, DC: American Psychiatric Publishing, Inc.

Maldonado, J. R., VanDerStarre, P. J., & Wysong, A. (2003). Postoperative sedation and the incidence of ICU delirium in cardiac surgery patients. *ASA Annual Meeting Abstracts: Anesthesiology, 99,* A465.

Margallo-Lana, M., Swann, A., O'Brien, J., et al. (2001). Prevalence and pharmacological management of behavioral and psychological symptoms amongst dementia sufferers living in care environments. *International Journal of Geriatric Psychiatry, 16,* 39-44.

Martin, R., Griffith, R., Belue, K., et al. (2008). Declining financial capacity in patients with mild Alzheimer's disease: A one-year longitudinal study. *American Journal of Geriatric Psychiatry, 16*(3), 209-219.

Martorana, A., Esposito, Z., & Koch, G. (2010). Beyond the cholinergic hypothesis: Do current drugs work in Alzheimer's disease? *Neuroscience & Therapeutics, 16,* 235-245.

Mattis, S. (1976). Mental status examination for organic mental syndrome in the elderly patient. In R. Bellack & B. Darasu (Eds.), *Geriatric psychiatry: A handbook for psychiatrists and primary care physicians* (pp. 77-121). New York: Grune & Stratton.

Maurer, K. (2006). Historical background of Alzheimer's research done 100 years ago. *Journal of Neural Transmission, 113,* 1597-1601.

McCurry, S. M., Gibbons, L. E., Logsdon, R. G., et al. (2005). Nighttime insomnia treatment and education for Alzheimer's disease. *Journal of American Geriatric Society, 53*(5), 793-802.

McKeage, K. (2010). Spotlight on memantine in moderate to severe Alzheimer's disease. *Drugs & Aging, 27*(2), 177-179.

McKee, A. C., Cantu, R. C., Nowinski, C. J., et al. (2009). Chronic traumatic encephalopathy in athletes: Progressive tauopathy after repetitive head injury. *Journal of Neuropathology and Experimental Neurology, 68,* 709-735.

McKeith, I. G., Del Ser, T., Spano, P., et al. (2000). Efficacy of rivastigmine in dementia with Lewy bodies: A randomized, double-blind, placebo-controlled international study. *Lancet, 356,* 2031-2036.

McKeith, I. G., Fairbairn, A., Perry, R., et al. (1992a). Neuroleptic sensitivity in patients with senile dementia of Lewy body type. *British Medical Journal, 305,* 673-678.

McKeith, I. G., Galaski, D., Kosaka, K., et al. (1996). Consensus guidelines for the clinical and pathologic diagnosis of dementia with Lewy bodies (DLB): Report of the consortium on DLB international workshop. *Neurology, 47,* 1113-1124.

McKeith, I. G., Perry, R. H., Fairbairn, A. F., et al. (1992b). Operational criteria for senile dementia of Lewy body type (SDLT). *Psychological Medicine, 22,* 911-922.

McMinn, B., & Draper, B. (2005). Vocally disruptive behavior in dementia: Development of an evidence based practice guideline. *Aging & Mental Health, 9*(1), 16-24.

McMurtray, A., Clark, D. G., Christine, D., et al. (2006). Early-onset dementia: Frequency and causes compared to late-onset dementia. *Dementia and Geriatric Cognitive Disorders, 21,* 59-64.

McQueen, M. B., & Blacker, D. (2008). Genetics of Alzheimer's disease. In J. W. Smoller, B. R. Sheidley, & M. T. Tsuang (Eds.), *Psychiatric genetics: Applications in clinical practice* (pp. 177-194). Washington, DC: American Psychiatric Publishing, Inc.

McShane, R., Areosa, S. A., & Minadaran, N. (2006). Memantine for dementia. *The Cochrane Database Systematic Review,* (2). CD003154. doi:10.1002/14651858.CD003154.pub.5.

Memory and Aging Center, University of California at San Francisco. (2010a). *Basic biology of FTD.* Retrieved from University of California at San Francisco Web site: http://memory.ucsf.edu/ftd/overview/biology/

Memory and Aging Center, University of California at San Francisco. (2010b). *Living with FTD: Practical tips.* Retrieved from University of California at San Francisco Web site: http://memory.ucsf.edu/ftd/livingwithftd/practicaltips/

Mendez, M. F., & Lim, G. (2003). Seizures in elderly patients with dementia: Epidemiology and management. *Drugs & Aging, 20,* 791-803.

Mendez, M. F., Shapira, J. S., McMurtray, A., et al. (2007). Preliminary findings: Behavioral worsening on donepezil in patients with frontotemporal dementia. *American Journal of Geriatric Psychiatry, 15,* 84-87.

Merrilees, J., & Ketelle, R. (2010). Advanced practice nursing: Meeting the caregiving challenges for families of persons with frontotemporal dementia. *Clinical Nurse Specialist, 24*(5), 245-251.

Michaud, L., Bula, C., Berney, A., et al.; Delirium Guidelines Development Group. (2007). Delirium: Guidelines for general hospitals. *Journal of Psychosomatic Research, 62*(3), 371-383.

Milbrandt, E., Deppen, S., Harrison, P., et al. (2004). Costs associated with delirium on mechanically ventilated patients. *Critical Care Medicine, 33,* 226-229.

Miller, B. L., Boone, K., Mishkin, F., et al. (1998). Clinical and neuropsychological features of FTD. In A. Kertesz & D. Munoz (Eds.), *Pick's disease and Pick complex* (pp. 23-33). New York: Wiley-Liss.

Miller, B. L., Cummings, J. L., Villanueva-Meyer, J., et al. (1991). Frontal lobe degeneration: Clinical, neuropsychological, and SPECT characteristics. *Neurology, 41,* 1374-1382.

Mitchell, S. L., Kiely, D. K., & Hamel, M. B. (2004). Dying with advanced dementia in the nursing home. *Archives of Internal Medicine, 164,* 321-326.

Mitrou, P. N., Kipnis, V., Thiebaut, A. C., et al. (2007). Mediterranean dietary pattern and prediction of all-cause mortality in a US population: Results from the NIHAARP Diet and Health Study. *Archives of Internal Medicine, 167*(22), 2462-2468.

Mitsuyama, Y., & Inoue, T. (2009). Clinical entity of frontotemporal dementia with motor neuron disease. *Neuropathology, 29,* 640-654.

Modrego, P. J., & Ferrández, J. (2004). Depression in patients with mild cognitive impairment increases the risk of developing dementia of Alzheimer type: A prospective cohort study. *Archives of Neurology, 61*(8), 1290-1293.

Monte, R., Rabunal, R., Casariego, E., et al. (2009). Risk factors for delirium tremens in patients with alcohol withdrawal syndrome in a hospital setting. *European Journal of Internal Medicine, 20,* 690-694.

Moretti, R., Torre, P., Antonello, R. M., et al. (2003). Frontotemporal dementia: Paroxetine as a possible treatment of behavior symptoms: A randomized, controlled, open 14 month study. *European Neurology, 49,* 13-19.

Moretti, R., Torre, P., Antonello, R. M., et al. (2004). Rivastigmine in frontotemporal dementia: An open-label study. *Drugs & Aging, 21,* 931-937.

Morley, J. E., & Tumosa, N. (2002). Saint Louis University Mental Status Examination (SLUMS). *Aging Successfully: A News Letter Publication, XII,* (1). Retrieved from Echo.unm.edu/PDFsdementia/SLUMS5%20form.pdf

Morris, J., & Volicer, L. (2001). Nutritional management of individuals with Alzheimer's disease and other progressive dementias. *Nutrition in Clinical Care, 4,* 148-155.

Morris, M. C., Evans, D. A., Tangney, C. C., et al. (2006). Associations of vegetable and fruit consumption with age-related cognitive change. *Neurology, 67,* 1370-1376.

Mosimann, U. P., & McKeith, I. G. (2003). Dementia with Lewy bodies—diagnosis and treatment. *Swiss Medical Weekly, 133,* 131-142.

Mowla, A., Mosavinasab, M., Haghshenas, H., et al. (2007). Does serotonin augmentation have an effect on cognition and activities of daily living in Alzheimer's dementia? A double-blind, placebo-controlled clinical trial. *Journal of Clinical Psychopharmacology, 27*(5), 484-487.

Mukamal, K. J., Kuller, L. H., Fitzpatrick, A. L., et al. (2003). Prospective study of alcohol consumption and risk of dementia in older adults. *Journal of the American Medical Association, 289,* 1405-1413.

Mychack, P., Kramer, J. H., Boone, K. B., et al. (2001). The influence of right frontotemporal dysfunction on social behavior in frontotemporal dementia. *Neurology, 56*(11 Suppl 4), S11-S15.

Nadkarni, N. K., Mawji, E., McIlroy, W. E., et al. (2009). Spatial and temporal gait parameters in Alzheimer's disease and aging. *Gait & Posture, 39*(4), 452-454.

National Institute on Aging. (2011). *Alzheimer's disease genetics fact sheet.* Retrieved from Alzheimer's Disease Education & Referral (ADEAR) Center Web site: www.nia.nih.gov/Alzheimers/Publications/geneticsfs.htm

National Institute of Neurological Disorders and Stroke. (2010). *NINDS Kuru Information Page* http://www.ninds.nih.gov/disorders/kuru/kuru.htm. Retrieved 7/27/2011.

Naughton, B. J., Moran, M. B., Kadah, H., et al. (1995). Delirium and other cognitive impairment in older adults in an emergency department. *Annals of Emergency Medicine, 25*(6), 751-755.

Nebes, R. D., Pollock, B. G., Meltzer, C. C., et al. (2005). Cognitive effects of serum anticholinergic activity and white matter hyperintensities. *Neurology, 65,* 1487-1489.

Neef, D., & Walling, A. D. (2006). Dementia with Lewy bodies: an emerging disease. *American Family Physician, 73,* 1223-1230.

Newman, A. B., Fitzpatrick, A. L., Lopez, O., et al. (2005). Dementia and Alzheimer's disease incidence in relationship to cardiovascular disease in the Cardiovascular Health Study cohort. *Journal of American Geriatric Society, 53,* 1101-1107.

Ngandu, T. (2006). *Lifestyle-related risk factors in dementia and mild cognitive impairment: A population-based study.* Stockholm, Sweden: Karolinska Institute.

Nguyen, Q. A., & Paton, C. (2008). The use of aromatherapy to treat behavioral problems in dementia. *International Journal of Geriatric Psychiatry, 23,* 337-346.

O'Brien, J. T., Colloby, S., Fenwick, J., et al. (2004). Dopamine transporter loss visualized with FP-CIT SPECT in the differential diagnosis of dementia with Lewy bodies. *Archives of Neurology, 61,* 919-925.

Orgogozo, J. M., Dartigues, J. F., Lafont, S., et al. (1997). Wine consumption and dementia in the elderly: A prospective community study in the Bordeaux area. *Revue Neurologique, 153*(3), 185-192.

Ott, A., Andersen, K., Dewey, M. D., et al. (2004). Effect of smoking on global cognitive function in non-demented elderly. *Neurology, 62,* 920-924.

Ownby, R. L., Crocco, E., Acevedo, A., et al. (2006). Depression and risk for Alzheimer disease: Systematic review, meta-analysis, and meta-regression analysis. *Archives of General Psychiatry, 63*(5), 530-538.

Palmer, K., Backman, L., Winblad, B., et al. (2008). Mild cognitive impairment in the general population: Occurrence and progression to Alzheimer's disease. *American Journal of Geriatric Psychiatry, 16*(7), 603-611.

Pandharipande, P., Cotton, B. A., Shintani, A., et al. (2008). Prevalence and risk factors for development of delirium in surgical and trauma intensive care unit patients. *The Journal of Trauma, Injury, Infection and Critical Care, 65,* 34-41.

Pandharipande, P., Shintani, A., Peterson, J., et al. (2006). Lorazepam is an independent risk factor for transitioning to delirium in intensive care unit patients. *Anesthesiology, 104*(1), 21-26.

Patel, L., & Grossberg, G. T. (2011). Combination therapy for Alzheimer's disease. *Drugs & Aging, 28*(7), 539-546.

Patterson, C., Feightner, J., Garcia, A., et al. (2007). Primary prevention of dementia. *Alzheimer's & Dementia, 3*(4), 348-354.

Paukert, A. L., Calleo, J., & Kraus-Schuman, C. (2010). Peaceful Mind: An open trial of cognitive behavioral therapy for anxiety in persons with dementia. *International Psychogeriatrics, 22*(6), 1012-1021.

Peila, R., White, L. R., Masaki, K., et al. (2006). Reducing the risk of dementia: Efficacy of long-term treatment of hypertension. *Stroke, 37*(5), 1165-1170.

Persson, J., Sylvester, C. Y., Nelson, J. K., et al. (2004). Selection requirements during verb generation: Differential recruitment in older and younger adults. *Neuroimage, 23,* 1382-1390.

Peters, R. (2009). The prevention of dementia. *International Journal of Geriatric Psychiatry, 24,* 452-458.

Peters, R., Poulter, R., Warner, J., et al. (2008). Smoking, dementia and cognitive decline in the elderly: A systematic review. *BMC Geriatrics, 8*(1), 36.

Petersen, R. C., Smith, G., Kokmen, E., et al. (1997). Memory function in normal aging. *Neurology, 42,* 396-401.

Petersen, R. C., Thomas, R. G., Grundman, M., et al. (2005). Vitamin E and donepezil for the treatment of mild cognitive impairment. *The New England Journal of Medicine, 352,* 2379-2388.

Peterson, J. F., Pun, B. T., Dittus, R. S., et al. (2006). Delirium and its motoric subtypes: A study of 724 critically ill patients. *Journal of American Geriatric Society, 54,* 479-484.

Pfeffer, R. I., Kurosaki, T. T., Harrah, C. H., et al. (1982). Measurement of functional activities of older adults in the community. *Journal of Gerontology, 37*(3), 323-329.

Pinquart, M., & Sorensen, S. (2006). Helping caregivers of persons with dementia: Which interventions work and how large are their effects? *International Psychogeriatrics, 18*(4), 577-595.

Plassman, B. L., Havlik, R. J., Steffens, D. C., et al. (2000). Documented head injury in early adulthood and risk of Alzheimer's disease and other dementias. *Neurology, 55,* 1158-1166.

Podewils, L. J., Guallar, E., Kuller, L. H., et al. (2005). Physical activity, APOE genotype, and dementia risk: Findings from the Cardiovascular Health Cognition Study. *American Journal of Epidemiology, 161,* 639-651.

Pollock, B. G., Mulsant, B. H., Rosen, J., et al. (2007). A double-blind comparison of citalopram and risperidone for the treatment of behavioral and psychotic symptoms associated with dementia. *American Journal of Geriatric Psychiatry, 15,* 942-952.

Porter, V. R., Buxton, W. G., Fairbanks, L. A., et al. (2003). Frequency and characteristics of anxiety among patients with Alzheimer's disease and related dementias. *Journal of Neuropsychiatry Clinical Neuroscience, 15,* 180-186.

Prvulovic, D., Hampel, H., & Pantel, J. (2010). Galantamine for Alzheimer's disease. *Expert Opinion on Drug Metabolism & Toxicology, 6*(3), 345-354.

Pun, B. T., & Ely, E. W. (2007). The importance of diagnosing and managing ICU delirium. *Recent Advances in Chest Medicine, 132,* 624-635.

Qiu, C., Kivipelto, M., & von Strauss, E. (2009). Epidemiology of Alzheimer's disease: Occurrence, determinants, and strategies toward intervention. *Dialogues in Clinical Neuroscience, 11*(2), 111-128.

Raaphorst, J., Grupstra, H. F., Linssen, W. H. J., et al. (2010). Amyotrophic lateral sclerosis en frontotemporal dementia: Overlapping characteristics. *Nederlands Tijdschrift voor Geneeskunde, 154*(1), A631.

Rabinowitz, J., Katz, I. R., DeDeyn, P. P., et al. (2004). Behavioral and psychological symptoms in patients with dementia as a target for pharmacotherapy with risperidone. *Clinical Psychiatry, 65,* 1329-1334.

Rabins, P. V. (2007). Do we know enough to begin prevention interventions for dementia? *Alzheimer's and Dementia, 3*(2 Suppl 1), S56-S88.

Ramakers, I. H., Visser, P. J., Aalten, P., et al. (2007). Symptoms of preclinical dementia in general practice up to five years before dementia diagnosis. *Dementia and Geriatric Cognitive Disorders, 24,* 300-306.

Rao, V., & Lyketsos, C. G. (1998). Delusion in Alzheimer's disease: A review. *Journal of Neuropsychiatry and Clinical Neuroscience, 10,* 373-382.

Rascovsky, K., Salmon, D. P., Lipton, A. M., et al. (2005). Rate of progression differs in frontotemporal dementia and Alzheimer disease. *Neurology, 65*(3), 397-403.

Raskind, M. A., Peskind, E. R., Wessel, T., et al. (2000). Galantamine in Alzheimer's disease: A 6-month randomized, placebo-controlled trial with a 6-month extension. The Galantamine USA-1 Study Group. *Neurology, 54,* 2261-2268.

Ravaglia, G., Forti, P., Maioli, F., et al. (2006). Conversion of mild cognitive impairment to dementia: Predictive role of mild cognitive impairment subtypes and vascular risk factors. *Dementia and Geriatric Cognitive Disorders, 21,* 51-58.

Rea, T. D., Breitner, J. C., Psaty, B. M., et al. (2005). Statin use and the risk of incident dementia: The Cardiovascular Health Study. *Archives of Neurology, 62,* 1047-1051.

Redeling, M. D., Lee, N. E., & Sorvillo, F. (2005). Pressure ulcer: More lethal than we thought? *Advanced Skin Wound Care, 18,* 367-372.

Reisberg, B., Borenstein, J., Salob, S. P., et al. (1987). Behavioral symptoms in Alzheimer's disease: Phenomenology and treatment. *Journal of Clinical Psychiatry, 48*(Suppl), 9-15.

Reisberg, B., Doody, R., Stoffler, A., et al. (2003). Memantine in moderate-to-severe Alzheimer's disease. *The New England Journal of Medicine, 348*(14), 1333-1341.

Reistad-Long, S. (2008, May 20). Older brain really may be a wiser brain. *New York Times.* Retrieved from http://www.nytimes.com/2008/05/20/health/research/20brai.html?incamp=article_popular

Reitz, C., den Heijer, T., van Duijn, C., et al. (2007). Relation between smoking and risks of dementia and Alzheimer disease: The Rotterdam Study. *Neurology, 69,* 988-1005.

Reyes, P. F., & Shi, J. (2006). Dementias: Etiologies and differential diagnoses. *Barrow Quarterly, 22*(1), *4-22.*

Rippon, G. A., & Marder, K. S. (2005). Dementia in Parkinson's disease. *Advanced Neurology, 96,* 95-113.

Roberts, G. W., Allsop, D., & Bruton, C. (1990). The occult aftermath of boxing. *Journal of Neurology, Neurosurgery and Psychiatry, 53,* 373-378.

Rogaeva, E., Meng, Y., Lee, J. H., et al. (2007). The neuronal sortilin-related receptor SORL1 is genetically associated with Alzheimer disease. *Nature Genetics, 39,* 168-177.

Roman, G. C., Salloway, S., Black, S. E., et al. (2010). Randomized, placebo-controlled, clinical trial of donepezil in vascular dementia. *Stroke, 41,* 1213-1221.

Roose, S. P., Pollock, B. G., & Devanand, D. P. (2009). Treatment during late life. In A. F. Schatzberg & C. B. Nemeroff (Eds.), *The American psychiatric publishing textbook of psychopharmacology* (4th ed.) (pp. 1430-1440). Washington, DC: American Psychiatric Publishing, Inc.

Rosness, A., Haugen, P. K., Passant, U., et al. (2008). Frontotemporal dementia—a clinically complex diagnosis. *International Journal of Geriatric Psychiatry, 23,* 837-842.

Rosenberg, R. N. (2004). The molecular and genetic basis of Alzheimer's disease. In M. F. Weiner & A. M. Lipton (Eds.), *The American psychiatric publishing textbook of Alzheimer disease and other dementias* (pp. 423-433). Washington, DC: American Psychiatric Publishing, Inc.

Rosness, A., Haugen, P. K., Passant, U., et al. (2008). Frontotemporal dementia—a clinically complex diagnosis. *International Journal of Geriatric Psychiatry, 23,* 837-842.

Rosso, S. M., Kaat, L. D., Baks, T., et al. (2003a). Frontotemporal dementia in The Netherlands: Patient characteristics and prevalence estimates from a population-based study. *Brain, 126,* 2016-2022.

Rosso, S. M., Landweer, E. J., Houterman, M., et al. (2003b). Medical and environmental risk factors for sporadic frontotemporal dementia: A retrospective case-control study. *Journal of Neurology, Neurosurgery, and Psychiatry, 74,* 1574-1576.

Roth, D. L., Mittelman, M. S., Clay, O. J., et al. (2005). Changes in social support as mediators of the impact of a psychosocial intervention for spouse caregivers of persons with Alzheimer's disease. *Psychological Aging, 20,* 634-644.

Roth, R. M., Flashman, L. A., & McAllister, T. W. (2007). Apathy and its treatment. *Current Treatment Options in Neurology, 9,* 363-370.

Rovio, S., Kareholt, I., Helkala, E. L., et al. (2005). Leisure-time physical activity at midlife and risk of dementia and Alzheimer's disease. *Lancet Neurology, 4,* 705-710.

Royall, D. R., Mulroy, A. R., Chiodo, L. K., et al. (1999). Clock drawing is sensitive to executive control: A comparison of six methods. *The Journals of Gerontology. Series B, Psychological Science and Social Science, 54*(5), 328-333.

Rush, A. J., First, M. B., & Blacker, D. (2008). *Handbook of psychiatric measures* (2nd ed.). Washington, DC: American Psychiatric Publishing, Inc.

Saczynski, J. S., Pfeifer, L. A., Masaki, K., et al. (2006). The effect of social engagement on incident dementia: The Honolulu-Asia Aging Study. *American Journal of Epidemiology, 163,* 433-440.

Salzman, C., & Tariot, P. N. (2009). Treatment of agitation and aggression in the elderly. In A. F. Schatzberg & C. B. Nemeroff (Eds.), *The American psychiatric publishing textbook of psychopharmacology* (4th ed.) (pp. 1201-1211). Washington, DC: American Psychiatric Publishing, Inc.

Sampson, E. L., Warren, J. D., & Rossor, M. N. (2004). Young onset dementia. *Postgraduate Medicine Journal, 80,* 125-139.

Samuels, S. C., & Evers, M. M. (2002). Delirium: Pragmatic guidance for managing a common, confounding, and sometimes lethal condition. *Geriatrics, 57*(6), 33-38.

Santoro, A., Siviero, P., Minicuci, N., et al. (2010). Effects of donepezil, galantamine and rivastigmine in 938 Italian patients with Alzheimer's disease: A prospective, observational study. *CNS Drugs, 24*(2), 163-176.

Savva, G. M., & Brayne, C. (2009). Epidemiology and impact of dementia. In M. F. Weiner & A. M. Lipton (Eds.), *The American psychiatric publishing textbook of Alzheimer disease and other dementias* (pp. 17-35). Washington, DC : American Psychiatric Publishing, Inc.

Saykin, A. J., Wishart, H. A., Rabin, L. A., et al. (2004). Cholinergic enhancement of frontal lobe activity in mild cognitive impairment. *Brain, 127*(Pt 7), 1574-1583.

Scarmeas, N., Levy, G., Tang, M-X., et al. (2001). Influence of leisure activity on the incidence of Alzheimer's disease. *Neurology, 57,* 2236-2242.

Scarmeas, N., Stern, Y., Tang, M-X., et al. (2006). Mediterranean diet and risk for Alzheimer's disease. *Annals of Neurology, 59,* 912-921.

Schneider, J. A., Arvanitakis, Z., Bang, W., et al. (2007). Mixed brain pathologies account for most dementia cases in community-dwelling older persons. *Neurology, 69*(24), 2197-2204.

Schneider, L. S., Dagerman, K. S., & Insel, P. (2005). Risk of death with atypical antipsychotic drug treatment for dementia: Meta-analysis of randomized placebo-controlled trials. *Journal of the American Medical Association, 294*(15), 1934-1943.

Schneider, L. S., Dagerman, K., & Insel, P. S. (2006b). Efficacy and adverse effects of atypical antipsychotics for dementia: Meta-analysis of randomized, placebo-controlled trials. *American Journal of Geriatric Psychiatry, 14*(3), 191-210.

Schneider, L. S., Tariot, P. N., Dagerman, K. S., et al.; CATIE-AD Study Group. (2006c). Effectiveness of atypical antipsychotic drugs in patients with Alzheimer's disease. *The New England Journal of Medicine, 355*(15), 1525-1538.

Schofield, I. (1997). A small exploratory study of the reaction of older people to an episode of delirium. *Journal of Advanced Nursing, 25,* 942-952.

Scholzel-Dorenbos, C. J., Meeuwsen, E. J., & Olde Rikkert, M. G. (2010). Integrating unmet needs into dementia health-related quality of life research and care: Introduction of the Hierarchy Model of Needs in Dementia. *Aging & Mental Health, 14*(1), 113-119.

Schubert, C. C., Boustani, M., Callahan, C. M., et al. (2006). Comorbidity profile of dementia patients in primary care: Are they sicker? *Journal of American Geriatric Society, 54,* 104-109.

Schulz, D., Kopp, B., Kunkel, A., et al. (2006). Cognition in the early stages of multiple sclerosis. *Journal of Neurology, 253,* 1002-1010.

Schulz, R., Boerner, K., Shear, K., et al. (2006). Predictors of complicated grief among dementia caregivers: A prospective study of bereavement. *American Journal of Geriatric Psychiatry, 14,* 650-658.

Schulz, R., & Martire, L. M. (2004). Family care-giving of persons with dementia: Prevalence, health effects, and support. *American Journal of Geriatric Psychiatry, 12,* 240-249.

Seltzer, B. (2007). Is long-term treatment of Alzheimer's disease with cholinesterase inhibitors justified? *Drugs & Aging, 24,* 881-890.

Seltzer, B. (2010). Galantamine-ER for the treatment of mild-to-moderate Alzheimer's disease. *Clinical Interventions in Aging, 5,* 1-6.

Sensonics, Inc. (n.d.). *The Pocket Smell Test.* Haddon Heights, NJ: Sensonics, Inc.

Serwach, J. (2008, April 28). Brain-training to improve memory boosts fluid intelligence. *Michigan Today.* Retrieved from http://michigantoday.umich.edu/2008/05/memoryphp?tr=y&ouid=3689376

Shigeta, H., Yasui, A., Nimura, Y., et al. (2001). Postoperative delirium and melatonin levels in elderly patients. *American Journal of Surgery, 182*(5), 449-454.

Shub, D., Darvishi, R., & Kunik, M. E. (2009). Non-pharmacologic treatment of insomnia in persons with dementia. *Geriatrics, 64*(2), 22-26.

Shulman, K. L. (2000). Clock-drawing: Is it the ideal cognitive screen test? *International Journal of Geriatric Psychiatry, 15,* 548-561.

Simard, M. (2007). *The end-of-life Namaste care program for people with dementia.* Baltimore, MD: Health Professions Press.

Simard, M., & van Reekum, R. (2004). The acetylcholinesterase inhibitors for treatment of cognitive and behavioral symptoms in dementia with Lewy bodies. *Journal of Neuropsychiatry and Clinical Neuroscience, 16,* 409-425.

Sink, K. M., Holden, K. F., & Yaffe, K. (2005). Pharmacological treatment of neuropsychiatric symptoms of dementia: A review of the evidence. *Journal of the American Medical Association, 293,* 596-608.

Sloane, P. D., Williams, C. S., & Mitchell, M. (2007). High-intensity environmental light on dementia: Effect on sleep and activity. *Journal of the American Geriatrics Society, 55,* 1524-1533.

Small, B. J., Rosnick, C. B., Fratiglioni, L., et al. (2004). Apolipoprotein E and cognitive performance: A meta-analysis. *Psychology & Aging, 19*(4), 592-600.

Smith, J. D. (2000). Apolipoprotein E4: An allele associated with many diseases. *Annals of Medicine, 32,* 118-127.

Smith, M., Samus, Q. M., Steele, C., et al. (2008). Anxiety symptoms among assisted living residents: Implications of the "no difference" finding for participants with dementia. *Research in Gerontological Nursing, 1*(2), 97-104.

Smith, M., Hall, G., Gerdner, L., et al. (2006). Application of the progressively lowered stress threshold model across the continuum of care. *Nursing Clinics of North America, 41*(1), 57-81.

Smith, M., Kolanowski, A., Buettner, L., et al. (2009). Beyond bingo: Meaningful activities for persons with dementia in nursing homes. *Annals of Long-term Care,* July, 22-30

Smoller, J. W., Sheidley, B. R., & Tsuang, M. T. (2008). *Psychiatric genetics; Applications in clinical practice.* Washington, DC: American Psychiatric Publishing, Inc.

Sorrell, J. M. (2008). Remembering: Forget about forgetting and train your brain instead. *Journal of Psychosocial Nursing, 46*(9), 25-27.

Sortland, O., & Tysvaer, A. T. (1989). Brain damage in former association football players. An evaluation by cerebral computed tomography. *Neuroradiology, 31*(1), 44-48.

Spar, J. E., & LaRue, A. (2006). *Clinical manual of geriatric psychiatry.* Washington, DC: American Psychiatric Publishing, Inc.

Starkstein, S. E., & Jorge, R. (2005). Dementia after traumatic brain injury. *International Psychogeriatrics, 17*(Suppl 1), S93-S107.

Steinberg, M., & Lyketsos, C. G. (2009). Psychiatric disorders in people with dementia. In M. F. Weiner & A. M. Lipton (Eds.), *The American psychiatric publishing textbook of Alzheimer disease and other dementias* (pp. 263-281). Washington, DC: American Psychiatric Publishing, Inc.

Suh, G. H., Son, H. G., Ju, Y. S., et al. (2006). Comparative efficacy of risperidone versus haloperidol on behavioural and psychological symptoms of dementia. *International Journal of Geriatric Psychiatry, 21,* 654-660.

Swanberg, M. M., & Cummings, J. L. (2002). Benefit-risk considerations in the treatment of dementia with Lewy bodies. *Drug Safety, 25,* 511-523.

Swearer, J. (1994). Behavioral disturbances in dementia. In J. C. Morris (Ed.), *Handbook of dementing illnesses.* New York: Marcel Dekker Inc.

Szoeke, C. E., Campbell, S., Chiu, E., et al. (2009). Vascular cognitive disorder. In M. F. Weiner & A. M. Lipton (Eds.), *The American psychiatric publishing textbook of Alzheimer disease and other dementias* (pp. 181-193). Washington, DC: American Psychiatric Publishing, Inc.

Tabert, M. H., Liu, X., Doty, R. L., et al. (2005). A 10-item smell identification scale related to risk for Alzheimer's disease. *Annals of Neurology, 58,* 155-160.

Tabert, M. H., Manley, J. J., Liu, X., et al. (2006). Neuropsychological prediction of conversion to Alzheimer disease in patients with mild cognitive impairment. *Archives of General Psychiatry, 63,* 916-924.

Tanios, M. A., Epstein, S. K., & Teres, D. (2004). Are we ready to monitor for delirium in the intensive care unit? *Critical Care Medicine, 32*(1), 295-296.

Tanzi, R. E., Kovacs, D. M., & Kim, T. W. (1996). The gene defects responsible for familial Alzheimer's disease. *Neurobiological Disorders, 3,* 159-168.

Tarawneh, R., & Galvin, J. E. (2009). Dementia with Lewy Bodies and other synucleinopathies. In M. F. Weiner & A. M. Lipton (Eds.), *The American psychiatric publishing textbook of Alzheimer disease and other dementias* (pp. 195-217). Washington, DC: American Psychiatric Publishing, Inc.

Tariq, S. H., Tumosa, N., Chibnall, J. T., et al. (2006). Comparison of the Saint Louis University Mental Status Examination and the Mini-Mental State Examination for detecting dementia and mild neurocognitive disorder—A pilot study. *American Journal of Geriatric Psychiatry, 14*(11), 900-910.

Teri, L., Gibbons, L. E., McCurry, S. M., et al. (2003). Exercise plus behavioral management in patients with Alzheimer disease. *Journal of the American Medical Association, 290*(15), 2015-2022.

Teri, L., Logsdon, R. G., Peskind, E., et al. (2000). Treatment of agitation in Alzheimer's disease: A randomized, placebo-controlled clinical trial. *Neurology, 52,* 1271-1278.

Thomas, F. P., & Roos, K. L. (2010). Variant Creutzfeldt-Jakob disease and bovine spongiform encephalopathy. *Medscape Drugs, Disease and Procedures.* Retrieved from Emedicine.medscape.com/article/1169688-overview. Retrieved July 27, 2011.

Tractenberg, R. E., Weiner, M. F., & Patterson, M. B. (2002). Emergent psychopathology in Alzheimer's disease patients over 12 months associated with functional, not cognitive, changes. *Journal of Geriatric Psychiatry and Neurology, 15*(2), 110-117.

Tractenberg, R. E., Weiner, M. F., & Thal, L. J. (2002). Estimating prevalence of agitation and behavioral disturbance in community dwelling person with Alzheimer's disease. *Journal of Neuropsychiatry and Clinical Neuroscience, 14,* 11-18.

Trzepacz, P. T., Baker, R. W., & Greenhouse, J. (1988). A symptom rating scale for delirium. *Psychiatry Research, 23*(1), 89-97.

Trzepacz, P., Breitbart, W., Franklin, J., et al. (2006). Practice guideline for the treatment of patients with delirium. In American Psychiatric Association (Ed.), *American psychiatric association practice guidelines for the treatment of psychiatric disorders: Compendium 2006* (pp. 65-100). Washington, DC: American Psychiatric Publishing, Inc.

Trzepacz, P. T., & Meagher, D. J. (2010). Neuropsychiatric aspects of delirium. In S. C. Yudofsky & R. E. Hales (Eds.), *Essential of neuropsychiatry and behavioral neurosciences* (2nd ed.) (pp. 149-221). Washington, DC: American Psychiatric Publishing, Inc.

Tsuang, D. W., & Bird, T. D. (2002). Genetics of dementia. *Medical Clinics of North America, 86*(3), 591-614.

Tuokko, H., Hadjistavropoulos, T., Miller, J. A., et al. (1995). The clock test: A sensitive measure to differentiate normal elderly from those with Alzheimer disease. *Journal of American Geriatric Society, 40*, 584.

Valenzuela, M. J. (2008). Brain reserve and the prevention of dementia. *Current Opinion in Psychiatry, 21*, 296-302.

Valenzuela, M. J., Breakspear, M., & Sachdev, P. (2007). Complex mental activity and the aging brain: Molecular, cellular, and cortical network mechanisms. *Brain Research Reviews, 56*, 198-213.

Valenzuela, M. J., & Sachdev, P. (2006). Brain reserve and dementia: A systematic review. *Psychological Medicine, 36*, 441-454.

Van Munster, B. C., Korevaar, J. C., Zwinderman, A. H., et al. (2009). The association between delirium and the Apolipoprotein E Epsilon 4 allele: New study results and a meta-analysis. *American Journal of Geriatric Psychiatry, 17*, 856-862.

Vecchierini, M. F. (2010). Sleep disturbances in Alzheimer's disease and other dementias. *Psychology & Neuropsychiatrie du Viellissement, 8*(2), 15-23.

Verghese, J., Lipton, R. B., Katz, M. J., et al. (2003). Leisure activities and the risk of dementia in the elderly. *The New England Journal of Medicine, 348*, 2508-2526.

Vidan, M. T., Sanchez, E., Alonso, M., et al. (2009). An intervention integrated into daily clinical practice reduces the incidence of delirium during hospitalization in elderly patients. *Journal of American Geriatric Society, 57*, 2029-2036.

Vitiello, M. V., & Borson, S. (2001). Sleep disturbances in patients with Alzheimer's disease. *CNS Drugs, 25*(10), 777-796.

Volicer, L. (2007). Goals of care in advanced dementia: Quality of life, dignity and comfort. *Journal of Nutrition, Health & Aging, 11*(6), 481.

Volicer, L., Harper, D. G., Manning, B. C., et al. (2001). Sundowning and circadian rhythms in Alzheimer's disease. *American Journal of Psychiatry, 158*, 704-711.

Volicer, L., Lane, P., Panke, J., et al. (2005). Management of constipation in residents with dementia: Sorbitol effectiveness and cost. *Journal of the American Medical Directors Association, 6*(Suppl 3), S32-S34.

Volicer, L., & Simard, J. (2009). Management of advanced dementia. In M. F. Weiner & M. Lipton (Eds.), *The American psychiatric publishing textbook of Alzheimer disease and other dementias* (pp. 333-349). Washington, DC: American Psychiatric Publishing, Inc.

Wagner, C., Popp, W., Posch, M., et al. (2003). Impact of pneumococcal vaccination on morbidity and mortality of geriatric patients: A case-control study. *Gerontology, 49*, 246-250.

Walker, M. P., Ayre, G. A., Cummings, J. L., et al. (2000). The clinician assessment of fluctuation and the one day fluctuation assessment scale. *British Journal of Psychiatry, 177*, 252-256.

Walker, Z., Allen, R. I., Shergill, S., et al. (2000). Three years survival in patients with a clinical diagnosis of dementia with Lewy bodies. *International Journal of Geriatric Psychiatry, 15*, 267-273.

Wang, H-X., Karp, A., Winblad, B., et al. (2002). Late-life engagement in social and leisure activities is associated with a decreased risk of dementia: A longitudinal study from the Kungsholmen Project. *American Journal of Epidemiology, 155*(12), 1081-1087.

Warner, M., & Warner, E. (1996). *The caregiver's guide to home modification.* Retrieved from http://www.ec-online.net/knowledge/articles/homemodify.html Retrieved 6/12/2010.online.net

Warshaw, G., & Mechlin, M. (2009). Prevention and management of postoperative delirium. *International Anesthesiology Clinics, 47*(4), 137-149.

Waszynski, C. M. (2007). Detecting delirium. *American Journal of Nursing, 107*(12), 50-59.

Weigel, M. B., Purselle, D. C., D'Orio, B. (2009). Treatment of psychiatric emergencies. In A. F. Schatzberg & C. B. Nemeroff (Eds.), *The American psychiatric publishing textbook of psychopharmacology* (4th ed.) (pp. 1287-1308). Washington: DC: American Psychiatric Publishing, Inc.

Weih, M., Wiltfang, J., & Kornhuber, J. (2007). Non-pharmacologic prevention of Alzheimer's disease: Nutritional and life-style risk factors. *Journal of Neural Transmission, 114*, 1187-1197.

Weiner, M. F. (2009). Dementia and Alzheimer disease: Ancient Greek medicine to modern molecular biology. In M. F. Weiner & A. M. Lipton (Eds.), *The American psychiatric publishing textbook of Alzheimer disease and other dementias* (pp. 3-16). Washington, DC: American Psychiatric Publishing, Inc.

Weiner, M. F., Garrett, R., & Bret, M. E. (2009). Neuropsychiatric assessment and diagnosis. In M. F. Weiner & A. M. Lipton (Eds.), *The American psychiatric publishing textbook of Alzheimer disease and other dementias* (pp. 39-70). Washington, DC: American Psychiatric Publishing, Inc.

Weinhouse, G. L., Schwab, R. J., Watson, P. L., et al. (2009). Bench-to-bedside review: Delirium in ICU patients-importance of sleep deprivation. *Critical Care, 13*(6), 234.

Wentzel, C., Rockwood, K., McKnight, C., et al. (2001). Progression of impairment in patients with vascular cognitive impairment without dementia. *Neurology, 57*, 714-716.

Werner, P., Stein-Shvachman, I., & Korczyn, A. D. (2009). Early onset dementia: Clinical and social aspects. *International Psychogeriatrics, 21*(4), 631-636.

Wesnes, K., McKeith, I., Ferrara, R., et al. (2002). Effects of rivastigmine on cognitive function in dementia with Lewy bodies: A randomized placebo-controlled international study using the cognitive drug research computerized assessment system. *Dementia and Geriatric Cognitive Disorders, 13*, 183-192.

Weuve, J., Kang, J. H., Manson, J. E., et al. (2004). Physical activity, including walking, and cognitive function in older women. *Journal of the American Medical Association, 292*, 1454-1461.

Whitaker, R. A., Sidney, S., Selby, J., et al. (2005). Midlife cardiovascular risk factors and risk of dementia in late life. *Neurology, 64*(2), 277-281.

Whitmer, R. A., Gunderson, E. P., Quesenberry, C. P., Jr., et al. (2007). Body mass index in midlife and risk of Alzheimer disease and vascular dementia. *Current Alzheimer Research, 4*, 103-109.

Williamson, J. D., Espeland, M., Kritchevsky, S. B., et al. (2009). Changes in cognitive function in a randomized trial of physical activity: Results of the lifestyle interventions and independence for elders pilot study. *The Journals of Gerontology. Series A, Biological Sciences and Medical Sciences, 64*(6), 688-694.

Willis, S. L., Tennstedt, S. L., Marsiske, M., et al. (2006). Long-term effects of cognitive training on everyday functional outcomes in older adults. *Journal of the American Medical Association, 296*, 2805-2814.

Wilson, R. S., Arnold, S. E., Schneider, J. A., et al. (2007a). Chronic distress, age-related neuropathology, and late-life dementia. *Psychosomatic Medicine, 69*, 47-53.

Wilson, R. S., Arnold, S. E., & Schneider, J. A. (2009). Olfactory impairment in presymptomatic Alzheimer's disease. *Annals of the New York Academy of Sciences, 1170*, 730-735.

Wilson, R. S., Bennett, D. A., Mendes de Leon, C. F., et al. (2005). Distress proneness and cognitive decline in a population of older persons. *Psychoneuroendocrinology, 30*, 11-17.

Wilson, R. S., Krueger, K. R., Arnold, S. E., et al. (2007b). Loneliness and risk of Alzheimer disease. *Archives of General Psychiatry, 64*, 234-240.

Wilson, R. S., Mendes de Leon, C. F., Barnes, L. L., et al. (2002). Participation in cognitively stimulating activities and risk of incident Alzheimer Disease. *Journal of the American Medical Association, 287*, 742-748.

Wilson, R. S., Scherr, P. A., Schneider, J. A., et al. (2007c). Relation of cognitive activity to risk of developing Alzheimer disease. *Neurology, 69*(20), 1911-1920.

Wilson, R. S., Schneider, J. A., Boyle, P. A., et al. (2007d). Chronic distress and incidence of mild cognitive impairment. *Neurology, 68*(24), 2085-2092.

Winblad, B., Black, S. E., Homma, A., et al. (2009). Donepezil treatment in severe Alzheimer's disease: A pooled analysis of three clinical trials. *Current Medical Research & Opinion, 25*(11), 2577-2587.

Winblad, B., Palmer, K., Kivipelto, M., et al. (2004). Mild cognitive impairment—beyond controversies, towards a consensus: Report of the

International Working Group on mild cognitive impairment. *Journal of Internal Medicine, 256,* 24-246.

Winblad, B., Wimo, A., Engedal, K., et al. (2006). 3-Year Study of donepezil therapy in Alzheimer's disease: Effects of early and continuous therapy. *Dementia and Geriatric Cognitive Disorders, 21,* 353-363.

Wood, S., Cummings. J. L., Hsu, M. A., et al. (2000). The use of the neuropsychiatric inventory in nursing home residents: Characterization and measurement. *American Geriatric Psychiatry, 8,* 75-83.

Woodruff, B. K., Graff-Radford, N. R., Ferman, T. J., et al. (2006). Family history of dementia is a risk factor for Lewy body disease. *Neurology, 66,* 1949-1950.

Xu, W. L., Qiu, C. X., Winblad, B., et al. (2007). The effect of borderline diabetes mellitus on the risk of dementia and Alzheimer's disease. *Diabetes, 56,* 211-216.

Yaari, R., Tariot, P. N., & Richards, D. (2009). Pharmacological treatment of neuropsychiatric symptoms. In M. F. Weiner & A. M. Lipton (Eds.), *The American psychiatric publishing textbook of Alzheimer disease and other dementias* (pp. 285-300). Washington, DC: American Psychiatric Publishing, Inc.

Yaffe, K., Blackwell, T., Gore, R., et al. (1999). Depressive symptoms and cognitive decline in non-demented elderly women: A prospective study. *Archives of General Psychiatry, 56,* 435-440.

Yaffe, K., Fiocco, A. J., Lindquist, K., et al. (2009). Predictors of maintaining cognitive function in older adults: The Health ABC Study. *Neurology, 72,* 2029-2035.

Yang, F. M., Marcantonio, E. R., Inouye, S. K., et al. (2009). Phenomenological subtypes of delirium in older persons: Patterns, prevalence, and prognosis. *Psychosomatics, 50*(3), 248-254.

Yao, L., & Algase, D. (2006). Environmental ambiance as a new window on wandering. *Western Journal of Nursing Research, 28*(1), 89-104.

Yoneyama, T., Yoshida, M., Ohrui, T., et al. (2002). Oral care reduces pneumonia in older patients in nursing homes. *Journal of American Geriatric Society, 50,* 430-433.

Yuhas, N., McGowan, B., Fontaine, T., et al. (2006). Psychosocial interventions for disruptive symptoms of dementia. *Journal of Psychosocial Nursing and Mental Health Services, 44*(11), 34-42.

Zaccai, J., McCracken, C., & Brayne, C. (2005). A systematic review of prevalence and incidence studies of dementia with Lewy bodies. *Age and Ageing, 34,* 562-566.

Zamrini, E., & Quiceno, M. (2009). Other causes of dementia. In M. F. Weiner & A. M. Lipton (Eds.), *The American psychiatric publishing textbook of Alzheimer disease and other dementias* (pp. 247-262). Washington, DC: American Psychiatric Publishing, Inc.

Zhang, Y. J., Xu, Y. F., Dickey, C. A., et al. (2007). Progranulin mediates caspase-dependent cleavage of TAR DNA binding protein-43. *Journal of Neuroscience, 27,* 10530-10534.

Zubenko, G. S., Zubenko, W. N., McPherson, S., et al. (2003). A collaborative study of the emergence and clinical features of the major depressive syndrome of Alzheimer's disease. *American Journal of Psychiatry, 160*(5), 857-866.

Answers to Case Study 16-1 Questions

1. Factors that increased Mrs. Keen's risk for developing delirium included advanced age, hearing deficit, lack of orientation to time, pain, sleep disturbance, limited mobility, possible head trauma related to a fall, and lack of family support.
2. Interventions that might be used to prevent another episode of delirium include preventing dehydration, promoting sleep with sleep hygiene strategies, reorienting the patient to place, time, and situation several times during the day, encouraging mobilization, limiting the number of medications, and enlisting the Parish nurse's help in arranging for a known person to sit with the patient during her recovery.

UNIT VII

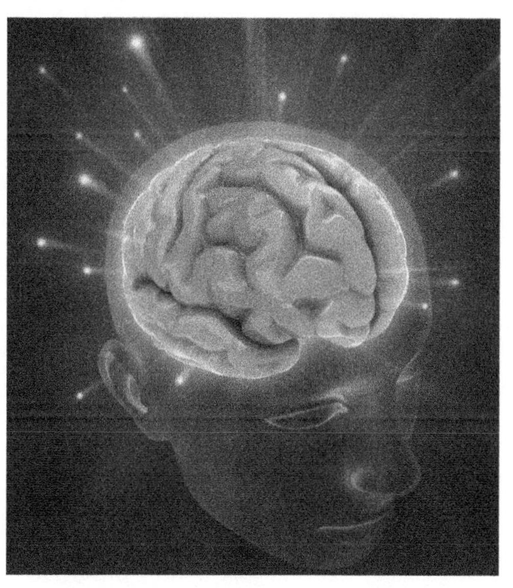

Psychiatric Disorders: Co-occurring Substance Use and Psychiatric Disorders

CHAPTER 17

Co-occurring Substance Use and Psychiatric Disorders

Kathleen A. H. Vertino, MSN, RN, PMHNP-BC, CARN-AP

One of the most challenging clinical situations that will confront the psychiatric advanced practice nurse is caring for the complex needs of an individual with co-occurring disorders (CODs). While the literature addressing "dual diagnosis" is voluminous, it is marred by a lack of standardized terminology (Sims, Woods, & Guppy, 2001). Further, with adoption of the recovery model by many behavioral health organizations, previously used terms such as *dually diagnosed, dually disordered, doubly troubled, dually recovering, MICA (mentally ill chemical abuser)*, and *MISA (mentally ill substance abuser)* that focus on illness are now considered derogatory and inappropriate.

When terms are unclearly defined, not standardized, and used interchangeably, studies will fail to capture an accurate epidemiological picture, which could cause misappropriation of funds and encouragement of treatment silos (Fornili & Baird, 2008). Compounding the problem, statistics on the scope of CODs vary, and the best methods to capture quantitative and qualitative data regarding treatment fidelity (Bellg, Borrelli, Resnick, et al., 2004) and treatment/recovery outcomes have been debated. Hence, in order to provide the best patient-centered care possible, practitioners must remain cognizant of the complexity of individuals with COD and of the diversity of subpopulations with COD. Because study terminology and foci vary, practitioners should scrutinize and integrate recommended evidence-based practice changes into the plan of care only after careful analysis of the research.

It is equally concerning that the literature reports that individuals with CODs frequently fall through the cracks of the health-care system. Studies indicate that health-care providers are not screening, diagnosing, and addressing the aforementioned problems—that diagnoses are frequently overlooked, patients are misdiagnosed, or providers have failed to document potential risks as part of routine assessments (Breakey, Calabrese, Rosenblatt, et al., 1998; Monroe, Levy, & McQuade, 1997). For example, an earlier study retrospectively reviewed records of 200 hospitalized psychiatric patients to assess whether substance abuse was being adequately identified and treated. Approximately 43% of patients admitted had a substance abuse history, but only about 33% had any documentation of this, and 50% of the patients had received no treatment for substance abuse (Milling, Faulkner, & Craig, 1994). More recently, Manning, Strathdee, Best, et al. (2002) compared patients receiving community mental health treatment services with patients receiving treatment for substance misuse. Results indicated that when mental health clients were screened, approximately 64% were positive for dual diagnosis, and in the same group, approximately 92% were positive for alcohol use and 87% were positive for drug use. Among those receiving substance abuse services, 38% were positive for mental health symptoms.

Figure 17-1 depicts treatment of adults ages 18 or older with "serious psychological distress and a substance use disorder in 2005," as reported by the Substance Abuse and Mental Health Services Administration (2006). In brief: 4.1% participated in substance use treatment only; 34.3% participated in mental health treatment only; 8.5% participated in treatment for both mental health and substance use problems; and 53% *received no treatment*, suggesting that providers have failed to identify and address CODs adequately. Magura, Rosenblum, & Betzler (2009) believed that in psychiatric day treatment programs, "virtually all patients may be at risk (for relapse)..." and that "typical clinical interviews identified *only a fraction* of the patients with drug use at admission [italics added]" (p. 6).

The literature addressing various aspects and problems in the development of treatment and recovery programs for individuals with COD has burgeoned in the last decade; thus, this chapter cannot encompass a full review of all published sources. Rather, it is a focused review covering many aspects of caring for individuals with COD and addresses some

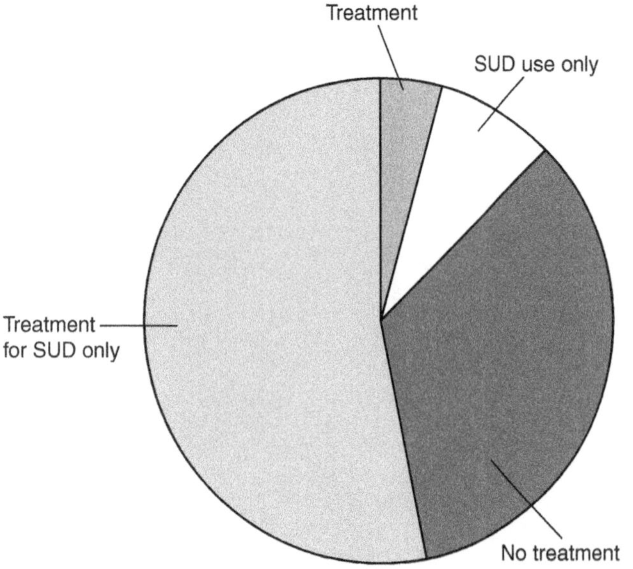

Treatment
SUD use only
Treatment for SUD only
No treatment

FIGURE 17-1: 5.2 Million Adults With Co-Occurring Serious Psychological Distress and Substance Use Disorder. Source: Substance Abuse and Mental Health Services Administration. (2006). *Results from the 2005 national survey on drug use and health: National findings.* Office of Applied Studies, NSDUH Series H-30, DHHS Publication No. SMA 06-4194. Rockville, MD: Substance Abuse and Mental Health Services Administration. Retrieved from http://www.oas.samhsa.gov/nsduh/2k5nsduh/2k5Results.pdf

specific, pragmatic implementation problems encountered in clinical practice settings and health-care delivery systems. It emphasizes implementation of evidence-based treatment for individuals diagnosed with COD (Miller, 2006; Willenbring, Kivlahan, Kenny, et al., 2004). Because much research is devoted either (1) to evidence-based treatment of substance use disorders (SUD) and substance related disorders (SRD) or (2) to evidence-based treatment of psychiatric disorders but not COD, the primary aim of this discussion is focused on literature that describes specific issues related to caring for individuals who are diagnosed with COD.

Definition of Co-occurring Disorder

An individual is diagnosed with a COD when one or more psychiatric diagnoses coexist or co-occur (are comorbid) with one or more substance abuse or substance dependence disorders. Specifically, COD is present "...when at least one disorder of each type can be established independent of the other and is not simply a cluster of symptoms resulting from the one disorder" (Center for Substance Abuse Treatment, 2007a, p. 3). Many individuals are cross-addicted (dependent on two substances in the last 12 months) or poly-addicted (dependent on three or more substances) and may have more than one psychiatric diagnosis (American Psychiatric Association, 2000). The clinical picture is further complicated when there is a coexisting Axis II diagnosis, such as personality disorder or mental retardation, or a psychiatric disorder that is the result of an Axis III general medical condition such as traumatic brain injury (TBI).

Economic and Health-care System Resource Considerations

Costs reported by the U.S. Department of Health and Human Services and National Institute on Drug Abuse (NIDA) approximate $110 billion annually for substance abuse or dependence treatment alone. The National Institute on Alcohol Abuse and Alcoholism (NIAAA) reported a $184.6 billion expenditure for alcohol abuse or dependence treatment in 1998, with an expected incidental growth of 3.8% per year (Harwood, 2000; Harwood, Fountain, & Livermore, 1998).

Indirect costs related to substance or alcohol abuse or addiction—such as medical or psychiatric care for victims of sexual assault and domestic violence, legal or court fees, incarceration, forensic services, or costs of marital or family therapy—largely go unmeasured. Occupational costs to employers for sick time, work-related accidents, compensation, disability, and the provision of employee assistance programs can be burdensome. Federal and state tax dollars cover costs of providing public assistance, welfare, food stamps, and health care to those who cannot work. A percentage of recipients of social service monies are individuals with substance-related disorders who have lost employment owing to addiction or may be additionally disabled owing to mental illness.

Finally, the presently overburdened U.S. health-care system is not producing enough new providers to keep up with current needs, and the nursing shortage in this country is now reaching a crisis point. Furthermore, the full impact of implementation of the Patient Protection and Affordable Care Act of 2010, which will require more health-care services, has not been fully realized (http://docs.house.gov/energycommerce/ppacacon.pdf). Health-care services will be scarcer, and prudent utilization will no longer be optional, but necessary. Existing programs and services must be able to demonstrate evidence-based clinical outcomes in order to remain fiscally sound and clinically viable.

Epidemiology

Prevalence

An estimated 47% to 86% of individuals diagnosed with a psychiatric disorder have an SUD. Estimates have ranged from 4.7% to 9% of the U.S. population, or between 5 and 8 million people (Brooner, King, Kidorf, et al., 1997; Center for Substance Abuse Treatment, 2007c; Hastings-Vertino, 1996; Little, 2001; Sonne & Brady, 2002; Teplin, O'Connell, Daiter, et al., 2004). The Drug and Alcohol Services Information System (DASIS) report (Substance Abuse and Mental Health Services Administration, 2004) states that admissions for COD increased from 12% in 1995 to 16% in 2001, and according to the Agency for Healthcare

Research and Quality (2004), nearly one out of four hospital stays for adults in U.S. community hospitals involved mental health substance abuse (MHSA) disorders—about 7.6 million hospitalizations. Of these, 1.9 million hospitalizations (6% of adult hospital stays) were for a principal MHSA diagnosis, and 5.7 million (18%) were primarily for non-MHSA diagnoses but had a "secondary" mental health or substance abuse diagnosis (Owens, Myers, Elixhauser, et al., 2007, p. 1).

Besides episodes of recurring psychiatric symptoms, relapse, and frequent hospitalization, individuals with COD experience quality of life issues in many life domains, including but not limited to emotional and psychological distress of everyday living, social problems, financial difficulties, complications with social service agencies, housing issues or homelessness, legal system involvement including incarceration, managing appointments with providers, transportation issues, organizing medications, and simply meeting basic needs and accessing health care.

Prevalence in Adolescents

Depressive symptoms and alcohol or drug use are strongly correlated, especially for female youths. Among "street youths"—defined as "adolescents who lived by themselves on the street" (Obando, Kliewer, Murrelle, et al., 2004, p. 39)—males have been shown to have more drug problems than females.

An estimated 62% of adolescents who are abusing substances are diagnosed with a co-occurring psychiatric condition, usually conduct disorder, and adolescents with CODs have many more service and treatment needs. Conduct disorder puts youths between the ages of 13 and 15 at risk for the later development of SUD, with as high as 11% prevalence (Grella, Joshi, & Hser, 2004; Sung, Erkanli, Angold, et al., 2004).

Boys with a history of depression are at an increased risk of developing SUD, whereas anxiety disorders put girls at an increased risk of developing SUD. According to Sung et al. (2004, p. 294), "...although onsets of most substances were less common in girls than boys, the risk of transition to SUD's by age 16 was equal once a child had begun to use any drugs." Early use seems to be a partial predictor of later SUDs in adolescents, whether or not there is a comorbid psychiatric illness (Sung et al.). The same holds true for alcoholism: *for each year* that an adolescent or young adult does not drink, he or she reduces the risk of becoming alcohol dependent by 14% (Substance Abuse and Mental Health Services, 2008). Furthermore, 15- to 21-year-olds are reported to have more severe anxiety, use more illicit drugs, and be more likely to relapse than older individuals (Farren & McElroy, 2008). Additionally, this age group is at a much greater risk of suicide than the general population, and unfortunately, despite ongoing, pressing needs, research indicates that current treatment programs remain ill-equipped and are not adequately treating adolescents with COD (Hawkins, 2009).

Prevalence in Older Adults

The Agency for Healthcare Research and Quality found that there were more mental health substance-related (MHSR) hospitalizations for older adult women than for men (Owens et al., 2007). The most frequent diagnoses for older women were mood disorders, while the most frequent diagnoses for older men were substance-related disorders. Other frequent diagnoses for which patients were hospitalized include delirium or dementia (the most common diagnosis for adults 80 years and older), anxiety disorders, and schizophrenia. In a study by Owens et al. (2007), among older adults, delirium or dementia accounted for 21% of hospital stays in the MHSA group, the top diagnostic category, while the second most common diagnosis in this group was mood disorders.

In addition to the aforementioned psychiatric disorders, approximately 17% of older adults are reported to be affected by alcohol and prescription drug misuse, and this issue is overlooked far too often by health-care providers. For example, among older adults, a positive history for psychiatric problems has been reported in 14%, and alcohol problems have been reported in 6% (Levkoff, Chen, Coakley, et al., 2004). Therefore, all elderly or older adults (adults older than 60 years) should be screened for psychiatric illness and alcohol abuse. The National Institute on Aging (2010) has made the following recommendations regarding alcohol consumption in older adults: "...individuals over age 65 have no more than *one drink per day* (which is 12 oz. beer or wine cooler, 5 oz. glass of wine, or 1.5 oz. of 80 proof spirits) as drinking at this level is usually not associated with health risks."

Alcohol use has been highly correlated with an increased risk of suicide, not only in older adults but in all age groups (Davis, Rush, Wisniewski, et al., 2005). Because of older adults' ongoing medical and nutrition problems; decreased liver, kidney, heart, and brain functioning; and numerous medications, their physical health, in addition to their risk for suicide, should be monitored especially carefully. Unmarried or widower elderly males, in particular, who are reported to have more alcohol problems than women in the same age group, are at an increased risk for suicide (Davis et al.). The National Institute of Mental Health (2010) reported that "older Americans are disproportionately likely to die by suicide." Over 70% of older suicide victims have seen their primary medical provider within 30 days prior to their death; this finding indicates that depression can be masked by or mistaken for a physical health problem and hence not properly diagnosed or treated. Contrary to what some may believe, depression is *not* a normal part of aging.

Ethnicity

Empirical evidence addressing COD in specific ethnic/racial populations is sparse and an area in need of future research. Hesselbrock, Hesselbrock, Segal, et al. (2003) reported that ethnic differences in individuals with CODs are salient among Alaskan Natives, Caucasians, African Americans, and Hispanics. There seem to be differences in the types of SUDs found in African Americans and Caucasians, but not as many differences in the types of psychiatric disorders found. For example, a significantly larger proportion of African Americans were found in drug treatment versus mental health treatment. This finding should alert providers to perform important screening, diagnostic, and treatment planning in these settings (Alvidrez & Havassy, 2005). Alcohol abuse or dependence with comorbid psychiatric disorders has a lifetime prevalence of 7.5% for Mexican-born adult males; these rates are higher for U.S.-born Mexican Americans versus those with Mexican ancestry who have immigrated to the United States (Vega, Sribney, & Achara-Abrahams, 2003). In a study with 972 school-based youths in Puerto Rico, higher severity of alcohol use and alcohol problems was more strongly correlated with higher rates of marijuana use, increased prevalence of sexual intercourse, and trouble with the law in the past year (Latimer, Rojas, & Mancha, 2008).

In 2001, the racial/ethnic distributions of admissions for individuals with COD were 74% white, 15% black, and 7% Hispanic, in comparison with all other admissions, which were 57% white, 23% black, and 15% Hispanic (Drug and Alcohol Services Information System, 2004). The National Survey on Drug Use and Health (2010) reported, "Among persons aged 12 or older, the rate of substance dependence or abuse was the lowest among Asians (3.5 percent). The rates for the other racial/ethnic groups were 15.5 percent for American Indians or Alaska Natives, 13.2 percent for persons reporting two or more races, 10.1 percent for Hispanics, 9.0 percent for whites, and 8.8 percent for blacks. These rates in 2009 were similar to the rates in 2002 through 2008."

Gender

Historically, individuals with COD were reported to be more often male, younger, less stable, unemployed, diagnosed with more than one psychiatric comorbidity or personality disorder, and more likely to lead a crisis-oriented, risky lifestyle (Virgo, Bennett, Higgins, et al., 2001). For substance dependence alone, the National Survey on Drug Use and Health (2010) reported, "As was the case from 2002 through 2008, the rate of substance dependence or abuse for males aged 12 or older in 2009 was about twice as high as the rate for females. For males in 2009, the rate was 11.9 percent, which was similar to the 11.5 percent in 2008, while for females, it was 6.1 percent in 2009, which did not differ significantly from the 6.4 percent in 2008."

Women with schizophrenia and co-occurring substance abuse were found to differ in several ways from men with CODs. Women are reported to have more children, are viewed as more socially competent, are more often victims of violence, have more medical illnesses, and are diagnosed more often with anxiety and depression than men (Brunette & Drake, 1998). Women "problem drinkers" with a history of childhood sexual abuse are more likely to have a lifelong diagnosis of depressive, anxious, or eating disorders, as well as comorbid post-traumatic stress disorder (PTSD) and borderline personality disorders. Males with COD who are considered to be alcohol dependent have more social problems. These men are more likely to be single, divorced, or widowed, be diagnosed with PTSD, and have borderline personality disorder (Martinez-Rega, Keaney, Marshall, et al., 2002).

Between 1995 and 2001, hospital admissions for females with COD increased from 38% to 44%. In 2001, females with COD represented 44% of hospital admissions as compared with a 30% admission rate of the general population (Substance Abuse and Mental Health Services Administration, Office of Applied Studies, 2004).

In 2007, Becker, Fiellen, and Desai examined data from the 2002-2004 National Survey on Drug Use and Health for the purposes of identifying demographic and clinical characteristics associated with nonmedical use of sedatives and tranquilizers in order to elucidate potential risk factors for such use. They reported overall prevalence of past-year nonmedical use of sedatives and tranquilizers to be 2.3% (N = 92,020) among women and reported that 9.8% of that group met criteria for substance abuse or dependence. Panic symptoms and scores on serious mental illness measures were elevated in those with past-year nonmedical use of the medications as well. Other variables associated with nonmedical use of these medications were female sex, criminal arrest, unemployment, lack of health insurance, alcohol abuse or dependence, cigarette use, illicit drug use, younger age when initiating illicit substance use, and history of intravenous drug use. The results of the 2009 National Survey on Drug Use and Health (2010) showed that the average rate of illicit drug use in the past month among pregnant women ages 15 to 44 years in 2008-2009 was 4.5%. Although this rate is lower than that in women who were not pregnant, rates of drug use increased among women in that age group from 9.7% in 2006-2007 to 10.6% in 2008-2009.

Women have complex treatment needs, and although they are more likely to seek help than men, they present special challenges to providers, especially when they have children. Evidence-based treatment now strongly encourages family involvement (Fornili, 2008). Further, according to social role theory, women with CODs and a history of abuse who adopt more positive, "valued" social roles have demonstrated increased self-esteem, confidence, and happiness (Stenius, Veysey, Hamilton, et al., 2005). Best practices based on expert consensus and empirical evidence recommend that programs be tailored specifically to treatment needs of women with children and that programs be trauma informed. In sum, the complex service and treatment needs of women with COD, especially those with children in the home and those with histories of abuse, are not being adequately met (Brown & Melchior, 2008; Finkelstein, Rechberger, Russell, et al., 2005; Fornili, 2008; National Abandoned Infants Assistance Resource Center, 2008; Savage & Russell, 2005).

Etiology

A number of etiological theories regarding CODs have been proposed (Mueser, Drake, & Wallach, 1998). The first set of theories attempts to answer the question, "What came first—the psychiatric illness or substance use/abuse?" The second set of theories addresses causation and includes research on childhood abuse, organic brain disorders, neurological considerations, and medical illnesses.

What Came First?

There appear to be three separate ideas regarding the "What came first?" etiology of COD:

1. Psychiatric symptoms lead to substance use or abuse.
2. Substance use or abuse leads to psychiatric symptoms.
3. Psychiatric symptoms and substance use or abuse coexist, and both are primary diagnoses.

The first idea proposes that psychiatric illness is considered the *primary diagnosis* and substance abuse is *secondary* (Kessler, 2004). These researchers believe that drugs or alcohol are used to self-medicate either symptoms that accompany psychiatric illness or side effects of psychiatric medication, such as anxiety, depression, panic, tension, racing thoughts, agitation, jumpiness, jitteriness, anger, insomnia, paranoia, sadness, irritability, suicidal thoughts, akathisia, dyskinesias, or hallucinations.

The second idea proposes that *primary* SUDs can lead to *secondary* psychiatric symptoms and thus mimic psychiatric disorders, such as in substance-induced psychoses, delirium, anxiety, and mood disorders. These substance-induced symptoms can be present during intoxication, during withdrawal, and after detoxification is completed (American Psychiatric Association, 2000; Rosenblum, Fallon, Magura, et al., 1999; Suppes & Keck, 2005).

Both the first and second etiologies require clear evidence either that a substance or medication produced the psychiatric symptoms or vice versa; this evidence can be obtained from a comprehensive evaluation that includes a reliable history, laboratory studies, and a physical or mental status examination. However, if this evidence is not present, the psychiatric advanced practice nurse must consider the third answer to the "Which came first?" question: simultaneous SUD and psychiatric illness. Commonly, the conditions co-occur or are comorbid. (Interested readers should review the article by Hastings-Vertino [1996], which discusses in detail the interactive diseases model first described by Bricker [1994]). This model purports that CODs interact and overlap, and indeed each can contribute to the course and outcome of each respective problem, singularly or in concert (Zimberg, 1999).

To complicate the clinical picture even further, the terms "dual diagnosis" and "co-occurring disorders" imply that there are *two* problems: *one* psychiatric illness and *one* substance dependence. However, in real-world clinical practice, individuals can meet diagnostic criteria for a number of problems simultaneously. For example, attention deficit-hyperactivity disorder (ADHD), bipolar disorder, opiate dependence, and alcohol dependence can all co-occur. Treatment programs for COD have historically failed, likely because treatment approaches have attempted to compartmentalize these problems instead of treating them simultaneously. If one disorder pre-dates another disorder or is considered "primary" and thus "more important," providers are tempted to treat the "primary" problem first and ignore the "secondary" problem or problems. Compartmentalization of CODs is an approach that is largely responsible for failures related to nonadherence, as individuals want to feel better *fast* and cannot wait for their "primary" problem to be treated first while their "secondary" problem hangs in abeyance. The literature reports serious access and barriers to care, such as patients' being refused admission to substance abuse programs while taking psychotropic medication and being told to come back when their other problem is under control (Drake, Essock, Carey, et al., 2001; van Wamel, Kroon, & van Roojen, 2009). Laker (2007) stated, "Current dual diagnosis policy advocates for a process of change from the old system of separate services for mental health problems and substance misuse problems to an integrated service" (p. 725).

In order to take a "multitargeted" or integrated approach and incorporate evidenced-based modalities into practice, psychiatric advanced practice nurses must conceptualize and embrace the interactive diseases model[1] rather than the primary medical disease/secondary medical disease model. The interactive diseases model considers both (or all) of the diagnosed conditions as "primary" and directs the treatment plan accordingly (Bricker, 1994; Douaihy, Jou, Gorske, et al., 2003; Drake, Mercer-McFadden, Mueser, et al., 1998; Drake, Yovetich, Bebout, et al., 1998; Herman, Frank, Mowbray, et al., 2000; Jerrell, 1996; Sitharthan, Singh, Kranitis, et al., 1999; Van den Bosch, Verheul, Schippers, et al., 2002). Figure 17-2, based on Vertino's multidirectional

[1]Indeed, terminology such as "disease and treatment" is now being replaced with recovery models that use language that reflects wellness versus illness, such as "co-occurring recovery." When quoting earlier sources, however, I will use the language that was written.

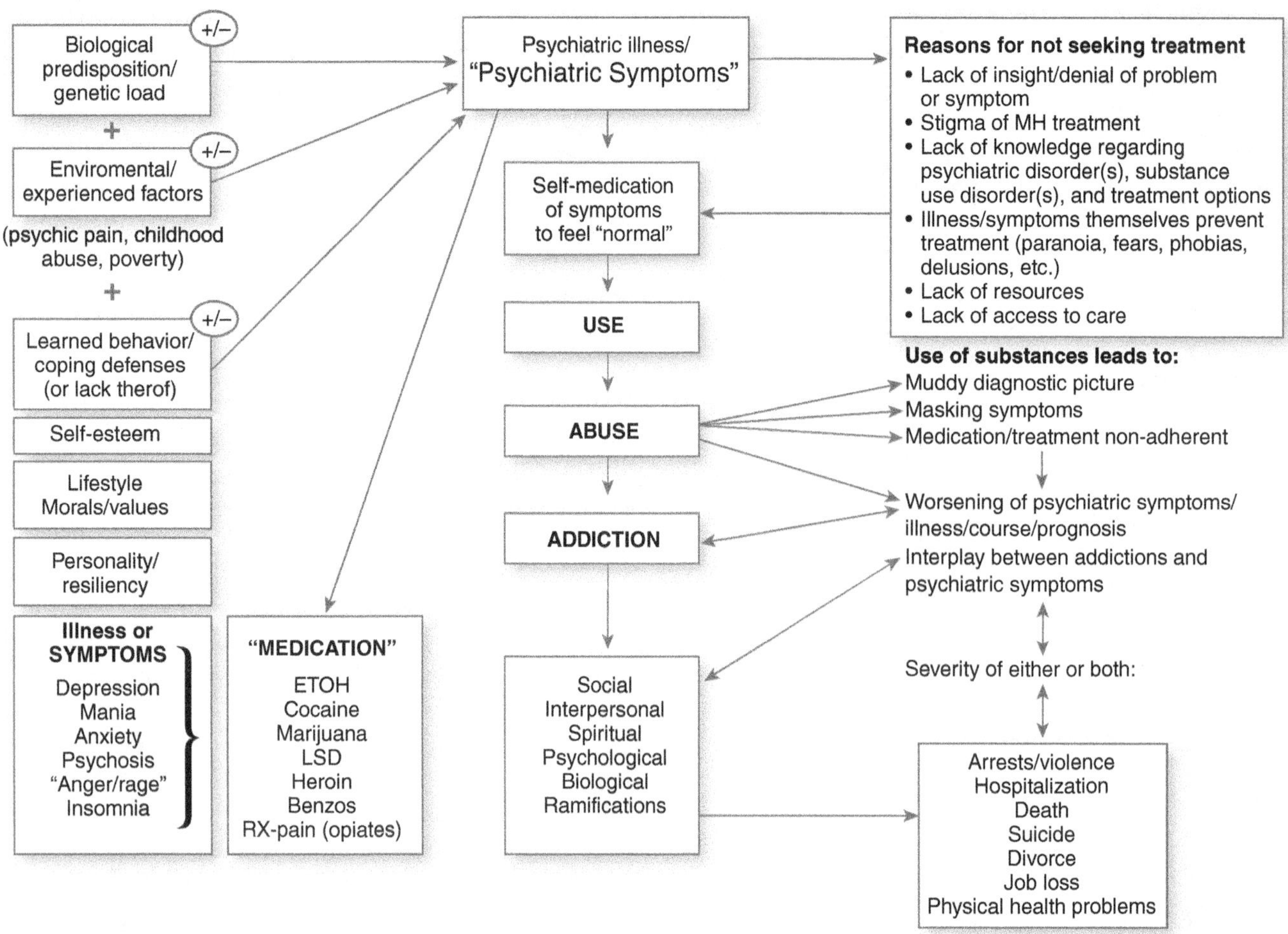

FIGURE 17-2: Vertino's Multidirectional Schemata of Co-Occurring Disorders. Benzos, benzodiazepines; ETOH, alcohol; MH, mental health; Rx, prescription pain medication, e.g., opiates.

schemata of co-occurring disorders, depicts the interaction and complex relationships between and among variables that may influence course, progression, and recovery of individuals with COD.

Factors Contributing to the Development of Co-occurring Disorders

Factors contributing to the development of COD may include (1) exposure to childhood abuse and environmental adversities and (2) neurodevelopmental, neurological, and medical factors.

Exposure to Childhood Abuse and Environmental Adversities

Approximately 30% of females and 6% of males experience child abuse (physical and sexual abuse), and a strong connection has been found between childhood abuse and subsequent development of SUDs and psychiatric disorders, particularly PTSD, other anxiety disorders, and major depressive disorder (Kasten, 1997, p. 237; Martinez-Rega et al., 2002). Among those who have experienced violent or traumatic events and have SUD, approximately 30% meet the criteria for PTSD, and PTSD-related symptoms are associated with more severe drug abuse (Bohn, 2003; Clark, Masson, Delucchi, et al., 2001).

Severity of childhood abuse of females has been linked to PTSD and more suicide attempts, whereas childhood abuse of males has been linked to PTSD, social phobia, agoraphobia, and dysthymia (Langeland, Draijer, & Van Den Brink, 2004). Affective disorders and suicide attempts in those with alcohol dependence have also been strongly linked to an inadequate or dysfunctional maternal figure (Langeland et al.).

Exposure to environmental and social adversities during childhood has been linked to adult development of CODs. These adversities include substance abuse in the childhood home; poverty in the childhood home; nonfunctioning and noncontributing household members; abusive caregivers; and serious psychiatric illness in a member of the child's household (Alverson, Alverson, & Drake, 2000; Taylor & Barusch, 2004).

Neurodevelopmental, Neurological, and Medical Factors

Cognitive deficits—such as diminished frontal lobe activity—can be disabling and can create impairment in executive functioning and other cognitive domains, which can compound problems related to drug abuse or alcoholism and psychiatric illness. Up to two-thirds of individuals with CODs are reported to have cognitive deficits, with impaired memory and judgment as the most significant predictors of functional difficulty (Harrison & Precin, 1996; Hibbard, Uysal, & Keppler, 1998).

Neurological disorders are highly correlated with COD; in particular, frontal lobe or subcortical disorders (trauma, tumors or masses, normal pressure hydrocephalus, or infections) have been associated with cognitive, emotional, personality, or behavioral changes, such as pathological laughing and crying (Wortzel, Anderson, & Arciniegas, 2007). Individuals with TBI will be covered in more detail in the discussion of COD in special populations.

In addition to brain disorders, many medical illnesses, some medical treatments, and a number of medications can cause personality changes, delirium, and psychiatric symptoms, These factors will be discussed in the Comorbidity section of this chapter. Cognitive impairments with attention, concentration, processing, and memory deficits; emotional changes; impairment of functioning; and behavioral changes may confound the process of generating differential diagnoses, prolong the course of the illness, and make recovery complex. Therefore, a thorough psychiatric evaluation should include (1) screening for neuropsychiatric, metabolic, or medical problems, particularly in children, young adolescents, and the elderly, and (2) a discussion with the patient regarding a referral to an appropriate specialist for further investigation if needed.

Biological Basis

It is thought that the biological basis of COD may include genetic influences and abnormalities of prenatal neurodevelopment of the central nervous system.

Heredity and Genetic Factors

Alcoholism and psychiatric disorders—in particular, schizophrenia, bipolar disorder, ADHD, panic disorder, Alzheimer's disease, and autism—have been reported to have high rates of heritability (Malaspina, Corcoran, & Hamilton, 2002). Genetic tendencies for heritable illnesses have been postulated to be multifactorial. Biological problems such as susceptible alleles, other cellular abnormalities, or neurochemical dysregulation can be present in genetically vulnerable individuals. Problems with synaptic transmission can create molecular and cellular adaptations, such as structural changes in neurons in the ventral tegmental area and nucleus accumbens (Malaspina et al.). In addition, it is postulated that illnesses may result from the brain's having experienced structural and functional changes with environmental or other psychosocial stressors (Suppes & Dennehy, 2005). Horsfall, Cleary, Hunt, et al. (2009) concluded that "There is no evidence that substance abuse and psychosis have a common genetic basis. However, the emotional, social, and biological sequelae of early childhood trauma may constitute an increased vulnerability to both conditions" (p. 26).

Heritability of Bipolar Disorder

Epidemiological studies report that the lifetime risk of developing bipolar disorder is sevenfold for family members, and that risk and severity of bipolar disorder can increase as the number of psychiatrically ill relatives increases (Malaspina et al., 2002). More on the genetics of bipolar disorder can be found in Chapter 14.

Heritability of Alcoholism and Psychiatric Illness

Certain biological markers that suggest heritability of SUDs and psychiatric illness have been identified. For example, studies have shown that

- Children of alcoholic parents can have abnormal electroencephalograms when given alcohol infusions (Sadock & Sadock, 2003).
- The cerebrospinal fluid of individuals with alcohol-related disorders has demonstrated abnormal concentrations of neurotransmitters: in particular, low amounts of serotonin, dopamine, gamma-aminobutyric acid, and their metabolites (Sadock & Sadock, 2003).
- Neurotransmitter receptors such as D_2 may be involved in the inheritance of alcohol disorders (Sadock & Sadock, 2003, p. 398).
- Decreased overall metabolic cortical activity is noted on brain positron emission tomography scans of individuals with alcohol dependence; e.g., the left parietal and right frontal cortexes are noted to be more affected than normal controls (Volkow, Hitzeman, Wang, et al., 1992).
- Neuronal kindling and the involvement of dopamine-releasing neurons in the mesolimbic region are thought to be involved in psychiatric illnesses (Goldsmith & Garlapati, 2004).
- Mood and the urge to drink have been linked to rapid depletion of tryptophan (the precursor of serotonin), and the role of serotonergic neurotransmission in modulating mood and the urge to drink has been supported (Pierucci-Lagha, Feinn, Modesto-Lowe, et al., 2004).

Heritability of Attention Deficit-Hyperactivity Disorder

Childhood ADHD, which has been found to have a genetic basis (Abrantes, Brown, & Tomlinson, 2003), appears to be a risk factor for later development of an SUD (Wilens, 2006). SUDs that begin in adolescence and continue into adulthood affect 15% to 20% of adults. Interestingly, treatment of ADHD has been shown to reduce the risk of later substance abuse (Biederman, Wilens, Mick, et al., 1999). Co-occurring psychiatric illness has been estimated to be as high as 70% in children with ADHD.

Prenatal Neurodevelopmental Factors

Exposure to toxins during pregnancy—such as nicotine, alcohol, "crack" cocaine, radiation, and some prescription medications such as certain antibiotics (tetracyclines), anticonvulsants (valproate [Depakote], carbamazepine, and phenytoin), progesterones, lithium, benzodiazepines, and warfarin (Coumadin)—are known to cause birth defects. It has been reported that boys are more vulnerable to developmental damage prenatally; by contrast, girls are more "biologically vigorous" (Sadock & Sadock, 2003, p. 21).

Fetal alcohol syndrome affects approximately one-third of all babies born to alcoholic mothers. The degree of resultant disability can be mild to severe and has been linked to later development of hyperactivity or attention deficits, learning disability, low IQ or intellectual development, and seizure disorders (Sadock & Sadock, 2003, p. 24). Whether babies exposed to drugs or alcohol in utero are more predisposed to development of SUDs or CODs later in life is an area requiring further research.

Chapter 3 of this text provides further discussion on the effect of substances on prenatal and fetal brain development.

Although information on COD is not covered on this Web site, detailed information on the biological basis of addictions can be obtained from McGill University's "The Brain From Top to Bottom" at http://thebrain.mcgill.ca/flash/index_d.html.

Clinical Presentation

Individuals with CODs, regardless of the type of psychiatric disorders or the substances that have been abused, exhibit more severe symptoms and suffer more distress than individuals without co-morbidities. Individuals with CODs are more functionally and cognitively limited, and the interaction between CODs in terms of severity and persistence of both disorders can create severe episodic exacerbations of psychiatric symptoms (Kessler, 2004; Zauszniewski, 1995). Historically, individuals with COD have been reported to be more often hospitalized, behaviorally disruptive, medication nonadherent, homeless, and considered more "disabled" and to have experienced poorer treatment outcomes (Siegfried, 1998). Unfortunately, these prognostic indicators have not changed in recent years. For example, individuals with schizophrenia tend to have minimal change in substance abuse over time. Reports state that low motivation to change is a key factor contributing to poor outcomes in this population (Horsfall et al., 2009; Siegfried, 1998). Individuals with CODs have a history of accidents (patients with COD are six to eight times more likely to die from accidents than the general population [Dickey, Dembling, Azeni, et al., 2004]). In addition to the psychiatric and behavioral symptoms associated with COD, they have more health problems, dental problems, sleep disruptions, vocational problems, social problems (housing, finances, and relationships), and legal problems.

Comorbidity

Oppositional defiant disorder, conduct disorder, mood disorders, anxiety disorders, substance abuse, and learning disability are documented as the most common comorbid conditions. CODs with comorbid ADHD, SUDs, or psychiatric illness in young people often lead to a difficult course, more severe illness, and more disability (particularly in occupational, educational, and interpersonal functioning), making treatment for the individual as well as his or her family much more challenging (Wilens, 2006).

The discussion of special populations in this chapter provides more information specific to the following:

- Individuals with co-occurring PTSD, sexual trauma, and SUD
- Individuals with co-occurring TBI, psychiatric illness, and SUD
- Individuals with co-occurring bipolar affective disorder and SUD
- Individuals with co-occurring personality disorder and SUD

Differential Diagnosis

With many possible co-morbidities—both medically and psychiatrically—differential diagnosis can be difficult. This chapter addresses differential diagnosis in subsequent Treatment and Management sections.

Treatment

This section discusses assessment, psychopharmacology, and management and recovery strategies for treating persons with CODs, including integrated treatment programs, application of a recovery model for persons with COD in a partial hospital setting, and self-help recovery groups.

Assessment

A thorough diagnostic evaluation is the first step. When interacting with the patient, the clinician should establish straightforward, open communication with a warm, accepting approach while maintaining a professional demeanor. The clinician should ask the individual to report everything that he or she is comfortable disclosing; the individual may not say much at first, but patience and acceptance can go a long way toward development of a collaborative therapeutic bond. *Destigmatization* of the presenting problem is critical. The clinician should expect that there will be numerous questions, particularly if the clinician is the first psychiatric professional that the individual has ever seen or if this is a first-time diagnosis, whether it is a psychiatric diagnosis, an SUD diagnosis, or both. During the initial consultation, the clinician should be prepared to provide information such as patient education materials, Web sites, and printouts about medications to be prescribed. The clinician should ask the individual to come back with questions and offer to include a significant other in the session if the person being seen is comfortable with this. At the initial psychiatric evaluation, diagnostic studies should be ordered and goals discussed, including a plan for follow-up and the initiation of pharmacological therapy, if warranted. At the follow-up session, the clinician should review diagnostic test results and refer as indicated if medical or neurological findings are significant.

Laboratory Studies

Laboratory studies of electrolytes, glucose, blood urea nitrogen, creatinine clearance, urinalysis, and urine toxicology screen are beneficial and appropriate for an initial psychiatric evaluation. If there are cognitive concerns, thyroid studies and B_{12} deficiency assessment should be performed. Serum medication levels can be measured to obtain a baseline. If an alcohol use disorder is suspected, the following tests may be useful: blood or breath alcohol tests; gamma-glutamyltransferase; liver function tests, including serum aspartate aminotransferase; complete blood cell count; and testing for vitamin deficiencies.

For patients of childbearing age, a pregnancy test is recommended, especially prior to starting any psychotropic medication. Structural neuroimaging—such as computed tomography or magnetic resonance imaging of the brain, electroencephalogram, or functional imaging studies such as single-photon emission computed tomography or positron emission tomography—may be needed depending on the differential diagnoses being considered. Although electrocardiography is not part of the usual psychiatric work-up, it should be considered (1) if there is any cardiac history or (2) before ordering tricylic antidepressants (TCAs) or other drugs that may affect cardiac conduction. In addition, a complete medication list with dosages and the schedule for each medication should be compiled at the initial visit. Following this, a multi-check for potential drug interactions may be considered to rule out or prevent medication-induced confusion, falls, delirium, psychosis, anxiety, depression, and suicidal ideation, particularly in the elderly and young children.

As noted earlier, individuals can present with more than two diagnoses: for example, an individual could have ADHD plus bipolar disorder plus personality disorder plus a substance use disorder. Furthermore, polysubstance dependence can occur, such as with alcohol, benzodiazepines, marijuana, opiates, or heroin. Individuals report that certain drugs and alcohol can calm nerves, slow down racing thoughts, and promote sleep. Others use cocaine, methamphetamines, caffeine, stimulants, methylenedioxymethamphetamine (MDMA, also known as ecstasy), or steroids to promote wakefulness or medicate a depressed mood. This pattern of use can become a troubling seesaw-type phenomenon. Typically, individuals do not readily admit to substance or alcohol abuse. When asked directly, individuals may deny, minimize, rationalize, or lie, even when they are confronted with factual data, such as a positive toxicology screen or drug arrest. Thus, corroboration from a significant other is *crucial* in terms of eliciting past history and events leading up to the current presenting problem or chief complaint.

Screening instruments—such as the *Mood Disorder Questionnaire (MDQ)* developed by Hirshfeld, Williams, Spitzer, et al. (2000); the *CAGE questionnaire* (Ewing, 1984); the NIAAA *Guide to Alcohol Screening;* the *Mini-mental state examination (MMSE)* (Folstein, Folstein, & McHugh, 1975); the *Alcohol Use Disorders Identification Test (AUDIT)* (Babor, de la Fuente, Saunders, et al., 1992); the *Michigan Alcohol Screening Test (MAST)* (Selzer, 1971); and the *Screening, Brief Intervention, and Referral to Treatment (SBIRT)* (Substance Abuse and Mental Health Services Administration, 2011)—can be helpful diagnostically, but screening instruments are meant to supplement, not replace, good clinical acumen and experience. The art and practice of therapeutic engagement must be done early and well: establishing trust and rapport with the individual is an essential first step that can lay the foundation for all future treatment efforts.

Psychopharmacotherapy

This discussion assumes that the reader is familiar with psychopharmacological agents, Food and Drug Administration (FDA) indications and uses, appropriate dosing, side effects, potential drug interactions, all potential risks and benefits, and, in particular, all FDA black box warnings on certain psychotropic medications. (See FDA warnings at www.fda.gov/Drugs/DrugSafety/default.htm for review of important prescribing information. For additional reading, refer to the textbook by Stahl [2008].)

General Considerations

Following is a brief overview and some general considerations for the psychiatric advanced practice nurse who is prescribing medications for individuals with CODs. Because of the rapid changes in availability of new agents, this review is not meant to be comprehensive or all-inclusive.

Since 1990, psychopharmacological agents have proliferated, with new medications continuously under development. With the implementation of parity laws for mental health care, psychotropic medication may become more accessible, which could ultimately lead to more research in the area of psychotherapeutic agents that may be more specifically geared toward treatment of CODs. In psychiatry, some medications are used off-label (without FDA approval for that particular indication), and numerous anecdotal reports describe serendipitous results when prescribing medications for SUDs, such as antidepressants, mood stabilizers, or antipsychotics. However, off-label use of medications will not be discussed here.

Individuals with CODs generally need more than one medication to maintain psychiatric stability and sobriety. Individuals with recurrent psychiatric illnesses may need a combination of psychotropics (any combination of antidepressants, antipsychotics, mood stabilizers, and relapse-prevention agents) to maintain psychiatric stability and to prevent hospitalization, drug or alcohol relapse, and suicides.

Insomnia is probably the most common complaint. Sleep history, a review of sleep hygiene practices, and an account of daytime functioning are necessary elements of the psychiatric work-up, as poor daytime functioning may be related to exacerbation of the psychiatric disorder, active substance or alcohol use, or both. Although drugs, alcohol, and sleep aids may promote initial relaxation, they can also result in poorer sleep quality and rebound insomnia, which can exacerbate or evoke psychiatric symptoms. Prescribing sleep aids (hypnotics) or benzodiazepines for anxiety or insomnia for any individual who has a past or present diagnosis of substance abuse is not recommended except in special justifiable circumstances with a clear clinical rationale. For example, individuals with chronic unrelenting panic disorder may be able to participate more socially if given a few doses of a benzodiazepine to carry in a pocket or purse. Some individuals will carry the medication around for months and never use it, but they are reassured knowing that they have it in case of an acute panic attack. Another appropriate use of a benzodiazepine is for acute alcohol withdrawal to prevent withdrawal seizures.

If a benzodiazepine is deemed appropriate to use, longer-acting agents—such as clonazepam (Klonopin), which has a half-life of 18 to 50 hours, or lorazepam (Ativan), which has a half-life of approximately 12 hours—are preferred in an outpatient setting. Individuals who have been prescribed benzodiazepines must be monitored carefully; they should be given only small supplies of the drug, and the agent should be tapered down and discontinued as soon as possible. In general, for sleep difficulties, trazodone (Desyrel) can be used safely in this population (Minkoff, 2005). The possibility of priapism should be discussed with the patient as well as a strategy to manage this rare side effect.

Selective serotonin reuptake inhibitors (SSRIs) have been associated with lower alcohol use in some alcohol-dependent patients, whether or not they were depressed (Minkoff, 2005). For example, sertraline (Zoloft) at 200 mg a day has been reported to reduce drinking in alcohol-dependent individuals without lifelong depression (Pettinati, Volpicelli, Luck, et al., 2001). Sertraline and other SSRIs are reported to be effective for post-TBI depression if dosed slowly and if agents with anticholinergic side effects are avoided (as anticholinergic effects can further impair attention, concentration, and memory, especially in those with brain lesions) (Alderfer, Arciniegas, & Silver, 2005).

Fluoxetine (Prozac) failed to demonstrate a positive treatment response in cocaine-dependent individuals with major depressive disorder (Schmitz, Averill, Stotts, et al., 2001), but it demonstrated a positive reduction in marijuana use in individuals with depression and alcohol dependence, and in earlier studies it also demonstrated a reduction in depressive symptoms and alcohol consumption in individuals with comorbid disorders (Cornelius, Salloum, Ehler, et al., 1997; Cornelius, Salloum, Haskett, et al., 1999). Paroxetine (Paxil) at 20 to 60 mg/day as a target dose has shown some efficacy in reducing social anxiety and drinking behavior (Randall, Johnson, Thevos, et al., 2001). Imipramine (Tofranil), a TCA, was reported to improve mood, but the results were inconclusive for improvement of substance use in opiate-dependent individuals with depression (Nunes, Quitkin, Donovan, et al., 1998). Similar results were shown with desipramine (Norpramin), which was reported to afford a great reduction in depressive symptoms but was not associated with great reductions in cocaine use (Carroll, Nich, & Rounsaville, 1995). However, TCAs and monoamine oxidase inhibitors (MAOIs) should be used with caution in this population owing to the risk of suicide, as they can be fatal in overdose (Minkoff, 2005).

Pemoline (Cylert)—which was removed from the U.S. market in 2005 owing to serious risks of liver toxicity—was shown to have efficacy in reducing the severity of ADHD, but no changes in substance abuse or chemical dependency symptoms were noted in substance-abusing adolescents (ages 13 to 19) with comorbid conduct disorder (Riggs, Hall, Milkulich-Gilbertson, et al., 2004). However, another report stated that treatment of ADHD with pharmacotherapy (versus treatment of ADHD without pharmacotherapy) in 15-year-old males reduced the risk of their developing an SUD by up to 85% (Biederman et al., 1999).

Nefazodone (Serzone) was reported to significantly decrease the number of heavy drinking days in depressed individuals with alcohol dependence (Hernandez-Avila, Modesto-Lowe, Feinn, et al., 2004); however, because it has been associated with hepatotoxicity, it is recommended that liver function tests be monitored. As of this writing, the trademark drug Serzone is no longer available, but generic nefazodone is still available in the United States.

Venlafaxine (Effexor) at a median dose of 150 mg per day was reported in a small sample to reduce cocaine use by 75% in depressed individuals (McDowell, Levin, Seracini, et al., 2000).

Bupropion (Wellbutrin) was reported to ameliorate cocaine cravings and in some cases to decrease cocaine use in adults with comorbid ADHD and opiate dependence; however, it did not significantly affect cravings for alcohol (Avants, Margolin, DePhilippis, et al., 1998; Levin, Evans, McDowell, et al., 2002). Lithium was reported to be efficacious in treating both "secondary" substance dependency and bipolar disorder in adolescents when the mean blood level of lithium was maintained at 0.9 mEq/L and when the substances of dependence were most commonly alcohol and marijuana (Geller, Cooper, Sun, et al., 1998).

Clozapine has been reported to have a direct effect on reducing substance abuse in CODs (Minkoff, 2005).

To date, no single agent addresses psychiatric symptoms and SUDs simultaneously. Comprehensive studies on medications that include individuals with COD in study samples, and projections regarding possible prognostic benefits and efficacy of agents with this population, are needed. However, certain medication strategies may be employed to aid in stabilizing one or both conditions. Some general guidelines are as follows:

1. Always treat psychosis. Depot medications may be helpful to promote adherence. If oral medications are needed, once-daily dosing is preferred.
2. Benzodiazepines, sedatives-hypnotics, and pain medications that are known to be habit forming are generally not recommended in patients with any kind of substance abuse history, but there are exceptions to this rule, as discussed above.
3. For ADHD, noncontrolled agents such as bupropion or atomoxetine (Strattera) are the first-line choice, and avoid stimulants if there is a risk that the patient may be actively using substances or drinking.

Finally, adherence to medication is known to be problematic in individuals with COD: up to 50% non-adherence has been reported. Non-adherence is particularly common when the medications have troublesome side effects. It is extremely important to continuously work with individuals and discuss possible side effects up front. If possible adverse reactions or side effects are not addressed early and directly, the individual may be surprised or frightened by an untoward effect and may stop the medication without consulting the provider.

Medications Used to Reduce Relapse

Studies specifically examining the efficacy of medication with the COD population are sparse, but a few promising results were found, including decreases in cocaine cravings, decreases in actual use of cocaine, reduction of psychiatric symptoms, some evidence of reduction of alcohol consumption and cravings, a possible role in ameliorating alcohol withdrawal symptoms, substantial improvement in psychiatric stability, a decrease in cocaine cravings in bipolar outpatients, and adherence to medication that may contribute to completion of substance abuse treatment (Albanese & Suh, 2006; Brown, Nejtek, Perantie, et al., 2002; Brown, Nejtek, Perantie, et al., 2003; Kalyoncu, Mirsal, Pektas, et al., 2005; Margolin, Avants, DePhilippis, et al., 1998).

As mentioned earlier, mood-stabilizing medications are paramount in the treatment of individuals with bipolar disorder and co-occurring SUDs. At the same time, controlling cravings for alcohol or drugs may assist in adherence to psychotropic medication. Head-to-head placebo-controlled studies comparing mood stabilizers such as lithium and valproate with other agents to examine long-term efficacy in individuals with bipolar disorder and SUDs are needed.

Medications Used to Reduce Relapse in Alcohol Dependence

Alcohol consumption can worsen mood symptoms; in particular, it can contribute to mixed mood states, worsening of mania, rapid cycling, and suicidal ideation and attempts. Thus, psychopharmacological agents used for abstinence from alcohol may be a necessary adjunct to psychiatric medication for individuals with COD.

Disulfiram (Antabuse), oral naltrexone (Revia, Depade), injectable naltrexone (Vivitrol), and acamprosate (Campral) are available for alcohol dependence. Tables 17-1 and 17-2 compare medications, indications, actions, and contraindications of these drugs.

Disulfiram interferes with alcohol metabolism via alcohol dehydrogenase, and in its action as a dopamine betahydroxylase inhibitor, it can occasionally evoke psychosis, necessitating an adjustment in antipsychotic medication (Minkoff, 2005).

Both naltrexone and acamprosate are FDA-approved medications designed to decrease cravings for alcohol. Naltrexone is reported to be effective in preventing alcoholic relapse after 12 weeks, but longer-term studies are needed (Morris, Hopwood, Whelan, et al., 2001). Studies with naltrexone report that approximately 80% of study participants maintained compliance for approximately 8 weeks, thereby curbing their alcohol use for a significant period of time (Maxwell & Shinderman, 2000). Petrakis, Poling, Levinson, et al. (2006) conducted a medication study (n = 254) at three outpatient Veterans Administration clinics. Study participants who met *DSM-IV* criteria of PTSD and alcohol dependence were randomized into four groups—disulfiram alone, naltrexone alone, disulfiram and naltrexone together, and placebo—for 12 weeks. These authors concluded that subjects had better alcohol outcomes on medication versus placebo; psychiatric symptoms (of PTSD) improved over time; disulfiram-treated patients showed greater improvement in PTSD symptoms over time than naltrexone-treated patients; and more side effects emerged when patients were treated with combined agents. Individuals have been known to discontinue naltrexone owing to intolerable side effects such as insomnia, headache, nausea, vomiting, muscle aches, and liver problems (Sonne & Brady, 2000).

The exact mechanism of action of acamprosate is unknown; however, it is postulated that it lowers neuronal excitability and exerts an inhibitory effect on excitatory amino acids and may modulate glutamate and gamma-aminobutyric acid (GABA) neurotransmitter systems, thus decreasing the individual's urge to drink (Paille, Guelfi, Perkins, et al., 1995; Pelc, Verbanck, Le Bon, et al., 1997; Sass, Soyka, Mann, et al., 1996). Acamprosate is reported to be "safer" than its predecessors because most individuals do not become ill if they drink while taking it; however, studies on the effectiveness of acamprosate as a solo agent

TABLE 17-1 ALCOHOL USE DISORDERS MEDICATION DECISION GRID

Pretreatment Indicators	Acamprosate (Campral)	Disulfiram (Antabuse)	Oral Naltrexone (Revia, Depade)	Injectable Naltrexone (Vivitrol)
Renal failure	X	A	A	A
Significant liver disease	A	C	C	C
Coronary artery disease	A	C	A	A
Chronic pain	A	A	C	C
Current opiate use	A	A	X	X
Psychosis	A	C	A	A
Unwilling or unable to sustain total abstinence	A	X	A	A
Risk factors for poor medication adherence	C	C	C	A
Diabetes	A	C	A	A
Obesity that precludes intramuscular injection	A	A	A	X
Family history of alcohol use disorders	A	A	+	+
Bleeding/other coagulation disorders	A	A	A	C
High level of craving	A	A	+	+
Opiate dependence in remission	A	A	+	+
History of post-acute withdrawal syndrome	+	A	A	A
Cognitive impairment	A	X	A	A

A, Appropriate to use; C, Use with caution; X, Contraindicated; +, Particularly appropriate.

Adapted from Center for Substance Abuse Treatment. (2009). Incorporating alcohol pharmacotherapies into medical practice (p. 52).Treatment Improvement Protocol (TIP) Series 49. HHS Publication No. (SMA) 09-4380. Rockville, MD: Substance Abuse and Mental Health Services Administration.

TABLE 17-2 COMPARISON OF FDA-APPROVED MEDICATIONS FOR MAINTENANCE OF ABSTINENCE FROM ALCOHOL*

	Acamprosate	Disulfiram	Oral Naltrexone	Extended-Release Injectable Naltrexone
Mechanism of action	Not clearly understood; appears to restore to normal the altered balance of neuronal excitation and inhibition induced by chronic alcohol exposure, possibly through interaction with the glutamate neurotransmitter system	Inhibits aldehyde dehydrogenase, causing a reaction of flushing, sweating, nausea, and tachycardia when alcohol is ingested	Not clearly understood; opiate antagonist; blocks the effects of endogenous opiate peptides; appears to attenuate euphoria associated with alcohol use; may make alcohol use less rewarding; may reduce craving	Same as oral naltrexone
Examples of drug interactions	No clinically relevant interactions	Metronidazole; medications containing alcohol; anticoagulants such as warfarin; amitriptyline; isoniazid; diazepam	Opiate medications; cough/cold medications; antidiarrheal medications; thioridazine; yohimbine	Presumed same as oral naltrexone; clinical drug interaction studies have not been performed
Common side effects	Diarrhea and somnolence	Transient mild drowsiness; metallic taste; dermatitis; headache; impotence	Nausea; vomiting; anxiety; headache; dizziness; fatigue; somnolence	Same as oral naltrexone, plus injection-site reactions; joint pain; muscle aches or cramps
Contraindications	Severe renal impairment (creatinine clearance ≤ 30 mL/min)	Hypersensitivity to rubber derivatives; significant liver disease; alcohol still in system; coronary artery disease	Currently using opiates or in acute opiate withdrawal; anticipated need for opiate analgesics; acute hepatitis or liver failure	Same as oral naltrexone, plus inadequate muscle mass for deep intramuscular injection; body mass that precludes deep intramuscular injection; rash or infection at injection site
Cautions	Dosage may be modified for moderate renal impairment (creatinine clearance 30–50 mL/ min); pregnancy category C†	Hepatic cirrhosis or insufficiency; cerebrovascular disease; psychoses; diabetes mellitus; epilepsy; renal impairment; pregnancy category C†	Renal impairment; chronic pain; pregnancy category C†	Same as oral naltrexone, plus hemophilia or other bleeding problems

TABLE 17-2 COMPARISON OF FDA-APPROVED MEDICATIONS FOR MAINTENANCE OF ABSTINENCE FROM ALCOHOL*—continued

	Acamprosate	Disulfiram	Oral Naltrexone	Extended-Release Injectable Naltrexone
Serious adverse reactions	Rare events include suicidal ideation; severe persistent diarrhea	Disulfiram–alcohol reaction; hepatotoxicity; peripheral neuropathy; psychotic reactions; optic neuritis	Precipitates opiate withdrawal if the patient is dependent on opiates; hepatotoxicity (although it does not appear to be a hepatotoxin at recommended doses)	Same as oral naltrexone plus inadvertent subcutaneous injection may cause a severe injection-site reaction; depression; rare events including allergic pneumonia and suicidal ideation and behavior

*Based on information in the FDA-approved product labeling or published literature.

†FDA pregnancy category C: Animal studies have indicated potential fetal risk OR have not been conducted and no or insufficient human studies have been done. The drug should be used with pregnant or lactating women only when potential benefits justify potential risk to the fetus or infant.

Adapted from Center for Substance Abuse Treatment. (2009). Incorporating alcohol pharmacotherapies into medical practice (p. 53).Treatment Improvement Protocol (TIP) Series 49. HHS Publication No. (SMA) 09-4380. Rockville, MD: Substance Abuse and Mental Health Services Administration.

are limited and dated. Combining acamprosate and naltrexone has been reported to be more effective than use of either agent alone (Minkoff, 2005). Finally, Krupitsky, Rudenko, Burakov, et al. (2007) published promising results hailing the first systematic clinical evidence of an antiglutamatergic approach for treating alcohol withdrawal symptoms with lamotrigine, memantine, or topiramate as compared with diazepam and placebo.

In the aforementioned studies, some individuals with severe psychiatric illnesses or those taking prescribed psychiatric medications were excluded from study samples, making plausible comparability of these studies questionable. Again, studies conducted with persons with CODs, especially those with serious and persistent psychiatric disorders, are needed to assess the true efficaciousness of relapse-prevention medications for this population. A separate but noteworthy concern is that when studies are funded by pharmaceutical companies, they must be scrutinized with a keen eye and compared with other studies not so funded to rule out potentially biased outcome data and other general study issues.

Medications Used to Reduce Relapse in Opiate Dependence

Psychiatric comorbidity in opiate-dependent individuals is as high as 47% in women and 48% in men. Antisocial personality disorder has been reported in at least 25% of opiate abusers, whereas major depression is reported in only 15% of opiate abusers (Brooner et al., 1997). Axis II, Cluster B personality disorders—in particular, antisocial and borderline personality disorders—are reported to be as high as 69% in those with opiate dependence (Teplin et al., 2004).

Naltrexone, a moderately long acting opiate blocker, has been used effectively in three times per week dosing, and is reported to be effective in treating opiate dependence, especially when combined with other supportive therapies (Minkoff, 2005).

Methadone has been widely prescribed and has been the mainstay of opiate treatment for years. Briefly, methadone is a synthetic opiate with actions resembling heroin and morphine. It has a well-established reputation for successful treatment of opiate addiction in programs that are regulated by the federal government. Levo-alpha-acetylmethadol (LAAM) is a synthetic compound closely resembling methadone with a longer duration of action than methadone. The goal of treatment for narcotic addiction is to substitute methadone or LAAM for drugs with a shorter duration of action, such as heroin or other narcotics.

Because diversion of medication is possible with methadone, LAAM, and buprenorphine, and because entry into treatment is largely voluntary, individuals should expect to be closely monitored, especially in the early phase of treatment for opiate addiction. Treatment contracts are recommended whether or not the person has co-occurring personality disorder. If treated in an office-based setting, individuals on methadone (in particular, buprenorphine/naloxone [Suboxone]) should be required to sign a treatment contract at the first visit. Suggested items for possible inclusion in a treatment contract are

- Adherence to all appointments
- Random urine testing
- Substance abuse counseling and 12-step or recovery meetings
- Proper use and storage of medication
- Random spot-checks of medication bottles

The ultimate goal is to retain the individual in treatment. Contracts are *not* meant to set up a conflicted or confrontational relationship; rather, they are initiated to clearly explain that there will be certain behavioral expectations during treatment. In my clinical experience, if the treatment contract is explained up front and there are no surprises, and if the patient is serious about recovery and has truly "hit bottom," then most individuals are willing to sign a treatment contract and will comply with the "rules" of their treatment.

For individuals experiencing opiate withdrawal symptoms, clonidine (an α_2-adrenergic agonist) calms the overactivation of the locus ceruleus neurons. While clonidine is generally palliative, it can be helpful for ameliorating uncomfortable withdrawal symptoms; however, supervised medical detoxification is usually necessary and prudent for opiate or alcohol withdrawal for individuals with chronic or long-standing chemical dependencies.

Previously, individuals who were addicted to opiates could not be treated safely on an outpatient basis. This is no longer the case: buprenorphine/naloxone (Suboxone) is now available for office-based (outpatient) opiate dependence treatment owing to the Drug Addiction Treatment Act of 2000 (DATA 2000). In double-blind, placebo-controlled studies, Suboxone, a partial opiate receptor agonist, was shown to be safe in office-based settings. Suboxone (buprenorphine/naloxone) and Subutex (buprenorphine without naloxone) sublingual preparations are the only medications approved by the FDA for office-based opiate addiction (induction and maintenance) treatment.

Studies report that treatment of individuals with Suboxone has resulted in controlling of opiate cravings and has produced drug-free urine samples in 35.2% to 67.4% of samples (Fudala, Bridge, Herbert, et al., 2003) and as high as 75% of samples negative for illicit substances after 1 year (Kakko, Svanborg, Kreek, et al., 2003).

Individuals on maintenance Suboxone who had abused both opiates and cocaine are reported to have shown some improvement in depressive symptoms when treated with desipramine in addition to buprenorphine, but only if their depression had not been chronic or lifelong. Other studies have yielded mixed results, as (1) the addition of antidepressant medication did not seem to make a difference in decreasing cravings for drugs and (2) behavioral interventions, in some groups, were just as effective (Gonzalez, Feingold, Oliveto, et al., 2003). Again, in studies with Suboxone, individuals with serious psychiatric illnesses, individuals on medication for psychiatric problems, and individuals considered to be less than psychiatrically "stable" were largely excluded from the aforementioned studies; however, although buprenorphine has not been well studied in the COD population, Minkoff (2005) reported that it has demonstrated efficacy but cautions that there may be interactions with enzymatic systems that metabolize psychotropic medications.

Traditional substance abuse treatment models encourage the practitioner to place the entire burden of maintaining a clean, sober lifestyle squarely on the shoulders of the recovering person in order to encourage self-responsibility and to facilitate facing the consequences of the addiction. However, individuals with co-occurring psychiatric illness who are on prescription medication must be monitored and supported throughout all attempts to reduce or eliminate substance use, especially if there is a past history of lethality. As stated by Finnell (2003), "...quitting substance use does not mean that individuals with co-occurring disorders have completed treatment and are ready to be self-reliant. Rather, it appears that continued alliance with a clinician, self-help groups, and other tangible support systems are critical to support and sustain the behavioral change and to ensure that there is prompt intervention should psychiatric symptoms emerge or worsen" (p. 13). In other words, individuals need ongoing encouragement and emotional support from their clinician, family, and friends/recovery circle to maintain a clean and sober lifestyle. This supportive but firm approach diverges from the "traditional" substance abuse treatment approach, which espouses the accepted rule of "confront and hold accountable." Seasoned clinicians with solid clinical skills and who are cross-trained or certified in both psychiatry and addictions can generally maintain the necessary balance between the two extremes of confrontation and enabling, and they are capable of introducing into their therapeutic stance some "gray" in terms of flexibility.

Management and Recovery Strategies

Vertino's multidirectional schemata of CODs (see Fig. 17-2) illustrates a complex interaction of multiple variables. Genetic vulnerability, manifestation of symptoms, course, severity, prognosis, and outcomes will vary among individuals. Environment, socioeconomic status, psychological and emotional resources, strengths, resiliency, spirituality, interpersonal relationships, and prior treatment and recovery experiences can affect eventual outcomes. To refer to processes as unidirectional or bidirectional is a vast oversimplification, as outcomes are not linear, but cyclical. Individuals with CODs may go through many treatment episodes until measurable gains are made, but *there is hope that gains can be made,* which is the point to underscore.

Intervention points provide optimal opportunities for engagement. An intervention point is defined as a specific point in time when a teachable moment can occur. Teachable moments can happen at any time, in any situation. For example, they could occur during a brief encounter during an ER visit or walk-in clinic. As evident in Figure 17-2, teachable moments generally occur during periods of transition or crisis, such as progression from drug abuse to drug addiction or a life-changing event that forces the individual to seek help (bottom right corner of Fig. 17-2). The 12-Step/Alcoholics Anonymous recovery models refer to their members' first opportunity for intervention as "hitting bottom." A brief motivational intervention can be especially therapeutic when an individual is suffering and reaching out for help, even though he or she may not follow through. Providers can "plant a seed" that may encourage treatment or recovery later on.

Common roadblocks to seeking care (upper right corner of Fig. 17-2) include but are not limited to

1. *Lack of insight or denial of the problem,* which occurs when the individual simply does not believe that he or she

has a psychiatric illness or addiction, and therefore is not willing to seek help or does not see the need for it.
2. *Stigma of psychiatric illness or substance dependence,* which may be enough to keep an individual from treatment.
3. *Lack of knowledge,* which occurs when an individual may be aware that a problem exists but has no idea that help is available or how to go about getting help.
4. *System failures,* which occur when individuals are aware and know they need help, but health-care delivery "system failures" prevent timely or appropriate linkage. Many organizations still adhere to rigid admission criteria rather than embracing the concept of "NO WRONG DOOR," meaning that individuals should be able to gain entrance to any part of "the system" even when self-referred, and that internal collaboration should make transitions to care in other parts of the system easy.
5. *Individual issues,* which occur when symptoms such as anxiety, depression, agoraphobia, delusions, paranoia, insomnia, severe depression, or relapse into substance abuse can prevent individuals from attending appointments, or even from getting out of bed. Individuals may cancel or be no-shows. A crisis-oriented lifestyle may lead an individual to present only when completely out of medication or severely symptomatic.

Once treatment is initiated, further hurdles—such as the difficulty in obtaining medication posed by limited resources, tier structures, and the impact of managed care on certain prescription drug programs—must be navigated. Through the entire aforementioned hoop jumping—that is, "...persistent administrative, funding and structural barriers that limit access..." (Fornili, 2008, p. 111)—individuals are expected to maintain a 100% drug- and alcohol-free lifestyle or risk getting "kicked out of" or terminated from a program, losing housing opportunities, losing social service benefits, and so on. Of course, the goal of abstinence is desirable, but it is not always realistic for individuals with COD, particularly in the early phases of recovery. Further, current evidence based practices, such as motivational interviewing, advocate the goal of *harm reduction* or *reduction in substance use*—rather than complete abstinence—in order to encourage individuals in this population to remain engaged in recovery (Cleary, Hung, Matheson, et al., 2009; Laker, 2007; Minkoff, 2005; Tiet & Mausbach, 2007; van Wamel et al., 2009). Proactive strategies and contingency management should be spelled out in the recovery plan; however, expectations may need to be somewhat flexible early on. It is possible to convey a firm yet supportive approach coupled with unconditional positive regard without becoming punitive or judgmental. It is imperative to take a balanced approach by setting limits and avoiding enabling behavior in order to ward off any potential transference/countertransference issues. Clark, Becker, Giard, et al. (2005) looked at the perceptions of women with CODs and trauma histories and patterns of coercion used to keep them in treatment, the argument being that "mandatory treatment rests on the assumption that required interventions would increase treatment compliance and thus ultimately improve client outcomes" (p. 168). According to the findings of these authors and their review of the evidence, this assumption is flawed for a number of methodological reasons. Further, they noted that women who have been physically and/or sexually abused are a special population and present "important concerns to be considered in any discussion of coercive practices in behavioral healthcare" (p. 170). The psychodynamics of addiction are complex. Individuals with SUDs can consciously (or subconsciously) evoke negative emotions and reactions from service providers. Inexperienced or unseasoned providers may not possess the maturity level, clinical skills, or knowledge of evidence-based practice needed to be optimally effective with this population. Indeed, the literature dictates that "current policy recommends integrated treatment for co-morbidity, coordinated by dual diagnosis specialists" (Laker, 2007, p. 720) and that "Clients receive care from experienced integrated treatment specialists serving on a multidisciplinary team" (Center for Mental Health Services, 2003; Fornili, 2008, p. 115). Therefore, it is incumbent upon health-care systems to recruit experienced personnel who hold appropriate certifications and are clinically astute enough to address the multitudinous care management issues that so commonly sabotage and undermine treatment efforts. Limited access and follow-up to medical and psychiatric care, poverty, homelessness, parenting issues, domestic violence, suicide, child abuse, criminal activity, and vocational/occupational deficits that constantly plague individuals with COD will challenge providers. Furthermore, practitioners are expected to be role models and educators for individuals, family members, and the public with regard to mental health and recovery from addictions.

Integrated Treatment Programs and Recovery Models

Integrated, multifaceted treatment models that focus on *concomitant* recovery have a higher success rate over time than traditional programs. Integrated treatment programs report improvement of psychiatric symptoms and substance abuse, improved quality of life, decreased involvement with the criminal justice system, and decreases in certain health-care costs (Drake & Mueser, 2000; Drake et al., 1998; Judd, Thomas, Schwartz, et al., 2003; Moggi, Brodbeck, Koltzsch, et al., 2002; Siegfried, 1998). Roadblocks to (1) implementing new models into clinical practice and (2) achieving system transformation include lack of adequate training for providers, inability to find and recruit cross-trained professional staff, and a variety of philosophical, administrative, financial, and policy encumbrances (Brems, Johnson, Bowers, et al., 2002; Grella & Gilmore, 2002; National Abandoned Infants Assistance Resource Center, 2008, p. 94; Willenbring et al., 2004). Barriers to implementation of "integrated dual disorders treatment" as identified by Brunette, Asher, and Whitley (2008) included "...administrative leadership, consultation and training, supervisor mastery and supervision, chronic staff turnover, and finances" (p. 989).

Quality of treatment and clinical outcomes in integrated programs—in which care is provided by cross-trained professionals who are comfortable and clinically equipped to address both mental illness and substance dependence problems simultaneously—are far superior to "parallel treatment programs" and Mentally Ill Chemical Abuse (MICA) programs (terminology now considered archaic, as it is disease focused rather than recovery focused). In a parallel treatment model, the individual is burdened with the difficult task of negotiating two disparate systems: substance abuse treatment services and mental health treatment services. Often excluded from both, individuals are rarely engaged in concurrent mental health and substance abuse treatment programs. A MICA program, which is a substance abuse treatment program that simply admits individuals with psychiatric disorders and expects chemical dependency counselors to effectively treat psychiatrically ill individuals with substance abuse problems, is inadequate. Such disconnectedness confuses individuals, prevents them from becoming fully integrated into *either* program, reinforces overutilization of services, and contributes to unnecessary costs.

Seigfreid (1998) stated that "*Central* to all integrated treatment models is the principle that mental health and drug and alcohol treatments are simultaneously (not sequentially) provided by the *same person, team or organization*" (pp. 712-713, emphasis added). Individuals are not shuffled back and forth among providers, programs, or agencies. Individuals seeking treatment or recovery should not be pigeonholed into existing programs because these programs have staff. Rather, patient-centered programs that meet the individual's treatment or recovery needs should be developed.

Systemic barriers to the integration of mental health and substance abuse treatment are difficult and longstanding. These barriers include different administrative structures, funding mechanisms, priority populations, philosophies, clinician competencies, and eligibility criteria. Among the most significant barriers to the provision of integrated, comprehensive service systems are (1) inadequate resources for both mental health services and substance abuse treatment, (2) lack of staff who are educated and trained in COD treatment (Substance Abuse and Mental Health Services Administration, 2002), and (3) lack of trauma-informed care for women with abuse histories.

Since the 1980s, much literature has been written on integrated treatment programs and the key program components (Box 17-1) that are necessary for successful outcomes. Cognitive behavioral and motivational therapies; case management models; intensive community-based programs, such as a partial hospital setting; psychopharmacological interventions; family models; supported employment; self-help; and empowerment models are some examples of evidence-based therapies that have been described. These programs and modalities have met with varying levels of success (Bogenschutz, Geppart, & George, 2006; Brooks & Penn, 2003; Center for Substance Abuse Treatment, 2007b; Cleminshaw, Shepler, & Newman, 2005; Fisher & Bentley, 1996; Goldsmith & Garlapati, 2004; Graeber, Moyers, Griffith, et al., 2003; Kleber, 2003; Polgar, Johsen, Starrett, et al., 2000; Ridgely & Jerrell, 1996). Though many viable models have been implemented, huge gaps in service remain, and reports do not agree as to which approach is best practice.

Graham (2004) examined impediments to implementation of an integrated treatment program that were related to staff issues. The study looked at the lack of mental health staff confidence and motivation to work with individuals with COD. Ninety percent of the study participants were community psychiatric nurses. Staff were evaluated before and after training and at 18- and 36-month follow-up. Staff concerns were "Perceived difficulties in accessing specialist services and carrying out assessments, attending necessary training sessions, safety concerns when conducting home visits with substance abusing clients, and concern about implementing techniques with difficult to engage substance abusing clients" (p. 467). Results demonstrated that teams who received necessary support and training "experienced significant improvements in their self-reported confidence

BOX 17-1 Key Components of an Integrated Treatment Program

- Management of finances and provision for basic needs
- Safe housing: availability of residential long-term care
- Strategies for harm reduction and management of symptoms
- Availability of comprehensive medical and psychiatric care, including medication management and monitoring
- Vocational services
- Decreasing or eliminating substance use; relapse prevention
- Promoting positive family and social relationships and support
- Psychoeducation for patient and family or significant others
- 12-step, modified, or specialized support groups including a spiritual component
- Case management or home-based model on long-term basis
- Flexible scheduling or 24/7 coverage by staff
- Small caseloads
- Services are provided by master's-level cross-trained professionals who provide an empathic, motivational, engaging, persuasive, and supportive (nonthreatening, nonpunitive, nonjudgmental) stance

Source: Center for Substance Abuse Treatment, 2005, 2007.

and skills relevant to working with combined problems," and that these "gains were maintained over time" (p. 467). There is no question that even if all key components are present but the staff is not adequately trained, treatment outcomes will very likely falter.

Certain provider characteristics are ideal and most likely to result in positive outcomes for individuals with COD. These characteristics are

1. Having a solid working knowledge of both psychiatric illness and addictions
2. Fully understanding how CODs interact and impact one another, and that this interaction is not a smooth or sequential process
3. Having a mature attitude, being able to maintain appropriate boundaries while being flexible, warm, nonjudgmental, patient, and tolerant
4. Not being easily manipulated, intimidated, or frightened
5. Not needing to receive positive feedback from clients in order to work effectively with them, and being good at conflict management
6. Willingness to be firm, even when his or her decisions or strategies are unpopular

Psychiatric advanced practice nurses with certification in both psychiatric/mental health and addictions are well positioned to provide comprehensive quality care to individuals with COD. In fact, Kendall (2004) wrote: "The APN improves access to health services by providing *integrated* mental health and substance abuse services. *An expert clinician,* the APN provides services that include psychiatric assessment, medication prescription and management, individual and family therapy, and health education. Further the APN serves as liaison among multidisciplinary team members in disciplines that include medicine, social work, pharmacy, and others within the community" (pp. 185-186, emphasis added).

Application of a Recovery Model in a Partial Hospital Setting

The following statement was developed by expert panelists following the National Consensus Conference on Mental Health Recovery and Mental Health Systems Transformation in December, 2004.

> *Mental health recovery is a journey of healing and transformation enabling a person with a mental health problem to live a meaningful life in a community of his or her choice while striving to achieve his or her full potential (Substance Abuse and Mental Health Services Administration, 2006b).*

"Recovery" is a model that was introduced in 2006. A program based on the recovery model is a structured, evidence-based intervention program that encompasses various therapeutic modalities and a specific philosophy of care that involves and empowers the care recipient as an equal partner in goal setting and recovery planning. Behavioral health programs that use a recovery model focus on teaching and learning (didacticism) rather than on traditional psychotherapy (process). Client empowerment, wellness, medication management, and proactive planning are key elements of recovery.

A *partial hospital* is a safe place for recovery, provided that there is a high staff-to-patient ratio, intensive monitoring, support, and medication management. It is an ideal environment for implementation of a recovery-based model and realization of the ten fundamental components of recovery, listed in Box 17-2. In a partial hospital program, individuals participate in evidence-based modalities (classes, psychoeducation, evidence-based staff-led groups, and self-help groups) at least 3 to 4 hours per day, 5 days per week:

- *Evidence-based modalities* offered include social skills training, motivational interviewing, relapse prevention, contingency planning, recovery and 12-step groups, cognitive behavioral therapy, psychiatric assessment and evaluation, medication management, health and wellness, family psychoeducational and educational programs, peer support services, supported employment services, and community integration activities.
- *Optional adjunctive services* offered include occupational/recreational therapy, spirituality (individual or group), case management services, linkage to primary care/women's health services, and ongoing adjunctive individual and group therapy as deemed necessary for additional support.
- *Goals of recovery* in an evidence-based partial hospital program include increased independence, increased problem-solving ability, increased coping mechanisms, social competence (through community integration and social skills training), self-advocacy, and decreased feelings of stigmatization.

Because individuals' needs vary, the recovery program must be flexible, adaptive, and creative in order to provide structure and learning while supporting each individual's specific needs and place along the recovery continuum. Box 17-3 provides the phases of recovery in an integrated treatment program. Current evidence supports individualized, creatively developed, flexible treatment and recovery plans in which the care recipient is actively involved as a partner in the planning process.

Finally, the importance of early detection and screening of adolescents, adults, and the elderly for substance abuse problems is critical. Thus, screening processes and brief interventions that can be administered by nurses in primary or specialty care may facilitate early diagnosis and treatment, encourage engagement and retention in programs, and foster education and prevention, which are major foci of all recovery programs (Substance Abuse and Mental Health Services Administration, 2002; Substance Abuse and Mental Health Services Administration, 2006a). Laker (2007, p. 724) stated, "...delivery of a focused intervention by nurses that draws on skills of therapeutic engagement and effective communication could show

BOX 17-2 The 10 Fundamental Components of Recovery

Self-Direction: Consumers lead, control, exercise choice over, and determine their own path of recovery by optimizing autonomy, independence, and control of resources to achieve a self-determined life. By definition, the recovery process must be self-directed by the individual, who defines his or her own life goals and designs a unique path towards those goals.

Individualized and Person-Centered: There are multiple pathways to recovery based on an individual's unique strengths and resiliencies as well as his or her needs, preferences, experiences (including past trauma), and cultural background in all of its diverse representations. Individuals also identify recovery as being an ongoing journey and an end result as well as an overall paradigm for achieving wellness and optimal mental health.

Empowerment: Consumers have the authority to choose from a range of options and to participate in all decisions—including the allocation of resources—that will affect their lives, and are educated and supported in so doing. They have the ability to join with other consumers to collectively and effectively speak for themselves about their needs, wants, desires, and aspirations. Through empowerment, an individual gains control of his or her own destiny and influences the organizational and societal structures in his or her life.

Holistic: Recovery encompasses an individual's whole life, including mind, body, spirit, and community. Recovery embraces all aspects of life, including housing, employment, education, mental health and healthcare treatment and services, complementary and naturalistic services, addictions treatment, spirituality, creativity, social networks, community participation, and family supports as determined by the person. Families, providers, organizations, systems, communities, and society play crucial roles in creating and maintaining meaningful opportunities for consumer access to these supports.

Non-Linear: Recovery is not a step-by step process but one based on continual growth, occasional setbacks, and learning from experience. Recovery begins with an initial stage of awareness in which a person recognizes that positive change is possible. This awareness enables the consumer to move on to fully engage in the work of recovery.

Strengths-Based: Recovery focuses on valuing and building on the multiple capacities, resiliencies, talents, coping abilities, and inherent worth of individuals. By building on these strengths, consumers leave stymied life roles behind and engage in new life roles (e.g., partner, caregiver, friend, student, and employee). The process of recovery moves forward through interaction with others in supportive, trust-based relationships.

Peer Support: Mutual support—including the sharing of experiential knowledge and skills and social learning—plays an invaluable role in recovery. Consumers encourage and engage other consumers in recovery and provide each other with a sense of belonging, supportive relationships, valued roles, and community.

Respect: Community, systems, and societal acceptance and appreciation of consumers—including protecting their rights and eliminating discrimination and stigma—are crucial in achieving recovery. Self-acceptance and regaining belief in one's self are particularly vital. Respect ensures the inclusion and full participation of consumers in all aspects of their lives.

Responsibility: Consumers have a personal responsibility for their own self-care and journeys of recovery. Taking steps towards their goals may require great courage. Consumers must strive to understand and give meaning to their experiences and identify coping strategies and healing processes to promote their own wellness.

Hope: Recovery provides the essential and motivating message of a better future—that people can and do overcome the barriers and obstacles that confront them. Hope is internalized; but can be fostered by peers, families, friends, providers, and others. Hope is the catalyst of the recovery process. Mental health recovery not only benefits individuals with mental health disabilities by focusing on their abilities to live, work, learn, and fully participate in our society, but also enriches the texture of American community life. America reaps the benefits of the contributions individuals with mental disabilities can make, ultimately becoming a stronger and healthier Nation.

Source: National Consensus Statement on Mental Health Recovery, 2004, U.S. Dept of Health and Human Services; Substance Abuse and Mental Health Services Administration; Center for Mental Health Services. Retrieved from http://www.co.marion.or.us/HLT/CAPS/resources/SAMHSA.htm

benefits to patients [with COD]." The Screening, Brief Intervention, and Referral to Treatment (SBIRT) is an example of a comprehensive screening approach applicable for use in primary care to aid in detection and early intervention for those at risk for developing substance abuse problems (Substance Abuse and Mental Health Services Administration, 2011).

Finally, the Substance Abuse and Mental Health Services Administration's main concerns for delivery of services to individuals with CODs will be measured by the following performance indicators:

- *Percentage of persons with co-occurring disorders who receive appropriate treatment services that address both disorders (documented by responses on the National Survey on Drug Use and Health—NSDUH);*
- *Percentage of prevention and treatment settings that screen for COD, assess for COD, and provide treatment to clients through collaborative, consultative and integrated models of care (documented by the administrative records of SAMHSA's Co-Occurring State Incentive Grants for infrastructure development—COSIG);*
- *Number of people trained to implement appropriate co-occurring prevention and integrated treatments among States, communities, providers and consumers (documented by administrative records of SAMHSA's Co-Occurring Center for Excellence—COCE) (Fornili, 2008, pp. 113-114).*

BOX 17-3 Phases of Recovery in an Integrated Treatment Program

1. **Acute Stabilization—**Short term focused intervention to stabilize the acute manifestation of the disorder.
2. **Engagement and Motivational Enhancement—** Interventions designed to establish a primary clinical relationship and to facilitate the person's ability and motivation to initiate and maintain participation in a program of stabilizing treatment.
3. **Active Treatment to Maintain Stabilization—**Interventions of any type which are designed to stabilize the symptoms of the disorder, prevent relapse, and help individuals to maintain a stable baseline and optimal level of functioning.
4. **Rehabilitation and Recovery—**Interventions designed to help individuals to develop new skills, reacquire old skills, and achieve personal growth and serenity, once prolonged stabilization has been consistently established.

Source: American Association of Community Psychiatrists. (2000). Principles for the care and treatment of individuals with co-occurring psychiatric and substance disorders. Retrieved from www.comm.psych.pitt.edu/finds/dualdx.html

Self-Help Recovery Groups

Comparison studies that include self-help models for individuals with COD have emerged in recent years (Bellack & Gearon, 1998; Bogenschutz, 2005; Bogenschutz et al., 2006; Brooks & Penn, 2003; Dinitto, Webb, Rubin, et al., 2001; Galanter, Dermatis, Egelko, et al., 1998; Humphreys, Huebsch, Finney, et al., 1999; Jordan, Davidson, Herman, et al., 2002; Kelly, McKellar, Moos, et al., 2003; Meissen, Powell, Wituk, et al., 1999; Moos, Moos, & Andrassy, 1999; Ouimette, Gima, Moos, et al., 1999; Pristach & Smith, 1999; Tsuang & Fong, 2004). For example, the 12-step-based "self-help fellowship" recovery program has been both criticized and applauded, and even now it competes with traditional approaches in programs in which the concept of client empowerment has not been embraced. Brooks and Penn (2003) compared 12-step self-help with a therapist-led cognitive behavioral therapy approach for "dual diagnosis." They found the treatment approaches to be similar and complementary: "Each approach has different benefits and a blending of the strengths of each approach may be necessary in treating dually diagnosed individuals" (p. 379).

Questions have been raised as to whether an individual with a psychiatric diagnosis such as schizophrenia has the social wherewithal to fully participate in self-help groups. Although self-help groups have been known to help those with SUDs *without* comorbid psychiatric disorders, little is known about whether self-help groups actually help individuals *with* COD. Bogenschutz et al. (2006) reported, however, that individuals with COD attended 12-step meetings at comparable rates to those without COD (with the exception of individuals with active psychosis), and involvement in these groups has been consistently associated with positive outcomes.

Alcoholics Anonymous (AA)

AA has been called "the largest self-help recovery movement in this country" (Bristow-Braitman, 1995, p. 414) and "one of the *most important and valuable social movements of the 20th century*" (Smith, 1994, p. 111, emphasis added). But barriers to full immersion in the 12 steps and the spiritual concept of "*surrendering to a higher power*"—a core belief in AA that requires humility and letting go (in essence, powerlessness)—can be very difficult for some (Alcoholics Anonymous "The Big Book," 2001), especially those with PTSD and comorbid substance abuse (Satel, Becker, & Dan, 1993). However, another study found that individuals with PTSD and SUDs who participated in 12-step recovery groups benefited from their involvement (Ouimette, Humphries, Moos, et al., 2001).

Peteet (1993) revealed one explanation for the success of AA: "Twelve step programs...stress the need to acknowledge moral failure, begin restitution, repair defects of character and begin to be of service to others...[convert] guilt to altruism.... [T]hrough this process of repentance [members] report a renewed sense of integrity" (p. 265). Twelve-step "fellowships" are also successful in filling a void for some, in that they "offer what intact families, religious communities and other institutions provided at an earlier time" (Peteet, p. 266). Some individuals fear that AA will try to force religion on participants, which is not the case; however, spiritual growth is an expected part (and a generally serendipitous benefit) of 12-step programs, and members without religious beliefs have benefitted. Many who enter AA as atheists or agnostics renew their religious faith and reconnect to God, although participation is not reserved for any particular denomination or religious group: the "only requirement for membership is a desire to stop drinking" (AA Preamble, n.d.).

Gonzalez & Rosenheck (2002) compared a large cohort of over 5,000 homeless individuals with serious and persistent mental illness (SPMI) with and without a co-occurring SUD. The individuals with SPMI and a co-occurring SUD were more ill at baseline; however, the individuals with SPMI and a co-occurring alcohol use disorder who participated extensively in self-help groups had "superior" outcomes as compared with other individuals with COD. These authors concluded, "Adequate treatment of this population seems to demand the availability of both intensive clinical services and the facilitation of referrals to self-help groups" (p. 445). Self-help models are considered valuable and are associated with consistently positive outcomes (Jerrell & Ridgely, 1995; Laudet, Magura, Cleland, et al., 2003; Laudet, Magura, Cleland, et al., 2004; Magura, Knight, Vogel, et al., 2003a; Timko & Sempel, 2004; Vogel, Knight, Laudet, et al., 1998), such as "increased abstinence from 54% at baseline to 72% at follow-up" (Magura, Laudet, Mamood, et al., 2003b, p. 408) and better adherence to medication regimens (Magura, Laudet, Mahmood, et al., 2002).

AA participants report that prescription medications are no longer a taboo subject for discussion, as was the case in the past, because more individuals recovering from alcohol dependence take psychotropic medication than previously. In one study of 125 contact individuals representing AA, 93% reported that they would encourage other recovering individuals to continue to take medication (Meissen et al., 1999). And contrary to popular belief, AA is not opposed to properly supervised and prescribed medication by a licensed health-care provider (Decker & Ries, 1993).

Case Study 17-1 presents a patient with COD.

Co-occurring Disorder Special Populations

As discussed earlier in this chapter, navigating life can be especially difficult for individuals with complex psychiatric and physical comorbidities (Mannynsalo, Putkonen, Lindberg, et al., 2009). We have discussed how CODs such as substance abuse, psychiatric illness, personality disorders, intellectual or cognitive deficits, and medical problems can overlap, compound, and complicate diagnosis

CASE STUDY 17-1

A Patient with Co-occurring Disorder

The patient is a 28-year-old single white female who is referred for psychiatric evaluation at the request of her primary care provider owing to ongoing depressed mood and intermittent suicidal ideation.

Chief complaint

"I am miserable."

History of Presenting Illness (HPI)

Patient presents with depressed mood that is accompanied by marked anhedonia that lasts 2 weeks at a time. She also reports intermittent suicidal ideation, but no plan or intent because of religious convictions. She reports two or three periods in the last year (or maybe longer) when she has experienced rapid speech, racing thoughts, flight of ideas, and marked irritability that is exacerbated around the time of menses. During these periods she has trouble sleeping, which causes difficulty with focus and concentration the next day. She reports periods of anger that borders on rage when she feels like impulsively throwing things. She denies assaulting people or harming animals. She has been having increasing trouble at work with coworkers and her supervisor. She reports that certain coworkers give her assignments, which she resents because "they are not the boss," and she has become angry, resentful, passive-aggressive, and sullen at work. Her supervisor, noticing the behavior, suggested that she see an outside counselor or the company employee assistance representative. She resents this suggestion and being forced to come in for the evaluation.

Past Psychiatric History (PPH)

No history of inpatient psychiatric admissions or drug/ETOH rehabs. She reports at least two prior outpatient psychiatric treatment providers. She reports outpatient counseling as a teenager for "self-injurious behavior." She has had many medication trials that she claims have had little or no effect or have had intolerable side effects.

Developmental History

Normal birth by vaginal delivery, no complications, no developmental delays. She grew up in a suburb outside of Chicago in an intact home. She is the second youngest of six children, the youngest girl. She was raised by devout Roman Catholic parents and has a brother who is a priest and a sister who is a nun. Reports a happy childhood. Mom was the disciplinarian, Dad more quiet and reserved. Denies physical or sexual abuse. In her late teens, she became somewhat rebellious. She reports heavy drinking, acquisition of tattoos and piercings, riding motorcycles, and at one time owning a gun.

Educational/Occupational History

Attended Catholic elementary and secondary schools and college. Received a BA in Business. Reports good grades throughout academic career. Denies school failures or learning disability. Reports that one psychiatrist diagnosed her with ADD as an adult, but Ritalin had no effect. Since graduation from college she has worked as an Administrative Assistant to the Bishop in her local diocese.

Medical History

Essentially negative, denies chronic illness, surgeries, allergies, head injuries, or seizure history. No medications at this time. Denies any sexual activity and has not seen an OB-GYN for routine testing due to "embarrassment." Nonsmoker, nondrinker, denies illicit substance use.

Legal History

No arrests or incarcerations.

Family Psychiatric History

Father treated for depression. One sister treated for depression and is described as alcohol dependent. Denies family history of suicides.

Mental Status Examination (MSE)

Medium tall (5′6″), Caucasian female. Dark, well-kept conservative hairstyle. Wears glasses. Tattoo on R upper arm of an angel, shows through under shawl and short-sleeved dress. Appropriate dress for weather and situation. Good eye contact throughout examination. Soft-spoken, articulates well. Answers questions but speech is mostly nonspontaneous. Mood—"depressed." Affect—constricted. Thoughts—goal directed. Thought content—no delusions, illusions, paranoia, but admits "suspiciousness" with coworkers. Denies a/v hallucinations, admits to occasional suicidal ideation. Cognition is overall intact, can abstract and calculate, but responses are slowed. Short- and long-term memory within normal limits, can recall 3/3 after 5 minutes. Insight—poor, has no understanding of symptoms or illness.

Questions

1. What are your diagnostic impressions?
2. How would you proceed with a treatment/recovery plan for this patient?

Answers to these questions can be found at the end of this chapter.

and treatment for each disorder. We will now discuss how CODs can affect special population groups.

Some subgroups of individuals are more severely ill, both in terms of psychiatric illness and substance use. These individuals require specialized intensive treatment modalities to achieve and maintain stability and work toward recovery goals. It is not possible within the scope of this chapter to address each subgroup in detail; however, an introductory discussion is offered below.

Individuals With Co-occurring Post-traumatic Stress Disorder, Sexual Trauma, and Substance Use Disorder

The correlation between PTSD and substance abuse has been well documented. Individuals with co-occurring PTSD and SUDs are reported to have 25% to 50% lifetime prevalence of SUDs, lower functionality, poorer well-being, and poorer outcomes on a number of measures (Najavits, 2007; Schafer & Najavits, 2007). In addition, the relationship between combat-related PTSD, military sexual trauma, co-occurring SUDs, and suicide has become a salient issue and an area in need of further study (Substance Abuse and Mental Health Services Administration, 2007). Research has supported that individuals with the foregoing CODs are in need of highly specialized evidence-based treatment programs, such as "Seeking Safety" (Najavits, 2007). Indeed, treatment of PTSD and co-occurring SUDs with or without a history of sexual abuse requires planned programming and appropriate clinical supervision of staff, and it should be undertaken only by therapists who are specifically trained in both PTSD and SUD. Well-meaning therapists who are not adequately prepared and encourage exploration of traumatic memories can destabilize individuals, which may lead to re-traumatization and a cascade of symptoms resulting in psychiatric decompensation, increased substance use or relapse, suicidal thoughts, and possible hospitalization (Najavits, 2007). Fornili (2008) stated that treatment outcomes for women with COD may be influenced by whether the program has adopted a "trauma informed treatment philosophy" (p. 116). *Trauma informed* is an environment that adheres to boundaries, uses empowering language, and avoids shaming and punitive approaches (Fornili). According to the findings by Clark et al. (2005), staff should avoid coercive or controlling measures to retain women with CODs and abuse histories in treatment.

Individuals With Co-occurring Traumatic Brain Injury, Psychiatric Illness, and Substance Use Disorder

The prevalence of Axis I diagnoses after TBI is estimated to be 44%, with the most frequent diagnoses being major depression and anxiety disorders (Alderfer et al., 2005; Hibbard et al., 1998). In addition, an estimated 49% to 74% of individuals report personality changes after TBI (Arciniegas & Silver, 2006; Arciniegas, Topkoff, & Silver, 2000).

Individuals who have suffered a TBI are irritable, impulsive, and subject to angry outbursts, seemingly unprovoked. In addition, these individuals may struggle with depression, PTSD, headaches, or constant pain. As a result of pain and depression, they are not sleeping and thus may begin to drink and develop alcohol dependence. These actions have ramifications on family and marital relationships. Family members may not understand why there are changes in their loved one's personality; they may not understand why their afflicted family member becomes unpredictably angry or irritable, and why the family member has no interest in doing things that the family used to enjoy together. In addition to emotional and psychological changes, problematic behaviors ranging from inappropriate touching to assault owing to disinhibition and aggressiveness can manifest. Excessive acute neurotransmitter release at the time of injury can be responsible for problems with memory, attention, slowed processing, anxiety, depression, irritability, agitation, disinhibition, apathy, mania, or psychosis.

Interestingly, an estimated 38% of individuals with brain injury had SUDs and CODs, including sociopathic and behavioral problems, *before* brain injury. In addition, it has been reported that alcohol or drug use *causes* 50% of all TBIs in individuals who are under 40 years of age (Hibbard et al., 1998; Silver, Kramer, Greenwald, et al., 2001; Silver, Hales, & Yudofsky, 2002). According to Silver et al. (2002), "...a history of substance abuse has been associated with increased morbidity and mortality" after TBI (p. 633). The sequence and severity of events could be important prognostic indicators, could impact rehabilitation, and could create vulnerabilities to complex comorbidities after brain injury; thus, thorough chronological medical and psychiatric histories are essential.

Individuals With Co-occurring Bipolar Affective Disorder and Substance Use Disorder

Approximately 40% to 60% of individuals diagnosed with bipolar disorder have a co-occurring SUD. Anxiety disorders and bipolar disorder co-occur approximately 24% to 42% of the time, and personality disorders and bipolar disorder co-occur approximately 30% of the time (Suppes & Keck, 2005, pp. 5-14).When any of these conditions co-occur in addition to substance dependence, patients can be in crisis until the condition(s) stabilize. Moreover, substance abuse can contribute to rapid cycling in individuals with bipolar disorder (Brown et al., 2002; Suppes & Keck). Rapid cycling is defined as four mood episodes within a 12-month period that comprise symptoms that are distinct from the individual's usual functioning, and these episodes meet criteria for a major depressive, manic, hypomanic, or mixed state. Alcohol abuse—which occurs in as many as 50% in those diagnosed with bipolar disorder—may worsen the course, severity, and prognosis of bipolar disorder (Suppes & Dennehy, 2005) and put individuals at high risk for suicide, because individuals with bipolar disorder have 10% to 15% lifetime suicide rates (Suppes & Keck, pp. 4-19), even without the added risk of alcohol use and the mood changes it can produce. Individuals with bipolar disorder and co-occurring SUDs are reported to be significantly more impaired than individuals with other psychiatric illnesses and SUDs (Pollack, Cramer, & Varner, 2000; Suppes & Keck). Bipolar disorder and SUDs are reported to manifest in a cyclical fashion: psychiatric symptoms can precipitate relapse into drug or alcohol use, or drug or alcohol use can evoke psychiatric symptoms, and the cycling continues. For example, an estimated 92% of individuals with bipolar disorder describe a relapse prodrome of heightened anxiety, sleep disturbance, and irritability leading to medication nonadherence, drug or alcohol relapse, or both. Individuals with co-occurring alcohol dependence and bipolar depression are a subgroup that has a poorer prognosis overall than those who have bipolar disorder or SUD alone (Farren & McElroy, 2008).

Aggressive pharmacological intervention or hospitalization may be required to stabilize acute psychiatric symptoms, such as severe mania, depression, or psychosis. Because mood stabilization is the priority for an individual experiencing a cycling mood disorder, a mood stabilizer is the treatment of choice for bipolar disorder and co-occurring SUD (provided that the medication can be safely prescribed and that there are no contraindications). There are a number of FDA-approved mood stabilizing agents from which to choose, including anticonvulsants, lithium, and atypical antipsychotics. Studies that examine the efficacy of medication for individuals with bipolar disorder who have co-occurring SUDs are needed. One such study conducted by Kosten and Kosten (2004) reviewed the literature on pharmacological agents and suggested valproate as an efficacious agent for this population owing to its GABA-enhancing properties. Psychopharmacological interventions that may be useful in treating individuals with CODs were discussed earlier in this chapter, and general information on psychopharmacology can be found in Chapter 6 of this text.

Individuals With Co-occurring Personality Disorder and Substance Use Disorder

Active substance use coupled with a personality disorder—in particular, an Axis II, Cluster B personality disorder—will present great challenges to the psychiatric advanced practice nurse. In the absence of an Axis I psychiatric diagnosis, medication is generally not indicated; however, it can be useful for certain target symptoms, such as impulsivity, aggression, lability, mood symptoms, and transient intermittent psychosis (Stern & Herman, 2004).

Depending on the type of personality disorder and the individual's current stage of organization, certain therapeutic models of psychotherapy can be used. Interventions will likely be time- and labor-intensive, and gains may be minimal. Individuals with personality disorders—even in the absence of a co-occurring SUD—can be extremely challenging, can take up inordinate amounts of staff time, and can contribute to strong feelings of countertransference, particularly anger, frustration, and helplessness. Burnout among care professionals is very possible when working with individuals diagnosed with personality disorders. Sacks, Skinner, Sacks, et al. (2002) stated that when "antisocial personality features are present in (homeless) MICA individuals" there can be "personality disturbance characterized by poor frustration tolerance, poor impulse control, and problems with authority" (p. 5).

One longitudinal study completed on 750 adolescents collected data on subjects at a mean age of 16 and at a mean age of 22 to compare the effects of Axis I psychiatric disorders and Axis II personality disorders on quality of life in this population. The authors reported that personality disorders—especially those in Cluster B—had lasting negative effects on quality of life that were sustained over time in this study population. Also, those youths with comorbid Axis I and Axis II disorders had the worst outcomes as compared to those with either an Axis I or Axis II disorder (Chen, Cohen, Kasen, et al., 2006). Individuals with Axis II, Cluster B personality disorders, especially when "drug-seeking," present special challenges that require intervention by a seasoned provider. Individuals with an Axis II, Cluster B personality disorder have been noted to use intimidation tactics, emotional or psychological abuse, manipulation, or the threat of violence in order to have their needs met or wants fulfilled. In general, many individuals with Cluster B antisocial personality disorder and co-occurring SUDs are found in the forensic setting. To be effective and therapeutic with this subpopulation of individuals, the psychiatric advanced practice nurse needs to be experienced, clinically competent, able to set limits, able to maintain clear boundaries, and impervious to intimidation. See Chapter 18 of this text for further reading on Personality Disorders.

Summary

Individuals with COD will present to practitioners in every area of health care. Their needs are diverse and challenging. These men, women, and children represent all racial, religious, and cultural groups. Costs to care for them are burdensome, and delivery of services will continue to be under budgetary scrutiny. Therefore, evidence-based programs and research to support and document ongoing clinical and performance outcomes are necessary. As Tiet and Mausbach

(2007) described, "The current status of the literature, unfortunately is so poor that urgent attention by researchers and funding agencies is needed to conduct more and more methodologically rigorous research in this area given the high prevalence of dual diagnosis patients " (p. 534).

In sum, psychiatric advanced practice nurses must embark on a multifaceted campaign to secure funding and develop creative, *integrated* treatment (and recovery) programs. We must work for change in the behavioral health-care delivery systems to provide positive, desirable, and sustainable evidence-based outcomes. Most importantly, we must provide *hope* for our fellow human beings who are diagnosed with COD.

Key Points

- Although biology can account for much in the field of psychiatric disorders, the evidence for an emphasis on the psychosocial aspects of CODs cannot be understated.
- Because the research on CODs, though voluminous, covers very diverse foci, multiple intervention strategies, and heterogeneous populations, it is difficult to generalize results of studies to determine which interventions are most effective in real-world practice.
- Clearly, some interventions show promise (e.g., evidence-based modalities such as cognitive behavioral therapy and motivational interviewing), but more studies are needed, especially to determine long-term positive clinical outcomes.
- Evidence-based studies based on nursing science are seriously lacking in the literature.
- Persons with CODs must be offered integrated treatment programs staffed by certified cross-trained professionals who are clinically competent to address both the individual's psychiatric disorder and his or her chemical dependence. These services should be delivered by the same team, in the same program, at the same site. To deliver best care, ongoing clinical supervision and collaboration with an expert who is also credentialed is paramount.
- Psychiatric advanced practice nurses who are board certified in psychiatry and addictions are competent and well positioned to take the lead on Substance Abuse and Mental Health Services Administration's initiatives (http://www.samhsa.gov/about/strategy.aspx) to address the needs, develop and evaluate programs, and influence policy for the COD population in their respective agencies or states or at the national level.
- Integrated treatment and recovery programs must be patient centered, must be delivered in a systematic manner, and must address all the patient's needs concurrently: crisis intervention/acute psychiatric stabilization or detoxification, long-term maintenance of psychiatric stability, and relapse prevention.
- The biopsychosocial, spiritual, holistic, health-promoting, disease-prevention, and teaching orientation of psychiatric advanced practice nurses makes them particularly suited to work with this challenging group of patients.

Resources

Organizations

Double Trouble in Recovery
c/o Mental Health Empowerment Project
271 Central Avenue
Albany, NY 12209
518-434-1393
www.doubletroubleinrecovery.org

Dual Diagnosis Anonymous
320 North E. Street, Suite 207
San Bernardino, CA 92401
909-888-9282

Dual Disorders Anonymous
PO Box 681264
Schaumburg, IL 60168
847-781-1553

Dual Recovery Anonymous World Services, Inc
PO Box 8107
Prairie Village, KS 66208
877-833-2332
www.draonline.org

Dual Diagnosis Recovery Network (DDRN)
220 Venture Circle
Nashville, TN 37228
888-869-9230
www.dualdiagnosis.org

The National GAINS Center for People with Co-occurring Disorders in the Justice System
http://gainsctr.com

Substance Abuse and Mental Health Services Administration (SAMHSA) http://www.samhsa.gov/index.aspx

- Center for Substance Abuse Prevention, http://prevention.samhsa.gov
- Center for Substance Abuse Treatment, http://csat.samhsa.gov
- Co-occurring dialogues electronic discussion list, http://www.treatment.org/Topics/DualDialogues.html
- Substance Abuse and Mental Health Services Administration Co-Occurring Center for Excellence, http://coce.samhsa.gov

Support Together for Emotional and Mental Serenity and Sobriety (STEMSS)
Michael G. Bricker, Executive Director
STEMSS Institute and Bricker Clinic
140 E. Dekora Street
Saukville, WI 53080
414-268-0899

Consumer Organization and Networking Technical Assistance Center (CONTAC)

1036 Quarrier Street, Suite 208A
Charleston, WV 25891
304-346-9992 or 888-825-8324
www.contac.org

National Council on Alcoholism and Drug Dependence (NCADD)
20 Exchange Place, Suite 2902
New York, NY 10005
Tel 212-269-7797; Fax: 212-269-7510

National Empowerment Center
599 Canal Street
Lawrence, MA 01840
800-769-3728
www.power2u.org

National Mental Health Association
1021 Prince Street
Alexandria, VA 22314-2971
800-969-6642; TTY: 800-433-5959
www.nmha.org

National Mental Health Consumers' Self-Help Clearinghouse
1211 Chestnut Street, Suite 1207
Philadelphia, PA 19107
800-553-4KEY
www.mhselfhelp.org

Movies

Mangold, J. (Director). (2005). *Walk the line* [Motion picture]. United States: 20th Century Fox.

MacGillivray, W. D. (Director). (2010). *The man of a thousand songs* [Documentary]. United States.

Frappier, R., & Vandal, L. (Producers) & Aubert, R. (Director). (2010). *Crying out* [Motion picture]. Canada: TVA Films. (Source: http://www.siff.net/festival/film/detail.aspx?id=44340&fid=206)

References

Abrantes, A. M., Brown, S. A., & Tomlinson, K. L. (2003). Psychiatric co-morbidity among inpatient substance-abusing adolescents. *Journal of Child and Adolescent Substance Abuse, 13*(2), 83-101.

Albanese, M., & Suh, J. (2006). Risperidone in cocaine-dependent patients with co-morbid psychiatric disorders. *Journal of Psychiatric Practice, 12*(5), 306-311.

Alcoholics Anonymous. (2001). *Alcoholics Anonymous: The story of how many thousands of men and women have recovered from alcoholism* ["The Big Book"] (4th ed.). New York: Alcoholics Anonymous World Service Inc.

Alcoholics Anonymous. (n.d.) Preamble. Retrieved from www.aa.org/lansg/en/en_pdfs/smf-92_en.pdf

Alderfer, B., Arciniegas, D., & Silver, J. (2005). Treatment of depression following traumatic brain injury. *Journal of Head Trauma Rehabilitation, 20*(6), 544-562.

Alverson, H., Alverson, M., & Drake. R. E. (2000). An ethnographic study of the longitudinal course of substance abuse among people with severe mental illness. *Community Mental Health Journal, 36*(6), 557-569.

Alvidrez, J., & Havassy, B. E. (2005). Racial distribution of dual-diagnosis clients in public sector mental health and drug treatment settings. *Journal of Health Care for the Poor and Under-Served, 16*(1), 53-62.

American Association of Community Psychiatrists. (2000). *Principles for the care and treatment of individuals with co-occurring psychiatric and substance disorders.* Retrieved from www.comm.psych.pitt.edu/finds/dualdx.html

American Psychiatric Association. (2000). *Diagnostic and statistical manual of mental disorders* (4th ed., text rev.). Washington, DC: American Psychiatric Publishing, Inc.

Arciniegas, D., & Silver, J. (2006). Pharmacotherapy of post-traumatic cognitive impairments. *Behavioral Neurology, 17*(1), 25-42.

Arciniegas, D., Topkoff, J., & Silver, J. (2000). Neuropsychiatric aspects of traumatic brain injury. *Current Treatment Options in Neurology, 2*(2), 169-186.

Avants, S., Margolin, A., DePhilippis, D., et al. (1998). A comprehensive pharmacologic-psychosocial treatment program for HIV-seropositive cocaine and opioid dependent patients. *Journal of Substance Abuse Treatment, 15*, 261-265.

Babor, T. F., de la Fuente, J. R., Saunders, J., et al. (1992). *AUDIT, The Alcohol Use Disorders Identification Test: Guidelines for use in primary health care.* Geneva: World Health Organization.

Becker, W., Fiellen, D., & Desai, R. (2007). Non-medical use, abuse and dependence on sedatives and tranquilizers among U.S. adults: Psychiatric and socio-demographic correlates. *Drug and Alcohol Dependence, 90*(2-3), 280-287.

Bellack, A., & Gearon, J. (1998). Substance abuse treatment for people with schizophrenia. *Addictive Behaviors, 23*(6), 749-766.

Bellg, A., Borrelli, B., Resnick, B., et al. (2004). Enhancing treatment fidelity in health behavior change studies: Best practices and recommendations from the NIH behavior change consortium. *Health Psychology,* 23(5), 443-451.

Biederman, J., Wilens, T., Mick, E., et al. (1999). Pharmacotherapy of attention-deficit/hyperactivity disorder reduces risk for substance-use disorder. *Pediatrics, 104*(2), e20.

Bogenschutz, M. (2005). Specialized 12-step programs and 12-step facilitation for the dually diagnosed. *Community Mental Health Journal, 41*(1), 7-20.

Bogenschutz, M., Geppart, C., & George, J. (2006). The role of twelve-step approaches in dual-diagnosis treatment and recovery. *The American Journal on Addictions, 15*, 50-60.

Bohn, D. K. (2003). Lifetime physical and sexual abuse, substance abuse, depression and suicide attempts among Native-American women. *Issues in Mental Health Nursing, 24*(3), 333-352.

Breakey, W. R., Calabrese, L., Rosenblatt, A., et al. (1998). Detecting alcohol use disorders in the severely mentally ill. *Community Mental Health Journal, 34*(2), 165-174.

Brems, C., Johnson, M. E., Bowers, L., et al. (2002). Co-morbidity training needs at a state psychiatric hospital. *Administration & Policy in Mental Health, 30*(2), 109-120.

Bricker, M. G. (1994). The STEMSS supported self-help model for dual diagnosis recovery: Applications for rural settings. In M. Groves, et al. (Eds.). *Treating alcohol and other drug abusers in rural and frontier areas* (pp. 93-108). Technical Assistance Publication (TAP) Series 17. Awards for Excellence Papers. Rockville, MD: U.S. Department of Health and Human Services/Substance Abuse and Mental Health Services Administration. Available at http://kap.samhsa.gov/products/manuals/taps/17k.htm

Bristow-Braitman, A. (1995). Addiction recovery: 12-Step programs and cognitive-behavioral psychology. *Journal of Counseling and Development, 73*, 414-418.

Brooks, A., & Penn, P. (2003). Comparing treatments for dual diagnosis: Twelve-step and self-management and recovery training. *American Journal of Drug and Alcohol Abuse, 29*(2), 359-383.

Brooner, R., King, L., Kidorf, M., et al. (1997). Psychiatric and substance use comorbidity among treatment-seeking opioid abusers. *Archives of General Psychiatry, 54*(1), 71-80.

Brown, E. S., Nejtek, V. A., Perantie, D. C., et al. (2002). Quetiapine in bipolar disorder and cocaine dependence. *Bipolar Disorders, 4*(6), 406-411.

Brown, E. S., Nejtek, V. A., Perantie, D. C., et al. (2003). Lamotrigine in patients with bipolar disorder and cocaine dependence. *Journal of Clinical Psychiatry, 64*(2), 197-201.

Brown, V., & Melchior, L. (2008). Women with co-occurring disorders (COD): Treatment settings and service needs. *Journal of Psychoactive Drugs, Nov*(Suppl 5), 365-376.

Brunette, M., Asher, D., & Whitley, R. (2008). Implementation of integrated dual disorders treatment: A qualitative analysis of factors and barriers. *Psychiatric Services, 59*, 989-995.

Brunette, M., & Drake, R. E. (1998). Gender differences in homeless individuals with schizophrenia and substance abuse. *Community Mental Health Journal, 34*(6), 627-642.

Carroll, K., Nich, C., & Rounsaville, B. (1995). Differential symptom reduction in depressed cocaine abusers treated with psychotherapy and pharmacotherapy. *The Journal of Nervous and Mental Disease, 183*(4), 251-259.

Center for Mental Health Services. (2003). *Integrated dual disorders treatment fidelity scale. Co-occurring disorders: Integrated dual disorders treatment implementation resource kit.* Rockville, MD: Substance Abuse and Mental Health Services Administration.

Center for Substance Abuse Treatment. (1998). *Substance abuse among older adults.* Treatment Improvement Protocol (TIP) Series 26. Retrieved from http://www.ncbi.nlm.nih.gov/books/bv.fcgi?rid=hstat5.chapter.48302

Center for Substance Abuse Treatment. (2005). *Substance abuse treatment for persons with co-occurring disorders.* Treatment Improvement Protocol (TIP) Series 42. DHHS Publication No. (SMA) 08-3992. Rockville, MD: Substance Abuse and Mental Health Services Administration. Available at http://www.fadaa.org/services/resource_center/PD/WebEx/Tip42.pdf

Center for Substance Abuse Treatment. (2007a). *Definitions and terms relating to co-occurring disorders.* COCE Overview Paper 1. DHHS Publication No. (SMA) 07-4163. Rockville, MD: Substance Abuse and Mental Health Services Administration, and Center for Mental Health Services. Available at http://www.atforum.com/addiction-resources/documents/OP1-DefinitionsandTerms-8-13-07.pdf

Center for Substance Abuse Treatment. (2007b). *Understanding evidence-based practices for co-occurring disorders.* COCE Overview Paper 5. DHHS Publication No. (SMA) 07-4278. Rockville, MD: Substance Abuse and Mental Health Services Administration, and Center for Mental Health Services. Available at http://store.samhsa.gov/shin/content/SMA07-4278/SMA07-4278.pdf

Center for Substance Abuse Treatment. (2007c). *The epidemiology of co-occurring substance use and mental disorders.* COCE Overview Paper 8. DHHS Publication No. (SMA) 07-4308. Rockville, MD: Substance Abuse and Mental Health Services Administration, and Center for Mental Health Services. Available at http://www.samhsa.gov/co-occurring/topics/data/OP8Epidemiology10-03-07.pdf

Center for Substance Abuse Treatment. (2009). *Incorporating alcohol pharmacotherapies into medical practice.* Treatment Improvement Protocol (TIP) Series 49. DHHS Publication No. (SMA) 09-4380. Rockville, MD: Substance Abuse and Mental Health Services Administration, and Center for Mental Health Services. Available at http://kap.samhsa.gov/products/manuals/tips/pdf/TIP49.pdf

Chen, H., Cohen, P., Kasen, S., et al. (2006). Adolescent axis I and personality disorders predict quality of life during young adulthood. *Journal of Adolescent Health, 39*(1), 14-19.

Clark, C., Becker, M., Giard, J., et al. (2005). The role of coercion in the treatment of women with co-occurring disorders and histories of abuse. *Journal of Behavioral Health Services and Research, 32*(2), 167-181.

Clark, H. W., Masson, C. L., Delucchi, K. L., et al. (2001). Violent traumatic events in drug abuse severity. *Journal of Substance Abuse Treatment, 20*(2), 121-127.

Cleary, M., Hunt, G., Matheson, S., et al. (2009). Psychosocial treatments for people with co-occurring severe mental illness and substance misuse: Systematic review. *Journal of Advanced Nursing, 65*(2), 238-258.

Cleminshaw, H., Shepler, R., & Newman, I. (2005). The Integrated Co-Occurring Treatment (ICT) model: A promising practice for youths with mental health and substance abuse disorders. *Journal of Dual Diagnosis, 1*(3), 85-94.

Cornelius, J., Salloum, I., Ehler, J., et al. (1997). Fluoxetine in depressed alcoholics: A double-blind, placebo-controlled trial. *Archives of General Psychiatry, 54*(8), 700-705.

Cornelius, J., Salloum, I., Haskett, R., et al. (1999). Fluoxetine versus placebo for the marijuana use of depressed alcoholics. *Addictive Behaviors, 24*(1), 111-114.

Davis, L., Rush, J., Wisniewski, S., et al. (2005). Substance use co-morbidity in major depressive disorder: An exploratory analysis of the sequenced treatment alternatives to relieve depression (STAR-D) cohort. *Comprehensive Psychiatry, 46*, 81-89.

Decker, K., & Ries, R. (1993). Differential diagnosis and psychopharmacology of dual disorders. *Psychiatric Clinics of North America, 16*(4), 703-718.

Dickey, B., Dembling, B., Azeni, H., et al. (2004). Externally caused deaths for adults with substance use and mental disorders. *Journal of Behavioral Health Services and Research, 31*(1), 75-85.

Dinitto, D., Webb, D., Rubin, A., et al. (2001). Self-help group meeting attendance among clients with dual diagnosis. *Journal of Psychoactive Drugs, 33*(3), 263-272.

Douaihy, A. B., Jou, R. J., Gorske, T., et al. (2003). Triple diagnosis: Dual diagnosis and HIV disease, part 2. *The AIDS Reader, 13*(8), 375-382.

Drake, R. E., Essock, S. M., Carey, K. B., et al. (2001). Implementing dual diagnosis services for clients with severe mental illness. *Psychiatric Services, 52*, 469-476.

Drake, R. E., Mercer-McFadden, C., Mueser, K. T., et al. (1998). Review of integrated mental health and substance abuse treatment for patients with dual disorders. *Schizophrenia Bulletin, 24*(4), 589-608.

Drake, R. E., & Mueser, K. T. (2000). Psychosocial approaches to dual diagnosis. *Schizophrenia Bulletin, 26*(1), 105-118.

Drake, R. E., Mueser, K. T., Brunette, M. F., et al. (2004). A review of treatments for people with severe mental illnesses and co-occurring substance use disorders. *Psychiatric Rehabilitation Journal, 27*(4), 360-374.

Drake, R. E., O'Neal, E. L., & Wallach, M. A. (2008). A systematic review of psychosocial research on psychosocial interventions for people with co-occurring severe mental and substance use disorders. *Journal of Substance Abuse Treatment, 34*, 123-138.

Drake, R. E., Yovetich, N. A., Bebout, R. R., et al. (1997). Integrated treatment for dually diagnosed homeless adults. *The Journal of Nervous and Mental Disease, 185*(5), 298-305.

Ewing, J. (1984). Detecting alcoholism: The CAGE questionnaire. *Journal of the American Medical Association, 254*(14), 1905-1907.

Farren, C., & McElroy, S. (2008). Treatment response of bipolar and unipolar alcoholics to an inpatient dual diagnosis program. *Journal of Affective Disorders, 106*(3), 265-272.

Finkelstein, N., Rechberger, E., Russell, L. A., et al. (2005). Building resilience in children of mothers who have co-occurring disorders and histories of violence: Intervention model and implementation issues. *Journal of Behavioral Health Services and Research, 32*(2), 141-154.

Finnell, D. (2003). Use of the transtheoretical model for individuals with co-occurring disorders. *Community Mental Health Journal, 39*(1), 3-15.

Fisher, M. S., & Bentley, K. J. (1996). Two group therapy models for clients with a dual-diagnosis of substance abuse and personality disorder. *Psychiatric Services, 47*(11), 1244-1250.

Folstein, M., Folstein, S., & McHugh, P. (1975). Mini-mental state: A practical method for grading the cognitive state of patients for the clinician. *Journal of Psychiatric Research, 12*, 189-198.

Fornili, K. (2008). Integrated treatment for women with co-occurring disorders and an explanatory model for policy analysis and evaluation. *Journal of Addictions Nursing, 19*(2), 109-118.

Fornili, K., & Baird, C. (2008). Effective health care delivery and integrated behavioral health screening. *Journal of Addictions Nursing, 19*(3), 174-177.

Fudala, P., Bridge, T., Herbert, S., et al. (2003). Office-based treatment of opiate addiction with sublingual-tablet formulation of buprenorphine and naloxone. *The New England Journal of Medicine, 349*(10), 949-958.

Galanter, M., Dermatis, H., Egelko, S., et al. (1998). Homelessness and mental illness in a professional and peer-led cocaine treatment clinic. *Psychiatric Services, 49*(4), 533-535.

Geller, B., Cooper, T., Sun, K., et al. (1998). Double-blind and placebo-controlled study of lithium for adolescent bipolar disorders with secondary substance dependency. *Journal of the American Academy of Child and Adolescent Psychiatry, 37*(2), 171-178.

Goldsmith, R., & Garlapati, V. (2004). Behavioral interventions for dual-diagnosis patients. *Psychiatric Clinics of North America, 27*(4), 709-725.

Gonzalez, G., Feingold, A., Oliveto, A., et al. (2003). Co-morbid major depressive disorder as a prognostic factor in cocaine-abusing buprenorphine-maintained patients treated with desipramine and contingency management. *The American Journal of Drug and Alcohol Abuse, 29*(3), 497-514.

Gonzalez, G., & Rosenheck, R. (2002). Outcomes and service use among homeless individuals with serious mental illness and substance use. *Psychiatric Services, 53*(4), 437-446.

Graeber, D., Moyers, T., Griffith, G., et al. (2003). A pilot study comparing motivational interviewing and educational intervention in patients with schizophrenia and alcohol use disorders. *Community Mental Health Journal, 39*(3), 189-202.

Graham, H. (2004). Implementing integrated treatment for co-existing substance use and severe mental health problems in assertive outreach teams: Training issues. *Drug and Alcohol Review, 23*, 463-470.

Grella, C. E., & Gilmore, J. (2002). Improving service delivery to the dually diagnosed in Los Angeles County. *Journal of Substance Abuse Treatment, 23*(2), 115-122.

Grella, C. E., Joshi, V., & Hser, Y. (2004). Effects of co-morbidity on treatment processes and outcomes among adolescents in drug treatment programs. *Journal of Child and Adolescent Substance Abuse, 13*(4), 13-31.

Harrison, D. S., & Precin, P. (1996). Cognitive impairments in clients with dual-diagnoses (chronic psychotic disorders and substance abuse): Considerations for treatment. *Occupational Therapy International, 3*(2), 122-141.

Harwood, H. (2000). *Updating estimates of the economic costs of alcohol abuse in the United States: Estimates, update methods, and data.* Report prepared by The Lewin Group for the National Institute on Alcohol Abuse and Alcoholism. Retrieved from http://pubs.niaaa.nih.gov/publications/economic-2000/

Harwood, H., Fountain, D., & Livermore, G. (1998). *The economic costs of alcohol and drug abuse in the United States, 1992.* Report prepared for the National Institute on Drug Abuse and the National Institute on Alcohol Abuse and Alcoholism, National Institutes of Health, Department of Health and Human Services. NIH Publication No. 98-4327. Rockville, MD: National Institutes of Health.

Hastings-Vertino, K. A. (1996). STEMSS (Support Together for Emotional and Mental Serenity and Sobriety): An alternative to traditional forms of self-help for the dually diagnosed consumer. *Journal of Addictions Nursing, 8*(1), 20-28.

Hawkins, E. H. (2009). A tale of two systems: Co-occurring mental health and substance abuse disorders treatment for adolescents. *Annual Review of Psychology, 60*, 197-227.

Herman, S. E., Frank, K. A., Mowbray, C. T., et al. (2000). Longitudinal effects of integrated treatment on alcohol use for individuals with serious mental illness and substance use disorders. *The Journal of Behavioral Health Services and Research, 27*(3), 286-302.

Hernandez-Avila, C., Modesto-Lowe, V., Feinn, R., et al. (2004). Nefazodone treatment of co-morbid alcohol dependence and major depression. *Alcoholism, Clinical and Experimental Research, 28*(3), 433-440.

Hesselbrock, M. N., Hesselbrock, V. M., Segal, B., et al. (2003). Ethnicity and psychiatric co-morbidity among alcohol-dependent individuals who receive in-patient treatment: African-Americans, Alaskan Natives, Caucasians and Hispanics. *Alcoholism, 27*(8), 1368-1373.

Hibbard, M. R., Uysal, F., & Keppler, K. (1998). Axis I psychopathology in individuals with traumatic brain injury. *Journal of Head Trauma Rehabilitation, 13*(4), 24-39.

Hirschfeld, R., Williams, J., Spitzer, R., et al. (2000). Development and validation of a screening instrument for bipolar spectrum disorder: The mood disorder questionnaire. *American Journal of Psychiatry, 157*(11), 1873-1875.

Horsfall, J., Cleary, M., Hunt, G., et al. (2009). Psychosocial treatments for people with co-occurring severe mental illnesses and substance use disorders (dual diagnosis): A review of empirical evidence. *Harvard Review of Psychiatry, 17*, 24-34.

Humphreys, K., Huebsch, P. D., Finney, J. W., et al. (1999). A comparative evaluation of substance abuse treatment: V. Substance abuse treatment can enhance the effectiveness of self-help groups. *Alcoholism, Clinical and Experimental Research, 23*(3), 558-563.

Jerrell, J. M. (1996). Toward cost-effective care for individuals with dual diagnoses. *Journal of Mental Health Administration, 23*(3), 329-337.

Jerrell, J., & Ridgely, M. (1995). Evaluating changes in symptoms and functioning of dually diagnosed clients in specialized treatment. *Psychiatric Services, 46*(3), 233-238.

Jordan, L., Davidson, W., Herman, F., et al. (2002). Involvement in 12-step programs among individuals with dual diagnosis. *Psychiatric Services, 53*(7), 894-896.

Judd, P. H., Thomas, N., Schwartz, T., et al. (2003). A dual diagnosis demonstration project: Treatment outcomes and cost analysis. *Journal of Psycho-Active Drugs, 35*(Suppl 1), 181-192.

Kakko, J., Svanborg, K., Kreek, M., et al. (2003). 1-year retention and social function after buprenorphine–assisted relapse treatment for heroin dependents in Sweden: A randomized, placebo-controlled trial. *Lancet, 361*(9358), 662-668.

Kalyoncu, A., Mirsal, H., Pektas, O., et al. (2005). Use of lamotrigine to augment clozapine in patients with resistant schizophrenia and co-morbid alcohol dependence: A potent anti-craving effect? *Journal of Psychopharmacology, 19*(3), 301-305.

Kasten, B. P. (1997). *Experience of mentally-ill adults with co-occurring substance-use disorders* (Doctoral Dissertation). University of California, San Francisco.

Kelly, J., McKellar, J., & Moos, R. (2003). Major depression in patients with substance use disorders: Relationship to 12-step self-help involvement and substance use outcomes. *Addiction, 98*(4), 499-508.

Kendall, C. (2004). Treatment of mental illness and comorbid substance abuse: Concepts for evidence-based practice. *Journal of Addictions Nursing, 15*, 183-186.

Kessler, R. C. (2004). The epidemiology of dual-diagnosis. *Biological Psychiatry, 56*(10), 730-737.

Kleber, H. (2003). Pharmacologic treatments for heroin and cocaine dependence. *The American Journal on Addictions, 12*, S5-S18.

Kosten, T., & Kosten, T. (2004). New medication strategies for co-morbid substance use and bipolar effective disorders. *Biological Psychiatry, 56*(10), 771-777.

Krupitsky, E. M., Rudenko, A. A., Burakov, A. M., et al. (2007). Antiglutamatergic strategies for ethanol detoxification: Comparison with placebo and diazepam. *Alcoholism, Clinical and Experimental Research,* 31(4), 604-611.

Laker, C. (2007). How reliable is the current evidence looking at the efficacy of harm reduction and motivational interviewing interventions in the treatment of patients with a dual diagnosis? *Journal of Psychiatric and Mental Health Nursing, 14*, 720-726.

Langeland, W., Draijer, N., & Van Den Brink, W. (2004). Psychiatric co-morbidity in treatment-seeking alcoholics: The role of childhood trauma and perceived parental dysfunction. *Alcoholism, Clinical and Experimental Research, 28*(3), 441-447.

Latimer, W., Rojas, V., & Mancha, B. (2008). Severity of alcohol use and problem behaviors among school-based youths in Puerto Rico. *Pan American Journal of Public Health, 23*(5), 325-332.

Laudet, A., Magura, S., Cleland, C., et al. (2003). Predictors of retention in dual-focus self-help groups. *Community Mental Health Journal, 39*(4), 281-297.

Laudet, A., Magura, S., Cleland, C., et al. (2004). The effect of 12-step based fellowship participation on abstinence among dually diagnosed individuals: A two-year longitudinal study. *Journal of Psychoactive Drugs, 36*(2), 207-216.

Levin, F., Evans, F., McDowell, D., et al. (2002). Bupropion treatment for cocaine abuse and adult attention-deficit/hyperactivity disorder. *Journal of Addictive Diseases, 21*(2), 1-16.

Levkoff, S. E., Chen, H., Coakley, E., et al. (2004). Design and sample characteristics of the PRISM-E multisite randomized trial to improve behavioral health care for the elderly. *Journal of Aging and Health, 16*(1), 3-27.

Little, J. (2001). Treatment of dually diagnosed clients. *Journal of Psychoactive Drugs, 33*(1), 27-31.

Magura, S., Knight, E., Vogel, H., et al. (2003a). Mediators of effectiveness in dual-focus self-help groups. *American Journal of Drug and Alcohol Abuse, 29*(2), 301-322.

Magura, S., Laudet, A., Mahmood, D., et al. (2002). Adherence to medication regimens and participation in dual-focus self-help groups. *Psychiatric Services, 53*(3), 310-316.

Magura, S., Laudet, A., Mahmood, D., et al. (2003b). Role of self-help processes in achieving abstinence among dually diagnosed individuals. *Addictive Behaviors, 28*(3), 399-413.

Magura, S., Rosenblum, A., & Betzler, T. (2009). Substance use and mental health outcomes for comorbid patients in psychiatric day treatment. *Substance Abuse, 28*(3), 71-78.

Malaspina, D., Corcoran, C., & Hamilton, S. (2002). Epidemiologic and genetic aspects of neuropsychiatric disorders. In S. Yudofsky & R. Hales (Eds.). *The American Psychiatric publishing textbook of neuropsychiatry and clinical neurosciences* (4th ed.). Washington, DC: American Psychiatric Publishing, Inc.

Manning, V. C., Strathdee, G., Best, D., et al. (2002). Dual-diagnosis screening: Preliminary finding on the comparison of 50 clients attending community mental health services and 50 clients attending community substance misuse services. *Journal of Substance Use, 7*(4), 221-228.

Mannynsalo, L., Putkonen, H., Lindberg, N., et al. (2009). Forensic psychiatric perspective on criminality associated with intellectual disability: A nationwide register-based study. *Journal of Intellectual Disability Research, 53*(Part 3), 279-288.

Margolin, A., Avants, S., DePhilippis, D., et al. (1998). A preliminary investigation of lamotrigine for cocaine abuse in HIV-seropositive patients. *American Journal of Drug and Alcohol Abuse, 24*, 85-101.

Martinez-Rega, J., Keaney, F., Marshall, E. J., et al. (2002). Positive or negative history of childhood sexual abuse among problem drinkers: Relationship to substance use disorders and psychiatric co-morbidity. *Journal of Substance Use, 7*(1), 34-40.

Maxwell, S., & Shinderman, M. (2000). Use of naltrexone in the treatment of alcohol use disorders in patients with concomitant major mental illness. *Journal of Addictive Disease, 19*, 61-69.

McDowell, D., Levin, F., Seracini, A., et al. (2000). Venlafaxine treatment of cocaine abusers with depressive disorders. *The American Journal of Drug and Alcohol Abuse, 26*(1), 25-31.

Meissen, G., Powell, T., Wituk, S., et al. (1999). Attitudes of AA contact individuals toward group participation by individuals with a mental illness. *Psychiatric Services, 50*(8), 1079-1081.

Miller, W. R. (2006). Motivational factors in addictive behaviors. In W. R. Miller & K. M. Carroll (Eds.), *Rethinking substance abuse: What the science shows and what we should do about it* (pp. 134-152). New York: Guilford Press.

Milling, R., Faulkner, L., & Craig, J. (1994). Problems in the recognition and treatment of patients with dual diagnosis. *Journal of Substance Abuse Treatment, 11*, 267-271.

Minkoff, K. (2005). *Comprehensive Continuous Integrated System of Care (CCISC): Psychopharmacology practice guidelines for individuals with co-occurring psychiatric and substance use disorders (COD)*. Developed for Illinois Behavioral Health Recovery Management Project. Retrieved 11/1/10 from www.kenminkoff.com

Moggi, F., Brodbeck, J., Koltzsch, K., et al. (2002). One-year follow-up of dual diagnosis patients attending a 4-month integrated inpatient treatment. *European Addiction Research, 8*(1), 30-37.

Monroe, A. D., Levy, S., & McQuade, W. (1997). Effects of gender on documentation of alcohol use in patients with psychiatric symptoms. *Substance Abuse, 18*(2), 79-87.

Moos, R., Moos, B., & Andrassy, J. (1999). Outcomes of four treatment approaches in community residential programs for patients with substance use disorders. *Psychiatric Services, 50*(12), 1577-1583.

Morris, P., Hopwood, M., Whelan, G., et al. (2001). Naltrexone for alcohol dependence: A randomized controlled trial. *Addiction, 96*(11), 1565-1573.

Mueser, K. T., Drake, R. E., & Wallach, M. A. (1998). Dual-diagnosis: A review of etiological theories. *Addictive Behaviors, 23*(6), 717-734.

Najavits, L. (2007). Seeking safety: An evidence-based model for substance abuse and trauma/PTSD. In K. Witkiewitz & G. Marlatt (Eds.), *Therapist's guide to evidence-based relapse prevention* (pp. 141-167). San Diego: Elsevier Academic Press.

National Abandoned Infants Assistance Resource Center (NAIA). (2008). Women with co-occurring mental illness and substance abuse. *Journal of Addictions Nursing, 19*, 93-100.

National Consensus Statement on Mental Health Recovery. (2004). U.S. Department of Health and Human Services, Substance Abuse and Mental Health Services Administration, Center for Mental Health Services. Retrieved from http://www.co.marion.or.us/HLT/CAPS/resources/SAMHSA.htm

National Institute on Aging. (2009). *Alcohol use in older people*. Retrieved from http://www.nia.nih.gov/HealthInformation/Publications/alcohol.htm

National Institute of Mental Health. (2010). *Suicide in the U.S.: Statistics and prevention*. Retrieved from http://www.nimh.nih.gov/health/publications/suicide-in-the-us-statistics-and-prevention/index.shtml#adults

National Survey on Drug Use and Health. (2010). Results from the 2009 National Survey on Drug Use and Health: Volume I. Summary of National Findings. Retrieved from http://oas.samhsa.gov/NSDUH/2k9NSDUH/2k9Results.htm#7.3

Nunes, E., Quitkin, F., Donovan, S., et al. (1998). Imipramine treatment of opiate-dependent patients with depressive disorders. A placebo-controlled trial. *Archives of General Psychiatry, 55*(2), 153-160.

Obando, P., Kliewer, W., Murrelle, L., et al. (2004). The co-morbidity of substance abuse and depressive symptoms in Costa Rican adolescents. *Drug and Alcohol Dependence, 76*(1), 37-44.

Ouimette, P., Gima, K., Moos, R., et al. (1999). A comparative evaluation of substance abuse treatment: IV - The effect of co-morbid psychiatric diagnoses on amount of treatment, continuing care, and one-year outcomes. *Alcoholism, Clinical and Experimental Research, 23*(3), 552-557.

Ouimette, P., Humphries, K., Moos, R., et al. (2001). Self-help group participation among substance-use disorder patients with post traumatic stress disorder. *Journal of Substance Abuse Treatment, 20*(1), 25-32.

Owens, P., Myers, M., Elixhauser, A., et al. (2007). *Care of adults with mental and substance abuse disorders in U.S. community hospitals, 2004*. Healthcare Research and Quality, 2007. HCUP Fact Book No. 10. AHRQ Publication No. 07-0008. Available at http://www.ahrq.gov/data/hcup/factbk10/

Paille, F., Guelfi, J., Perkins, A., et al. (1995). Double-blind randomized multicentre trial of acamprosate in maintaining abstinence from alcohol. *Alcohol and Alcoholism, 30*(2), 239-247.

Pelc, I., Verbanck, P., Le Bon, O., et al. (1997). Efficacy and safety of acamprosate in the treatment of detoxified alcohol-dependent patients. *British Journal of Psychiatry, 171*, 73-77.

Peteet, J. (1993). A closer look at the role of a spiritual approach in addictions treatment. *Journal of Substance Abuse Treatment, 10*, 263-267.

Petrakis I. L., Poling, J., Levinson, C., et al. (2006). Naltrexone and disulfiram in patients with alcohol dependence and comorbid post-traumatic stress disorder. *Biological Psychiatry, 1*, 60(7), 777-783.

Pettinati, H., Volpicelli, J., Luck, G., et al. (2001). Double-blind clinical trial of sertraline treatment for alcohol dependence. *Journal of Clinical Psychopharmacology, 21*(2), 143-153.

Pierucci-Lagha, A., Feinn, R., Modesto-Lowe, V., et al. (2004). Effects of rapid tryptophan depletion on mood and urge to drink in patients with co-morbid major depression alcohol dependence. *Psychopharmacology, 171*(3), 340-348.

Polgar, M. F., Johsen, M. C., Starrett, B. E., et al. (2000). New patterns of community care: Coordinated services for dually diagnosed adults in North Carolina. *Journal of Health & Human Services Administration, 23*(1), 50-64.

Pollack, L. E., Cramer, R. D., & Varner, R. V. (2000). Psychosocial functioning of people with substance abuse and bipolar disorders. *Substance Abuse, 21*(3), 193-203.

Pristach, C., & Smith, C. (1999). Attitudes towards alcoholics anonymous by dually diagnosed psychiatric in-patients. *Journal of Addictive Diseases, 18*(3), 69-76.

Randall, C., Johnson, M., Thevos, A., et al. (2001). Paroxetine for social anxiety and alcohol use in dual-diagnosed patients. *Depression and Anxiety, 14*(4), 255-262.

Ridgely, M. S., & Jerrell, J. M. (1996). Analysis of three interventions for substance abuse treatment of severely mentally ill people. *Community Mental Health Journal, 32*(6), 561-572.

Riggs, P., Hall, S., Milkulich-Gilbertson, S., et al. (2004). A randomized control trial of pemoline for attention-deficit/hyperactivity disorder in substance-abusing adolescents. *Journal of the American Academy of Child and Adolescent Psychiatry, 43*(4), 420-429.

Rosenblum, A., Fallon, B., Magura, S., et al. (1999). The autonomy of mood disorders among cocaine-using methadone patients. *The American Journal of Drug and Alcohol Abuse, 25*(1), 67-80.

Sacks, D., Skinner, J., Sacks, A., et al. (2002). Manual for engaging homeless mentally ill chemical abusers in a modified TC shelter program. New York: National Development and Research Institutes (NDRI). Retrieved from www.ndri.org

Sadock, B. J., & Sadock, V. A. (2003). *Kaplan and Sadock's synopsis of psychiatry: Behavioral sciences/clinical psychiatry* (9th ed.). Philadelphia: Lippincott, Williams & Wilkins.

Sass, H., Soyka, M., Mann, K., et al. (1996). Relapse prevention by acamprosate: Results from a placebo-controlled study on alcohol dependence. *Archives of General Psychiatry, 53*, 673-680.

Satel, S., Becker, B., & Dan, E. (1993). Reducing obstacles to affiliation with alcoholics anonymous among veterans with PTSD and alcoholism. *Hospital and Community Psychiatry, 44*(11), 1061-1065.

Savage, A., & Russell, L. A. (2005). Tangled in a web of affiliation: Social support networks of dually diagnosed women who are trauma survivors. *Journal of Behavioral Health Services & Research, 32*(2), 199-214.

Schafer, I., & Najavits, L. M. (2007). Clinical challenges in the treatment of patients with posttraumatic stress disorder and substance abuse. *Current Opinions in Psychiatry, 20*(6), 614-618.

Schmitz, J., Averill, P., Stotts, A., et al. (2001). Fluoxetine treatment of cocaine-dependent patients with major depressive disorder. *Drug and Alcohol Dependence, 63*(3), 207-214.

Selzer, M. L. (1971). The Michigan alcoholism screening test: The quest for a new diagnostic instrument. *American Journal of Psychiatry, 127*(12), 1653-1658.

Siegfried, N. (1998). A Review of co-morbidity: Major mental illness and problematic substance use. *Australian and New Zealand Journal of Psychiatry, 32*(5), 707-717.

Silver, J. M., Hales, R. E., & Yudofsky, S. C. (2002). Neuropsychiatric aspects of traumatic brain injury. In S. Yudofsky & R. Hales (Eds.), *The American psychiatric publishing textbook of neuropsychiatry and clinical neurosciences* (4th ed.). Washington, DC: American Psychiatric Publishing, Inc.

Silver, J., Kramer, R., Greenwald, S., et al. (2001). The association between head injuries and psychiatric disorders: Findings from the New Haven NIMH Epidemiologic Catchment Area Study. *Brain Injury, 15*(11), 935-945.

Sims, J., Woods, S., & Guppy, A. (2001). Mental health in illicit drug users. *Mental Health Nursing, 21*(5), 18-22.

Sitharthan, T., Singh, S., Kranitis, P., et al. (1999). Integrated drug and alcohol intervention: Development of an opportunistic intervention program to reduce alcohol and other substance use among psychiatric patients. *The Australian and New Zealand Journal of Psychiatry, 33*(5), 676-683.

Smith, D. (1994). AA recovery and spirituality: An addiction medicine perspective. *Journal of Substance Abuse Treatment, 11*(2), 111-112.

Sonne, S., & Brady, K. (2000). Naltrexone for individuals with co-morbid bipolar disorder and alcohol dependence. *Journal of Psychopharmacology, 20*, 114-115.

Sonne, S., & Brady, K. (2002). Bipolar disorder and alcoholism. *Alcohol Research and Health, 26*(2), 103-109.

Stahl, S. (2008). *Essential psychopharmacology: Neuroscientific basis and practical applications* (3rd ed.). Oxford, UK: Cambridge University Press.

Stenius, V. M., Veysey, B. M., Hamilton, Z., et al. (2005). Social roles in women's lives: Changing conceptions of self. *Journal of Behavioral Health Services and Research, 32*(2), 182-198.

Stern, T., & Herman, J. (2004). *Massachusetts General Hospital psychiatry update and board preparation* (2nd ed.). New York: McGraw-Hill, Inc.

Substance Abuse and Mental Health Services Administration. (2002). *Report to Congress on the prevention and treatment of co-occurring substance abuse disorders and mental disorders*. Rockville, MD: Substance Abuse and Mental Health Services Administration. Retrieved from http://www.samhsa.gov/reports/congress2002/index.html

Substance Abuse and Mental Health Services Administration, Office of Applied Studies. (2004). *Admissions with co-occurring disorders: 1995-2001*. Drug and Alcohol Services Information System, Rockville, MD: Substance Abuse and Mental Health Services Administration. Retrieved from http://oas.samhsa.gov/2k4/dualTX/dualTX.htm

Substance Abuse and Mental Health Services Administration, Office of Applied Studies. (2006a). *Results from the 2005 national survey on drug use and health: National findings*. NSDUH Series H-30, DHHS Publication No. SMA 06-4194. Rockville, MD: Substance Abuse and Mental Health Services Administration. Retrieved from http://www.oas.samhsa.gov/nsduh/2k5nsduh/2k5Results.pdf

Substance Abuse and Mental Health Services Administration. (2006b). *SAMHSA Issues Consensus Statement on Mental Health Recovery*. Retrieved from http://www.power2u.org/downloads/SAMHSA%20Recovery%20Statement.pdf

Substance Abuse and Mental Health Services Administration, Office of Applied Studies. (2007). *The NSDUH [National Survey on Drug Use and Health] report: Serious psychological distress and substance use disorder among veterans*. Rockville, MD: Substance Abuse and Mental Health Services Administration.

Substance Abuse and Mental Health Services Administration, Office of Applied Studies. (2008). *On-Line Analysis of Alcohol, Tobacco, and Drug Use: Part 1*. Retrieved from http://www.oas.samhsa.gov/samhda.htm

Substance Abuse and Mental Health Services Administration. (2011). *Screening, Brief Intervention, and Referral to Treatment (SBIRT)*. Retrieved from http://www.samhsa.gov/prevention/SBIRT/

Sung, M., Erkanli, A., Angold, A., et al. (2004). Effects of age at first substance use and psychiatric co-morbidity on the development of substance use disorders. *Drug and Alcohol Dependence, 75*(3), 287-299.

Suppes, T., & Dennehy, E. (2005). *Bipolar disorder: The latest assessment and treatment strategies*. Kansas City, MO: Dean Psych Press Corp.

Suppes, T., & Keck, P. (2005). *Bipolar disorder: Treatment and management*. Kansas City, MO: Dean Psych Press Corp.

Taylor, M. J., & Barusch, A. S. (2004). Personal, family, and multiple barriers of long-term welfare recipients. *Social Work, 49*(2), 175-183.

Teplin, D., O'Connell, T., Daiter, J., et al. (2004). A psychometric study of the prevalence of DSM-IV personality disorders among office-based methadone maintenance patients. *American Journal of Drug and Alcohol Abuse, 30*(3), 515-524.

Tiet, Q., & Mausbach, B. (2007). Treatments for patients with dual diagnosis: A review. *Alcoholism, Clinical and Experimental Research, 31*(4), 513-536.

Timko, C., & Sempel, J. (2004). Intensity of acute services, self-help attendance and one-year outcomes among dual-diagnosis patients. *Journal of Studies on Alcohol, 65*(2), 274-282.

Tsuang, J., & Fong, T. (2004). Treatment of patients with schizophrenia and substance abuse disorders. *Current Pharmaceutical Design, 10*(18), 2249-2261.

Van den Bosch, L. M., Verheul, R., Schippers, G. M., et al. (2002). Dialectical behavior therapy of borderline patients with and without substance use problems: Implementation and long term effects. *Addictive Behaviors, 27*(6), 911-923.

Van Wamel, A., Kroon, H., & van Roojen, S. (2009). Systematic implementation of integrated dual disorders treatment in The Netherlands. Mental health and substance abuse. *Journal of Dual Diagnosis, 2*(2), 101-110. Retrieved from http://www.tandfonline.com/doi/abs/10.1080/17523280902932649

Vega, W. A., Sribney, W. N., & Achara-Abrahams, I. (2003). Co-occurring alcohol, drug and other psychiatric disorders among Mexican-origin people in the United States. *American Journal of Public Health, 93*(7), 1057-1064.

Virgo, N., Bennett, G., Higgins, D., et al. (2001). The prevalence and characteristics of co-occurring Serious Mental Illness (SMI) and substance abuse or dependence in the patients of adult mental health and addiction services in Eastern Dorset. *Journal of Mental Health, 10*(2), 175-188.

Vogel, H., Knight, E., Laudet, A., et al. (1998). Double-trouble in recovery: Self-help for people with dual diagnosis. *Psychiatric Rehabilitation Journal, 21*(4), 356-364.

Volkow, N. D., Hitzeman, R., Wang, G. J., et al. (1992). Decreased brain metabolism in neurologically intact healthy alcoholics. *American Journal of Psychiatry, 149*, 1016-1022.

Wilens, T. E. (2006). Attention deficit hyperactivity disorder and substance use disorder. *The American Journal of Psychiatry, 163*(12), 2059-2063.

Willenbring, M. L., Kivlahan, D., Kenny, M., et al. (2004). Beliefs about evidence-based practices in addiction treatment: A survey of Veterans Administration program leaders. *Journal of Substance Abuse and Treatment, 26*(2), 79-85.

Wortzel, H., Anderson, C., & Arciniegas, D. (2007). Treatment of pathological laughing and crying. *Current Treatment Options in Neurology, 9*(5), 371-380.

Zauszniewski, J. A. (1995). Severity of depression, cognitions, and functioning among depressed inpatients with and without coexisting substance abuse. *Journal of the American Psychiatric Nurses Association, 1*(2), 55-60.

Zimberg, S. (1999). A dual diagnosis typology to improve diagnosis and treatment of dual disordered patients. *Journal of Psychoactive Drugs, 31*(1), 47-51.

Answers to Case Study 17-1 Questions

1. Diagnostic impressions:
   - Axis I: Bipolar Disorder, Type I, currently depressed; Alcohol Abuse, by history
   - Axis II: R/O Personality Disorder
   - Axis III: Exacerbation of psychiatric symptoms around time of menses
   - Axis IV: Occupational stress: conflict with coworkers
   - Axis V: GAF 48
2. Discussion and plan: The patient reports suicidal ideation and past history of "self-injurious behavior," so a full suicide assessment must be completed and interventions planned accordingly. Although the patient reports that she is not currently using drugs or alcohol, she endorses a history of "heavy drinking" in her teens; therefore, active alcohol use and/or risk of relapse must be explored in more depth and should be ruled out. Particularly because alcohol use and suicide are highly correlated, if she is drinking or relapses, she will be at a higher risk for self-harm. Further, because she has had a gun in the past, the clinician must determine if the gun is in her possession now, and if so, negotiate a plan with the patient to have it secured, locked, or removed from her possession. In addition to concerns over suicidal ideation, homicidal ideation must be thoroughly explored, in particular with respect to coworkers and supervisor. Safety for self and others must be ensured, or inpatient admission must be discussed. If the patient is deemed to be safe and not in need of admission at this time, close follow-up will be necessary on an outpatient basis. The clinician may consider a referral to a partial hospital program for acute stabilization, observation, initiation of mood-stabilizing medication and monitoring, and evidence-based group interventions. Mood-stabilizing medication, such as divalproex (Depakote) or an atypical antipsychotic, is indicated at this time. Baseline lab work-up, including pregnancy test and liver panel, should be ordered if divalproex is being considered. For atypical antipsychotics, baseline labwork including HgA_{1c}, fasting lipids and glucose, and weight would be prudent practice to aid in future monitoring of possible side effects.

Acknowledgment

The author would like to acknowledge and thank Janet K. Cole for her generous donation of time and editorial assistance in the preparation of this manuscript.

[Note: The use of the terms "addict" and "addiction" remain somewhat emotionally laden and are considered by some to be harsh. However, there are a number of scientific journals, papers, publications, and clinical treatment programs that use the term "addiction" in their titles; thus, use of these terms in this text is not meant to be pejorative.]

UNIT VIII

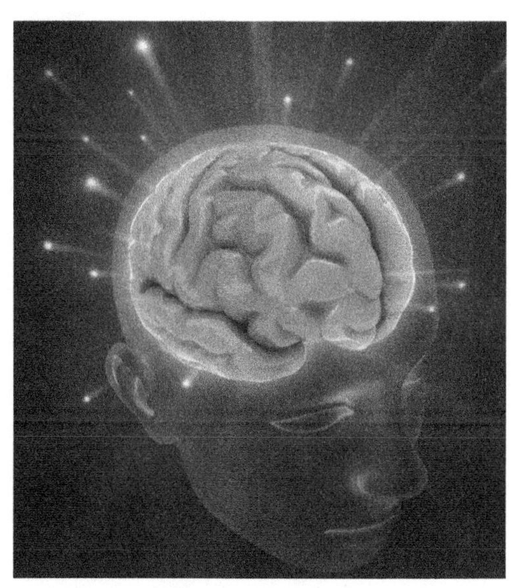

Personality Disorders

CHAPTER 18

Personality Disorders

Eris F. Perese, APRN-PMH

All humans have personality traits, which are established ways of thinking about things, responding emotionally, behaving, and interacting with others. Each human has specific personality traits that form his or her unique personality style (Oldham, 2009). Personality disorders can be viewed as extremes of normal personality traits, distinguished from personality traits by the presence of a rigid maladaptive pattern of responding to all interpersonal interactions and experiences (Knutson & Heinz, 2004; O'Connor & Dyce, 2001; Paris, 2003). These severe maladaptive patterns result in the emotional distress, disruptions of interpersonal relationships, and impairments of family, social, and vocational functioning that characterize personality disorders (Oldham, Skodol, & Bender, 2009). Personality disorders are maladaptations of personality styles that are created by the interaction of genetically influenced temperament, neurodevelopmental abnormalities of the brain with resulting compromised functioning, and stressful life experiences (Oldham et al., 2009).

The ten personality disorders are as follows:

- Antisocial personality disorder (ASPD)
- Avoidant personality disorder (AVPD)
- Borderline personality disorder (BPD)
- Dependent personality disorder (DPD)
- Histrionic personality disorder (HPD)
- Narcissistic personality disorder (NPD)
- Obsessive-compulsive personality disorder (OCPD)
- Paranoid personality disorder (PPD)
- Schizoid personality disorder (SZPD)
- Schizotypal personality disorder (STPD)

Personality disorders affect the individual, the family, and society (Ruegg & Francis, 1995). Individuals with personality disorders are affected by failed relationships, problems with school or work, suicide attempts, self-injurious behaviors, sexually transmitted diseases, delayed recovery from medical and psychiatric disorders, and diminished quality of life (Chen, Cohen, Crawford, et al., 2006). Families of patients with personality disorders are affected by conflict and disruptions, irresponsible and aggressive behaviors, child neglect and maltreatment, unemployment, and poverty. For society, the impact of personality disorders is seen in increased use of health-care services and the justice system, loss of productivity, and need for financial assistance. Personality disorders often require lengthy treatment with a variety of modalities. They are viewed as more difficult to treat than Axis I psychiatric disorders, and the benefits achieved are often more limited than those for Axis I disorders (Paris, 2003; Simeon & Hollander, 2009).

Whereas personality disorders occur in 10% to 20% of the general population, approximately 50% of patients with Axis I psychiatric disorders will have a co-occurring personality disorder (Torgersen, 2009). Because patients with personality disorders constitute a large percentage of patients seen in clinical practice, an understanding of the biological, psychological, and social factors that underlie the development and maintenance of personality disorders is essential for psychiatric advanced practice nurses.

Personality

Magnavita (2004) defined personality as "an individual's habitual way of thinking, perceiving, and reacting to the world" (p. 16). Personality is formed by temperament and character and is honed by life experiences and societal and cultural expectations.

Temperament

Temperament is present at birth and refers to inborn tendencies to react in certain ways to new experiences or challenges (see Chapter 3 for discussion of temperament). About 50% of the variance of temperament is genetically influenced (Magnavita, 2002; Plomin, 1990). Temperament becomes stable by 2 years of age, and stability of personality traits is evident by 3 years of age (Rothbart, Ahadi, & Evans, 2000). Personality becomes more stable over time, reaching a plateau by age 50 with only slight change after that age

(Caspi, Roberts, & Shiner, 2005; Lewis, 2001; Paris, 2003). Stability of personality traits is involved (1) in the process of forming and maintaining self-identity and (2) in the process of "niche building," in which people create, seek out, or find themselves in environments that fit with their personality traits (Caspi et al., p. 469). Environments that fit with individuals' personality traits tend to reinforce those traits and limit opportunities for change (Roberts & Wood, 2004). Genetically influenced choice of environment may also increase individuals' chances of victimization and exposure to risky living situations and drug use (Vaughn, Fu, Delisi, et al., 2010).

Character

Unlike temperament, character is not present at birth. It accrues from relationships with caregivers, experiences, and the expected, valued, and rewarded responses to new experiences and challenges. According to Cloninger, Svrakic, & Przybeck (1993, p. 979), character includes three dimensions:

1. Self-directedness (responsibility, purposefulness, and self-acceptance)
2. Cooperativeness (empathy, compassion, and helpfulness)
3. Self-transcendence (spirituality, idealism, and enlightenment)

Cloninger et al. (1993) believed that self-directedness was the "major determinant of the presence or absence of personality disorder" (p. 979). Whereas temperament is associated with procedural learning, character is associated with insight learning (Cloninger, Van Eerdewegh, Goate, et al., 1998). Character is not as strongly genetically influenced as temperament (Coccaro & Siever, 2009).

Personality Structure

Personality structure is thought to comprise five factors (five categories of traits) that exist in varying degrees (Digman, 1990; Heim & Westen, 2009; McCrae & John, 1992). Each of the five factors shows strong genetic influence (Bourchard, 1994; Bourchard & Loehlin, 2001). The five factors are

1. Extraversion (warmth, outgoingness, assertiveness, energetic activity, excitement-seeking, and positive emotions such as enthusiasm and humor)
2. Agreeableness (trust, soft-heartedness, compliance, and sympathy)
3. Neuroticism (anxiety, hostility, depression, self-consciousness, impulsivity, and vulnerability)
4. Conscientiousness (organization, efficiency, dutifulness, goal-directedness, and self-discipline)
5. Openness (imaginativeness, wide interests, sense of humor, and unconventional values) (Costa & McCrae, 1992; Livesley, Jackson, & Schroeder, 1992; Skodol & Gunderson, 2008).

Relationship Between Personality and Personality Disorders

Personality disorders can be thought of as dysfunctional exaggerations of normal ways of interacting with others and responding to experiences and challenges (Paris, 2004; Skodol & Gunderson, 2011). For example, individuals with personality disorders tend to use immature defense mechanisms, such as projection, withdrawal, splitting, and dissociation, to control feelings of anxiety, depression, inadequacy, and anger (Sadock & Sadock, 2007). In treating patients with personality disorders, the psychiatric advanced practice nurse must help them to give up immature, maladaptive defense mechanisms that may serve to control anxiety but often interfere with relationships and with social and vocational functioning. Patients must be helped to learn more adaptive defense mechanisms, such as anticipation, problem-solving, humor, suppression, altruism, and sublimation (Sadock & Sadock).

Personality Disorders (General)

Early concepts of personality disorders were influenced by psychodynamic theory, which proposed that personality is co-determined by temperament and internalized value systems—the id, the ego, and the superego (Heim & Westen, 2009; Kernberg, 2004). Another theory was to consider personality disorders in relation to major psychiatric disorders, such as being on a continuum with schizophrenia, anxiety disorders, or mood disorders (Akiskal, 1981; Fanous, Neale, Aggen, et al., 2007; Simeon & Hollander, 2009).

In 2007, Gunderson described two significant advances in understanding personality disorders:

1. Personality disorders have been found to have a strong genetic influence, and components within each personality disorder—such as responsive/reactive components like self-harm and trait-like components like shyness—have been found to have distinctive genetic influences.
2. Contrary to earlier beliefs that personality disorders are stable, enduring disorders, personality disorders have been found to improve, thus bringing into question the concept of stability as a characteristic of personality disorders (Grilo & McGlashan, 2009; Skodol, 2008; Skodol, Oldham, Bender, et al., 2005b).

Gunderson (2007) said that personality traits are less stable than the description of them in the *Diagnostic and Statistical Manual of Mental Disorders*, 4th edition, Text Revision *(DSM-IV-TR)* (American Psychiatric Association, 2000), which states that they have an "enduring pattern of perceiving, relating to and thinking about the environment and oneself that are exhibited in a wide range of social and personal contexts" (p. 686). These two advances—knowledge that personality traits and responses or behaviors have different genetic foundations and thus different responses to treatment, and evidence that personality disorders improve—are influencing how psychiatric advanced practice nurses care for patients with personality disorders.

Definition of Personality Disorders

As the *Diagnostic and Statistical Manual of Mental Disorders*, 4th edition *(DSM-IV)* (American Psychiatric Association, 1994) was being developed, personality disorders were placed on Axis II with mental retardation because it was thought that the development of personality disorders began at an early age and lasted for a lifetime; that is, they are stable and enduring (Knutson & Heinz, 2004). The *DSM-IV-TR* (American Psychiatric Association, 2000) also describes personality disorders as having stable, enduring patterns of experience or behaviors that deviate markedly from the expectations of the person's culture, but it adds to the previous guide's explanation by stating that personality disorders have an onset in adolescence or early adulthood and cause unhappiness, distress, and impaired functioning.

Impairment of functioning of patients with personality disorders is evidenced by a lack of educational attainment and problems with marital relationships, interpersonal relationships, employment, and social functioning (Skodol, 2009). For example, those with personality disorders are more likely to be separated, divorced, or never married and have more job changes, unemployment, and periods of disability than patients with no personality disorders (Skodol & Gunderson, 2008). To a varying extent, individuals with personality disorders see their unhappiness, distress, and impaired functioning as being caused by others, by fate, or by the way the world works. They do not see their life problems as their fault or resulting from their behaviors (Freedman, 2002).

Epidemiology

Prevalence

The estimated rate of personality disorders among the general population of the United States ranges from 7% to 13% with a median prevalence of 10% (Torgersen, 2009). The prevalence of personality disorders among inpatient and outpatient psychiatric populations has been estimated to be between 15% and 20% (Knutson & Heinz, 2004); however, a more recent study found that the prevalence of specific personality disorders among patients seen in outpatient psychiatric settings was 31%, and when the diagnosis of "personality disorder not otherwise specified" was included, the prevalence was 45.5% (Zimmerman, Rothschild, & Chelminski, 2005).

Among patients meeting criteria for a specific personality disorder, approximately 50% had more than one personality disorder, with some having two personality disorders and a few having more than two personality disorders (Torgersen, 2009). Evidence from clinical practice suggests that there is an increase in the number of adolescents and young adults entering treatment for personality dysfunction and that they are presenting with greater severity of symptoms and with less support from family and community (Magnavita, 2004). There is also evidence that personality disorders have increased in North America during the past 50 years (Perez, Santos, Molina, et al., 2001), with a greater increase among the more severe personality disorders, such as BPD and ASPD (Paris, 1998, 2003).

Sociocultural Factors

In addition to genetic influence and the effect of psychosocial adversities, the development of personality disorders is influenced by conflict between individuals' personality traits and the demands of the culture in which they live. The broad dimensions of personality are similar in many cultures, but some personality traits are socially sensitive; i.e., they are enhanced, contained, or buffered by culture (Paris, 2004). These socially sensitive personality traits tend to be externalizing behaviors, such as those seen in ASPD, BPD, and substance-related disorders. Personality traits that are socially insensitive or less affected by culture are more likely to be internalizing behaviors, such as depression and anxiety, and they are more stable across cultures (Paris, 2003).

Traditional cultures that have high social cohesion, fixed social roles, and continuity between the generations tend to buffer or contain behaviors that are socially sensitive. In traditional cultures, people tend to be strongly influenced by the extended family and the community. There are expectations that young people will follow the same work as their parents and live and marry in the same area. In traditional families, fathers are strong and authoritarian. There are high expectations for achievement by the children, and family loyalty is valued. In traditional cultures, the family and the community may protect unusually shy individuals, find employment and marriage partners that fit with each individual's traits, channel selfish or self-centered behaviors to more productive behaviors, and constrain antisocial behaviors or exclude the nonconforming individual from the community (Paris, 2004). For example, there are low rates of ASPD in China and Japan, two countries that still have traditional cultures, although they are changing.

In contrast, in nontraditional cultures or modern societies, the level of social cohesion is lower. There is greater diversity of roles and less continuity between generations (Paris, 2004). Adolescents are expected to develop their own personality. They do not have the protection of assigned roles and networks. They usually learn a new occupation from strangers and they are expected to find their own jobs, housing, and spouses. Individuality is valued over the family and community (Paris, 2004). In nontraditional cultures, the forces that buffer personality traits that lead to shyness and social isolation and that contain externalizing behaviors may be weaker.

Etiology

Genetics

Heritability refers to the degree to which genetic factors influence the development of a disorder (Glatt, Faraone, & Tsuang, 2007). The heritability for personality disorders ranges from 30% to 80% depending on the specific personality disorder (Simeon & Hollander, 2009), with many personality disorders having a stronger degree of genetic influence than many of the Axis I psychiatric disorders. (The heritability of each personality disorder is presented later in this chapter.)

Although genes influence the development of the brain and neurotransmitter systems and may establish predispositions or vulnerabilities to certain responses or behaviors, experienced factors such as neglect and abuse are also involved in determining if the vulnerabilities develop into personality disorders (Oldham, 2009; Silk, 1998). It is the interaction of genetic vulnerabilities and experiences (positive and negative) that shapes human behavior, including the behaviors that constitute the personality disorders (Oldham; Widiger & Sankis, 2000).

Genes also influence the likelihood of exposure to adverse experiences that contribute to the development of personality disorders. Genes influence how individuals select experiences and the degree to which they place themselves in high-risk or low-risk situations (Torgersen, 2005). Based on their unique genetic makeup, individuals choose from a range of stimuli, events, experiences, and relationships and create their own unique environment (Scarr & McCartney, 1983).

Experienced Factors

Among the general population, adults who had experienced childhood abuse or neglect had a rate of personality disorders four times higher than did those who had not experienced abuse or neglect (Johnson, Cohen, Brown, et al., 1999). Studies of the effect of early trauma on the developing brain suggest that stress may have a detrimental effect on the functioning of the hypothalamic-pituitary-adrenal (HPA) axis, on the hippocampus, and on brain lateralization; e.g., childhood neglect and abuse may make the HPA axis and the autonomic nervous system hyper-reactive and may result in long-term neurobiological and neuroendocrine alterations (Lee, Geracioti, Kasckow, et al., 2005). Childhood maltreatment has been found to be related to abnormal levels of corticotropin-releasing factor, which is associated with production of the stress hormone cortisol.

Early childhood *emotional neglect* has been found to have a stronger relationship with changes in corticotropin-releasing factor and levels of cortisol than childhood emotional abuse or physical abuse have (Lee et al., 2005). Lee et al. believed that early emotional neglect, such as lack of maternal care, has a greater effect because it occurs at an earlier time of brain development than abuse.

Some studies have shown reduced hippocampal and amygdala volume—nearly 16% less volume of the hippocampus and 8% less volume of the amygdala—in patients with BPD who experienced trauma in childhood (Driessen, Herrmann, & Stahl, 2000). Schmahl, Vermetten, Elzinga, et al. (2003) reported an even greater loss of volume of the amygdala: a 21.9% smaller amygdala.

Early trauma may also promote lateralization of functioning of the right and left brain hemispheres, limiting integration of right and left hemisphere functioning. It has been found that abused children use the left hemisphere when thinking about neutral memories and the right hemisphere for frightening memories. Nonabused children used both the left and right hemispheres for both types of memory (Schiffer, Teicher, & Papanicolaou, 1995). Gabbard (2005) suggested that lack of hemispheric integration may be reflected in the use of splitting as a defense mechanism in patients with BPD. (Splitting is a mental action in which individuals see themselves and others as all good or all bad. Because they cannot integrate positive and negative qualities into a whole image, they may rapidly shift from idealizing a person to completely devaluing that same person [Black & Andreasen, 2011].)

Different forms of childhood maltreatment are associated with later development of different forms of psychopathology. For example:

- Children who experienced maternal verbal abuse are more than three times as likely as those who do not experience maternal verbal abuse to develop PPD, BPD, NPD, and OCPD during adolescence or early adulthood. The influence of maternal verbal abuse was still present after controlling for temperament, physical and sexual abuse, neglect, and physical punishment during childhood (Johnson, Cohen, Smailes, et al., 2001).
- Childhood emotional neglect—lack of parental affection—is associated with ASPD, PPD, BPD, DPD, AVPD, and SZPD (Carter, Joyce, Mulder, et al., 1999; Norden, Klein, Donaldson, et al., 1995).
- Childhood supervision neglect is associated with increased risk for passive-aggressive behaviors and with BPD and PPD (Johnson, Smailes, Cohen, et al., 2000).
- Childhood physical abuse is associated with ASPD, BPD, and STPD and with the development of depressive, paranoid, schizoid, and passive-aggressive traits (Johnson, Bromley, & McGeoch, 2009).
- Childhood sexual abuse is associated with BPD, HPD, NPD, STPD, and PPD and may contribute to AVPD (Johnson et al., 2009).

Protective factors associated with the development of adaptive personality traits include ones within the individual and family: hardiness, resiliency, family warmth (empathy and supportive nurturing), and family support by others. Protective factors outside the family include the presence of mentors, godparents, adult role models, and peers. Protective factors within the community include availability of opportunities to engage in arts and crafts, athletic activities, hobbies, music, and projects (Johnson et al., 2009).

Biological Basis

Some researchers believe that the source of personality disorders is brain based, i.e., that the cause of personality disorders lies in neural networks rather than in temperament or personality (Lee & Coccaro, 2009). Panksepp (2004) proposed that gene expression influences protein expression, which alters neurophysiological functioning; this altered neurophysiological functioning is manifested in behavioral tendencies that, over time, become traits that may convey vulnerability to the development of a personality disorder. Panksepp's model suggests that there are physiological correlates of personality disorder symptoms that are linked to behavioral traits (Knutson & Heinz, 2004). The biological basis of personality disorders has not been well established, but there is consensus that neurobiological deficits are involved in the dimensions of personality disorders (Goodman, New, & Siever, 2004).

Physiological Correlates

Links between low serotonin activity and traits of aggressive behavior and impulsivity have been described (Coccaro, Kavoussi, Hauger, et al., 1998; Frankle, Lombardo, New, et al., 2005; Knutson, Wolkowitz, Cole, et al., 1998). For example, there is evidence of a link between low serotonin levels and impulsive behavior among violent offenders, among those who have committed murder or serious assaults (Linnoila, Virkkunen, Scheinin, et al., 1983), and among impulsive arsonists (Virkkunen, Nuutila, Goodwin, et al., 1987). The evidence points to a strong relationship between dysfunction of serotonin systems and impulsivity (Coccaro & Siever, 2009).

The neurotransmitter dopamine, which is modulated by serotonin, may be involved in aggression as well as psychotic symptoms (Coccaro, 1996). For example, higher levels of dopamine appear to be associated with psychotic-like symptoms, such as the suspiciousness and magical thinking, which are symptoms of STPD (Coccaro et al., 1998). Recent evidence suggests a positive relationship between dopamine and the personality trait of extroversion, which encompasses positive emotionality, novelty seeking, and excitability (Knutson & Heinz, 2004).

In sum, dopamine and serotonin are two neurotransmitters that may affect the dimensions of personality. Knutson and Heinz (2004) suggested that introversion (inhibition) is linked with low levels of dopamine activity, and neuroticism (anxiety, fear, irritability, and depression) and disagreeableness are linked with low levels of serotonin activity. Both neuroticism and disagreeableness have been found to improve with the use of selective serotonin reuptake inhibitor (SSRI) medications, which increase levels of serotonin (Kuntson & Heinz). In addition, norepinephrine and vasopressin may be involved in aggression, and acetylcholine appears to be involved in affective sensitivity or rapid shifts of emotions (Coccaro et al., 1998; Coccaro & Siever, 2009).

Comorbidity

Among patients who have been diagnosed as having one personality disorder, half will meet the criteria for two or three other personality disorders. Comorbidity frequently but not always is within the same cluster. For example, there is a high rate of comorbid DPD with BPD (Skodol, 2009). There is also a high comorbidity of Axis I psychiatric disorders that follows a pattern (Dolan-Sewell, Krueger, & Shea, 2001). For example, Cluster A personality disorders (odd-eccentric) tend to occur with psychotic disorders (Oldham, 2009); Cluster B personality disorders (dramatic-emotional) with major depressive disorder, other mood disorders, anxiety disorders, substance abuse, and bulimia nervosa (Oldham); and Cluster C personality disorders (anxious-fearful) with anxiety disorders, major depressive disorder, social phobia, and obsessive-compulsive disorder (OCD) (Oldham). Suicidality, which is comorbid in some of the personality disorders, has been found to be associated with exposure to negative life events such as those relating to love, marriage, crime, and legal matters (Yen, Pagano, Shea, et al., 2005).

Treatment

The goal of treatment is to help patients achieve better adaptation in their lives (1) by changing their dysfunctional interpersonal relationships and their use of immature coping mechanisms and (2) by reducing the distressing symptoms that they experience. The foundation of treatment for personality disorders is psychotherapy (Simeon & Hollander, 2009).

Some researchers believe that personality disorders are more difficult to treat than many of the Axis I psychiatric disorders (Paris, 2003; Simeon & Hollander, 2009). Stone (2006) considered treatability of personality disorders to be determined by patients' capacity to participate in psychotherapy, motivation to change, ability to reflect, and ability to develop a therapeutic alliance. For example, Stone has recognized that

- Patients who are *most amenable* to treatment are those with Cluster C personality disorders (AVPD, DPD, and OCPD); those with BPD with anxious or depressive features; and those with milder forms of HSD.
- Patients with *intermediate amenability* to treatment include those with NPD, PPD, STPD, and SZPD; those with milder forms of ASPD; and those with BPD who are less able to engage in treatment.

- Patients with *low amenability* to treatment include those with BPD with persistent anger, chaotic life situations, paranoid trends, and persistent substance use; those with PPD with religious fanaticism; those with ASPD with predatory traits, violence, callousness, and lack of motivation; and those with NPD with extreme manipulative and paranoid features.
- Patients *at the edge of treatability* include those who have traits that are offensive or repugnant to others such as bigotry, bullying, greed, querulousness, and spitefulness.
- *Untreatable* patients are those at the most severe ends of NPD and ASPD who have extreme entitlement, exploitativeness, and sadism and those who are serial killers.

In treating patients with personality disorders, psychiatric advanced practice nurses must formulate biopsychosocial plans for treatment that address patients' needs in all domains—safety, physical health problems, psychiatric symptoms, interpersonal distress, and impairment of social and vocational functioning (Gabbard, 2005).

Psychotherapy

Although psychotherapy is the "cornerstone of treatment for personality disorders," there have been few empirical studies of psychotherapy for personality disorders other than for the BPD (Stone, 2006, p. 4). Paris (2003) said that while psychotherapy does not change personality, the modification of personality traits may be reflected in the behavioral expression of impulsivity, affective lability, and anxiety. Two types of psychotherapy—psychodynamic therapy and cognitive behavioral therapy (CBT)—have been found to be effective as treatment for personality disorders (Leichsenring & Leibing, 2003). Research-generated data suggest that different types of psychotherapy are indicated for different personality disorders (Nathan & Gorman, 1998; Leichsenring & Leibing).

Cognitive therapy has been found to be effective for eight of the ten personality disorders. The results are mixed for patients with BPD and are not available for patients with STPD (Pretzer, 2004). Studies have shown that

- *Dialectical behavioral therapy* is effective for patients with the parasuicidal behaviors that frequently are present among patients with BPD.
- *Psychodynamic therapy* is effective for patients with BPD and for patients with mixed personality disorders.
- *Behavior therapy* is effective for patients with AVPD.
- *CBT* may be useful for patients with ASPD.
- *Psychotherapy in combination with structured activities, group activities, and use of step-down community-based programs* has been found to bring about beneficial changes earlier than a 1-year residential program or standard community-based treatment consisting of medication and case management, and the benefits continue over time (Chiesa, Fonagy, & Holmes, 2006).

Pharmacotherapy

There is no medication with a Food and Drug Administration (FDA) indication for treatment for any of the personality disorders (Grossman, 2004; Simeon & Hollander, 2009). Neither are there medications that change personality traits (Paris, 2004) or medications that change character traits or maladaptive behaviors (Simeon & Hollander; Soloff, 2000). Nevertheless, medications are used to reduce symptoms associated with personality disorders based on the symptoms-focused model (Simeon & Hollander). In this model, the principle is to treat the symptoms without focusing on the etiology. Pharmacotherapy is used to target four symptoms clusters: cognitive-perceptual, impulsivity and aggression, mood instability, and anxiety-behavioral inhibition (Simeon & Hollander). Symptoms become the outcome measures:

- For symptoms that reflect cognitive-perceptual disturbances, such as dissociative symptoms, low-dose antipsychotic medications are the first choice.
- For symptoms of mood dysregulation, antidepressants in the SSRI class are the first choice, followed by atypical antipsychotics and, less often, by antidepressants in the monoamine oxidase inhibitor (MAOI) class (Gunderson & Links, 2007).
- For symptoms of impulsivity, the SSRIs and atypical antipsychotics are the most beneficial, followed by lithium and other mood stabilizers (Gunderson & Links, 2007; Links, Heslegrave, & Villella, 1998; Soloff, 2009).
- For symptoms of anxiety and behavioral inhibition, the SSRIs and MAOIs have been found to be effective (Deltito & Stam, 1989).

A medication targeted at one symptom, such as an atypical antipsychotic used for psychotic-like symptoms, may also improve anxiety, obsessive-compulsive symptoms, mood, and suicidal behaviors (Gunderson & Links, 2007). For example, SSRIs used to treat specific symptoms of patients with BPD, such as depression and anxiety, have been found to improve interpersonal sensitivity and global functioning (Gunderson & Links, 1995).

Because patients with one personality disorder often have symptoms of other personality disorders, the psychiatric advanced practice nurse needs to understand the underlying psychodynamics and neurobiological correlates of each personality disorder, not just the symptoms. For example, both patients with SZPD and patients with AVPD may lack friends, but their needs for medications—based on the neurobiological correlates of their disorders—will be different.

Issues in Management of Patients with Personality Disorders

Suicide attempts and completed suicide are serious problems in the management of patients with personality disorders. For example, approximately 75% of patients with BPD will make a suicide attempt (Grossman, 2004). Risk factors for suicide attempts among individuals with personality disorders include negative life events, such as problems with love relationships or marriage; legal problems; a diagnosis of BPD and comorbid major depression or substance-related disorders; and a history of childhood sexual abuse (Yen et al., 2005).

Measuring outcomes of personality disorders remains an issue, with the criteria for some personality disorders being symptom based, some trait based, and some a combination (Stone, 2006). Because personality disorders are described as having stable and enduring patterns of inner experiences and behaviors, the question arises as to what are anticipated treatment outcomes (Sanislow & McGlashan, 1998).

In contrast to treatment outcomes of Axis I psychiatric disorders, which are usually measured in terms of syndromal variation (that is, whether the patient still meets the criteria for the disorder or is in remission), treatment outcomes of personality disorders are usually measured in terms of symptoms, attitudes, behaviors, and functioning. Treatment with pharmacotherapy targets the *symptoms* that are indicators of specific personality disorders; treatment with psychotherapy targets the *behaviors* associated with specific personality disorders; and treatment with psychosocial interventions targets *distress and impaired functioning* (Stone, 2006).

Measurement of treatment outcome is influenced by

- Need to measure outcome of multidisciplinary team interventions (Woods & Richards, 2003)
- Patients' nonadherence to treatment or discontinuation of treatment
- Problems between patients and the treatment team caused by the team's being inconsistent in responses to patients' behaviors, the team's anger with patients, and the patients' use of immature defense mechanisms, such as splitting (Duff, 2003)

Overall, the strongest response to treatment is seen in the area of symptoms, and the second strongest is in social functioning. Amount of use of services is the next strongest response to treatment, and change in personality disorder status is weakest (Woods & Richards).

Course

Recent follow-up studies of personality disorders have shown significant improvement in psychopathology over time (Grilo & McGlashan, 2009; Gunderson & Links, 2007). According to Skodol, Gunderson, Shea, et al. (2005a), more than half of patients with personality disorders achieved remission within the first 2 years of follow-up, with remission defined as "at least 12 consecutive months with no more than two criteria of their baseline disorder" (pp. 494-495).

Of the two components of personality disorders—(1) dysfunctional personality traits and (2) the dysfunctional behaviors (such as self-injury or avoiding people) that are attempts at adapting, coping, or compensating for the dysfunctional personality traits—personality traits are more stable, more enduring. Skodol et al. (2005b) suggested that their greater stability may reflect their genetic and biological components. Behaviors, which are less stable, may reflect developmental and learning experiences, life situations, and stress. As such, they may be more responsive to psychotherapy, changes in life situations, and management of stressors. Although the psychopathology of personality disorders may improve, there is often persistent impairment of functioning, behavioral problems, and diminished quality of life (Skodol, 2008; Skodol et al., 2005a).

Classification

The two most frequently used systems are classification by *dimension* and classification by *category*. Classification by dimension, which was proposed by Siever and Davis (1991), groups personality disorders by four dimensions: cognitive-perceptual organization, impulse control, affect regulation, and anxiety modulation Based on the evidence provided by research in the neurosciences, there has been a trend to accept the concept of personality disorders in terms of underlying dimensions (Skodol, 2009). However, currently the most used system of classification is the categorical, multiaxial *DSM-IV-TR* system (American Psychiatric Association, 2000). It is used in research, in clinical settings, and as a way of obtaining reimbursement for clinical services. Each classification system has its supporters and detractors (Livesley, 1998; Magnavita, 2004). For example, Krueger (2010) said that the classification by category is based on arbitrary thresholds of severity and length of time of symptoms, and he recommended that the dimensional model be used in the revised *DSM-V*. Other researchers are also recommending that classification by dimension be accepted for personality disorders in the *DSM-V* (Oldham, 2009; Widiger, 1991).

Personality disorders classified by dimension will be introduced, but because psychiatric advanced practice nurses are more likely to use the *DSM-IV-TR* system of classification in their practice, descriptions of the specific personality disorders as classified by category will be the focus of this chapter.

Personality Disorders by Dimensional Theory

Some researchers view the ten personality disorders and their physiology not only as being linked to each other by their symptoms but also as being linked to Axis I psychiatric disorders (Table 18-1). So far, research has not supported either the connection between Cluster B personality disorders and mood disorders or the

TABLE 18-1 DIMENSIONAL CATEGORIES: CHARACTERISTICS, EXAMPLES OF PERSONALITY DISORDERS, AND POSSIBLE LINK WITH *DSM-IV-TR* AXIS I DISORDERS

Dimensional Category	Characteristics	Examples of Personality Disorders	Possible Link with DSM-IV-TR Axis I Disorders
Cognitive-perceptual organization	Impairment of ability to perceive and process information from the environment in relation to past experiences and to select an appropriate response	Schizoid personality disorder: detachment, indifference, and isolation Schizotypal personality disorder: odd beliefs, speech, and ideas Paranoid personality disorder: read hidden meanings into remarks or events	Psychotic disorders, such as schizophrenia
Impulse control	Action-oriented; impulsive, aggressive, and novelty-seeking behaviors (Fossati et al., 2007)	Antisocial personality disorder: irritability, recklessness, and lack of concern for others Borderline personality disorder: outbursts of intense anger, suicidal ideation, and self-injurious behaviors Narcissistic personality disorder: aggressive, assertive, domineering, and manipulative behaviors Histrionic personality disorder: activities may be impulsive with emphasis on attracting attention	Impulse-control disorders
Affect regulation	Instability of emotions	Antisocial personality disorder: irritability and anger Borderline personality disorder: unstable relationships, unstable self-image, anger, and feelings of emptiness Narcissistic personality disorder: rage in response to failure of others to acknowledge the patient's uniqueness and superiority Histrionic personality disorder: shallow emotions	Mood disorders
Anxiety modulation	Anxiety and inhibition involve the ability to anticipate future danger or the consequences of immediate behaviors	Avoidant personality disorder: anxiety and inhibition are shown in fear of rejection and of being criticized Dependent personality disorder: anxiety is seen in reluctance to assume responsibility for decision-making Obsessive-compulsive personality disorder: anxiety and inhibition are seen in reluctance to make changes	Anxiety disorders

Sources: Coccaro & Siever, 2009; Lee & Coccaro, 2009; Siever & Davis, 1991.

connection between Cluster C personality disorders and anxiety disorders. There is support for the connection between STPD within Cluster A and schizophrenia (an Axis I disorder), some support for a connection between PPD and schizophrenia, but little support for a connection between SZPD and schizophrenia (Dolan-Sewell et al., 2001). Thus, at this time, there is little evidence that the personality disorders are on a continuum with Axis I psychiatric disorders.

Personality Disorders by Category

Classification by category is based on the premise that personality disorders are distinct clinical syndromes. It relies on establishing the presence of observable criteria to determine the presence of a psychiatric disorder. General characteristics of each of the ten *DSM-IV-TR* personality disorder diagnoses can be found in Table 18-2. The ten personality disorders are arranged in three categories: Cluster A is called the odd-eccentric; Cluster B, the dramatic-emotional; and Cluster C, the anxious-fearful (American Psychiatric Association, 2002).

Cluster A Personality Disorders: Odd-Eccentric

Cluster A includes PPD, STPD, and SZPD. These personality disorders are characterized by cognitive distortions, disturbances of perception, emotional flatness, and suspiciousness (Simeon & Hollander, 2006). Patients with Cluster A personality disorders share certain characteristics. They are guarded, are unlikely to interact with others, are uncomfortable in intimate relationships, have difficulty reading social cues, and lack empathy (Skodol & Gunderson, 2008; Stone, 2007). However, their symptoms result from different biological, developmental, and experienced factors.

Paranoid Personality Disorder (PPD)

The word *paranoia* comes from old Greek: it means "a mind beside itself" and was originally used to describe insanity (Robinson, 1996, p. 75). The key characteristics of PPD are suspiciousness and a pervasive and unwarranted distrust of others (Oldham, 2009; Skodol & Gunderson, 2008).

TABLE 18-2 CHARACTERISTICS OF THE TEN *DSM-IV-TR* PERSONALITY DISORDER DIAGNOSES

Personality Disorder	Characteristics
Antisocial	Criminal activities; aggressive, impulsive, irresponsible behaviors. Disregards rights of others. History of conduct disorder before age 15 years.
Avoidant	Avoids occupational activities that involve significant interpersonal contact because of fear of criticism, disapproval, or rejection.
Borderline	Instability of interpersonal relationships. Impulsivity. Frantic efforts to avoid real or imagined abandonment.
Dependent	Needs other to assume responsibility for most major areas of his or her life. Wants someone to take care of him or her. Clinging behaviors. Unable to make decisions.
Histrionic	Excessive display of emotions. Is uncomfortable in situations in which he or she is not the center of attention.
Narcissistic	Has a grandiose sense of self-importance and entitlement. Has a need for constant admiration. Lacks empathy.
Obsessive-compulsive	Preoccupation with orderliness. Desire to be in control. Unable to delegate work. Shows perfectionism that interferes with task completion. Can't discard worn-out or useless items.
Paranoid	Suspects, without sufficient basis, that others are exploiting, harming, or deceiving him or her (e.g., spousal jealousy without cause).
Schizoid	Pattern of detachment from social relationships. Neither desires nor seeks close relationships.
Schizotypal	Cognitive and perceptual distortions. Odd or eccentric behavior, beliefs, and speech; constricted emotional expression; ideas of reference. Limited capacity for close relationships.

Sources: Allnutt & Links, 1996, Skodol, 2009.

Epidemiology and Etiology

PPD has been found to occur in 1.25% to 1.5% of the general population (Torgersen, 2005), but others have reported a much higher rate of 4.41% of the general population (Grant, Hasin, Stinson, et al., 2004). PPD is more common in men (First & Tasman, 2004). The heritability of PPD is 28% (Smoller, Sheidley, & Tsuang, 2008; Torgersen et al., 2000). Because PPD occurs frequently in families of patients with schizophrenia or delusional disorder, it is thought that there may be some link with these disorders (Coccaro & Siever, 2009). Childhood emotional abuse (verbal abuse, shaming, and humiliation), physical abuse, and sexual abuse have been found to be associated with the development of PPD (Bierer, Yehuda, Schmeidler, et al., 2003), and patients with PPD have been found to have insecure attachment patterns of the dismissive/avoidant type (Stone, 2006).

It is thought that patients with PPD may have experienced parenting that was sadistic, hostile, or controlling and included the use of harsh punishment. As infants, patients may have been handled harshly and punished for crying. The parents may have viewed crying as the baby's criticizing them or demanding something from them (Benjamin, 1996). Children who have experienced maternal verbal abuse and neglect of supervision are at increased risk of developing PPD as adults (Johnson et al., 2000; Johnson et al., 2001). From these experiences, it is thought that the child learns to be fearful, mistrusting, and vigilant for cues to possible abusive treatment from caregivers. Other studies have found that among adolescents, symptoms of PPD are associated with increased exposure to maltreatment and bullying (Natsuaki, Cicchetti, & Rogosch, 2009).

Biological Basis

There is no information available at this time about the biological basis of PPD.

Clinical Presentation

Patients with PPD often do not seek treatment for the symptoms associated with the disorder. They may seek treatment for anxiety, depression, or substance-related disorders, or they may come for treatment because of marital, work, or legal conflicts. Often they come at the urging of spouses or family members. They view suspiciousness and distrust as realistic based on their view of the world as a dangerous, unsafe place (First & Tasman, 2004; Skodol & Gunderson, 2008). On presentation, they are suspicious without cause, and often the suspiciousness is focused on the faithfulness of their spouse or partner. They may be reluctant to reveal information about themselves because they are afraid that it could be used against them. They believe that others are exploiting or deceiving them. They read hidden meaning into benign remarks and are unforgiving of slights. They hold onto grudges. In addition, they may be hypersensitive, feel mistreated and misjudged, and lack a sense of humor and empathic feelings (Robinson, 1996; Skodol, 2009). They may appear sullen, abrasive, or cynical and are unable to read social cues (Skodol & Gunderson). More severe symptoms include pathological jealousy, persecutory beliefs, and litigiousness (Stone, 2007). They do not usually have delusions or hallucinations, but they may have transient psychotic symptoms when under severe stress (First & Tasman, 2004; Lee & Coccaro, 2009). They may use protective behaviors such as locking doors, closing windows and curtains, being unwilling to sign papers, and displaying hypervigilance and self-isolation (Hayward, 2007).

Differential Diagnosis

Paranoid behaviors can be thought of as being on a continuum, from normal vigilance, to PPD, to delusional disorder, to paranoid schizophrenia. Whereas an individual with delusional disorder has an encapsulated, nonbizarre delusion but his or her activities outside the delusion are not obviously unusual, individuals with PPD are hypervigilant and suspicious at all times and in all circumstances. They do not have delusions and their behavior is not encapsulated; rather, their paranoia is pervasive throughout their interactions with others (First & Tasman, 2004). Unlike patients with paranoid schizophrenia, patients with PPD do not have bizarre delusions, hallucinations, and formal thought disorder. Other differential diagnoses that must be considered include mood disorders, which manifest with paranoid elements, and use of amphetamines, marijuana, or cocaine, which can induce paranoid reactions in individuals without psychiatric disorders (Skodol & Gunderson, 2008).

Treatment

The cardinal features of treatment for patients with PPD are respect, integrity, tact, and patience. Psychiatric advanced practice nurses should use a straightforward, nonintrusive style. Recommended treatment strategies include the following:

- Be honest, and be precise.
- Provide detailed information.
- Do *not* challenge negative views or patients' recollection of events; instead, get details and empathize with feelings.
- Do *not* deflate grandiosity, because behind it is often low self-esteem.
- Provide care and information in a nonemotional and matter-of-fact manner (First & Tasman, 2004; Skodol & Gunderson, 2011).

Treatment includes supportive individual psychotherapy and antipsychotic medications for transient psychosis or psychotic decompensation (Skodol & Gunderson, 2008). Patients with PPD do not do well with group therapy because of their suspiciousness and hypersensitivity (Piper & Ogrodniczuk, 2009). The principles of pharmacotherapy for patients with PPD follow the general principles of pharmacotherapy for cognitive-perceptual difficulties. For example, atypical antipsychotic medications, which are the first-line treatment for patients with cognitive-perceptual difficulties, may also improve deficits in attention, learning, and working memory (Ichikawa, Ishii, Bonaccorso, et al., 2001). The antipsychotic pimozide (Orap) has been found to reduce paranoid ideation for some patients (Sadock & Sadock, 2007). Lithium carbonate may also be effective for PPD (Schatzberg, Cole, & DeBattista, 2007). Patients with PPD are often reluctant to take medications for paranoia but may be willing to take medications for co-occurring symptoms of anxiety and depression (Skodol & Gunderson, 2008). There are no controlled studies of pharmacotherapy for PPD (Grossman, 2004; Simeon & Hollander, 2009).

Course

There may be early signs in adolescence of hypersensitivity, hypervigilance, social anxiety, social isolation, anger, hostility, and peculiar thoughts (First & Tasman, 2004). For example, individuals who later developed PPD were judged by their peers, when they were adolescents, to be less cooperative, to have poor leadership skills, and to be more likely to instigate fighting (Natsuaki et al., 2009). As adults, individuals with PPD frequently have poor interpersonal relationships, and although they are usually able to work, they may have difficulty with coworkers (First & Tasman, 2004). They tend to have lifelong problems with working and living with others. Older adults with PPD often make accusations of theft or may barricade themselves in their rooms or homes. Older adults with PPD and physical health problems, sensory decline, and dependence on others find it difficult to accept help from others such as home health-care workers (Segal, Coolidge, & Rosowsky, 2006). PPD runs a chronic course and is generally resistant to therapeutic efforts. Patients with PPD may be at increased risk of developing schizophrenia (Sadock & Sadock, 2007).

Resources

Movies

Kramer, S. (Producer), & Dmytryk, E. (Director). (1954). *The Caine mutiny* [Motion picture]. United States: Columbia Pictures.

Warner, J. L. (Producer), & Huston, J. (Director). (1948). *The treasure of the Sierra Madre* [Motion picture]. United States: Warner Bros.

SOURCE: WEDDING & BOYD, 1999.

Schizoid Personality Disorder (SZPD)

The word *schizoid* means "representing splitting or cleaving" (Robinson, 1996, p. 57). Other terms used in the past to describe patients with SZPD are *shut-in* or *reclusive*. SZPD is characterized by aloofness or a lack of interest in forming relationships with others, detachment from social relationships, restricted range of emotional expressions when with others, and little or no desire for friendships (Skodol & Gunderson, 2008).

Epidemiology and Etiology

The prevalence of SZPD is less than 1% of the general population (Torgersen, 2009). It is one of the least common of the personality disorders and occurs more frequently in men (Skodol & Gunderson, 2008). The heritability of SZPD has been estimated as 28% (Torgersen et al., 2000). The fact that families of patients with SZPD have a higher rate of schizophrenia and STPD than the general population supports the possibility of a genetic link with schizophrenia (Coccaro & Siever, 2009).

Biological Basis, Developmental Influences, and Experienced Factors

Research supporting the link with schizophrenia has shown that patients with SZPD have abnormal functioning in the prefrontal area of the brain that is believed to account for symptoms that are similar to the negative symptoms of schizophrenia (affective flattening, poverty of speech, apathy, lack of energy, and anhedonia) (First & Tasman, 2004). Patients with SZPD have structural abnormalities of the brain—enlarged ventricles and smaller temporal lobe. They have impairment of cognitive functioning, such as problems with sustained attention, verbal learning, working memory, and staying focused. They also have problems with interpreting verbal and facial cues (Coccaro & Siever, 2009). They have the impaired smooth pursuit eye movement that is frequently present in patients with schizophrenia. An indication that brain development of patients with SZPD has been compromised has been provided by the study by Hoek, Susser, Buck, et al. (1996), in which they found an increased rate of SZPD among individuals who had been exposed to nutritional deprivation in utero. Hoek et al. concluded that the developing brains of the infants had not received enough nutrients to develop normally. Other studies have found that SZPD is associated with a history of childhood neglect (Oldham, Skodol, Gallagher, et al., 1996), emotional abuse (Johnson, Bromley, & McGeoch, 2009), physical abuse (Bierer et al., 2003), and sexual abuse (Johnson et al.).

Clinical Presentation

Patients with SZPD present with symptoms that include lack of a desire to be in close relationships, not even part of the family; tendency to choose solitary activities (computer games or puzzles); and an indifference to approval or criticism of others. They have few friends, do not date, seldom marry, and work at jobs that do not require interacting with others (Skodol & Gunderson, 2011). They may be described as cold, aloof loners with no close friends or as daydreamers (Oldham, 2009; Robinson, 1996). Often they do not respond to social cues, and they structure their lives to avoid the necessity of interacting with others (Hayward, 2007). Although they may appear to be socially isolated or lonely to their families, they may not come for treatment because their social isolation does not bother them. An acute stressor that causes anxiety or depression or insistence of a family member may bring them in for treatment (Sadock & Sadock, 2007). On evaluation, they often appear ill at ease and avoid eye contact. They frequently provide short answers to questions, do not engage in spontaneous conversation, and demonstrate poverty of thought and concrete thinking (Hayward). Work history is likely to show that they have worked in noncompetitive, lonely jobs. Their social support network may be limited to relatives, and a history of leisure activities may reveal that they choose activities with limited social contact such as mathematics, astronomy, or animals.

Differential Diagnosis

Differential diagnoses that should be considered include

1. *Avoidant personality disorder.* Patients with AVPD desire relationships but avoid them because of fear of rejection, but patients with SZPD have no desire for social relationships (First & Tasman, 2004).
2. *Schizotypal personality disorder.* Patients with SZPD lack the cognitive and perceptual distortions associated with STPD (Skodol & Gunderson, 2008).
3. *Paranoid personality disorder.* Patients with SZPD lack suspiciousness and distrust seen in patients with PPD (Skodol & Gunderson, 2011).
4. *Schizophrenia.* Although patients with SZPD have symptoms that are similar to the negative symptoms of schizophrenia, they usually do not have the delusions and hallucinations that are associated with schizophrenia, although an acute stressor may cause transient psychotic symptoms that do not last more than 24 hours (Robinson, 1996).
5. *Autistic disorder and Asperger's disorder.* Patients with SZPD do not have as severe impairment of social interactions and do not have stereotyped behaviors and interests, such as fascination with numbers or train schedules (First, Frances, & Pincus, 2002; Skodol & Gunderson, 2011).

Treatment

The goals of treatment for patients with SZPD are modest: reduce social isolation, improve coping, and make their lives more rewarding through the introduction of activities that they can do alone, hobbies, or attending community events (Stone, 2007). Treatment interventions include supportive individual psychotherapy, psychodynamic individual psychotherapy, CBT, and group psychotherapy (Skodol & Gunderson, 2008). The boundaries of therapy—such as time limits, professional setting, ethical restrictions against social relationships, and a therapeutic contract—are comforting for patients with SZPD. They reduce the patient's fear of engulfment or of being dominated. Helpful techniques include the following:

- Be supportive of the patient.
- Use active, warm, empathic, and even humorous approaches.
- Use inanimate bridges, such as writing and artistic productions, to ease the patient into therapy (Coen, 2005; Skodol & Gunderson, 2011).

Very little information is available about pharmacotherapy for patients with SZPD. One study of patients who were thought to have SZPD suggests that use of the atypical antipsychotic risperidone (Risperdal) improves negative symptoms, makes the patient feel more at ease socially, increases interest in social activities, and improves memory and attention (Tsuang, Stone, Tarbox, et al., 2002). Low doses of antipsychotics, antidepressants, and psychostimulants have benefited some patients. Benzodiazepines help to reduce interpersonal anxiety for some (Sadock & Sadock, 2007).

Psychosocial interventions such as support, education about building interpersonal skills, and training in effective communication have been found to be helpful (Stone, 1993). Cognitive adaptation training (which has been used to teach patients with schizophrenia compensatory strategies to improve skills in communication, social interactions, leisure activities, and work) may also be helpful for patients with SZPD (Velligan & Bow-Thomas, 2000).

Course

There tends to be an early childhood onset with symptoms of social isolation. SZPD tends to be stable over time (Paris, 2003). Older adults with SZPD may experience great distress if health problems or impairment of functioning necessitates their living with others such as in a rehabilitation unit or an assisted living situation (Segal et al., 2006).

Resources

Movies

Engel, F. (Producer), & Gries, T. (Director). (1968). *Will Penny* [Motion picture]. United States: Paramount Pictures.

Wizan, J. (Producer), & Pollack, S. (Director). (1972). *Jeremiah Johnson* [Motion picture]. United States: Warner Bros.

Kasdan, L. (Director). (1988). *The accidental tourist* [Motion picture]. United States: Warner Bros.

SOURCE: WEDDING & BOYD, 1999.

Parker, J. (Director). (2001). *Bartleby* [Motion picture]. United States: Outrider Pictures.

Coen, J. (Director). (2001). *The man who wasn't there* [Motion picture]. United States: USA Films.

SOURCE: WEDDING, BOYD & NIEMIEC, 2010, P. 73.

Schizotypal Personality Disorder (STPD)

The word *schizotypal* is an abbreviation for "schizophrenic genotype." Black and Andreasen (2011) considered STPD to be part of the schizophrenia spectrum, which includes "schizophreniform disorder, schizoaffective disorder, and perhaps psychotic mood disorders." STPD is characterized by deficits in interpersonal relationships and distortions in cognition and perception, such as magical thinking or strange ideas. The symptoms associated with STPD are similar to the positive symptoms of schizophrenia but are expressed to a lesser degree (First & Tasman, 2004). The symptoms that are most frequent and stable over time are paranoid ideation, ideas of reference (interpreting incidents and events as having direct reference to them), odd beliefs, and unusual experiences such as telepathy or clairvoyance (McGlashan, Grilo, Sanislow, et al., 2005; Oldham, 2009). Patients with STPD suffer impaired functioning in many domains, including employment, household duties, academic work, interpersonal relationships, and socialization. The degree of impairment is less than that experienced by patients with schizophrenia (Skodol, Gunderson, McGlashan, et al., 2002).

Epidemiology and Etiology

The prevalence of STPD is 0.7% to 1.2% of the general population (Torgersen, 2005). It may occur slightly more often in men (Corbitt & Widiger, 1995), although Black and Andreasen (2011) found the rate to be similar for men and women. Heritability accounts for 61% of the variance of STPD (Torgersen et al., 2000). SZPD has a strong genetic link to schizophrenia (Gooding, Tallent, & Matts, 2007; Raine, Lencz, & Mednick, 1995). In addition to strong genetic influence, the etiology of STPD appears to be associated with abnormalities of brain development, adverse circumstances of birth, and neglect and abuse.

Biological Basis and Other Influences

Patients with STPD have structural brain abnormalities, impairments of functioning, and abnormalities of neurochemistry that are similar to those of patients with schizophrenia. They have multiple deficits in the frontal lobe, subcortical areas, temporal area, and to some degree the thalamus, which serves as the primary transport of information from the subcortical brain structures to the cortical brain areas (McCloskey, Phan, & Coccaro, 2005). Patients with STPD have cognitive impairment, such as abnormalities of executive functioning, working memory, and sustaining attention (Gold & Harvey, 1993; Grossman, 2004; Raine, Sheard, Reynolds, et al., 1992). They show hyperarousal to external stimuli, as do patients with schizophrenia. They have impairment of smooth pursuit eye movement, which is also found in patients with schizophrenia. Siever, Keefe, Bernstein, et al. (1990) wrote that abnormal eye movements are linked with the negative symptoms (flat affect, apathy, poverty of speech, asociality, and inattentiveness) that are found in patients with schizophrenia and found to a lesser degree in patients with STPD. Abnormalities of neurochemistry include elevated levels of dopamine (Coccaro & Siever, 2009) and increased cortisol levels (Walker, Logan, & Waller, 1999).

Developmental Influences

Similarly to schizophrenia, prenatal exposure to famine is associated with increased risk for STPD (Hoek et al., 1996). Also similar to schizophrenia, patients with STPD have increased rates of minor physical anomalies, which are external marks of abnormal fetal development (see Chapter 3 for discussion of minor physical anomalies). Adolescents with STPD have more abnormal involuntary motor movements—such as writhing, facial grimacing, twitching, and lip/tongue movements—than controls or than adolescents with other personality disorders. This finding suggests the possibility of prenatal damage to the motor circuitry of the brain.

Adverse Circumstances of Birth

Patients with STPD often have histories of birth complications, such as problems with breathing, need for oxygen, breech delivery, and induced labor.

Experienced Factors

Neglect, physical abuse, and sexual abuse in childhood have been found to be associated with increased risk for the development of STPD (Bierer et al., 2003; Johnson et al., 1999; Johnson et al., 2009).

Clinical Presentation

Patients with STPD do not usually seek treatment, but exposure to a severe stressor may increase their symptoms or may cause transient psychotic symptoms that prompt others to seek treatment for them. They have a pattern of difficulty with social and interpersonal relationships and often are anxious in social situations. They tend to believe that there is a reason for everything that happens. They often view themselves as defective (Hayward, 2007). They exhibit disturbances of thinking and communication, such as odd beliefs or magical thinking. They are often superstitious or paranoid or claim powers of clairvoyance. They may believe that they have a sixth sense and may demonstrate odd behaviors, such as rubbing small smooth stones. They may also describe ideas of reference and unusual perceptual experiences. They may behave in an eccentric manner, talk to themselves in public, dress in a peculiar or unkempt way, and use metaphorical or circumstantial patterns of speech. They are socially uncomfortable and withdrawn (Skodol & Gunderson, 2011). Although they have symptoms that are similar to the positive symptoms of schizophrenia, they usually do not have delusions and hallucinations. Any transient psychotic symptoms of delusions and hallucinations usually do not last longer than 24 hours. They often do not have friends, and their social network is limited to family members.

Differential Diagnosis

Differential diagnoses include other personality disorders, delusional disorder, and schizophrenia. STPD differs from schizophrenia, delusional disorder, and mood disorder with psychotic features because it lacks long-lasting psychosis. The social detachment in STPD differs from that of PPD and SZPD by the presence of cognitive or perceptual distortions and eccentricity or odd beliefs or perceptions (First et al., 2002; Skodol & Gunderson, 2008). The social detachment differs from that of AVPD, in which there is a desire for relationships but a fear of rejection if relationships are attempted (First et al.).

Treatment

Treatment may focus on the feelings or situations that brought the patient for treatment such as depression, paranoia, suspiciousness, or social isolation (Black & Andreasen, 2011). Treatment includes supportive individual psychotherapy and cognitive psychotherapy. Pharmacotherapy in the form of low-dose antipsychotic medications may be useful in dealing with anxiety, ideas of reference, or psychotic-like features. Psychosocial interventions, such as psychoeducation and social skills training, are beneficial (Skodol & Gunderson, 2011).

Psychotherapy and Cognitive Therapy

Group therapy can increase socialization and may function as a surrogate family for the patient; however, because patients with STPD often have strange beliefs and practices, they may be ridiculed by other members of a group (Piper & Orgrodniczuk, 2009). Cognitive therapy has the potential to change basic cognitive distortions such as mistrust, suspiciousness, ideas of reference, emotional reasoning (automatically thinking that things will go wrong), and personalization (e.g., the patient's belief that he or she is responsible for situations) (Robinson, 1996). Cognitive therapy teaches patients to look for objective evidence to evaluate their automatic assumptions. It increases coping skills that do not rely on emotional responses, and it teaches effective communication skills.

Pharmacotherapy

Atypical antipsychotics, such as olanzapine (Zyprexa) and risperidone, have been found to be effective for the positive and negative symptoms of STPD (Grossman, 2004; Schatzberg et al., 2007; Soloff, 2009). SSRIs have been found to be effective in reducing depression, anxiety, interpersonal sensitivity, paranoia, and psychotic symptoms. It has been reported that tricyclic antidepressants make the symptoms of STPD worse (Grossman).

Course

Patients with STPD may have had symptoms in childhood, such as social isolation, peculiar behaviors, problems with school, and fantasies. As adults, patients with STPD are at increased risk of developing depression, dysthymia, and anxiety disorders. Unlike some personality disorders, the symptoms of STPD do not decrease with age (First & Tasman, 2004; Paris, 2003), and some older adults experience an increase in bizarre behaviors and social isolation (Segal et al., 2006). Because of its overlap genetically with schizophrenia, 10% to 20% of patients with STPD may develop schizophrenia. Predictors for development of schizophrenia include the presence of magical thinking, paranoid ideation, and social isolation. Ten percent of patients with STPD commit suicide (Sadock & Sadock, 2007). Among patients with STPD, positive achievement experiences and positive interpersonal relationships during childhood or adolescence are significantly associated with better outcomes and remission. The greater the number of positive experiences and the broader the developmental period they covered, the better the prognosis (Skodol, Bender, Pagano, et al., 2007). In the Collaborative Longitudinal Personality Disorders Study (CLIPS), 33% of patients with STPD achieved remission within 24 months (Grilo, Sanislow, Gunderson, et al., 2004).

Resources

Movies

Scorsese, M. (Director). (1976). *Taxi driver* [Motion picture]. United States: Columbia Pictures.

Source: Wedding & Boyd, 1999.

Burton, T. (Director). (2005). *Charlie and the chocolate factory* [Motion picture]. United States: Warner Bros.

Binder, M. (Director). (2007). *Reign over me* [Motion picture]. United States: Columbia Pictures.

Source: Wedding, Boyd, & Niemiec, 2010, p. 73.

Cluster B Personality Disorders: Impulsive-Dramatic

Cluster B includes ASPD, BPD, HBD, and NPD. Patients with Cluster B personality disorders tend to show dramatic, emotional, and impulsive behaviors. These disorders tend to be comorbid with major depressive disorders, substance use disorders, bulimia nervosa, and anxiety disorders (panic disorder and post-traumatic stress disorder) (Oldham, 2009).

Antisocial Personality Disorder (ASPD)

ASPD is the oldest and best-validated of the personality disorders. The terms "moral insanity" and "psychopathic personality" have been used in the past to describe ASPD. The key features of ASPD are a pattern of exploitative and irresponsible behaviors, attitudes that deny or violate the rights of others, and history of conduct disorder before the age of 15 years (Skodol, 2009). There is a lifelong tendency to commit crimes and other acts forbidden by society. Patients with ASPD are often reckless in their behaviors, do not anticipate the consequences of their behaviors, and do not learn from their mistakes. They lack remorse for the harm that they cause to others and may be irresponsible as parents, unfaithful as spouses, and dishonest and deceitful as employees (Paris, 2003; Skodol & Gunderson, 2011). They crave constant novelty and excitement and have difficulty controlling their aggressive impulses (Oldham, 2009). Some are glib and charming and use these attributes to seduce or exploit others (Skodol & Gunderson).

Epidemiology and Etiology

Estimates of the prevalence of ASPD are 1.1% of the general population. It is more common among men than women (Torgersen, 2009). Prevalence is much higher in psychiatric hospitals, among the homeless, among individuals addicted to alcohol or drugs, and among those who are incarcerated (Black & Andreasen, 2011). For example, among the prison population, the rate of ASPD is estimated to be 50% (Robins & Regier, 1991), although more recent estimates are as high as 75% (Sadock & Sadock, 2007). On the other hand, some individuals with ASPD are high achievers. For example, studies of top business executives show that 15% have misrepresented their educational achievements and 33% have lied on their resumes. Individuals with ASPD do not do well in organizations where there are rigid policies and procedures, but they do very well in companies that are undergoing rapid change. They thrive amid chaos (Sherman, 2000).

The etiology of ASPD is believed to be a combination of genetic predisposition, abnormalities of brain development, childhood maltreatment, adverse experiences within the family, negative social influences, and absence of protective factors. The heritability of ASPD is 68% (Smoller et al., 2008), and the rate of concordance in identical twins is 67%. The genetic risk is high; for children with one parent with ASPD, the risk of developing ASPD is 16%.

The genetic influence for antisocial behaviors and for alcohol dependence seems to be similar in that the two disorders appear to share susceptibility genes. This shared susceptibility may explain why alcohol dependence in late adolescence has been found to be associated with persistence of antisocial behaviors, i.e., alcohol dependence potentiates and maintains the antisocial behaviors (Malone, Taylor, Marmorstein, et al., 2004).

Abnormalities of prenatal development of the brain also appear to be involved in the development of ASPD. Among patients with ASPD, 38% have been found to have minimal brain damage, suggesting abnormalities of brain development (Van Reekum, 1993). Abnormalities of brain development are indicated by the increased rate of soft neurological signs among patients with ASPD and increased rate of minor physical anomalies (Lindberg, Tani, Stenberg, et al., 2004) (see Chapter 3 for discussion of soft neurological signs and minor physical anomalies).

Adverse factors within the family also play a role in the development of ASPD. In families of patients with ASPD, there is often a history of alcoholism, paternal criminality, family conflict, divorce, and poverty. Parenting is characterized by the use of physical punishment, rejection, lack of parental supervision, poorly regulated schooling, and little emphasis on communication within the family. During the first 5 years of childhood, patients who later develop ASPD experience high rates of traumatic abandonment and physical and sexual abuse (Johnson et al., 2009; Paris, 2004).

Protective factors (factors that promote the development of adaptive personality traits) were discussed earlier in the chapter. Protective factors specific to ASPD are believed to include a sense of anxiousness about consequences of wrongdoing (a conscience), ability for self-regulation of behaviors (constraint), intelligence that enables the individual to consider other options, and absence of substance use (Sutker & Allain, 2001).

Biological Basis

Individuals with ASPD have been found to have reductions in whole-brain volume, in the volume of the temporal lobe (Barkataki, Kumari, Das, et al., 2006), and in the volume of the prefrontal cortex (Raine, Lencz, Bihrle, et al., 2000). The prefrontal area of the brain is involved in modulating emotion, arousal (thrill-seeking), and attention, and a consequence of its impairment of functioning may be the individual's failure to develop a conscience. This speculation is supported by the finding that exposure to a fear stimulus in psychopathic criminal offenders results in deficient brain activation of the prefrontal-limbic circuit (Birbaumer, Veit, Lotze, et al., 2005).

In addition to lower volume, the brain scans of patients with ASPD show lower than average activity in the frontal lobes, which govern judgment and decision making

(McCloskey et al., 2005). Compromised functioning of the prefrontal area is evidenced by impaired learning and problem-solving, insensitivity to the emotional connotations of language, failure to develop normal fearfulness, and inability to learn from rewards and punishment (Paris, 1996). Patients with ASPD have also been found to have dysfunction of the amygdala (Schwerdtner, Sommer, Weber, et al., 2004), which, together with the prefrontal cortex, modulates aggression. The prefrontal cortex modulates reactive aggression (the aggression that is elicited in response to frustration such as that seen in patients with BPD) by interpreting other social cues from the environment. The amygdala is involved in regulating instrumental aggression (the aggression that is goal directed and is seen in patients with ASPD) (Blair, 2004). Patients with ASPD also have abnormalities of the autonomic nervous system, e.g., reduced autonomic activity during exposure to stress. Autonomic activity is thought to be involved in experiencing emotional states, in guiding pro-social behavior, and in making good decisions. In addition, patients with ASPD have abnormal physiological signs that suggest altered regulation of both the dopamine system, which regulates aggression, and the serotonin system, which modulates aggression and depression.

Clinical Presentation

Patients with ASPD may give a childhood history starting at age of 5 years of bedwetting, hitting others, lying, behaving aggressively toward others, fire-setting, being cruel to animals, and running away. As adults, there may be a history of irresponsibility, impulsiveness, reckless behaviors, and exploitation and manipulation of others. They may appear self-centered, demanding, cocky, irritable, and angry (Robinson, 1996) or glib, charming, ingratiating, and manipulative (Sadock & Sadock, 2007; Skodol & Gunderson, 2011). They do not usually show anxiety, depression, or irrational thinking. Robinson described the common themes in the lives of individuals with ASPD as having had behavioral problems as a child and as an adult engaging in criminal activities, having parole or probation violations, engaging in sexually promiscuous behaviors, conning others, having poor impulse control, avoiding responsibility for actions, and abusing substances. Patients with ASPD may display or give a history of aggression in which violence is accompanied by high levels of sympathetic arousal and emotions, usually anger or fear. They may also display or give a history of predatory aggression in which the violence is emotionless, planned, and purposeful (Melroy, 2007). Comorbid alcohol or drug use disorders, mood disorders, anxiety disorders, and suicide attempts are frequently present (Black & Andreasen, 2011).

Differential Diagnosis

Antisocial behavior occurs in other psychiatric disorders, in other personality disorders, and in substance-related disorders. In differentiating ASPD from schizophrenia and bipolar disorder, patients with ASPD will have a history of conduct disorder and early onset of antisocial behavior. In schizophrenia, there are often prolonged psychotic episodes that are not present in ASPD. In bipolar disorder, behaviors are related to mood changes.

In differentiating ASPD from other personality disorders, NPD and HPD usually do not have a history of conduct disorder and are not characterized by aggressiveness and impulsivity. In PPD, antisocial behavior is motivated by revenge (First et al., 2002). In BPD, there are often symptoms of fear of abandonment that are not present in individuals with ASPD. In substance-related disorders, antisocial behaviors are episodic and associated with alcohol or drug intake (Skodol & Gunderson, 2011).

Treatment

ASPD is one of the most difficult of the personality disorders to treat (Melroy, 2007; Stone, 1993, 2006). Melroy recommended that the level of psychopathy be measured in order to determine the likelihood of response to treatment. Psychopathy can be measured with the *Psychopathy Checklist-Revised Manual* (Hare, 1991), which is a scale that has 20 items with a range of response from 0 to 2. A score in the 10-to-19 range indicates a mild level of psychopathy; a score of 20 to 29 indicates moderate psychopathy; and a score of 39 or more indicates severe psychopathy. Patients with ASPD with severe psychopathy have a poor response to treatment and are generally considered by clinical and legal professionals to be untreatable (Melroy, 2007; Stone, 2006).

Patients with ASPD often lack motivation and commitment to change (Stone, 2006), and motivation for treatment may be related to a court order, a requirement of an employer, or the insistence of a relative or spouse (First & Tasman, 2004). Principles of treatment for individuals with ASPD include being respectful and using unwavering honesty, keeping promises, and addressing the reality of the patient's situation.

Psychotherapy

Although psychotherapy for patients with ASPD is often thought to be ineffective, Salekin (2002) found that therapy such as CBT provided four times a week in individual sessions for 1 year was associated with a decrease in lying, an increase in remorse and empathy, and improvement in relationships. Salekin recommended that psychotherapy include helping patients with ASPD to consider the long-term consequences of antisocial behaviors and the material value and advantages to be gained from pro-social behavior.

Pharmacotherapy

Although the core features of ASPD are not responsive to pharmacotherapy, explosive, impulsive aggression that causes interpersonal and social problems can be treated with medication. Some patients benefit from anticonvulsants for impulsive behaviors or repetitive, violent behaviors (Schatzberg et al., 2007). The atypical antipsychotic risperidone has been found to decrease aggression

(Hirose, 2001). Irritability, impulsivity, and aggression have been found to respond to quetiapine (Seroquel) (Walker, Thomas, & Allen, 2003). Some patients respond to lithium and anticonvulsants such as phenytoin (Dilantin). For example, lithium has been found to reduce anger, threatening behavior, and assaultiveness in prisoners (Black & Andreasen, 2011). Beta blockers may reduce aggression (Grossman, 2004). Medications such as SSRIs may be used for co-occurring depression and anxiety. Because patients with ASPD have a high rate of comorbid substance abuse, medications must be used with caution.

Psychosocial Interventions

Psychosocial interventions that have been tried include milieu or residential therapy, token therapy, therapeutic community, and wilderness programs. Reports of effectiveness of these approaches are inconclusive.

Course

The impulsive behaviors of ASPD can be seen in childhood in the behaviors that meet the criteria for conduct disorder: aggression to people and animals, destruction of property, deceitfulness or theft, and failure to follow rules (American Psychiatric Association, 2000; Caspi, Moffitt, Newman, et al., 1996; Simonoff, Elander, Holmshaw, et al., 2004). Among children with conduct disorder, 40% of boys and 25% of girls go on to develop ASPD. Those with a greater degree of conduct deviance and greater severity, especially before the age of 10 years, are at greater risk of developing ASPD (Lynam, 1996). As teenagers, they may engage in shoplifting and automobile theft. As young adults, they may be impoverished, homeless, or incarcerated (Robins & Regier, 1991). As 30-year-olds, they may be unable to maintain employment or relationships and may be involved in robbery or rape. As 40-year-olds, they may drink too much and cheat their employers. Conversely, they may be charming and successful in their careers (Widiger & Lynam, 1998).

Patients with ASPD may have co-occurring depressive disorders, alcohol use disorders, substance abuse disorders, suicide attempts, and legal problems (Black & Andreasen, 2011). Over time, patients with ASPD may experience long prison terms, physical injuries, loss of speed and strength, and substance abuse; they may also experience positive life events, such as marriage or employment. There is a decrease in impulsivity by age 38, but the problems with interpersonal relationships and employment remain (Andreasen & Black, 2006). As older adults they are often socially isolated because they have been cut off by their family, and although they may no longer be involved in antisocial activities, they may continue to be exploitative, deceitful, and irresponsible (Segal et al., 2006).

In one follow-up study of men with ASPD, 25% had died prematurely, 61% had married (39% had married more than once), and 91% had had children. Few had been involved in raising the children, and among the children, one-third had psychiatric disorders (Black, Baumgard, Bell, et al., 1996). In another report of the outcome of patients with a diagnosis of ASPD, 94% had work-related problems, 85% had problems with violence, 72% had moving traffic accidents, and 67% had marital problems (Black, 1999). Thus, the cost to society of ASPD is high: crime, swindling, assault, abuse of family, failure to pay child support, and scams that victimize others.

Case Study 18-1 illustrates a comprehensive assessment of a patient with ASPD including a legal history; the generation of diagnoses and use of the five axes of the *DSM-IV-TR*; development of a treatment plan; nonadherence of the patient to treatment; and outcome.

CASE STUDY 18-1

Comprehensive Assessment of a Patient With Antisocial Personality Disorder

James is a 27-year-old Caucasian male who presented at interview with expansive mood. Affect was friendly, engaging, and initially appropriate to words. He appeared well groomed, tall, and very muscular, wearing clean, expensive name-brand athletic wear, jeans, and sneakers. He was tanned, with large dark eyes and long eyelashes, highlighted by a single, blackish-blue, teardrop-shaped tattoo under one eye. (Interviewer aware that literature shows that some gang members have one tattooed teardrop under their eye as a symbol for each person's life they have taken.)

James reported that last month he had been court ordered to go to counseling but skipped a few appointments, as he believed he knew more about life than the counselor. In a matter-of-fact way, he stated that because he missed counseling and had a fight with the mother of his 4-year-old son, he was arrested. He then presented as very remorseful, with intrusive eye contact, and stated, "The judge told me I had to resume counseling, so I'm ready to work on improving myself." He then leaned forward in his chair and stated, "I was in a gang for awhile but I gave up that life for the sake of my son."

Chief Complaint

"When I'm very angry I don't always know what happened...I'm afraid I might someday hurt someone." "I have periods in my life when I think I'm 10 feet tall and bulletproof." (Smilingly), he described history of "misunderstandings and unfairness with the legal system."

History

History of Present Illness: James reported that he was visiting his 4-year-old son at his girlfriend's house, and they had an argument over her dating another guy; she infuriated him to the point that he put a knife to her throat, but only to scare her.

CASE STUDY 18-1—continued

She then called the police and, before the police arrived, he took more than 50 tablets of his prescribed muscle relaxant. He relayed he had no intention of dying, but realized he would be referred to psychiatry after his arrest.

After arrest, he was seen by a psychiatrist. He told the psychiatrist that he had suicidal ideation and was placed on an antidepressant. He went on to say that he had read the antidepressant side effects, which showed that an antidepressant could increase suicidal ideation, so—after 3 days of taking this—he waited until bedtime and loosely tied a plastic bag around his head and went to sleep. He added that he knew the jail staff would find him. Subsequently, he was transferred to the Psychiatric floor of a local hospital.

Later, he again went before the judge, and was again mandated to continue psychiatric treatment and anger management counseling. He added that his prior counselor had spoken to him about "guilt," but he stated that he feels no guilt for protecting himself from his girlfriend's actions and the police.

In a matter-of-fact way, James briefly reported that he had brought home a puppy for his son a few months ago, and it kept barking so he punched it and it died. James stated that his mother "overreacted" and told him he needs help. He verbalized that he didn't like to see his mother upset, but that he can always get another dog.

Past Psychiatric History:

- Inpatient: First admission 2 months ago, as described above.
- Outpatient: One year ago, drug counseling. Attempted court-ordered counseling last month.

Drug and ETOH History:

- Cannabis: Occasionally since age 12 until about 3 weeks ago.
- While in college (attended for 3 years), used cocaine daily. Last use was the end of the last year in college.
- In college, injected HGH, steroids, and illegal use of testosterone.
- After college for about 3 years, used crack cocaine daily, with occasional weekend use of heroin (IV and snort). Also social ETOH use, then he claims he "got clean for his son."

Family Psychiatric History:

- Father: lifelong use of cocaine, cannabis, "pharmaceutical drugs, acid, painkillers." He recalls, as a young boy, observing his father using cocaine. His father was incarcerated for 10 years for selling cocaine at their family-owned restaurant.
- He further recalled both parents' use of drugs and gambling, and often his parents hired prostitutes to babysit him.
- At age 4, his parents enrolled him in wresting and hockey as an outlet, and he has a black belt in Tae Kwon Do.

History of Suicidality:

Recent history of overdose just before arrest (as described above).

Soon after, made suicidal gesture in order to be transferred from jail to psychiatric hospital.

Medical History:

- Chronic lumbar pain related to injury while briefly working as roofer. He reported that this occurred 1 month before he was scheduled to sign Pro-Hockey contract. (Primary Medical Doctor verified injury and contract opportunity.)
- He is currently under care of MD Pain Specialist and has been prescribed muscle relaxer as needed.
- Upon Initial Interview, height is 6′ and weight is 218 lb.

Allergies

- NKDA
- He reported hx side effect: brand-name antidepressant caused suicidal ideation. (Questionable due to 3-day trial.)

Legal History

- First arrest age 12 for vandalism and breaking and entering.
- Age 14, arrested for criminal mischief, shooting out neighbor's picture window with BB gun.
- Age 20, arrested for attempted murder, pled down to self-defense.
- Attempted to join military, but when ordered to do exercises, punched officer, led to dishonorable discharge.
- Age 25, arrested for cannabis possession.
- Age 26, arrested for endangering the welfare of a minor.
- Age 26, joined gang, running/selling drugs, violence, using/selling guns. He claims he "left for his son, and as most of the members went to prison." He admitted he continues to have contact with some of the members.

Marital Status

- Single, never married.
- Has 4-year-old son with girlfriend of 7 years; she has custody of son. Tenuous relationship with girlfriend, he stated he has never lived with her.
- Lives with mother, who takes care of his son during visitation.
- Father incarcerated.

Occupational History

- Periodically works as welder.

Mental Status Examination

- Mood: expansive. Affect friendly, engaging, calm, and initially appropriate to words.
- Alert, oriented all spheres. No psychomotor agitation present. Speech rapid at times, normal rate/tone.
- Thought process tangential at times, able to return to topic. Coherent. No psychosis or delusions present at this interview.
- Concentration: fair. Insight: limited. Judgment: poor. Appetite: good. He is conscientious and knowledgeable of proper diet.
- Sleep: about 4 to 5 hours per night, and awakens feeling rested. He does not believe he requires more sleep.
- He denies any suicidal ideation, is future oriented, and stated he works hard to stay in good shape.

Diagnoses

- Axis I: Bipolar 1 Disorder, MRE hypomanic; Cannabis abuse, episodic; Cocaine dependence, sustained full remission; Opioid abuse, sustained full remission
- Axis II: Antisocial Personality Disorder
- Axis III: Chronic lumbar pain related to injury while briefly working as roofer. Currently under care of MD Pain Specialist and has been prescribed muscle relaxer as needed.
- Axis IV: Psychosocial stressors: severe—primary support group, physical/legal altercations with girlfriend (mother of 4-year-old son).
- Axis V: GAF 55

Continued

CASE STUDY 18-1—continued

Treatment Plan

1. After assessment and discussion of the risks and benefits of lamotrigine, including Stevens-Johnson syndrome, he would like to begin taking Lamictal ODT, as directed per Orange Starter pack, for mood stabilization. Reassess in 3 weeks for efficacy, and titrate upward.
2. Begin Vistaril 50 mg PO bid for relief from tension and impulsivity. Monitor for efficacy.
3. Monitor suicidality. He has contracted to contact service or clinic if any suicidal ideation.
4. Linked to Counselor, for individual and group therapy, with emphasis on anger (triggers, what to do for early warning signs of anger), avoidance of repetition of family of origin patterns of behavior, life-planning goals.
5. He asked for book shown in office, *Anger Management*, and this was given to him.
6. Encourage him to explore coaching in Hockey as outlet.
7. He has agreed to consent for last physical examination and lab work.
8. Ordered urine toxicology screen.
9. Rtc for f/u in 3 weeks. He is encouraged to rtc sooner if needed.

Outcome

1. James did not phone or show for next three appointments. NP received letter from Parole officer regarding treatment progress. James had signed consent.
2. James' mother phoned office to ask about his progress, and as James had refused to sign consent for his mother, no information was provided.
3. NP attempted to phone client. His provided cell phone number was disconnected.
4. NP phoned client's Pharmacy to check on status of his prescribed medications, and Pharmacist reported that client's medications had not been filled for 2 months, since his mother had picked up his medications for the first time.
5. Case-closed letter was mailed to client for noncompliance with Treatment Plan, and he was offered linkage to area clinics for continuity of care and medication follow-up.
6. Unfortunately, James did not continue contact for treatment.

Source: Lorraine A. Lopez, PMHNP-BC

Resources

Movies

Foley, J. (Director). (1992). *Glengarry Glen Ross* [Motion picture]. United States: New Line Cinema.

Demme, J. (Director). (1991). *Silence of the lambs* [Motion picture]. United States: Orion Pictures.

McNaughton, J. (Director). (1990). *Henry: Portrait of a serial killer* [Motion picture]. United States: Maljack Productions.

Fleischer, R. (Director). (1986). *The Boston strangler* [Motion picture]. United States: 20th Century Fox.

Kubrick, S. (Director). (1971). *A clockwork orange* [Motion picture]. United States: Warner Bros.

Brooks, R. (Director). (1967). *In cold blood* [Motion picture]. United States: Columbia Pictures.

Hitchcock, A. (Director). (1951). *Strangers on the train* [Motion picture]. United States: Warner Bros.

SOURCE: WEDDING & BOYD, 1999.

Borderline Personality Disorder (BPD)

In 1884, Hughes described patients with symptoms of BPD as being in the borderlands between sanity and insanity (p. 297), sometimes crossing the line into one side or the other side. Later, patients with symptoms of BPD were considered as being on the border between neurosis and psychosis (Sadock & Sadock, 2007), and terms such as "borderline schizophrenia" were used (Black & Andreasen, 2011). Now, patients with similar symptoms are diagnosed as having a BPD.

BPD is characterized by a pattern of emotional dysregulation, mood instability, intense interpersonal relationships, impulsivity, intense anger, recurrent suicidal threats, self-mutilating behaviors, problems with sense of identity, feelings of emptiness, and frantic efforts to avoid abandonment (American Psychological Association, 2000; Black & Andreasen, 2011; Paris, 2008).

McGlashan et al. (2005) found that all the criteria listed in the *DSM-IV-TR* (American Psychological Association, 2000) for BPD were highly prevalent at the baseline assessment of patients with the disorder (all symptoms were present in at least 60% of the patients). Affective instability, anger, and impulsivity were the most frequent symptoms, and identity disturbance, abandonment fears, and self-injury were the least frequent symptoms. After 2 years, the criteria that were the most frequent and most stable among these patients were impulsivity, anger, and affective instability. Identity disturbance, abandonment fears, and self-injurious behaviors were less stable symptoms (McGlashan et al.). McGlashan et al. suggested that the stable symptoms may be more closely related to genetically influenced temperament traits and the less stable symptoms may be related to symptomatic behaviors that are associated with stress, are habitual, or are learned. The stable symptoms may be more responsive to pharmacotherapy and the less stable symptoms may be more responsive to psychotherapy and other psychosocial interventions (McGlashan et al.).

Epidemiology

Prevalence

The prevalence of BPD is estimated to be 1% to 1.6% of the general population (Torgersen, 2009). The prevalence is as high as 20% of hospital and clinic admissions (Gunderson & Links, 2007). It is believed that there has been an increase in the prevalence of BPD in the United States (Paris, 1996). Millon (1987) attributed that increase to two sociocultural trends. The first is the emergence of social customs that exacerbate rather than remediate early maladaptive parent-child relationships—e.g., rapid industrialization, changing roles for men and women, increased rate of divorce, poor role models in the media, and increased availability of illegal drugs. The second trend is the diminished power of formerly protective institutions, such as the reduced influence of community schools and religious institutions on families and communities, the absence of nurturing surrogates, and the scattering of extended families.

Gender

Although the rate of BPD has been found to be higher among women in clinical settings (Morey, Alexander, & Boggs, 2005), Torgersen, Kringlen, and Cramer (2001) reported no significant gender differences in community-based studies. Another view is that the same symptoms are diagnosed differently in men and women. For example, whereas approximately 75% of individuals with BPD are female (Gunderson, 2001), men with similar symptoms are often diagnosed as having ASPD or NPD (Sadock & Sadock, 2007). Women with BPD often have co-occurring eating disorders, identity disturbance, and post-traumatic stress disorder, and men who are diagnosed with BPD often have co-occurring substance-related disorders and PPD, STPD, NPD, and ASPD (Johnson, Shea, Yen, et al., 2003).

Onset

The symptoms of BPD begin in adolescence. The mean age of first clinical presentation is 18 years (Paris, 2008).

Etiology

The etiology of BPD is related to a complex interaction of at least four factors:

1. Genetic influence. The heritability of BPD is 69% (Torgersen et al., 2000).
2. Abnormalities of brain development present at birth, which may adversely affect brain cells, brain chemistry, neuroendocrine functioning, and developing neuronal circuits.
3. Poor fit between the child's temperament and the parents' ability to meet their child's needs.
4. Adverse childhood experiences, such as neglect and physical abuse (Herman, Perry, & van der Kolk, 1981; Johnson et al., 2001; Robinson, 1996) and sexual abuse (Judd & McGlashan, 2003; Links, Boiago, Huxley, et al., 1990).

In addition to the interaction of the four factors listed above, development of BPD appears to be strongly influenced by the presence of

- Unstable early environments (chaos in families, separations, relocations, and poverty)
- Parental psychopathology (BPD, ASPD, depression, anxiety, and substance abuse)
- Absence of protective factors, such as having an above-average level of intelligence; achieving well in school; possessing talents in music, art, or other areas; and having special interests (Helgeland & Torgersen, 2004).

Genetic Influence

The genetic transmission appears to be through genetically influenced traits such as affective instability, impulsivity, self-harm, and identity problems (Judd & McGlashan, 2003; Siever & Frucht, 1997; Torgersen, 2000; van Reekum, Links, & Boiago, 1993). The heritability of BPD is 69% (Smoller et al., 2008). The families and the extended families of individuals with BPD also have increased rates of BPD and other psychopathology, such as substance use, ASPD, conduct disorder, learning disabilities, and mood disorders (Oldham, Gabbard, Goin, et al., 2004).

Temperament

Both genetics and abnormalities of brain development shape temperament and personality traits (see Chapter 3 for discussion of temperament). The temperament of patients with BPD is characterized both by high harm avoidance (pessimism and fearfulness) and by high novelty seeking (impulsivity and exploration). The temperament of patients with BPD may create a poor fit between their needs as infants and the capacity of their parents to meet those needs, resulting in inconsistent, inadequate, unpredictable, or abusive parenting. Poor parenting may also be related to parental psychopathology or to conflicted relationships of the parents (Judd & McGlashan, 2003).

Childhood Adversities

Patients with BPD have often experienced multiple separations, emotional discord in the family, neglect of their feelings and needs, and verbal, emotional, physical, or sexual abuse, which prevent the child from developing a secure pattern of attachment (Lyons-Ruth & Block, 1996; Paris, 2008; Zanarini, Williams, Lewis, et al., 1997) (see Chapter 3 for discussion of experienced factors associated with compromised brain development). For example, among patients with BPD, 81% have experienced childhood abuse (Zanarini, 1997; Zanarini et al., 1997). Those who had experienced sexual abuse were more likely to develop BPD than those who had experienced physical abuse (Johnson et al., 2001; Zelkowitz, Paris, Guzder, et al., 2001).

Early childhood maltreatment alters neurotransmitter and neuroendocrine functioning (Nemeroff, 2004; Teicher, Anderson, Polcari, et al., 2003). Thus, patients with BPD may have an alteration in brain chemistry due not only to genetic influences and developmental abnormalities that occur before birth but also to postnatal environment or experiences such as neglect and abuse. Research findings suggest a relationship between specific types of maltreatment and symptoms of psychopathology. For example:

- Chronic self-mutilation, such as cutting, is strongly associated with a childhood history of neglect.

- Children who have been physically abused may become violent, but they are less likely to be self-destructive.
- Repeated suicide attempts are associated with histories of childhood sexual abuse.
- Sexual abuse that involved incest causes rage and guilt, whereas physical abuse does not cause guilt. The deception and dishonesty associated with incest affects the person's entire life and causes a distortion of all interactions (Johnson et al., 2009).

Biological Basis

Patients with BPD have been found to have reduced volumes of subcortical structures of the brain, such as the amygdala, hippocampus, orbitofrontal cortex, and anterior cingulate cortex, that are involved in emotional information processing. Reduced volume was associated with diminished glucose metabolism, indicating less activity (Coccaro & Siever, 2009).

Approximately 60% of individuals with BPD have neurological soft signs that indicate diffuse brain damage, which may be evidenced later as developmental delays (sitting, walking, talking) and learning disabilities (Judd & McGlashan, 2003; van Reekum, 1993). In addition to prenatal brain damage, patients with BPD have an increased rate of birth complications (17.8% for individuals with BPD vs. 4% for individuals with mood disorders) that may be accompanied by postnatal anoxia, which may cause further brain damage. They also have a high rate of childhood-acquired brain injuries (head injuries, trauma, seizures, anoxia, and encephalitis), which may compromise brain development (Van Reekum, 1993). By altering brain development, adverse experienced factors compromise the brain's capacity for functioning, which is manifested in the symptoms of BPD. Abnormalities of the amygdala and other regions of the brain that are involved in modifying fear, modulating aggression, and creating socially appropriate responses to fear (e.g., the anterior cingulate cortex) have been demonstrated in patients with BPD (Minzenberg, Fan, New, et al., 2008; Siever & Frucht, 1997).

Experienced stressors that may alter the development of the prefrontal cortex area and destroy the hippocampal cells that are associated with learning and memory include physical and sexual abuse, parental separations and divorce before age 6, and witnessing violence (Zelkowitz et al., 2001). Childhood abuse may also cause abnormalities of functioning of the HPA axis (Gollan, Lee, & Coccaro, 2005; Nemeroff, 2004). Abnormal functioning is associated with the increased HPA axis response to later stressors that is seen as anxiety and depression (Heim, Newport, Bonsall, et al., 2001). The hyper-responsiveness of the HPA axis in patients with BPD is believed to be due to childhood abuse rather than pathology related to the BPD (Rinne, de Kloet, Wouters, et al., 2002).

Patients with BPD who self-mutilate tend to be more antisocial, impulsive, angry, and anxious than patients with BPD who do not. Many who self-mutilate have underlying serotonergic system dysfunction that is due to low levels of serotonin (Simeon, Stanley, Frances, et al., 1992). Based on the finding that the painful stimulation of self-mutilation results in a release of endorphins (the body's natural painkillers), some researchers believe that there may be impairment of the opiate system in patients with BPD.

Clinical Presentation

Patients with BPD presenting for treatment are often in crisis (Sadock & Sadock, 2007). They may present with cognitive impairment; emotional dysregulation; fragile self-concept; chaotic relationships and interpersonal dependency; and behavioral dysregulation.

Cognitive Impairment

Patients may present with symptoms and behaviors indicating impairment of cognitive functioning, such as odd reasoning (superstitiousness, magical thinking), all-black or all-white thinking ("you are for me or you are against me"), unusual perceptions, dissociation, paranoia, and transient psychotic thoughts (Zanarini, Gunderson, & Frankenburg, 1990). They may demonstrate problems in information processing and memory that are manifested as forgetfulness or missed appointments (Judd & McGlashan, 2003).

Emotional Dysregulation

Because emotional dysregulation is a core feature of BPD, patients with BPD may use verbal outbursts of intense anger; describe feelings of frustration, hurt, and disappointment; or complain of feeling bored or empty (Judd & McGlashan, 2003). Approximately half of adult patients with BPD use transitional objects, such as stuffed animals or pillows that are often present from childhood, to soothe themselves and to manage anxiety at times of stress, separation, or tension (Cardasis, Hochman, & Silk, 1997; Morris, Gunderson, & Zanarini, 1986).

Fragile Self-Concept, Chaotic Relationships, and Interpersonal Dependency

Patients with BPD often display a fragile self-concept and high levels of interpersonal dependency. Patients with BPD often have an unstable sense of self or self-identity. Their values, types of friends, career goals, and ideas of what they want to be in life are unstable (Oldham et al., 2004). Patients with BPD have chaotic relationships because they tend to see people as all good or all bad, e.g., as all-nurturing or as threatening to abandon them. They can be close to someone and then become very angry if something happens in the relationship that frustrates them. They have difficulty tolerating being alone and fear that they will be abandoned. High levels of interpersonal dependency are evidenced by clinginess, neediness, seeking approval of others, viewing themselves as powerless or ineffective, and anxiety when faced with the need to do something alone (Bornstein, Becker-Matero, Winarick, et al., 2010).

Behavioral Dysregulation

Behavioral dysregulation is another core feature of BPD, and patients with BPD often engage in impulsive behaviors such as substance use, promiscuity, self-injurious acts such as wrist-cutting, and suicidal or homicidal behaviors. Self-injurious acts are associated with a childhood history of neglect and occur among approximately 69% of adults with BPD (Dubo, Zanarini, Lewis, et al., 1997). The purpose of self-injurious acts such as cutting is to relieve negative emotions, and patients report feeling better after the act (Paris, 2008). Patients with BPD may give a history of repeated suicide attempts, which are frequently associated with a history of childhood sexual abuse. Patients with BPD often use maladaptive defense mechanisms, such as splitting, dissociation, denial, distortion, and projective identification.

In summary, patients with BPD will present with symptoms related to cognitive dysfunction; emotional and behavioral dysregulation; intense, unstable interpersonal relationships; and interpersonal dependency (Bornstein et al., 2010).

Comorbidity

Among patients with BPD, 75% will have a comorbid Axis I psychiatric disorder (Zanarini et al., 1998). The comorbid prevalence rate is 56% for generalized anxiety disorder, 41% for major depressive disorder, 37% for social phobia, 34% for post-traumatic stress disorder, and 22% for substance abuse (Swartz, Blazer, George, et al., 1990). The most common comorbid personality disorder is DPD, which is present in 30% to 40% of patients with BPD (Bornstein et al., 2010). HPD, ASPD, and STPD have also been found to coexist with BPD (Links et al., 1998). Suicidality is a frequent comorbidity (Paris, 2008). Medical comorbidities include hypertension, arteriosclerosis, cardiovascular disease, liver disease, and gastrointestinal disorders (El-Gabalawy, Katz, & Sareen, 2010).

Differential Diagnosis

The symptoms of BPD are similar to features of bipolar disorder; however, in BPD, the mood swings are often triggered by interpersonal stressors (such as rejection or termination of a relationship) and are not as sustained as in bipolar disorder. In contrast to major depressive disorder, the depression of BPD has features of emptiness, fears of abandonment, and self-destructiveness (Oldham et al., 2004). Post-traumatic stress disorder is often comorbid with BPD. Patients with post-traumatic stress disorder have specific memories of the trauma. Their symptoms are triggered by something that reminds them of the event. In contrast, patients with BPD have experienced multiple traumas that they may minimize. In differentiating BPD from schizophrenia, patients with BPD do not have prolonged psychotic episodes or thought disorder.

BPD must also be differentiated from HPD, STPD, PPD, NPD, DPD, and ASPD. HPD, STPD, PPD, NPD, and DPD are not characterized by self-destructive behaviors, anger in relationships that leads to termination of relationships, and feelings of emptiness. In ASPD, manipulative behavior is related to a desire for power or gain rather than for obtaining nurturance, as in BPD (First et al., 2002).

Treatment

The cornerstone of treatment for patients with BPD is psychotherapy—individual psychotherapy, supportive psychotherapy, group therapy, psychodynamic psychotherapy, CBT, and dialectical behavioral therapy (Gunderson & Links, 2007). Other treatment interventions include pharmacotherapy, hospitalization, partial hospitalization, and psychosocial interventions such as social skills training, vocational rehabilitation, and Assertive Community Treatment (ACT). Paris (2008) wrote, "The most important principle is to take a systematic approach to core problems" (p. 169). The focus is not on support or exploring childhood maltreatment but instead on teaching patients skills to manage emotional dysregulation and impulsivity. Each treatment intervention can be thought of as a building block to recovery (Gunderson & Links).

Psychotherapy

According to Gunderson and Links (2007), treatment should be based on the following principles:

- Therapy should be regular, consistent, and reliable.
- Structure is essential, and expectations of both the patient and the clinician should be clear.
- Patients with BPD need stable relationships, and therefore treatment should help patients to attain and maintain supportive relationships.
- Self-destructive acts and suicidality require attention but should not be the entire focus of therapeutic interventions.
- A team approach is beneficial.
- Treating co-occurring substance-related disorders will improve the course of BPD.

Two psychotherapeutic approaches that have been proven to be effective—psychoanalytic/psychodynamic therapy and CBT, particularly dialectical behavior therapy—share three features: weekly meetings with a therapist, one or more weekly group sessions, and regular meetings of therapists for consultation and supervision. These approaches have been associated with improvement in self-harm, violent behaviors, use of drugs, and hospital admissions (Hofmann & Tompson, 2002; Oldham et al., 2004; Stevenson & Meares, 1992). Improvement may take as long as a year and a half, and many patients may require longer (Leichsenring & Leibing, 2003). More on psychodynamic therapy, dialectical behavior therapy, and group therapy can be found in Box 18-1.

Pharmacotherapy

In considering pharmacotherapy, psychiatric advanced practice nurses should keep in mind Soloff's (2009) words, "the U.S. Food and Drug Administration has not approved any medication for treatment of any personality disorder" (p. 269). However, for patients with BPD receiving psychotherapy, pharmacotherapy is often used as an additive intervention to target symptoms in four areas:

1. Cognitive-perceptual symptoms (paranoia, suspiciousness, derealization, depersonalization, ideas of reference, and transient psychotic episodes)
2. Affective dysregulation (depression, mood lability, rejection sensitivity, and intense emotions such as anger)
3. Impulsive-behavioral dyscontrol (impulsive-aggressiveness, self-injurious behaviors, suicide attempts, binge-eating, risk-taking, and substance abuse)
4. Anxiety (Gunderson & Links, 2007; Soloff, 2009)

Atypical antipsychotics are used for cognitive-perceptual symptoms. Improvement of cognitive dysregulation and also of other symptoms such as interpersonal functioning, affective dysregulation, and impulsivity has been reported with the use of atypical antipsychotics such as olanzapine (Zanarini, Frankenburg, Parachini, 2004) and risperidone (Chengappa, Sheth, Brar, et al., 1999; Rocca, Marchiaro, Cocuzza, et al., 2000). Olanzapine is associated with decrease in anger, paranoia, anxiety, irritability, and suicidality and improvement of global functioning (Simeon & Hollander, 2009). Clozapine (Clozaril) is associated with overall improvement of 33% (Simeon & Hollander). Aripiprazole (Abilify) has been found to be associated with improvement of insecurity in social contacts, depression, anxiety, aggressiveness/hostility, and paranoid thinking (Nickel, Muehlbacher, Nickel, et al., 2006). Quetiapine is associated with improvement of impulsivity (Simeon & Hollander).

The first line of pharmacotherapy for affective dysregulation and impulse-behavioral dyscontrol is the use of the SSRIs (Gunderson & Links, 2007; Soloff, 2009). Use of SSRIs for patients with BPD is associated with improvement in anger, impulsive-aggressive behavior, and affective lability (Gabbard, 2005); improvement in overall functioning (Salzman, Wolfson, Schatzberg, et al., 1995; Simeon & Hollander, 2009); and reduction of suicidality (Simeon & Hollander). There is evidence that SSRIs may stimulate neurogenesis in the hippocampus. This new growth of neurons has been seen in improved memory, cognition, and work performance (Bremner & Vermetten,

BOX 18-1 Psychotherapies Used to Help Patients Who Have Borderline Personality Disorder

Psychodynamic Therapy

According to Oldham et al. (2004), "Psychodynamic psychotherapy draws from three major theoretical perspectives: ego psychology, object relations, and self psychology" (p. 793). The goals of psychodynamic psychotherapy for patients with BPD are to bring patterns of thinking, emotions, and behaviors to the patient's awareness, to increase the patient's ability to tolerate emotions, to increase the patient's ability to delay impulsive actions, to help the patient gain an understanding of relationship problems, and to increase the patient's ability to reflect on his or her motivations and the motivations of others (Oldham et al.). Other goals are to help the patient see others as having both positive and negative qualities and to help the patient to gain a more cohesive sense of self.

Dialectical Behavior Therapy (DBT)

DBT is a form of cognitive behavioral psychotherapy that balances change strategies with acceptance and validation techniques (Stanley & Brodsky, 2009). It usually consists of weekly group and individual sessions for 1 year:

- In the group sessions, a psychoeducational approach is used to teach interpersonal skills, distress tolerance, reality acceptance, and emotion regulation skills.
- The individual therapy sessions involve problem-solving techniques and supportive techniques (Crits-Christoph, 1998).

Two assumptions of Linehan's (1987) DBT are that (1) the primary dysfunction of BPD is inadequate affect regulation and (2) inadequate affect regulation causes instability of cognitive functioning, sense of self-identity, and behavior that contributes to chaotic interpersonal relations and suicidal behavior (Stanley & Brodsky). One goal of DBT is to decrease self-destructive behaviors, cognitive dysregulation, interpersonal chaos, labile emotions and moods, impulsiveness, and confusion about self. Another goal is to increase interpersonal skills such as communication skills, emotion regulation, ability to tolerate distress or frustration, and use of self-soothing strategies. DBT has been found to decrease parasuicidal behaviors, reduce hospital admissions, and increase adherence to treatment (Koons, Robins, Tweed, et al., 2001; Verheul, van den Bosch, Koeter et al., 2003). Patients who received DBT were found to have less substance abuse and problems with anger than a control group (Linehan, Schmidt, Dimeff, et al., 1999).

Group Therapy

The goals of group therapy for patients with BPD are to stabilize the patient, manage impulsiveness, and provide opportunities for social support. Group interventions can reduce the intensity of the interaction in individual therapy, provide an opportunity to teach the patient limit-setting, and give the patient an opportunity to help others (Oldham et al.). However, some patients' tendency to express anger and other emotions suddenly and loudly may cause other group members to reject them (Piper & Orgrodniczuk, 2009).

2004; Vermetten, Vythilingam, Southwick, et al., 2003). SSRIs may also reduce the hyperactivity of the HPA axis (Gabbard, 2005). Rinne et al. (2002) found that the SSRI fluvoxamine (Luvox) reduced HPA hyper-responsiveness in patients with BPD who had a history of sustained childhood abuse. The SSRIs fluoxetine (Prozac, Sarafem), sertraline (Zoloft), and venlafaxine (Effexor) have been found to decrease impulsive-behavioral dyscontrol, such as self-injurious behaviors (Kavoussi, Liu, & Coccaro, 1994; Markovitz & Wagner, 1995). Sertraline has been found to decrease anxiety, depression, and suicidality (Simeon & Hollander), and venlafaxine has been found to be associated with overall reduction of symptoms (Simeon & Hollander).

In patients with BPD, tricyclic antidepressants may make hostility, depression, anxiety, agitation, irritability, impulsivity, and suicidality worse, and the use of MAOIs is limited by the necessity of close adherence to dietary restrictions and avoidance of other contraindicated substances (Gunderson & Links, 2007). The use of mood stabilizers such as lithium and divalproex sodium (Depakote) has been studied for patients with BPD and has been found to be effective in reducing interpersonal sensitivity, anger/hostility, and anxiety (Schatzberg et al., 2007; Soloff, 2009). Lamotrigine (Lamictal) has been found to improve functioning and impulsive behaviors (Tritt, Nickel, Lahmann, et al., 2005).

In summary, SSRIs may be effective for anger, anxiety, chronic emptiness, temper outbursts, and impulsive behaviors. SSRIs have been found to decrease suicidal behavior by 90%. In addition, SSRIs appear to facilitate psychotherapy by reducing symptoms such as intense anger, hypervigilance, anxiety, and dysphoria that get in the way of therapy (Gabbard, 2005). Lithium, divalproex, and carbamazepine (Tegretol) may be used for irritability, impulsivity, and mood swings. Some patients with BPD have a good response to lamotrigine (Pinto & Akiskal, 1998; Tritt et al., 2005). Antipsychotics, usually atypical antipsychotics, may be used for transient psychotic symptoms (Schatzberg, Cole, & DeBattista, 2003) and also for impulsive/behavioral symptoms such as anger, hostility, and recklessness (Gunderson & Links, 2007; Oldham et al., 2004). There has been a shift from considering SSRIs as the frontline treatment for BPD to greater use of anticonvulsants and atypical antipsychotics (Abraham & Calabrese, 2008).

Other Therapeutic Interventions

Hospitalization or *partial hospitalization* is often a needed intervention for patients with BPD to provide safety for the patient; these interventions provide a structured, supportive, and consistent environment, set limits, and help patients to take responsibility for the consequences of their actions (Gunderson & Links, 2007). To prevent recurrent hospitalizations, Gunderson, Gratz, Neuhaus, et al. (2009, p. 169) said that the hospital experience should be businesslike and practical, with the focus directed toward the problem that brought the patient to the hospital and the necessity of the patient's coping with the problem after discharge. They said that a milieu that encourages long one-to-one talks or bonding among patients is harmful. The emphasis should be on the impending discharge and making plans for coping with the problem and for ongoing care in settings other than hospitals.

Education for patients is also beneficial. The psychiatric advanced practice nurse teaches patients about a nutritious diet, good sleep habits, physical activity, abstaining from alcohol and drugs, safe sex practices, and the danger of self-injurious behaviors (infections, HIV, coma, paralysis, and death). The psychiatric advanced practice nurse also teaches patients

- Problem-solving
- Responsibility and accountability
- What behaviors may cause interpersonal problems, work problems, and legal problems
- How to access and maintain social support

Patients are also taught specific self-management strategies, such as how to express feelings, use self-soothing techniques, engage in activity to relieve tension, delay gratification, and use adaptive coping strategies.

Cognitive Adaptation Training teaches patients how to use strategies to compensate for cognitive deficits (Velligan & Bow-Thomas, 2000). Because patients with BPD have problems with memory, the following strategies that compensate for impairment of memory may be helpful:

- Using a keychain-type small tape recorder such as "Memo Mate" for remembering brief information such as phone numbers or the need to buy a specific item
- Carrying a card with personal phone numbers, addresses, medications, and phone numbers of health-care providers
- Using a pocket calendar and recording all appointments, treatments, and meetings, crossing off each day that the items were accomplished

Course

As children, patients with BPD are likely to have been impulsive, angry, or hostile; they may also have had learning problems, particularly problems with concentration. Friendships may have been jeopardized or terminated because of episodes of out-of-control behavior. They may have experienced social alienation. As adolescents, their symptoms increase, and some do not complete their education or vocational training. They may leave home and may become involved in relationships and activities that are problematic. Substance abuse is common, and in late adolescence there are increased attempts at self-harm, hospital admissions, difficulties in relationships, and emotional instability. As adults, they continue to experience unstable emotions with many crises resulting from impulsive decisions. Relationships are unstable and employment is affected (Gunderson, 2001). The suicide rate is 10%, with the highest risk in the first 6 years of treatment (Paris, 2008; Stone, 1990). Risk for suicide is highest among those with depressive symptoms and substance abuse. There is some reduction of mood instability and impulsivity after 30 years of age (Stone, 2001). Older adults with BPD in assisted living or nursing homes have difficulty with relationships with other patients and with caregivers. They tend to create chaos by their tendency to form intense attachments and then suddenly to reject other patients or staff. Because they have not been able to make and keep friends and often have worn out their families, they are often socially isolated (Segal et al., 2006).

With treatment, approximately half of patients with BPD will have significant remission of their symptoms within 2 years (Skodol & Gunderson, 2008) and approximately three-quarters (74%) after 6 years (Zanarini, Frankenburg, Hennen, et al., 2006). The 10-year course of patients with BPD was summarized by Gunderson, Stout, McGlashan, et al. (2011) as characterized by high rates of remission (85%), low rates of relapse, and severe and persistent impairment of social functioning. Follow-up studies of patients with BPD are included in Box 18-2. Issues in management can be found in Box 18-3.

BOX 18-2 Follow-up Studies of Patients with Borderline Personality Disorder

- Patients with BPD gain something from each therapist, and therapy seems to speed up the process of recovery.
- Patients gradually learn to modulate behaviors and to find more adaptive solutions to problems (Paris & Zweig-Frank, 2001).
- Paris and Zweig-Frank found that improvement (defined as the lessening of severe symptoms) begins 10 years after the first hospitalization.
- Fifteen years after initial diagnosis, the majority of patients no longer meet the criteria for BPD.
- Improvement is most striking in the domain of impulsivity.
- By age 40 years about half will be functioning normally, and at 50 years or older only 10% of patients with BPD will still meet the criteria for the disorder.
- However, one-third will still have significant role dysfunction and psychopathology, and many will have given up trying to have intimate personal relationships (Paris, 1996).
- The Chestnut Ridge Follow-up Study reported on the outcome of patients with BPD 15 years after discharge (Judd & McGlashan, 2003). Most were living independently and had good work records. They were moderately active socially. Among the women, many had tried intimate relationships, but over time they stopped engaging in relationships. Work and outpatient treatment teams became their source of social contact and provided structure and stability in their lives. Male patients tended to avoid social activities and had little contact with the mental health care system. Work, church, or Alcoholics Anonymous made up their social support system.
- Gunderson, Daversa, Grilo, et al. (2006) found that certain factors present at baseline were predictive of outcome at 2-year follow-up. Poorer outcome was associated with greater severity of dysfunction and psychopathology at baseline, presence of more OCPD criteria, and history of early childhood abuse and neglect.
- Gunderson et al. (2011) found that over the course of 10 years, 85% of patients with BPD achieved remission. Impairment of social functioning persisted.

Resources

Movies

Lyne, A. (Director). (1987). *Fatal attraction* [Motion picture]. United States: Paramount Pictures.

SOURCE: WEDDING & BOYD, 1999.

Mangold, J. (Director). (1999). *Girl, interrupted* [Motion picture]. United States: Columbia Pictures.

Eyre, R. (Director). (2006). *Notes on a scandal* [Motion picture]. United Kingdom: Fox Searchlight.

Baumbach, N. (Director). (2007). *Margot at the wedding* [Motion picture]. United States: Paramount Vantage.

SOURCE: WEDDING, BOYD, & NIEMIEC, 2010, P. 73.

Histrionic Personality Disorder (HPD)

HPD is characterized by excessive emotionality, attention-seeking behavior, concern for appearance, flighty thinking, dramatic behaviors, and attention-seeking behavior in interpersonal relationships (Millon, Grossman, Millon, et al., 2004; Skodol & Gunderson, 2011). These patients experience rapidly shifting intense emotions and may show self-dramatization and theatrical or exaggerated expression of their emotions. They tend to act on these emotions without stopping to think (Grossman, 2004). Their behaviors may be flirtatious and focused on their physical attractiveness or may include somatic complaints and many physical symptoms. Patients with HPD will often take on the interests and values of others in order to develop new relationships. Temper tantrums and outbursts of anger as overreactions to minor events are common, and they may engage in self-destructive behaviors (Skodol & Gunderson, 2008). They have a poor understanding of cause and effect, and they experience disturbances in emotional, behavioral, and interpersonal domains (Nestadt, Kromanoski, Chahal, et al., 1990).

Epidemiology and Etiology

HPD is one of the most frequently occurring of the personality disorders (Sokol & Gunderson, 2008). The prevalence of HPD is 1.5% of the general population (Torgersen, 2009). It is diagnosed more frequently in women, but it may be underdiagnosed in men. For example, when a structured interview is used, the rate is the same for men and women (Paris, 1997). The age of onset is often before 25 years. Common comorbid Axis I psychiatric disorders

BOX 18-3 Borderline Personality Disorder: Issues in Management

Psychiatric advanced practice nurses should not target the treatment approach to the experience of early abuse. Focusing on early abuse may precipitate psychosis and may reactivate the trauma. Instead, the focus of treatment should be on helping the patient to learn new ways of coping. In managing the care of patients with BPD, psychiatric advanced practice nurses should

- Be constantly aware of their own reactions to the patient's behavior.
- Have patience, persistence, consistency, flexibility, and trust (i.e., the belief that the patient will improve) when interacting with the patient.
- Use a direct and matter-of-fact approach in confronting behavior.
- Model appropriate problem-solving, interpersonal, and social skills.
- Reinforce appropriate behaviors.
- Set clear limits.
- Establish clear rules, regulations, and consequences.

include somatization disorder, conversion disorder, and hypochondriasis. Common comorbid personality disorders include BPD, NPD, and DPD.

The heritability of HPD is 67% (Smoller et al., 2008) and the genetic influence is illustrated by the higher prevalence of HPD in the first-degree relatives of patients with HPD. Some studies suggest the possibility of a genetic link between HPD and the impulsivity and novelty seeking that is present in individuals with ASPD (Lilienfeld & Hess, 2001). The development of HPD is also thought to be due to abnormalities of brain functioning. For example, individuals with HPD appear to have hyper-responsiveness of the noradrenergic system (involved in emotional reactions) that may contribute to sensitivity to rejection (Markovitz, 2001).

The development of HPD is also thought to be influenced by experienced factors such as the family environment and maltreatment (Johnson et al., 2009). For example, sexual abuse has been found to be associated with the development of HPD (Norden et al., 1995). The individual who later develops HPD may have been loved for his or her good looks and entertainment value. The family did not value competence or signs of personal strength; instead, the child's value was dependent on how attractive, how pleasant, and how entertaining he or she could be. Family life was chaotic in an interesting and dramatic way, and frequently the family was involved in the performing arts. In some instances, the charm of the child who later develops HPD may distract the father from abusing the mother and siblings. If the child is not pretty or entertaining enough to control the father, the family situation could become dangerous. Thus, the child learns the survival value of being pretty, distracting, and entertaining. Women with HPD have often been "Daddy's girls," and men have often been "Mama's boys" (Gabbard, 2009, p. 201).

Biological Basis

In relation to cognitive processing, individuals with HPD are thought to be right-brain dominant. For example, when responding to questions, they describe vivid impressions such as "He's wonderful" rather than facts (Skodol & Gunderson, 2008, p. 844). Infants who later develop HPD are extremely alert and emotionally responsive. They appear to find more gratification from external stimuli in the early months of life than other infants do. It is thought that they may receive brief, highly charged, and irregular reinforcement from multiple caregivers. From that experience, they learn to receive gratification from short, concentrated reinforcement and to seek it from different sources (Robinson, 1996).

Clinical Presentation

Individuals with HPD may exaggerate their thoughts and feelings and make things sound more important than they are. They may present with complaints of depression and somatic symptoms. Their style of speech is often dramatic, impressionistic, and lacking in detail. Expression of emotions is often exaggerated or theatrical. They use physical appearance to draw attention to themselves. They prefer to be the center of attention and they are uncomfortable and may have temper tantrums or cry when they are not. Their behavior and interactions with others may be inappropriate, e.g., coy, flirtatious, provocative, or seductive (Skodol & Gunderson, 2011). They do not like to follow routines and tend not to attend to details. They may be unable to analyze problems or generate solutions (Skodol & Gunderson, 2008). They prefer to seek new experiences and thrills, and they become excited by new ideas, relationships, or activities. They may judge new, quickly formed relationships to be more intimate than they are (Fossati, Barratt, Borroni, et al., 2007).

HPD exists on a continuum, with the milder end having a neurotic organization of personality (once called hysterical) and the more severe end having a primitive organization of personality. The neurotically organized patient displays a subtle form of seduction, is likely to fall in love with unavailable partners, and has good impulse control. The patient with a primitively organized personality is more dramatic emotionally, is more aggressive in seduction, is more likely to seek caretaking from others, and has poor impulse control under stress (Gabbard & Allison, 2007). There is a risk for suicide when patients with HPD are overwhelmed by losses or abandonment. They may become anxious or depressed and may have hysterical rages. On the other hand, they may display a defensive form of emotional detachment, "la belle indifference" (lack of concern).

Differential Diagnosis

Differential diagnoses include mania, hypomania, mood swings (cyclothymia), dysthymia that has a similar feature of rejection sensitivity, eating disorders, somatization disorder, and other personality disorders. Patients with HPD differ from those with DPD—which is characterized by need for attention from others, inability to make decisions, and need for others to make decisions for them—by their belief that others will find their dependency to be attractive or seductive (Skodol & Gunderson, 2011). HPD differs from BPD in that patients with HPD do not usually experience multiple crises in intimate relationships and do not have problems maintaining a sense of self-identity (Skodol & Gunderson). In contrast to NPD, individuals with HPD are characterized by the need to be the center of attention rather than the need for praise and support for their sense of entitlement and superiority (First et al., 2002).

Treatment

There is little research on the treatment of patients with HPD (Gabbard & Allison, 2007). The accepted goals of treatment are to attend to practical ways of coping with the immediate problems in the patient's life and to promote the ability to think before acting (First & Tasman, 2004). Treatment interventions include cognitive therapy (Pretzer, 2004), supportive psychotherapy, CBT, and problem-solving therapy (Black & Andreasen, 2011). Skodol and Gunderson (2008) recommended the use of individual psychodynamic psychotherapy.

There are no pharmacological trials reported for HPD. Because patients with HPD have rapid, intense, shifting emotions and because they act on these emotions without thinking about them logically, SSRIs may decrease emotional reactivity and rejection sensitivity and give them the opportunity to think before acting. If SSRIs are not effective, mood stabilizers can be used (Grossman, 2004).

Course

Little is known about the childhood of patients with HPD. As adults, they are able to form new relationships easily but have difficulty maintaining them. They fall in and out of love quickly (First & Tasman, 2004). Employment may be adversely affected by their emotional instability and tendency to become emotionally involved with coworkers. As individuals with HPD age, they may complain of more physical symptoms, develop dysthymia, abuse substances, and act promiscuously (Paris, 2003; Sadock & Sadock, 2007). Older adults with HPD have difficulty adjusting to changes in their appearance and sexual appeal and to others' diminished response to their attempts to attract attention. Their self-centeredness may lead to others' avoiding them and to loneliness and isolation (Segal et al., 2006).

Resources

Movies

Kasan, E. (Director). (1951). *A streetcar named Desire* [Motion picture]. United States: Warner Bros.

DaCosta, M. (Director). (1958). *Auntie Mame* [Motion picture]. United States: Warner Bros.

Lumet, S. (1962). *Long day's journey into night* [Motion picture]. United States: Embassy Pictures.

SOURCE: WEDDING & BOYD, 1999.

Narcissistic Personality Disorder (NPD)

Narcissus was a mythological person who was unable to love others. He fell in love with his reflection in a pool, became fixed on what he saw, pined away, and died. NPD stems from this myth. Patients with NPD are characterized by a high sense of self-importance and grandiose beliefs that they are special, unique, and entitled. They have an inexhaustible need for admiration. They lack empathy, are egotistical, inflate their accomplishments, cannot accept the success of others, and often exploit others (Black & Andreasen, 2011; Ritter & Lammers, 2006). Common narcissistic characteristics include:

- A condescending attitude
- Arrogance
- A desire to be admired
- Hypersensitivity to criticism and feeling injured easily
- Difficulty maintaining a sense of self-esteem
- Having many fantasies, but few accomplishments
- Readily blaming others
- A conspicuous lack of empathy
- Being highly self-referential (Millon et al., 2004; Robinson, 1996; Ritter & Lammers, 2006)

Epidemiology and Etiology

NPD is one of the least frequently occurring of the personality disorders, estimated to be prevalent in less than 1% of the population (Skodol & Gunderson, 2008). Men are diagnosed with NPD almost three times as often as women. The diagnosis of NPD is uncommon in Europe and in Eastern countries where traditional societies are structured to suppress narcissism, e.g., where children are taught to put family and community ahead of their own personal goals (First & Tasman, 2004). NPD is more likely to develop in families that allow or actively encourage their children to be self-centered.

The heritability of NPD is 67% (Smoller et al., 2008). Genetic influence for NPD appears to be through genetically influenced temperament traits such as high energy, overconscientiousness, and low tolerance for anxiety. NPD does not seem to be genetically linked to any of the Axis I psychiatric disorders.

Early experienced factors are believed to be involved in the development of NPD. Individuals with NPD are thought to have arrested psychosocial development. In infancy, the child is given noncontingent adoration. Parents may exaggerate the child's perfection and believe that the child is entitled to a better life than the parents had, e.g., the child deserves to have it all. The toddler stage is normally the time when the child clashes with reality. It is the time when most parents burst the baby's sense of noncontingent entitlement. The child must learn that others have needs, wants, and feelings. Some researchers believe that NPD results from overgratification during childhood that does not allow for the development of self-regulation and normal maturation (Fernando, 1998) and that reinforces traits of self-centeredness and entitlement (Paris, 2003). Parents do not mirror that which is inappropriate behavior back to the child and instead send the message to the child that he or she is valued because he or she is perfect.

Biological Basis

Biological, neuropsychological, or brain structure deviations have not been reported for individuals with NPD (Grossman, 2004). The symptoms of NPD are attitudes—attitude toward self (grandiosity and entitlement) and attitude toward others (belittling, callous, and lacking in empathy)—rather than symptoms arising from impairment of cognition, mood modulation, anxiety, or impulsivity.

Clinical Presentation

Patients with NPD do not usually seek treatment, as they do not see anything wrong with their attitudes or behaviors. They are likely to come or are brought for treatment after an acute crisis such as a work problem, personal failure or loss, a confrontation or ultimatum from family or employer, or onset of an Axis I psychiatric disorder such as depression, bipolar disorder, or substance-related disorder (Ronningstam & Maltsberger, 2007).

Patients with NPD may appear arrogant, needing constant admiration and recognition of their superiority. They may display an attitude of entitlement, use exploitative behaviors, and are often grandiose about their importance and achievements. They consider themselves to be special and deserving of special treatment. They often lack empathy and are preoccupied with power, beauty, or love. They want to have fame and fortune and believe that they are entitled to have them. They tend to view others as either superior or inferior. When criticized, they may react with rage, shame, or humiliation, but mask these feelings with cool indifference. Their relationships with others seem shallow but may be maintained because they enhance the patient's self-esteem. They may fish for compliments and express envy of those they view as being more successful. They may even destroy others' rewards. They have problems with interpersonal relationships, but they make friends if they perceive the friendship as one from which they can benefit. They may present with physical or marital complaints or with co-occurring mood and anxiety disorders that may increase the use of maladaptive behaviors (Grossman, 2004; Miller, Campbell, & Pilkonis, 2007; Ritter & Lammers, 2006).

Impairment of functioning is seen in problems with intimate relationships, work, and social life and in the distress they cause others (Miller et al., 2007). When not supported in their belief of entitlement, patients with NPD may become angry, despondent, or dejected. Suicidality is linked with job loss, failure to obtain a promotion, divorce, loss of a significant source of emotional support, and increased use of alcohol or drugs (Ronningstam & Maltsberger, 2007). Older patients with NPD tend to have more problems with their work and social relationships.

Differential Diagnosis

Some of the traits of hypomania overlap with NPD. These include grandiosity, a sense of entitlement, increased goal-directed activity, and involvement in risky yet pleasurable activities. NPD is distinguished from hypomania by lack of mood symptoms and a long-standing rather than an episodic course. Major depressive episode and dysthymia must be considered as differential diagnoses. The grief, shame, and withdrawal after a narcissistic injury—which is humiliation experienced because the patient did not get what he or she thought he or she was entitled to have—resemble some of the criteria of a major depressive episode or dysthymic disorder. However, in NPD, there is an obvious stressor and less severity and duration than is seen in mood disorders (Andreasen & Black, 2006). Substance-related disorders, especially with stimulants (cocaine or amphetamines), can produce a clinical picture resembling NPD (American Psychiatric Association, 2000).

BPD, HPD, and ASPD often co-occur with NPD. In ASPD, there is a long history of impulsive behaviors, higher rates of substance abuse, and more encounters with the justice system. Patients with NPD are differentiated from those with ASPD by their grandiosity and their belief that they are unique and superior (Gunderson & Ronningstam, 2001). In comparison to patients with BPD, patients with NPD have less anxiety, less chaotic lives, less fear of abandonment, and less likelihood of suicide attempts. Patients with HPD are more likely to use exhibitionist behaviors to meet their need for attention and are less likely to have feelings of anger, emptiness, and boredom and self-destructive behaviors (First et al., 2002).

Treatment

The goal of treatment is to help patients with NPD to accept themselves without grandiosity or devaluing others; however, patients with NPD have a fragile self-esteem, limited capacity to tolerate distress, and a tendency to ignore or sabotage others' knowledge or efforts, including those of the clinician. Their character style of grandiosity, superiority, lack of empathy, and exploitation of others is a protective armor that holds them together. Without their armor, they feel anxious and ashamed. Psychotherapy in the form of CBT or therapy similar to that used for patients with BPD can help. Cognitive therapy can be used to address basic cognitive distortions, such as self-righteousness ("I did it correctly—I always do"), grandiosity ("Can you meet my standards?"), or exploitation ("I'll find someone with better training next time"). Psychotherapy includes education to teach the patient about NPD in a supportive way; validation that identifies aspects of their childhood that may have molded their attitudes and behaviors; and identification of target behaviors that can be changed for more adaptive behaviors (Ronningstam & Maltsberger, 2007). Group psychotherapy may be helpful, but patients with NPD may dominate the group.

Because comorbid anxiety disorders or mood disorders may cause increased use of maladaptive behaviors, pharmacotherapy for anxiety or depression may indirectly improve NPD symptoms (Grossman, 2004). Pharmacotherapy that includes the use of lithium and serotonergic drugs may help with mood swings and intolerance of rejection.

In general, the psychiatric advanced practice nurse should be careful of being perceived as critical while helping patients with NPD to change their attitudes of entitlement and grandiosity.

Course

Beginning in childhood, individuals with NPD believe that they are special, unique, and superior and that others should recognize that. In adolescence, they may appear self-centered, assertive, domineering, and arrogant (Cooper & Ronningstam, 1992). They often have difficulty accepting the success of others. As adults, they may be high achievers, but they often have difficulty in their relationships with others. Because patients with NPD value beauty, strength, and youthful attributes, they struggle to stay young and are vulnerable to midlife crises (First & Tasman, 2004). Patients with NPD may seek treatment later in life, but by then they have a pattern of using and discarding other people (Andreasen & Black, 2006). Among older adults with NPD, retirement may be accompanied by loss of power and prestige. Relationships with family and friends may be strained owing to lifelong behaviors of being demanding, reacting angrily to imagined slights, and belittling others. Responses to age-related changes often include depression and rage that they have not been given what they believed they were entitled to have in life (Segal et al., 2006). However, positive changes do occur sometimes in midlife owing to an achievement, a new durable friendship, or improvement of their ability to manage disappointments (Paris, 2003).

Resources

Movies

Wilder, B. (Director). (1950). *Sunset Boulevard* [Motion picture]. United States: Paramount Pictures.

Haines, R. (Director). (1991). *The doctor* [Motion picture]. United States: Touchstone Pictures.

Levinson, B. (Director). (1991). *Bugsy* [Motion picture]. United States: TriStar Pictures.

Van Sant, G. (Director). (1995). *To die for* [Motion picture]. United States: Columbia Pictures.

Source: Wedding & Boyd, 1999.

McKay, A. (Director). (2004). *Anchorman: The legend of Ron Burgundy* [Motion picture]. United States: DreamWorks.

Source: Wedding, Boyd, Niemiec, 2010, p. 73.

Cluster C Personality Disorders: Anxious-Fearful

Cluster C includes the avoidant, dependent, and obsessive-compulsive personality disorders (Gooding et al., 2007). Patients with Cluster C personality disorders tend to show anxious and fearful behaviors. They tend to be comorbid with Axis I anxiety disorders (Oldham, 2009). Patients with Cluster C personality disorders have less impairment than those with Cluster A or Cluster B personality disorders (Perry, 2007). Overall, patients with Cluster C personality disorders benefit most from psychodynamic and cognitive psychotherapy, although they also benefit from interpersonal psychotherapy and supportive psychotherapy. There is little evidence of sustained long-term benefits from pharmacotherapy (Perry, 2007).

Avoidant Personality Disorder (AVPD)

The central theme in AVPD is that of shame, guilt, and fear of being rejected (Skodol & Gunderson, 2008). Patients with AVPD view themselves as unworthy of love, as defective (Robinson, 1996). Shame involves the sense of not living up to an internal standard and of being seen as bad or defective. Shame causes feelings of impotence or helplessness. Guilt is the belief that one has violated an internal rule and merits punishment. AVPD is characterized by marked avoidance of social activities because of feelings of shyness, inadequacy, and fear of being ridiculed (Perry, 2007). Patients with AVPD often experience hypersensitivity and feelings of inadequacy, social ineptness, and defectiveness. The symptoms that are the most stable over time are feelings of inadequacy, social ineptness, and a need to be certain of being liked before making social contacts (McGlashan et al., 2005). Patients with AVPD tend to avoid employment and activities that involve contact with other people because of their fear of rejection or criticism or disapproval.

Epidemiology and Etiology

The prevalence of AVPD is 3% of the general population (Torgersen, 2005). Patients with AVPD have high rates of co-occurring social phobia (Rettew, Zanarini, Yen, et al., 2003). They also have co-occurring post-traumatic stress disorder, major depression, BPD, PBD, and STPD. The heritability of AVPD is low, at 28% (Smoller et al., 2008). There are no studies suggesting clear genetic influence; however, traits such as introversion, social anxiousness, shyness, and inhibition have strong heritability (Jang & Vernon, 2001), and there is some evidence of a link with generalized social anxiety that is believed to be genetically influenced (Skodol, 2009).

In combination with genetically influenced temperament, traits of inhibition, and timidity, children who have experienced rejection, belittlement, and criticism by their parents may be at increased risk for developing AVPD (First & Tasman, 2004). Childhood emotional abuse in the form of intolerant and shaming parental behavior and childhood neglect has been found to be associated with AVPD (Johnson et al., 2001). Meyer and Carver (2000) reported childhood histories of isolation and rejection. In the study by Rettew et al. (2003), patients with AVPD reported that during childhood and adolescence they had poor athletic performance and few hobbies, did not take on leadership roles, and were not popular.

Biological Basis

There is some evidence that the right hemisphere of the brain, which is involved in emotional stability and nonverbal interpersonal skills, has experienced damage or abnormality of development in patients with AVPD. Patients with AVPD have hyperarousal of the sympathetic nervous system, tachycardia, dilation of the pupils, and laryngeal tightness. Their baseline levels of cortisol are often abnormally high. Lee et al. (2005) studied the relationship of childhood trauma, personality disorders, and corticotropin-releasing factor, which is linked to cortisol, and found that although all forms of childhood trauma were associated with increased levels of corticotropin-releasing factor, the strongest relationship with corticotropin-releasing factor was not physical or sexual abuse but *emotional neglect*. Thus, an early life stress such as emotional neglect or lack of maternal caregiving leads to alterations of HPA axis functioning, with resulting increased levels of cortisol; increases in cortisol are known to have detrimental effects on the hippocampus, which is involved in learning, memory, and inhibiting behavioral responses. In patients with AVPD, cognitive processing abnormalities are evidenced by decreased flexibility when they are presented with new situations (Lee et al.).

Clinical Presentation

Patients with AVPD show extreme sensitivity to rejection. This sensitivity causes them to lead socially withdrawn lives (Millon et al., 2004). They yearn for a warm, secure relationship, but they stay hidden within themselves, avoiding interaction with others and involvement with the outside world because of their feelings of being inept, unattractive, or inferior and because of their fears of rejection (Millon et al.). Because they fear disapproval or criticism at work, they avoid work situations in which they would need to have contact with others. Patients with AVPD are often the first-born or an only child, unmarried, and male. Frequently, they have had no sexual experience and live alone or with their parents. They tend not to have had childhood friends and as adults are often socially isolated because they fear being shamed or ridiculed. They have problems interacting with peers and strangers unless they are sure that they are going to be liked and accepted.

Differential Diagnosis

In considering the differential diagnosis of DPD, the patient with DPD has difficulty with separations whereas the person with AVPD has difficulty in initiating interactions. Patients with AVPD are hypersensitive to rejection, shy, timid, and unwilling to enter into relationships, and their desire for acceptance is coupled with low self-esteem. Individuals with DPD, on the other hand, need a new relationship as soon as one ends: they need someone to take care of them (First et al., 2002). Patients with AVPD are unlike patients with SZPD, who prefer social isolation, because patients with AVPD are not emotionally cold; rather, they crave relationships (Skodol & Gunderson, 2008).

Treatment

Because of the fear of rejection experienced by patients with AVPD, initial therapy may be supportive psychotherapy (Skodol & Gunderson, 2011). In time, these patients are able to respond to other types of psychotherapy (Gabbard, 2005), such as cognitive therapy that challenges their belief that they are inept (Beck, Freeman, Davis, et al., 2004). Group therapy has also been found to be helpful (Black & Andreasen, 2011; Piper & Ogrodniczuk, 2009).

Pharmacotherapy has been little studied for patients with AVPD, and there is no evidence that it is beneficial. However, because there is a high level of comorbidity with social anxiety disorder, it is thought that medications that are effective for social anxiety disorder may be helpful for patients with AVPD. Thus, the first-line medications for anxiety and rejection sensitivity are SSRIs (Grossman, 2004). The SSRIs seem to decrease interpersonal hypersensitivity and to improve social and performance anxiety. One-third of patients with AVPD who receive SSRIs will be very much improved, and another third will be improved (Grossman, 2004). Second-line medications include gabapentin (Neurontin), bupropion (Wellbutrin), and some benzodiazepines. The beta blocker atenolol (Tenormin) may be used to manage autonomic nervous system hyperactivity, which tends to be high in patients with AVPD. It has been found that when patients with AVPD received antidepressant medications for a comorbid Axis I diagnosis of anxiety or depression, some of the core features of AVPD—shyness, rejection sensitivity, and distress—improved. Patients with AVPD improve more with a combination treatment of medications and therapy (Kool, Dekker, Kuijsens, et al., 2003).

Among psychosocial interventions, both short-term social skills training and social skills training combined with cognitive interventions have been found to reduce social anxiety and increase social interactions (Stravynski, Marks, & Yule, 1982). Graded exposure, social skills training, and intimacy-focused social skills training have all been found to be effective (Alden, 1989). In a later study, patients receiving manual-based supportive psychodynamic therapy improved after 1 year of treatment to the point that 61% of the patients no longer met the criteria for AVPD (Barber, Morse, Krakauer, et al., 1997).

Course

Patients with AVPD may be able to function in a protected environment. Some marry and have children, but many limit their social network to their family of origin. They may develop social anxiety disorder. They may become depressed and anxious if their social support system fails. Severity of the symptoms of AVPD may lessen with age (First & Tasman, 2004); however, older adults with AVPD, because of their small social networks, are particularly vulnerable to the deaths of spouses, family members, and friends that further reduce their social support (Segal et al., 2006). Among patients with AVD, positive achievement experiences and positive interpersonal relationships during childhood or adolescence are associated with remission. The greater the number of positive experiences and the broader the developmental period they cover, the better the prognosis (Skodol et al., 2007).

Resources

Movies

Van Sant, G. (Director). (2000). *Finding Forrester* [Motion picture]. United States: Columbia Pictures.

SOURCE: WEDDING, BOYD, & NIEMIEC, 2010, P. 87.

Allen, W. (1983). *Zelig* [Motion picture]. United States: Orion Pictures.

Dependent Personality Disorder (DPD)

Individuals with DPD feel inadequate, incompetent, and helpless. They lack self-confidence and put their needs after the needs of others. They have difficulty making decisions. They rely on others to manage their lives and believe that someone else must take care of them. Even a temporary separation from a spouse or the one who takes care of them is very frightening. The strategies that they use to maintain relationships include appearing helpless and vulnerable; being ingratiating; providing help to others and then making the other person feel indebted; and frightening others by using threats of self-harm (Bornstein, 2007). Because they are afraid that any disagreement may lead to rejection, they often stay in bad or abusive situations, refuse to leave a bad marriage, tolerate exploitive roommates or coworkers, and perform demeaning jobs simply to be part of the group (Bornstein; First & Tasman, 2004).

Among women, the combination of emotional dependence (need for nurturing, protection, and support) and economic dependency (lack of money, access to financial resources, alternative housing, and support for their children) and, among men, a combination of emotional dependence (fears of rejection and abandonment), feelings of jealousy, and problems with anger management are associated with increased risk for domestic violence (Bornstein, 2006). Among women with DPD, severity of abuse has been found to correlate with the severity of the symptoms of DPD. Economic dependency in women is associated with more severe abuse (life-threatening violence) than emotional dependency (Watson, Barnett, Nikunen, et al., 1997).

Epidemiology and Etiology

The prevalence of DPD is 0.7% of the general population (Torgersen, 2009), and it is more common among women (Grant et al., 2004). Individuals who have had chronic physical illnesses in childhood appear to be at increased risk of developing DPD (Sadock & Sadock, 2007). Childhood depression also increases the risk for developing DPD (Kasen, Cohen, Skodol, et al., 2001). DPD often co-occurs with other personality disorders—such as BPD, AVPD, HPD, and STPD (Lyons, 1995)—and with mood disorders, anxiety disorders, eating disorders, somatization disorder (Bornstein, 2007), and panic attacks (Grossman, 2004).

The heritability of DPD is 57%, in the moderate range (Smoller et al., 2008). Lack of parental affection and childhood neglect have been found to be associated with DPD (Johnson et al., 2009). In contradistinction, it is thought that parental overprotectiveness and authoritarianism may foster the development of dependency in a child and may prevent the child from developing independent, autonomous behaviors (Bornstein, 1992). Some cultures value dependency and may reward the child who displays dependency traits (Skodol & Gunderson, 2011).

Biological Basis

There has been very little neurobiological research with patients with DPD. There appears to be a reduction of dopamine activity and an increase of serotonergic activity (Coccaro & Siever, 2009).

Clinical Presentation

The core feature of DPD is the patient's need to obtain and maintain nurturing, supportive relationships. Patients experience distress if alone. They are often preoccupied with fears of being left to care for themselves because they believe that they are unable to look after themselves. They may appear submissive or passive and they may express self-doubts about their ability to make decisions or to manage their own affairs. They have difficulty starting projects because of lack of confidence in their ability. They find it difficult to disagree with others and may tolerate an abusive relationship in order not to disturb the attachment (Bornstein, 1992; Skodol & Gunderson, 2011). Although a key feature of DPD is neediness that is manifested in clinging behaviors, patients with DPD often wish that they were more independent and autonomous (Stone, 2006).

Differential Diagnosis

Traits of dependency are present in many psychiatric disorders. Fear of abandonment is present in BPD, and need for reassurance and approval is present in HSD. In differentiating DPD from HSD and BPD, patients with DPD have a history of *a long-term* relationship with one person, which is unlike patients with HSD and BPD. The fear of abandonment of patients with DPD is not characterized by rage and demands as in BPD, and their need for approval and reassurance is not related to need for being the center of attention as in HSD (First et al., 2002; Skodol & Gunderson, 2011).

Treatment

Treatment includes psychotherapy—psychodynamic individual psychotherapy, CBT, family therapy, couples therapy, and group psychotherapy (Black & Andreasen, 2011; Skodol & Gunderson, 2008). Psychotherapeutic interventions that have been found to be useful for patients with DPD include identifying relationships from the past and present that reinforce dependent behavior; helping patients to examine their view of themselves as helpless; challenging patients' self-denigrating statements; helping patients to gain insight into the ways they express dependency needs; helping them to think of alternative ways to meet their needs; and building coping skills (Bornstein, 2007).

No psychotropic medications—antidepressants, anxiolytics, or antipsychotics—have been found to be more effective than placebo in the treatment of DPD (Bornstein, 2007). Pharmacotherapy has been used for co-occurring symptoms of anxiety and depression, and patients with DPD and co-occurring depression have been found to respond to antidepressant medications with some improvement of the DPD features (Kool et al., 2003). Psychosocial interventions that have been found to be helpful include assertiveness training and social skills training (Skodol & Gunderson, 2011).

Course

Patients with DPD may have limited vocational achievement and social relationships and are at risk for depression if they lose the person they depend on. If they lose a relationship that provided care for them, they may rush into another relationship that they hope will protect and nurture them (Skodol & Gunderson, 2011). In doing so, they may expose themselves to physical and sexual abuse and exploitation (Sadock & Sadock, 2007). As they age, their increasing dependence on their spouse or children may become burdensome and create stressful family relationships (Segal et al., 2006). With treatment, prognosis is favorable.

Resources

Movies

Oz, F. (Director). (1991). *What about Bob?* [Motion picture]. United States: Touchstone Pictures.

SOURCE: WEDDING & BOYD, 1999.

Kosminsky, P. (Director). (2002). *White oleander* [Motion picture]. United States: Warner Bros.

SOURCE: WEDDING, BOYD, & NIEMIEC, 2010.

Obsessive-Compulsive Personality Disorder (OCPD)

Sigmund Freud (1908) said that individuals with OCPD had three peculiarities of orderliness—cleanliness, parsimony, and obstinacy. Nearly a hundred years later, the *DSM-IV-TR* (American Psychiatric Association, 2000) described the criteria for OCPD as a preoccupation with orderliness, perfectionism, control, and details; overconscientious; reluctance to delegate tasks; miserliness; and rigidity. The symptoms that are most prevalent and most stable over time are rigidity, problems with delegating work or tasks, and perfectionism. Miserliness was the least prevalent and least stable over time (McGlashan et al., 2005). Individuals with OCPD often demonstrate a degree of perfectionism that interferes with their completing a task and reaching their goals, and it impairs their functioning in interpersonal relationships, social relationships, and vocational situations (Skodol & Gunderson, 2011; Stone, 1993).

Epidemiology and Etiology

The prevalence of OCPD is estimated to be 2.1% of the general population (Torgersen, 2009). Men are diagnosed with OCPD twice as often as women. It is more common in the oldest child in the family (Sadock & Sadock, 2007). OCPD frequently co-occurs with major depressive disorder and anxiety disorders. The heritability of OCPD is 78% (Smoller et al., 2008). There is evidence of heritability of some of the traits of OCPD. For example, there is heritability of the trait of obsessionality (Nigg & Goldsmith, 1994), conscientiousness (Widiger, Trull, Clarkin, et al., 2002), and self-regulation of attention (Jang & Vernon, 2001). There are conflicting views on a genetic link between OCD and OCPD. They often coexist. It is thought that in response to excessive parental disapproval and pressure to perform correctly and to follow rules, the child focuses on being perfect so as to win parental approval (Sadock & Sadock).

Biological Basis

There is little information available about the biological basis of OCPD. It is thought that abnormalities of dopamine and serotonin may be involved in OCPD (Lee & Coccaro, 2009). For example, it is known that the trait of perfectionism is associated with abnormalities of dopamine functioning and that patients with OCPD have been found to have abnormalities of the dopamine D_3 receptor gene (Light, Joyce, Luty, et al., 2006). Serotonin deficits have been found to be associated with inhibition of flexibility of approach to goals. For example, low levels of serotonin in the prefrontal area of the brain may contribute to a narrow focus on arbitrary or inappropriate goals (Clarke, Walker, Dalley, et al., 2007).

Clinical Presentation

Patients with OCPD view their traits of rigidity, obstinacy, excessive orderliness, and parsimony as ego-syntonic. They see no reason to seek treatment for these traits; however, they may seek treatment for an Axis I disorder, such as depression or substance-related disorder, or because they have no interest in life.

In response to a severe stressor, such as failure to achieve a goal, their view of themselves may become critical and self-devaluating, and they may develop depression and suicidality (Perry, 2007). Patients with OCPD often present with a stiff or rigid manner. During the psychiatric interview, they may seek to control the evaluation, and their responses to questions will be detailed. They are preoccupied with lists, rules, regulations, orderliness, neatness, details, and perfection. They may have difficulty completing a task because it must be perfect. Their overconscientiousness may result in devoting so much time to work that it limits time for leisure activities and interpersonal relationships. They often have difficulty delegating work to others or working with others. They may have an inability to throw away worn-out or useless things, and they often hoard money. Their behavior is characterized by rigidity and stubbornness (Skodol & Gunderson, 2008).

Patients with OCPD tend to be well educated and able to maintain employment. Their daily activities are rigidly structured. Even their hobbies and leisure activities are organized. They are unable to compromise and have limited interpersonal skills and few friends. They often have difficulty controlling anger (Grossman, 2004). Because they fear making mistakes, they are indecisive and ruminate about making decisions. Patients with OCPD see themselves as conscientious and responsible. They do not see the effect of their perfectionism and rigidity on others.

Differential Diagnosis

Differential diagnoses include OCD and NPD. Unlike OCD, OCPD is not characterized by obsessions and compulsions. Whereas patients with OCD consider their symptoms to be ego-dystonic and unwanted, patients with OCPD consider their characteristics to be ego-syntonic—acceptable and not problematic (Skodol & Gunderson, 2008); they see themselves as conscientious, responsible, and dutiful workers. Both NPD and OCPD are characterized by assertiveness, domination, achievement, and perfectionism, but whereas patients with OCPD will have doubts, worries, and self-criticism, patients with NPD usually will not (First & Tasman, 2004).

Treatment

Primary treatment for OCPD is psychotherapy, such as psychodynamic individual psychotherapy; psychoanalysis; CBT; and psychodynamic group psychotherapy (Skodol & Gunderson, 2008). Among patients with OCPD who were treated with supportive-expressive psychodynamic therapy for 1 year, 85% no longer met the criteria for the syndrome (Barber et al., 1997). Most of them had a good response to treatment at the end of 4 months, with improvement in depression, anxiety, general function, and interpersonal problems.

Symptoms such as depression may be treated with pharmacotherapy such as the SSRIs. The SSRIs may also modify behaviors. For example, when healthy volunteers were given SSRIs, there was an increase in cooperation and socializing behaviors and a decrease in hostile and aggressive behaviors (Allgulander, Cloninger, Przybeck et al., 1998; Tse & Bond, 2002). Similarly, Grossman (2004) found that the use of the SSRIs citalopram (Celexa) and paroxetine (Paxil) was associated with an increase in cooperating with others and in socializing with others and a decrease in hostility and aggressive behaviors. Based on these studies and on reports from clinical practice, it is assumed that SSRIs would be beneficial for patients with OCPD. In clinical practice, it has been found that patients with OCPD and depression respond to antidepressants with improvement of depression and some improvement in OCPD symptoms (Ekselius & von Knorring, 1998). Black and Andreasen (2011) said that the SSRIs fluoxetine, paroxetine, and citalopram may reduce patients' need for perfection and the rituals used to try to attain perfection. Clonazepam (Klonopin), a benzodiazepine, has been found to reduce symptoms in OCD, but its use in OCPD is not known.

Course

The course of OCPD is unpredictable. Some patients may develop OCD with obsessions and compulsions. Some adolescents evolve into warm, open, and loving adults. In others, OCPD can be the prodromal stage of schizophrenia or, decades later, major depressive disorder. Some older adults with OCPD become more rigid and have difficulty adjusting to the new routines of retirement or different living situations. They may also increase their hoarding behaviors (Segal et al., 2006). However, in a recent prospective study, 55% of patients with OCPD who received treatment were able to achieve remission at 2-year follow-up (Grilo et al., 2004).

Resources

Movies

Saks, G. (Director). (1968). *The odd couple* [Motion picture]. United States: Paramount Pictures.

SOURCE: WEDDING & BOYD, 1999.

DiCillo, T. (Director). (1996). *Box of moonlight* [Motion picture]. United States: Trimark Pictures.

SOURCE: WEDDING, BOYD, & NIEMIEC, 2010.

Summary

Effective treatment for patients with personality disorders depends on knowledge of the biopsychosocial foundation of the personality disorders. Effective treatment includes (1) a supportive alliance between the psychiatric advanced practice nurse and the patient, (2) psychotherapy, such as CBT, (3) pharmacotherapy, and (4) psychosocial interventions such as education about the illness and treatment, social support, rehabilitation, collaboration with other disciplines, and case management to coordinate care and access to supports and resources (Knutson & Heinz, 2004).

Key Points

- Personality disorders develop from maladaptive personality styles that have resulted from the interaction of genetically influenced temperament, abnormalities of brain development and functioning, and exposure to adverse experiences such as neglect and abuse.
- Risk factors for the development of maladaptive personality traits include lack of parental affection, neglect, and emotional, physical, and sexual abuse.
- Protective factors that promote development of adaptive personality traits include parental empathy; support and warmth; supportive communities; participation in sports, hobbies, and other activities; resiliency; hardiness; and self-efficacy.
- Personality disorders are present in 10% of the general population.
- The heritability varies among the personality disorders from 28% to 78%.
- Personality disorders can be classified by dimensions and by categories.
- Dimensions of personality disorders include cognitive-perceptual, impulse control, affect regulation, and anxiety.
- Categories of personality disorders include Cluster A (paranoid, schizoid, and schizotypal personality disorders); Cluster B (antisocial, borderline, histrionic, and narcissistic personality disorders); and Cluster C (avoidant, dependent, and obsessive-compulsive personality disorders).
- Personality disorders are currently classified by category (*DSM-IV-TR* categories). Classification by dimension (cognitive-perceptual, impulse control, affect regulation, and anxiety) is a change being recommended for the revision of the current *DSM-IV-TR*.
- Treatment includes hospitalization, psychotherapy, pharmacotherapy, and psychosocial interventions (support groups, assertive community treatment, and community resources).
- Psychotherapy targets problems of character, behavior, and interpersonal relationships.
- Pharmacotherapy targets symptoms of cognitive-perceptual disturbance, affective dysregulation, and impulsive-behavioral dyscontrol.
- Psychosocial interventions target problems related to home, work, and daily life.
- Personality disorders are less stable than was once thought.
- Impulsive and aggressive features may decrease with age, and introverted traits may increase as people get older.

References

Abraham, P. F., & Calabrese, J. R. (2008). Evidence-based pharmacologic treatment of borderline personality disorder: A shift from SSRIs to anticonvulsants and atypical antipsychotics? *Journal of Affective Disorders, 111*, 21-30.

Akiskal, H. S. (1981). Sub-affective disorders: Dysthymic, cyclothymic, and bipolar II disorders in the "borderline" realm. *Psychiatric Clinics of North America, 4*, 25-46.

Alden, L. E. (1989). Short-term structured treatment for avoidant personality disorder. *Journal of Consulting and Clinical Psychology, 57*, 756-764.

Allgulander, C., Cloninger, C. R., Przybeck, T. R., et al. (1998). Changes on the Temperament and Character Inventory after paroxetine treatment in volunteers with generalized anxiety disorder. *Psychopharmacology Bulletin, 34*(2), 165-166.

Allnutt, S., & Links, P. S. (1996). Diagnosing specific personality disorders, and the optimal criteria. In P. S. Links (Ed.), *Clinical assessment and management of severe personality disorders (clinical practice 35)* (pp. 21-47). Washington, DC: American Psychiatric Publishing, Inc.

American Psychiatric Association. (1994). *Diagnostic and statistical manual of mental disorders* (4th ed.). Washington, DC: American Psychiatric Publishing, Inc.

American Psychiatric Association. (2000). *Diagnostic and statistical manual of mental disorders* (4th ed., text rev.). Washington, DC: American Psychiatric Publishing, Inc.

Andreasen, N. C., & Black, D. W. (2006). *Introductory textbook of psychiatry* (4th ed.). Washington, DC: American Psychiatric Publishing, Inc.

Barber, J. P., Morse, J. Q., Krakauer, I. D., et al. (1997). Change in obsessive-compulsive and avoidant personality disorders following time-limited supportive-expressive therapy. *Psychotherapy, 34*, 133-143.

Barkataki, I., Kumari, V., Das, M., et al. (2006). Volumetric structural brain abnormalities in men with schizophrenia or antisocial personality disorder. *Behavior and Brain Research, 169*, 239-247.

Beck, A. T., Freeman, A., Davis, D. D., et al. (2004). *Cognitive therapy of personality disorders* (2nd ed.). New York: Guilford Press.

Benjamin, L. (1996). *Interpersonal diagnosis and treatment of personality disorders* (2nd ed.). New York: Guilford Press.

Bierer, L. M., Yehuda, R., Schmeidler, J., et al. (2003). Abuse and neglect in childhood: Relationship to personality disorder diagnoses. *CNS Spectrum, 8*, 737-754.

Birbaumer, N., Veit, R., Lotze, M., et al. (2005). Deficient fear conditioning in psychopathy: A functional magnetic resonance imaging study. *Archives of General Psychiatry, 78*, 373-388.

Black, D. W. (1999). *Bad boys, bad men*. New York: Oxford University Press.

Black, D. W., & Andreasen, N. C. (2011). *Introductory textbook of psychiatry* (5th ed.). Washington, DC: American Psychiatric Publishing, Inc.

Black, D. W., Baumgard, C. H., Bell, S. E., et al. (1996). Death rates in 71 men with antisocial personality disorder: A comparison with general population mortality. *Psychosomatics, 37*, 131-136.

Blair, R. J. (2004). The roles of orbital frontal cortex in the modulation of antisocial behavior. *Brain & Cognition, 55*(1), 198-208.

Bornstein, R. F. (1992). The dependent personality: Developmental, social, and clinical perspectives. *Psychological Bulletin, 112*(1), 3-23.

Bornstein, R. F. (2006). The complex relationship between dependency and domestic violence. *American Psychologist, 61*(6), 595-606.

Bornstein, R. F. (2007). Dependent personality disorder: Effective time-limited therapy. *Current Psychiatry, 6*(1), 37-44.

Bornstein, R. F., Becker-Matero, N., Winarick, D. J., et al. (2010). Interpersonal dependency in borderline personality disorder: Clinical context and empirical evidence. *Journal of Personality Disorders, 24*(1), 109-127.

Bouchard, T. J. (1994). Genes, environment, and personality. *Science, 264*(5166), 1700-1701.

Bouchard, T. J., & Loehlin, J. C. (2001). Genes, evolution, and personality. *Behavioral Genetics, 31*, 243-273.

Bremner, J. D., & Vermetten, E. (2004). Neuroanatomical changes associated with pharmacotherapy in posttraumatic stress disorder. *Annals of the New York Academy of Sciences, 1032*, 154-157.

Cardasis, W., Hochman, J., & Silk, K. (1997). Transitional objects and borderline personality disorder. *The American Journal of Psychiatry, 154*(2), 250-255.

Carter, J. D., Joyce, P. R., Mulder, R. T., et al. (1999). Early deficient parenting in depressed outpatients is associated with personality dysfunction and not with depression subtypes. *Journal of Affective Disorders, 54*, 29-37.

Caspi, A., Moffitt, T. E., Newman, D. L., et al. (1996). Behavioral observations at age 3 years predict adult psychiatric disorders. *Archives of General Psychiatry, 53*(11), 1033-1039.

Caspi, A., Roberts, B. W., & Shiner, R. (2005). Personality development: Stability and change. *Annual Review of Psychology, 56*, 453-484.

Chen, H., Cohen, P., Crawford, T. N., et al. (2006). Relative impact of young adult personality disorders on subsequent quality of life: Findings of a community-based longitudinal study. *Journal of Personality Disorders, 20*(5), 510-523.

Chengappa, K. N., Sheth, S., Brar, J. S., et al. (1999). Risperidone use at a state hospital: A clinical audit 2 years after the first wave of risperidone prescriptions. *Journal of Clinical Psychiatry, 60*(6), 373-378.

Chiesa, M., Fonagy, P., & Holmes, J. (2006). Six-year follow-up of three treatment programs to personality disorder. *Journal of Personality Disorders, 20*, 493-509.

Clarke, H. F., Walker, S. C., Dalley, J. W., et al. (2007). Cognitive inflexibility after prefrontal serotonin depletion is behaviorally and neurochemically specific. *Cerebral Cortex, 17*, 18-27.

Cloninger, C. R., Svrakic, D. M., & Przybeck, T. R. (1993). A biopsychosocial model of temperament and character. *Archives of General Psychiatry, 50*(12), 975-990.

Cloninger, C. R., Van Eerdewegh, P., Goate, A., et al. (1998). Anxiety proneness linked to epistatic loci in genome scan of human personality traits. *American Journal of Medical Genetics, 81*, 313-317.

Coccaro, E. F. (1989). Central serotonin and impulsive aggression. *British Journal of Psychiatry, 155*, 52-62.

Coccaro, E. F. (1996). Neurotransmitter correlates of impulsive aggression in humans. *Annals of the New York Academy of Sciences, 795*, 82-89.

Coccaro, E. F., Kavoussi, R. J., Hauger, R. L., et al. (1998). Cerebrospinal fluid vasopressin levels. Correlates with aggression and serotonin function in personality disordered subjects. *Archives of General Psychiatry, 55*, 708-714.

Coccaro, E. F., & Siever, L. J. (2009). Neurobiology. In J. M. Oldham, A. E. Skodol, & D. S. Bender (Eds.), *Essentials of personality disorders* (pp. 103-122). Washington, DC: American Psychiatric Publishing, Inc.

Coen, S. J. (2005). How to play with patients who would rather remain remote. *Journal of the American Psychoanalytic Association, 53*(3), 811-834.

Cooper, A. M., & Ronningstam, E. (1992). Narcissistic personality disorder. In A. Tasman & M. B. Riba (Eds.), *Review of psychiatry* (Vol. 11, pp. 80-97). Washington, DC: American Psychiatric Publishing, Inc.

Corbitt, E. M., & Widiger, T. A. (1995). Sex differences among the personality disorders: An exploration of the data. *Clinical Psychological Science Practice, 2*, 225-238.

Costa, P. T., & McCrae, R. R. (1992). *Revised NEO Personality Inventory (NEO-PI-R), and the NEO Five-Factory Inventory (NEO-FFI) professional manual.* Odessa, FL: Psychological Assessment Resources.

Crits-Christoph, P. (1998). Psychosocial treatments for personality disorders. In P. E. Nathan & J. M. Gorman (Eds.), *A guide to treatments that work* (pp. 544-553). New York: Oxford University Press.

Deltito, J. A., & Stam, M. (1989). Psychopharmacological treatment of avoidant personality disorder. *Comprehensive Psychiatry, 30*, 498-504.

Digman, J. M. (1990). Personality structure: Emergence of the five-factor structure. *American Review of Psychology, 41*, 417-440.

Dolan-Sewell, R. T., Krueger, R. F., & Shea, M. T. (2001). Co-occurrence with syndrome disorders. In W. J. Livesley (Ed.), *Handbook of personality disorders.* New York: Guilford Press.

Driessen, M., Herrmann, J., Stahl, K., et al. (2000). Magnetic resonance imaging volumes of the hippocampus and the amygdala in women with borderline personality disorder and early traumatization. *Archives of General Psychiatry, 57*(12), 1115-1122.

Dubo, E., Zanarini, M., Lewis, R., et al. (1997). Childhood antecedents of self-destructiveness in borderline personality disorder. *Canadian Journal of Psychiatry, 42*, 63-69.

Duff, A. (2003). Managing personality disorders: Making positive connections. *Nursing Management, 10*(6), 27-30.

Ekselius, L., & von Knorring, L. (1998). Personality disorder comorbidity with major depression and response to treatment with sertraline or citalopram. *International Clinics of Psychopharmacology, 13*, 205-211.

El-Gabalawy, R., Katz, L., & Sareen, J. (2010). Comorbidity-associated severity of BPD and physical health conditions in a nationally representative sample. *Psychosomatic Medicine, 72*(7), 647-700.

Fanous, A. H., Neale, M. C., Aggen, S. H., et al. (2007). A longitudinal study of personality and major depression in a population-bases sample of male twins. *Psychological Medicine, 37*, 1163-1172.

Fernando, J. (1998). The etiology of the narcissistic personality disorder. *The Psychoanalytic Study of the Child, 53*, 141-158.

First, M. B., Frances, A., & Pincus, H. A. (2002). *DSM-IV-TR handbook of differential diagnosis.* Washington, DC: American Psychiatric Publishing, Inc.

First, M. B., & Tasman, A. (2004). *DSM-IV-TR mental disorders: Diagnosis, etiology, and treatment.* West Sussex, UK: John Wiley & Sons, Inc.

Fossati, A., Barratt, E. S., Borroni, S., et al. (2007). Impulsivity, aggressiveness, and DSM-IV personality disorders. *Psychiatric Research, 149*, 157-167.

Frankle, W. G., Lombardo, I., New, A. S., et al. (2005). Brain serotonin transport distribution in subjects with impulsive aggressivity: A positron emission study with (11C) McN5652. *American Journal of Psychiatry, 162*, 915-923.

Freedman, A. (2002). Cognitive-behavioral therapy for severe personality disorders. In S. G. Hofman & M. C. Tompson (Eds.), *Treating chronic and severe mental disorders: A handbook of empirically supported interventions* (pp. 382-402). New York: Guilford Press.

Freud, S. (1908). Character and anal eroticism. In J. Strachey (Ed.). *The standard edition of the complete psychological works of Sigmund Freud* (Vol. 9) (pp. 168-175). London: Hogarth Press.

Gabbard, G. O. (2005). Mind, brain, and personality disorders. *The American Journal of Psychiatry, 162*(4), 648-655.

Gabbard, G. O. (2009). Psychoanalysis and psychodynamic psychotherapy. In J. M. Oldham, A. E. Skodol, & D. S. Bender (Eds.), *Essentials of personality disorders* (pp. 185-207). Washington, DC: American Psychiatric Publishing, Inc.

Gabbard, G. O., & Allison, S. E. (2007). Histrionic personality disorder. In G. O. Gabbard (Ed.), *Gabbard's treatment of psychiatric disorders* (4th ed.) (pp. 823-833). Washington, DC: American Psychiatric Publishing, Inc.

Glatt, S. G., Faraone, S. V., & Tsuang, M. T. (2007). Genetic risk factors for mental disorders. In M. T. Tsuang, W. S. Stone, & M. J. Lyons (Eds.), *Recognition and prevention of major mental and substance use disorders* (pp. 3-20). Washington, DC: American Psychiatric Publishing, Inc.

Gold, J. M., & Harvey, P. D. (1993). Cognitive deficits in schizophrenia. *Psychiatric Clinics of North America, 16*, 295-312.

Gollan, J. K., Lee, R., & Coccaro, E. F. (2005). Developmental psychopathology and neurobiology of aggression. *Development and Psychopathology, 17*, 1151-1171.

Gooding, D. C., Tallent, K. A., & Matts, C. W. (2007). Rates of avoidant, schizotypal, schizoid, and paranoid personality disorders in psychometric high-risk groups at 5-year follow-up. *Schizophrenia Research, 94*, 373-374.

Goodman, M., New, A., & Siever, L. (2004). Trauma, genes, and the neurobiology of personality disorders. *Annals of New York Academy of Sciences, 1032*, 104-116.

Grant, B. F., Hasin, D. S., Stinson, F. S., et al. (2004). Prevalence, correlates, and disability of personality disorders in the United States: Results from the national epidemiologic survey on alcohol and related conditions. *Journal of Clinical Psychiatry, 65*(7), 948-958.

Grilo, C. M., & McGlashan, T. H. (2009). Course and outcome. In J. M. Oldham, A. E. Skodol, & D. S. Bender (Eds.), *Essential of personality disorders* (pp. 63-79). Washington, DC: American Psychiatric Publishing, Inc.

Grilo, C. M., Sanislow, C. A., Gunderson, J. G., et al. (2004). Two year stability and change of schizotypal, borderline, avoidant, and obsessive-compulsive personality disorders. *Journal of Consulting and Clinical Psychology, 72*, 767-775.

Grossman, R. (2004). Pharmacotherapy of personality disorders. In J. J. Magnavita (Ed.), *Handbook of personality disorders: Theory and practice* (pp. 331-355). Hoboken, NJ: Wiley.

Gunderson, J. G. (2001). *Borderline personality disorder: A clinical guide.* Washington, DC: American Psychiatric Publishing, Inc.

Gunderson, J. G. (2007). Introduction. In G. O. Gabbard (Ed.), *Gabbard's treatment of psychiatric disorders* (4th ed.) (pp. 759-761). Washington, DC: American Psychiatric Publishing, Inc.

Gunderson, J. G., Daversa, M. T., Grilo, C., et al. (2006). Predictors of 2-year outcome for patients with borderline personality disorder. *The American Journal of Psychiatry, 163*(5), 822-826.

Gunderson, J. G., Gratz, K. L., Neuhaus, E. C., et al. (2009). Levels of care in treatment. In J. M. Oldham, A. E. Skodol, & D. S. Bender (Eds.), *Essentials of personality disorders* (pp. 161-183). Washington, DC: American Psychiatric Publishing, Inc.

Gunderson, J. G., & Links, P. S. (1995). Borderline personality disorder. In G. O. Gabbard (Ed.), *Treatments of psychiatric disorders* (2nd ed.) (pp. 2291-2309). Washington, DC: American Psychiatric Publishing, Inc.

Gunderson, J. G., & Links. P. S. (2007). Borderline personality disorder. In G. O. Gabbard (Ed.), *Gabbard's treatment of psychiatric disorders* (4th ed.) (pp. 805-821). Washington, DC: American Psychiatric Publishing, Inc.

Gunderson, J. G., & Ronningstam, E. (2001). Differentiating narcissistic and antisocial personality disorders. *Journal of Personality Disorders, 15*(2), 103-109.

Gunderson, J. G., Stout, R. L., McGlashan, T. H., et al. (2011). Ten-year course of borderline personality disorder. *Archives of General Psychiatry, 68*(8), 827-837.

Hare, R. D. (1991). *The Hare psychopathy checklist—Revised manual.* Toronto, Ontario, Canada: Multi Health Systems.

Hayward, B. A. (2007). Cluster A personality disorders: Considering the "odd-eccentric" in psychiatric nursing. *International Journal of Mental Health Nursing, 16,* 15-21.

Heim, A., & Westen, D. (2009). Theories of personality and personality disorders. In J. M. Oldham, A. E. Skodol, & D. S. Bender (Eds.), *Essentials of personality disorders* (pp. 13-34). Washington, DC: American Psychiatric Publishing, Inc.

Heim, C., Newport, D. J., Bonsall, R., et al. (2001). Altered pituitary-adrenal axis responses to provocative challenge tests in adult survivors of childhood abuse. *American Journal of Psychiatry, 158*(4), 575-581.

Helgeland, M. I., & Torgersen, S. (2004). Developmental antecedents of borderline personality disorder. *Comprehensive Psychiatry, 45*(2), 138-147.

Herman, J. L., Perry, J. C., & van der Kolk, B. A. (1989). Childhood trauma in borderline personality disorder. *American Journal of Psychiatry, 146,* 490-495.

Hirose, S. (2001). Effective treatment of aggression and impulsivity in antisocial personality disorder with risperidone. *Psychiatry and Clinical Neuroscience, 55*(2), 161-162.

Hoek, H. W., Susser, E., Buck, K. A., et al. (1996). Schizoid personality disorder after prenatal exposure to famine. *American Journal of Psychiatry, 153*(12), 1637-1639.

Hoffman, S. G., & Tompson, M. C. (2002). Preface. In S. G. Hofmann & M. C. Tompson (Eds.), *Treating chronic and severe mental disorders: A handbook of empirically supported interventions* (pp. XI-XIII). New York: Guilford Press.

Hughes, C. H. (1884). Moral (affective) insanity: Psycho-sensory insanity. *Alienist and Neurologist, 5,* 296-315.

Ichikawa, J., Ishii, H., Bonaccorso, S., et al. (2001). 5-HT 2A and D2 receptor blockade increases cortical DA release via 5-HT1A receptor activation: A possible mechanism of atypical antipsychotic induced cortical dopamine release. *Journal of Neurochemistry, 5*(5), 1521-1531.

Jang, K. L., & Vernon, P. A. (2001). Personality disorder traits, family environment, and alcohol misuse: A multivariate behavioral genetic analysis. *Addiction, 95,* 873-888.

Johnson, D. M., Shea, M. T., Yen. S., et al. (2003). Gender differences in BPD: Finding from the Collaborative Longitudinal Personality Disorders Study. *Comprehensive Psychiatry, 44*(4), 284-292.

Johnson, J. G., Bromley, E., & McGeoch, P. G. (2009). Childhood experiences and development of maladaptive and adaptive personality traits. In J. M. Oldham, A. E. Skodol, & D. S. Bender (Eds.), *Essentials of personality disorders* (pp. 143-157). Washington, DC: American Psychiatric Publishing, Inc.

Johnson, J. G., Cohen, P., Brown, J., et al. (1999). Childhood maltreatment increases risk for personality disorders during early adulthood. *Archives of General Psychiatry, 56,* 600-606.

Johnson, J. G., Cohen, P., Smailes, E. M., et al. (2001). Childhood verbal abuse and risk for personality disorders during adolescence and early adulthood. *Comprehensive Psychiatry, 42*(1), 16-23.

Johnson, J. G., Smailes, E. M., Cohen, P., et al. (2000). Associations between four types of childhood neglect and personality disorder symptoms during adolescence and early adulthood: Findings of a community-based longitudinal study. *Journal of Personality Disorders, 14*(2), 171-187.

Judd, P. H., & McGlashan, T. H. (2003). *A developmental model of borderline personality disorder: Understanding variations in course and outcome* (pp. 51-90). Washington, DC: American Psychiatric Publishing, Inc.

Kasen, S., Cohen, P., Skodol, A. E., et al. (2001). Childhood depression and adult personality disorder: Alternative pathways of continuity. *Archives of General Psychiatry, 58,* 231-236.

Kavoussi, R. J., Liu, J., & Coccaro, E. F. (1994). An open trial of sertraline in personality disordered patients with impulsive aggression. *Journal of Clinical Psychiatry, 55*(4), 137-141.

Kernberg, O. (2004). Borderline personality disorder and borderline personality organization: Psychopathology and psychotherapy. In J. J. Magnavita (Ed.), *Handbook of personality disorder: Theory and Practice* (pp. 92-119). Hoboken, NJ: Wiley.

Knutson, B., & Heinz, A. (2004). Psychobiology of personality disorders. In J. Panksepp (Ed.), *Textbook of biological psychiatry* (pp. 145-166). Hoboken, NJ: Wiley-Liss, Inc.

Knutson, B., Wolkowitz, O. M., Cole, S., et al. (1998). Selective alteration of personality and social behavior by serotonergic intervention. *American Journal of Psychiatry, 155,* 373-379.

Kool, S., Dekker, J., Kuijsens, I. J., et al. (2003). Changes in personality pathology after pharmacotherapy and combined therapy for depressed patients. *Journal of Personality Disorders, 17,* 60-72.

Koons, C., Robins, C. J., Tweed, J. L., et al. (2001). Efficacy of dialectical behavior therapy in women veterans with borderline personality disorder. *Behavioral Therapy, 32,* 371-390.

Krueger, R. (2010). Personality pathology is dimensional, So what shall we do with the DSM-IV personality categories? The case of NPD: Comment on Miller and Campbell: 2010. *Personality Disorders, 1*(3), 195-196.

Lee, R., & Coccaro, E. F. (2009). Neurobiology of personality disorders. In A. F. Schatzberg & C. B. Nemeroff (Eds.), *Essentials of clinical psychopharmacology* (pp. 1045-1060). Washington, DC: American Psychiatric Publishing, Inc.

Lee, R., Geracioti, T. D., Kasckow, J. W., et al. (2005). Childhood trauma and personality disorder: Positive correlation with adult CSF corticotropin-releasing factor concentrations. *The American Journal of Psychiatry, 162*(5), 995-997.

Leichsenring, F., & Leibing, E. (2003). The effectiveness of psychodynamic therapy and cognitive behavior therapy in the treatment of personality disorders: A meta-analysis. *The American Journal of Psychiatry, 160*(7), 1223-1232.

Lewis, M. (2001). Issues in the study of personality development. *Psychological Inquiry, 12,* 67-83.

Light, K. J., Joyce, P. R., Luty, S. E., et al. (2006). Preliminary evidence for an association between a dopamine D3 receptor gene variant and obsessive-compulsive personality disorder in patients with major depression. *American Journal of Medical Genetics. Part B, Neuropsychiatric Genetics, 141,* 409-413.

Lilienfeld, S. O., & Hess, T. H. (2001). Psychopathic personality traits and somatization: Sex differences and the mediating role of negative emotionality. *Journal of Psychopathological Behavioral Assessment, 23,* 11-24.

Lindberg, N., Tani, P., Stenberg, J. J. H., et al. (2004). Neurological soft signs in homicidal men with antisocial personality disorder. *European Psychiatry: The Journal of the Association of European Psychiatrists, 19*(7), 433-437.

Linehan, M. M. (1987). Dialectical behavior therapy for borderline personality disorder. Theory and method. *Bulletin of the Menninger Clinic, 51*(3), 261-276.

Linehan, M. M., Schmidt, H. III., Dimeff, J. A., et al. (1999). Dialectical behavior therapy for patients with borderline personality disorder and drug dependence. *American Journal of Addictions, 8,* 279-292.

Links, P. S., Boiago, I., Huxley, G., et al. (1990). Sexual abuse and biparental failure as etiologic models in borderline personality disorder. In P. S. Links (Ed.), *Family environment and borderline personality disorder* (pp. 105-120). Washington, DC: American Psychiatric Publishing, Inc.

Links, P. S., Heslegrave, R., & Villella, J. (1998). Psycho-pharmacological management of personality disorders: An outcome-focused model. In K. Silk (Ed.), *Biology of personality disorders* (pp. 93-127). Washington, DC: American Psychiatric Publishing, Inc.

Linnoila, M., Virkkunen, M., Scheinin, M., et al. (1983). Low cerebrospinal fluid 5-hydroxyindoleacetic acid concentration differentiates impulsive from non-impulsive violent behavior. *Life Sciences, 33,* 2609-2614.

Livesley, W. J. (1998). Suggestions for a framework for an empirically based classification of personality disorder. *Canadian Journal of Psychiatry, 43,* 137-147.

Livesley, W. J., Jackson, D. N., & Schroeder, M. L. (1992). Factorial structure of traits delineating personality disorders in clinical and general population samples. *Journal of Abnormal Psychology, 101,* 32-44.

Lynam, D. R. (1996). The early identification of chronic offenders: Who is the fledgling psychopath? *Psychological Bulletin, 120,* 209-234.

Lyons, M. (1995). Epidemiology of personality disorders. In M. Tsuang, M. Tohen, & G. Zahner (Eds.), *Textbook in psychiatric epidemiology.* New York: Wiley-Liss.

Lyons-Ruth, K., & Block, D. (1996). The disturbed care-giving system: Relations among childhood trauma, maternal care-giving and infant affect and attachment. *Infant Mental Health Journal, 17,* 257-275.

Magnavita, J. J. (2002). *Theories of personality: Contemporary approaches to the science of personality.* New York: John Wiley & Sons.

Magnavita, J. (2004). Classification, prevalence, and etiology of personality disorders: Related issues and controversy. In J. Magnavita (Ed.), *Handbook of personality disorder: Theory and practice* (pp. 3-23). Hoboken, NJ: Wiley.

Malone, S. M., Taylor, J., Marmorstein, N. R., et al. (2004). Genetic and environmental influences on antisocial behavior and alcohol dependence from adolescence to early adulthood. *Developmental Psychopathology, 16*(4), 943-966.

Markovitz, P. (2001). Pharmacotherapy. In W. J. Livesley (Ed.), *Handbook of personality disorders: Theory, research, and treatment* (pp. 475-493). New York: Guilford Press.

Markovitz, P. J., & Wagner, S. C. (1995). Venlafaxine in the treatment of borderline personality disorder. *Psychopharmacology Bulletin, 31*(4), 773-777.

McCloskey, M. S., Phan, K. L., & Coccaro, E. F. (2005). Neuroimaging and personality disorders. *Current Psychiatry Reports, 7*(1), 65-72.

McCrae, R. R., & John, O. P. (1992). An introduction to the five-factor model and its applications. *Journal of Personality, 54,* 430-446.

McGlashan, T. H., Grilo, C. M., Sanislow, C. A., et al. (2005). Two-year prevalence and stability of individual DSM-IV criteria for schizotypal, borderline, avoidant, and obsessive-compulsive personality disorders: Toward a hybrid model of Axis II disorders. *The American Journal of Psychiatry, 162*(5), 883-889.

Melroy, J. R. (2007). Antisocial personality disorder. In G. O. Gabbard (Ed.), *Gabbard's treatment of psychiatric disorders* (4th ed.) (pp. 775-789). Washington, DC: American Psychiatric Publishing, Inc.

Meyer, B., & Carver, C. S. (2000). Negative childhood accounts, sensitivity, and pessimism: A study of avoidant personality disorder features in college students. *Journal of Personality Disorders, 14*(3), 233-248.

Miller, J. D., Campbell, W. K., & Pilkonis, P. A. (2007). Narcissistic personality disorder: Relations with distress and functional impairment. *Comprehensive Psychiatry, 48*(2), 170-177.

Millon, T. (1987). On the genesis and prevalence of the borderline personality disorder: Asocial learning thesis. *Journal of Personality Disorders, 1,* 354-372.

Millon, T., Grossman, S. D., Millon, C., et al. (2004). *Personality disorders in modern life* (2nd ed.). Hoboken, NJ: John Wiley & Sons.

Minzenberg, M. J., Fan, J., New, A. S., et al. (2008). Frontolimbic structural changes in borderline personality disorder. *Journal of Psychiatric Research, 42*(9), 727-733.

Morey, L. C., Alexander, G. M., & Boggs, C. (2005). Gender. In J. M. Oldham, A. E. Skodol, & D. S. Bender (Eds.), *The American psychiatric publishing textbook of personality disorders* (pp. 541-559). Washington, DC: American Psychiatric Publishing, Inc.

Morris, H., Gunderson, J., & Zanarini, M. (1986). Transitional object use and borderline psychopathology. *American Journal of Psychiatry, 143*(12), 1534-1538.

Nathan, P. E., & Gorman, J. M. (Eds.) (1998). *A guide to treatments that work.* New York: Oxford University Press.

Natsuaki, M. N., Cicchetti, D., & Rogosch, F. A. (2009). Examining the developmental history of child maltreatment, peer relations, and externalizing problems among adolescents with symptoms of paranoid personality disorder. *Development and Psychopathology, 21*(4), 1181-1193.

Nemeroff, C. B. (2004). Neurobiological consequences of childhood trauma. *Journal of Clinical Psychiatry, 65*(Suppl 1), 18-28.

Nestadt, G., Kromanoski, A., Chahal, R., et al. (1990). An epidemiological study of histrionic personality disorder. *Psychological Medicine, 20,* 413-422.

Nickel, M. K., Muehlbacher, M., Nickel, C., et al. (2006). Aripiprazole in the treatment of patients with borderline personality disorder: A double blind placebo-controlled study. *American Journal of Psychiatry, 163,* 833-838.

Nigg, J. T., & Goldsmith, H. H. (1994). Genetics of personality disorders: Perspectives from personality and psychopathology research. *Psychological Bulletin, 115,* 346-380.

Norden, K. A., Klein, D. N., Donaldson, S. K., et al. (1995). Reports of the early home environment in DSM-III-R personality disorders. *Journal of Personality Disorders, 9,* 213-233.

O'Connor, B. P., & Dyce, J. A. (2001). Rigid and extreme: A geometric representation of personality disorders in five-factor model space. *Journal of Personality and Social Psychology, 81,* 1119-1130.

Oldham, J. M. (2009). Personality disorders: Recent history and the DSM system. In J. M. Oldham, A. E. Skodol, & D. S. Bender (Eds.), *Essentials of personality disorders* (pp. 3-11). Washington, DC: American Psychiatric Publishing, Inc.

Oldham, J. M., Gabbard, G. O., Goin, M. K., et al. (2004). Practice guideline for the treatment of patients with borderline personality disorder. In American Psychiatric Association (Ed.), *American Psychiatric Association practice guidelines for the treatment of psychiatric disorders: Compendium 2004* (pp. 745-833). Washington, DC: American Psychiatric Publishing, Inc.

Oldham, J. M., Skodol, A. E., & Bender, D. S. (2009). Introduction. In J. M. Oldham, A. E. Skodol., & D. S. Bender (Eds.), *Essentials of personality disorders* (pp. XV-XVIII). Washington, DC: American Psychiatric Publishing, Inc.

Oldham, J. M., Skodol, A. E., Gallaher, P. E., et al. (1996). Relationship of borderline symptoms to histories of abuse and neglect: A pilot study. *The Psychiatric Quarterly, 67*(4), 287-295.

Panksepp, J. (2004). Biological psychiatry sketched—past, present, and future. In J. Panksepp (Ed.), *Textbook of biological psychiatry* (pp. 3-32). Hoboken, NJ: Wiley-Liss, Inc.

Paris, J. (1996). *Social forces in the personality disorders.* Cambridge, UK: Cambridge University Press.

Paris, J. (1997). Antisocial and borderline personality disorders: Two separate diagnoses or two aspects of the same psychopathology. *Comprehensive Psychiatry, 38*(4), 237-242.

Paris, J. (1998). Does childhood trauma cause personality disorders in adults? *Canadian Journal of Psychiatry, 43,* 148-153.

Paris, J. (2003). *Personality disorders over time: Precursors, course, and outcome.* Washington, DC: American Psychiatric Publishing, Inc.

Paris, J. (2004). Sociocultural factors in the treatment of personality disorders. In J. J. Magnavita (Ed.), *Handbook of personality disorders: Theory and practice* (pp. 135-147). Hoboken, NJ: Wiley.

Paris, J. (2008). *Treatment of borderline personality disorder: A guide to evidence-based practice.* New York: Guilford Press.

Paris, J., & Zweig-Frank, H. (2001). A 27-year follow-up of patients with borderline personality disorder. *Comprehensive Psychiatry, 42*(6), 482-487.

Perez, U. A., Santos, G., Molina, R. R., et al. (2001). Sociocultural aspects of the genesis of personality disorders. *Actas Españolas de Psiquiatría, 29*(1), 45-57.

Perry, J. C. (2007). Cluster C Personality disorders: Avoidant, obsessive-compulsive, dependent. In G. O. Gabbard (Ed.), *Gabbard's treatment of psychiatric disorders* (4th ed.) (pp. 835-854). Washington, DC: American Psychiatric Publishing, Inc.

Pinto, O. C., & Akiskal, H. S. (1998). Lamotrigine as a promising approach to borderline personality: An open case series without concurrent DSM-IV major mood disorder. *Journal of Affective Disorders, 51,* 333-343.

Piper, W. E., & Ogrodniczuk, J. S. (2009). Group treatment. In J. M. Oldham, A. E. Skodol, & D. S. Bender (Eds.), *Essentials of personality disorders* (pp. 253-266). Washington, DC: American Psychiatric Publishing, Inc.

Plomin, R. (1990). The role of inheritance in behavior. *Science, 248,* 283-288.

Pretzer, J. (2004). Cognitive therapy of personality disorders. In J. J. Magnavita (Ed.), *Handbook of personality disorders: Theory and practice* (pp. 169-193). Hoboken, NJ: Wiley.

Raine, A., Lencz, T., Bihrle, S., et al. (2000). Reduced prefrontal gray matter volume and reduced autonomic activity in antisocial personality disorder. *Archives of General Psychiatry, 57*(2), 119-127.

Raine, A., Lencz, T., & Mednick, S. A. (Eds.) (1995). *Schizotypal personality.* New York: Cambridge University Press.

Raine, A., Sheard, C., Reynolds, G. P., et al. (1992). Prefrontal structural and functional deficits associated with individual differences in schizotypal personality. *Schizophrenia Research, 7,* 237-247.

Rettew, D. C., Zanarini, M. C., Yen, S., et al. (2003). Childhood antecedents of avoidant personality disorder: A retrospective study. *Journal of the American Academy of Child & Adolescent Psychiatry, 42*(9), 1122-1130.

Rinne, T., de Kloet, E. R., Wouters, L., et al. (2002). Hyperresponsiveness of hypothalamic-pituitary-adrenal axis to combined dexamethasone/corticotrophin-releasing hormone challenge in female borderline personality disorder subjects with a history of sustained childhood abuse. *Biological Psychiatry, 52*(11), 1102-1112.

Ritter, K., & Lammers, C. H. (2006). Narcissistic personality disorder. *MMW forschritte der Medizin, 148*(8), 39-42.

Roberts, B. W., & Wood, D. (2004). Personality development in the context of the neosocioanalytic model of personality. In D. Proczek & T. Little (Eds.), *Handbook of personality development.* Hillsdale, NJ: Lawerence Erlbaum Associates.

Robins, L. N., & Regier, D. A. (Eds.) (1991). *Psychiatric disorders in America.* New York: Free Press.

Robinson, D. (1996). *Disordered personalities: A primer.* London, Ontario, Canada: Rapid Psychler Press.

Rocca, P., Marchiaro, L., Cocuzza, E., et al. (2000). Treatment of borderline personality disorder with risperidone. *Journal of Clinical Psychiatry, 65,* 241-244.

Ronningstam, E. F., & Maltsberger, J. T. (2007). Narcissistic personality disorder. In G. O. Gabbard (Ed.), *Gabbard's treatment of psychiatric disorders* (4th ed.) (pp. 791-803). Washington, DC: American Psychiatric Publishing, Inc.

Rothbart, M. K., Ahadi, S. A., & Evans, D. E. (2000). Temperament and personality: Origins and outcomes. *Journal of Personality and Social Psychology, 78*(1), 122-135.

Ruegg, R., & Francis, A. (1995). New research in personality disorders. *Journal of Personality Disorders, 9*(1), 1-48.

Sadock, B. J., & Sadock, V. A. (Eds.) (2007). *Kaplan & Sadock's synopsis of psychiatry: Behavioral sciences/clinical psychiatry* (10th ed.). Philadelphia: Wolters Kluwer/Lippincott, Williams & Wilkins.

Salekin, R. T. (2002). Psychopathy and therapeutic pessimism: Clinical lore or clinical reality? *Clinical Psychology Review, 22*(1), 79-112.

Salzman, C., Wolfson, A. N., Schatzberg, A., et al. (1995). Effect of fluoxetine on anger in symptomatic volunteers with borderline personality disorder. *Journal of Clinical Psychopharmacology, 15,* 23-29.

Sanislow, C. A., & McGlashan, T. H. (1998). Treatment outcome of personality disorders. *Canadian Journal of Psychiatry, 43,* 237-250.

Scarr, S., & McCartney, K. (1983). How people make their own environments: A theory of genotype to environment effects. *Child Development, 54,* 424-435.

Schatzberg, A. F., Cole, J. O., & DeBattista, C. (2003). *Manual of clinical psychopharmacology* (4th ed.). Washington, DC: American Psychiatric Publishing, Inc.

Schatzberg, A. F., Cole, J. O., & DeBattista, C. (2007). *Manual of clinical psychopharmacology* (6th ed.). Washington, DC: American Psychiatric Publishing, Inc.

Schiffer, F., Teicher, M. H., & Papanicolaou, A. C. (1995). Evoked potential evidence for right brain activity during the recall of traumatic memories. *Journal of Neuropsychiatry and Clinical Neuroscience, 7*(2), 169-175.

Schmahl, C. G., Vermetten, E., Elzinga, B. M., et al. (2003). Magnetic resonance imaging of hippocampal and amygdale volume in women with childhood abuse and borderline personality disorder. *Psychiatry Research, 122*(3), 193-198.

Schwerdtner, J., Sommer, M., Weber, T., et al. (2004). Functional neuroanatomy of emotions [German]. *Psychiatrische Praxis, 31*(Suppl 1), S66-S67.

Segal, D. L., Coolidge, F. L., & Rosowsky, E. (2006). *Personality disorders and older adults: Diagnosis, assessment, and treatment.* Hoboken, NJ: John Wiley & Sons, Inc.

Sherman, C. (2000). "Industrial Psychopaths" can thrive in business. *Clinical Psychiatry News, 28*(5), 38.

Siever, L. J., & Davis, K. L. (1991). A psychobiological perspective on the personality disorders. *American Journal of Psychiatry, 148,* 1647-1658.

Siever, L. J., & Frucht, W. (1997). The new view of self: How genes and neurotransmitters shape your mind, your personality and your mental health. Darby, PA: Diane Publishing Company.

Siever, L. J., Keefe, R., Bernstein, D. P., et al. (1990). Eye-tracking impairment in clinically identified patients with schizotypal personality disorder. *American Journal of Psychiatry, 147,* 740-745.

Silk, K. R. (Ed.) (1998). *Biology of personality disorders.* Washington, DC: American Psychiatric Publishing, Inc.

Simeon, D., & Hollander, E. (2006). Treatment of personality disorders. In A. F. Schatzberg & C. B. Nemeroff (Eds.), *Essentials of clinical psychopharmacology* (pp. 689-705). Washington, DC: American Psychiatric Publishing, Inc.

Simeon, D., & Hollander, E. (2009). Treatment of personality disorders. In A. F. Schatzberg & C. B. Nemeroff (Eds.), *The American psychiatric publishing textbook of psychopharmacology* (pp. 1267-1285). Washington, DC: American Psychiatric Publishing, Inc.

Simeon, D., Stanley, B., Frances, A., et al. (1992). Self-mutilation in personality disorders: Psychological and biological correlates. *American Journal of Psychiatry, 149*(2), 221-226.

Simonoff, E., Elander, J., Holmshaw, J., et al. (2004). Predictors of antisocial personality: Continuities from childhood to adult life. *British Journal of Psychiatry, 184,* 118-127.

Skodol, M. E. (2008). Longitudinal course and outcome of personality disorders. *Psychiatric Clinics of North America, 31*(3), 495-503.

Skodol, M. E. (2009). Manifestations, clinical diagnosis, and comorbidity. In J. M. Oldham, A. E. Skodol, & D. S. Bender (Eds.), *Essentials of personality disorders* (pp. 37-61). Washington, DC: American Psychiatric Publishing, Inc.

Skodol, M. E., Bender, D. S., Pagano, M. E., et al. (2007). Positive childhood experiences: Resilience and recovery from personality disorder in early adulthood. *Journal of Clinical Psychiatry, 68*(7), 1102-1108.

Skodol, M. E., & Gunderson, J. G. (2008). Personality disorders. In R. E. Hales, S. C. Yudofsky, & G. O. Gabbard (Eds.), *The American psychiatric publishing textbook of psychiatry* (5th ed.) (pp. 821-859). Washington, DC: American Psychiatric Publishing, Inc.

Skodol, A. E., & Gunderson, J. G. (2011). Personality disorders. In R. E. Hales, S. C. Yudofsky, & G. O. Gabbard (Eds.), *Essentials of psychiatry* (3rd ed.) (pp. 293-323). Washington, DC: American Psychiatric Publishing, Inc.

Skodol, A. E., Gunderson, J. G., McGlashan, T. H., et al. (2002). Functional impairment in patients with schizotypal, borderline, avoidant or obsessive-compulsive personality disorder. *The American Journal of Psychiatry, 159*(2), 276-283.

Skodol, A. E., Gunderson, J. G., Shea, M. T., et al. (2005a). The Collaborative Longitudinal Personality Disorders Study (CLPS): Overview and implications. *Journal of Personality Disorders, 19*(5), 487-504.

Skodol, A. E., Oldham, J. M., Bender, D. S., et al. (2005b). Dimensional representations of DSM-IV personality disorders: Relationships to functional impairment. *American Journal of Psychiatry, 162,* 1919-1925.

Smoller, J. W., Sheidley, B. R., & Tsuang, M. T. (2008). *Psychiatric genetics: Applications in clinical practice.* Washington, DC: American Psychiatric Publishing, Inc.

Soloff, P. H. (2000). Psychopharmacological treatment for borderline personality disorder. *Psychiatric Clinics of North America, 23,* 169-192.

Soloff, P. H. (2009). Somatic treatments. In J. M. Oldham, A. E. Skodol, & D. S. Bender (Eds.), *Essentials of personality disorders* (pp. 267-268). Washington, DC: American Psychiatric Publishing, Inc.

Stanley, B., & Brodsky, B. S. (2009). Dialectical behavior therapy. In J. M. Oldham, A. E. Skodol, & D. S. Bender (Eds.), *Essentials of personality disorders* (pp. 235-252). Washington, DC: American Psychiatric Publishing, Inc.

Stevenson, J., & Meares, R. (1992). An outcome study of psychotherapy for patients with borderline personality disorder. *American Journal of Psychiatry, 149,* 358-362.

Stone, M. H. (1990). *The fate of borderline patients: Successful outcome and psychiatric practice.* New York: Guilford Press.

Stone, M. H. (1993). *Abnormalities of personality: Within and beyond the realm of treatment.* New York: W. W. Norton.

Stone, M. H. (2001). Natural history and long-term outcomes. In W. J. Livesley (Ed.), *Handbook of personality disorders* (pp. 250-273). New York: Guilford Press.

Stone, M. H. (2006). *Personality-disordered patients: Treatable and untreatable.* Washington, DC: American Psychiatric Publishing, Inc.

Stone, M. H. (2007). Cluster A personality disorders: Paranoid, schizoid, and schizotypal. In G. O. Gabbard (Ed.), *Gabbard's treatment of psychiatric disorders* (4th ed.) (pp. 763-773). Washington, DC: American Psychiatric Publishing, Inc.

Stravynski, A., Marks, I., & Yule, W. (1982). Social skills problems in neurotic outpatients: Social skills training with and without cognitive modification. *Archives of General Psychiatry, 39,* 1378-1385.

Sutker, P. B., & Allain, A. N. (2001). Antisocial personality disorder. In P. B. Sutker & H. E. Adams (Eds.), *Comprehensive handbook of psychopathology* (3rd ed.) (pp. 445-490). New York: Kluwer Academic/Plenum Publishers.

Swartz, M., Blazer, D., George, L., et al. (1990). Estimating the prevalence of borderline personality disorder in the community. *Journal of Personality Disorders, 4,* 257-272.

Teicher, M. H., Anderson, S. L., Polcari, A., et al. (2003). The neurobiological consequences of early stress and childhood maltreatment. *Neuroscience and Behavioral Review, 27,* 33-44.

Torgersen, S. (2000). Genetics of patients with borderline personality disorder. *Psychiatric Clinics of North America, 23,* 1-9.

Torgersen, S. (2005). Epidemiology. In J. M. Oldham, A. E. Skodol, & D. S. Bender (Eds.), *The American psychiatric publishing textbook of personality disorders* (pp. 129-141). Washington, DC: American Psychiatric Publishing, Inc.

Torgersen, S. (2009). Prevalence, sociodemographics, and functional impairment. In J. M. Oldham, A. E. Skodol, & D. S. Bender (Eds.), *Essentials of personality disorders* (pp. 83-102). Washington, DC: American Psychiatric Publishing, Inc.

Torgersen, S., Kringlen, E., & Cramer, V. (2001). The prevalence of personality disorders in a community sample. *Archives of General Psychiatry, 58*(6), 590-596.

Torgersen, S., Lygren, S., Oien, P. A., et al. (2000). A twin study of personality disorders. *Comprehensive Psychiatry, 41*(6), 416-425.

Tritt, K., Nickel, C., Lahmann, C., et al. (2005). Lamotrigine treatment of aggression in female borderline patients: A randomized, double-blind, placebo-controlled study. *Journal of Psychopharmacology, 19,* 287-291.

Tse, W. S., & Bond, A. J. (2002). Serotonergic intervention affects both social dominance and affiliative behavior. *Psychopharmacology, 161*(3), 324-330.

Tsuang, M. T., Stone, W. S., Tarbox, S. I., et al. (2002). An integration of schizophrenia with schizotypy: Identification of schizotaxia and implications for research on treatment and prevention. *Schizophrenia Research, 54,* 169-175.

Van Reekum, R. (1993). Acquired and developmental brain dysfunction in borderline personality disorder. *Canadian Journal of Psychiatry, 38*(Suppl 1), S4-S10.

van Reekum, R., Links, P. S., & Boiago, I. (1993). Constitutional factors in borderline personality disorder: Genetics, brain dysfunction, and biological markers in borderline personality disorder. In J. Paris (Ed.), *Borderline personality disorder: Etiology and treatment* (pp. 13-38). Washington, DC: American Psychiatric Publishing, Inc.

Vaughn, M. G., Fu, Q., Delisi, M., et al. (2010). Criminal victimization and comorbid substance use and psychiatric disorders in the United States: Results from NESARC. *Annals of Epidemiology, 20*(4), 281-288.

Velligan, D. I., & Bow-Thomas, C. C. (2000). Two case studies of cognitive adaptation training for outpatients with schizophrenia. *Psychiatric Services, 51*(1), 25-29.

Verheul, R., van den Bosch, L. M. C., Koeter, M. W. J., et al. (2003). Dialectical behavior therapy for women with borderline personality disorder. *British Journal of Psychiatry 182,* 135-140.

Vermetten, E., Vythilingam, M., Southwick, S. M., et al. (2003). Long-term treatment with paroxetine increases verbal declarative memory and hippocampal volume in posttraumatic stress disorder. *Biological Psychiatry, 54*(7), 693-702.

Virkkunen, M., Nuutila, A., Goodwin, F. K., et al. (1987). Cerebrospinal fluid monoamine metabolite levels in male arsonists. *Archives of General Psychiatry, 44,* 241-247.

Walker, C., Thomas, J., & Allen, T. S. (2003). Treating impulsivity, irritability, and aggression of antisocial personality disorder with quetiapine. *International Journal of Offender Therapy & Comparative Criminology, 47*(5), 556-567.

Walker, E. F., Logan, C. B., & Waller, D. (1999). Indicators of neurodevelopmental abnormality in schizotypal personality disorder. *Psychiatric Annals, 29*(3), 132-136.

Watson, C. G., Barnett, M., Nikunen, L., et al. (1997). Lifetime prevalence of nine common psychiatric/personality disorders in female domestic abuse survivors. *Journal of Nervous and Mental Disorders, 185,* 645-647.

Wedding, D., & Boyd, M. A. (1999). *Movies & mental illness: Using films to understand psychopathology.* Boston: McGraw-Hill College.

Wedding, D., Boyd, M. A., & Niemiec, R. M. (2010). *Movies and mental illness 3: Using films to understand psychopathology* (3rd ed.). Cambridge, MA: Hogrefe Publishing.

Widiger, T. A. (1991). Personality disorder dimensional models proposed for DSM-V. *Journal of Personal Discord, 5,* 386-398.

Widiger, T., & Lynam, D. R. (1998). Psychopathy from the perspective of the five-factor model of personality. In T. Millon, E. Simonsen, M. Birket-Smith, et al. (Eds.), *Psychopathy: Antisocial, criminal, and violent behaviors* (pp. 171-187). New York: Guilford Press.

Widiger, T., & Sankis, L. (2000). Adult psychopathology: Issues and controversies. *Annual Review of Psychology, 51,* 377-404.

Widiger, T., Trull, T. J., & Clarkin, J. F., et al. (2002). A description of the DSM-IV personality disorders with the five-factor model of personality. In P. T. Costa & T. A. Widiger (Eds.), *Personality disorders and the five-factor model of personality* (pp. 899-909). Washington, DC: American Psychological Association.

Woods, P., & Richards, D. (2003). Effectiveness of nursing interventions in people with personality disorders. *Journal of Advanced Nursing, 44*(2), 154-172.

Yen, S., Pagano, M. E., Shea, M. T., et al. (2005). Recent life events preceding suicide attempts in a personality disorder sample: Findings from the collaborative longitudinal personality disorders study. *Journal of Consulting & Clinical Psychology, 73*(1), 99-105.

Zanarini, M. (1997). *Role of sexual abuse in the etiology of borderline personality disorder.* Washington, DC: American Psychiatric Publishing, Inc.

Zanarini, M. C., Frankenburg, F. R., Dubo, E. D., et al. (1998). Axis I comorbidity of borderline personality disorder. *American Journal of Psychiatry, 155,* 1733-1739.

Zanarini, M. C., Frankenburg, F. R., Hennen, J., et al. (2006). Prediction of the 10-year course of borderline personality disorder. *American Journal of Psychiatry, 163,* 827-832.

Zanarini, M. C., Frankenburg, F. R., & Parachini, F. A. (2004). A preliminary, randomized trial of fluoxetine, olanzapine, and the olanzapine-fluoxetine combination in women with borderline personality disorder. *Journal of Clinical Psychiatry, 65,* 903-907.

Zanarini, M. C., Gunderson, J., & Frankenburg, F. (1990). Cognitive features of borderline personality disorder. *American Journal of Psychiatry, 147,* 57-63.

Zanarini, M., Williams, A., Lewis, R., et al. (1997). Reported pathological childhood experiences associated with the development of borderline personality disorder. *American Journal of Psychiatry, 154*(8), 1101-1106.

Zelkowitz, P., Paris, J., Guzder, J., et al. (2001). Diathesis and stressors in borderline pathology of childhood: The role of neuropsychological risk and trauma. *Journal of American Academy of Child and Adolescent Psychiatry, 40,* 100-105.

Zimmerman, M., Rothschild, L., & Chelminski, I. (2005). The prevalence of DSM-IV personality disorders in psychiatric outpatients. *American Journal of Psychiatry, 162,* 1911-1918.

UNIT IX

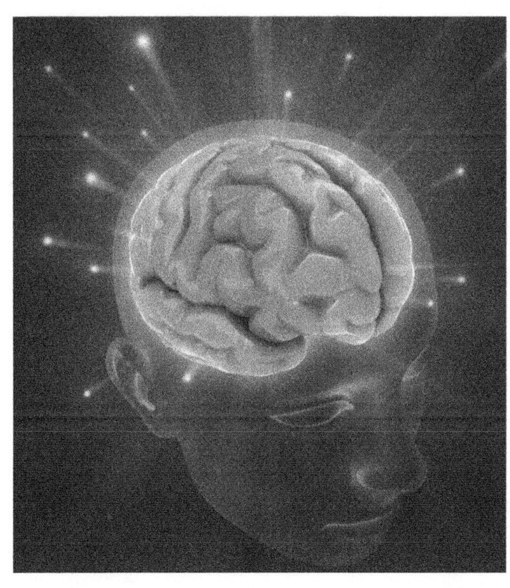

Prevention of Psychiatric Disorders

CHAPTER 19

Prevention of Psychiatric Disorders

Eris F. Perese, APRN-PMH

In a given year, 14% to 20% of American youth—children, adolescents, and young adults—experience mental, emotional, and behavioral disorders (O'Connell, Boat, & Warner, 2009), and 26.2% of American adults have a diagnosable psychiatric disorder (Braithwaite, 2006). Psychiatric disorders have the earliest age of onset of all health problems (Compton, 2008). Fifty percent of adults with psychiatric disorders first experienced symptoms by 14 years of age, and 75% met the criteria for the disorder before 18 years of age (Compton, Koplan, Oleskey, et al., 2010; Kim-Cohen, Caspi, Moffitt, et al., 2003). Most did not receive treatment until the age of 24 years (Kessler, Berglund, Demler, et al., 2005a; Kim-Cohen et al.; Maughan & Kim-Cohen, 2005).

The presence of psychiatric disorders in childhood and adolescence increases the risk of adverse outcomes for America's youths. Children with mental health problems are likely to perform poorly in class, miss school, drop out of school, and abuse alcohol and drugs (Compton, 2008), and as adults they often experience lower levels of employment, lower salaries when employed, problems with personal relationships, increased contact with the criminal justice system, increased rates of psychiatric disorders, and a shortened life span (Chen, Cohen, Kasen, et al., 2006; Fergusson, Grant, & Horwood, 2005).

The most common psychiatric disorders in the United States—depression, anxiety, and substance use disorders—account for three-quarters of the burden generated by all the mental disorders (Andrews & Wilkinson, 2002, p. S97). Psychiatric disorders place a heavy burden on the individuals who experience them, on their families, and on society (O'Connell et al., 2009). They affect individuals' sense of self-identity; their ability to carry out their roles as partner, parent, and employee; and their ability to relate to others, including their families. Society is affected by the cost of providing mental health care; increased need for medical care for comorbid physical illnesses; the cost of providing special educational services; costs related to involvement with the justice system; lack of productivity due to impairment of functioning; and diminished productivity of family members, who often must limit their work hours to provide care for a family member with a psychiatric disorder (O'Connell et al.). Psychiatric disorders also place a heavy burden on nations. They account for 22% of the global burden of disease, with anxiety disorders, depression, and substance-related disorders accounting for three-fourths of that burden (Eaton, Martins, Nestadt, et al., 2008; Murray & Lopez, 1997). The burden associated with psychiatric disorders is magnified by their frequent onset early in life (Akil, Brenner, Kandel, et al., 2010), often in childhood (Insel, 2009; Ursano, Kartheiser, & Barnhill, 2008), and by their persistence across the life span.

Prevention of Psychiatric Disorders

Even if treatment were provided at maximum efficacy for all of those seeking treatment, only half of the burden of psychiatric disorders could be prevented with current treatment—psychotherapy, pharmacotherapy, and psychosocial interventions (Andrews & Wilkinson, 2002). Reducing the burden of psychiatric disorders would require either developing new treatments that are more effective than current ones or preventing the occurrence of new cases of psychiatric disorders (Cuijpers, van Straten, & Smit, 2005. Insel (2009) pointed out that despite the heavy use of antipsychotic and antidepressant medications during the last two decades, there is no evidence that the morbidity or mortality of psychiatric disorders has decreased. According to Hosman, Jane-Llopis, and Saxena (2005), *prevention* is key to reducing the rapidly increasing global burden of psychiatric disorders, and in 2003, the President's New Freedom Commission on Mental Health called for research that would promote recovery, resilience, and prevention of mental illness (Boyce, Heinssen, Ferrell, et al., 2007).

Prevention of mental illness cannot be achieved at the level proposed in the President's New Freedom Commission's report (2003), which is to screen all citizens, identify psychopathology or risk of developing psychopathology, and provide appropriate treatment (Albee, 2005). Even in developed countries, there are not enough professional resources to accomplish what the New Freedom Commission proposed. Andrews and Wilkinson (2002) estimated that even if the competencies of all clinicians were maximized and if all patients seeking treatment for these disorders adhered to treatment, only half of the burden of psychiatric disorders could be averted. Beekman, Cuijpers, van Marwijk, et al. (2006) have taken a different view: prevention. They estimated that the incidence of psychiatric disorders—the number of new cases—could be reduced by at least 25% through the use of preventive interventions.

Prevention has not had a prominent role in psychiatry or psychiatric nursing (Compton, 2010a). Traditionally, managing psychiatric disorders has entailed treatment with medications and psychotherapy after the disorder developed. Although there are treatments for many of the psychiatric disorders—including anxiety disorders, mood disorders, schizophrenia, substance-related disorders, dementia, and personality disorders—patients respond in varying degrees to treatment, and not everyone who needs treatment receives it (Shonkoff, Boyce, & McEwen, 2009). For example, the gap between those who need treatment and those who receive it is 32% for patients with schizophrenia, 50% for patients with bipolar disorder, 55.9% for patients with panic disorder, 56% for patients with dysthymia, 56.3% for patients with depression, 57.3% for patients with obsessive-compulsive disorder (OCD), and 78% for patients with alcohol abuse and dependence (Kohn, Saxena, Levay, et al., 2004). The gap between patients' need for mental health care and the availability of care is expected to increase with the aging of America and the accompanying increased burden of psychiatric disorders such as dementia, unless ways can be found to reduce the incidence of new cases of psychiatric disorders.

Preventive Interventions Across the Life Span

In the past, preventing psychiatric disorders focused on identifying and providing treatment for individuals who were at high risk for developing a psychiatric disorder. More recently, the approach has been to think of prevention across the life span. Psychiatric disorders, which often emerge in childhood and adolescence and continue into adulthood, develop from

- The interaction of genetic vulnerabilities with other risk factors
- Deficits of development of brain structures and neural circuitry
- Insecure attachment formed during infancy that failed to foster trust, security, and self-regulation of emotions, stress response, and behavior
- The sequelae of exposure to adverse childhood maltreatment, including neglect and emotional, physical, and sexual abuse (Maughan & Kim-Cohen, 2005; World Health Organization, 2002).

Advances in the neurosciences are indicating that early experiences and exposures to adversities are biologically embedded and have lifelong consequences. This new information supports the need to prevent psychiatric disorders by focusing on preconception, prenatal, and early childhood periods of life (Shonkoff et al., 2009; Waddell, Hua, Garland, et al., 2007a).

Based on research-generated information, new interventions target the preconceptual period. The focus is on promoting the health of the mother and father before conception. Preventive interventions that focus on the prenatal and perinatal periods of life are directed toward reducing risk factors such as poor prenatal nutrition and prenatal exposure to toxins, infections, and maternal depression and stress. For example, research studies suggest that prenatal exposure to maternal stress is associated with later vulnerability to stress-related mental disorders (Kjoer, Wegener, Rosenberg, et al., 2010). During the postnatal period, the focus of prevention is on fostering protective factors, such as emotional self-regulation and secure attachment, and on preventing exposure to neglect, abuse, harsh parenting practices, and exposure to parental psychopathology, which are known to have negative influences on the child's brain development and are associated with the increased risk for developing psychiatric disorders (see Chapter 3).

During childhood and adolescence, prevention is directed toward reducing (1) specific childhood emotional and behavioral problems and (2) psychiatric disorders that have their onset in childhood and adolescence and that have a high risk of persisting into adulthood, e.g., depression, anxiety disorders, and substance-related disorders (Andrews & Wilkinson, 2002). Among adults and older adults, the focus of prevention is on either preventing the occurrence of new cases of psychiatric disorders such as mood disorders or delaying the onset of psychiatric disorders such as dementia. The goal of prevention is to use evidence generated in neurodevelopmental neuroscience research to develop interventions that can reduce the incidence of new cases across the life span (O'Connell et al., 2009).

Models of Prevention

The model of prevention of psychiatric disorders has shifted from the earlier medical model of primary prevention (preventing the occurrence of new cases), secondary prevention (early identification and treatment), and tertiary prevention (prevention of disability associated with a disease or prevention or recurrence) to a model of *primary prevention with three levels* (Mrazek & Haggerty, 1994):

1. Universal prevention
2. Selective prevention
3. Indicated prevention

In this new model, *prevention* is defined as preventing the occurrence of new cases of psychiatric disorders (Schrecker, Acosta, Somerville, et al., 2001) and depends on brain plasticity (the brain's ability to change in response to new experiences) and on preventive interventions (such as cognitive behavioral therapy) to change gene expression, neurons, and neuronal networks and thus change brain functioning (thinking, emotions, and behaviors) (see Chapter 1 for theory of brain plasticity).

Universal Prevention

Universal prevention is founded on the premise that the development of psychiatric disorders is multifactorial, with factors other than genetic factors influencing development. Mojtabai, Malaspina, and Susser (2003) suggested that universal preventive interventions—interventions similar to the universal preventive interventions of fluorination of water, childhood immunizations, and seat-belt laws—have the potential to reduce the incidence of psychiatric disorders. Mojtabai et al. stated that universal preventive interventions should include promotion of prenatal health through adequate maternal nutrition and maternal immunizations; prevention of childhood trauma and abuse; prevention of head injuries through the use of helmets and availability of safe playing conditions; and preventive programs that target the reduction of childhood and adolescence substance use. Psychiatric nurse researchers Laraia (2005) and Saugstad (2004) suggested that including omega-3 fatty acids in the diet has the potential for not only increasing cognitive functioning but also decreasing the incidence of psychiatric disorders such as Alzheimer's disease, depression, schizophrenia, and attention deficit-hyperactivity disorder (ADHD) and reducing suicidality. They recommended that the general population be educated about the benefits of choosing a diet that has the potential to enhance brain development and functioning, which is a diet that includes foods containing omega-3 fatty acids: avocados, cod, salmon, tuna, nuts, oils (olive, sesame, and canola), soybeans, walnuts, and pumpkin or sunflower seeds.

Universal preventive interventions also include programs to improve public housing, to provide access to health care, to reduce smoking, and to provide greater access to education (Hosman et al., 2005). An example of universal prevention is *Mental Health First Aid* (www.mhfa.com.au). This intervention was developed by Kitchener and Jorm (2008) to improve mental health literacy, reduce stigmatizing attitudes, and encourage appropriate and early help-seeking by people with mental health problems. The intervention includes activities such as assessing risk for suicide or harm, listening nonjudgmentally, giving reassurance and information, encouraging the person to get appropriate professional help, and encouraging self-help and other support strategies from peers, family members, and friends. Outcomes of the intervention are improved recognition of mental disorders by the clinician, diminished stigma for the patient, the clinician's greater confidence in his or her ability to provide help, and more assistance provided by family, friends, and others (Kitchener & Jorm). Because universal preventions target the whole population, they use interventions such as public education, stigma reduction, teaching of parenting skills, and promotion of resilience to reduce the occurrence of new cases of psychiatric disorders among the general population.

Selective Prevention

Selective preventive interventions target individuals or subgroups of the population that are at increased risk of developing a specific psychiatric disorder. The risk may be immediate or in the future. It may be biological, psychological, or social. Examples of populations at risk include children of depressed parents, postpartum mothers, individuals who have been exposed to a traumatic occurrence, and individuals who have lost a loved one (Evans, Foa, Gur, et al., 2005). An example of a selective program is *Keeping Families Strong (KFS)* (Riley, Valdez, Barrueco, et al., 2008), which focuses on families in which the mother is depressed. The goal of the program is to reduce risk for development of psychiatric disorders in children of parents with depression.

Indicated Prevention

Indicated preventive interventions target high-risk individuals who are already having subthreshold symptoms of a psychiatric disorder, such as children with high levels of anxiety symptoms, adolescents with symptoms of depression, or individuals with premorbid or prodromal symptoms of schizophrenia (Evans et al., 2005). Indicated prevention may also begin treatment to prevent or delay the development of a disorder such as schizophrenia.

Based on a meta-analytic review of the three preventive interventions, Cuijpers et al. (2005, p. 119) concluded that prevention of new cases of psychiatric disorders is possible. They found that indicated prevention has the strongest preventive effect.

Preventive Interventions Across the Life Span: Protective Factors and Risk Factors

An accepted principle of prevention is that it should be founded on evidence-based knowledge of protective factors and risk factors that contribute to the development of psychiatric disorders (Glatt, Faraone, & Tsuang, 2008; Hosman et al., 2005).

Protective factors are characteristics at the individual, family, or community level that are associated with decreasing the likelihood of an individual's developing a psychiatric disorder or with reducing the impact of a risk factor. Protective factors may be biological, such as optimal brain development and functioning; emotional, such as the capacity for modulating emotions; or cognitive, such as the ability to interpret information accurately. Protective factors may also be part of the overall family environment or they may arise from the community. The greater the number of protective factors available to an individual, the lower the risk of his or her developing a psychiatric disorder (O'Connell et al., 2009).

Risk factors can be biological, psychological, or social and may occur at the level of the individual, the family, the community, or society (Durlak, 1998; O'Connell et al., 2009; Hosman et al., 2005). They can be fixed, such as gender, or variable, such as exposure to abuse. The strength of the contribution of risk factors to the development of psychiatric disorders varies among different populations, at different windows of time, and in relation to the presence of other risk factors and protective factors. Risk factors have a cumulative effect, with the occurrence of multiple risk factors having the strongest effect (Chartier, Walker, & Naimark, 2010; Copeland, Shanahan, Costello, et al., 2009b; Durlak, 1998; Rutter, 1989; Sameroff, Gutman, & Peck, 2003; O'Connell et al., 2009). (Risk and protective factors for specific psychiatric disorders are discussed in Chapters 9 through 18.)

According to Albee (2005), the main risk factors for psychiatric disorders are exposure to stressors such as poverty and childhood maltreatment and having been born unwanted. Albee advocated for reduction of the gap in income between the nation's poorest citizens and richest citizens. He pointed out that maltreatment of children—neglect and emotional, physical, and sexual abuse—is associated with increased risk for developing psychopathology; additionally, being born unwanted—in contrast to being born into a welcoming, caring, supportive family and community—is a risk factor for poor mental health in adulthood (David, Dytych, & Matejcek, 2003). (See Chapter 3 for a discussion of prenatal, perinatal, and postnatal risk factors.)

While the distal goal of preventive programs is to prevent psychiatric disorders, the proximal goals are to increase protective factors and to reduce risk factors at crucial windows of time across the life span. Some risk factors, such as genetic influences that are considered to have a causative link to the development of psychiatric disorders, are present at conception. Although genetic vulnerability may not be directly modifiable by preventive interventions, how genes are expressed may be modified. Other risk factors—circumstances, occurrences, and situations that have been found to be associated with increased rates of psychiatric disorders—may be modifiable by preventive interventions.

Genetic Vulnerability for Psychiatric Disorders

Genetic influence has long been believed to be associated with psychiatric disorders. Research has identified genes that increase an individual's risk for developing a phenotype, which is defined as the symptoms, neurochemistry, and behaviors that constitute a psychiatric disorder. These genes are called "risk genes" (Glatt et al., 2008, p. 4) because, at this time, there are no single genes that cause a specific psychiatric disorder, only genes that appear to increase risk (O'Connell et al., 2009). Genes supply a general plan for brain development and functioning with room for many options. They account for the heritability of a disorder, which Glatt et al. described as "...a measure of the degree to which genetic factors influence variability in the manifestation of the phenotype" (p. 9). That is, heritability is the proportion of variance in the disorder that is accounted for by genetic factors. For example, a heritability of 1.0 indicates that all of the variance in the disorder is due to genetic factors alone, and a heritability of 0 indicates that all of the variation in the disorder is due to environmental factors. Heritability varies in different psychiatric disorders and is described as high, medium, or low. Examples of heritability include the following:

- High heritability: autism, Tourette's syndrome, bipolar disorder, and schizophrenia
- Medium heritability: ADHD, conduct disorder (CD), oppositional defiant disorder (ODD), OCD, Alzheimer's disease, and antisocial, borderline, narcissistic, and histrionic personality disorders
- Low heritability: panic disorder, major depressive disorder (MDD), alcohol abuse, generalized anxiety disorder (GAD), and paranoid, avoidant, and schizotypal personality disorders (Glatt et al., 2008). Low heritability is also associated with exposure to stressful life events that is linked to individuals' selection of their environment based on their genetically influenced behavior.

However, genes do not operate independently. Rutter, Moffitt, and Caspi (2006) have demonstrated that early childhood maltreatment interacts with genetic vulnerability to increase one's risk for developing psychopathology. Recent research has focused on the interaction of genetic and environmental factors. For example, a gene in the serotonin neurotransmitter system that is known to be associated with development of depressive symptoms, major depressive disorder, and suicidality was found to increase the risk *only* in the presence of a history of stressful life events (Caspi, Sugden, Moffitt, et al., 2003). Another example of gene and environment interactions is provided by the finding that positive social supports were protective against the risk for developing depression among children who had a genetic risk for developing depression (Kaufman, Yang, Douglas-Palumberi, et al., 2004, 2006). It is believed that even psychiatric disorders with high heritability may be influenced by environmental factors, such as preventive interventions (Smoller & Korf, 2008). One way of thinking about the genetic effect on the development of psychopathology is the concept of genetic influence on dimensions such as emotional modulation, response to stress, and temperament. Genetic effect may be reinforced later by adverse circumstances of birth, by parenting, and by other experiences such as attachment, learning, illnesses, abuse, and traumas (Rutter, 1989).

The brain is plastic and continues to change throughout life. It is in response to experiences and environmental influences that the brain undergoes changes, such as the birth of new neurons, the death of neurons, epigenetic changes (how a gene will be expressed) (Nasrallah, 2011), and how connections are formed and maintained between neurons (Dayer, Cleaver, Abouantoun, et al., 2005; Stahl, 2000). These changes are ultimately reflected in perception, thinking, emotions, behaviors, and the presence or absence of psychopathology (Boyce et al., 2007, p. 45). Thus, although genes are not modifiable, the way genes are expressed is influenced by experience and environmental factors. Changing of risk factors or protective factors has the potential to change how genes are expressed and ultimately to influence the development of psychiatric disorders (Akil et al., 2010).

Periods of risk and opportunities for prevention can occur across the life span: in the preconception period, the prenatal period, childhood, adolescence, adulthood, and older adulthood. The remainder of this chapter will discuss the risks and prevention opportunities for each of these life stages.

Risks and Prevention Opportunities in the Preconception Period

The brain begins to develop 2 to 3 weeks after conception (O'Connell et al., 2009). (See Chapter 2 for information on brain development.) By the time a woman goes for her first prenatal visit, usually when she is 10 to 12 weeks pregnant, birth defects and abnormalities of brain development that may increase vulnerability to the development of psychiatric disorders have already happened (Rabin, 2006). A very early preventive intervention is for prospective parents to prepare for pregnancy at least 3 months before conception. The immediate goal of preconception care is to modify biomedical, behavioral, and social risks to a woman's health and pregnancy outcome (Lu & Geffen, 2007). A longer-term goal of preconception care is to promote life span biopsychosocial health for women, children, and families (Atrash, Jack, Johnson, et al., 2008).

The recommendations of the Centers for Disease Control and Prevention (CDC) to improve preconception health have been described by Johnson, Posner, Biermann, et al. (2006). The CDC's recommendations and the recommendations of other researchers are summarized as follows:

Recommendations for Women:

- Take 400 to 800 mcg (0.4 to 0.8 mg) of folic acid daily to lower risk of birth defects of the brain and spine.
- Stop smoking, drinking alcohol, and using drugs.
- Get sufficient sleep.
- Reduce stress.
- Increase resilience.
- Treat medical conditions such as asthma, diabetes, oral health problems, obesity, and epilepsy.
- Talk to the doctor about any over-the-counter and prescription medicines taken. These include dietary or herbal supplements.
- Be sure vaccinations—hepatitis B, rubella, varicella, influenza, human papillomavirus, and Tdap (tetanus, diphtheria, and pertussis) are up to date.
- Avoid contact with toxic substances or materials that could cause infection at work and at home such as solvents, pesticides, heavy metals, and allergens.
- Stay away from cat or rodent feces.

Recommendations for Men:

- Be tested for sexually transmitted infections and have them treated to prevent passing infections to female partners.
- Limit intake of alcohol.
- Stop smoking and using illegal drugs.
- Eat a healthy diet.
- Reduce stress.
- Be careful not to expose the female partner to any toxins or chemicals that the man has been working with or to clothes that might have toxins on them (Berghella, Buchanan, Pereira, et al., 2010; Johnson et al., 2006; Lu & Geffen, 2007).

The CDC also recommends that women and men formulate a life plan that includes a timetable for having children. Women with planned pregnancies are more likely to change their lifestyle to benefit their unborn child than women with unplanned pregnancies. They often decrease coffee intake and discontinue the use of tobacco, alcohol, and illicit drugs, and they are more likely to seek and follow prenatal health-care recommendations (Verbiest & Holliday, 2009; Xaverius, Tenkku, & Salas, 2009). In contrast, pregnancies among adolescents—which are often unplanned—are associated with risks for the infant, such as preterm birth and perinatal complications, and with adverse circumstances for the mother, such as single motherhood, low levels of academic achievement, and poverty (Ayoola, Brewer, & Nettleman, 2006). Children who are planned are less likely to be born unwanted, which is associated with increased risk for the development of psychiatric disorders (David et al., 2003; Henry, 2006).

Risks and Prevention Opportunities in the Prenatal, Perinatal, and Infancy Period

Prenatal and perinatal factors that interact to cause less than optimal development of the brain and compromised brain functioning include genetic vulnerability, neurodevelopmental deficits, adverse obstetrical events, and difficult temperament (see Chapter 3). The brain that has been molded by these factors continues to be molded after birth by its interaction with both positive and negative experiences and environmental factors. This molding process may result in either (1) optimal brain functioning or (2) compromised brain functioning that is manifested later in cognitive impairment; impaired ability to self-regulate emotions, behaviors, and response to stress; impaired functioning of the immune system; and maladaptive interpersonal and social behaviors.

Protective Factors

Parents who have support from their family, friends, neighbors, and the community are more likely to provide a safe, health-promoting environment prenatally and in infancy. Protective factors—factors associated with lower incidence of child neglect and abuses—include

- Secure attachment: strong, warm feelings between child and parents
- Parental understanding of child development and what are normal behaviors at specific ages
- Parents who have positive attitudes and use problem-solving skills
- Social connectedness: parents who have trusted and caring family friends
- Concrete support: parents who have consistently available basic resources—food, clothing, housing, transportation, employment, and health care ("Preventing Child Abuse and Neglect," 2008)

Risk Factors

Risk factors during the prenatal and perinatal periods associated with later development of psychiatric disorders include exposure to "prenatal adversities" (McGuiness, 2010, p. 16) such as inadequate nutrition or famine; exposure to alcohol, drugs, toxins, infections, and stress; and adverse circumstance of birth, such as hypoxia, low birth weight, and premature birth (Seed & Higgins, 2003). For example, the rate of psychiatric disorders was 23.3% among 11-year-old children who had experienced extremely preterm birth (less than 26 weeks), in comparison to 8.6% for classmates born at term. The most frequent diagnosis was ADHD (12%), followed by emotional disorders (anxiety disorders and depression) (9%) and autism spectrum disorders (8%) (Hack, Taylor, Schluchter, et al., 2009; Johnson, Hollis, Kochhar, et al., 2010).

Risk factors during infancy associated with later development of psychiatric disorders include having a difficult temperament (irritability and impulsivity), lacking emotional self-regulation, developing insecure attachment patterns, and experiencing neglect and abuse (Seed & Higgins, 2003) (see Chapter 3 for description of prenatal, perinatal, and postnatal factors associated with increased risk of developing psychopathology).

Preventive Interventions

Early preventive interventions include promoting good prenatal care, fostering secure attachment patterns, and assisting parents to help their children develop the ability to self-regulate their emotions, their response to stress, and their behaviors and to engage in social activities (O'Connell et al., 2009).

Early preventive interventions are supported by developmental neuroscience, which proposes that genes encode proteins, proteins build cells, cells create neural circuits, and neural circuits determine emotions and behavior. Interactions with the environment, such as preventive interventions, cause changes in gene expression that cause changes in cells and neural circuitry. These changes result in alterations of emotions and behavior. For example, early exposure to stress causes epigenetic changes of the gene involved in the stress response, and these epigenetic changes can be transmitted across generations. Early interventions have a greater potential for modifying deficits or malfunctioning of brain circuits that control emotions and behavior than interventions provided when the child is older (Evans et al., 2005).

Maternal *sensitivity* refers to a mother's ability to engage with the infant at the mental level as well as at physical and emotional levels (Bigelow, MacLean, Proctor, et al., 2010). It is the mother's (or the primary caregiver's) sensitivity to the infant's needs and behaviors that promotes the infant's development of cognitive, emotional, and social self-competencies; secure attachment patterns; easy, warm socializing behaviors; language fluency; and resilience. This sensitivity also buffers the deleterious effects of poverty and family stress (Beckwith, 2002). Maternal facial, vocal, and physical responsiveness to the infant's movements, sounds, and expressions teaches the infant what is valued and what is not, and the infant gains a sense of self-competence from eliciting maternal responses. Maternal *insensitivity*, neglect, and abuse underlie the development of insecure attachment patterns (see Chapter 1 for a description of attachment patterns and maternal characteristics). Disorganized attachment—the most severe of the insecure attachment patterns—has been linked to the caregiver's feeling of unresolved loss or to experienced trauma; to high levels of emotion toward the child, such as anger or hostility; and to abuse or harsh treatment of the child (Green, Stanley, & Peters, 2007). Disorganized attachment is associated with psychopathology in childhood, such as oppositional defiant disorder (Green et al.; Wilson, 2009).

Preventive interventions are designed to promote the infant's successful achievement of age-appropriate developmental tasks, which include regulating physiological processes, mastering emotional self-regulation, and developing a sense of self-identity and autonomy (Beckwith, 2002). Preventive interventions that have the goal of increasing maternal sensitivity and improving attachment include the *Circle of Security* program (Marvin, Cooper, Hoffman, et al., 2002) and the *Nurse Home Visitation* program (Olds,

Eckenrode, Henderson, et al., 1997; Olds, Henderson, Chamberlin, et al., 1986; Olds, Henderson, Cole, et al., 1998; Olds, Henderson, Tatelbaum, et al., 1988; Olds, Robinson, O'Brien, et al., 2002) (Table 19-1). Interventions to increase maternal sensitivity and infant attachment have been found to be moderately successful, especially in relatively well functioning families, but multiproblem families may need broader preventive interventions (Bakermans-Kranenburg, van Ijzendoorn, & Juffer, 2003).

There are preventive intervention programs that support families, foster improvement of socializing behaviors, and promote self-regulation; reduce childhood neglect and abuse; and provide counseling for parents with psychiatric disorders or substance-related disorders. The most effective preventive programs

- Intervene with children and families very early on
- Are based on the risk and protective factors of the families
- Are long-term and intensive
- Provide parents with concrete help in areas such as housing, employment, completing education, finances, and health care (Beckwith, 2002)

See Table 19-1 for more information on these programs. The programs have been arranged from those that focus on the infancy period to those that focus on older children.

Risks and Prevention Opportunities in Childhood

Children develop within the context of their interactions with their families, friends, schools, communities, and cultures. During childhood, they experience both protective factors that promote healthy development and reduce the risk of their developing psychiatric disorders, and risk factors that increase the likelihood of their developing psychiatric disorders. Approximately 20% of U.S. children experience mental health problems with minimal impairment of

TABLE 19-1 PROGRAMS DESIGNED TO PREVENT MENTAL DISORDERS IN CHILDREN

Intervention	Population	Goals	Characteristics	Outcomes
The Prenatal/ Early Infancy Project (Olds et al., 1986, 1988, 1997, 1998, 2002)	Pregnant women from a low-income urban area	Improve health behaviors and parenting; provide social support for mothers; help mothers achieve more education and better employment; reduce unwanted pregnancies; improve cognition and language development of children; decrease psychological and behavioral problems of children	Home visits by nurse through pregnancy and until child was 2 years old	Reduced maternal smoking; improved social support; reduced child abuse; improved vocational adjustment for mothers; and improved educational achievement in children
Nurse Home Visitation (Olds et al., 1998)	Young women (19 years of age) pregnant for the first time, who were unmarried or of low socioeconomic status	Reduce antisocial behavior in their children	Home visits by nurses during mother's pregnancy and for first 2 years of child's life Nurses promote positive health behaviors during pregnancy; competent care of children; and maternal personal development	Improved pregnancy outcomes; improved childcare; improved mother's life Reduced physical abuse, aggression, and harsh parenting Prevented development of antisocial behavior (O'Connell et al., 2009)
Nurse-Family Partnership (NFP) program (Olds, 2006)	First-time mothers who are low income, single, or adolescents	Prevent negative outcomes for children and improve mothers' life course	Three components: 1. Promote healthy pregnancy, health and development of child, and parents' life course 2. Assist mothers in building social relationships 3. Link mothers and their families with health and social services (MacMillan, 2008)	Improved prenatal health of mother, parenting, and progress toward life goals Less physical abuse of child (Gonzalez & MacMillan, 2008) Prevented development of antisocial behavior and reduced substance use among children at age 15 years (O'Connell et al., 2009)
The Infant Health and Development Programme (Ramey, Bryant, Wasik, et al., 1992)	Low birth weight infants and comparison group of normal-weight infants	Prevent health problems, developmental disabilities, and learning and behavioral problems associated with infants with low birth weights	Parents were taught child development activities and parenting skills	At 36 months, experimental group showed better cognitive competence and lower rate of behavioral problems

Continued

TABLE 19-1 PROGRAMS DESIGNED TO PREVENT MENTAL DISORDERS IN CHILDREN—continued

Intervention	Population	Goals	Characteristics	Outcomes
Perry Preschool (Schweinhart & Weikart, 1989)	Children ages 3 to 4 years with low IQ and conduct symptoms, and families with low incomes		Comprehensive early education program: focus on child's cognitive, language, and social skills Intervention for parents	Less child maltreatment; less use of special education; higher rates of high school graduation and college attendance; fewer arrests; higher rates of employment (O'Connell et al., 2009)
Circle of Security (Marvin, Cooper, Hoffman, et al., 2002)	Preschool children and caregiver dyads	Promote secure attachment to prevent neglect and abuse	Helps caregivers to understand attachment theory and how to read the child's cues.	Increase of positive interactions between caregiver and child More caregiver affection and less rejection Increase in secure child attachment patterns (Marvin et al., 2002)
Dare to be You (Developed by Jan Miller-Heyl, Program Director, in 1979, as a grant-funded program under Colorado State University Extension 4-H Youth Development)	High-risk families positive for alcohol use with children ages 2 to 5 years	Improve parent's self-esteem, decision-making skills, and communication skills; stress management; improve social isolation and awareness of child development	Program objectives focus on children's developmental attainments and aspects of parenting that contribute to youth resilience to later substance abuse, including parental self-efficacy, effective childrearing, social support, and problem-solving skills	Improvement of child development and decrease of oppositional behaviors Parental improvement of self-esteem, communication, and reasoning skills (Miller-Heyl, McPhee, & Fritz, 1998)
Healthy Families America (Duggan, Caldera, Rodriguez, et al., 2007)	A home visitation program by paraprofessionals; targets high-risk families		Visits begin after birth and extend 3 to 5 years Provide information about community resources; teach families about childhood milestones and appropriate expectations; promote child safety	No overall effects on child maltreatment have been reported (Gonzales & MacMillan, 2008)
Caring School Community (formerly *The Child Development Program*) (Solomon, Battistich, Watson, et al., 2000)	Kindergarten to 6th grade	Promote pro-social values and sense of school community	Promote positive youth development The program is designed to create a caring school environment characterized by kind and supportive relationships and collaboration among students, staff, and parents	Increase of pro-social and supportive behaviors but no discernible effects on knowledge, attitudes, values, and academic domains (What Works Clearinghouse, 2007)
Incredible Years BASIC Parent Training Program (Webster-Stratton, 1987, 1990; Webster-Stratton et al., 2001)	2- to 12-year-old children and their parents and teachers	A program to prevent conduct disorder; a comprehensive, multifaceted, and developmentally based curriculum	The parent, child, and teacher training interventions that compose *Incredible Years* are guided by developmental theory on the role of multiple interacting risk and protective factors in the development of conduct problems	Improved parent-child interactions, reduced criticism and violent discipline, reduced child conduct problems (Weisz et al., 2005)
Positive Parenting Program (Triple P) (Bor et al., 2002)		Focus is on effective parenting and solutions to common behavioral problems	Components are based on family needs and preferences Include common rearing problems; managing aggressive behavior; and managing parental depression, marital discord, and other family problems	Positive effects on parenting and on child disruptive behaviors (O'Connell et al., 2009; Thomas & Zimmer-Gembeck, 2007)

TABLE 19-1 PROGRAMS DESIGNED TO PREVENT MENTAL DISORDERS IN CHILDREN—continued

Intervention	Population	Goals	Characteristics	Outcomes
Project SafeCare (Gershater-Molko, Lutzker, & Wesch, 2001)	Home visiting program	Prevent abuse and maltreatment	SafeCare is a home-based behavioral intervention that focuses on changing parental behavior to address home safety, home cleanliness, child medical care, and parent-child interactions Education about parenting, child development, and safety is provided, and, in addition, counseling is provided for parents with mental illness and substance abuse	*Project SafeCare* has been found to be effective in reducing neglect and maltreatment of children (Gershater-Molko et al., 2001)
Tools of the Mind (Diamond, Barnett, Thomas, et al., 2007)	Preschool and school-age children	Build executive functioning skills	Curriculum focused on inhibitory control (resisting distractions); working memory (retaining and using information); and cognitive flexibility (adjusting to change)	Improvement of executive functioning and readiness for school (Diamond et al., 2007)
PATHS (Promoting Alternative Thinking Strategies) (Greenberg & Kusche, 1998)	Children in elementary school or preschool	Promote social and emotional competence	Focus is on social-emotional development (self-control, self-esteem, emotional awareness, social skills, friendships, and interpersonal problem-solving skills) while reducing aggression and other behavioral problems	Improvement of problem-solving skills and reductions of conduct problems
I Can Problem Solve program (Shure, 1997; Shure & Spivack, 1988)	School-age children and children with ADHD	Help child develop interpersonal cognitive problem-solving skills that relate to behavioral problems	Focus is on enhancing social skills Child is taught problem-solving vocabulary; how to listen; how to identify feelings; consequences of acts; and how to problem-solve Parents learn how to help children problem-solve	Improvement of thinking, problem-solving, and high-risk behaviors (Shure, 2000)
Family-school Partnership (Ialongo, Poduska, Werthamer, et al., 2001; Ialongo, Werthamer, Kellam, et al., 1999)	First-grade children	Reduce early aggression, shy behavior, and problems with concentration	Provide parents with effective teaching and child behavior management strategies	Improvement in reading and math Lower rates of behavioral problems Lower rates of aggression among boys
Good Behavior Game (Barrish, Saunders, & Wolfe, 1969)	First-grade children	Reduce conduct disorder	Focus on shy and aggressive behaviors Has four classroom rules: 1. Work quietly, e.g., no yelling 2. Be polite to others, e.g., no hitting or kicking 3. Get out of one's seat only with permission 4. Follow directions	Reduced disruptive behavior and increased time in academic activities; reduced incidence of conduct disorder (O'Connell et al., 2009)
Lions Quest Skills for Adolescence (SFA)	Middle school children	Help young people develop positive commitments to their families, schools, peers, and communities and to encourage healthy, drug-free lives	A multicomponent, comprehensive life skills education program designed for schoolwide use and classroom implementation in grades 6 to 8 (ages 10 to 14)	Marijuana use was significantly lowered Decrease of binge drinking (Eisen, Zellman, & Murray, 2003)

Continued

TABLE 19-1 PROGRAMS DESIGNED TO PREVENT MENTAL DISORDERS IN CHILDREN—continued

Intervention	Population	Goals	Characteristics	Outcomes
Norwegian Bullying Prevention Programme (Olweus, 1989; Olweus & Limber, 2010)	Elementary and junior high school children	Prevent bullying and reduce risk for disorders associated with bullying: depression, anxiety, poor self-esteem, and suicide	Multimodal school program that restructures school environment to reduce opportunities for bullying and builds a sense of community among students and school Focus is on development of pro-social behaviors	Decreased bullying (World Health Organization, 2005) Reduced bullying by 21% to 28% Reduced antisocial behaviors, e.g., theft, vandalism, and truancy (Olweus & Limber, 2010)
Fast Track (Conduct Problems Prevention Research Group, 2002)	Kindergarten to 10th grade		Social and problem-solving skills training, play sessions, academic tutoring	Reduced self-reported antisocial behavior; reduced incidence of conduct disorder among highest risk children; reduced incidence of ADHD among highest risk children (O'Connell et al., 2009)
FRIENDS (Dadds et al., 1997; Lowry-Webster, Barrett, & Dadds, 2001)	7- to 16-year-old children with elevated levels of anxiety		Focus is on prevention of anxiety by strengthening resilience and problem-solving and cognitive skills	Reduced rate of developing anxiety disorders
Coping Cat (Kendall, Aschenbrand, & Hudson, 2003)	8- to 13-year-old children with generalized anxiety disorder, separation anxiety disorder, or social phobia		Individual cognitive behavioral therapy	Reduced rates of anxiety disorders and improved scores on self-report and parent-report anxiety scales
The Safe Start Initiative (Kracke, 2001)	Prevention and early intervention for children at high risk of being exposed to violence and for those who have already been exposed		Universal school-based preventive intervention The Safe Start Initiative is funded by the Office of Juvenile Justice and Delinquency Prevention (OJJDP), Office of Justice Programs, U.S. Department of Justice	Review of universal school-based programs to prevent violent behavior found decreased rates of violent and aggressive behaviors among school-age children and youth (Hahn, Fuqua-Whitley, Wethington, et al., 2007)

functioning at any given time, and 10% to 15% experience more severe psychiatric disorders, such as CD, anxiety disorders, and depression (Waddell, McEwan, Peters, et al., 2007b). These childhood psychiatric disorders often persist into adulthood (Essex, Kraemer, Slattery, et al., 2009; Roza, Hofstra, van der Ende, et al., 2003).

Protective Factors and Risk Factors in Childhood

Protective Factors

Protective factors include factors at the child's level, the family level, the school level, and the community level. Although protective factors and risk factors may be on a continuum at times, protective factors are not the reverse or absence of risk factors. Protective factors in childhood are listed in Box 19-1.

Risk Factors

Risk factors that are associated with the development of psychiatric disorders are presented in Box 19-2. Although risk factors are often presented in specific categories (child, family, and social or environmental), their effects are cumulative and intertwined (Trentacosta, Hyde, Shaw, et al., 2008) and may occur in specific configurations that confer greater risk (Copeland, Shanahan, Costello, et al., 2009a). For example, the configuration of parental mental illness, parental criminal behavior, family conflict, and impairment of family functioning places children at the highest risk of developing psychiatric disorders (Copeland et al.).

Some risk factors are associated with the development of multiple disorders while other risk factors are associated with specific disorders. Risk factors associated with the development of multiple problems are discussed in the following section, and risk factors associated with specific disorders—such as depression, anxiety disorders, substance-related disorders, schizophrenia, and suicide—will be discussed later.

Risk Factors Associated With Multiple Disorders

As early as the 1970s, researchers Rutter and Quinton (1977) had identified six adverse factors associated with childhood mental disturbances: severe marital discord; low social class and income; large family size (more than four children spaced less than 2 years apart); paternal

BOX 19-1 Protective Factors: Child, Family, School, and Community

Child Protective Factors
- Easy temperament
- Good verbal and communication skills
- Good play skills and activities
- Self-efficacy
- Ability to realistically appraise situations
- Social problem-solving skills
- Special talent or interest
- Ability to respond to others
- Secure attachment
- Resilience

Family Protective Factors
- Parental mental health
- Intact family structure
- Consistent warm relationship with an adult in family
- A family that shows warmth, harmony, and cohesion
- Mother with good communication skills and positive self-concept
- High but realistic parental expectations
- Child has tasks and responsibilities within the family
- Positive role models
- Extended social support networks
- Secure family income

School Protective Factors
- High but realistic expectations for students
- Caring, supportive school environment

Community Protective Factors
- Community norms of caring, mutual protection, and nondrug use
- Resources for children: childcare programs, nutritional programs, recreational programs

Sources: Crews, Bender, Cook, et al., 2007; Dawson, Ashman, & Carver, 2000; Kaplan, Turner, Norman, et al., 1996; Rutter, 1989; Werner, 1995; Werner & Smith, 1982.

BOX 19-2 Risk Factors in Childhood Associated With Development of Psychiatric Disorders

Child Risk Factors
- Born unwanted
- Low birth weight
- Physiological or temperamental vulnerabilities
- Insecure attachment patterns
- Child maltreatment (neglect and physical or sexual abuse)
- Academic failure
- Bullying
- Loneliness
- Chronic medical illnesses
- Losses, e.g., bereavement or separation from a parent
- Poor social skills
- Stressful life events
- Exposure to violence
- Foster care placement

Family Risk Factors
- Teenage parents
- Parental insecure attachment patterns
- Single-parent household
- Step-parent household
- Large family size
- Poor family supervision of children
- Family conflict/arguments
- Lack of financial resources
- Parental unemployment
- Family disruptions (divorce, separations)
- Parental mental illnesses and substance-related disorders
- Paternal criminality
- Step-parent dysfunction (history of mental illness, substance abuse, or criminality)

Social and Environmental Risk Factors
- Failure during first 2 years of school
- Poverty; socioeconomic status accounts for 79% of the variation of mental illness rates (Albee, 2005)
- Exposure to violence and trauma
- Poor housing situations
- Unemployment

Sources: Copeland et al., 2009a; Greenberg et al., 2001b; Hosman et al., 2005; Kiesler, 1999; Repetti, Taylor, & Seeman, 2002; Rutter, 1985; Rutter & Quinton, 1977; Werner & Smith, 1992 (also see Chapter 3 for experienced/environmental risk factors associated with development of psychiatric disorders).

criminality; maternal mental disorder; and foster care placement. They reported that no single risk factor increased the likelihood of mental disorders in children, but that two risk factors increased the risk four times, and four risk factors increased the risk ten times. Later research has supported their findings and has added information about the exposure of children to maltreatment or adversities and the lifelong legacy of childhood maltreatment (Taylor, 1999).

Currently, risk factors that are associated with many disorders can be categorized as

1. Poverty
2. Community and school factors
3. Family disruptions
4. Child maltreatment/childhood adversities (O'Connell et al., 2009)

The broad adverse effects associated with these risk factors are believed to be due to disruptions of normal developmental trajectories. For example, family disruptions, such as divorce or incarceration, are often associated with decreased parental involvement with the child that may lead to academic failure, substance use, and antisocial behavior. Childhood maltreatment, which is often embedded in risk-laden living situations, leads to many adverse outcomes, including psychiatric disorders of depression, substance abuse, and suicide (O'Connell et al., 2009). It is thought that preventive interventions that target any of the risk factors will be associated with a reduced risk for more than one psychiatric disorder (O'Connell et al.).

Poverty

Over 18% of American children live in families whose income is below the poverty line, defined in 48 states as $22,050 a year for a family of four. The poverty line is higher in Hawaii ($25,360) and Alaska ($27,570) (United States Department of Health & Human Services, 2009). Parental lack of a high school education, unemployment, and mental health problems are strong risk factors for children's living in poverty. For example, among children of single mothers who have not completed high school and who are not employed, the poverty rate is 82% (Aber, Jones, & Cohen, 2002). Even families at the poverty line or slightly above often cannot meet the family's basic needs (Boushey, Brocht, Gundersen, et al., 2001).

Poverty is a risk factor for the development of psychiatric disorders (O'Connell et al., 2009). The effect of poverty is transmitted through different pathways, such as lack of parental investment in the child; parental stress, conflict, and violence; and inadequate living situations, child care, schools, and community resources (O'Connell et al.). The effect of poverty is manifested in children as low birth weight, lead poisoning, developmental delays, health problems, and academic problems early in life (Aber et al., 2002) (see Chapter 3 for discussion of childhood adversities, such as poverty, and the development of psychopathology). The effects of poverty often last a lifetime. Poor children, in comparison to financially advantaged children, experience more family conflict, more violence, greater instability of the family, more separations from the family, and lower social support (Evans, 2004). Albee (2005) emphasized the need to eradicate poverty as the first step in universal prevention of mental illness.

Preventive Interventions

Preventive interventions to reduce negative effects of poverty include programs to change life pathways, such as job training and education to increase parents' earning capacity; programs to encourage young women to postpone childbearing and to complete their education; income support programs; and supplemental programs, such as food for women, infants, and children, health insurance for children, and good child care. Some projects, such as *Head Start* and *Early Head Start,* focus on improving the child's development, the family's functioning and well-being, and availability of community resources (Beardslee, Hosman, Solantaus, et al., 2005). There have been several studies of preventive interventions for children in poverty. *Sure Start,* a preventive intervention that was implemented in England, targeted child poverty and social exclusion (Rutter, 2006). It provided five core services: outreach and home visiting; support for families and parents; good-quality play opportunities, learning, and child care; health care; and support for children and parents with specialized needs. The outcomes were inconclusive, but they suggest an increase of parental acceptance of the child (less scolding and slapping) and less family chaos. There was no evidence of effect on the children's behavior or health.

In a study that examined the effects of nurse home visiting on child development, it was found at 6-year follow-up that those who had received nurse home visits during the prenatal period and first months after birth were more likely to have higher intellectual functioning and fewer behavior problems than the control group (Olds, Kitzman, Cole, et al., 2004). Among the mothers who received the nurse home visit intervention, ability to adapt to stressful events with fewer mental health problems improved, binge drinking decreased, and the rate of better parenting practices was higher 15 years after the intervention than that of the mothers who did not receive the nurse home visit intervention (Izzo, Eckenrode, Smith, et al., 2005). After reviewing programs designed to reduce the incidence of health and developmental problems among young children, Olds, Sadler, and Kitzman (2007) concluded that programs such as nurse home visiting are effective among diverse populations.

The *Nurse-Family Partnership (NFP)* program is a nurse home visitation program that targets first-time mothers who are low income, single, or adolescent. The program is designed to improve birth outcomes; reduce child neglect, abuse, and injuries; and improve the mother's life course. Outcomes include improved prenatal health–related behaviors and pregnancy outcomes, reduced child injuries, and a trend toward reduced rates of child abuse and neglect. At 15-year follow-up, women in the NFP program were 48% less likely to be identified as perpetrators of child abuse and neglect; however, the presence of intimate partner violence lessened the effect of the program on maltreatment of the child. In some of the programs, the women tended to have a longer interval between births of their children, less intimate partner violence, longer relationships with current partners, and less use of welfare and food stamps (Olds et al., 1997); (see Table 19-1 for other programs).

Community and School Risk Factors

Risk factors for the development of psychiatric disorders that are associated with schools and communities include bullying, academic failure, and exposure to violence (O'Connell et al., 2009). For example, bullying is associated with depression, anxiety, poor self-esteem, and suicidal ideation (Olweus & Limber, 2010); academic failure is linked with increased rates of antisocial behavior and substance abuse (Dryfoos, 1990); and exposure to violence is linked with increased rates of post-traumatic stress disorder, other anxiety disorders, depression, antisocial behavior, and substance use (Gorman-Smith & Tolan, 1998; Turner, Finkelhor, & Ormrod, 2010).

Preventive Interventions

Preventive interventions that promote pro-social behavior, academic achievement, or positive bonding to the school have been found to reduce aggressive behavior in first grade and, later, are associated with reduced rates of alcohol and drug use (Muthen, Jo, & Brown, 2003) and reduced rates of antisocial personality disorder (Petras, Kellam, Brown, et al., 2008).

Family Disruptions

Disruption of the family can be due to death of a parent, separation or divorce, military deployment, or incarceration of a parent. It changes the structure of the family and the functioning of the family. Disruption of the family often results in

- Emotional upheaval
- Increased stress
- Reduced financial status of the family
- Poorer living conditions
- Changing schools
- New family roles
- Loss of family routines
- Fragmented child care
- Worry about safety
- Inability to plan for the future (O'Connell et al., 2009; Rentz, Marshall, Loomis, et al., 2007)

Death of a Parent

Death of a parent occurs in less than 4% of U.S. children under the age of 18. Children who experience the death of a parent are at increased risk for the development of emotional and behavioral problems, depression, and post-traumatic stress disorder for up to 2 years after the death (Melhem, Walker, Moritz, et al., 2008). There is some evidence that women who as children experienced death of a parent are at increased risk for depression (Maier & Lachman, 2000). Protective factors following the death of a parent are positive parenting by the surviving parent, few mental health problems in the surviving parent, good coping skills in the child, and the child's view that the parent's death does not threaten the child's well-being (Wolchik, Tein, Sandler, et al., 2006).

Divorce

Divorce is experienced by 34% of U.S. children before the age of 16 years. Divorce is an adversity that occurs in a matrix of family difficulties and that increases the likelihood of children's experiencing abuse or witnessing abuse (Dong, Anda, & Felitti, 2004). Following divorce, children experience many changes in their lives and may experience continued conflict between their parents (Amato, 2000). They have increased rates of both internalizing disorders, such as anxiety disorders and depression, and externalizing disorders, such as childhood disruptive disorders and substance abuse disorders (Barrett & Turner, 2006). As adults, in comparison to adults who did not experience parental divorce, they have increased rates of mood disorders, major depressive disorder, bipolar I disorder, and post-traumatic stress disorder. Among those who experienced both divorce and abuse in childhood, there is a higher rate of mood disorders and anxiety disorders and an increased rate of antisocial behavior, substance use, and suicidal behavior (Afifi, Boman, Fleisher, et al., 2009).

Military Deployment

Military deployment involves separation from a parent, changes of parental roles, daily uncertainty, and a sense of danger. It may involve a decrease in family finances and relocation (Flake, Davis, Johnson, et al., 2009). Deployment has been found to be associated with increased family stress (Rosen, Durand, & Martin, 2000), increased rates of divorce (Schumm, Bell, & Gade, 2000), spousal violence (McCarroll, Ursano, Liu, et al., 2000), and increased child maltreatment (Rentz et al., 2007). Children have been found to experience increased stress during parental deployment and also during reuniting after deployment. For example, in Operation Desert Storm, 1990-1991, children of deployed parents were found to have increased rates of anxiety, depression, and aggressive behaviors (Jensen, Martin, & Watanabe, 1996). In a recent study, it was found that one-third of children of deployed parents were at increased risk for internalized symptoms of anxiety, depression, and social withdrawal. When surveyed, teachers reported that although many children with a deployed parent did not seem to have problems, other such children looked to teachers for social and emotional support and considered school to be a "safe haven" from a stressful, unstable home life (Chandra, Martin, Hawkins, et al., 2010, p. 222). Children's response to parental deployment is related to the nondeployed parent's level of stress, which is often related to relocations, financial problems, and feeling detached from home, support networks, and religious congregations. When nondeployed parents are older, have higher levels of education, are employed, and receive support from family or from community, military, or religious organizations, the children have fewer psychosocial problems (Flake et al., 2009).

Incarceration

Children of parents who are incarcerated have been found to have increased rates of externalizing behaviors, such as aggression, defiance, and disobedience, and of internalizing behaviors, such as depression, anxiety, and withdrawal. They are often lonely and sad and have school problems and difficulties with other children. Children who experienced warm acceptance from the people caring for them have fewer behavioral problems (Hairston, 2007).

Impaired Functioning of the Family

Impaired family functioning may be due to changes in family status—such as unemployment, illness, and social isolation—and to disruptions of the family (Riley, Valdez, Barrueco, et al., 2008). Impaired family functioning is often related to multiple co-occurring factors (Chartier et al., 2010). Child maltreatment is an example of extreme impairment of family functioning. It occurs at higher rates in families in which there is poverty, domestic violence, mental health problems, substance abuse, and incarceration of a family member (Chartier et al.; Connell et al., 2009).

Child Maltreatment/Childhood Adversities

Rates of Adversities

The National Survey of Children's Exposure to Violence conducted in 2008 in the United States studied the occurrence of victimization—such as physical assault, maltreatment, sexual assault, witnessing of family violence, exposure to community violence, and bullying—in children ages 10 to 17 years. The data revealed that 80% of the children had experienced at least one type of victimization and that among these children, 66% had been exposed to more than one type and 30% to five or more types (Finkelhor, Turner, Ormrod, et al., 2009). In 2010, Chartier et al. reported similar findings among Canadian children: 72% of the children had experienced at least one adverse experience and 37% had experienced two or more. Dong et al. (2004) divided forms of victimization or adversities into categories, as presented in Table 19-2. Based on evidence-based research, two categories that may have been subsumed in the work of Dong et al. have been added as separate categories: bullying (Olweus & Limber, 2010) and institutional care (Zeanah, Egger, Smyke, et al., 2009).

Rates for some of the adversities included in the report "Children's Exposure to Violence: A Comprehensive National Survey" from the Office of Juvenile Justice and Delinquency Prevention (Finkelhor et al., 2009) are presented below:

- Physical abuse: 46.3% were physically assaulted within the previous year.
- Bullying: 13.2% reported physical bullying during the previous year; 19.7% reported being teased or emotionally bullied during the previous year; and 5.7% reported Internet harassment during the previous year.
- Maltreatment (physical abuse, psychological or emotional abuse, child neglect, and custodial interference): 10.2% reported maltreatment during the previous year and 18.6% during their lifetime.
- Sexual victimization: 6.1% report sexual victimization during the previous year and 9.8% reported lifetime sexual victimization.
- Witnessing violence: 25.3% had witnessed violence during the previous year and 37% during their lifetime.
- Multiple victimizations: 38.7% reported experiencing more than one direct episode of victimization within the previous year.

Clusters Related to Family Characteristics and Life Circumstances

From this survey, it appears that more than one-third of children who are maltreated are victims of multiple forms of abuse. The factors that place the child in harm's way occur in clusters related to family characteristics and life circumstances. Six clusters have been identified:

1. Maladaptive family functioning, which includes parental mental illness, substance abuse, and criminality; family violence; and child maltreatment (neglect, verbal abuse, emotional abuse, physical abuse, and sexual abuse)
2. Parental death
3. Parental divorce
4. Child's placement in foster care
5. Child's physical illness
6. Family economic hardship (Green, McLaughlin, Berglund, et al., 2010)

With the exception of parental death, all clusters increased the risk of psychopathology; however, among the

TABLE 19-2 CATEGORIES OF ADVERSITIES AND THEIR CHARACTERISTICS

Category of Adversity	Characteristics
Emotional abuse	Swearing at the child, insulting the child, or putting the child down
Physical abuse	Pushing, grabbing, slapping, or throwing something at the child
Sexual abuse	Touching, fondling, attempting any type of sexual intercourse, or having any type of intercourse (oral, anal, vaginal) with the child
Physical neglect	Not having enough to eat; not having clean clothes; no one available to care for them and protect them
Bullying (can be by words, physical contact, gestures, or intentional exclusion)	"Intentional, repeated, negative (unpleasant or hurtful) behavior by one or more persons directed against a person who has difficulty defending himself or herself" (Olweus & Limber, 2010, p. 125)
Institutional rearing as an adverse caregiving environment; e.g., Romanian orphanages	High ratios of caregivers to children; no individualized care; no opportunities to develop attachment; no psychosocial stimulation or learning opportunities (Zeanah, Egger, Smyke, et al., 2009)
Domestic violence	Physical pushing, hitting, slapping, biting, or threatening with a knife or gun between parents
Substance abuse	Parent who was a problem drinker or a drug user
Mental illness in the household	Parent who was depressed, was mentally ill, or had attempted suicide
Disruption of family structure	Parents separated or divorced
Criminality of parents	Parent in jail or prison

Sources: Dong et al., 2004; Olweus & Limber, 2010; Zeanah et al., 2009.

six clusters of adversities, maladaptive family functioning was found to have the strongest association with development of psychopathology (Green et al., 2010) and with persistence of mood disorders, anxiety disorders, and substance-related disorders across the life span, even into old age (Afifi, Enns, Cox, et al., 2008; McLaughlin, Green, Gruber, et al., 2010).

Protective Factors, Risk Factors, and Preventive Interventions

In planning preventive interventions, it is necessary to know specific protective factors and risk factors that can be targeted. Protective and risk factors for child abuse and neglect are presented in Table 19-3. Preventive interventions are also based on knowing what risk factors are associated with specific forms of abuse. Risk factors for physical abuse, sexual abuse, and neglect are presented in Table 19-4.

Outcomes of Childhood Adversities

The journey from childhood adversities to adult psychopathology is illustrated in Figure 19-1. A specific effect of exposure to childhood adversities is the alteration of the stress response of the hypothalamic-pituitary-adrenal axis that makes it more vulnerable to later stressors (Gunner & Donzella, 2002; Gunnar & Quevedo, 2008; McGowan, Sasaki, Alessio, et al., 2009), and a more generalized effect is interruption of the normal development of the child with subsequent impairment of emotional, social, and cognitive functioning (Cicchetti & Toth, 2005; Matz, Junghofer, Elbert, et al., 2010). In adulthood, the effect of childhood adversities is seen in problems with learning, cognition, self-regulation

TABLE 19-3 CHILD, FAMILY, AND SOCIETAL PROTECTIVE FACTORS AND RISK FACTORS FOR CHILDHOOD NEGLECT AND ABUSE

Child	Family	Societal
Protective Factors		
• Good health, normal development • Easy temperament • Above-average intelligence • Hobbies and interests • Ability to get along well with peers • Active coping style; resilience • Good social skills	• Secure attachment; warm parent-child relationship • Supportive family environment • Household rules; structure • Involvement of extended family • Parents model good coping skills • High level of parental education • Parents have reconciled their experienced childhood abuse and neglect	• Middle to upper socioeconomic status • Access to health care • Consistent employment • Adequate housing • Family participating in religious community • Good schools • Supportive adults outside of family who serve as role models or mentors
Risk Factors		
• Premature birth • Slow-to-warm-up or difficult temperament • Presence of physical or mental disabilities	• Presence of substance abuse • Parental history of childhood abuse • Arguing, high-conflict divorce, or domestic violence • Single parent with lack of material support • Social isolation • Parental psychopathology	• Poverty • Unemployment • Stressful life events • Lack of access to health care • Homelessness • Dangerous or violent neighborhood

Source: National Clearinghouse on Child Abuse and Neglect, 2004a.

TABLE 19-4 RISK FACTORS FOR CHILD PHYSICAL ABUSE, SEXUAL ABUSE, AND NEGLECT

Physical Abuse	Sexual Abuse	Neglect
Young mother (less than 20 years old), low level of educational achievement, and early separation from her own mother	Young mother	Young mother, low level of academic achievement, and early separation from her own mother
Single-parent family; if married, poor marital relationship; partner violence	Death of a parent Presence of stepfather doubles risk for girls (Smith, 2002; Child sexual abuse: Evaluation outcome, 2007)	Single-parent family
Limited finances	Stress associated with poverty (Botash, 2010)	Low family income
Parents lack social support and religious participation	Social isolation and family secrecy (Botash, 2010)	Parents lack social support
Parental psychopathology	Maternal psychopathology	Parental psychopathology
Parents have history of childhood maltreatment	Parents have history of childhood maltreatment	Parents have history of childhood maltreatment
Other: low level of parental involvement with child	Other: born of an unwanted pregnancy; use of harsh forms of punishment; female gender of child	Other: large family size; serious maternal illness; violence in the family; parental involvement in illegal activities

Sources: Botash, 2010; Lahoti, McClain, Girardet, et al., 2001; Gonzalez & MacMillan, 2008; MacMillan, 2009.

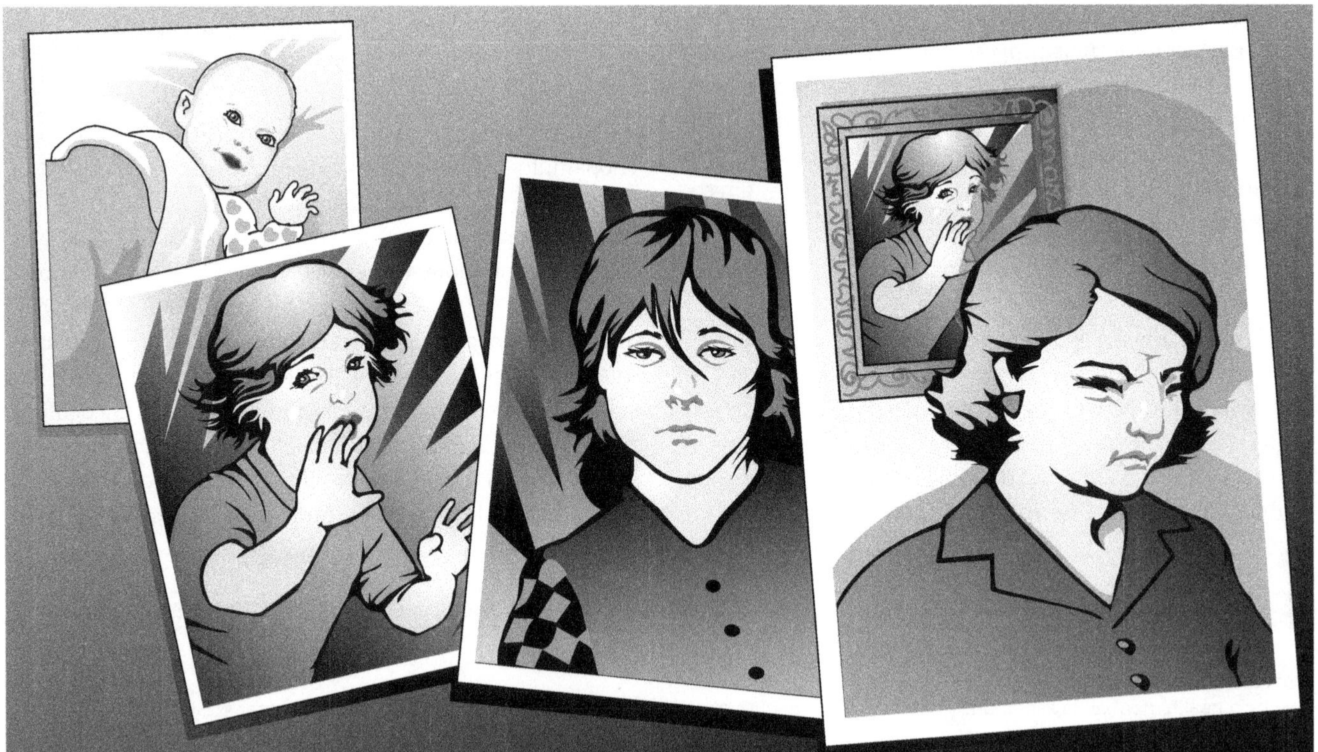

FIGURE 19-1: The Journey From Childhood Adversities to Adult Psychopathology.

of mood and anxiety, and interpersonal and social relationships (Anda, Felitti, Bremner, et al., 2006); a greater prevalence of physical health problems (coronary artery disease, liver disease, chronic pulmonary disease, obesity, and cancer) (Dube, Cook, & Edwards, 2010; Edwards, Holden, Felitti, et al., 2003; Felitti, Anda, Nordenberg, et al., 1998); lower levels of educational achievement, socioeconomic status, and stability of employment (Dube et al.); and the development of psychiatric disorders, such as anxiety disorders, depression, alcoholism, and drug abuse (Anda et al.; Matz et al.; National Clearinghouse on Child Abuse and Neglect Information, 2004b; Nemeroff, 2004; Shea, Walsh, MacMillan, et al., 2004). Childhood adversities increase the risk of early drug use two to four times and account for 50% to 66% of serious problems with drug use (Dube, Felitti, Dong, et al., 2003). Exposure to childhood adversities is also associated with increased risk for suicide in adulthood; that is, accumulated adversities are associated with suicide attempts and with completed suicides (Afifi et al., 2008).

Exposure to childhood adversities explains or predicts 32.4% of the onset of psychiatric disorders (Scott, Varghese, & McGrath, 2010). More specifically, childhood adversities predict 41.2% of disruptive behavioral disorders, 32.4% of anxiety disorders, 26.2% of mood disorders, and 21.0% of substance use disorders (Green et al., 2010). For example, among deployed military personnel, a history of two or more childhood adversities was associated with an increased risk for depression and post-traumatic stress disorder that was above the risk imposed by combat (Cabrera, Hoge, Bliese, et al., 2007).

In addition to increased rates of psychiatric disorders, children who have been maltreated experience more stressors throughout their lives. Negative life events—such as unemployment, being fired, poverty, homelessness, and arrests—and life changes—such as divorce and death of a parent, spouse, or child—are more common among adults who experienced childhood maltreatment (Horwitz, Widom, McLaughlin, et al., 2001). According to Horwitz et al., "The long-term mental health impacts of childhood victimization unfold within the context of a lifetime of stressors" (p. 197). Adults who have experienced severe maltreatment in childhood have described their lives as joyless and full of longing (Massie & Szajnberg, 2006).

Afifi et al. (2008, p. 950) said that one in four women with a mood disorder, one in five women with an anxiety disorder, and one in three women with a substance use disorder might not have had the disorder if childhood physical abuse, childhood sexual abuse, and witnessing domestic violence had not occurred. In men, 24% of psychopathology might have been reduced if they had not been exposed to physical abuse, sexual abuse, and witnessing domestic violence in childhood. If childhood adversities had not occurred, suicide attempts might be reduced by 50% in women and by 33% in men.

Preventive Interventions

Research-generated evidence that the effect of childhood adversities predicts the development of nearly *one-third* of psychiatric disorders sends a strong message that preventing psychiatric disorders must include preventing childhood adversities. Because adversities within the cluster of "maladaptive family functioning" have the strongest association with the onset of psychiatric disorders and with the persistence of psychiatric disorders over the life span, preventive interventions to target maladaptive family functioning must be developed (Scott et al., 2010). Interventions must address parental issues, such as mental illness, substance-related disorders, and criminality; family issues, such as conflict and violence; and child maltreatment. Additionally, based on the research of Gonzales and MacMillan (2008) it is evident that preventive interventions should address the mother's lack of education, early separation from her own mother, prior experiences with maltreatment, current abuse, and social isolation. Because psychiatric advanced practice nurses have a biopsychosocial approach and preparation for providing care across the life span, they are in a unique position among mental health care professionals to develop and implement interventions to prevent childhood adversities (Pearson, 2010).

Preventive Interventions for Childhood Mental Disorders

Preventive interventions are based on evidence-based knowledge of risk factors and protective factors (Kraemer, Kazdin, Offord, et al., 1997) and on knowledge that risk factors "work together" in sequential or parallel processes and that they may modify or mediate the effect of other risk factors (Kraemer, 2010, p. 38). Therefore, programs to prevent mental disorders in children are often broad based and target several risk factors and protective factors. Examples of broad preventive programs are included in Table 19-1.

Promoting the Protective Factor of Resilience in Children

Resilience has been described as the "power to recover" (Kiesler, 1999, p. 148). Factors associated with greater resilience have been identified as having a nurturing, supportive relationship with at least one adult, having external support from people in the community, and having an easy temperament (Ryff & Singer, 2000; Werner, 1989).

Families can be helped to nurture resilient children through the use of specific interventions, including communication, problem-solving, authoritative parenting style, and family fun time (Shenfeld, 2007). Families can be taught to encourage effective communication. They can learn to listen with empathy to everyone's emotions, points of view, and problems. They can be taught to use "I" statements, not to interrupt, and to ask appropriate questions. Families can be taught problem-solving skills that they can use in resolving conflicts rather than emotion-focused coping skills. Parents should be encouraged to use an authoritative parenting style, which has been found to be associated with well-being of children. Authoritative parenting includes being warm, nurturing, and loving, even when expressing disapproval of a child's behavior; providing firm, clearly defined rules, but being able to be flexible when needed; using discipline that is fair; having age-appropriate expectations for the child; and providing praise for efforts and accomplishments. Families can be encouraged to set aside time to do fun things together, such as playing games, learning new things, participating in physical activities, and sharing interests or hobbies, such as gardening or car maintenance. Families can be helped to identify their spiritual values, such as by connecting with religious institutions or by sharing their appreciation of music, art, or nature with their children (Shenfeld). Children who are helped to grow up resilient have a sense of belonging and security (DiClemente & Raczynski, 1999).

Preventing Specific Psychiatric Disorders in Childhood

Specific psychiatric disorders that might be prevented in childhood include disruptive behavioral disorders (DBDs), anxiety disorders, depression, and suicide.

Preventing Childhood Disruptive Behavioral Disorders (DBDs)

Childhood DBDs include

1. ADHD
2. CD
3. ODD

These disorders are a source of distress to the child and the family and a financial burden to society because of their prevalence, their need for special services, and their effects across the life span. DBDs are associated with diminished overall functioning and increased risks for problems during adolescence and adulthood, such as academic failure, dropping out of school, substance abuse, risky sexual behavior, and antisocial behavior (Petitclerc & Tremblay, 2009, p. 223). Three clusters of symptoms associated with DBDs—frequent and persistent symptoms of physical aggression, disregard for rules, and hyperactive-impulsive behavior—are evidenced very early in childhood (Petitclerc & Tremblay); that is, children who have high levels of DBD symptoms have the symptoms in the first 2 years of life. Therefore, preventive interventions should be offered before the age of 3 years. Ideally, preventive interventions should be provided for at-risk mothers starting during pregnancy.

Attention Deficit-Hyperactivity Disorder (ADHD)

ADHD affects 3% to 5% of American children under age 13, and in 40% of cases of ADHD the disorder persists into adulthood. ADHD is characterized by a triad of symptoms: inattention, impulsivity, and hyperactivity. Impairment of functioning of ADHD falls within the executive functioning of the frontal lobe—specifically the prefrontal lobe area—and is believed to originate from deviations of brain development that may have been under genetic influence.

Risk Factors

Risk factors associated with ADHD include

- Prenatal exposure to tobacco smoke (Braun, Kahn, Froehlich, et al., 2006), alcohol (Vaurio, Riley, & Mattson, 2008), drugs of abuse (Linares, Singer, Kirchner, et al., 2006), deficient diet (Gale, Robinson, Godfrey, et al., 2008), and stress (Rodrigues & Bohlin, 2005)
- Adverse circumstances of birth, such as hemorrhage, prolonged labor, hypoxia, and low birth weight (Ursano et al., 2008)
- Disorganized attachment patterns (Green et al., 2007)
- Extended periods of television watching (Christakos, Zimmerman, DiGiuseppe, et al., 2004), e.g., more than 2 hours a day (Hallowell, 1998)
- Parental discord (Ficks & Waldman, 2009)
- Low socioeconomic status (Ficks & Waldman)

Preventive Interventions

Because ADHD emerges from multiple underlying developmental processes, early preventive interventions that target developmental processes—such as deficient pre-academic skills, poor social skills, and problems establishing and maintaining close relationships—may change the trajectory of development of the disorder (Sonuga-Barke & Halperin, 2010). A program for preschool children with ADHD, *New Forest Parenting Programme (NFPP)* (Sonuga-Barke, Thompson, Abikoff, et al., 2006), includes components designed to improve attention, working memory, and general self-regulation. It has been found to have beneficial effects on ADHD symptoms (Thompson, Laver-Bradbury, Ayres, et al., 2009). Parent training programs based on social learning approaches such as *The Incredible Years BASIC Parent Training Program* (Webster-Stratton, Reid, & Hammond, 2001) or the *Positive Parenting Program (Triple P)* (Bor, Sanders, & Markie-Dadds, 2002) have been found to be associated with reduced levels of oppositionality, defiance, and conduct problems in children and improved mental health in parents. They can be adapted for children with ADHD (Sonuga-Barke & Halperin) (see Table 19-1 for descriptions of similar programs).

Conduct Disorder (CD)

A child diagnosed with CD often ignores the rights of others and displays unmanageable behavior. CD is a risk factor for later development of antisocial behavior (Tremblay, Pagani-Kurtz, Masse, et al., 1995). Approximately 40% of children with CD develop antisocial personality disorder in adulthood. Children with a history of drug use before age 15 years, who have experienced out-of-home placement such as foster care, and who are living in extreme poverty are at higher risk of developing antisocial personality disorders as adults (Ursano et al., 2008). It has been estimated that preventing one case of CD may save an estimated $1.5 million of accumulated lifetime costs (Cohen, 1998).

Risk Factors

Risk factors include

- Difficult temperament
- Impaired ability to interpret social cues, e.g., a neutral situation may be interpreted as hostile
- Deficits in social problem-solving skills
- Impaired ability to anticipate consequences
- Low academic achievement
- Reading disabilities
- Maternal depression
- Paternal alcoholism, antisocial behavior, and criminality
- Parental conflict around divorce
- Family violence and spousal abuse
- Poverty and unemployment
- Maternal lack of social support
- Critical or harsh discipline
- Exposure of children to violence through television and other media (Bushman & Huesmann, 2006; Duff, 2005; Ursano et al., 2008)

Specific risk factors or "signature sets of putative risk factors" for conduct disorders have been identified:

- Sexual abuse
- Problems with peers
- Poor sibling relationships
- Losses
- Poor parental supervision
- Parental unemployment
- Parental depression (Shanahan, Copeland, Costello, et al., 2008, p. 39)

Preventive Interventions

Preventive approaches that have been found to be effective for CD include those that build the child's self-competence. Self-competence includes the ability to get along with others, complete developmental tasks, play with others, develop friendships, and communicate effectively (Duff, 2005). Preventive intervention programs that have been found to be effective include *Fast Track, Perry Preschool, Incredible Years BASIC Parent Training Program,* and *Nurse-Family Partnership* (Gross, Fogg, & Tucker, 1995) (see Table 19-1 for more details about these programs).

Oppositional-Defiant Disorder (ODD)

Early symptoms of being touchy, easily annoyed, resentful, spiteful, and vindictive are associated with development of ODD (Greenberg, Speltz, DeKlyen, et al., 2001). The distinguishing features of ODD are a negative, hostile attitude and defiant behavior toward authority figures. The defiant behavior may include arguing, refusing to follow rules, blaming others, and displays of emotional dysregulation, such as temper tantrums (Petitclerc & Tremblay, 2009).

Risk Factors

Risk factors for the development of ODD include

- Child characteristics: prematurity, birth complications, exposure to toxins (alcohol, smoking, drugs) during pregnancy, and difficult temperament
- High-risk parenting practices: critical, controlling behaviors; harsh or abusive discipline; and physical abuse
- Insecure child-parent attachment: 58% of children with ODD were found to have a disorganized pattern of attachment, which is associated with abuse of the child (Green et al., 2007)
- Family adversities: family conflict and violence; parental mental illness; life stressors such as poverty, transitions, and negative life events; and lack of social support (Greenberg et al., 2001)

Key risk factors for ODD are

- Poor parental supervision
- Poor sibling relationships
- Scapegoating
- Sexual abuse
- Lack of friends
- Neglect (a key risk factor for females but not males) (Shanahan et al., 2008)

Children who have experienced high-risk parenting practices and two other risk factors are at greatest risk for developing ODD. It is believed that a developmental sequence of experiences may be involved in ODD. The experiences may start with ineffective parenting practices followed by difficulty with authority figures and poor peer interactions. In response to these experiences, a pattern of opposition and defiant behaviors may develop. Children who have experienced both perinatal risk factors and environmental risk factors such as high-risk parenting practices or family adversities have worse behavioral outcomes in middle childhood and adolescence (Greenberg et al., 2001; Werner & Smith, 1982).

Preventive Interventions

The focus of prevention of ODD is on building effective parenting skills and helping the child develop communication skills and social skills to reduce the use of opposition and defiance with adults, peers, and schools (Children's Hospital Boston, 2005). Traditionally, treatment of ODD has focused on family and parent training in effective parenting; however, Greenberg et al. (2001) found that half of the boys with ODD in their study (1) had characteristics that made them vulnerable, such as prematurity, insecure attachment patterns, and delays in achieving developmental milestones and (2) were living in a situation with a high level of family adversities, e.g., in situations with family conflict, violence, parental psychopathology, and poverty. Greenberg et al. pointed out that neither child vulnerabilities nor family adversities are modifiable by training in *effective parenting.*

Effectiveness of Disruptive Behavioral Disorders Prevention

In evaluating the effectiveness of programs ostensibly designed to prevent DBDs, Petitclerc and Tremblay (2009) found that few programs actually focused on prevention of the disorders. Rather, the focus was on parenting practices or reducing behavioral symptoms. The programs that were successful were indicated or selective intervention programs. Petitclerc and Tremblay reported that more information is needed about the causal risk factors for DBD that can be identified during the perinatal and early infancy periods. Preventive interventions must focus on prenatal and perinatal risk factors, insecure attachment, and family adversities in addition to parenting practices.

Preventing Anxiety Disorders in Childhood

Anxiety disorders are one of the most frequently occurring psychiatric disorders in childhood. They have a lifetime prevalence that ranges from 8% to 27% of children (Costello, Egger, & Angold, 2005). However, only 31% of children with anxiety disorders receive treatment (Chavira, Stein, Bailey, et al., 2004). Anxiety disorders frequently occurring in children include generalized anxiety disorder, separation anxiety disorder, and social anxiety disorder (Emslie, 2008). Separation anxiety and phobias tend to occur at 7 years of age, and social anxiety disorder tends to occur at 13 years (Kessler et al., 2005a). Because the symptoms of anxiety disorders usually precede symptoms of depressive disorders and substance-related disorders, it has been proposed that anxiety is a risk factor for depressive disorders and substance-related disorders (Wittchen, Beesdo, Bittner, et al., 2003). Others consider anxiety to be a prodromal phase of depressive disorders (Krueger, 1999). Untreated anxiety disorders early in life are associated with failure to achieve academically and with increased rates of anxiety disorders, depression, and substance-related disorders later in life (Emslie).

Risk Factors

Risk factors for anxiety disorders are presented in Box 19-3.

Preventive Interventions

A selective preventive cognitive behavioral therapy intervention, the *Queensland Early Intervention and Prevention of Anxiety Project* (Dadds, Spence, Holland, et al., 1997), was developed to teach children strategies for coping with anxiety, to help them to plan graduated exposure to feared stimuli, to teach them relaxation techniques, and to teach them how to use positive self-talk and reward for overcoming worries. The intervention was found to be effective in reducing symptoms of anxiety and in preventing the progression to an anxiety disorder among children with symptoms of anxiety. In comparison, in the group of children at risk for developing anxiety disorders who did not receive the intervention, more than half had progressed to a diagnosable anxiety disorder at the end of 6 months (Dadds et al., 1997). Similar results were reported

BOX 19-3 Risk Factors for Anxiety Disorders in Childhood

- An inhibited temperament (fearful and shy)
- Insecure attachment pattern
- Sensitivity to new situations (viewing new situations as sources of harm or danger)
- Use of avoidant coping strategies that focus on avoiding or escaping problems
- Having no friends
- Threatening life events: divorce, family conflict, frequent changes of schools
- Sexual abuse
- Parents with anxiety disorders, depression, or drug use
- Parental unemployment
- Financial difficulties
- Parental conflict
- Harsh discipline

Sources: Evans et al., 2005; O'Connell et al., 2009; Shanahan et al., 2008.

in another study of children at risk for developing anxiety disorders. Those who received ten sessions of cognitive behavioral therapy had half the risk of developing an anxiety disorder that the at-risk children who were on the wait list had (Dadds, Holland, Laurens, et al., 1999).

One preventive intervention that uses cognitive behavioral therapy and has been found to reduce symptoms of anxiety and depression is *FRIENDS* (Barrett & Turner, 2001). The acronym FRIENDS stands for Feeling worried, Relax and feel good, Inner thoughts, Explore plans of action, Nice work, Reward yourself, Don't forget to practice; and Stay cool. Benefits derived from the intervention were still present at 1-year follow-up.

A selective preventive intervention, the *Coping and Promoting Strength (CAP)* program, focused on high-risk children who did not have symptoms of anxiety but whose parents had anxiety disorders. The intervention was directed to the parents and included education about anxiety, reducing parents' anxiety levels, teaching parents to model coping behaviors for their children, and increasing family communication and coping skills. At 1 year, there were no anxiety disorders among the children of the parents receiving the intervention and a 30% rate among high-risk children whose parents did not receive the intervention (Ginsberg, 2009).

Preventive interventions provided early in life have the potential to reduce the incidence of anxiety disorders. Bienvenu, Siegel, and Ginsburg (2010) said that providing preventive interventions to two groups—anxious, expectant parents and 3- to 5-year-old children with symptoms of anxiety—may have the greatest impact.

Preventing Depression in Childhood

The rate of depression is 2% to 2.5% for U.S. children and 4.4% to 6.4% for adolescents (Gladstone & Beardslee, 2009). Depression may be evidenced in preschool-age children as intense irritability, social withdrawal, anhedonia, changes in sleep and play, and feelings of shame and guilt (Luby, Xuemei, Belden, et al., 2009). Preschool depression persists into childhood, adolescence, and adulthood (Luby et al.).

Risk Factors

The strongest risk factor for childhood depression is being the child of a depressed parent (Garber, 2006). It makes a child four times more likely to develop a mood disorder by the age of 20 (Beardslee, Versage, & Gladstone, 1998). Risk factors associated with depression are presented in Box 19-4.

Other risks include gateways to depression, such as anxiety disorders. Increased risk of developing depression has been found among children who were fearful at age 3 years (Caspi, Moffitt, Newman, et al., 1996) and among those who were socially withdrawn at age 8 years (Goodwin, Fergusson, & Horwood, 2004). The number of anxiety disorders that adolescents had experienced earlier in childhood was significantly related to the risk for major depressive disorder in early adulthood (Pine, Cohen, & Brook, 2001). From these studies, Bittner, Goodwin, Wittchen, et al. (2004) concluded that childhood anxiety disorders contribute to the risk of onset of major depressive disorder among adolescents and adults and that treating childhood anxiety disorders may prevent the development of depression.

Alterations in emotional development that result in deficits of ability to regulate emotions are believed to contribute to the development of depression. Emotion theory proposes that emotions and the interaction of emotions and cognition underlie the development of behavioral problems and psychopathology (Izard, Fine, Mostow,

BOX 19-4 Risk Factors for Depression in Childhood

- Difficult temperament
- Insecure attachment
- Depressive style of thinking
- History of a depressive episode
- High level of symptoms of depression
- Negative self-evaluation, poor interpersonal problem-solving, and low expectations for self-performance
- No friends
- Parental rejection
- Child maltreatment (exposure to sexual abuse in childhood doubles the lifetime risk for depression)
- Foster home placement
- Exposure to violence
- Single parent
- Parents with mood disorders
- Parental arrest
- Family conflict or breakup
- Social isolation of family
- Parents' loss of employment and financial problems

Sources: Evans et al., 2005; Gladstone & Beardslee, 2009; O'Connell et al., 2009; Shanahan et al., 2008.

et al., 2002). Emotions play a crucial role in adaptation and in survival. In the beginning of an infant's life, emotions function independently, without cognitive input. Thus, among infants, emotions have a direct effect on behavior, e.g., curiosity promotes learning; joy or pleasure reduces distress; sadness increases bonding behaviors; fear elicits protection; anger fuels courage and self-assertiveness; and mastery results in confidence (Izard, 1977). Starting in infancy, children learn to understand their emotions, how to modulate them, and how to use them in positive adaptation through the process of emotional development (Izard et al., 2002). Emotional development that includes acquiring emotional self-regulation involves the development of connections between emotions and cognition. Emotional development is influenced by the infant's characteristics, such as difficult temperament, and by family characteristics, such as harsh parenting practices. Optimal development of adaptive connections requires emotional coaching to modulate emotional arousal and to promote the use of adaptive emotional responses. The mother usually carries out emotional coaching through her face-to-face interactions with her infant, which help the infant to experience the positive, rewarding emotional experiences that are the foundation of mental health. Rewarding emotional experiences facilitate the development of a secure attachment pattern and help to prevent persistent negative emotions. Conversely, maladaptive emotion-cognition connections may result in the child's developing patterns of hostility, anger, and oppositionality that persist over time.

Preventive Interventions

The severity of symptoms of depression begins to increase by age 13, and there is a marked increase in diagnosed depressive disorders between ages 15 and 18 (Sutton, 2007). Therefore, Sutton recommended that preventive interventions be initiated before age 13. Some interventions based on cognitive behavioral and interpersonal models have been found to be effective in reducing depressive symptoms, although there is less evidence of their effectiveness in preventing depressive disorders (Gladstone & Beardslee, 2009). A preventive intervention that uses cognitive behavioral therapy, *Coping with Stress* (Clarke, Hornbrook, Lynch, et al., 2001), has been found to be effective in preventing depression, though its effect diminishes over time. Examples of preventive programs are presented in Table 19-5.

In evaluating approaches to preventing depression in children, selective programs that target members of a

TABLE 19-5 PROGRAMS DESIGNED TO PREVENT DEPRESSION

Intervention	Population	Goals	Characteristics	Outcomes
Emotion-Based Prevention Program (EBP) (Izard, King, Trentacosta, et al., 2008)	Children ages 2½ to 5 years old	Accelerate the development of emotional competence and decrease maladaptive behaviors and internalizing symptoms, such as depression	Part of Head Start program Children learn to identify and label emotions and emotional expressions Children learn what causes the emotion and how to regulate emotions	Decrease of negative emotional expressions, negative classroom encounters, externalizing behaviors, and anxious and depressed behaviors
New Beginnings Program (NBP) (Wolchik, West, Sandler, et al., 2000)	Divorced families	Prevent adjustment problems	Two components: A mother program and a program that targeted mother and child in separate but simultaneous interventions	At 6 years, children in the program in comparison to a control group had fewer diagnosed mental disorders and improvement of psychiatric symptoms, substance use, behavioral problems, and grades; mothers had a reduced number of sexual partners (Wolchik, Sandler, Millsap, et al., 2002)
Family Bereavement Program (Sandler, Ayers, Wolchik, et al., 2003; Tein, Sandler, Ayers, et al., 2006; Sandler, Ma, Tein, et al., 2010)	Bereaved children ages 8 to 16 years	Prevent mental health problems	Two components: Separate groups for parents or caregivers and for bereaved children	No change in children's mental health problems immediately after the program At 11 months, girls showed improvement At 6 years, the children showed improvement of self-esteem and behavior problems (Tein et al., 2006)
Penn Resiliency Program (PRP) (Gillham, Jaycox, Reivich, et al., 1990)	School-age children	Targets cognitive and behavioral risk factors for depression	Based on cognitive behavioral therapy, PRP teaches the link between life events, child's interpretation of the events, and emotional consequences of their interpretations	Reduced depressive symptoms, but no reduction of depression diagnoses

Continued

TABLE 19-5 PROGRAMS DESIGNED TO PREVENT DEPRESSION—continued

Intervention	Population	Goals	Characteristics	Outcomes
Clarke Cognitive-Behavioral Prevention Intervention Program (Clarke et al., 2001)	Targets adolescents at risk for developing depression	Help adolescents gain control over negative moods, to resolve conflicts, and to change maladaptive thought patterns	Manual-based psychoeducational program	Fewer depressive symptoms, fewer symptoms of suicide, and improved overall functioning Reduced rate of developing depression (O'Connell et al., 2009)
Interpersonal Psychotherapy Model (IPT-AST) (Mufson, Dorta, Wickramaratne, et al., 2004)	High-risk teens	Prevent onset of depressive disorders	Psychoeducation regarding depression and prevention, skill-building to manage interpersonal role disputes, role transitions, and interpersonal deficits	Fewer symptoms of depression and better overall functioning Lower rate of developing depression than the control group (Mufson et al., 2004; Young, Mufson, Davies, et al., 2006)
Problem-solving for Life (Spence, Sheffield, & Donovan, 2003)	Universal school-based intervention for youth ages 12 to 14 years	Reduce symptoms of depression	Weekly sessions that taught cognitive restructuring and problem-solving, e.g., identify and connect thoughts and feelings	Students in the program showed fewer symptoms of depression at the end of the program Differences were not maintained over time No change in rate of depressive disorders
Keeping Families Strong (KFS) (Riley et al., 2008)	Families in which mother is depressed	Promote resilience and reduce risk for development of psychiatric disorders in children of parents with depression	Education about depression; cognitive restructuring for children, e.g., ill parent is not mad at them and does love them; building family problem-solving skills and communication skills; positive family activities; increasing social support	Preliminary findings suggest positive changes in mood of depressed parent, fewer stressful life events, more togetherness, and improvement of emotional and behavioral problems of the children (Riley et al., 2008)
Preventive Interventions for Parental Depression (Beardslee, Gladstone, Wright, et al., 2007)	Families of children with a parent with depression Family-based preventive intervention	Get treatment for parent with depression Reduce risk factors that often accompany parental depression, such as poor problem-solving and family conflict Increase protective factors for children, such as outside activities, support from family, and understanding that they are not to blame for their parent's depression		Improved family functioning Improvement of children's behavior Children's symptoms of depression and anxiety decreased

high-risk group and indicated approaches that target individuals with subclinical symptoms of the disorder have been found to be more effective than universal programs (Horowitz & Garber, 2006; MacMillan, 2009; Merry, 2007; Sutton, 2007). Garber (2006) stated that because depression is associated with stress, most children will benefit from learning stress-reduction strategies such as problem-solving, adaptive coping, conflict resolution, and effective communication, Because adverse family circumstances have a high correlation with depression in children, programs for decreasing childhood depression should include interventions that improve the family environment (Gladstone & Beardslee, 2009).

Preventing Suicide in Childhood

Young children do think about suicide, make plans for committing suicide, and make suicide attempts (Dervic, Brent, & Oquendo, 2008; Foley, Goldston, Costello, et al., 2006; Steele & Doey, 2007). In fact, suicide is the 12th leading cause of death in children 12 years old or younger (Tishler, Reiss, & Rhodes, 2007). In the United States, approximately 1% of school-age children attempt to harm themselves (Goldman & Beardslee, 1999). Family and school problems that may be actual or *anticipated* play a major role in childhood suicide (Dervic et al.).

Risk Factors

Risk factors include characteristics of the child, family risk factors, and negative life events. Risk factors also include beliefs and desires that motivate a child to commit suicide, such as the belief that the child will be reunited with a parent who has died; the desire for the child's suicide to distract the family from acting on conflicts; or the desire to act out a perceived wish of a parent to be rid of the child (Centre for Suicide Prevention, 2000). Risk factors for childhood suicide are presented in Box 19-5.

Preventive Interventions

Children's suicidal behaviors are not impulsive, and their reasons are similar to those of adults. Parents, teachers, and health-care providers must listen carefully to what children are saying about suicide and must be aware that they may act on suicidal ideas. Prevention starts with the family. Parents should be encouraged to take an active part in their children's lives, to be aware of their feelings and problems, and to remove tools of suicide or opportunities for suicide. Gatekeepers—teachers, coaches, school nurses, and religious leaders—should be taught how to identify children at risk for suicide.

BOX 19-5 Risk Factors for Childhood Suicide

- Exposure to adversities: physical and sexual abuse; witnessing violence against the mother; living in a home where there is substance abuse, a parent with psychopathology, or where a parent is incarcerated
- Previous suicide attempt
- Presence of psychiatric disorders: depression, bipolar disorder, disruptive/conduct disorders, schizophrenia, and psychotic or delusional thinking
- Presence of feelings of hopelessness
- Comorbidity: conduct disorder and depression or anxiety disorder and depression
- Preoccupation with death, e.g., pathological preoccupation with death
- Family history of suicidal behavior: children of parents who have attempted suicide are at a six times higher risk of attempting suicide (Brent, Oquendo, Birmaher, et al., 2002)
- Presence of family psychopathology: mood disorders, personality disorders, violent behavior, and substance abuse
- Home environment of poverty, divorce, multiple changes of family structure, witnessing or experiencing violence, and child maltreatment such as physical or sexual abuse
- Negative school environment: peer problems, poor academic performance, loneliness, bullying, and extortion
- Poor coping skills and poor social adjustment

Sources: Foley et al., 2006; O'Connell et al., 2009; Steele & Doey, 2007; Tishler et al., 2007.

Summary of Psychiatric Disorders in Childhood

In summary, there is often a continuation of childhood psychiatric disorders into adulthood as the same disorder or in the form of other psychiatric disorders. For example, anxiety disorders, depression, and CD are likely to persist in the same form into adulthood (Waddell et al., 2007b), but ODD has a broader influence. ODD is a risk factor for a variety of adult disorders—depression, generalized anxiety disorder, and panic disorder without agoraphobia (Copeland et al., 2009a). Because of their persistence into adulthood, psychiatric disorders in children must be prevented in order to achieve the goal of preventing psychiatric disorders.

Risks and Prevention Opportunities in Adolescence

Adolescence is a transitional period of many changes—brain development, endocrine functioning, emotions, cognition, behavior, and interpersonal relationships. It is also the time of onset of many of the major psychiatric disorders. Approximately half of the major psychiatric disorders begin in adolescence (by age 15 years), and many continue into adulthood as chronic illnesses (Evans & Seligman, 2005). Adolescence is also the time of developing lifestyle practices that influence the development of psychiatric disorders (Evans & Seligman). Promoting healthy development requires that adolescents be provided with the support, relationships, experiences, resources, opportunities, and role models needed for them to develop into healthy, competent, successful adults (Durlak, 1998; Seligman, Berkowitz, Catalano, et al., 2005).

Threats to healthy development, risk factors that increase the likelihood of negative outcomes, protective factors that increase the likelihood of positive outcomes, factors that support healthy development, and interventions are presented in Box 19-6.

BOX 19-6 Adolescent Healthy Development: Threats, Risk Factors, Protective Factors, Supportive Factors, and Interventions

Threats

- Poverty
- Substance use
- Violence
- Unsafe sexual practices
- Mental health problems
- Suicide
- Poor-quality schools (schools characterized by low achievement, low expectations, a nondemanding curriculum, and poor relationships between teachers, parents, and students)
- Living in impoverished neighborhood

Continued

BOX 19-6 Adolescent Healthy Development: Threats, Risk Factors, Protective Factors, Supportive Factors, and Interventions—continued

Risk Factors

- Low academic achievement
- Impairment of intellectual functioning
- Health problems
- Having only one parent
- Peer rejection
- Family's low socioeconomic status
- Parental psychopathology
- Marital discord
- Harsh childrearing practices
- Abuse

Protective Factors

- Academic achievement
- Extracurricular activities
- Volunteerism
- Effective parenting
- Connections to adults other than parents
- Being appealing to others, especially adults
- Talent or hobby valued by others
- Self-efficacy, self-worth, and hopefulness
- Religious beliefs

Supportive Factors

- Having a close relationship with a role model or caregiver
- Having friends and interests
- Having good language and communication skills
- Having the ability to reason and problem-solve
- Having positive peer relationships
- Having good parent/child relationships
- Having personal and social skills
- Having a strong sense of self-efficacy
- Availability of social support
- Living in a community with social norms (enforcing laws that prohibit smoking; drug prevention programs; antibullying programs)
- Living in a community with effective social policies
- Attending high-quality schools

Interventions

- Programs that promote connectedness with family and school (they stimulate the reward center of the brain)
- Promotion of self-identity, self-efficacy, belief in the future, and spirituality
- Programs that promote competencies by development of new skills that they can use to help others
- Promotion of resilience (Bernat & Resnick, 2006)
- Programs such as "Going for the Goal" that increase health-promoting behaviors and decrease health-compromising behaviors (Danish, 1997)
- Interventions such as *Penn Resilience Program* (Gillham & Reivich, 2004) and *Promoting Alternative Thinking Strategies (PATHS)* (Greenberg & Kusche, 1998)

Sources: Bernat & Resnick, 2006; Durlak, 1998; Seligman et al., 2005.

Protective Factors and Risk Factors in Adolescence

Protective Factors

Protective factors for healthy development include a high sense of self-esteem and self-worth, a strong sense of purpose, and parental monitoring and involvement (Copeland-Linder, Lambert, & Ialongo, 2010).

Risk Factors

The presence of adversities is associated with increased rates of academic problems, social withdrawal, depression, anxiety disorders, antisocial personality disorder, substance abuse, and suicide (Lambert, Copeland-Linder, & Ialongo, 2008). The most frequent adversities reported by adolescents include

- Parents separating
- Unemployment of parents with accompanying financial hardships
- Parents abusing alcohol or drugs
- Experiencing sexual abuse or assault
- Witnessing violence, injury, or murder (among adolescents living in urban areas, between 50% and 96% have witnessed community violence) (Copeland-Linder et al., 2010)

Preventing Specific Psychiatric Disorders in Adolescence

The most frequently occurring psychiatric disorders among adolescents are depression, anxiety disorders, substance-related disorders, conduct disorder, schizophrenia, and suicide. The rate of psychiatric disorders differs between female and male adolescents. Most frequently occurring psychiatric disorders among female adolescents ages 14 to 17 years include simple phobias (17.9%); social phobia (social anxiety disorder) (11.7%); major depressive disorder (9.1%); dysthymia (5.9%); overanxious disorder (5.4%); and agoraphobia (4.4%). Most frequently occurring psychiatric disorders among male adolescents ages 14 to 17 years include CD (9.1%); social phobia (social anxiety disorder) (6.2%); simple phobias (4.1%); major depressive disorder (1.4%); and agoraphobia (1.4%) (Romano, Tremblay, Vitaro, et al., 2001).

Preventing Depression in Adolescence

Adolescents with depression describe their feelings as thinking about suicide; feeling as though nothing will work out; feeling sad most of the time; hating oneself; feeling alone; not feeling loved; and feeling like crying most of the time. Depression is experienced by 10% of girls and 7% of boys in grades 5 through 12. Among older adolescents (seniors in high school) who had been exposed to adversities—such as parents separating, parental unemployment, parental alcohol and drug abuse, and being the victim of physical abuse, sexual abuse, or both—the rate of depression was the same for boys and girls (Schilling, Aseltine, & Gore, 2007). One-half of all first episodes of depression occur during adolescence (Kessler, Chiu, Demler, et al., 2005b), and adolescent-onset major depressive disorder is associated with increased risk for suicide and for recurrence of depression in adulthood (Williams, O'Connor, Eder, et al., 2009). The effects of depression are seen in impairment of school, family, and social functioning; higher rates of early pregnancies; and diminished quality of life. Unfortunately, treatment for depression—psychotherapy and pharmacotherapy—has been found to be effective for only 50% to 60% of children and adolescents (March, Silva, Petrycki, et al., 2004).

Risk Factors

Similar to depression in childhood, one of the strongest risk factors for depression in adolescence is being the child of a depressed parent (Beardslee et al., 1998; Institute of Medicine, 1994). Other risk factors include dysfunctional parenting; conflicted family interactions; the adolescent's personality, temperament, cognitive vulnerabilities, and internal and external stress; negative life events; poor interpersonal relationships; poverty; and exposure to violence (Evans et al., 2005).

Preventive Interventions

Prevention of depression is focused on reducing the risk for developing the first episode of depression in order to (1) prevent the recurrence of episodes and (2) prevent the sequelae of depression—academic problems, impaired social functioning, substance abuse, and suicide (Evans et al., 2005). Preventive programs for adolescents are based on cognitive behavioral therapy and family education that targets risk factors and promotes resiliency (see Table 19-5).

Preventing Anxiety Disorders in Adolescence

Separation anxiety disorder and specific phobias, which are common in childhood, occur less frequently in adolescence, and panic disorder and agoraphobia, which are uncommon in childhood, increase in adolescence (Evans et al., 2005). Reports of prevalence of anxiety disorders in adolescents range from 12.4% among adolescents with a mean age of 16 years (Chen, Cohen, Johnson, et al., 2009) to 26.9% among adolescents and young adults (ages 14 years to 24 years) (Zimmermann, Wittchen, Hofler, et al., 2003). Frequently occurring anxiety disorders are phobias, social anxiety disorder, generalized anxiety disorder, panic attacks, and panic disorder with and without agoraphobia. Social anxiety disorder and panic disorder are predictors of alcohol problems among adolescents and young adults (Zimmermann et al.). The National Alliance on Mental Illness stated that anxiety disorders affect one in ten young adults and that the most frequently occurring include panic disorder, OCD, post-traumatic stress disorder, phobias, and generalized anxiety disorder (National Alliance on Mental Illness, 2002).

Risk Factors

Risk factors for the development of anxiety disorders include symptoms of anxiety; impaired functioning at home and at school; insecure attachment of ambivalent or disorganized type; parenting that is low in affection, rejecting, or controlling; smoking, alcohol, and drug use; exposure to trauma; and poor social support (Evans et al., 2005).

Preventive Interventions

Prevention of anxiety disorders includes the use of universal programs that target all adolescents, such as FRIENDS (Dadds et al., 1997), which is based on cognitive behavioral therapy principles. Children ages 10 to 13 years who were in the FRIENDS program reported less anxiety symptoms in comparison with those not in the program (see Table 19-1 for other programs).

Preventing Schizophrenia in Adolescents and Young Adults

The rate of onset of schizophrenia is highest during adolescence and early adulthood. However, indications of schizophrenia are evident very early in life and include difficulty in achieving age-appropriate developmental tasks and problems with attention and language (Weiser, Reichenberg, Rabinowitz, et al., 2001). Later, premorbid signs include cognitive, social, and academic problems (Evans et al., 2005). In adolescence or early adulthood, the symptoms progress to prodromal signs that include strange thoughts, odd perceptions, paranoia, and more severe social and academic problems. Prodromal symptoms of schizophrenia are discussed in Chapter 15.

Risk Factors

Risk for developing schizophrenia begins prenatally (Harvard Mental Health Letter, 2009). Risk factors specific for schizophrenia include genetic influences and the effect of exposure to adverse prenatal circumstances—deficits of nutrition and exposure to toxins, infections, and stress. Specific risk factors for schizophrenia are presented in Box 19-7.

Preventive Interventions

There is little information about preventive interventions for schizophrenia in the premorbid stage. Compton (2010b) suggested that prevention of schizophrenia should include universal preventive interventions, such as provision of prenatal care for all women; reduction of poverty, discrimination, and childhood maltreatment; and cessation of marijuana smoking in adolescence. Prevention has tended to be of the indicated type, focusing on preventing the prodromal stage from converting to the full syndrome of schizophrenia. Because antipsychotics reduce the symptoms of psychosis, it

BOX 19-7 Specific Risk Factors for the Development of Schizophrenia

- Genetic influence. Having one parent with schizophrenia conveys a risk of 5% to 15%, and having two parents with schizophrenia conveys a risk of 50% (Bromet & Fennig, 1999). However, 90% of patients with new onset of schizophrenia do not have a relative with schizophrenia (Brown & Faraone, 2004).
- Prenatal exposure to toxins (see Chapter 3).
- Obstetrical complications: malnutrition, hypoxia, or infection (Balloon, Dean, & Cadenhead, 2008; Pearce, 2001).
- Male gender: more frequent and more severe in males (Aleman, Kahn, & Selten, 2003).
- Older age of father (Brown, Schaefer, Wyatt, et al., 2002; Fisch, 2009; Malaspina, Harlap, Fennig, et al., 2001). There was a four times greater rate when the fathers were 50 years old or older than when fathers were 25 years old or younger. Malaspina et al. (2001) and Brown et al. (2002) suggested that the risk factor of advanced paternal age may be due to the fact that spermatocytes divide every 16 days. Thus, there is an ever-increasing opportunity for genetic mutations resulting from replication errors.
- Childhood sexual abuse. Approximately one-third of patients with schizophrenia experienced childhood sexual abuse (Lysaker, Meyer, Evans, et al., 2001).
- Cannabis use. Use of cannabis on a weekly or daily basis increases risk for psychotic disorders including schizophrenia by two to three times (Moore, Zammit, Lingford-Hughes, et al., 2007).
- Lower socioeconomic status. In industrial societies, an increased rate of schizophrenia is found among those in lower socioeconomic groups (Dohrenwend & Egri, 1981; Sadock & Sadock, 2007). Stresses associated with lower socioeconomic status may contribute to the development of schizophrenia (Sadock & Sadock, 2007).
- Urban living. An excess of patients with schizophrenia are born in cities in comparison to those born in rural areas (Marcelis, Navarro-Mateu, Murray, et al., 1998).
- Season of birth. Higher rates of schizophrenia are found among people born in late winter or early spring (Torrey, Bowler, Rawlings, et al., 1993). In the United States, people who develop schizophrenia are likely to have been born in the months from January through April (Sadock & Sadock, 2007). Maximal risk period is February and March, and minimal risk period is August and September (Mortensen, Pedersen, Westergaard, et al., 1999).

was hoped that administering antipsychotics before the syndrome developed might prevent schizophrenia. More recently, approaches to preventing conversion from the prodromal stage to the syndrome have included combinations of antipsychotic medications and psychotherapy; antipsychotics alone; cognitive therapy; antidepressants; psychosocial interventions; omega-3 fatty acids; and comprehensive programs.

- ***Antipsychotic medication plus cognitive therapy.*** A trial with the antipsychotic risperidone (Risperdal) and cognitive behavioral therapy was more effective in preventing conversion than usual case management during the initial 6-month period, but in the 6 months that followed it was no more effective than usual case management, perhaps because patients did not take the antipsychotic medication consistently (McGorry, Yung, Phillips, et al., 2002).
- ***Antipsychotic medication.*** A trial with olanzapine (Zyprexa) was no more effective than placebo (McGlashan, Zipursky, Perkins, et al., 2006).
- ***Cognitive therapy.*** Because patients in the prodromal stage of schizophrenia already have the problems with attention, memory, and social skills that patients with schizophrenia have, it was proposed that cognitive behavioral therapy might provide the coping skills that would prevent the progression to the full syndrome of schizophrenia. Cognitive therapy was associated with greater reduction of conversion than the control intervention and a greater reduction of psychiatric symptoms (Morrison, French, Walford, et al., 2004).
- ***Antidepressant medications.*** The use of antidepressants as a preventive intervention is based on the belief that they might improve mood and thinking ability and reduce stress. Early results have suggested that antidepressants are effective in preventing the progression to schizophrenia (Cornblatt, Lencz, Smith, et al., 2007).
- ***Psychosocial interventions.*** Family-targeted interventions, such as Family-Aided Assertive Community Treatment (FACT), and family education and crisis intervention groups that focus on reducing stress in young adults with prodromal symptoms of schizophrenia have been found to reduce symptoms, improve functioning, and reduce conversion (McFarlane, Cook, Downing, et al., 2010; McFarlane, Dushay, Stastny, et al., 1996). Supportive therapy has been found to be as effective as antipsychotic medication plus cognitive behavioral therapy or cognitive behavioral therapy alone in reducing conversion (Phillips, Nelson, Yuen, et al., 2009).
- ***Omega-3 fatty acids.*** Patients with schizophrenia have been found to have lower than normal levels of polyunsaturated fats (Horrobin, Al, & Vaddadi, 1994). Patients in the prodromal stage of schizophrenia who took omega-3 supplements had a much lower rate of progression to schizophrenia than those taking a placebo pill of coconut oil. They also experienced greater improvement of the positive and negative symptoms of schizophrenia and improved functioning (Amminger, Schafer, Papageorgiou, et al., 2010).

- ***Comprehensive programs with universal, selective, and targeted interventions,*** such as the *Portland Identification and Early Referral (PIER)* program. The PIER program reaches out to educate family practitioners, college health services, mental health clinicians, military bases and recruiters, clergy, emergency and crisis services, the general public, employers, schoolteachers, guidance counselors, school nurses, and pediatricians. It has four components: (1) education for professionals and the community, (2) clinical services (extensive assessment and psychosocial interventions), (3) pharmacological treatment, and (4) outreach (www.preventmentalillness.org/pier_home.html).
  1. The education component focuses on
     - Reducing stigma
     - Providing information about modern concepts of psychotic disorders
     - Increasing understanding of early stages of mental illnesses and prodromal symptoms
     - Describing how to get consultation, specialized assessments, and treatment quickly
     - Encouraging ongoing interprofessional collaborations
  2. In the clinical services component, clinical assessment includes the use of screening tools and instruments for assessing prodromal signs. The treatment component of the PIER program is described as family-aided assertive community treatment and includes
     - Rapid crisis-oriented initiation of treatment
     - Education: teaches families how to help their children deal with problems and stressors, adhere to treatment, and achieve scholastic or employment goals
     - Multifamily groups: focus is on practical, incremental problem-solving steps for each family
     - Supported employment and educational programs
     - Strengthening family relationships
     - Creating an optimal protective home environment
  3. The pharmacological component includes low-dose atypical antipsychotic medications, mood stabilizers, or antidepressants, as indicated by symptoms.
  4. The outreach component includes case management using key Assertive Community Treatment (ACT) methods (integrated treatment, multidisciplinary team, outreach as needed, rapid response, and continuous case review).

The rate of conversion of the prodromal stage to schizophrenia has dropped from an earlier rate of 40% to 50% to about 12% and appears to be continuing to decline. It is not known why the rate is dropping, but it may be due to earlier detection and treatment or more effective psychosocial interventions (Yung, Yuen, Berger, et al., 2007). However, although there has been a drop in conversion to schizophrenia, many patients with prodromal signs of psychosis develop psychiatric disorders other than schizophrenia, such as depression and anxiety disorders. Therefore, McGorry, Nelson, Amminger, et al. (2009) have recommended a conservative approach during the prodromal stage, offering safe interventions such as supportive therapy, cognitive behavioral therapy, or omega-3 therapy rather than antipsychotics.

Preventing Substance Abuse–Related Disorders in Adolescence

Underage drinking occurs as young as 10 to 12 years of age and occurs in approximately 18% of youths 12 to 17 years of age (Li, Witt, & Hewitt, 2007). Adolescent substance abuse is associated with unwanted pregnancy, juvenile delinquency, and school failure (Donaldson, Thomas, Graham, et al., 2000), and it predicts substance abuse and also depression in adulthood (Copeland et al., 2009a). Adolescent substance-related disorders are thought to be due to multiple factors, including the interaction of genetic vulnerability, parenting, and environmental influences, and the absence of protective factors (Evans et al., 2005).

Protective Factors

Protective factors include

- Feeling close to their parents
- Feeling that their parents care about them and love them
- Feeling that they are a part of their school
- Feeling that they are treated fairly by their teachers (Resnick, Bearman, Blum, et al., 1997)
- Succeeding in school
- Having strong bonds with pro-social institutions, such as religious organizations
- Living in a community that enforces responsible beverage services and availability to minors and that enforces drunk driving laws (Powers, 2010)

Risk Factors

Risk factors for adolescents' developing substance-related disorders are presented in Box 19-8.

Preventive Interventions

Preventative interventions can be universal, selective, indicated, or multilevel.

Universal Preventive Interventions

Universal preventive interventions are programs that are designed to reach all students and include the following:

- *Drug Abuse Resistance Education (DARE).* The early version of *DARE* was not found to be effective in reducing alcohol and drug use (Donaldson et al., 2000; Dukes, Ullman, & Stein, 1996; Ennent, Tobler, Ringwalt, et al., 1994; United States Department of Health and Human Services, 2001). A second version, *DARE Plus,* included parental involvement, youth-led activities, community adult action teams,

BOX 19-8 Risk Factors for Substance-Related Disorders in Adolescence

Risk Factors in the Adolescent

- Genetic vulnerability (Mayes & Suchman, 2006)
- Difficult temperament as an infant
- Friends who engage in the problem behavior
- Poor impulse control; sensation-seeking behaviors; negative emotionality; antisocial behavior; and early drug use (O'Connell et al., 2009)
- Alienation and rebelliousness
- Rejection by peers and association with substance-using peers (Mayes & Suchman, 2006)
- Victim of trauma, neglect, or abuse (Evans et al., 2005)
- Attention-deficit hyperactivity disorder, conduct disorder, or aggression problems (Powers, 2010)

Risk Factors in the Family

- Substance-abusing parents (Evans et al., 2005)
- Family conflict
- Family violence
- Crowded, noisy, and disorderly home
- Lack of rules or religion
- Parents who are absent from the home, separated, or divorced
- Poor parenting and lack of parental supervision (Powers, 2010)

Risk Factors in School

- School problems or academic failure (Hawkins, Catalano, & Miller, 1992)
- Lack of commitment to school

Risk Factors in the Community

- Extreme economic deprivation
- Living in a dangerous, drug-using community

and postcard mailings to parents. The *DARE Plus* program was associated with a reduction of alcohol, tobacco, and multidrug use among boys but not among girls (Perry, Komro, Veblen-Mortenson, et al., 2003).

- *Life Skills Training Program* (Botvin, Baker, Dusenbury, et al., 1995). The Life Skills Training Program focuses on teaching drug-resistance skills, self-management skills, and general social skills in junior high school. The program is associated with reduced drug experimentation among the students (Evans et al., 2005).
- *Strengthening Families Program: For Parents and Youth 10-14 (SFP 10-14).* SFP 10-14 is a family-focused universal preventive intervention that has been found to be effective (Evans et al., 2005).
- *Project STAR (Students Taught Awareness and Resistance)* (Pentz, Dwyer, MacKinnon, et al., 1989). *Project STAR* involves parents and the community and has been effective in reducing drug use behavior in high school among youths who were in the program in junior high (Evans et al., 2005). There was 30% less use of marijuana, 25% less use of tobacco, and 20% less use of alcohol. The strongest preventive factor was the perception of friends' intolerance to drug use (see Table 19-1 for description of several programs).

Selective Preventative Interventions

Selective preventative interventions are designed to target adolescents at risk, such as those with school problems or those who have parents with substance-related problems. Examples of selective preventive interventions are as follows:

- *Strengthening Families Program* (Kumpfer & Alvardo, 1995), which focuses on parent training to reduce substance abuse; child skills training to decrease socially unacceptable behavior; and family skills training to improve the family environment. Outcomes include reduction of family conflict and youth conduct problems, aggression, and substance use, and improvement of family functioning (Kumpfer, Molraard, & Spoth, 1996).
- *Focus on Families Program* (Catalano, Gainey, Fleming, et al., 1999), which is for parents receiving methadone maintenance. Parents are taught parenting skills and family management skills.

Indicated Preventive Interventions

Indicated preventive interventions are targeted toward adolescents already experimenting with drugs or other risky behaviors or who are in danger of dropping out of school. Examples include

- *Reconnecting Youths Program* (Eggert, Thompson, Herting, et al., 1995), which focuses on enhancing self-esteem, decision making, and personal control; building interpersonal communication skills; school bonding; social activities; and suicide prevention. Outcomes include better school performance, less involvement with drugs, increased school bonding and social support, and improvement of aggression, anger, depression, hopelessness, stress, and suicidal behavior (Eggert et al.).
- *Gatehouse Project* (Bond, Patton, Glover, et al., 2004) for youths ages 13-14 years, which has as a goal to reduce involvement with drugs. Outcomes included a reduction of drinking and smoking but no significant change in depressive symptoms or improvement of social and school relationships (Bond et al.).

Multilevel Intervention Programs

Multilevel intervention programs include components of universal, selective, and indicated preventive programs. One such program is the ecological approach to family intervention and treatment, *EcoFIT,* which targets risk factors such as problem behaviors in school, substance use, deviant peer affiliations, and family management deficits (Dishion & Stormshak, 2007). The intervention is school based, family centered, and culturally sensitive. It is tailored to fit the young person's and the family's circumstances and the family's level of skill in limit setting, parental monitoring, and communicating. The key feature of the program is the intervention "Family Check-Up," which asks parents to identify their concerns, their goals, and their motivation to change (Shaw, Dishion, Supplee, et al., 2006). It includes an assessment and provides information about intervention options that are available to meet the needs of the family and to help the family achieve its goals. Intervention options include skill building, parental management training, using positive reinforcement, limit setting, monitoring, problem-solving, and building communication skills. The program also provides brief interventions during times of transitions that may increase the risk of behavioral problems, academic failure, and drug use. In 11th grade, in comparison to students not enrolled in the EcoFIT program, students who had been enrolled in the program were six times less likely to have been arrested; five times less likely to use marijuana; and nearly three times less likely to have been absent from school (Stormshak & Dishion, 2009).

Preventing Suicide in Adolescence

Suicide is the third leading cause of death among adolescents in the United States (Heron, 2007), following accidents and homicide (MacManus, 2002). The suicide rate among American adolescents is higher than rates for adolescents in other industrialized countries, and it is increasing in the 15- to 24-year-old age group (MacManus). At the present time, adolescent suicide is the driving force behind increases in the overall suicide rate in the United States. There had been a decrease in suicide in U.S. youth from 1990 until 2003 that may have been related to more frequent treatment of depression with medication, reduction of alcohol use, and tighter gun control laws (Pirruccello, 2010). Between 2003 and 2004, the suicide rate among U.S. youth increased by 18% (Hamilton, Minino, Martin, et al., 2007). Possible reasons include higher rates of untreated depression related to black box warnings on antidepressants; increased participation in Internet social networks; and suicide among young people in the military (Cash & Bridge, 2009). Black and Andreasen (2010) suggested that the changing social norms regarding use of drugs and sexual activity, the increased use of mood-altering drugs, the disruption of family (divorce and remarriage), and media influences are contributing to the increase. It has also become easier to get the means for committing suicide, such as handguns and pills for self-poisoning (Cash & Bridge).

In a study of youths in grades 9 through 12, 14.5% reported having ideas of suicide; 11.3% made a suicide plan; and 6.9% had made at least one suicide attempt (Cash & Bridge, 2009; Eaton, Kann, Kinchen, et al., 2008). Among older high school students, 20% have considered suicide in the previous 12 months. They have often experienced recent stressful family events, such as divorce, moving, unemployment, or death of a parent. Other stressful events in their lives include having trouble with a girlfriend or boyfriend; problems with academic achievement; pregnancy; alcohol or substance use; and trouble getting along with parents. However, 80% to 90% of teenagers who die by suicide have a diagnosable mental illness, with depression, anxiety disorders, CD, and substance-related disorders being the most frequently occurring psychiatric disorders (Bridge, Goldstein, & Brent, 2006).

Protective Factors

Factors that have been identified as protective against suicide may be indicators of mental health and not specifically protective against suicide (Evans et al., 2005). Factors that are associated with a reduced incidence of suicidal behaviors are presented in Box 19-9.

Populations at Risk

Adolescent females are three times more likely than males to attempt suicide, and adolescent males are four times more likely to commit suicide. In the United States, the highest rates of attempted and completed adolescent suicide are among Native Americans.

Levels of Risk: Ideators, Attempters, and Completers

Suicidal thoughts are an indicator of adolescent psychopathology. Among adolescents, 15% to 20% think about suicide. Among those who attempt suicide, 88% report prior suicidal thoughts. Thus, only about 12% of attempted suicides occur unexpectedly. Those who attempt suicide are at a higher risk of committing suicide than those who just think about suicide (attempters go on to commit suicide about 14% of the time). Attempters have higher rates of risk factors, such as psychopathology, adjustment problems, and family problems. They are twice as likely to report depression, to use alcohol, and to run away from home. They often use over-the-counter drugs to attempt suicide and may make the attempt when they know that a loved one will find them. In adolescents, the act of suicide is usually associated with

BOX 19-9 Factors Associated With Reduced Incidence of Suicide in Adolescence

- Student's connectedness to school (Resnick et al., 1997)
- Academic achievement (Resnick et al., 1997)
- Social skills, problem-solving skills, and decision-making skills (Jessor, 1991)
- Cohesive families (Resnick et al., 1997)
- Emotionally involved, supportive families (McKeown, Garrison, Cuffe, et al., 1998)
- Parental expectations of high academic achievement and appropriate behavior (Borowsky, Ireland, & Resnick, 2001)
- Religious beliefs (Greening & Stoppelbein, 2002)
- Restriction of availability of lethal agents: Keeping guns locked and unloaded and storing ammunition in a separate place reduces risk of use of firearms (Grossman, Mueller, Riedy, et al., 2005)

feelings of hopelessness and worthlessness and may occur in the first episode of a mental illness, as self-punishment, or in response to parental fighting.

Risk Factors.

Risk factors for suicide are listed in Box 19-10. Indicators that suicide is imminent include the following:

- Preoccupation with suicide or death
- Verbal hints or statements suggesting hopelessness, despair, or imminent departure
- Complaints of being "rotten inside"
- Giving away favorite possessions
- Cleaning room, putting affairs in order
- Sudden cheerfulness following depression (Granello & Granello, 2007)

Preventive Interventions

Preventative interventions include those that are general and could be provided by parents, caregivers, educators, and community members and those that are more likely to be implemented by psychiatric advanced practice nurses.

General preventive interventions include

- Reassuring adolescents that they are loved and, no matter how awful they think a situation is, it can be worked out and you will help or get help
- Using peer-group interventions (break the "code of silence" of classmates)
- Improving adolescents' coping and problem-solving
- Restricting access to guns. Guns are the primary suicide weapons for adolescents: 64.9% of suicides in children, adolescents, and young adults were accomplished using guns.
- Restricting access to other suicide tools, such as pills, knives, and ropes
- Restricting access to information. Sensationalistic accounts of teen suicide apparently lead to copycat attempts. Media coverage leads to "cluster effect" of adolescent suicide (Garland & Zigler, 1993).

BOX 19-10 Risk Factors for Suicide in Adolescence

Key Risk Factors (Gould, Greenberg, Velting, et al., 2003)

- Presence of a psychiatric disorder, such as depression or disruptive behavior disorder. Combination of depression and anxiety or depression and oppositional defiant disorder increases risk of suicide (Foley et al., 2006; Gould et al., 2003).
- Maltreatment. Physical and sexual abuse increase risk for suicidal behaviors. Sexual abuse has greater effect than physical abuse (Cash & Bridge, 2009).
- Stressful events—separations, loss of a parent, and being incarcerated (Ash, 2008).
- Family history of suicide and psychiatric disorders (Gould et al., 2003; Spirito & Esposito-Smythers, 2006).
- Availability of lethal agents. Firearms in the house increase risk of suicide for adolescents with suicidal ideation (Bridge et al., 2006)

Other Risk Factors

- Presence of health-risk behaviors: binge eating, binge drinking, weapon carrying, and having unprotected sex (Bridge et al., 2006).
- Current cigarette smoking: associated with increased risk for feeling sad and hopeless, considering suicide, planning suicide, attempting suicide, and requiring medical treatment for suicide attempt (Jiang, Perry, & Hesser, 2010).
- Substance abuse (Chatterji, Dave, Kaestner, et al., 2004; Dunn, Goodrow, Givens, et al., 2008).
- Sleep disturbances: increasing problems with insomnia or hypersomnia (Goldstein, Bridge, & Brent, 2008).
- Self-perception of being overweight (Eaton, Lowry, Brener, et al., 2005); associated with feeling sad and hopeless, considering suicide, and planning suicide, but not with attempting suicide (Jiang et al., 2010).
- Sexual orientation (Clements-Nolle, Marx, & Katz, 2006). Lesbian/gay/bisexual/unsure orientations were associated with feeling sad and hopeless, considering suicide, planning suicide, attempting suicide, and requiring medical treatment for suicide attempt (Jiang et al., 2010).
- Low academic achievement. Having Cs and Ds was associated with feeling sad and hopeless and considering suicide, and having Ds and Fs was associated with planning suicide (Jiang et al., 2010).
- Being pregnant and not knowing how to cope (Preventing Teen Suicide, n.d.).
- Having a friend who attempted or completed suicide (Steele & Doey, 2007).
- Frequent change of residence. Youths who had moved 10 times were 3.3 times more likely to attempt suicide (Qin, Mortensen, & Pedersen, 2009).
- Bullying; associated with increased risk of suicidal behaviors for both boys and girls, but girls have higher rates of suicidal behaviors (Barker, Arseneault, Brendgen, et al., 2008).
- Disconnection from family, school, and community; dropping out of school or living apart from family (Bridge et al., 2006).
- Family discord (Bridge et al., 2006).
- Immigrant status. Not speaking English at home is associated with feeling sad and hopeless, considering suicide, planning suicide, attempting suicide, and requiring medical treatment for suicide attempt (Jiang et al., 2010).
- Feeling unsafe to go to school: associated with feeling sad and hopeless, considering suicide, and planning suicide but not with attempting suicide (Jiang et al., 2010).

Interventions implemented by psychiatric advanced practice nurses include

- Providing an immediate psychiatric assessment of adolescents expressing suicidal intent
- Identifying and treating psychiatric disorders, including alcohol- and drug-related disorders
- Increasing suicide awareness training for primary health-care providers
- Increasing family and adult suicide education
- Increasing public awareness
- Increasing access to services

Preventive Interventions

Based on knowledge of threats, protective factors, and risk factors in adolescence, preventive interventions should offer multicomponent programs that target multiple risk factors and promote protective factors. A list of suicide prevention intervention programs can be found in Table 19-6.

A recent intervention, the *Community Suicide Prevention Project,* was developed by nurses to prevent adolescent suicide in a rural community that had seen an increase in suicide among its adolescents. The goals of the program were to eliminate adolescent suicide in the community (to have no adolescent suicides recorded in the annual coroner's report); improve collaboration among community agencies; increase community awareness of factors associated with risk or high risk for suicide; and increase awareness about available crisis help and referral resources (Pirruccello, 2010). The project had three components:

1. A wallet-size card that was developed and given to all high school students. It had three 24/7 crisis phone numbers:
   - Services offering support for substance abuse, mental health issues, homelessness, and runaways
   - Sexual assault crisis intervention
   - Unplanned pregnancy help

   At the bottom of the card was written, "Remember prayer and your spiritual community" (Pirruccelo, 2010, p. 38).
2. A local resource brochure that provided information about services, including physical and mental health care services, social services, substance abuse treatment, sexual assault and physical abuse help, homeless shelters, employment and transportation services, and leisure activities.
3. Community education about risk and protective factors for suicide that was made available to students, parents, teachers, community members, and other professionals.

Students found the card useful and easy to carry. They liked having the referral numbers easily available. At the end of a year, the coroner's report listed no adolescent suicides.

Risks and Prevention Opportunities in Adulthood

Protective Factors and Risk Factors in Adulthood

Protective factors and risk factors for each of the major psychiatric disorders are described in Chapters 9 through 18 (which are devoted to specific disorders).

Protective Factors

Other factors that have been identified as being present among individuals who have not developed psychiatric disorders in adulthood can be considered to be protective. These protective factors are summarized in Box 19-11.

TABLE 19-6 SUICIDE PREVENTIVE INTERVENTION PROGRAMS

Intervention	Goals	Characteristics	Outcomes
All Stars (SAMHSA's National Registry of Evidence-based Programs and Practices, 2007)	Prevent and delay onset of high-risk behaviors, such as drug use, violence, and premature sexual activity	Multiyear school-based program for middle school students (ages 11 to 14 years) Fosters pro-social attitudes and attachment to school	Program had impact on perceptions of high-risk behaviors but not on behaviors (Harrington, Giles, Hoyle, et al., 2001)
Personal Growth Class (PGC) (Thompson, Eggert, & Herting, 2000)	Reduce depression, suicide, drug involvement, and dropping out of school	Life skills training; teacher and peer support; goal setting; and monitoring mood, school performance, and drug involvement	Decrease in suicide behaviors and depression
CARE (Care, assess, respond, empower) (Thompson, Eggert, Randell, et al., 2001)	Reduce depression, anger, and suicide risk	High school–based suicide prevention program; components of PGC program with added one-on-one with counselors and skills building	Decrease in suicide behaviors and depression Improved coping and problem-solving
Dialectical Behavioral Therapy (DBT) (Linehan, Armstrong, Suarez, et al., 1991)	Reduce suicidal and self-injurious behaviors associated with borderline personality disorder Intermediate goal is to increase ability to tolerate distress	A comprehensive treatment based on cognitive and behavioral principles that includes mindfulness strategies	Decrease of suicide and self-harm behaviors (Linehan et al., 1991)

BOX 19-11 Factors Associated With Nondevelopment of Psychiatric Disorders in Adulthood

- Few adverse life events (Wilhelm, Wedgwood, Parker, et al., 2010)
- Strong social support (Huppert & Whittington, 2003)
- High self-esteem; self-esteem is related to a sense of being included or excluded and is inversely related to loneliness (Wilhelm et al., 2010)
- Not being critical of self when life goals were not met (Wilhelm et al., 2010)
- Optimism (Fredrickson, Tugade, Waugh, et al., 2003; Vaillant, 2003)
- Satisfaction with work situation (Wilhelm et al., 2010)
- Having social roles (Huppert & Whittington, 2003)
- Problem-solving skills (Dumont & Provost, 1999)
- Resilience; resilience is protective against the stress associated with adverse events (Goldstein & Brooks, 2006).
- Presence of low neuroticism (prone to worry, nervous, high-strung), high extroversion, and openness to new experiences (Fredrickson et al., 2003; Hettema, Neale, Myers, et al., 2006; Jorm, Christensen, Henderson, et al., 2000).

Five broad categories of protective factors that are amenable to modification are conscientiousness, stress management, social support, religion and spirituality, and resilience.

Conscientiousness

The personality trait of conscientiousness encompasses being able to control impulses, being goal oriented, and being dependable. It has been found to be associated with reduced risk for developing mental and physical disorders among adults in the general population (Goodwin & Friedman, 2006). Conscientiousness is shaped by genetic influences and also by experience. It is a trait that psychiatric advanced practice nurses can encourage parents to foster in their children because it will serve them as a protective factor against the development of medical illnesses and psychiatric disorders in adulthood. Conscientiousness can be promoted through the following activities:

- Building strong and positive family bonds
- Providing parental monitoring of children's activities and peers
- Having clear rules of conduct that are consistently enforced within the family
- Being involved in the lives of their children
- Developing strong ties with schools and religious organizations
- Adopting conventional norms about non-drug use

Stress Management

Each individual's response to stress is modulated by genetic influences and environmental factors (Duhault, 2002) and is achieved through the process of brain plasticity. Brain plasticity, which is activated by stress-producing experiences and events, is also activated by stress management interventions (McEwen, 2007, 2009). Esch and Stefano (2010) said that when a stress reduction strategy is effective, increased activity of the reward system in the limbic area of the brain makes the individual feel good and reinforces the behavior that brought about the good feeling.

Across the life span, individuals are constantly exposed to social and environmental experiences that are processed by the brain. Brain plasticity allows the brain to change its structure and functioning in response to its determination of experiences as a threat (and thus stressful) or not a threat (and thus nonstressful). The acute stress response promotes adaptation by activating systems involved in survival—the central nervous system, cardiovascular system, autonomic system, and immune system (see Chapter 9 for more information on the stress response). However, there are stressors or accumulation of stressors that exceed an individual's ability to adapt. Cumulative stressors have a chronic adverse effect on health owing to the body's failure to adapt. Failure to adapt results in prolonged activation of the hypothalamic-pituitary-adrenal axis, which is associated with depression and other psychopathology. Excessive or prolonged exposure to stress has an adverse effect across the life span on the development of the brain and also on brain functioning, on maintenance of brain structures, and on cognition, emotions, and behavior (Lupien, McEwen, Gunnar, et al., 2009).

Chronic or prolonged stress may result in behaviors that are designed to reduce the continuing sensation of stress (frustration and anxiety) such as smoking, overeating or eating comforting foods, drinking alcohol, reducing physical exercise, and curtailing social activities (McEwen, 2008). These changes in behavior may interact with genetic vulnerability and result in an increase of health problems and psychiatric disorders. Among adults, the most common chronic stressors are those related to work overload, job strain, problems in the workplace and living situation, life losses, transitions or crises, extremely demanding professional or educational responsibilities, economic insecurity, and the emphasis on acquisition of material goods as the mark of success and happiness (Duhault, 2002; Flannery, 2004).

Stress management consists of the use of activities that Esch and Stefano (2010, p. 22) have identified as being effective in managing stress:

- Behaviors: pleasurable activities, social interactions, social support, friendship, love, healthy communication, arts and creativity, cognitive behavioral therapy, and motivational and positive psychology
- Exercise: aerobic and anaerobic physical activity
- Relaxation: meditation, spirituality/belief, and sleep hygiene
- Nutrition: a healthy diet, including supplements if indicated

Stress management also involves accessing and using social support, religion, spirituality, meditation, and resilience. Interventions include the use of home visitors, neighbors, religious institutions, ready-made companions such as provided by Befriending (Andrews, Gavin, & Begley, 2003), mentors, support groups, and parish nurses (Gottlieb, 2000; Hosman et al., 2005) (see Chapter 8 for discussion of psychosocial interventions).

Social Support

Loneliness, often associated with social isolation and lack of social support, has been found to be associated with increased stress as manifested in sleep problems and elevated levels of morning cortisol, the stress hormone (Steptoe, Owen, Kunz-Ebrecht, et al., 2004; Steptoe, Wardlaw, & Marmot, 2005), and with depression (Cattan, White, Bond, et al., 2005). Social support interventions associated with reduction of loneliness and social isolation include discussion groups, group activities that combined health education with exercise, group social activation interventions, and ongoing self-help groups. Direct support provided in the home or by telephone and problem-solving therapy was not effective (Cattan et al., 2005). It is known that social support buffers the effect of stress (Spiegel, 1999) and that social support reduces depression and suicidal behaviors (Dervic, Oquendo, Grunebaum, et al., 2004). However, social support that is limited to one source, such as a family member, is less effective in reducing stress than social support coming from several sources; having three or more regular social contacts has been found to be associated with lower levels of stress (Seeman, Singer, Ryff, et al., 2002). Prevention of psychiatric disorders includes building or restructuring social support networks in order to improve the quantity, quality, and suitability of support that will buffer stress; promote healthy behaviors, optimal functioning, and well-being; and reduce loneliness and social isolation.

Religion and Spirituality

People often use religion and spirituality to cope with stress. Ninety percent of the world population is involved in some form of religious or spiritual practice (Barrett, Kurian, & Johnson, 2001). Among individuals hospitalized with medical illnesses, 90% said that they used religion to cope (Koenig, 1998), and among patients with severe mental illness, 80% said that they used religion to cope (Tepper, Rogers, Coleman, et al., 2001). Religion involves beliefs, practices, and rituals related to something that is held sacred—God, Religious Traditions, Ultimate Truth, or Reality (Koenig, 2009). Religion is an established tradition of a group of people with the same beliefs and who follow the same practices in relation to what they believe is sacred. Religions often have beliefs about life after death and rules that guide behaviors within a group. Spirituality is sometimes defined as having the spirit of God; or more frequently, it is something that individuals define for themselves. It does not have rules, regulations, responsibilities, or rituals. It is sometimes accepted as including a meaning or purpose in life, connectedness with others, acceptance of a higher power, peacefulness, and well-being (Baetz, Bowen, Jones, et al., 2006; Koenig, 2009).

Religion is a powerful coping strategy that enables individuals to deal with suffering and stress. Religion provides a sense of meaning and purpose to life during difficult times. It promotes behaviors that facilitate getting along with people and providing mutual support, and it reduces isolation and loneliness (Koenig, 2009). It has been found that there are lower rates of depression among individuals who are religious and lower rates of suicide attempts (Dervic et al., 2004).

Religious beliefs can also comfort individuals who are experiencing anxiety by increasing their sense of security and self-confidence or confidence in what they hold sacred. For example, among patients with schizophrenia, who often experience high levels of anxiety, nondelusional religiosity such as regular church attendance has been found to be associated with improved outcomes. Overall, religious involvement has been found to be related to better coping with stress and less depression, anxiety, substance abuse, and suicide (Koenig, 2009).

Resilience

Resilience implies that the individual has the capacity both to endure stressful events without adverse reactions and to go on to develop improved functioning (McEwen, 2009; New, Keegan, & Charney, 2007; Wagnild & Collings, 2009). Resilience is an innate attribute of individuals, but it also involves behaviors, thoughts, and actions that can be learned and developed. Strategies for building resilience include fostering self-efficacy, increasing ability to realistically appraise situations, improving social problem-solving skills, and developing a sense of direction in life, e.g., talents, dreams, spirituality, or religious faith (Edward, 2005; Kaplan, Turner, Norman, et al., 1996; Shenfeld, 2007).

Risk Factors

Risk factors that are associated with many major psychiatric disorders include

- Female gender
- Family history of psychopathology
- History of childhood abuse (physical abuse increases the risk of adult depression three times, and sexual abuse increases the risk of depression four times)
- Comorbid medical illnesses
- Lack of social support
- Active alcohol or substance abuse
- Lower socioeconomic status
- Lower educational achievement
- Stressful life events that cause a sense of loss, humiliation, diminished self-esteem, or feelings of entrapment
- History of family conflict, discord, or violence (Paradis, Reinherz, Giaconia, et al., 2009)

Preventing Specific Psychiatric Disorders in Adulthood

Prevention of psychiatric disorders in adulthood is hampered by established vulnerabilities related to childhood exposure to maltreatment and other adversities; difficulty in changing behavior and lifestyle as individuals age; and the tendency both to focus on the adult's thinking and behaviors as the main health risk factor for developing psychiatric disorders and to ignore the fact that the risk factors may have occurred very early in life (Shonkoff et al., 2009). Preventive interventions for psychiatric disorders in adulthood have traditionally focused on

- Indicated preventive interventions, such as early identification of symptoms and treatment
- Universal preventive interventions that encourage health-promoting activities, such as healthy diet, exercise, and sufficient sleep
- Cessation of risk-generating behaviors, such as smoking, excessive alcohol consumption, and use of illicit drugs (Shonkoff et al., 2009)

Preventing Anxiety Disorders in Adulthood

In the past, critical incident stress debriefing was used immediately after exposure to a stressful event, such as a shooting or a disaster. The debriefing process encouraged the individual exposed to the traumatic event to recall, describe, and rework the trauma within 24 to 72 hours of the event. It was thought that debriefing would reduce the risk for developing an anxiety disorder. Not only has it been found to be ineffective (Rose, Bisson, & Wessely, 2003), but it is now known that debriefing can have adverse effects (Mayou, Ehlers, & Hobbs, 2000).

Using cognitive behavioral therapy as an early intervention reduces the risk of developing post-traumatic stress disorder from 67% to 15% (Bryant, Harvey, Dang, et al., 1998; Bryant, Sackville, Dang, et al., 1999). Another preventive intervention focuses on preventing the consolidation of traumatic memories. The emotional impact associated with memories causes the release of neurotransmitters such as norepinephrine and cortisol, which consolidate and strengthen the memories. Blocking these neurotransmitters produces the opposite effect. A beta-adrenergic receptor blocker, such as propranolol, has been found to block the memory-enhancing effect of norepinephrine and cortisol (Cahill, Prins, Weber, et al., 1994) and is being used after traumatic events to reduce the patient's risk of developing post-traumatic stress disorder (Pitman & Delahanty, 2007). Other preventive interventions include reducing stress by teaching stress management and problem-solving strategies; cognitive restructuring and reframing of the stressor; and enhancing self-regulation of thinking, emotions, and behaviors in response to stressors (see Chapter 8 for a discussion of stress management).

Preventing Depression in Adulthood

Evidence that the rate of depression is increasing among children, adolescents, and adults (Achenbach, Dumenci, & Rescorla, 2003; Kessler et al., 2005a) supports the urgent need to prevent depression across the life span. Research on prevention of depression through the use of interventions that focus on cognitive factors and social problem-solving skills has shown inconsistent results. Overall, these interventions appear to be ineffective in preventing depression (Flannery-Schroeder, 2006).

Reducing Anxiety to Prevent Depression

Because anxiety and depression share similar biological, genetic, and psychological vulnerability factors, some researchers believe that anxiety is the prodromal stage of depression and that treating anxiety may prevent depression (Flannery-Schroeder, 2006; Krueger, 1999). In one study, patients who received treatment for an anxiety disorder (specifically, panic disorder) had half the rate of developing depression of those who did not receive treatment for the anxiety disorder (Goodwin & Olfson, 2001). Similarly, ongoing untreated social anxiety disorder has been found to be associated with higher rates of depression, whereas treated social anxiety that was in remission was not associated with higher rates of depression. In 1999, Kessler, Stang, Wittchen, et al. reported that early interventions for social anxiety disorder reduced the rate of developing depressive disorders by 10%. Now it is believed that treating childhood anxiety disorders has the potential to prevent adult anxiety disorders, depression, and substance abuse disorders (Emslie, 2008).

Selective Preventive Intervention for Postpartum Depression

Risk factors associated with the development of postpartum depression include a stressful life, marital conflict, maternal low self-esteem, and lack of social support. Based on that information, selective preventive interventions are directed at either the risk factors or the mechanisms through which the risk factors increase the likelihood of the patient's developing postpartum depression. Preventive interventions—such as antenatal and postnatal classes; early postpartum follow-up; home visits by professionals and nonprofessionals; debriefing before discharge that focuses on labor, birth, and experiences after delivery; and interpersonal psychotherapy—have not demonstrated consistent efficacy (Dennis, 2005). The only intervention to consistently show a preventive effect was intensive postpartum support provided by a health-care professional. For example, home visits by nurses were protective during the first 6 weeks, but the benefit did not last beyond 16 weeks, at which time the visits were reduced to monthly visits (Dennis).

Other researchers have reported a decrease in depressive symptoms among women at risk for developing postpartum depression using other preventive interventions. In England, a group intervention, *Preparation for Parenthood,* was found to be associated with lower levels of depressive symptoms postpartum than standard care (Elliot, Leverton, Sanjack, et al., 2000). In France, a 1-hour preventive intervention for women at increased risk for developing postpartum depression that was provided during the second or third day postpartum was associated with a reduction of depressive symptoms in comparison to a control group. The preventive intervention included

1. Education about normal infant development and problems
2. Support for the mothers to talk about their negative feelings
3. Interpretation of ambivalence as normal
4. A cognitive behavioral component that focused on problem-solving skills and on reducing the expectation of needing to be a perfect mother (Chabrol, Teissedre, Saint-Jean, et al., 2002)

In a recent Australian study of prenatal preventive interventions, women were assessed for risk for symptoms of depression and for risk of developing postpartum depression using structured instruments. Among those who had been identified as having mild symptoms of depression or of being at risk for developing postpartum depression, one group was randomly assigned to receive cognitive behavioral group therapy and the other group to receive an information booklet. Both the cognitive behavioral therapy intervention—which focused on prevention and management of stress, education about the needs and behaviors of newborn infants, relaxation training, goal setting, problem-solving, assertiveness training, and information about developing a social support network—and the information-booklet intervention were associated with a reduction of symptoms of depression and anxiety in the perinatal period. The two interventions were equally effective (Austin, Frillingos, Lumley, et al., 2008).

It should be noted that these preventive interventions were provided in countries with government-provided health care, so participation of at-risk mothers was not limited by financial constraints. Although these three successful interventions provided different amounts of education, cognitive behavioral therapy, and supportive therapy, they all influenced one of the risk factors for the development of postpartum depression: limited social networks. The interventions increased the participants' social networks through the assessment process, the interventions, and the follow-up evaluation process.

Indicated Prevention for Depression

Short-term psychotherapy that targets individuals with subsyndromal depressive symptoms (symptoms that do not meet the full criteria for depressive disorder) has been found to reduce the incidence of depression by 30% (Cuijpers et al., 2005). Other therapeutic interventions that have been found to be effective in reducing the incidence of depression are bibliotherapy (Cuijpers, 1997) and the use of a self-help manual that teaches individuals how to cope with depression (Cuijpers, 1998). There are also low-cost computerized interventions that have been proven to be effective (Christensen, Griffiths, & Jorm, 2004; McCrone, Knapp, Proudfoot, et al., 2004). Indicated prevention has the potential to prevent the development of depression, but it requires that patients be identified by screening for risk factors and early signs of depression.

Psychosocial Interventions to Prevent Depression

Psychosocial interventions that have been found to be associated with reduced risk of developing depression include

- Teaching stress management
- Enhancing social support
- Promoting resilience
- Teaching self-regulation
- Maintaining consistent amounts of sleeping hours, waking hours, eating, socializing, physical activity, and mental activity (Edward, 2005)
- Promoting daily reward experiences. Patients who were able to generate multiple positive emotions throughout the day from pleasant events, such as talking with friends or watching a movie, reduced their depressive symptoms (Geschwind, Peeters, Jacobs, et al., 2010) (see Chapter 8 for discussion of psychosocial interventions).

In summary, based on their meta-analytic review of interventions to prevent depression, Cuijpers, van Straten, Smit, et al. (2008) concluded that preventive interventions could reduce the incidence of depressive disorders by 22%. They found evidence that universal interventions were less effective than either (1) selective interventions that focused on individuals at risk for developing depression or (2) targeted interventions that focused on individuals with early symptoms of the disorder. Selective interventions and targeted interventions demonstrated equal effectiveness.

Preventing Schizophrenia in Adulthood

Two levels of prevention—universal, which targets the whole population, and indicated, which targets individuals at risk for developing schizophrenia—have been proposed for reducing the incidence of schizophrenia (Mojtabai et al., 2003).

Universal prevention includes interventions that focus on reducing risk factors associated with the development of schizophrenia:

- Maternal infections (use of vaccinations for measles, mumps, and rubella to prevent infections during pregnancy)
- Prenatal malnutrition (optimal nutrition and multivitamins during pregnancy)

- Prenatal exposure to toxins (avoidance of toxins)
- Maternal physical and mental health problems and stress
- Adverse circumstances of birth
- Childhood head injuries
- Cannabis use in adolescents and young adulthood (Compton, 2010b)

There are no studies of the use of universal prevention to reduce the incidence of schizophrenia (Mojtabai et al., 2003).

Indicated preventive interventions have been found to be effective in reducing the incidence of schizophrenia in high-risk individuals. For example, high-risk individuals who received an intervention consisting of (1) supportive psychotherapy that focused on social relationships, work issues, and family concerns; (2) case management; (3) cognitive behavioral therapy that focused on learning how to control symptoms and reduce distress; and (4) a low-dose antipsychotic medication had lower rates of developing schizophrenia than high-risk individuals who received supportive psychotherapy and case management but did not receive antipsychotic medication or cognitive behavioral therapy (McGorry et al., 2002).

Preventing Personality Disorders in Adulthood

Personality disorders reflect maladaptive, rigid traits and behaviors that are derived from the interaction of genetically influenced temperaments with adverse, stressful, or non-supportive life experiences (Oldham, 2009). Personality disorders occur among approximately 10% to 16% of the general population (Black & Andreasen, 2010). They are associated with great distress for patients and their families; delayed recovery from medical illnesses and psychiatric disorders; and high use of medical services and community services (police, jails, homeless shelters, and courts).

Protective Factors

Factors that promote the development of *adaptive* personality traits rather than *maladaptive* personality traits include family warmth and affection; support from outside the family (teachers, godparents, friends, and mentors); participation in community activities, sports, and hobbies; social skills; and resiliency.

Risk Factors

The genetic influence and other risk factors vary among the ten personality disorders (antisocial personality disorder, avoidant personality disorder, borderline personality disorder, dependent personality disorder, histrionic personality disorder, narcissistic personality disorder, obsessive-compulsive personality disorder, paranoid personality disorder, schizoid personality disorder, and schizotypal personality disorder) and are presented in Chapter 18. In general, patients with personality disorders have often experienced childhood maltreatment—emotional and physical neglect and emotional, physical, and sexual abuse—that is associated with long-term neurobiological and neuroendocrine alterations and later impairment of ability to self-regulate responses. Parenting may have lacked warmth and affection and discipline may have been harsh. Patients with personality disorders have high rates of other adversities: parental death, parental separation or divorce, poverty, assault, or bullying (Johnson, Bromley, & McGeoch, 2009).

Preventive Interventions

There are no studies of preventive interventions. Johnson et al. (2009) suggested that clinicians promote the development of adaptive personality traits during childhood and adolescence and assist parents in developing supportive relationships with their children.

Preventing Substance-Related Disorders in Adulthood

Substance-related disorders include the use of alcohol, sedatives, opioids, stimulants, hallucinogens, phencyclidine, cannabis, and other substances such as nicotine, caffeine, anabolic steroids, and nitrate inhalants (Black & Andreasen, 2010). Among American adults, 66% drink alcohol occasionally and 12% are heavy drinkers. Blazer and Wu (2009) found that 60% of American adults used alcohol, 2.6% used marijuana, and 0.41% used cocaine. However, they cautioned that this information was obtained from 10,953 participants by self-report and the prevalence is probably higher.

In relation to preventing alcohol use disorders, Li et al. (2007, p. 297) suggested that the focus should be on preventing the high-risk drinking behaviors—drinking too young, too much, too fast, and too much too often—that occur in three out of ten adults and are associated with increased risk of alcohol abuse and dependence. Li et al. stated that primary care clinicians can reduce problem drinking (1) by screening to identify those at risk and (2) by providing brief interventions to individual patients who are engaging in high-risk drinking behaviors. Brief interventions, such as giving advice or encouragement to change the high-risk behaviors, have been found to be effective (Wilk, Jensen, & Havighurst, 1997).

Anthony (2007) pointed out that the U.S. government spends over $17 billion a year on prevention and control of illegal drugs, and when the expenditures of states and local communities are included, the total is over $30 billion. The outcomes of universal preventive interventions are mixed and may even be negative. Li et al. (2007) stated that adolescence and early adulthood are critical windows of time for preventing alcohol use disorders, and Volkow and Li (2007) affirmed that prevention of substance-related disorders in adulthood must start in childhood.

Preventing Suicide in Adulthood

In the United States, suicide is the 11th leading cause of death, with over 30,000 Americans dying by suicide each year (Nock, Borges, Bromet, et al., 2008). Adolescence and early adulthood are the peak times for the first onset of suicidal behaviors. The rate of onset is highest at age 16 years and it remains high through the early 20s and then stabilizes in early middle life (Nock et al.). Among individuals with suicidal ideation, 34% go on to make a plan, and 72% of individuals with a suicide plan make a suicide attempt. This progression takes place during the first year after ideation onset in 60% of the cases (Nock et al.). Suicide attempts are the strongest predictors of death by suicide (Nock, Hwang, Sampson, et al., 2009).

Protective Factors and Risk Factors

Recognizing risk factors for suicide and also factors that reduce the risk can help psychiatric advanced practice nurses to reduce suicide among adults. Protective factors and risk factors and are presented in Box 19-12.

To summarize, 90% to 95% of suicides are believed to be associated with the presence of a psychiatric disorder (Cavanagh, Carson, Sharpe, et al., 2003). In an analysis by Nock et al. (2009), a history of a prior psychiatric disorder was present among 50% of individuals who had considered killing themselves and among 66% of those who made a suicide attempt. Mood disorders, impulse control disorders, alcohol or substance use, psychotic disorders, and personality disorders carry the highest risk of suicide. The disorders associated with progression from suicidal ideation to suicide attempt are anxiety disorders, such as post-traumatic stress disorder, and disorders with problems with impulse control, such as bipolar disorder and substance-related disorders. Presence of more than one psychiatric disorder increases the risk of suicide (Nock et al.).

BOX 19-12 Protective Factors and Risk Factors Associated With Suicide in Adulthood

Factors Associated With Decreased Risk of Suicide

- Having religious beliefs and practices; spirituality
- Having positive social support
- Being connected to family and others
- Being pregnant or having young children in the family
- Having a sense of responsibility to family
- Having good reality-testing skills
- Having positive coping skills
- Using problem-solving skills
- Having a positive therapeutic relationship with health-care providers
- Satisfaction with life

Factors Associated With Increased Risk of Suicide

- Male gender
- Young adulthood
- Being unmarried, unemployed, and having a lower level of academic achievement
- Suicidal ideation; intent, plan, access to means
- Previous suicide attempts (strong predictors)
- Presence of a psychiatric disorder such as mood, impulse control, psychotic, or personality or alcohol or substance abuse disorders
- Prior history of psychiatric diagnosis
- Psychological distress such as hopelessness, helplessness, anhedonia, and loneliness
- Stressful life events such as family conflicts, problems with romantic relationships, work problems, or legal problems
- Recent losses
- Family history of suicide
- Comorbid health problems

Adapted from Nock et al., 2008.

Preventive Interventions

Universal preventive programs that target the general population or school populations have not been found to reduce the incidence of suicide. However, an example of a universal preventive intervention that has been found to be effective is the United States Air Force's suicide prevention program. In order to reduce the rate of suicide and other psychosocial problems, such as family violence, in Air Force personnel, the Air Force changed its policies and social norms regarding mental health problems. It focused on removing the stigma associated with seeking help for mental health problems. At a 5-year follow-up, the rate of suicides had been reduced by 33% and other problems had been reduced 18% to 54% (Knox, Litts, Talcott, et al., 2003). Other universal interventions that have been recommended by the World Health Organization include detoxification of domestic gas and car exhaust, safety guards on high buildings and bridges, control of access to sedatives and painkillers, and reduction of access to means of suicide such as handguns (Hosman et al., 2005).

Indicated preventive interventions that target the patient with early signs of suicide risk could be effective. For example, 83% of individuals who commit suicide had contact with a primary care physician in the year before their death, and 66% had contact a month before their death. This suggests that opportunities for prevention are present but not used (Luoma, Martin, & Pearson, 2002).

The most effective approaches for preventing suicide appear to be those that restrict access to lethal means, such as firearms and pesticides, and those that train primary care physicians to recognize and treat depression and suicidal behavior. Training "gatekeepers"—clergy, first responders, pharmacists, geriatric caregivers, personnel staff, and workers in schools, prisons, and the military—to identify at-risk individuals and refer them for assessment and treatment is believed to reduce risk of suicide (Mann, Apter, Bertolote, et al., 2005, p. 2067).

Risk and Prevention Opportunities in Older Adults

It is estimated that 16.3% of older adults have psychiatric disorders other than dementia (Jeste, Alexopoulos, Bartels, et al., 1999). However, the prevalence may be underestimated because psychiatric disorders among older adults are often unrecognized or the symptoms are interpreted as signs of normal aging. Increased age is a risk factor for the development of certain psychiatric disorders (such as anxiety disorders, depression, dementias, Alzheimer's disease, and suicide) that cannot be changed. However, there is evidence that (1) identification and early interventions for anxiety may prevent or delay the development of depression and (2) identification and early intervention for depression may prevent or delay the onset of dementia, as older adults with depressive symptoms have approximately twice the risk of developing dementia as those without depressive symptoms.

Protective Factors and Risk Factors in Older Adulthood

Protective Factors

Older adults continue to face the lifelong process of adapting to challenges, changes, and losses (Cole, 2004). Successful adaptation consists of obtaining maximum positive outcomes, such as well-being, and minimal negative outcomes, such as psychopathology (Bohlmeijer, Roemer, Cuijpers, et al., 2007). Obtaining maximum positive outcomes depends on having multiple protective factors and few risk factors. Factors that protect against the development of psychopathology include

- Marriage. Married status protects health (Spar & La Rue, 2006).
- Physical activity. Physical activity has been linked with positive mental health and decreased rates of depression (Blow, Bartels, Brockmann, et al., 2005). Individuals who maintain activities, such as walking long distances, climbing stairs, and lifting objects, are more likely to maintain memory and cognitive functioning than those who are inactive (Albert & McKhann, 2006).
- Mental activity. Individuals who maintain memory and cognitive functioning have been found to participate daily in more mental activities that are stimulating, such as working on crossword puzzles, playing board games, reading books, and attending lectures or conferences (Albert & McKann, 2006; Fillit, Butler, O'Connell, et al., 2002).
- Education and income. Higher levels of education and financial resources are protective (Albert & McKann, 2006).
- Social engagement. Social engagement refers to how people feel about their connectedness to members of their family and to the community. Social engagement is associated with feelings of self-worth and self-efficacy. It is thought that social engagement reduces the level of stress hormones in the brain and may protect neurons. (Elevated levels of the stress hormone cortisol have been found to lead to loss of cells in the hippocampus, which is the area of the brain involved in learning and memory) (Albert & McKann, 2006).
- Optimal physical health. Controlling hypertension, lowering cholesterol, controlling weight, avoiding smoking, and treating medical conditions such as diabetes prevent damage to the brain (Albert & McKann, 2006).

Risk Factors

Risk factors that occur frequently among older adults include

- Poor physical health
- Multipharmacy adverse drug reactions or drug interactions
- Bereavement and loss; women lose their spouses at a younger age than men
- Poverty; financial problems have been linked to the development of depression in older adults
- Lack of social support, which has been linked to suicide in older adults (Waern, Rubernowitz, & Wilhelmson, et al., 2003)
- Undernutrition (Bhat, Chiu, & Jeste, 2005)
- Elder maltreatment; a shared living environment is associated with an increased risk for abuse (Bonnie & Wallace, 2002)

Preventing or Delaying Onset of Specific Psychiatric Disorders in Older Adulthood

Keys to preventing or delaying onset of psychiatric disorders are identification of older adults at risk for developing mental disorders; providing selective preventive interventions for those at risk; and providing indicated preventive interventions for those who have early symptoms of mental disorders and substance-related disorders. It has been said that preventing or delaying the onset of Alzheimer's disease by just 5 years could decrease the number of people with Alzheimer's disease by 50% in one generation because, within those 5 years, many older adults are likely to die from other disorders before developing Alzheimer's disease (Thal, 1996) (see Chapter 16 for information on preventing or delaying onset of dementia).

Among older adults, preventive interventions frequently target loneliness, depression, and suicide.

Preventing Loneliness in Older Adults

It has been found that loneliness is greater among older adults living in senior housing than among those living in a single dwelling or with their children (McInnis, 1999) and that the loneliness of older adults has themes that are different from loneliness in other stages of life. Common themes among older adults include

- Absence of important relationships
- Lost sense of self-identity

- Loss of connectedness with loved ones
- Anxiety and sadness related to fear of dependency on others that is often not expressed (Bohlmeijer et al., 2007; McInnis & White, 2001)

Loneliness creates emotional, physical, spiritual, and social distress and is associated with increased risk of depression, Alzheimer's-like dementia, and medical problems (McInnis & White, 2001; Wilson, Krueger, Arnold, et al., 2007). In fact, loneliness is believed to be a precursor of depression (Barg, Huss-Ashmore, Wittink, et al., 2006). Loneliness can be reduced by helping older adults to maintain established relationships with family members, neighbors, and members of their religious community and by encouraging them to maintain a diverse social network. Loneliness with loss of self-identity can be reduced through the use of reminiscence therapy (Bohlmeijer et al., 2007). Interventions that have been found to reduce loneliness include (1) group interventions with educational input, combined health education and exercise (swimming, dancing, walking), and a social support element, such as discussion groups; (2) bereavement groups; and (3) reminiscence groups (Adams, Sanders, & Auth, 2004).

Preventing Depression in Older Adults

Late-life depression occurs in approximately 13.5% of older adults (Cole, 2008; Schoevers, Smit, Deeg, et al., 2006). Late-life depression is associated with reduced quality of life, poorer prognosis of recovery from medical conditions, and earlier death (Smit, Ederveen, Cuijpers, et al., 2006; Whyte & Rovner, 2006). One in every five cases of late-life depression is a new or recurrent case (Smit et al.); older adults constitute the majority of new cases of depression in the general population (Smit, Smit, Schoevers, et al., 2008). Therefore, prevention of depression among older adults is key to reducing the overall incidence of depression (Cole, 2008).

Risk Factors

Among older adults, risk factors associated with the development of depression include

- Female gender
- Lower educational achievement
- Presence of two or more chronic illnesses
- Impaired functioning
- Recent loss of spouse
- Insomnia or disruptions of sleep
- Generalized anxiety disorder
- History of depression or anxiety
- Small social networks (Rovner & Casten, 2008; Schoevers, Beekman, Deeg, et al., 2000; Smit et al., 2008)

Preventive Interventions

The risk factors for late-onset depression are well known, but evidence about interventions that reduce the incidence of late-life depression is sparse (Smit et al., 2006). In reviewing interventions used to prevent the development of depression in older adults, four appear to be effective (Cole, 2008):

- Individual therapy for bereaved individuals (Raphael, 1977)
- Educational interventions for subjects with chronic illnesses (Gilden, Hendryx, Clare, et al., 1992; Phillips, 2000)
- Cognitive behavioral therapy to change negative thinking (Rovner, Casten, Hegel, et al., 2007; Willemse, Smit, Cuijpers, et al., 2004)
- Life review and reminiscence therapy for loneliness (Haight, Michek, & Hendrix, 1998)

A home-based program to prevent depression, the *Program to Encourage Active, Rewarding Lives for Seniors (PEARLS)*, was able to reduce symptoms of depression by 50% and also improve quality of life and functioning (Ciechanowski, Wagner, Schmaling, et al., 2004) (Table 19-7). There is some evidence that Befriending programs that increase social support and reduce loneliness and depression in older women prevent depression (Stevens, 2001). Problem-solving therapy has been found to be effective as a short-term preventive treatment, but the benefits did not persist over time (Rovner & Casten, 2008). According to Schoevers et al. (2006), indicated prevention is the most effective way to reduce the incidence of depression in older adults, and they suggested the use of bibliotherapy, coping skills training, and self-help groups. Smit et al. (2008) believed that providing the indicated preventive intervention of treatment for anxiety or anxiety disorders would reduce the number of cases of depression among older adults by almost 50%.

Preventing Suicide in Older Adults

Suicide risk is high in older adults, with males at a much higher risk—a ten times higher risk for males over 75 years of age (Conwell, 2009). Older white males account for 80% of suicides occurring among people ages 65 years and older (Schmutte, O'Connell, Weiland, et al., 2009). Three-fourths of older adults who commit suicide visited their primary care physician in the last month of their life (Conwell & Thompson, 2006). Older adults who commit suicide are less likely to have made previous suicide attempts, less likely to tell anyone about their ideas of suicide, and more likely to plan the suicide carefully to avoid anyone's knowing what they intend to do (Conwell, Duberstein, Conner, et al., 2003).

Protective Factors

Protective factors against suicide in older adults include

- Belonging to a religious community
- Having a caring family or supportive community network
- Having access to a caring health-care provider

TABLE 19-7 PREVENTIVE PROGRAMS FOR OLDER ADULTS

Intervention	Goals	Characteristics	Outcomes
PACE (Program of All-Inclusive Care for the Elderly, a Medicare option)	Prevent need for nursing home admission	A program of all-inclusive care	Not available
PEARLS (Program to Encourage Active, Rewarding Lives for Seniors)	Encourage active rewarding lives for older adults who have dysthymia or depression	Eight 50-minute counseling sessions are provided over 19 weeks in patients' homes Content: Depression is linked with unsolved problems, so focus is on problem-solving, increasing socialization, and reinstating participation in pleasurable activities	Reduction of severity of depressive symptoms; improvement of functional and emotional well-being; reduced use of health care services (Ciechanowski et al., 2004)
PROSPECT (Prevention of suicide in primary care elderly: Collaborative trial)	Prevent suicide by reducing suicidal ideation and depression	Recognition of suicidal ideation and depression by primary care physicians Treat depression with medication or psychotherapy Manage health problems	Reduction of depression, suicidal ideation, and death by suicide over a 24-month period (Alexopoulos, Reynolds, Bruce, et al., 2009)
PRISM-E (Primary Care Research in Substance Abuse and Mental Health for the Elderly)	Reduce suicide risk by reducing risk factors of depression and substance use	Referral to a specialty mental health clinic	Reduction of drinking and depressive symptoms compared with standard care (Oslin et al., 2004)
Project IMPACT (Improving Mood: Promoting Access to Collaborative Treatment) (Unutzer, Katon, Williams, et al., 2001)	Reduce depression and suicide risk	Collaborative care by primary care clinician and mental health provider trained to provide care for depression	Improvement of depression and reduction of suicidal thoughts (Unutzer, Tang, Oishi, et al., 2006) Patients over the age of 75 with depression also responded to IMPACT (Van Leeuwen Williams, Unutzer, Lee, et al., 2009)
Project GOAL (Guiding Older Adult Lifestyles) (www.niaaa.nih.gov/NewsEvents/NewsReleases/Pages/drinker.aspx)	Older adults with problem drinking behaviors	Counseling sessions by physicians that included advice, education, and a workbook; follow-up telephone call by a nurse	34% reduction of alcohol use; 74% reduction of episodes of binge drinking; 62% reduction of frequency of excessive drinking (Fleming, 1999)

- Having a past history of successful transitions to life changes
- Having a sense of meaning in life (Spar & La Rue, 2006)

Risk Factors

Risk factors for suicide among older adults include

- Presence of a psychiatric disorder; among older adults who died by suicide, 50% to 75% had a depressive disorder (Schmutte et al., 2009)
- Sleep disturbances
- Current or previous alcohol abuse
- Poor social supports
- Social isolation
- Feeling unimportant, not needed by anyone, or disconnected from others
- Being widowed or divorced
- Lacking relatives or friends in whom to confide (Conwell & Thompson, 2006)

Life events or circumstances that are often present among older adults who die by suicide include physical illnesses, impairment of functioning, retirement, financial difficulties, relocation, and a large number of daily hassles (Schmutte et al., 2009). Among older men, those who are married have the lowest suicide rate and those who are widowed or divorced are at high risk. Having a handgun in the home is associated with increased risk for suicide among older adults (Schmutte et al.). Although some of these factors cannot be changed, others can be modified to reduce the risk of suicide.

Preventive Interventions

Meta-analysis of 100 studies of suicide prevention in 15 countries provides evidence that two preventive interventions are effective in reducing the incidence of suicide: education of physicians about detecting suicide, and restriction of lethal means in patients' homes. Educating physicians to recognize and treat depression was included because depression is such a strong risk factor for suicide among older adults. This intervention was associated with 22% to 73% reduction of annual suicide rates. The other effective preventive intervention was restricting access to lethal means, such as firearm control. Approximately 28% of older adults have some type of firearm in their home (Oslin, Zubritsky, Brown, et al., 2004), and handguns are used in 80% of suicides committed by older men (Centers for Disease Control and Prevention, 2006). Limiting access to handguns is a crucial preventive intervention. Examples of preventive programs for older adults for loneliness, depression, substance abuse, and suicide are presented in Table 19-7.

Conclusion

The goal of prevention of psychiatric disorders lies within the broader goal of health and well-being for families, communities, and societies. The current model for prevention of psychiatric disorders is based on evidence that origins of many psychiatric disorders are linked to adversities experienced early in life. These adversities create biological memory traces, impairment of physiological systems, and vulnerabilities for the development of psychiatric disorders in adulthood (Shonkoff et al., 2009). Therefore, prevention of adult psychiatric disorders begins with (1) promoting preconception health of men and women who plan to have children and (2) providing optimal conditions for prenatal development of the child after conception (Brown & Sturgeon, 2005). The next crucial step is the prevention of childhood exposure to adversities, such as marital conflict and violence; deficits of income, housing, educational opportunities, and health care; and neglect and abuse. During adolescence, prevention of psychiatric disorders includes remediation of the effects of exposure to childhood adversities, promotion of a sense of self-worth and purpose in life, and building resilience. In adulthood, the goals of prevention are (1) to reduce risk factors that increase likelihood of the first incidence of a psychiatric disorder or relapse of a disorder in remission, and (2) to increase protective factors, such as social support, adaptive coping, resilience, and spirituality. Among older adults, the goal of preventive interventions is to foster positive adaptation by bolstering protective factors and reducing risk factors or mediating their influence.

Does Prevention Work?

Preventive programs that are carefully designed and implemented can be effective in preventing many of the problems of children and adolescents. Effective programs tend to

- Be comprehensive, with several interventions targeting the problem
- Provide enough of the intervention to bring about change
- Promote strong relationships with adults and peers
- Be implemented at a time when they will have the maximum impact and before the child is exhibiting unwanted behaviors
- Be tailored to the family, community, and culture
- Have clear goals
- Provide staff training and support (Nation, Crusto, Wandersman, et al., 2003)

In a meta-analytic review of prevention programs for children and adolescents, it was found that the programs were associated with reduced rates of social, behavioral, and academic problems. The outcomes of the programs ranged from small effect size to large effect size. For example, indicated preventive interventions that targeted specific problems such as child abuse, negative effects of divorce, and drug abuse were found to have a medium effect size (Weisz, Sandler, Durlak, et al., 2005). In their meta-analytic review of prevention of new cases of mental disorders, Cuijpers et al. (2005) found that all preventive interventions, with the exception of debriefing, were associated with a reduced incidence of new cases of psychiatric disorders.

Implications for Psychiatric Advanced Practice Nurses

Knowledge of both brain development and functioning and the factors that influence brain development and functioning provides the foundation for developing preventive interventions (Cicchetti & Cohen, 1995). This knowledge is foundational to the education and preparation of psychiatric advanced practice nurses. Based on this preparation, they have the knowledge, expertise, and competencies to build the bridges that will connect knowledge of risk and protective factors associated with the development of psychiatric disorders with specific preventive interventions across the life span (Staten, 2008).

Psychiatric advanced practice nurses must advocate for the use of evidence-based preventive interventions in prenatal care and primary care settings, in schools, in the workplace, in housing for older adults, and in religious and spiritual settings. They must promote nationwide internalization of the norm that all children should be provided with prenatal care, food, adequate housing, good schools, and freedom from exposure to childhood adversities in order that they may become contributing, successful adults. We must stop the occurrence of childhood maltreatment that, according to Felitti (2002), turns our nation's gold into lead.

Key Points

- Childhood adversities explain or predict 32.4% of the onset of psychiatric disorders.
- Childhood adversities predict 41.2% of childhood disruptive behaviors, such as conduct disorder, which is a risk factor for adult antisocial personality disorder.
- Exposure to childhood adversities is associated with specific adverse effects across the life span—changes of brain structures and functioning, impairment of coping or adaptation, physical health problems, relationship and social problems, and development of psychiatric disorders.
- Risk and protective factors at the level of the patient, family, and environment should be assessed routinely in clinical practice.
- Prevention of psychiatric disorders includes reducing factors associated with their development, such as bullying, substance use, maltreatment, and lack of social support.

- Preventive interventions for conduct disorder and oppositional defiant disorder are effective and have the potential to reduce depression, substance-related disorders, and suicide in adulthood.
- Anxiety disorders are associated with later development of depressive disorders and substance-related disorders.
- Reducing new cases of anxiety disorders requires providing preventive interventions in childhood.
- Reducing new cases of depression requires providing preventive interventions for children of depressed parents and older adults at risk for developing depression.
- Prevention of schizophrenia starts very early in life with good prenatal care; prevention of adverse obstetrical events; meeting the family's needs for sufficient income, adequate housing, and social support; and providing warm, nurturing care to build secure attachment patterns.
- Prevention of substance-related disorders should focus on adolescents and should take into consideration risk factors such as family history of substance abuse, relationships with family and with peers, and school and community influences.
- Prevention of suicide involves (1) training health-care providers and gatekeepers—clergy, emergency responders, pharmacists, and schoolteachers—to detect depression and early signs of suicide, such as suicidal thoughts, and to facilitate access to care, and (2) restricting means of committing suicide in the household, such as firearms, drugs, poisons, and items that could be used for hanging.

Resources

Child Abuse and Neglect

Child Welfare Information Gateway
www.childwelfare.gov/can/index/cfm
Preventing Child Abuse and Neglect
www.childwelfare.gov/preventing/
National Clearinghouse on Child Abuse and Neglect Information
http://nccanch.acf.hhs.gov
Prevent Mental Illness with Early Detection
www.preventmentalillness.org/pier_home.html

Childhood Disorders

American Academy of Child and Adolescent Psychiatry
www.aacap.org
Children and Adults with Attention Deficit/Hyperactivity Disorder
www.chadd.org

Adult Disorders

Schizophrenia.com
http://www.schizophrenia.com

Suicide Prevention among Young Adults and College Students

Campus Blues: Provides information on mental health, anxiety, loneliness, alcohol abuse, gambling and other social and emotional problems
http://www.campusblues.com
Go Ask Alice!: Provides information about relationships, sexuality, emotional health, alcohol, and other drugs (Bernat & Resnick, 2006)
http://www.goaskalice.columbia.edu/

Suicide Prevention

Suicide Prevention Resource Center (SPRC)
http://www.sprc.org/
SPRC Library Catalog: A database of information on suicide and suicide prevention
http://library.sprc.org/
American Foundation for Suicide Prevention
http://www.afsp.org
National Center for Injury Prevention and Control
http://www.cdc.gov/ncipc/
National Suicide Prevention Lifeline
http://www.suicidepreventionlifeline.org/

References

Aber, J. L., Jones, S., & Cohen, J. (2002). The impact of poverty on the mental health and development of very young children. In C. H. Zeanah, Jr. (Ed.), *Handbook of infant mental health* (2nd ed.) (pp. 113-128). New York: Guilford Press.

Achenbach, T. M., Dumenci, L., & Rescorla, L. A. (2003). Are American children's problems still getting worse? A 23-year comparison. *Journal of Abnormal Child Psychology, 31*(1), 1-11.

Adams, K. B., Sanders, S., & Auth, E. A. (2004). Loneliness and depression in independent living retirement communities: Risk and resilience factors. *Aging & Mental Health, 8*(6), 475-485.

Afifi, T. O., Boman, J., Fleisher, W., et al. (2009). The relationship between child abuse, parental divorce, and lifetime mental disorders and suicidality in a nationally representative adult sample. *Child Abuse & Neglect, 33*, 139-147.

Afifi, T. O., Enns, M. W., Cox, B. J., et al. (2008). Population attributable fractions of psychiatric disorders and suicide ideation and attempts associated with adverse childhood experiences. *American Journal of Public Health, 98*(5), 946-952.

Akil, H., Brenner, S., Kandel, E., et al. (2010). The future of psychiatric research: Genomes and neural circuits. *Science, 327*, 1580-1581.

Albee, G. W. (2005). Call to revolution in the prevention of emotional disorders. *Ethical Human Psychology and Psychiatry, 7*(1), 37-44.

Albert, M., & McKhann, G. (2006). The aging brain. In *Progress report on brain research* (pp. 11-15). New York: The Dana Alliance for Brain Initiatives.

Aleman, A., Kahn, R. S., & Selten, J. P. (2003). Sex differences in the risk of schizophrenia: Evidence from meta-analysis. *Archives of General Psychiatry, 60*(6), 565-571.

Alexopoulos, G. S., Reynolds, C. F., Bruce, M. L., et al. (2009). The PROSPECT Group: Reducing suicidal ideation and depression in older primary care patients: 24 month outcomes of the PROSPECT Study. *American Journal of Psychiatry, 166*, 883-890.

Amato, P. R. (2000). The consequences of divorce for adults and children. *Journal of Marriage and the Family, 62*(4), 628-640.

American Academy of Pediatrics. (n.d.). *Preventing teen suicide.* Retrieved from http://www.aap.org/advocacy/childhealthmonth/prevteensuicide.htm

Amminger, G. P., Schafer, M. R., Papageorgiou, K., et al. (2010). Long-chain omega-3 fatty acids for indicated prevention of psychotic disorders: A randomized, placebo-controlled trial. *Archives of General Psychiatry, 67*(2), 146-154.

Anda, R. F., Felitti, V. J., Bremner, D., et al. (2006). The enduring effects of abuse and related adverse experiences in childhood. *Archives of Psychiatry and Clinical Neuroscience, 256,* 174-186.

Andrews, G. J., Gavin, N., Begley, S., et al. (2003). Assisting friendships, combating loneliness: Users' views of a "befriending" scheme. *Ageing & Society, 23,* 349-362.

Andrews, G., & Wilkinson, D. D. (2002). The prevention of mental disorders in young people. *Medical Journal of Australia, 177,* S97-S100.

Anthony, J. C. (2007). Five facts about preventing drug dependence. In M. T. Tsuang, W. S. Stone, & M. J. Lyons (Eds.), *Recognition and prevention of major mental and substance use disorders* (pp. 329-346). Washington, DC: American Psychiatric Publishing, Inc.

Ash, P. (2008). Suicidal behavior in children and adolescents. *Journal of Psychosocial Nursing, 46*(1), 26-30.

Atrash, H., Jack, B., Johnson, K., et al. (2008). Where is the "W"oman in MCH? *American Journal of Obstetrics and Gynecology, 199*(Suppl 2), S259-S265.

Austin, M., Frillingos, M., Lumley, J., et al. (2008). Brief antenatal cognitive behavior therapy group intervention for the prevention of postnatal depression and anxiety: A randomized controlled trial. *Journal of Affective Disorders, 105*(1-3), 35-44.

Ayoola, A., Brewer, J., & Nettleman, M. (2006). Epidemiology and prevention of unintended pregnancy in adolescents. *Primary Care: Clinics in Practice, 33,* 391-403.

Baetz, M., Bowen, R., Jones, G., et al. (2006). How spiritual values and worship attendance relate to psychiatric disorders in the Canadian population. *Canadian Journal of Psychiatry, 51*(10), 654-661.

Balloon, J. S., Dean, K. A., & Cadenhead, K. S. (2008). Obstetrical complications in people at risk for developing schizophrenia. *Schizophrenia Research, 98*(1-3), 307-334.

Barg, F. K., Huss-Ashmore, R., Wittink, M. N., et al. (2006). A mixed-methods approach to understanding loneliness and depression in older adults. *The Journals of Geronotology. Series B, Psychological Sciences & Social Sciences, 61*(6), S329-S339.

Barker, E. D., Arseneault, L., Brendgen, M., et al. (2008). Joint development of bullying and victimization in adolescence: Relations to delinquency and self-harm. *Journal of American Academy of Child and Adolescent Psychiatry, 47,* 1030-1038.

Barrett, D. B., Kurian, G. T., and Johnson, T. M. (2001). *World Christian encyclopaedia: A comparative survey of churches and religions in the modern world* (2nd ed.). New York: Oxford University Press.

Barrett, P., & Turner, C. (2001). Prevention of anxiety symptoms in primary school children: Preliminary results from a universal school-based trial. *British Journal of Clinical Psychology, 40*(Pt 4), 399-410.

Barrett, A. E., & Turner, R. J. (2006). Family structure and substance use in adolescence and early adulthood: Examining explanations for the relationship. *Addiction, 101,* 109-120.

Barrish, H. H., Saunders, M., & Wolfe, M. D. (1969). Good behavior game. Effects of individual contingencies for group consequences and disruptive behavior in a classroom. *Journal of Applied Behavior Analysis, 2,* 119-124.

Beardslee, W. R., Gladstone, T. R. G., Wright, E. J., et al. (2007). Long-term effects from a randomized trial of two public health preventive interventions for parental depression. *Journal of Family Psychology, 21*(4), 703-713.

Beardslee, W. R., Versage, E., & Gladstone, T. R. G. (1998). Children of affectively ill parents: A review of the past 10 years. *Journal of the American Academy of Child and Adolescent Psychiatry, 37,* 1134-1141.

Beckwith, L. (2002). Prevention science and prevention programs. In C. H. Zeanah, Jr. (Ed.), *Handbook of infant mental health* (2nd ed.) (pp. 439-456). New York: Guilford Press.

Beekman, A. T., Cuijpers, P., van Marwijk, H. W., et al. (2006). The prevention of psychiatric disorders. *Nederlands Tijdschrift voor Geneeskunde, 150*(8), 419-423.

Berghella, V., Buchanan, E., Pereira, L., et al. (2010). Preconception care. *Obstetrical and Gynecological Survey, 65*(2), 119-131.

Bernat, D. H., & Resnick, M. D. (2006). Healthy youth development: Science and strategies. *Journal of Public Health Management and Practice, 12*(Suppl 6), S10-S16.

Bhat, R. S., Chiu, E., & Jeste, D. V. (2005). Nutrition and geriatric psychiatry: A neglected field. *Current Opinion in Psychiatry, 18*(6), 609-614.

Bienvenu, O. J., Siegel, D. J., & Ginsburg, G. S. (2010). Prevention of anxiety disorders. In M. T. Compton (Ed.), *Clinical manual of prevention in mental health* (pp. 83-103). Washington, DC: American Psychiatric Publishing, Inc.

Bigelow, A. E., MacLean, K., Proctor, J., et al. (2010). Maternal sensitivity throughout infancy: Continuity and relation to attachment security. *Infant Behavior and Development, 33,* 50-60.

Bittner, A., Goodwin, R. D., Wittchen, H-U, et al. (2004). What characteristics of primary anxiety disorders predict subsequent major depressive disorder? *Journal of Clinical Psychiatry, 65,* 618-626.

Black, D. W., & Andreasen, N. C. (2011). *Introductory textbook of psychiatry* (5th ed.). Washington, DC: American Psychiatric Publishing, Inc.

Blazer, D. G., & Wu, L-T. (2009). The epidemiology of substance use and disorders among middle aged and elderly community adults: National survey on drug use and health. *American Journal of Geriatric Psychiatry, 17*(3), 237-245.

Blow, F. C., Bartels, S. J., Brockmann, L. M., et al. (2005). Evidence-based practices for preventing substance abuse and mental health problems in older adults. SAMHSA Older Americans Substance Abuse and Mental Health Technical Assistance Center. Retrieved from http://gsa-alcohol.fmhi.usf.edu/Evidence-Based%20Practices%20for%20Preventing%20Substance%20Abuse%20and%20Mental%20Health%20Problems%20in%20Older%20Adults.pdf

Bohlmeijer, E., Roemer, M., Cuijpers, P., et al. (2007). The effects of reminiscence on psychological well-being in older adults: A meta-analysis. *Aging & Mental Health, 11*(3), 291-300.

Bond, L., Patton, G., Glover, S., et al. (2004). The Gatehouse Project: Can a multilevel school intervention affect emotional well-being and health risk behaviors? *Journal of Epidemiology and Community Health, 58,* 997-1003.

Bonnie, R., & Wallace, R. (2002). *Elder maltreatment: Abuse, neglect and exploitation in an aging America.* Washington, DC: The National Academies Press.

Bor, W., Sanders, M. R., & Markie-Dadds, C. (2002). The effects of the Triple P-Positive Parenting Program on preschool children with co-occurring disruptive behavior and attentional/hyperactive difficulties. *Journal of Abnormal Child Psychology, 30,* 571-587.

Borowsky, I. W., Ireland, M., & Resnick, M. D. (2001). Adolescent suicide attempts: Risks and protectors. *Pediatrics, 107*(3), 485-493.

Botash, A. S. (2010). Child sexual abuse in emergency medicine. *Medscape Drugs, Disease and Procedures.* Retrieved from http://emedicine.medscape.com/article/800770-overview

Botvin, G. J., Baker, E., Dusenbury, L., et al. (1995). Long-term follow-up results of a randomized drug abuse prevention trial in a white middle-class population. *Journal of the American Medical Association, 273,* 1106-1112.

Boushey, H., Brocht, C., Gundersen, B., et al. (2001). *Hardships in America: The real story of working families.* Washington, DC: Economic Policy Institute.

Boyce, C. A., Heinssen, R., Ferrell, C. B., et al. (2007). Prospects for the prevention of mental illness: Integrating neuroscience and behavior. In M. T. Tsuang, W. S. Stone, & M. J. Lyons (Eds.), *Recognition and prevention of major mental and substance use disorders* (pp. 241-260). Washington, DC: American Psychiatric Publishing, Inc.

Braithwaite, K. (2006). Mending our broken mental health systems. *American Public Health Association, 96*(10), 1724.

Braun, J. M., Kahn, R. S., Froehlich, T., et al. (2006). Exposures to environmental toxicants and attention deficit hyperactivity disorder in U.S. children. *Environmental Health Perspectives, 114*(12), 1904-1909.

Brent, D. A., Oquendo, M., Birmaher, B., et al. (2002). Familial pathways to early-onset suicide attempts: Risk for suicidal behavior in offspring of mood-disordered suicide attempters. *Archives of General Psychiatry, 59,* 801-907.

Bridge, J. A., Goldstein, T. R., & Brent, D. A. (2006). Adolescent suicide and suicidal behavior. *Journal of Child Psychology and Psychiatry, 47,* 372-394.

Bromet, E. J., & Fennig, S. (1999). Epidemiology and natural history of schizophrenia. *Biological Psychiatry, 46,* 871-881.

Brown, A. S., Schaefer, C. A., Wyatt, R. S., et al. (2002). Paternal age and risk of schizophrenia in adult offspring. *American Journal of Psychiatry, 159,* 1528-1533.

Brown, C. H., & Faraone, S. V. (2004). Prevention of schizophrenia and psychotic behavior: Definitions and methodologic issues. In W. S. Stone, S. V. Faraone, & M. T. Tsuang (Eds.), *Early clinical intervention and prevention in schizophrenia* (pp. 255-284). New York: Humana Press.

Brown, C. H., & Sturgeon, S. (2005). Promoting a healthy start of life and reducing early risks. In C. Hosman, E. Jane-Llopis, & S. Saxena (Eds.), *Prevention of mental disorders: Effective interventions and policy options* (pp. 27-30). Oxford, UK: Oxford University Press.

Bryant, R. A., Harvey, A. G., Dang, S. T., et al. (1998). Treatment of acute stress disorder: A comparison of cognitive-behavioral therapy and supportive counseling. *Journal of Consulting and Clinical Psychology, 66,* 862-866.

Bryant, R. A., Sackville, T., Dang, S. T., et al. (1999). Treating acute stress disorder: An evaluation of cognitive-behavioral therapy and counseling techniques. *American Journal of Psychiatry, 156,* 178-186.

Bushman, B. J., & Huesmann, L. R. (2006). Short-term and long-term effects of violent media on aggression in children and adults. *Archives of Pediatric Adolescent Medicine, 160,* 348-352.

Cabrera, O. A., Hoge, C. W., Bliese, P. D., et al. (2007). Childhood adversity and combat as predictors of depression and post-traumatic stress in deployed troops. *American Journal of Preventive Medicine, 33*(2), 77-82.

Cahill, L., Prins, B., Weber, M., et al. (1994). Impaired memory consolidation in rats produced with adrenergic blockade. *Neurobiology of Learning and Memory, 74,* 259-266.

Cash, S. J., & Bridge, J. A. (2009). Epidemiology of youth suicide and suicidal behavior. *Current Opinion in Pediatrics, 21,* 613-619.

Caspi, A., Moffitt, T. E., Newman, D. L., et al. (1996). Behavioral observations at age 3 predict adult psychiatric disorders: Longitudinal evidence from a birth cohort. *Archives of General Psychiatry, 53,* 1033-1039.

Caspi, A., Sugden, K., Moffitt, T. E., et al. (2003). Influence of life stress on depression: Moderation by polymorphism in the 5-HTT gene. *Science, 301,* 386-389.

Catalano, R. F., Gainey, R. R., Fleming, C. B., et al. (1999). An experimental intervention with families of substance abusers: One-year follow-up of the focus on families project. *Addiction, 94*(2), 241-254.

Cattan, M., White, M., Bond, J., et al. (2005). Preventing social isolation and loneliness among older people: A systematic review of health promotion interventions. *Ageing & Society, 25,* 41-67.

Cavanagh, J. T., Carson, A. J., Sharpe, M., et al. (2003). Psychological autopsy studies of suicide: A systematic review. *Psychological Medicine, 33,* 395-405.

Centers for Disease Control and Prevention. (2006). National Center for Injury Prevention and Control Fatal Injury Reports. Retrieved from http://webapp.cdc.gov/sasweb/ncipc/mortrate.html

Centre for Suicide Prevention. (2000). *Children and suicide.* SIEC Alert#39. Retrieved from www.suicideinfo.ca

Chabrol, H., Teissedre, F., Saint-Jean, M., et al. (2002). Prevention and treatment of post-partum depression: A controlled randomized study on women at risk. *Psychological Medicine, 32*(6), 1039-1047.

Chandra, A., Martin, L. T., Hawkins, S. A., et al. (2010). The impact of parental deployment on child social and emotional functioning: Perspectives of school staff. *Journal of Adolescent Health, 46,* 218-223.

Chartier, M. J., Walker, J. R., & Naimark, B. (2010). Separate and cumulative effects of adverse childhood experiences in predicting adult health and health care utilization. *Child Abuse & Neglect, 34,* 454-464.

Chatterji, P., Dave, D., Kaestner, R., et al. (2004). Alcohol abuse and suicide attempts among youth. *Economics and Human Behavior, 2*(2), 159-180.

Chavira, D. A., Stein, M. B., Bailey, K., et al. (2004). Child anxiety in primary care: Prevalent but untreated. *Depression and Anxiety, 20,* 155-164.

Chen, H., Cohen, P., Johnson, J. G., et al. (2009). Psychiatric disorders during adolescence and relationships with peers from age 17 to age 27. *Social Psychiatry and Psychiatric Epidemiology, 44,* 223-230.

Chen, H., Cohen, P., Kasen, S., et al. (2006). Adolescent axis I and personality disorders predict quality of life during young adulthood. *Journal of Adolescent Health, 39*(1), 14-19.

Child sexual abuse: Evaluation outcomes. (2007). *Child Welfare News, 30, Summer.* Center for Advanced Studies in Child Welfare, University of Minnesota.

Children's Hospital Boston. (2005). Oppositional defiant disorder. Retrieved from http://www.childrenshospital.org/az/Site1385/mainpageS1385P0.html

Christakos, D. A., Zimmerman, F. J., DiGiuseppe, D. L., et al. (2004). Early television exposure and subsequent attentional problems in children. *Pediatrics, 113,* 708-713.

Christensen, H., Griffiths, K. M., & Jorm, A. F. (2004). Delivering interventions for depression by using the Internet: Randomized controlled trial. *British Medical Journal, 328,* 265-268.

Cicchetti, D., & Cohen, D. J. (Eds.). (1995). *Developmental psychopathology* (Vol I. Theory and methods). New York: John Wiley & Sons, Inc.

Cicchetti, D., & Toth, S. L. (2005). Child maltreatment. *Annual Review of Clinical Psychology, 1,* 409-438.

Ciechanowski, P., Wagner, E., Schmaling, K., et al. (2004). Community-integrated home-based depression treatment in older adults: A randomized controlled trial. *Journal of the American Medical Association, 291*(13), 1569-1577.

Clarke, G. N., Hornbrook, M., Lynch, F., et al. (2001). A randomized trial of a group cognitive intervention for preventing depression in adolescent offspring of depressed parents. *Archives of General Psychiatry, 58,* 1127-1134.

Clements-Nolle, K., Marx, R., & Katz, M. (2006). Attempted suicide among transgender persons: The influence of gender-based discrimination and victimization. *Journal of Homosexuality, 51,* 53-69.

Cohen, M. A. (1998). The monetary value of saving a high risk youth. *Journal of Quantitative Criminology, 4,* 3-35.3.

Cole, M. G. (2008). Brief interventions to prevent depression in older subjects: A systematic review of feasibility and effectiveness. *American Journal of Geriatric Psychiatry, 16,* 435-443.

Cole, T. (2004, June). *After the life cycle: The moral challenges of later life.* Paper presented at the President's Council on Bioethics, Washington, DC. Retrieved from http://bioethics.georgetown.edu/pcbe/background/cole.html

Compton, M. T. (2008, June). Highlights of the 2008 Mental Health America Conference: Inaugural Promotion and Prevention Summit, Washington, DC. Retrieved on 9/11/2008 from http://www.medscape.com/viewarticle/576983

Compton, M. T. (2010a). Preface. In M. T. Compton (Ed.), *Clinical manual of prevention in mental health* (pp. XXV-XXXII). Washington, DC: American Psychiatric Publishing, Inc.

Compton, M. T. (2010b). Applying prevention principles to schizophrenia and other psychotic disorders. In M. T. Compton (Ed.), *Clinical manual of prevention in mental health* (pp. 125-161). Washington, DC: American Psychiatric Publishing, Inc.

Compton, M. T., Koplan, C., Oleskey, C., et al. (2010). Prevention in mental health. In M. T. Compton (Ed.), *Clinical manual of prevention in mental health* (pp. 1-28). Washington, DC: American Psychiatric Publishing, Inc.

Conduct Problems Prevention Research Group. (2002). Predictor variables associated with positive Fast Track outcomes at the end of third grade. *Journal of Abnormal Child Psychology, 30*(1), 37-52.

Conwell, Y. (2009). Suicide prevention in later life: A glass half full, or half empty? *American Journal of Psychiatry, 166*(8), 845-848.

Conwell, Y., Duberstein, P. R., Conner, K. R., et al. (2003). *Suicide in the second half of life—A psychological autopsy study.* Presented at the 11th International Congress of the International Psychogeriatrics Association, Chicago, IL.

Conwell, Y., & Thomson, C. (2006). Suicidal behavior in elders. *Psychiatric Clinics of North America, 31,* 333-356.

Copeland, W. F., Shanahan, L., Costello, J., et al. (2009a). Childhood and adolescent psychiatric disorders as predictors of young adult disorders. *Archives of General Psychiatry, 66*(7), 764-772.

Copeland, W. F., Shanahan, L., Costello, J., et al. (2009b). Configurations of common childhood psychosocial risk factors. *The Journal of Child Psychology and Psychiatry, 50*(4), 451-459.

Copeland-Linder, N., Lambert, S. F., & Ialongo, N. S. (2010). Community violence, protective factors and adolescent mental health: A profile analysis. *Journal of Clinical Child & Adolescent Psychology, 39*(2), 176-186.

Cornblatt, B. A., Lencz, T., Smith, C. W., et al. (2007). Can antidepressants be used to treat the schizophrenia prodrome? Results of a prospective, naturalistic treatment study of adolescents. *Journal of Clinical Psychiatry, 68*(4), 546-557.

Costello, E. J., Egger, H., & Angold, A. (2005). The developmental epidemiology of anxiety disorders: Phenomenology, prevalence, and comorbidity. *Child and Adolescent Psychiatric Clinics of North America, 14*, 631-648.

Crews, S. D., Bender, H., Cook, C. R., et al. (2007). Risk and protective factors of emotional and/or behavioral disorders in children and adolescents. A mega-analytic synthesis. *Behavioral Disorders, 32*(2), 64-77.

Cuijpers, P. (1997). Bibliotherapy in unipolar depression: A meta-analysis. *Journal of Behavioral Therapy and Experimental Psychiatry, 28*, 139-147.

Cuijpers, P. (1998). Psychoeducational approach to the treatment of depression: A meta-analysis of Lewinsohn's "Coping With Depression" course. *Behavioral Therapy, 29*, 521-533.

Cuijpers, P., van Straten, A., & Smit, F. (2005). Preventing the incidence of new cases of mental disorders: A meta-analytic review. *Journal of Nervous and Mental Disorders, 193*(1), 119-125.

Cuijpers, P., van Straten A., Smit, F., et al. (2008). Preventing the onset of depressive disorders: A meta-analytic review of psychological interventions. *American Journal of Psychiatry, 165*(10), 1272-1280.

Dadds, M. R., Holland, D. E., Laurens, K. R., et al. (1999). Early intervention and prevention of anxiety disorders in children: Results at 2-year follow-up. *Journal of Consulting Clinical Psychology, 67*, 145-150.

Dadds, M. R., Spence, S. H., Holland, E. E., et al. (1997). Prevention and early intervention for anxiety disorders: A controlled trial. *Journal of Consulting and Clinical Psychology, 65*(4), 627-635.

Danish, S. J. (1997). Going for the goal: A life skills program for adolescents. In G. W. Albee & T. P. Gullotta (Eds.), *Primary prevention works* (pp. 291-312). Thousand Oaks, CA: Sage Publications.

David, H. P., Dytych, Z., & Matejcek, Z. (2003). Born unwanted. Observations from the Prague study. *American Psychologists, 58*(3), 224-229.

Dawson, G., Ashman, S. B., & Carver, L. J. (2000). The role of early experience in shaping behavioral and brain development and its implications for social policy. *Development and Psychopathology, 12*, 695-712.

Dayer, A. G., Cleaver, K. M., Abouantoun, T., et al. (2005). New GABAergic interneurons in the adult neocortex and striatum are generated from different precursors. *Journal of Cell Biology, 168*(3), 415-427.

Dennis, C-L. (2005). Psychosocial and psychological interventions for prevention of postnatal depression: Systematic review. *British Medical Journal, 331*, 1-8.

Dervic, K., Brent, D. A., & Oquendo, M. A. (2008). Completed suicide in childhood. *Psychiatric Clinics of North America, 31*(2), 271-291.

Dervic, K., Oquendo, M. A., Grunebaum, M. F., et al. (2004). Religious affiliation and suicide attempt. *American Journal of Psychiatry, 161*(12), 2303-2308.

Diamond, A., Barnett, W. S., Thomas, J., et al. (2007). Preschool program improves cognitive control. *Science, 318*, 1387-1388.

DiClemente, R. J., & Raczynski, J. M. (1999). The importance of health promotion and disease prevention. In J. M. Raczynski & R. J. DiClemente (Eds.), *Handbook of health promotion and disease prevention* (pp. 3-11). New York: Kluwer Academic/Plenum.

Dishion, T. J., & Stormshak, E. A. (2007). *Intervening in children's lives: An ecological family-centered approach to mental health care.* Washington, DC: APA Books.

Dohrenwend, B. P., & Egri, G. (1981). Recent stressful life events and episodes of schizophrenia. *Schizophrenia Bulletin, 7*(1), 12-23.

Donaldson, S. I., Thomas, C. W., Graham, J. W., et al. (2000). Verifying drug abuse prevention program effects using reciprocal best friend reports. *Journal of Behavioral Medicine, 23*(6), 585-601.

Dong, M., Anda, R. F., & Felitti, V. J. (2004). The interrelatedness of multiple forms of childhood abuse, neglect, and household dysfunction. *Child Abuse & Neglect, 28*, 771-784.

Dryfoos, J. (1990). *Adolescents at risk: Prevalence and prevention.* New York: Oxford University Press.

Dube, S. R., Cook, M. L., & Edwards. V. J. (2010). Health-related outcomes of adverse childhood experiences in Texas, 2002. *Preventing Chronic Disease, 7*(3), A52.

Dube, S. R., Felitti, V. J., Dong, M., et al. (2003). Childhood abuse, neglect and household dysfunction and the risk of illicit drug use: The Adverse Childhood Experiences Study. *Pediatrics, 111*, 564-572.

Duff, J. (2005). Disruptive behaviour disorders. *Behavioural Neurotherapy Clinic.* Retrieved from http://www.adhd.com.au/conduct.htm

Duggan, A., Caldera, D., Rodriguez, K., et al. (2007). Impact of a statewide home visiting program to prevent child abuse. *Child Abuse and Neglect, 31*, 801-827.

Duhault, J. L. (2002). Stress prevention and management: A challenge for patients and physicians. *Metabolism, 51*(6 Suppl 1), 46-48.

Dukes, R., Ullman, J., & Stein, J. (1996). Three-year follow-up of drug abuse resistance education (DARE). *Evaluation Review, 20*, 49-66.

Dumont, M., & Provost, M. (1999). Resilience in adolescents: Protective role of social support, coping strategies, self-esteem and social activities on experience of stress and depression. *Journal of Youth and Adolescence, 28*, 343-363.

Dunn, M. S., Goodrow, B., Givens, C., et al. (2008). Substance use behavior and suicide indicators among rural middle school students. *Journal of School Health, 78*(1), 26-31.

Durlak, J. A. (1998). Primary prevention mental health programs for children and adolescents are effective. *Journal of Mental Health, 7*, 463-469.

Eaton, D. K., Kann, L., Kinchen, S., et al. (2008). Youth risk behavior surveillance—United States, 2007. *Morbidity and Mortality Weekly Report Surveillance Summaries, 57*(4), 1-131.

Eaton, D. K., Lowry, R., Brener, N. D., et al. (2005). Associations of body mass index and perceived weight with suicide ideation and suicide attempts among US high school students. *Archives of Pediatric and Adolescent Medicine, 159*(6), 513-519.

Eaton, W. W., Martins, S. S., Nestadt, G., et al. (2008). The burden of mental disorders. *Epidemiologic Review, 30*, 1-14.

Edward, K. (2005). Resilience: A protector from depression. *Journal of the American Psychiatric Nurses Association, 11*(4), 241-243.

Edwards, V. J., Holden, G. W., Felitti, V. J., et al. (2003). Relationship between multiple forms of childhood maltreatment and adult mental health in community respondents: Results from the adverse childhood experiences study. *American Journal of Psychiatry, 160*(8), 1453-1460.

Eggert, I. L., Thompson, E. A., & Herting, J. R. (1995). Reducing suicidal potential among high-risk youth: Tests of a school-based program. *Suicide and Life-Threatening Behavior, 25*(2), 276-296.

Eisen, M., Zellman, G., & Murray, D. M. (2003). Evaluating the Lions-Quest "Skills for Adolescence" drug education program: Second-year behavior outcomes. *Addictive Behaviors, 28*, 883-897.

Elliott, S. A., Leverton, T. J., Sanjack, M., et al. (2000). Promoting mental health after childbirth: A controlled trial of primary prevention of postnatal depression. *British Journal of Clinical Psychology, 39*(Pt 3), 223-241.

Emslie, G. J. (2008). Pediatric anxiety—under recognized and undertreated. *The New England Journal of Medicine, 359*(26), 2835-2836.

Ennent, S. T., Tobler, N. S., Ringwalt, C. L., et al. (1994). How effective is drug abuse resistance education? A meta-analysis of Project DARE outcome evaluations. *American Journal of Public Health, 84*, 1394-1401.

Esch, T., & Stefano, G. B. (2010). The neurobiology of stress management. *Neuroendocrinology Letters, 31*(1), 19-39.

Essex, M. J., Kraemer, H. C., Slattery, M. J., et al. (2009). Screening for childhood mental health problems: Outcomes and early identification. *Journal of Child Psychology and Psychiatry, 50*(5), 562-570.

Evans, D. L., Foa, E. B., Gur, R. E., et al. (2005). *Treating and preventing adolescent mental health disorders: What we know and what we don't know.* Oxford, UK: Oxford University Press.

Evans, D. L., & Seligman, M. E. P. (2005). Introduction. In D. L. Evans, E. B. Foa, R. E. Gur, et al. (Eds.), *Treating and preventing adolescent mental health disorders: What we know and what we don't know* (pp. XXV-XL). Oxford, UK: Oxford University Press.

Evans, G. W. (2004). The environment of childhood poverty. *American Psychologist, 59*(2), 77-92.

Felitti, V. J. (2002). The relation between adverse childhood experiences and adult health: Turning gold into lead. *The Permantente Journal, Winter, 5*(1), 44-47.

Felitti, V. J., Anda, R. F., Nordenberg, D., et al. (1998). Relationship of childhood abuse and household dysfunction to many of the leading causes of death in adults: The adverse childhood experiences (ACE) Study. *American Journal of Preventive Medicine, 14*(4), 245-258.

Fergusson, D. M., Grant, H., Horwood, L. J., et al. (2005). Randomized trial of the Early Start program of home visitation. *Pediatrics, 116,* 803-809.

Ficks, C. A., & Waldman, I. D. (2009). Gene-environment interactions in attention-deficit/hyperactivity disorder. *Current Psychiatry Reports, 11*(5), 387-392.

Fillit, H. M., Butler, R. N., O'Connell, A. W., et al. (2002). Achieving and maintaining cognitive vitality with aging. *Mayo Clinic Proceedings, 77,* 681-696.

Finkelhor, D., Turner, H., Ormrod, R., et al. (2009). Poly-victimization in a national sample of children and youth. *American Journal of Preventive Medicine, 38*(3), 323-330.

Fisch, H. (2009). Older men having children, but the reality of a male biological clock makes this trend worrisome. *Geriatrics, 64*(1), 14-17.

Flake, E. M., Davis, B. E., Johnson, P. L., et al. (2009). The psychosocial effects of deployment on military children. *Journal of Developmental and Behavioral Pediatrics, 30,* 271-278.

Flannery, R. B. (2004). Managing stress in today's age: A concise guide for emergency services personnel. *International Journal of Emergency Mental Health, 6*(4), 205-209.

Flannery-Schroeder, E. C. (2006). Reducing anxiety to prevent depression. *American Journal of Preventive Medicine, 31*(6 Suppl 1), S136-S142.

Fleming, M. F. (1999). Brief physician advice for alcohol problems in older adults: A randomized community-based trial. *Journal of Family Practice, 48*(5), 378-384.

Foley, D. L., Goldston, D. B., Costello, E. J., et al. (2006). Proximal psychiatric risk factors for suicidality in youth: The Great Smoky Mountains Study. *Archives of General Psychiatry, 63,* 1017-1024.

Fredrickson, B. L., Tugade, M. M., Waugh, C. E., et al. (2003). What good are positive emotions in crises? A prospective study of resilience and emotions following the terrorist attacks on the United States on September 11, 2001. *Personality Process and Individual Differences, 84,* 365-376.

Gale, C. R., Robinson, S. M., Godfrey, K. M., et al. (2008). Oily fish intake during pregnancy—association with lower hyperactivity but not with higher full-scale IQ in offspring. *Journal of Child Psychology and Psychiatry, 49,* 1061-1068.

Garber, J. (2006). Depression in children and adolescents: Linking risk, research, and prevention. *American Journal of Preventive Medicine, 31*(6 Suppl 1), S104-S125.

Garland, A. F., & Zigler, E. (1993). Adolescent suicide prevention: Current research and social policy implications. *American Psychologist, 48,* 169-182.

Gershater-Molko, R. M., Lutzker, J. R., & Wesch, D. (2001). Project SafeCare: Improving health, safety, and parenting skills in families reported for, and at-risk for child maltreatment. *Journal of Family Violence, 18*(6), 377-386.

Geschwind, N., Peeters, F., Jacobs, N., et al. (2010). Meeting risk with resilience: High daily life reward experiences preserves mental health. *Acta Psychiatrica Scandinavica, 122*(2), 129-138.

Gilden, J. L., Hendryx, M. S., Clare, S., et al. (1992). Diabetes support groups improve health care of older diabetic patients. *Journal of the American Geriatrics Society, 40*(2), 147-150.

Gillham, J. E., Jaycox, L. H., Reivich, K. J., et al. (1990). The Penn Resiliency Program (also known as the Penn Depression Prevention Program and the Penn Optimism Program). (Unpublished manuscript.) University of Pennsylvania, Philadelphia, PA.

Gillham, J., & Reivich, K. (2004). Cultivating optimism in childhood and adolescence. *The Annals of the American Academy of Political and Social Science, 591,* 146-163.

Ginsberg, G. S. (2009). Parenting behaviors among anxious and non-anxious mothers: Relation with concurrent and long-term child outcomes. *Child and Family Behavior Therapy, 26,* 23-41.

Gladstone, T. R. G., & Beardslee, W. R. (2009). The prevention of depression in children and adolescents: A review. *Canadian Journal of Psychiatry, 54*(4), 212-221.

Glatt, S. J., Faraone, S. V., & Tsuang, M. T. (2008). Psychiatric genetics: A primer. In J. W. Smoller, B. R. Shedley, & M. T. Tsuang (Eds.), *Psychiatric genetics: Application in clinical practice* (pp. 3-26). Washington, DC: American Psychiatric Publishing, Inc.

Goldman, S., & Beardslee, W. (1999). Suicide in children and adolescents. *The Harvard Medical School guide to suicide assessment and intervention.* San Francisco, CA: Jossey-Bass.

Goldstein, S., & Brooks, R. B. (2006). Why study resilience? In S. Goldstein & R. B. Brooks (Eds.), *Handbook of resilience in children* (pp. 3-15). New York: Springer Science & Business Media, Inc.

Goldstein, T. R., Bridge, J. A., & Brent, D. A. (2008). Sleep disturbance preceding completed suicide in adolescents. *Journal of Counseling and Clinical Psychology, 76*(1), 84-91.

Gonzalez, A., & MacMillan, H. L. (2008). Preventing child maltreatment: An evidence-based update. *Journal of Postgraduate Medicine, 54*(4), 280-286.

Goodwin, R. D., Fergusson, D. M., & Horwood, L. (2004). Early anxious/withdrawn behaviors predict later internalizing disorders. *Journal of Child Psychology and Psychiatry, 45*(4), 874-883.

Goodwin, R. D., & Friedman, H. S. (2006). Health status and the five-factor personality traits in a nationally representative sample. *Journal of Health Psychology, 11*(5), 643-654.

Goodwin, R. D., & Olfson, M. (2001). Treatment of panic attack and risk of major depressive disorder in the community. *American Journal of Psychiatry, 158,* 1146-1148.

Gorman-Smith, D., & Tolan, P. (1998). The role of exposure to community violence and developmental problems among inner-city youth. *Development and Psychopathology, 10*(1), 101-116.

Gottlieb, F. (2000). Selecting and planning support interventions. In S. Cohen, L. G. Underwood, & B. H. Gotlieb (Eds.), *Social support measurement and intervention* (pp. 195-220). Oxford, UK: Oxford University Press.

Gould, M. S., Greenberg, T., Velting, D. M., et al. (2003). Youth suicide risk and preventive interventions: A review of the past 10 years. *Journal of American Academy of Child and Adolescent Psychiatry, 42*(4), 386-405.

Granello, D. H., & Granello, P. F. (2007). *Suicide: An essential guide for helping professionals and educators.* New York: Merrill, Pearson Education, Inc.

Green, J. G., McLaughlin, K. A., Berglund, P. A., et al. (2010). Childhood adversities and adult psychiatric disorders in the national Comorbidity Survey Replication I. *Archives of General Psychiatry, 67*(2), 113-123.

Green, J. G., Stanley, C., & Peters, S. (2007). Disorganized attachment representation and atypical parenting in young school age children with externalizing disorder. *Attachment and Human Development, 9*(3), 207-222.

Greenberg, M. T., & Kusche, C. A. (1998). *Promoting alternative thinking strategies. Blueprint for violence prevention (Book 10).* Boulder, CO: Institute of Behavioral Sciences, University of Colorado.

Greenberg, M. T., Speltz, M. L., DeKlyen, M., et al. (2001). Correlates of clinic referral for early conduct problems: Variable-and person-oriented approaches. *Development and Psychopathology, 13,* 255-276.

Greening, L., & Stoppelbein, L. (2002). Religiosity, attributational style, and social support as psychosocial buffers for African American and white adolescents' perceived risk for suicide. *Suicide & Life-Threatening Behavior, 29*(2), 105-118.

Gross, D., Fogg, L., & Tucker, S. (1995). The efficacy of parent training for promoting positive parent-toddler relationships. *Research in Nursing Health, 18,* 489-499.

Grossman, D. C., Mueller, B. A., Riedy, C., et al. (2005). Gun storage practices and risk of youth suicide and unintentional forearm injuries. *Journal of the American Medical Association, 293,* 707-714.

Gunnar, M. R., & Donzella, B. (2002). Social regulation of the cortisol levels in early human development. *Psychoneuroendocrinology, 27,* 199-220.

Gunnar, M. R., & Quevedo, K. M. (2008). Early care experiences and HPA axis regulation in children: A mechanism for later trauma vulnerability. *Progress in Brain Research, 167,* 137-149.

Hack, M., Taylor, H. G., Schulchter, M., et al. (2009). Behavioral outcomes of extremely low birth weight children at age 8 years. *Journal of Developmental & Behavioral Pediatrics, 30,* 122-130.

Hahn, R., Fuqua-Whitley, D., Wethington, H., et al. (2007). Effectiveness of Universal school-based programs to prevent violent and aggressive behavior. *American Journal of Preventive Medicine, 33*(2 Suppl), S114-S129.

Haight, B. K., Michek, Y., & Hendrix, S. (1998). Life review: Preventing despair in newly relocated nursing home residents short and long-term effects. *International Journal of Aging and Human Development, 47,* 119-142.

Hairston, C. F. (2007). *Focus on children with incarcerated parents: An overview of the research literature.* A report prepared for Annie E. Casey Foundation. Retrieved from http://www.fcnetwork.org/AECFOverview%20of%20the%20Research%20Literature.pdf

Hallowell, E. (1998). *Can you prevent your child from developing ADHD?* Retrieved from http://www.additudemag.com/adhd/article/695.html

Hamilton, B. E., Minino, A. M., Martin, J. A., et al. (2007). Annual summary of vital statistics: 2005. *Pediatrics, 119,* 345-360.

Harrington, N. G., Giles, S. M., Hoyle, R. H., et al. (2001). Evaluation of the All Stars character education and problem behavior prevention program: Effects on mediator and outcome variables for middle school students. *Health Education and Behavior, 28*(5), 533-546.

Harvard Mental Health Letter. (2009, December). *Challenges in preventing schizophrenia.* Retrieved from http://www.health.harvard.edu/newsletters/Harvard_Mental_Health_Letter/2009/December

Hawkins, J. D., Catalano, R. F., & Miller, J. Y. (1992). Risk and protective factors for alcohol and other drug problems in adolescence and early adulthood: Implications for substance abuse prevention. *Psychological Bulletin, 112,* 64-105.

Henry, D. P. (2006). Born unwanted, 35 years later: The Prague study. *Reproductive Health Matters, 14*(27), 181-190.

Heron, M. (2007). Deaths: Leading causes for 2004. *National Vital Statistics Reports, 56*(5), 1-96.

Hettema, J., Neale, M., Myers, J., et al. (2006). A population-based twin study of the relationship between neuroticism and internalizing disorders. *American Journal of Psychiatry, 163,* 857-864.

Horowitz, J. L., & Garber, J. (2006). The prevention of depressive symptoms in children and adolescents: A meta-analytic review. *Journal of Consulting and Clinical Psychology, 74*(3), 401-415.

Horwitz, A. V., Widom, C. S., McLaughlin, J., et al. (2001). The impact of childhood abuse and neglect on adult mental health: A prospective study. *Journal of Health and Social Behavior, 42*(2), 184-201.

Horrobin, D. F., Al, G., & Vaddadi, K. (1994). The membrane hypothesis of schizophrenia. *Schizophrenia Research, 13*(3), 195-207.

Hosman, C., Jane-Llopis, E., & Saxena, S. (Eds.). (2005). *Prevention of mental disorders; Effective interventions and policy options, Summary Report.* Geneva, Switzerland: World Health Organization.

Huppert, F. A., & Whittington, J. E. (2003). Evidence for the independence of positive and negative well-being: Implications for quality of life assessment. *British Journal of Health and Psychology, 9,* 107-122.

Ialongo, N., Poduska, J., Werthamer, L., et al. (2001). The distal impact of two first-grade preventive interventions on conduct problems and disorder in early adolescence. *Journal of Emotional and Behavioral Disorders, 9,* 146-160.

Ialongo, N. S., Werthamer, L., Kellam, S. G., et al. (1999). Proximal impact of two first-grade preventive interventions on the early risk behaviors for later substance abuse, depression, and antisocial behavior. *American Journal of Community Psychology, 27*(5), 599-641.

Insel, T. R. (2009). Disruptive insights in psychiatry: Transforming a clinical discipline. *The Journal of Clinical Investigation, 119*(4), 700-705.

Institute of Medicine (1994). *Reducing risks for mental disorders: Frontiers for preventive intervention research.* Washington, DC: National Academy Press.

Izard, C. E. (1977). *Human emotions.* New York: Plenum Press.

Izard, C. E., Fine, S., Mostow, A., et al. (2002). Emotion processes in normal and abnormal development and preventive intervention. *Development and Psychopathology, 14,* 761-787.

Izard, C. E., King, K. A., Trentacosta, C. J., et al. (2008). Accelerating the development of emotion competence in Head Start children: Effects on adaptive and maladaptive behavior. *Development and Psychopathology, 20,* 369-397.

Izzo, C. V., Eckenrode, J. J., Smith, E. G., et al. (2005). Reducing the impact of uncontrollable stressful life events through a program of nurse home visitation for new parents. *Prevention Science, 6*(4), 269-274.

Jensen, P. S., Martin, D., & Watanabe, H. (1996). Children's response to parental separation during Operation Desert Storm. *Journal of American Academy of Child Adolescent Psychiatry, 35,* 433-441.

Jessor, R. (1991). Risk behavior in adolescence: A psychosocial framework for understanding and action. *Journal of Adolescent Health, 12,* 597-605.

Jeste, D. V., Alexopoulos, G. S., Bartels, S., et al. (1999). Consensus statement on the upcoming crisis in geriatric mental health. *Archives of General Psychiatry, 56,* 848-853.

Jiang, Y., Perry, D. K., & Hesser, J. E. (2010). Adolescent suicide and health risk behaviors: Rhode Island's 2007 Youth Risk Behavior Survey. *American Journal of Preventive Medicine, 38*(5), 551-555.

Johnson, J. G., Bromley, E., & McGeoch, P. G. (2009). Childhood experiences and development of maladaptive and adaptive personality traits. In J. M. Oldham, A. E. Skodol, & D. S. Bender (Eds.), *Essentials of personality disorders* (pp. 143-157). Washington, DC: American Psychiatric Publishing, Inc.

Johnson, K., Posner, S. F., Biermann, J., et al. (2006). Recommendations to improve preconception health and health care—United States. A report of the CDC/ATSDR Preconception Care Work Group and the Select Panel on Preconception Care. *Morbidity and Mortality Weekly Reports: Recommended Reports,* 55(RR-6), 1-23. Retrieved from www.cdc.gov/mmwr/preview/mmwrhtml/rr5506a1.htm

Johnson, S., Hollis, C., Kochhar, P., et al. (2010). Psychiatric disorders in extremely preterm children: Longitudinal findings at age 11 years in the EPICure study. *Journal of American Academy of Child and Adolescent Psychiatry, 49,* 453-463.

Jorm, A., Christensen, H., Henderson, A., et al. (2000). Predicting anxiety and depression from personality: Is there a synergistic effect of neuroticism and extraversion. *Journal of Abnormal Psychology, 109,* 145-149.

Kaplan, C. P., Turner, S., Norman, E., et al. (1996). Promoting resilience strategies: A modified consultation model. *Social Works in Education, 18*(3), 158-168.

Kaufman, J., Yang, B. Z., Douglas-Palumberi, H., et al. (2004). Social supports and serotonin transporter gene moderation moderate depression in maltreated children. *Proceedings of the National Academy of Science, USA, 101,* 17316-17321.

Kaufman, J., Yang, B. Z., Douglas-Palumberi, H., et al. (2006). Brain-derived neurotropic factor-5HTTLPR gene interactions and environmental modifiers of depression in children. *Biological Psychiatry, 59,* 673-680.

Kendall, P. C., Aschenbrand, S. G., & Hudson, J. L. (2003). Child-focused treatment of anxiety. In A. E. Kazdin & J. R. Weisz (Eds.), *Evidence-based psychotherapies for children and adolescents* (pp. 81-100). New York: Guilford Press.

Kessler, R. C., Berglund, P., Demler, O., et al. (2005a). Lifetime prevalence and age-of-onset distributions of DSM-IV disorders in the National Comorbidity Replication. *Archives of General Psychiatry, 62,* 593-602.

Kessler, R. C., Chiu, W. T., Demler, O., et al. (2005b). Prevalence, severity, and comorbidity of 12-month DSM-IV disorders in the national co-morbidity survey replication. *Archives of General Psychiatry, 62*(6), 617-627.

Kessler, R. C., Stang, P., Wittchen, H-U, et al. (1999). Lifetime co-morbidities between social phobia and mood disorders in the US National Comorbidity Survey. *Psychological Medicine, 29*(3), 555-567.

Kiesler, D. J. (1999). *Beyond the disease model of mental disorders* (pp. 141-169). Westport, CT: Praeger Publishers.

Kim-Cohen, J., Caspi, A., Moffitt, T. E., et al. (2003). Prior juvenile diagnoses in adults with mental disorder: Developmental follow-back of a prospective-longitudinal cohort. *Archives of General Psychiatry, 60,* 709-717.

Kitchener, B. A., & Jorm A. F. (2008). Mental Health First Aid: An international programme for early intervention. *Early Intervention Psychiatry, 2,* 55-61.

Kjoer, S. L., Wegener, G., Rosenberg, R., et al. (2010). Prenatal and adult stress interplay—behavioral implications. *Brain Research, 1320,* 106-113.

Knox, K. L., Litts, D. A., Talcott, G. W., et al. (2003). Risk of suicide and related adverse outcomes after exposure to a suicide prevention programme in the U.S. Air Force: Cohort study. *British Medical Journal, 327*(7428), 1376.

Koenig, H. G. (1998). Religious beliefs and practices of hospitalized medically ill older adults. *International Journal of Geriatric Psychiatry, 13,* 213-224.

Koenig, H. G. (2009). Research on religion, spirituality, and mental health: A review. *The Canadian Journal of Psychiatry, 54*(5), 283-291.

Kohn, R., Saxena, S., Levay, I., et al. (2004). The treatment gap in mental health care. *Bulletin of the World Health Organization, 82*(11), 858-866.

Kracke, K. (2001). Children's exposure to violence: The Safe Start Initiative. Office of Juvenile Justice and Delinquency Prevention, April, 13, www.safestartcenter.org.

Kraemer, H. C. (2010). Epidemiological methods: About time. *International Journal of Environmental Research in Public Health, 7*, 29-45.

Kraemer, H. C., Kazdin, A. E., Offord, D. R., et al. (1997). Coming to terms with the terms of risk. *Archives of General Psychiatry, 54*, 337-343.

Krueger, R. F. (1999). The structure of common mental disorders. *Archives of General Psychiatry, 56*, 921-926.

Kumpfer, K., & Alvardo, R. (1995). Strengthening families to prevent drug use in multi-ethnic youth. In G. Botvin, S. Schinkle, & M. Orlandi (Eds.), *Drug abuse prevention with multi-ethnic youth* (pp. 253-292). Newbury Park, CA: Sage Publications.

Kumpfer, K., Molraard, V., & Spoth, R. (1996). The "Strengthening Families Program" for the prevention of delinquency and drug use. In R. Peters & R. McMahon (Eds.), *Preventing childhood disorders, substance abuse, and delinquency.* Thousand Oaks, CA: Sage Publications.

Lahoti, S. L., McClain, N., Girardet, R., et al. (2001). Evaluating the child for sexual abuse. *American Family Physician, 65*(5), 883-893.

Lambert, S. F., Copeland-Linder, N., & Ialongo, N. S. (2008). Longitudinal associations between community violence exposure and suicidality. *Journal of Adolescent Health, 43*, 380-386.

Laraia, M. T. (2005). Omega-3 fatty acids: A "fish Story" for mental health. *APNA News, 17*(4), 10-11, 16.

Li, T-K, Witt, E., & Hewitt, G. B. G. (2007). Alcoholism: Developmental patterns of drinking and prevention of alcohol use disorders. In M. T. Tsuang, W. S. Stone, & M. J. Lyons (Eds.), *Recognition and prevention of major mental and substance use disorders* (pp. 297-316). Washington, DC: American Psychiatric Publishing, Inc.

Linares, T. J., Singer, L. T., Kirchner, H. L., et al. (2006). Mental health outcomes of cocaine-exposed children at 6 years of age. *Journal of Pediatric Psychology, 31*, 85-97.

Linehan, M. M., Armstrong, H. E., Suarez, A., et al. (1991). Cognitive-behavioral treatment of chronically parasuicidal borderline patients. *Archives of General Psychiatry, 48*, 1060-1064.

Lowry-Webster, H. M., Barrett, P. M., & Dadds, M. R. (2001). A universal prevention trial of anxiety and depressive symptomatology in childhood: Preliminary data from an Australian study. *Behavior Change, 18*(1), 36-50.

Lu, M. C., & Geffen, D. (2007). Recommendations for preconception care. *American Family Physician, 76*, 397-400.

Luby, J. L., Xuemei, S., Belden, A. C., et al. (2009). Preschool depression: Homotypic continuity and course over 24 months. *Archives of Psychiatry, 66*(8), 897-905.

Luoma, J. B., Martin, C. E., & Pearson, J. L. (2002). Contact with mental health and primary care providers before suicide: A review of the evidence. *American Journal of Psychiatry, 19*, 909-916.

Lupien, S. J., McEwen, B. S., Gunnar, M. R., et al. (2009). Effects of stress throughout the lifespan on the brain, behaviour and cognition. *Nature Reviews and Neuroscience, 10*, 434-445.

Lysaker, P. H., Meyer, P. S., Evans, J. D., et al. (2001). Childhood sexual trauma and psychosocial functioning in adults with schizophrenia. *Psychiatric Services, 52*(11), 1485-1488.

MacManus, R. P. (2002). Adolescent care: Reducing risk and promoting resilience. *Primary Care and Clinical Office Practice, 29*, 557-569.

MacMillan, H. L. (2009). New insights into prevention of depression and disruptive behaviour disorders in childhood: Where do we go from here? *The Canadian Journal of Psychiatry, 54*(4), 209-211.

Maier, H., & Lachman, M. E. (2000). Consequences of early parental loss and separation for health and well-being in midlife. *International Journal of Behavioral Development, 24*(2), 183-189.

Malaspina, D., Harlap, S., Fennig, S., et al. (2001). Advancing paternal age and the risk of schizophrenia. *Archives of General Psychiatry, 58*(4), 361-367.

Mann, J. J., Apter, A., Bertolote, J., et al. (2005). Suicide prevention strategies: A systematic review. *Journal of the American Medical Association, 294*(16), 2064-2074.

Marcelis, M., Navarro-Mateu, F., Murray, R., et al. (1998). Urbanization and psychosis: A study of 1942-1978 birth cohorts in The Netherlands. *Psychological Medicine, 28*(4), 871-879.

March, J., Silva, S., Petrycki, S., et al. (2004). Fluoxetine, cognitive-behavioral therapy, and their combination for adolescents with depression: Treatment for Adolescents with Depression Study (TADS) randomized controlled trial. *Journal of the American Medical Association, 292*, 807-820.

Marvin, R., Cooper, G., Hoffman, K., et al. (2002). The Circle of Security project: Attachment-based intervention with care-giver preschool child dyads. *Attachment & Human Development, 4*, 107-124.

Massie, H., & Szajnberg, N. (2006). My life is longing: Child abuse and its adult sequelae. Results of the Brody longitudinal study from birth to age 30. *International Journal of Psychoanalysis, 87*, 471-496.

Matz, K., Junghofer, M., Elbert, T., et al. (2010). Adverse experiences in childhood influence brain responses to emotional stimuli in adult psychiatric patients. *International Journal of Psychophysiology, 75*, 277-286.

Maughan, B., & Kim-Cohen, J. (2005). Continuities between childhood and adult life. *British Journal of Psychiatry, 187*, 301-303.

Mayes, L. C., & Suchman, N. (2006). Developmental pathways to substance abuse. In D. Cicchetti & D. Cohen (Eds.), *Developmental psychopathology: Risk, disorders, and adaptation* (Vol. 3) (pp. 599-619). New York: Wiley.

Mayou, R. A., Ehlers, A., & Hobbs, M. (2000). Psychological debriefing for road traffic accident victims: Three-year follow-up of a randomized controlled trial. *British Journal of Psychiatry, 176*, 589-593.

McCarroll, J. E., Ursano, R. J., Liu, S., et al. (2000). Deployment and the probability of spousal aggression by U.S. Army soldiers. *Military Medicine, 165*, 41-44.

McCrone, P., Knapp, M., Proudfoot, J., et al. (2004). Cost-effectiveness of computerized cognitive-behavioral therapy for anxiety and depression in primary care: Randomized controlled trial. *British Journal of Psychiatry, 185*, 55-62.

McEwen, B. S. (2007). Physiology and neurobiology of stress and adaptation: Central role of the brain. *Physiology Review, 87*, 873-904.

McEwen, B. S. (2008). Central effects of stress hormones in health and disease: Understanding the protective and damaging effects of stress and stress mediators. *European Journal of Pharmacology, 583*, 174-185.

McEwen, B. S. (2009). The brain is the central organ of stress and adaptation. *NeuroImage, 47*(3), 911-913.

McFarlane, W. R., Cook, W. I., Downing, D., et al. (2010). Portland identification and early referral: A community-based system for identifying and treating youths at high risk of psychosis. *Psychiatric Services, 61*, 512-515.

McFarlane, W. R., Dushay, R. A., Stastny, P., et al. (1996). A comparison of two levels of family-aided assertive community treatment. *Psychiatric Services, 47*, 744-750.

McGlashan, T. H., Zipursky, R. B., Perkins, D. O., et al. (2006). Randomized, double-blind trial of olanzapine versus placebo in patients prodromally symptomatic for psychosis. *American Journal of Psychiatry, 163*(5), 790-799.

McGorry, P. D., Nelson, B., Amminger, P., et al. (2009). Intervention in individuals at ultra-high risk for psychosis: A review and future directions. *Journal of Clinical Psychiatry, 70*(9), 1206-1212.

McGorry, P. D., Yung, A. R., Phillips, L. J., et al. (2002). Randomized controlled trial of interventions designed to reduce the risk of progression to first-episode psychosis in a clinical sample with sub-threshold symptoms. *Archives of General Psychiatry, 59*, 921-928.

McGowan, P. O., Sasaki, A. D., Alessio, A. C., et al. (2009). Epigenetic regulation of the glucocorticoid receptor in human brain associated with childhood abuse. *Nature Neuroscience, 12*(3), 342-348.

McGuiness, T. M. (2010). Childhood adversities and adult health. *Journal of Psychosocial Nursing, 48*(8), 15-18.

McInnis, G. J., & White, J. H. (2001). A phenomenological exploration of loneliness in the older adult. *Archives of Psychiatric Nursing, 15*(3), 128-139.

McKeown, R. E., Garrison, C. Z., Cuffe, S. P., et al. (1998). Incidence and predictors of suicidal behaviors in a longitudinal sample of young adolescents. *Journal of the American Academy of Child and Adolescent Psychiatry, 37*, 612-619.

McLaughlin, K. A., Green, J. G., Gruber, M. J., et al. (2010). Childhood adversities and adult psychiatric disorders in the National Comorbidity Survey Replication II. *Archives of General Psychiatry, 67*(2), 124-132.

Melhem, N. M., Walker, M., Moritz, G., et al. (2008). Antecedents and sequelae of sudden parental death in offspring and surviving caregivers. *Archives of Pediatrics and Adolescent Medicine, 162*(5), 403-410.

Merry, S. N. (2007). Prevention and early intervention for depression in young people—a practical possibility? *Current Opinion in Psychiatry, 20*(4), 325-329.

Miller-Heyl, J., McPhee, D., & Fritz, J. (1998). DARE to be YOU: A family-support, early intervention program. *Journal of Primary Prevention, 18,* 251-258.

Mojtabai, R., Malaspina, D., & Susser, E. (2003). The concept of population prevention: Application to schizophrenia. *Schizophrenia Bulletin, 29*(4), 791-801.

Moore, T. H., Zammit, S., Lingford-Hughes, A., et al. (2007). Cannabis use and risk of psychotic or affective mental health outcomes: A systematic review. *Lancet, 370,* 319-328.

Morrison, A. P., French, P., Walford, L., et al. (2004). Cognitive therapy for the prevention of psychosis in people at ultra-high risk: Randomized controlled trial. *British Journal of Psychiatry, 185*(4), 291-297.

Mortensen, P. B., Pedersen, C. B., Westergaard, T., et al. (1999). Effects of family history and place and season of birth on the risk of schizophrenia. *The New England Journal of Medicine, 340*(8), 603-608.

Mrazek, P. J., & Haggerty, R. J. (Eds.). (1994). *Reducing risks for mental disorders: Frontiers for preventive intervention research.* Washington, DC: National Academies Press.

Mufson, L., Dorta, K. P., Wickramaratne, P., et al. (2004). A randomized effectiveness trial of interpersonal psychotherapy for depressed adolescents. *Archives of General Psychiatry, 61,* 577-584.

Murray, J. L., & Lopez, A. D. (1997). *The global burden of disease study.* Boston: World Health Organization.

Muthen, B. O., Jo, V., & Brown, C. H. (2003). Assessment of treatment effects using latent variable modeling: Comment on the Barnard, Frangakis, Hill and Rubin article—Principal stratification approach to broken randomized experiments: A case study of school choice vouchers in New York City. *Journal of the American Statistical Association, 98,* 311-314.

Nasrallah, H. A. (2011). Harassing epigenetics for psychiatry. *Current Psychiatry, 12,* 16.

Nation, M., Crusto, C., Wandersman, A., et al. (2003). What works in prevention: Principles of effective prevention programs. *American Psychologist, 58*(6/7), 449-456.

National Alliance on Mental Illness. (2002). *Anxiety disorders in children and adolescents.* Retrieved from http://www.nami.org/Content/ContentGroups/Helpline1/Anxiety_Disorders_in_Children_and_Adolescents.htm

National Clearinghouse on Child Abuse and Neglect Information. (2004a). *Risk and protective factors for child abuse and neglect.* Retrieved from http://www.nccanch.acf.hhs.gov/topics/prevention/emerging/report/index.cfm

National Clearinghouse on Child Abuse and Neglect Information. (2004b). *Long-term consequences of child abuse and neglect.* Retrieved from http://www.nccanch.acf.hhs.gov/pub/factsheets/long-term-consequences.cfm

Nemeroff, C. B. (2004). Neurobiological consequences of childhood trauma. *Journal of Clinical Psychiatry, 65*(Suppl 1), 18-28.

New, A. S., Keegan, K. A., & Charney, D. S. (2007). Psychobiology of resilience to stress. In M. T. Tsuang, W. S. Stone, & M. J. Lyons (Eds.), *Recognition and prevention of major mental and substance use disorders* (pp. 77-96). Washington, DC: American Psychiatric Publishing, Inc.

Nock, M. K., Borges, G., Bromet, E., et al. (2008). Suicide and suicidal behaviors. *Epidemiologic Review, 30,* 133-154.

Nock, M. K., Hwang, I., Sampson, N., et al. (2009). Cross-National analysis of the association among mental disorders and suicidal behavior: Findings from the WHO World Mental Health Surveys. *PloS Medicine, 6*(8), 1-17,

O'Connell, M. E., Boat, T., & Warner, W. E. (Eds.). (2009). *Preventing mental, emotional, and behavioral disorders among young people: Progress and possibilities.* Washington, DC, National Academies Press.

Oldham, J. M. (2009). Personality disorders. In J. M. Oldham, A. E. Skodol, & D. S. Bender (Eds.), *Essentials of personality disorders* (pp. 3-11). Washington, DC: American Psychiatric Publishing, Inc.

Olds, D. L. (2006). The nurse-family partnership: An evidence-based preventive intervention. *Infant Mental Health Journal, 27,* 5-25.

Olds, D. L., Eckenrode, J., Henderson, C. R., et al. (1997). Long-term effects of home visitation on maternal life course and child abuse and neglect. Fifteen-year follow-up of a randomized trial. *Journal of the American Medical Association, 278,* 637-643.

Olds, D. L., Henderson, C. R., Chamberlin, R., et al. (1986). Preventing child abuse and neglect: A randomized trial of nurse home visitation. *Pediatrics, 78,* 65-78.

Olds, D. L., Henderson, C. R., Cole, R., et al. (1998). Long-term effects of nurse home visitation on children's criminal and antisocial behavior. *Journal of the American Medical Association, 280*(14), 1238-1244.

Olds, D. L., Henderson, C. R., Jr., Tatelbaum, R., et al. (1988). Improving the life-course development of socially disadvantaged mothers: A randomized trial of nurse home visitation. *American Journal of Public Health, 78*(11), 1436-1445.

Olds, D. L., Kitzman, H., Cole, R., et al. (2004). Effects of nurse home-visiting on maternal life course and child development: Age 6 follow-up results of a randomized trial. *Pediatrics, 114*(6), 1550-1559.

Olds, D. L., Robinson, J., O'Brien, R., et al. (2002). Home visiting by paraprofessionals and by nurses: A randomized controlled trial. *Pediatrics, 110,* 486-496.

Olds, D. L., Sadler, L., & Kitzman, H. (2007). Programs for parents of infants and toddlers: Recent evidence from randomized trials. *Journal of Child Psychology and Psychiatry, 48*(3/4), 355-391.

Olweus, D. (1989). Bully/victim problems among schoolchildren: Basic facts and effects of a school-based intervention program. In K. Rubin & D. Heppler (Eds.), *The development and treatment of childhood aggression* (pp. 411-448). Hillsdale, NJ: Lawrence Erlbaum Associates.

Olweus, D., & Limber, S. P. (2010). Bullying in school: Evaluation and dissemination of the Olweus Bullying Prevention Program. *American Journal of Orthopsychiatry, 80*(1), 124-134.

Oslin, D. W., Zubritsky, C., Brown, G., et al. (2004). Managing suicide risk in late life: Access to firearms as a public health risk. *American Journal of Geriatric Psychiatry, 12,* 30-36.

Paradis, A. D., Reinherz, H. Z., Giaconia, R. M., et al. (2009). Long-term impact of family arguments and physical violence on adult functioning at age 30 years: Findings from the Simmons Longitudinal Study. *Journal of American Academy of Child and Adolescent Psychiatry, 48*(3), 290-298.

Pearce, B. D. (2001). Schizophrenia and viral infection during neurodevelopment: A focus on mechanisms. *Molecular Psychiatry, 6*(6), 634-646.

Pearson, G. S. (2010). The past defines the present. *Perspectives in Psychiatric Care, 46*(3), 169-170.

Pentz, M. A., Dwyer, J. H., MacKinnon, D. P., et al. (1989). A multicommunity trial for primary prevention of adolescent drug abuse. Effects on drug use prevalence. *Journal of the American Medical Association, 261,* 3259-3266.

Perry, C. L., Komro, K. A., Veblen-Mortenson, S., et al. (2003). A randomized controlled trial of the middle and junior high school D.A.R.E. and D.A.R.E. Plus programs. *Archives of Pediatrics and Adolescent Medicine, 157,* 178-184.

Petitclerc, A., & Tremblay, R. E. (2009). Childhood disruptive behaviour disorders: Review of their origin, development and prevention. *Canadian Journal of Psychiatry, 54*(4), 222-231.

Petras, H., Kellam, S. G., Brown, C. H., et al. (2008). Developmental epidemiological courses leading to antisocial personality disorder and violent and criminal behavior: Effects by young adulthood of a universal preventive intervention in first- and second-grade classrooms. *Drug and Alcohol Dependence, 95*(Suppl 1), S45-S59.

Phillips, L. J., Nelson, B., Yuen, H. P., et al. (2009). Randomized controlled trial of interventions for young people at ultra-high risk of psychosis: Study design and baseline characteristics. *Australian and New Zealand Journal of Psychiatry, 43*(9), 818-829.

Phillips, R. S. C. (2000). Preventing depression: A program for African American elders with chronic pain. *Family Community Health, 22,* 56-65.

Pine, D. S., Cohen, P., & Brook, J. (2001). Adolescent fears as predictors of depression. *Biological Psychiatry, 50*(9), 721-724.

Pirruccello, L. M. (2010). Preventing adolescent suicide: A community takes action. *Journal of Psychosocial Nursing, 48*(5), 34-41.

Pitman, R. K., & Delahanty, D. L. (2007). Conceptually driven pharmacological approaches to acute trauma. In M. T. Tsuang, W. S.

Stone, & M. J. Lyons (Eds.), *Recognition and prevention of major mental and substance use disorders* (pp. 371-387). Washington, DC: American Psychiatric Publishing, Inc.

Powers, R. A. (2010). Prevention of alcohol and drug abuse. In M. T. Compton (Ed.), *Clinical manual of prevention in mental health* (pp. 163-210). Washington, DC: American Psychiatric Publishing, Inc.

President's New Freedom Commission on Mental Health. (2003). *Achieving the promise: Transforming mental health care in America.* Washington, DC: Department of Health and Human Services.

Preventing Child Abuse and Neglect. (2008). Childwelfare Information Gateway. www.childwelfare.gov/pubs/factsheets/preveningcan.cfm

Qin, P., Mortensen, P. B., & Pedersen, C. B. (2009). Frequent change of residence and risk of attempted and competed suicide among children and adolescents. *Archives of General Psychiatry, 66,* 626-632.

Rabin, R. (2006, November 28). That prenatal visit may be months too late. *The New York Times.* Retrieved from http://query.nytimes.com/gst/fullpage.html?res=9C02EEDA103EF93BA15752C1A9609C8B63&scp=1&sq=That%20prenatal%20visit%20may%20be%20months%20too%20late&st=cse

Ramey, C., Bryant, D. M., & Wasik, B. H., et al. (1992). Infant health and development program for low birth weight, premature infants: Program elements, family participation and child intelligence. *Pediatrics, 89*(3), 454-465.

Raphael, B. (1977). Preventive intervention with the recently bereaved. *Archives of General Psychiatry, 34,* 1450-1454.

Rentz, E. D., Marshall, S. W., Loomis, D., et al. (2007). Effect of deployment on the occurrence of child maltreatment in military and nonmilitary families. *American Journal of Epidemiology, 165,* 1199-1206.

Repetti, R. L., Taylor, S. E., & Seeman, T. (2002). Risky families: Family social environments and the mental and physical health of offspring. *Psychological Bulletin, 128*(2), 330-366.

Resnick, M. D., Bearman, P. S., Blum, W. R., et al. (1997). Protecting adolescents from harm: Findings from the National Longitudinal Study on adolescent health. *Journal of the American Medical Association, 278,* 823-832.

Riley, A. W., Valdez, C. R., Barrueco, S., et al. (2008). Development of a family-based program to reduce risk and promote resilience among families affected by maternal depression: Theoretical basis and program description. *Clinical Child and Family Psychological Review, 11,* 12-29.

Rodriguez, A., & Bohlin, G. (2005). Are maternal smoking and stress during pregnancy related to ADHD symptoms in children? *Journal of Child Psychology and Psychiatry, 46,* 246-254.

Romano, E., Tremblay, R. E., Vitaro, F., et al. (2001). Prevalence of psychiatric diagnoses and the role of perceived impairment: Findings from an adolescent community sample. *Journal of Child Psychology and Psychiatry, 40*(4), 451-461.

Rose, S., Bisson, J., & Wessely, S. (2003). A systematic review of single-session psychological interventions ("debriefing") following trauma. *Psychotherapy and Psychosomatics, 72,* 176-184.

Rosen, L. N., Durand, D. B., & Martin, J. A. (2000). Wartime stress and family adaptation. In J. A. Martin, L. N. Rosen, & L. R. Sparacino (Eds.), *The military family: A practice guide for human service providers.* Westport, CT: Praeger Publishers.

Rovner, B. W., & Casten, R. J. (2008). Preventing late-life depression in age-related macular degeneration. *American Journal of Geriatric Psychiatry, 16,* 454-459.

Rovner, B. W., Casten, R. J., Hegel, M. T., et al. (2007). Preventing depression in age-related macular degeneration. *Archives of General Psychiatry, 64,* 886-892.

Roza, S. J., Hofstra, M. B., van der Ende, J., et al. (2003). Stable prediction of mood and anxiety disorders based on behavioral and emotional problems in childhood: A 14-year follow-up during childhood, adolescence and young adulthood. *American Journal of Psychiatry, 160,* 2116-2121.

Rutter, M. (1985). Resilience in the face of adversity. Protective factors and resistance to psychiatric disorders. *British Journal of Psychiatry, 147,* 598-611.

Rutter, M. (1989). Pathways from childhood to adult life. *Journal of Child Psychology and Psychiatry, 30*(1), 25-51.

Rutter, M. (2006). Is Sure Start an effective preventive intervention? *Child and Adolescent Mental Health, 11*(3), 135-141.

Rutter, M., Moffitt, T. C., & Caspi, A. (2006). Gene-environment interplay and psychopathology: Multiple varieties but real effects. *Journal of Child Psychological Psychiatry, 47,* 226-261.

Rutter, M., & Quinton, D. (1977). Psychiatric disorder. Ecological factors and concepts of causation. In H. McGurk (Ed.), *Ecological factors in human development* (pp. 173-187). Amsterdam: North-Holland Publishing.

Ryff, C. D., & Singer, B. (2000). Biopsychosocial challenges of the new millennium. *Psychotherapy and Psychosomatics, 69,* 170-177.

Sadock, B. J., & Sadock, V. A. (Eds.). (2007). *Kaplan & Sadock's synopsis of psychiatry* (10th ed.). Philadelphia: Walters Kluwer Health: Lippincott, Williams & Wilkins.

Sameroff, A. J., Gutman, I. M., & Peck, S. C. (2003). Adaptation among youth facing multiple risks: Prospective research findings. In S. S. Luthar (Ed.), *Resilience and vulnerability: Adaptation in the context of childhood adversities* (pp. 364-391). New York: Cambridge University Press.

SAMHSA's National Registry of Evidence-based Programs and Practices. (2007). Retrieved from http://www.nrepp.samhsa.gov/ViewIntervention.aspx?id=28

Sandler, I. N., Ayers, T. S., Wolchik., S. A., et al. (2003). The Family Bereavement Program: Efficacy evaluation of a theory-based prevention program for parentally bereaved children and adolescents. *Journal of Consulting and Clinical Psychology, 71,* 587-600.

Sandler, I. N., Ma, Y., Tein, J-Y, et al. (2010). Long-term effects of the Family Bereavement Program on multiple indicators of grief in parentally bereaved children and adolescents. *Journal of Consulting and Clinical Psychology, 78*(2), 131-143.

Saugstad, L. F. (2004). From superior adaptation and function to brain dysfunction—the neglect of epigenetic factors. *Nutrition and Health, 18,* 3-27.

Schilling, E. A., Aseltine, R. H., & Gore, S. (2007). Adverse childhood experiences and mental health in young adults: A longitudinal survey. *BMC Public Health, 7,* 30.

Schmutte, T., O'Connell, M., Weiland, M., et al. (2009). Stemming the tide of suicide in older white men: A call to action. *American Journal of Men's Health, 3*(3), 189-200.

Schoevers, R. A., Beekman, A. T., Deeg, D. J., et al. (2000). Risk factors for depression in later life: Results of a prospective community based study (AMSTEL). *Journal of Affective Disorders, 59,* 127-137.

Schoevers, R. A., Smit, F., Deeg, D. J., et al. (2006). Prevention of late-life depression in primary care: Do we know where to begin? *American Journal of Psychiatry, 163*(9), 1611-1621.

Schrecker, T., Acosta, L., Somerville, M. A., et al. (2001). The ethics of social risk reduction in the era of the biological brain. *Social Science & Medicine, 52,* 1677-1687.

Schumm, W. R., Bell, D. B., & Gade, P. A. (2000). Effects of military overseas peacekeeping deployment on marital quality, satisfaction, and stability. *Psychological Report, 87,* 815-821.

Schweinhart, I. J., & Weikart, D. P. (1989). The High/Scope Perry Preschool study: Implications for early childhood care and education. *Prevention in Human Services, 7,* 109-132.

Scott, J., Varghese, D., & McGrath, J. (2010). As the twig is bent, the tree inclines: Adult mental health consequences of childhood adversity. *Archives of General Psychiatry, 67*(2), 111-112.

Seed, M., & Higgins, S. (2003). Integrating mental illness prevention into community-based undergraduate education. *Journal of Nursing Education, 42*(1), 8-12.

Seeman, T. E., Singer, G. H., Ryff, C. D., et al. (2002). Social relationships, gender, and allostatic load across two age cohorts. *Psychosomatic Medicine, 64*(3), 395-406.

Seligman, M. E. P., Berkowitz, M. W., Catalano, R. F., et al. (2005). Beyond disorder: The positive perspective on youth development. In D. L. Evans, E. B. Foa, R. E. Gur, et al. (Eds.), *Treating and preventing adolescent mental health disorders: What we know and what we don't know* (pp. 498-527). Oxford, UK: Oxford University Press.

Shanahan, L., Copeland, W., Costello, E. J., et al. (2008). Specificity of putative psychosocial risk factors for psychiatric disorders in children and adolescents. *The Journal of Child Psychology and Psychiatry, 49*(1), 34-42.

Shaw, D. S., Dishion, T. J., Supplee, I., et al. (2006). Randomized trial of a family-centered approach to the prevention of early conduct problems:

2-year effects of the Family Check-Up in early childhood. *Journal of Consulting and Clinical Psychology, 74*(1), 1-9.

Shea, A., Walsh, C., MacMillan, H. L., et al. (2004). Child maltreatment and HPA axis dysregulation. Relationship to major depressive disorder and posttraumatic stress disorder in females. *Psychoneuroendocrinology, 30*, 162-178.

Shenfeld, K. (2007). CrossCurrents: From deficits to strengths: How to help families nurture resilient children. *Centre for Addiction and Mental Health.* Retrieved from http://www.camh.net/Publications/Cross_Currents/Summer_%202007/deficitsstrengths_crcusummer07.html

Shonkoff, J. P., Boyce, T., & McEwen, B. S. (2009). Neuroscience, molecular biology, and the childhood roots of health disparities: Building a new framework for health promotion and disease prevention. *Journal of the American Medical Association, 301*(21), 2252-2259.

Shure, M. B. (1997). Interpersonal cognitive problem solving: Primary prevention of early high-risk behaviors in the preschool and primary years. In G. W. Albee & T. P. Gullotta (Eds.), *Primary prevention works. Issues in children's and families' lives* (Vol. 6) (pp. 239-267). Thousand Oaks, CA: Sage Publications.

Shure, M. B. (2000). "I can Problem Solve." Retrieved from http://www.thinkingpreteen.com/icps.htm

Shure, M. B., & Spivack, G. (1988). Interpersonal cognitive problem-solving. In R. H. Price (Ed.), *14 ounces of prevention: A casebook for practitioners* (pp. 69-82). Washington, DC: American Psychological Association.

Smit, F., Ederveen, A., Cuijpers, P., et al. (2006). Opportunities for cost-effective prevention of late-life depression: An epidemiological approach. *Archives of General Psychiatry, 63*(3), 290-296.

Smit, F., Smit, N., Schoevers, R., et al. (2008). An epidemiological approach to depression prevention in old age. *American Journal of Geriatric Psychiatry, 16*, 444-453.

Smith, J. (2002). Evaluation, diagnosis and outcomes of child sexual abuse. *Child Sexual Abuse: Evaluation & Outcomes, The Child Advocate.* Retrieved from http://www.childadvocate.net/child_sexual_abuse.htm

Smoller, J. W., & Korf, B. R. (2008). The road ahead. In J. W. Smoller, B. R. Sheidley, & M. T. Tsuang (Eds.), *Psychiatric genetics: Application in clinical practice* (pp. 277-298). Washington, DC: American Psychiatric Publishing, Inc.

Solomon, D., Battistich, V., Watson, M., et al. (2000). A six-district study of educational change: Direct and mediated effects of the child development project. *Social Psychology of Education, 4*(1), 3–51.

Sonuga-Barke, E. J. S., & Halperin, J. M. (2010). Developmental phenotypes and causal pathways in attention deficit/hyperactivity disorder: Potential targets for early intervention? *The Journal of Child Psychology and Psychiatry, 51*(4), 368-389.

Sonuga-Barke, E. J. S., Thompson, M., Abikoff, H., et al. (2006). Non-pharmacological interventions for preschool ADHD: The case for specialized parent training. *Infants and Young Children, 19*, 142-153.

Spar, J. E., & La Rue, A. (2006). *Clinical manual of geriatric psychiatry.* Washington, DC: American Psychiatric Publishing, Inc.

Spence, S. H., Sheffield, J. K., & Donovan, C. I. (2003). Preventing adolescent depression: An evaluation of the problem-solving for life program. *Journal of Consulting Clinical Psychology, 7*, 3-13.

Spiegel, D. (1999). Healing words: Emotional expression and disease outcome. *Journal of the American Medical Association, 281*(4), 1328-1329.

Spirito, A., & Esposito-Smythers, C. (2006). Attempted and completed suicide in adolescence. *Annual Review of Clinical Psychology, 2*, 237-266.

Stahl, S. (2000). *Essential psychopharmacology* (2nd ed.). Cambridge, UK: Cambridge University Press.

Staten, R. (2008). Primary prevention: A call for advocacy and action: National Forum for Mental Health Promotion and Mental Illness Prevention. *Journal of Child & Adolescent Psychiatric Nursing, 21*(2), 121-122.

Steele, M. M., & Doey, T. (2007). Suicidal behaviour in children and adolescents, Part 1: Etiology and risk factors. *Canadian Journal of Psychiatry, 52*(6 Suppl 1), 21S-33S.

Steptoe, A., Owen, N., Kunz-Ebrecht, S. R., et al. (2004). Loneliness and neuroendocrine, cardiovascular, and inflammatory stress responses in middle-aged men and women. *Psychoneuroendocrinology, 29*, 593-611.

Steptoe, A., Wardlaw, J., & Marmot, M. (2005). Positive affect and health-related neuroendocrine, cardiovascular, and inflammatory processes. *Proceedings of the National Academy of Science, USA, 102*, 6508-6512.

Stevens, N. (2001). Combating loneliness: A friendship enrichment programme for older women. *Ageing & Society, 21*(2), 183-202.

Stormshak, E. A., & Dishion, T. J. (2009). A school-based, family-centered intervention to prevent substance use: The family check-up. *The American Journal of Drug and Alcohol Abuse, 35*, 227-232.

Sutton, J. M. (2007). Prevention of depression in youth: A qualitative review and future suggestions. *Clinical Psychology Review, 27*(5), 552-571.

Taylor, S. (1999). The lifelong legacy of childhood abuse. *The American Journal of Medicine, 107*(4), 399-400.

Tein, J. V., Sandler, I. N., Ayers, T. S., et al. (2006). Mediation of the effects of the Family Bereavement Program on mental health problems of bereaved children and adolescents. *Previews of Science, 7*, 179-195.

Tepper, L., Rogers, S. A., Coleman, E. M., et al. (2001). The prevalence of religious coping among persons with persistent mental illness. *Psychiatric Services, 52*, 660-665.

Thal, L. (1996). Potential prevention strategies for Alzheimer disease. *Alzheimer Disease and Associated Disorders, 10*, 6-8.

Thomas, R., & Zimmer-Gembeck, J. J. (2007). Behavioral outcomes of parent-child interaction therapy and Triple P-Positive Parenting Program: A review and meta-analysis. *Journal of Abnormal Child Psychology, 35*, 475-495.

Thompson, E. A., Eggert, L. L., & Herting, J. R. (2000). Mediating effects of an indicated prevention program for reducing youth depression and suicide-risk behaviors. *Suicide and Life Threatening Behavior, 30*, 252-271.

Thompson, E. A., Eggert, L. L., Randell, B. P., et al. (2001). Evaluation of indicated suicide-risk prevention approaches for potential high school dropouts. *American Journal of Public Health, 91*, 742-752.

Thompson, M. J. J., Laver-Bradbury, C., Ayres, M., et al. (2009). A small-scale randomized controlled trial of the revised New Forest Package for Preschoolers with Attention Deficit Hyperactivity Disorder. *European Child and Adolescent Psychiatry, 18*(10), 605-616.

Tishler, C. L., Reiss, N. S., & Rhodes, A. R. (2007). Suicidal behavior in children younger than twelve: A diagnostic challenge for emergency department personnel. *Academic Emergency Medicine, 14*, 810-818.

Torrey, E. F., Bowler, A. E., Rawlings, R., et al. (1993). Seasonality of schizophrenia and stillbirths. *Schizophrenia Bulletin, 19*(3), 557-562.

Tremblay, R. E., Pagani-Kurtz, L., Masse, L. C., et al. (1995). A bimodal preventive intervention for disruptive kindergarten boys: Its impact through mid-adolescence. *Journal of Counseling and Clinical Psychology, 63*(4), 560-568.

Trentacosta, C. J., Hyde, L. W., Shaw, D. S., et al. (2008). The relations among cumulative risk, parenting, and behavior problems during early childhood. *The Journal of Child Psychology and Psychiatry, 49*(11), 1211-1219.

Turner, H. A., Finkelhor, D., & Ormrod, R. (2010). Poly-victimization in a national sample of children and youth. *American Journal of Preventive Medicine, 38*(3), 323-330.

United States Department of Health and Human Services. (2001). *Youth violence: A report of the Surgeon General.* Retrieved from http://www.surgeongeneral.gov/library/youthviolence/youvioreport.htm

United States Department of Health and Human Services. (2009). *The 2009 HHS Poverty Guidelines.* Retrieved from http://aspe.hhs.gov/poverty/09poverty.shtml

Unutzer, J., Katon, W., Williams, J. W., Jr., et al. (2001). Improving primary care for depression in late life: The design of a multicenter randomized trial. *Medical Care, 39*, 785-799.

Unutzer, J., Tang, L., Oishi, S., et al.; for the IMPACT Investigators. (2006). Reducing suicidal ideation in depressed older primary care patients. *Journal of the American Geriatric Society, 54*(10), 1550-1556.

Ursano, A. M., Kartheiser, P. H., & Barnhill, L. J. (2008). Disorders usually first diagnosed in infancy, childhood, or adolescence. In R. E. Hales, S. C. Yudofsky, & G. O. Gabbard (Eds.), *The American psychiatric publishing textbook of psychiatry* (5th ed.) (pp. 861-920). Washington, DC: American Psychiatric Publishing, Inc.

Vaillant, G. E. (2003). Mental health. *American Journal of Psychiatry, 160*, 1373-1384.

Van Leeuwen Williams, E., Unutzer, J., Lee, S., et al. (2009). Collaborative depression care for the old-old: Findings from the IMPACT trial. *American Journal of Geriatric Psychiatry, 17*(12), 1040-1049.

Vaurio, L., Riley, E. R., & Mattson, S. N. (2008). Differences in executive functioning in children with heavy prenatal alcohol exposure or attention-deficit/hyperactivity disorder. *Journal of the International Neuropsychological Society, 14,* 119-129.

Verbiest, S., & Holliday, J. (2009). Preconception care: Building the foundation for healthy women, babies and communities. *North Carolina Medical Journal, 70*(5), 417-426.

Volkow, N. D., & Li, T-K. (2007). Drugs and alcohol: Treating and preventing abuse, addiction, and their medical consequences. In M. T. Tsuang, W. S. Stone, & M. J. Lyons (Eds.), *Recognition and prevention of major mental and substance use disorders* (pp. 263-266). Washington, DC: American Psychiatric Publishing, Inc.

Waddell, C., Hua, J. M., Garland, O. M., et al. (2007a). Preventing mental disorders in children. *Canadian Journal of Public Health, 98*(3), 166-173.

Waddell, C., McEwan, K., Peters, R., et al. (2007b). Preventing mental disorders in children: A public health priority. *Canadian Journal of Public Health, 98*(3), 174-178.

Waern, M., Rubernowitz, E., & Wilhelmson, K., et al. (2003). Predictors of suicide in the old elderly. *Gerontology, 49,* 328-334.

Wagnild, G. M., & Collins, J. A. (2009). Assessing resilience. *Journal of Psychosocial Nursing, 47*(12), 28-33.

Webster-Stratton, C. (1987). *Incredible years parents and children training series: BASIC manual,* Revised. Seattle, WA: Incredible Years.

Webster-Stratton, C. (1990). *The incredible years parent training program manual: Effective communication, anger management and problem-solving (ADVANCE).* Seattle, WA: Incredible Years.

Webster-Stratton, C., Reid, M. J., & Hammond, M. (2001). Preventing conduct problems, promoting social competence: A parent and teacher training partnership in Head Start. *Journal of Clinical Child Psychology, 30,* 283-302.

Weiser, M., Reichenberg, A., Rabinowitz, J., et al. (2001). Association between non-psychotic psychiatric diagnosis in adolescent males and subsequent onset of schizophrenia. *Archives of General Psychiatry, 58*(10), 959-964.

Weisz, J. R., Sandler, I. N., Durlak, J. A., et al. (2005). Promoting and protecting youth mental health through evidence-based prevention and treatment. *American Psychologist, 60*(6), 628-648.

Werner, E. E. (1989). High-risk children in young adulthood: A longitudinal study from birth to 32 years. *American Journal of Orthopsychiatry, 59,* 72-81.

Werner, E. E. (1995). Resilience in development. *Current Directions in Psychological Science, 4,* 81-85.

Werner, E. E., & Smith, R. S. (1982). *Vulnerable but invincible: A longitudinal study of resilient children and youth.* New York: McGraw-Hill Book Company.

Werner, E. E., & Smith, R. S. (1992). *Overcoming the odds: High risk children from birth to adulthood.* Ithaca, New York: Cornell University Press.

What Works Clearinghouse. (2007, April). *Intervention: Caring School Community.* Institute of Education Sciences, U.S. Department of Education. Retrieved from http://ies.ed.gov/ncee/wwc/reports/character_education/csc/

Whyte, E. M., & Rovner, B. (2006). Depression in late-life: Shifting the paradigm from treatment to prevention. *International Journal of Geriatric Psychiatry, 21,* 746-751.

Wilhelm, K., Wedgwood, L., Parker, G., et al. (2010). Predicting mental health and well-being in adulthood. *The Journal of Nervous and Mental Disease, 198*(2), 85-90.

Wilk, A. I., Jensen, N. M., & Havighurst, T. C. (1997). Meta-analysis of randomized control trials addressing brief interventions in heavy alcohol drinkers. *Journal of General Internal Medicine, 12,* 274-283.

Willemse, G. R., Smit, F., Cuijpers, P., et al. (2004). Minimal-contact psychotherapy for sub-threshold depression in primary care. *British Journal of Psychiatry, 185,* 416-421.

Williams, S. V., O'Connor, E. A., Eder, M., et al. (2009). Screening for child and adolescent depression in primary care settings: A systematic evidence review for the US Preventive Services Task Force. *Pediatrics, 123,* e716-e735.

Wilson, R. S., Krueger, K. R., Arnold, S. E., et al. (2007). Loneliness and risk of Alzheimer disease. *Archives of General Psychiatry, 64,* 234-240.

Wilson, S. L. (2009). Understanding and promoting attachment. *Journal of Psychosocial Nursing, 47*(8), 23-27.

Wittchen, H-U, Beesdo, K., Bittner, A., et al. (2003). Depressive episodes—evidence for a causal role of primary anxiety disorders? *European Psychiatry, 18,* 384-393.

Wolchik, S. A., Sandler, L., Millsap, R. E., et al. (2002). Six-year followup of a randomized controlled trial of preventive interventions for children of divorce. *Journal of the American Medical Association, 288,* 1847-1881.

Wolchik, S. A., Tein, J. Y., Sandler, I., et al. (2006). Self-system beliefs as mediators of the relations between positive parenting and children's adjustment problems after parental death. *Journal of Abnormal Child Psychology, 34,* 331-338.

Wolchik, S. A., West, S. G., Sandler, L., et al. (2000). An experimental evaluation of theory-based mother and mother-child programs for children of divorce. *Journal of Consulting and Clinical Psychology, 68*(5), 843-856.

World Health Organization. (2002). *Prevention and promotion in mental health. Mental health: Evidence and research. Department of Mental health and Substance Dependence,* Geneva, Switzerland: World Health Organization.

World Health Organization. (2005). *Mental health action plan for Europe: Facing the challenges, building solutions.* Copenhagen: World Health Organization.

Xaverius, P. K., Tenkku, L., & Salas, J. (2009). Differences between women at higher and lower risk for an unintended pregnancy. *Women's Health Issues, 19,* 306-312.

Young, J. F., Mufson, L., & Davies, M. (2006). Efficacy of interpersonal psychotherapy-adolescent skills training: An indicated preventive intervention for depression. *Journal of Child Psychology and Psychiatry, 47,* 1254-1262.

Yung, A. R., Yuen, H. P., Berger, G., et al. (2007). Declining transition rate in ultra high risk (prodromal) services: Dilution or reduction of risk? *Schizophrenia Bulletin, 33*(3), 673-681.

Zeanah, C. H., Egger, H. L., Smyke, A. T., et al. (2009). Institutional rearing and psychiatric disorders in Romanian preschool children. *American Journal of Psychiatry, 166,* 777-785.

Zimmermann, P., Wittchen, H-U, Hofler, M., et al. (2003). Primary anxiety disorders and the development of subsequent alcohol use disorders: A 4-year community study of adolescents and young adults. *Psychological Medicine, 33,* 1211-1222.

Index

Note: Page numbers followed by f refer to figures; page numbers followed by t refer to tables; page numbers followed by b refer to boxes.

C

D

E

H

I

M

P

Q

R

S

T

U

V

W